Clinical Periodontology and Implant Dentistry

Fifth Edition

Edited by

Jan Lindhe
Niklaus P. Lang
Thorkild Karring

Associate Editors
Tord Berglundh
William V. Giannobile
Mariano Sanz

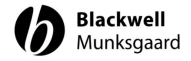

Blackwell
Munksgaard

Volume 2
CLINICAL CONCEPTS

Edited by

Niklaus P. Lang
Jan Lindhe

Blackwell Publishing editorial offices:
Blackwell Publishing Ltd, 9600 Garsington Road, Oxford OX4 2DQ, UK
Tel: +44 (0)1865 776868
Blackwell Publishing Professional, 2121 State Avenue, Ames, Iowa 50014-8300, USA
Tel: +1 515 292 0140
Blackwell Publishing Asia Pty Ltd, 550 Swanston Street, Carlton, Victoria 3053, Australia
Tel: +61 (0)3 8359 1011

First published 1983 by Munksgaard
Second edition published 1989
Third edition published 1997
Fourth edition published by Blackwell Munksgaard 2003
Reprinted 2003, 2005, 2006
Fifth edition 2008 by Blackwell Publishing Ltd
6 2012

ISBN: 978-1-4051-6099-5

Library of Congress Cataloging-in-Publication Data
Clinical periodontology and implant dentistry / edited by Jan Lindhe,
Niklaus P. Lang, Thorkild Karring. — 5th ed.
      p. ; cm.
Includes bibliographical references and index.
ISBN: 978-1-4051-6099-5 (hardback : alk. paper)
1. Periodontics. 2. Periodontal disease. 3. Dental implants. I. Lindhe, Jan.
II. Lang, Niklaus Peter. III. Karring, Thorkild.
[DNLM: 1. Periodontal Diseases. 2. Dental Implantation. 3. Dental Implants.
WU 240 C6415 2008]
RK361.C54 2008
617.6′32—dc22

                                                                2007037124

A catalogue record for this title is available from the British Library

Set in 9.5/12 pt Palatino by SNP Best-set Typesetter Ltd., Hong Kong
Printed and bound in Singapore by Fabulous Printers Pte Ltd

For further information on Blackwell Publishing, visit our website:
www.blackwellmunksgaard.com

Contents

Contributors, xvii

Preface, xxi

Volume 1: BASIC CONCEPTS
Editors: Jan Lindhe, Niklaus P. Lang, and Thorkild Karring

Part 1: Anatomy

1   The Anatomy of Periodontal Tissues, 3
Jan Lindhe, Thorkild Karring, and Maurício Araújo
Introduction, 3
Gingiva, 5
    Macroscopic anatomy, 5
    Microscopic anatomy, 8
Periodontal ligament, 27
Root cementum, 31
Alveolar bone, 34
Blood supply of the periodontium, 43
Lymphatic system of the periodontium, 47
Nerves of the periodontium, 48

2   The Edentulous Alveolar Ridge, 50
Maurício Araújo and Jan Lindhe
Clinical considerations, 50
    Remaining bone in the edentulous ridge, 52
    Classification of remaining bone, 53
Topography of the alveolar process, 53
Alterations of the alveolar process following tooth
    extraction, 54
    Intra-alveolar processes, 54
    Extra-alveolar processes, 62
Topography of the edentulous ridge, 66

3   The Mucosa at Teeth and Implants, 69
*Jan Lindhe, Jan L. Wennström, and
Tord Berglundh*
The gingiva, 69
    Biologic width, 69
    Dimensions of the buccal tissue, 69
    Dimensions of the interdental papilla, 71
The peri-implant mucosa, 71
    Biologic width, 72
    Quality, 76
    Vascular supply, 77
Probing gingiva and peri-implant mucosa, 78
Dimensions of the buccal soft tissue at implants, 80
Dimensions of the papilla between teeth and implants,
    81
Dimensions of the "papilla" between adjacent
    implants, 82

4   Bone as a Tissue, 86
*William V. Giannobile, Hector F. Rios, and
Niklaus P. Lang*
Basic bone biology, 86
    Bone cells, 86
    Modeling and remodeling, 87
    Growth factors and alveolar bone healing, 88
Local and systemic factors affecting bone volume and
    healing, 89
    Metabolic disorders affecting bone metabolism, 89
Bone healing, 93
    Bone grafting, 93
    Human experimental studies on alveolar bone
      repair, 94

5   Osseointegration, 99
Jan Lindhe, Tord Berglundh, and Niklaus P. Lang
The edentulous site, 99
Osseointegration, 99
Implant installation 99
    Tissue injury, 99
    Wound healing, 100
Cutting and non-cutting implants, 100
The process of osseointegration, 103

**6   Periodontal Tactile Perception and
    Peri-implant Osseoperception, 108**
Reinhilde Jacobs
Introduction, 108
Neurophysiological background, 109
    Afferent nerve fibres and receptors, 109
Trigeminal neurophysiology, 109
    Trigeminal neurosensory pathway, 109
    Neurovascularization of the jaw bones, 109
    Mandibular neuroanatomy, 110
    Maxillary neuroanatomy, 111
Periodontal innervation, 112
Testing tactile function, 113
    Neurophysiological assessment, 113
    Psychophysical assessment, 114
Periodontal tactile function, 115
    Active threshold determination, 115
    Passive threshold determination, 115
    Influence of dental status on tactile function, 116

Activation of oral mechanoreceptors during oral
   tactile function, 117
Functional testing of the oral somatosensory
   system, 117
   Oral stereognosis, 118
   Influence of dental status on stereognostic
      ability, 118
   Other compromising factors for oral stereognosis,
      118
   Receptor activation during oral stereognosis,
      119
From periodontal tactile function to peri-implant
   osseoperception, 119
   Tooth extraction considered as sensory
      amputation, 119
   Histological background of peri-implant
      osseoperception, 120
   Cortical plasticity after tooth extraction, 121
   From osseoperception to implant-mediated
      sensory motor interactions, 121
   Clinical implications of implant-deviated sensory
      motor interaction, 122
Conclusions, 122

Part 2: Epidemiology

7   Epidemiology of Periodontal Diseases, 129
   Panos N. Papapanou and Jan Lindhe
Introduction, 129
Methodological issues, 129
   Examination methods – index systems, 129
   Critical evaluation, 131
Prevalence of periodontal diseases, 133
   Introduction, 133
   Periodontitis in adults, 133
   Periodontal disease in children and
      adolescents, 138
Periodontitis and tooth loss, 141
Risk factors for periodontitis, 141
   Introduction – definitions, 141
   Non-modifiable background factors, 143
   Environmental, acquired, and behavioral
      factors, 145
Periodontal infections and risk for systemic disease,
   156
   Atherosclerosis – cardiovascular/cerebrovascular
      disease, 156
   Pregnancy complications, 159
   Diabetes mellitus, 162

Part 3: Microbiology

8   Oral Biofilms and Calculus, 183
   *Niklaus P. Lang, Andrea Mombelli, and
   Rolf Attström*
Microbial considerations, 183
General introduction to plaque formation, 184
Dental plaque as a biofilm, 187
Structure of dental plaque, 187
   Supragingival plaque, 187
   Subgingival plaque, 191
   Peri-implant plaque, 196

Dental calculus, 197
   Clinical appearance, distribution, and clinical
      diagnosis, 197
   Attachment to tooth surfaces and implants, 200
   Mineralization, composition, and structure, 201
   Clinical implications, 202

9   Periodontal Infections, 207
   Sigmund S. Socransky and Anne D. Haffajee
Introduction, 207
   Similarities of periodontal diseases to other
      infectious diseases, 207
   Unique features of periodontal infections, 208
Historical perspective, 209
   The early search, 209
   The decline of interest in microorganisms, 211
   Non-specific plaque hypothesis, 211
   Mixed anaerobic infections, 211
   Return to specificity in microbial etiology of
      periodontal diseases, 212
   Changing concepts of the microbial etiology of
      periodontal diseases, 212
Current suspected pathogens of destructive
   periodontal diseases, 213
   Criteria for defining periodontal pathogens, 213
   Periodontal pathogens, 213
   Mixed infections, 225
The nature of dental plaque – the biofilm way of life,
   226
   The nature of biofilms, 226
   Properties of biofilms, 227
   Techniques for the detection and enumeration of
      bacteria in oral biofilm samples, 229
   The oral biofilms that lead to periodontal
      diseases, 229
   Microbial complexes, 231
   Factors that affect the composition of subgingival
      biofilms, 232
   Microbial composition of supra- and subgingival
      biofilms, 238
   Development of supra- and subgingival biofilms,
      239
Prerequisites for periodontal disease initiation and
   progression, 242
   The virulent periodontal pathogen, 243
   The local environment, 243
   Host susceptibility, 244
Mechanisms of pathogenicity, 245
   Essential factors for colonization of a subgingival
      species, 245
Effect of therapy on subgingival biofilms, 249

10   Peri-implant Infections, 268
   *Ricardo P. Teles, Anne D. Haffajee, and
   Sigmund S. Socransky*
Introduction, 268
Early biofilm development on implant surfaces, 268
Time of implant exposure and climax community
   complexity, 271
The microbiota on implants in edentulous subjects, 273
The microbiota on implants in partially edentulous
   subjects, 275
The microbiota on implants in subjects with a history
   of periodontal disease, 276
The microbiota of peri-implantitis sites, 277

Part 4: Host–Parasite Interactions

11   Pathogenesis of Periodontitis, 285
Denis F. Kinane, Tord Berglundh, and Jan Lindhe
Introduction, 285
Clinically healthy gingiva, 286
Gingival inflammation, 287
    Histopathological features of gingivitis, 287
Different lesions in gingivitis/periodontitis, 289
    The initial lesion, 289
    The early lesion, 289
    The established lesion, 290
    The advanced lesion, 292
Host–parasite interactions, 294
    Microbial virulence factors, 294
Host defense processes, 295
    Important aspects of host defense processes, 295
    The innate defense systems, 297
    The immune or adaptive defense system, 299

12   Modifying Factors, 307
Richard Palmer and Mena Soory
Diabetes mellitus, 307
    Type 1 and type 2 diabetes mellitus, 307
    Clinical symptoms, 308
    Oral and periodontal effects, 308
    Association of periodontal infection and diabetic
        control, 309
    Modification of the host–bacteria relationship in
        diabetes, 310
    Periodontal treatment, 311
Puberty, pregnancy, and the menopause, 312
    Puberty and menstruation, 312
    Pregnancy, 312
    Menopause and osteoporosis, 314
    Hormonal contraceptives, 316
Tobacco smoking, 316
    Periodontal disease in smokers, 317
    Modification of the host–bacteria relationship in
        smoking, 319
    Smoking cessation, 322

13   Susceptibility, 328
*Bruno G. Loos, Ubele van der Velden, and
Marja L. Laine*
Introduction, 328
Evidence for the role of genetics in periodontitis, 331
    Heritability of aggressive periodontitis (early
        onset periodontitis), 331
    Heritability of chronic periodontitis (adult
        periodontitis), 332
A gene mutation with major effect on human disease
    and its association with periodontitis, 332
Disease-modifying genes in relation to periodontitis,
    333
    IL-1 and TNF-α gene polymorphisms, 334
    FcγR gene polymorphisms, 336
    Gene polymorphisms in the innate immunity
        receptors, 338
    Vitamin D receptor gene polymorphisms, 338
    IL-10 gene polymorphisms, 339
    Miscellaneous gene polymorphisms, 340
Disease-modifying genes in relation to implant failures
    and peri-implantitis, 340
    Early failures in implant dentistry, 341

Late failures in implant dentistry, 342
Conclusions and future developments, 342

Part 5: Trauma from Occlusion

**14   Trauma from Occlusion: Periodontal Tissues,
    349**
Jan Lindhe, Sture Nyman, and Ingvar Ericsson
Definition and terminology, 349
Trauma from occlusion and plaque-associated
    periodontal disease, 349
Analysis of human autopsy material, 350
Clinical trials, 352
Animal experiments, 353

**15   Trauma from Occlusion: Peri-implant Tissues,
    363**
Niklaus P. Lang and Tord Berglundh
Introduction, 363
Orthodontic loading and alveolar bone, 363
Bone reactions to functional loading, 365
Excessive occlusal load on implants, 365
Static and cyclic loads on implants, 366
Load and loss of osseointegration, 368
Masticatory occlusal forces on implants, 369
Tooth–implant supported reconstructions, 370

Part 6: Periodontal Pathology

**16   Non-Plaque Induced Inflammatory Gingival
    Lesions, 377**
Palle Holmstrup
Gingival diseases of specific bacterial origin, 377
Gingival diseases of viral origin, 378
    Herpes virus infections, 378
Gingival diseases of fungal origin, 380
    Candidosis, 380
    Linear gingival erythema, 381
    Histoplasmosis, 382
Gingival lesions of genetic origin, 383
    Hereditary gingival fibromatosis, 383
Gingival diseases of systemic origin, 384
    Mucocutaneous disorders, 384
    Allergic reactions, 392
    Other gingival manifestations of systemic
        conditions, 394
Traumatic lesions, 396
    Chemical injury, 396
    Physical injury, 396
    Thermal injury, 397
    Foreign body reactions, 398

17   Plaque-Induced Gingival Diseases, 405
Angelo Mariotti
Classification criteria for gingival diseases, 405
Plaque-induced gingivitis, 407
Gingival diseases associated with endogenous
    hormones, 408
    Puberty-associated gingivitis, 408
    Menstrual cycle-associated gingivitis, 409
    Pregnancy-associated gingival diseases, 409
Gingival diseases associated with medications, 410
    Drug-influenced gingival enlargement, 410

Oral contraceptive-associated gingivitis, 411
Gingival diseases associated with systemic diseases, 411
   Diabetes mellitus-associated gingivitis, 411
   Leukemia-associated gingivitis, 411
   Linear gingival erythema, 412
Gingival diseases associated with malnutrition, 412
Gingival diseases associated with heredity, 413
Gingival diseases associated with ulcerative lesions, 413
Treatment of plaque-induced gingival diseases, 414
The significance of gingivitis, 414

18   Chronic Periodontitis, 420
   Denis F. Kinane, Jan Lindhe, and
   Leonardo Trombelli
Clinical features of chronic periodontitis, 420
Overall characteristics of chronic periodontitis, 420
Gingivitis as a risk for chronic periodontitis, 422
Susceptibility to chronic periodontitis, 422
Prevalence of chronic periodontitis, 423
Progression of chronic periodontitis, 423
Risk factors for chronic periodontitis, 424
   Bacterial plaque, 424
   Age, 424
   Smoking, 424
   Systemic disease, 424
   Stress, 425
   Genetics, 426
Scientific basis for treatment of chronic periodontitis, 426

19   Aggressive Periodontitis, 428
   Maurizio S. Tonetti and Andrea Mombelli
Classification and clinical syndromes, 429
Epidemiology, 431
   Primary dentition, 432
   Permanent dentition, 432
   Screening, 433
Etiology and pathogenesis, 437
   Bacterial etiology, 437
   Genetic aspects of host susceptibility, 441
   Environmental aspects of host susceptibility, 445
   Current concepts, 445
Diagnosis, 445
   Clinical diagnosis, 445
   Microbiologic diagnosis, 448
   Evaluation of host defenses, 448
   Genetic diagnosis, 449
Principles of therapeutic intervention, 449
   Elimination or suppression of the pathogenic flora, 449

20   Necrotizing Periodontal Disease, 459
   Palle Holmstrup and Jytte Westergaard
Nomenclature, 459
Prevalence, 460
Clinical characteristics, 460
   Development of lesions, 460
   Interproximal craters, 461
   Sequestrum formation, 462
   Involvement of alveolar mucosa, 462
   Swelling of lymph nodes, 463
   Fever and malaise, 463
   Oral hygiene, 463

   Acute and recurrent/chronic forms of necrotizing gingivitis and periodontitis, 463
Diagnosis, 464
   Differential diagnosis, 464
Histopathology, 465
Microbiology, 466
   Microorganisms isolated from necrotizing lesions, 466
   Pathogenic potential of microorganisms, 466
Host response and predisposing factors, 468
   Systemic diseases, 468
   Poor oral hygiene, pre-existing gingivitis, and history of previous NPD, 469
   Psychologic stress and inadequate sleep, 469
   Smoking and alcohol use, 470
   Caucasian background, 470
   Young age, 470
Treatment, 470
   Acute phase treatment, 470
   Maintenance phase treatment, 472

21   Periodontal Disease as a Risk for Systemic Disease, 475
   Ray C. Williams and David W. Paquette
Early twentieth century concepts, 475
Periodontitis as a risk for cardiovascular disease, 476
   Biologic rationale, 479
Periodontitis as a risk for adverse pregnancy outcomes, 480
   Association of periodontal disease and pre-eclampsia, 486
Periodontitis as a risk for diabetic complications, 486
Periodontitis as a risk for respiratory infections, 488
Effects of treatment of periodontitis on systemic diseases, 489

22   The Periodontal Abscess, 496
   Mariano Sanz, David Herrera, and
   Arie J. van Winkelhoff
Introduction, 496
Classification, 496
Prevalence, 497
Pathogenesis and histopathology, 497
Microbiology, 498
Diagnosis, 498
   Differential diagnosis, 499
Treatment, 500
Complications, 501
   Tooth loss, 501
   Dissemination of the infection, 502

23   Lesions of Endodontic Origin, 504
   Gunnar Bergenholtz and Domenico Ricucci
Introduction, 504
Disease processes of the dental pulp, 504
   Causes, 504
   Progression and dynamic events, 505
   Accessory canals, 507
   Periodontal tissue lesions to root canal infection, 510
Effects of periodontal disease and periodontal therapy on the condition of the pulp, 516
   Influences of periodontal disease, 516
   Influence of periodontal treatment measures on the pulp, 518
   Root dentin hypersensitivity, 518

Part 7: Peri-implant Pathology

24 Peri-implant Mucositis and Peri-implantitis, 529
Tord Berglundh, Jan Lindhe, and Niklaus P. Lang
Definitions, 529
Ridge mucosa, 529
Peri-implant mucosa, 529
Peri-implant mucositis, 530
    Clinical features, 530
    Prevalence, 530
    Histopathology, 530
Peri-implantitis, 532
    Clinical features, 532
    Prevalence, 532
    Histopathology, 534

Part 8: Tissue Regeneration

25 Concepts in Periodontal Tissue Regeneration, 541
Thorkild Karring and Jan Lindhe

Introduction, 541
Regenerative periodontal surgery, 542
Periodontal wound healing, 542
    Regenerative capacity of bone cells, 547
    Regenerative capacity of gingival connective
        tissue cells, 547
    Regenerative capacity of periodontal ligament
        cells, 548
    Role of epithelium in periodontal wound healing,
        549
    Root resorption, 550
Regenerative concepts, 550
    Grafting procedures, 551
    Root surface biomodification, 557
    Growth regulatory factors for periodontal
        regeneration, 559
    Guided tissue regeneration (GTR), 559
Assessment of periodontal regeneration, 561
    Periodontal probing, 561
    Radiographic analysis and re-entry operations,
        562
    Histologic methods, 562

Index, i1

Volume 2: CLINICAL CONCEPTS
Editors: Niklaus P. Lang and Jan Lindhe

Part 9: Examination Protocols

26 Examination of Patients with Periodontal Diseases, 573
Giovanni E. Salvi, Jan Lindhe, and Niklaus P. Lang
History of periodontal patients, 573
    Chief complaint and expectations, 573
    Social and family history, 573
    Dental history, 573
    Oral hygiene habits, 573
    Smoking history, 574
    Medical history and medications, 574
Signs and symptoms of periodontal diseases, 574
    The gingiva, 574
    The periodontal ligament and the root cementum,
        577
    The alveolar bone, 583
Diagnosis of periodontal lesions, 583
Oral hygiene status, 584
Additional dental examinations, 585

27 Examination of the Candidate for Implant Therapy, 587
Hans-Peter Weber, Daniel Buser, and Urs C. Belser
Dental implants in periodontally compromised
    patients, 587
Patient history, 590
    Chief complaint and expectations, 590
    Social and family history, 590
    Dental history, 590
    Motivation and compliance, 591
    Habits, 591
    Medical history and medications, 591
Local examination, 591
    Extraoral, 591

    General intraoral examination, 592
    Radiographic examination, 592
    Implant-specific intraoral examination, 592
Patient-specific risk assessment, 597
    Risk assessment for sites without esthetic
        implications, 597
    Risk assessment for sites with esthetic
        implications, 597

28 Radiographic Examination of the Implant Patient, 600
Hans-Göran Gröndahl and Kerstin Gröndahl
Introduction, 600
Radiographic examination for implant planning
    purposes – general aspects, 601
    The clinical vs. the radiologic examination, 601
    What is the necessary radiographic information?,
        601
    Radiographic methods for obtaining the
        information required for implant planning, 603
Radiographic examination for implant planning
    purposes – upper jaw examination, 607
Radiographic examination for implant planning
    purposes – lower jaw examination, 610
Radiographic monitoring of implant treatment, 614
Radiation detectors for intraoral radiography, 618
Image-guided surgery, 621

29 Examination of Patients with Implant-Supported Restorations, 623
Urs Brägger
Identification of the presence of implants and implant
    systems, 623
    Screening, 623
    Implant pass, 623

x   Contents

Questionnaire for new patients, 625
Anamnestic information from patients on
maintenance, 625
The development of implant recognition software,
625
Clinical inspection and examination, 625
Characteristics of implant-supported restorations,
625
Characteristics of prosthetic components and
components of implant systems, 626
Technical failures/complications, 626
Function, 628
Functional analysis, 628
Articulation, phonetics, 628
Implant, 628
Clinical test of mobility, 629
Electronic tools to assess the quality of
osseointegration, 629
Bacterial deposits, 629
Soft tissues, 629
Mucosa, 629
Palpation/sensitivity, 629
Recession, pocket probing depth, probing
attachment level, bleeding on probing, 629
Esthetics, 630
Papillae, interdental space and type of mucosa,
630
Condition of adjacent teeth, 631
Color shades, 632

30   Risk Assessment of the Implant Patient, 634
Gary C. Armitage and Tord Lundgren
Principles of risk assessment, 634
Clinical information required for risk assessment,
636
Technical procedures to help minimize risk, 636
Local risk factors and conditions, 637
Presence of ongoing oral infections, 637
Systemic risk factors, 639
Age, 639
Smoking, 640
Medication history, 640
Immunosuppression, 642
History of radiation therapy to the jaws, 642
Diabetes mellitus, 642
Metabolic bone disease, 643
Connective tissue and autoimmune disorders, 643
Xerostomia, 644
Hematologic and lymphoreticular disorders, 644
Genetic traits and disorders, 644
Importance of behavioral considerations in risk
assessment, 645
Dental history of compliance behaviors, 645
Substance use/abuse, 645
Psychiatric/psychological issues, 645
Lack of understanding or communication, 645
Patient's expectations, 646
Interest and commitment to post-treatment care and
maintenance program, 646

Part 10: Treatment Planning Protocols

**31   Treatment Planning of Patients with
Periodontal Diseases, 655**
Giovanni E. Salvi, Jan Lindhe, and Niklaus P. Lang

Screening for periodontal disease, 656
Basic periodontal examination, 656
Diagnosis, 657
Treatment planning, 658
Initial treatment plan, 658
Pre-therapeutic single tooth prognosis, 660
Case presentation, 660
Case report, 667
Patient S.K. (male, 35 years old), 667

**32   Treatment Planning for Implant Therapy in
the Periodontally Compromised Patient, 675**
Jan L. Wennström and Niklaus P. Lang
Prognosis of implant therapy in the periodontally
compromised patient, 675
Strategies in treatment planning, 676
Treatment decisions – case reports, 676
Posterior segments, 676
Tooth versus implant, 679
Aggressive periodontitis, 680
Furcation problems, 682
Single-tooth problem in the esthetic zone, 683

33   Systemic Phase of Therapy, 687
Niklaus P. Lang and Hans-Rudolf Baur
Introduction, 687
Protection of the dental team and other patients
against infectious diseases, 687
Protection of the patient's health, 688
Prevention of complications, 688
Infection, specifically bacterial endocarditis, 688
Bleeding, 689
Cardiovascular incidents, 690
Allergic reactions and drug interactions, 690
Systemic diseases, disorders or conditions influencing
pathogenesis and healing potential, 690
Control of anxiety and pain, 690
Smoking counseling, 691

**Part 11: Initial Periodontal Therapy
(Infection Control)**

34   Motivational Interviewing, 695
*Christoph A. Ramseier, Delwyn Catley,
Susan Krigel, and Robert A. Bagramian*
The importance of behavioral change counseling in
periodontal care, 695
Development of motivational interviewing, 696
History of motivational interviewing, 697
What is motivational interviewing?, 697
Evidence for motivational interviewing, 697
Implementation of motivational interviewing into the
periodontal treatment plan, 698
Key principles of motivational interviewing, 698
Basic communication skills, 698
Giving advice, 700
Case examples for oral hygiene motivation, 700
Oral hygiene motivation 1, 700
Oral hygiene motivation 2, 701
Case example for tobacco use cessation, 702

**35   Mechanical Supragingival Plaque Control,
705**
*Fridus van der Weijden, José J. Echeverría,
Mariano Sanz, and Jan Lindhe*

Importance of supragingival plaque removal, 705
Self-performed plaque control, 706
  Brushing, 706
  Interdental cleaning, 714
  Adjunctive aids, 717
  Side effects, 718
Importance of instruction and motivation in
  mechanical plaque control, 719

36 Chemical Supragingival Plaque Control, 734
  Martin Addy and John Moran
Classification and terminology of agents, 734
The concept of chemical supragingival plaque control,
  735
  Supragingival plaque control, 736
  Chemical supragingival plaque control, 737
  Rationale for chemical supragingival plaque
    control, 738
  Approaches to chemical supragingival plaque
    control, 739
  Vehicles for the delivery of chemical agents, 740
Chemical plaque control agents, 742
  Systemic antimicrobials including antibiotics, 743
  Enzymes, 744
  Bisbiguanide antiseptics, 744
  Quaternary ammonium compounds, 744
  Phenols and essential oils, 745
  Natural products, 745
  Fluorides, 746
  Metal salts, 746
  Oxygenating agents, 746
  Detergents, 746
  Amine alcohols, 746
  Salifluor, 747
  Acidified sodium chlorite, 747
  Other antiseptics, 747
Chlorhexidine, 748
  Toxicology, safety, and side effects, 748
  Chlorhexidine staining, 749
  Mechanism of action, 750
  Chlorhexidine products, 750
  Clinical uses of chlorhexidine, 751
Evaluation of chemical agents and products, 754
  Studies *in vitro*, 755
  Study methods *in vitro*, 755
  Clinical trial design considerations, 757

37 Non-surgical Therapy, 766
  Noel Claffey and Ioannis Polyzois
Introduction, 766
Detection and removal of dental calculus, 766
Methods used for non-surgical root surface
  debridement, 768
  Hand instrumentation, 768
  Sonic and ultrasonic scalers, 770
  Reciprocating instruments, 770
  Ablative laser therapy, 771
  Choice of debridement method, 771
The influence of mechanical debridement on
  subgingival biofilms, 772
Implication of furcation involvement, 773
Pain and discomfort following non-surgical therapy,
  773
Re-evaluation, 774
  Interpretation of probing measurements at
    re-evaluation, 774

Average changes in measurements due to non-
  surgical therapy, 775
Interpretation of longitudinal changes at
  individual sites, 775
Prediction of outcome and evaluation of treatment, 775
Full-mouth disinfection, 776

Part 12: Additional Therapy

38 Periodontal Surgery: Access Therapy, 783
  Jan L. Wennström, Lars Heijl, and Jan Lindhe
Introduction, 783
Techniques in periodontal pocket surgery, 783
  Gingivectomy procedures, 784
  Flap procedures, 786
  Regenerative procedures, 793
Distal wedge procedures, 794
Osseous surgery, 795
  Osteoplasty, 796
  Ostectomy, 796
General guidelines for periodontal surgery, 797
  Objectives of surgical treatment, 797
  Indications for surgical treatment, 797
  Contraindications for periodontal surgery, 799
  Local anesthesia in periodontal surgery, 800
  Instruments used in periodontal surgery, 802
  Selection of surgical technique, 805
  Root surface instrumentation, 808
  Root surface conditioning/biomodification, 808
  Suturing, 808
  Periodontal dressings, 811
  Post-operative pain control, 812
  Post-surgical care, 812
Outcome of surgical periodontal therapy, 812
  Healing following surgical pocket therapy, 812
  Clinical outcome of surgical access therapy in
    comparison to non-surgical therapy, 814

39 Treatment of Furcation-Involved Teeth, 823
  *Gianfranco Carnevale, Roberto Pontoriero, and
  Jan Lindhe*
Terminology, 823
Anatomy, 824
  Maxillary molars, 824
  Maxillary premolars, 825
  Mandibular molars, 825
  Other teeth, 826
Diagnosis, 826
  Probing, 828
  Radiographs, 828
Differential diagnosis, 829
  Trauma from occlusion, 829
Therapy, 830
  Scaling and root planing, 830
  Furcation plasty, 830
  Tunnel preparation, 832
  Root separation and resection (RSR), 832
  Regeneration of furcation defects, 840
  Extraction, 843
Prognosis, 843

40 Endodontics and Periodontics, 848
  Gunnar Bergenholtz and Gunnar Hasselgren
Introduction, 848

Infectious processes in the periodontium of endodontic
    origin, 849
        General features, 849
        Clinical presentations, 850
        Distinguishing lesions of endodontic origin from
            periodontitis, 851
        Endo–perio lesions – diagnosis and treatment
            aspects, 856
        Endodontic treatments and periodontal lesions,
            858
Iatrogenic root perforations, 858
Vertical root fractures, 859
        Mechanisms, 860
        Incidence, 861
        Clinical expressions, 861
        Diagnosis, 862
        Treatment considerations, 863
External root resorptions, 865
        Mechanisms of hard tissue resorption in general,
            865
        Clinical presentations and identification, 866
        Different forms, 866

41   Treatment of Peri-implant Lesions, 875
    Tord Berglundh, Niklaus P. Lang, and Jan Lindhe
Introduction, 875
The diagnostic process, 875
Treatment strategies, 875
        Resolution of peri-implantitis lesions, 877
Cumulative Interceptive Supportive Therapy (CIST),
    878
        Preventive and therapeutic strategies, 878
        Mechanical debridement; CIST protocol A, 878
        Antiseptic therapy; CIST protocol A+B, 878
        Antibiotic therapy; CIST protocol A+B+C, 879
        Regenerative or resective therapy; CIST protocol
            A+B+C+D, 880

42   Antibiotics in Periodontal Therapy, 882
    Andrea Mombelli
Principles of antibiotic therapy, 882
        The limitations of mechanical therapy: can
            antimicrobial agents help?, 882
        Specific characteristics of the periodontal
            infection, 883
        Drug delivery routes, 884
Evaluation of antibiotics for periodontal therapy, 886
        Systemic antimicrobial therapy in clinical trials,
            888
        Systemic antibiotics in clinical practice, 889
        Local antimicrobial therapy in clinical trials, 890
        Local antibiotics in clinical practice, 893
        Overall conclusion, 893

Part 13: Reconstructive Therapy

43   Regenerative Periodontal Therapy, 901
    Pierpaolo Cortellini and Maurizio S. Tonetti
Introduction, 901
Classification and diagnosis of periodontal osseous
    defects, 901
Clinical indications, 903
Long-term effects and benefits of regeneration, 903
Evidence for clinical efficacy and effectiveness, 905
Patient and defect prognostic factors, 909

Patient factors, 911
        Defect factors, 911
        Tooth factors, 912
        Factors affecting the clinical outcomes of GTR in
            furcations, 913
The relevance of the surgical approach, 913
        Papilla preservation flaps, 916
        Modified papilla preservation technique, 917
        Simplified papilla preservation flap, 920
        Minimally invasive surgical technique, 922
        Post-operative regime, 925
        Post-operative morbidity, 926
Barrier materials for regenerative surgery, 928
        Non-absorbable materials, 928
        Bioabsorbable materials, 930
        Membranes in intrabony defects, 930
        Membranes for furcation involvement, 932
        Surgical issues with barrier membranes, 937
Bone replacement grafts, 938
Biologically active regenerative materials, 938
Membranes combined with other regenerative
    procedures, 940
Root surface biomodification, 943
Clinical strategies, 944

**44   Mucogingival Therapy – Periodontal Plastic
        Surgery, 955**
    *Jan L. Wennström, Giovanni Zucchelli, and
    Giovan P. Pini Prato*
Introduction, 955
Gingival augmentation, 955
        Gingival dimensions and periodontal health, 956
        Marginal tissue recession, 958
        Marginal tissue recession and orthodontic
            treatment, 961
        Gingival dimensions and restorative therapy, 964
        Indications for gingival augmentation, 965
        Gingival augmentation procedures, 965
        Healing following gingival augmentation
            procedures, 968
Root coverage, 970
        Root coverage procedures, 971
        Clinical outcome of root coverage procedures, 990
        Soft tissue healing against the covered root
            surface, 992
Interdental papilla reconstruction, 996
        Surgical techniques, 997
Crown-lengthening procedures, 997
        Excessive gingival display, 997
        Exposure of sound tooth structure, 1002
        Ectopic tooth eruption, 1005
The deformed edentulous ridge, 1008
        Prevention of soft tissue collapse following tooth
            extraction, 1009
        Correction of ridge defects by the use of soft
            tissue grafts, 1010
        Surgical procedures for ridge augmentation, 1011

45   Periodontal Plastic Microsurgery, 1029
    Rino Burkhardt and Niklaus P. Lang
Microsurgical techniques in dentistry (development of
    concepts), 1029
Concepts in microsurgery, 1030
        Magnification, 1030
        Instruments, 1035

Suture materials, 1035
Training concepts (surgeons and assistants), 1038
Clinical indications and limitations, 1039
Comparison to conventional mucogingival
   interventions, 1040

46   Re-osseointegration, 1045
Tord Berglundh and Jan Lindhe
Introduction, 1045
Is it possible to resolve a marginal hard tissue defect
   adjacent to an oral implant?, 1045
   Non-contaminated, pristine implants at sites with
      a wide marginal gap (crater), 1045
   Contaminated implants and crater-shaped bone
      defects, 1046
   Re-osseointegration, 1046
Is re-osseointegration a feasible outcome of
   regenerative therapy?, 1046
   Regeneration of bone from the walls of the defect,
      1046
   "Rejuvenate" the contaminated implant surface,
      1047
Is the quality of the implant surface important
   in a healing process that may lead to
   re-osseointegration?, 1048
   The surface of the metal device in the
      compromised implant site, 1048

Part 14: Surgery for Implant Installation

47   Timing of Implant Placement, 1053
*Christoph H.F. Hämmerle, Maurício Araújo, and
Jan Lindhe*
Introduction, 1053
Type 1: placement of an implant as part of the same
   surgical procedure and immediately following tooth
   extraction, 1055
   Ridge corrections in conjunction with implant
      placement, 1055
   Stability of implant, 1061
Type 2: completed soft tissue coverage of the tooth
   socket, 1061
Type 3: substantial bone fill has occurred in the
   extraction socket, 1062
Type 4: the alveolar ridge is healed following tooth
   loss, 1063
Clinical concepts, 1063
   Aim of therapy, 1063
   Success of treatment and long-term outcomes,
      1065

48   The Surgical Site, 1068
Marc Quirynen and Ulf Lekholm
Bone: shape and quality, 1068
   Clinical examination, 1068
   Radiographic examination, 1068
   Planning for implant placement, 1069
Implant placement, 1071
   Guiding concept, 1071
   Flap elevation, 1071
   Flapless implant insertion, 1071
   Model-based guided surgery, 1071
   Bone preparation, 1071
Anatomic landmarks with potential risk, 1072
Implant position, 1073

Number of implants, 1074
Implant direction, 1074
Healing time, 1076

Part 15: Reconstructive Ridge Therapy

49   Ridge Augmentation Procedures, 1083
Christoph H.F. Hämmerle and Ronald E. Jung
Introduction, 1083
Patient situation, 1084
Bone morphology, 1084
   Horizontal bone defects, 1084
   Vertical bone defects, 1084
Soft tissue morphology, 1085
Augmentation materials, 1085
   Membranes, 1085
   Bone grafts and bone graft substitutes, 1086
Long-term results, 1087
Clinical concepts, 1088
   Ridge preservation, 1088
   Extraction sockets (class I), 1089
   Dehiscence defects (classes II and III), 1090
   Horizontal defects (class IV), 1091
   Vertical defects (class V), 1092
Future developments, 1093
   Growth and differentiation factors, 1093
   Delivery systems for growth and differentiation
      factors, 1093
   Membrane developments, 1093
   Future outlook, 1094

50   Elevation of the Maxillary Sinus Floor, 1099
Bjarni E. Pjetursson and Niklaus P. Lang
Introduction, 1099
Treatment options in the posterior maxilla, 1099
Sinus floor elevation with a lateral approach, 1100
   Anatomy of the maxillary sinus, 1100
   Pre-surgical examination, 1101
   Indications and contraindications, 1102
   Surgical techniques, 1102
   Post-surgical care, 1105
   Complications, 1106
   Grafting materials, 1107
   Success and implant survival, 1108
Sinus floor elevation with the crestal approach
   (osteotome technique), 1110
   Indications and contraindications, 1111
   Surgical technique, 1111
   Post-surgical care, 1115
   Grafting material, 1115
   Success and implant survival, 1116
Short implants, 1117
Conclusions and clinical suggestions, 1118

Part 16: Occlusal and Prosthetic Therapy

51   Tooth-Supported Fixed Partial Dentures, 1125
Jan Lindhe and Sture Nyman
Clinical symptoms of trauma from occlusion, 1125
   Angular bony defects, 1125
   Increased tooth mobility, 1125
   Progressive (increasing) tooth mobility, 1125
Tooth mobility crown excursion/root displacement,
   1125

Initial and secondary tooth mobility, 1125
Clinical assessment of tooth mobility (physiologic
and pathologic tooth mobility), 1127
Treatment of increased tooth mobility, 1128
Situation I, 1128
Situation II, 1129
Situation III, 1129
Situation IV, 1132
Situation V, 1134

52   Implants in Restorative Dentistry, 1138
Niklaus P. Lang and Giovanni E. Salvi
Introduction, 1138
Treatment concepts, 1138
Limited treatment goals, 1139
Shortened dental arch concept, 1139
Indications for implants, 1139
Increase the subjective chewing comfort, 1141
Preservation of natural tooth substance and
existing functional, satisfactory reconstructions,
1143
Replacement of strategically important missing
teeth, 1144

53   Implants in the Esthetic Zone, 1146
*Urs C. Belser, Jean-Pierre Bernard, and
Daniel Buser*
Basic concepts, 1146
General esthetic principles and related guidelines,
1147
Esthetic considerations related to maxillary
anterior implant restorations, 1148
Anterior single-tooth replacement, 1149
Sites without significant tissue deficiencies, 1152
Sites with localized horizontal deficiencies, 1156
Sites with extended horizontal deficiencies, 1156
Sites with major vertical tissue loss, 1157
Multiple-unit anterior fixed implant restorations, 1161
Sites without significant tissue deficiencies, 1163
Sites with extended horizontal deficiencies, 1164
Sites with major vertical tissue loss, 1165
Conclusions and perspectives, 1165
Scalloped implant design, 1165
Segmented fixed implant restorations in the
edentulous maxilla, 1166

54   Implants in the Posterior Dentition, 1175
*Urs C. Belser, Daniel Buser, and
Jean-Pierre Bernard*
Basic concepts, 1175
General considerations, 1175
Indications for implant restorations in the load
carrying part of the dentition, 1177
Controversial issues, 1180
Restoration of the distally shortened arch with fixed
implant-supported prostheses, 1180
Number, size, and distribution of implants, 1180
Implant restorations with cantilever units, 1182
Combination of implant and natural tooth
support, 1183
Sites with extended horizontal bone volume
deficiencies and/or anterior sinus floor
proximity, 1184
Multiple-unit tooth-bound posterior implant
restorations, 1187
Number, size, and distribution of implants, 1187
Splinted versus single-unit restorations of

multiple adjacent posterior implants, 1189
Posterior single-tooth replacement, 1191
Premolar-size single-tooth restorations, 1191
Molar-size single-tooth restorations, 1191
Sites with limited vertical bone volume, 1192
Clinical applications, 1193
Screw-retained implant restorations, 1193
Abutment-level impression versus implant
shoulder-level impression, 1196
Cemented multiple-unit posterior implant
prostheses, 1197
Angulated abutments, 1198
High-strength all-ceramic implant restorations,
1199
Orthodontic and occlusal considerations related to
posterior implant therapy, 1200
Concluding remarks and perspectives, 1203
Early and immediate fixed implant restorations,
1203

**55   Implant–Implant and Tooth–Implant
Supported Fixed Partial Dentures, 1208**
Clark M. Stanford and Lyndon F. Cooper
Introduction, 1208
Initial patient assessment, 1208
Implant treatment planning for the edentulous arch,
1209
Prosthesis design and full-arch tooth replacement
therapy, 1210
Complete-arch fixed complete dentures, 1211
Prosthesis design and partially edentulous tooth
replacement therapy, 1211
Implant per tooth versus an implant-to-implant
FPD?, 1212
Cantilever pontics, 1213
Immediate provisionalization, 1215
Disadvantages of implant–implant fixed partial
dentures, 1215
Tooth–implant fixed partial dentures, 1216

**56   Complications Related to Implant-Supported
Restorations, 1222**
*Y. Joon Ko, Clark M. Stanford, and
Lyndon F. Cooper*
Introduction, 1222
Clinical complications in conventional fixed
restorations, 1222
Clinical complications in implant-supported
restorations, 1224
Biologic complications, 1224
Mechanical complications, 1226
Other issues related to prosthetic complications, 1231
Implant angulation and prosthetic complications,
1231
Screw-retained vs. cement-retained restorations,
1233
Ceramic abutments, 1233
Esthetic complications, 1233
Success/survival rate of implant-supported
prostheses, 1234

Part 17: Orthodontics and Periodontics

**57   Tooth Movements in the Periodontally
Compromised Patient, 1241**
Björn U. Zachrisson

Orthodontic tooth movement in adults with
  periodontal tissue breakdown, 1241
    Orthodontic treatment considerations, 1243
    Esthetic finishing of treatment results, 1248
    Retention – problems and solutions; long-term
      follow-up, 1248
    Possibilities and limitations; legal aspects, 1249
Specific factors associated with orthodontic tooth
  movement in adults, 1252
    Tooth movement into infrabony pockets, 1252
    Tooth movement into compromised bone areas,
      1253
    Tooth movement through cortical bone, 1253
    Extrusion and intrusion of single teeth – effects on
      periodontium, clinical crown length, and
      esthetics, 1255
    Regenerative procedures and orthodontic tooth
      movement, 1261
    Traumatic occlusion (jiggling) and orthodontic
      treatment, 1262
    Molar uprighting, furcation involvement, 1262
    Tooth movement and implant esthetics, 1263
Gingival recession, 1267
    Labial recession, 1267
    Interdental recession, 1271
Minor surgery associated with orthodontic therapy,
  1274
    Fiberotomy, 1274
    Frenotomy, 1274
    Removal of gingival invaginations (clefts), 1275
    Gingivectomy, 1275

**58 Implants Used for Orthodontic Anchorage,
      1280**
    Marc A. Schätzle and Niklaus P. Lang
Introduction, 1280
Evolution of implants for orthodontic anchorage, 1281
Prosthetic implants for orthodontic anchorage, 1282
    Bone reaction to orthodontic implant loading,
      1282
    Indications of prosthetic oral implants for
      orthodontic anchorage, 1283
    Prosthetic oral implant anchorage in growing
      orthodontic patients, 1283
Orthodontic implants as temporary anchorage devices,
  1284
    Implant designs and dimensions, 1284
    Insertion sites of palatal implants, 1286
    Palatal implants and their possible effect in
      growing patients, 1286
    Clinical procedures and loading time schedule for
      palatal implant installation, 1288
    Direct or indirect orthodontic implant anchorage,
      1288
    Stability and success rates, 1290
    Implant removal, 1290
    Advantages and disadvantages, 1290

Part 18: Supportive Care

**59 Supportive Periodontal Therapy (SPT),
      1297**
    *Niklaus P. Lang, Urs Brägger, Giovanni E. Salvi,
    and Maurizio S. Tonetti*
Definitions, 1297
Basic paradigms for the prevention of periodontal
  disease, 1297
Patients at risk for periodontitis without SPT, 1300
SPT for patients with gingivitis, 1302
SPT for patients with periodontitis, 1302
Continuous multi-level risk assessment, 1303
    Subject risk assessment, 1302
    Tooth risk assessment, 1309
    Site risk assessment, 1310
    Radiographic evaluation of periodontal disease
      progression, 1312
    Clinical implementation, 1312
Objectives for SPT, 1313
SPT in daily practice, 1314
    Examination, re-evaluation, and diagnosis (ERD),
      1314
    Motivation, reinstruction, and instrumentation
      (MRI), 1315
    Treatment of reinfected sites (TRS), 1315
    Polishing, fluorides, determination of recall
      interval (PFD), 1317

Part 19: Halitosis

60 Halitosis Control, 1325
    Edwin G. Winkel
Introduction, 1325
    Epidemiology, 1325
    Odor characteristics, 1326
    Pathogenesis of intraoral halitosis, 1326
    Pathogenesis of extraoral halitosis, 1327
Diagnosis, 1328
    Flowchart in a halitosis practice, 1328
    Before first consultation, 1328
    At the first examination, 1328
    Classification of halitosis, 1333
Therapy, 1333
    Pseudo-halitosis and halitophobia, 1333
    Temporary halitosis, 1334
    Extraoral halitosis, 1334
    Intraoral halitosis, 1334
    Physiologic halitosis, 1335
    Treatment planning, 1335
    Adjustment of therapy, 1337
    Future perspectives, 1337

Index, i1

Contributors

Martin Addy
Division of Restorative Dentistry (Periodontology)
Department of Oral and Dental Science
Bristol Dental School and Hospital
Bristol
UK

Maurício Araújo
Department of Dentistry
State University of Maringá
Maringá
Paraná
Brazil

Gary C. Armitage
Division of Periodontology
School of Dentistry
University of California San Francisco
San Francisco
CA
USA

Rolf Attström
Department of Periodontology
Centre for Oral Health Sciences
Malmö University
Malmö
Sweden

Robert A. Bagramian
Department of Periodontics and Oral Medicine
University of Michigan School of Dentistry
Ann Arbor
MI
USA

Hans-Rudolf Baur
Department of Internal Medicine
Spital Bern Tiefenau
Berne
Switzerland

Urs C. Belser
Department of Prosthetic Dentistry
School of Dental Medicine
University of Geneva
Geneva
Switzerland

Gunnar Bergenholtz
Department of Endodontology
Institute of Odontology
The Sahlgrenska Academy at Göteborg University
Göteborg
Sweden

Tord Berglundh
Department of Periodontology
Institute of Odontology
The Sahlgrenska Academy at Göteborg University
Göteborg
Sweden

Jean-Pierre Bernard
Department of Oral Surgery and Stomatology
School of Dental Medicine
University of Geneva
Geneva
Switzerland

Urs Brägger
Department of Periodontology and Fixed
    Prosthodontics
School of Dental Medicine
University of Berne
Berne
Switzerland

Rino Burkhardt
Private Practice
Zürich
Switzerland

Daniel Buser
Department of Oral Surgery and Stomatology
School of Dental Medicine
University of Berne
Berne
Switzerland

Gianfranco Carnevale
Private Practice
Rome
Italy

Delwyn Catley
Department of Psychology
University of Missouri – Kansas City
Kansas City
MO
USA

Noel Claffey
Dublin Dental School and Hospital
Trinity College
Dublin
Ireland

Lyndon F. Cooper
Department of Prosthodontics
University of North Carolina
Chapel Hill
NC
USA

Pierpaolo Cortellini
Private Practice
Florence
Italy

José J. Echeverría
Department of Periodontics
School of Dentistry
University of Barcelona
Barcelona
Spain

Ingvar Ericsson
Department of Prosthetic Dentistry
Faculty of Odontology
Malmö University
Malmö
Sweden

William V. Giannobile
Michigan Center for Oral Health Research
University of Michigan Clinical Center
Ann Arbor
MI
USA

Hans-Göran Gröndahl
Department of Oral and Maxillofacial Radiology
Institute of Odontology
The Sahlgrenska Academy at Göteborg University
Göteborg
Sweden

Kerstin Gröndahl
Department of Oral and Maxillofacial Radiology
Institute of Odontology
The Sahlgrenska Academy at Göteborg University
Göteborg
Sweden

Anne D. Haffajee
Department of Periodontology
The Forsyth Institute
Boston
MA
USA

Christoph H.F. Hämmerle
Clinic for Fixed and Removable Prosthodontics
Center for Dental and Oral Medicine and Cranio-
    Maxillofacial Surgery
University of Zürich
Zürich
Switzerland

Gunnar Hasselgren
Division of Endodontics
School of Dental and Oral Surgery
Columbia University College of Dental Medicine
New York
NY
USA

Lars Heijl
Department of Periodontology
Institute of Odontology
The Sahlgrenska Academy at Göteborg University
Göteborg
Sweden

David Herrera
Faculty of Odontology
University Complutense
Madrid
Spain

Palle Holmstrup
Department of Periodontology
School of Dentistry
University of Copenhagen
Copenhagen
Denmark

Reinhilde Jacobs
Oral Imaging Center
School of Dentistry, Oral Pathology and Maxillofacial
    Surgery
Catholic University of Leuven
Leuven
Belgium

Ronald E. Jung
Clinic for Fixed and Removable Prosthodontics
Center for Dental and Oral Medicine and Cranio-
    Maxillofacial Surgery
University of Zürich
Zürich
Switzerland

Thorkild Karring
Department of Periodontology and Oral Gerontology
Royal Dental College
University of Aarhus
Aarhus
Denmark

Denis F. Kinane
Oral Health and Systemic Disease Research Facility
School of Dentistry
University of Louisville
Louisville
KY
USA

Y. Joon Ko
Department of Prosthodontics
University of Iowa
Iowa City
IA
USA

Susan Krigel
Department of Psychology
University of Missouri – Kansas City
Kansas City
MO
USA

Marja L. Laine
Department of Oral Microbiology
Academic Centre for Dentistry Amsterdam (ACTA)
Amsterdam
The Netherlands

Niklaus P. Lang
Department of Periodontology and Fixed
  Prosthodontics
School of Dental Medicine
University of Berne
Berne
Switzerland

Ulf Lekholm
Department of Oral and Maxillofacial Surgery
Institute of Odontology
The Sahlgrenska Academy at Göteborg University
Göteborg
Sweden

Jan Lindhe
Department of Periodontology
Institute of Odontology
The Sahlgrenska Academy at Göteborg University
Göteborg
Sweden

Bruno G. Loos
Department of Periodontology
Academic Centre for Dentistry Amsterdam (ACTA)
Amsterdam
The Netherlands

Tord Lundgren
Department of Periodontics
School of Dentistry
Loma Linda University
Loma Linda
CA
USA

Angelo Mariotti
Section of Periodontology
Ohio State University College of Dentistry
Columbus
OH
USA

Andrea Mombelli
Department of Periodontology and Oral
  Pathophysiology
School of Dental Medicine
University of Geneva
Geneva
Switzerland

John Moran
Division of Restorative Dentistry (Periodontology)
Department of Oral and Dental Science
Bristol Dental School and Hospital
Bristol
UK

Sture Nyman
Deceased

Richard Palmer
Restorative Dentistry
King's College London Dental Institute
Guy's, King's and St Thomas' Hospitals
London
UK

Panos N. Papapanou
Division of Periodontics
Section of Oral and Diagnostic Sciences
Columbia University College of Dental Medicine
New York
NY
USA

David W. Paquette
Department of Periodontology
University of North Carolina School of Dentistry
Chapel Hill
NC
USA

Giovan P. Pini Prato
Department of Periodontology
University of Florence
Florence
Italy

Bjarni E. Pjetursson
Department of Periodontology and Fixed
  Prosthodontics
School of Dental Medicine
University of Berne
Berne
Switzerland

Ioannis Polyzois
Dublin Dental School and Hospital
Trinity College
Dublin
Ireland

Roberto Pontoriero
Private Practice
Milan
Italy

Marc Quirynen
Department of Periodontology
School of Dentistry
Catholic University of Leuven
Leuven
Belgium

Christoph A. Ramseier
Michigan Center for Oral Health Research
Department of Periodontics and Oral Medicine
University of Michigan School of Dentistry
Ann Arbor
MI
USA

Domenico Ricucci
Private Practice
Rome
Italy

Hector F. Rios
Department of Periodontics and Oral Medicine
University of Michigan School of Dentistry
Ann Arbor
MI
USA

Giovanni E. Salvi
Department of Periodontology
School of Dental Medicine
University of Berne
Berne
Switzerland

Mariano Sanz
Faculty of Odontology
University Complutense
Madrid
Spain

Marc A. Schätzle
Department of Orthodontics and Pediatric Dentistry
University of Zürich
Zürich
Switzerland

Sigmund S. Socransky
Department of Periodontology
The Forsyth Institute
Boston
MA
USA

Mena Soory
Restorative Dentistry
King's College London Dental Institute
Guy's, King's and St Thomas' Hospitals
London
UK

Clark M. Stanford
Dows Institute for Dental Research
University of Iowa
Iowa City
IA
USA

Ricardo P. Teles
Department of Periodontology
The Forsyth Institute
Boston
MA
USA

Maurizio S. Tonetti
Private Practice
Genoa
Italy

Leonardo Trombelli
Research Center for the Study of Periodontal
  Diseases
University of Ferrara
Ferrara
Italy

Ubele van der Velden
Department of Periodontology
Academic Centre for Dentistry Amsterdam (ACTA)
Amsterdam
The Netherlands

Fridus van der Weijden
Department of Periodontology
Academic Centre for Dentistry Amsterdam (ACTA)
Amsterdam
The Netherlands

Arie J. van Winkelhoff
Department of Oral Microbiology
Academic Centre for Dentistry Amsterdam (ACTA)
Amsterdam
The Netherlands

Hans-Peter Weber
Department of Restorative Dentistry and Biomaterials
  Science
Harvard School of Dental Medicine
Boston
MA
USA

Jan L. Wennström
Department of Periodontology
Institute of Odontology
The Sahlgrenska Academy at Göteborg University
Göteborg
Sweden

Jytte Westergaard
Department of Periodontology
School of Dentistry
University of Copenhagen
Copenhagen
Denmark

Ray C. Williams
Department of Periodontology
University of North Carolina School of Dentistry
Chapel Hill
NC
USA

Edwin G. Winkel
Department of Periodontology
Academic Centre for Oral Health
University Medical Centre Groningen
Groningen
The Netherlands

Björn U. Zachrisson
Department of Orthodontics
Dental Faculty
University of Oslo
Oslo
Norway

Giovanni Zucchelli
Department of Periodontology
Bologna University
Bologna
Italy

Preface

When the groundwork for the fifth edition of *Clinical Periodontology and Implant Dentistry* began in early 2007, it became clear that we had reached a fork in the road. It has always been my intention that each successive edition of this work should reflect the state of the art of clinical periodontology and, in doing such, should run the gamut of topics within this subject area. However, thorough coverage of an already large and now rapidly expanding specialty has resulted in a book of commensurate size and therefore for the fifth edition, the decision was taken to divide the book into two volumes: basic concepts and clinical concepts. The decision to make the split a purely physical one, and not an intellectual one, reflects the realization that over the past decade, implant dentistry has become a basic part of periodontology. The integrated structure of this latest edition of the textbook mirrors this merger.

In order for the student of dentistry, whatever his or her level, to learn how teeth and implants may function together as separate or connected units in the same dentition, a sound knowledge of the tissues that surround the natural tooth and the dental implant, as well as an understanding of the various lesions that may occur in the supporting tissues, is imperative. Hence, in both volumes of the textbook, chapters dealing with traditional periodontal issues, such as anatomy, pathology and treatment, are followed by similar topics related to tissues surrounding dental implants. In the first volume of the fifth edition, "basic concepts" as they relate to anatomy, microbiology and pathology, for example, are presented, while in the second volume ("clinical concepts"), various aspects of often evidence-based periodontal and restorative examination and treatment procedures are outlined.

It is my hope that the fifth edition of *Clinical Periodontology and Implant Dentistry* will challenge the reader intellectually, provide elucidation and clarity of information, and also impart an understanding of how the information presented in the text can, and should, be used in the practice of contemporary dentistry.

Jan Lindhe

Part 9: Examination Protocols

26 Examination of Patients with Periodontal Diseases, 573
Giovanni E. Salvi, Jan Lindhe, and Niklaus P. Lang

27 Examination of the Candidate for Implant Therapy, 587
Hans-Peter Weber, Daniel Buser, and Urs C. Belser

28 Radiographic Examination of the Implant Patient, 600
Hans-Göran Gröndahl and Kerstin Gröndahl

29 Examination of Patients with Implant-Supported Restorations, 623
Urs Brägger

30 Risk Assessment of the Implant Patient, 634
Gary C. Armitage and Tord Lundgren

Chapter 26

Examination of Patients with Periodontal Diseases

Giovanni E. Salvi, Jan Lindhe, and Niklaus P. Lang

History of periodontal patients, 573
   Chief complaint and expectations, 573
   Social and family history, 573
   Dental history, 573
   Oral hygiene habits, 573
   Smoking history, 574
   Medical history and medications, 574

Signs and symptoms of periodontal diseases, 574
   The gingiva, 574
   The periodontal ligament and the root cementum, 577
   The alveolar bone, 583
Diagnosis of periodontal lesions, 583
Oral hygiene status, 584
Additional dental examinations, 585

History of periodontal patients

The history of the patient is a revealing document as a basis for comprehensive treatment planning and understanding of the patient's needs, social and economic situation, as well as general medical conditions. In order to expedite history taking, a health questionnaire may be filled out by the patient prior to the initial examination. Such a questionnaire should be constructed in a way that the professional immediately realizes compromising or risk factors that may modify the treatment plan and, hence, may have to be discussed in detail with the patient during the initial visit. The assessment of the patient's history requires an evaluation of the following six aspects: (1) chief complaint, (2) social and family history, (3) dental history, (4) oral hygiene habits, (5) smoking history, and (6) medical history and medications.

Chief complaint and expectations

It is essential to realize the patient's needs and desires for treatment. If a patient has been referred for specific treatment, the extent of the desired treatment has to be defined and the referring dentist should be informed of the intentions for treatment.

Patients reporting independently, however, usually have specific desires and expectations regarding treatment outcomes. These may not be congruent with the true assessment of a professional with respect to the clinical situation. Optimal treatment results may only be achieved if the patient's demands are in balance with the objective evaluation of the disease and the projected treatment outcomes. There-fore, the patient's expectations have to be taken seriously and must be incorporated in the evaluation in harmony with the clinical situation.

Social and family history

Before assessing the clinical condition in detail, it is advantageous to elucidate the patient's social environment and to get a feeling for his/her priorities in life, including the attitude to dental care. Likewise, a family history may be important, especially with respect to aggressive forms of periodontitis.

Dental history

These aspects include an assessment of previous dental care and maintenance visits if not stated by a referring dentist. In this context, information regarding signs and symptoms of periodontitis noted by the patient, such as migration and increasing mobility of teeth, bleeding gums, food impaction, and difficulties in chewing have to be explored. Chewing comfort and the possible need for tooth replacement is determined.

Oral hygiene habits

In addition to the exploration of the patient's routine dental care, including frequency and duration of daily tooth brushing, knowledge about interdental cleansing devices and additional chemical supportive agents, and regular use of fluorides should be assessed.

Smoking history

Since cigarette smoking has been documented to be the second most important risk factor after inadequate plaque control (Kinane *et al.* 2006) in the etiology and pathogenesis of periodontal diseases, the importance of smoking counseling cannot be overestimated. Hence, determination of smoking status, including detailed information about exposure time and quantity, has to be gathered. Further aspects of smoking cessation programs are presented in Chapter 33.

Medical history and medications

General medical aspects may be extracted from the health questionnaire constructed to highlight the medical risk factors encountered for routine periodontal and/or implant therapy. The four major complexes of complications encountered in patients may be prevented by checking the medical history with respect to: (1) cardiovascular and circulatory risks, (2) bleeding disorders, (2) infective risks, and (4) allergic reactions. Further aspects are presented in Chapters 30 and 33.

In light of the increasing consumption of medications in the aging population, an accurate assessment of the patient's prescribed medications and their potential interactions and effects on therapeutic procedures has to be made. It may be necessary to contact the patient's physician for detailed information relevant to the planned dental treatment.

Signs and symptoms of periodontal diseases

Periodontal diseases are characterized by color and texture alterations of the gingiva, e.g. redness and swelling, as well as an increased tendency to bleeding upon probing in the gingival sulcus/pocket area (Fig. 26-1). In addition, the periodontal tissues may exhibit reduced resistance to probing perceived as increased probing depth and/or tissue recession. Advanced stages of periodontitis may also be associated with increased tooth mobility as well as drifting or flaring of teeth (Fig. 26-2).

In radiographs, periodontitis may be recognized by moderate to advanced loss of alveolar bone (Fig. 26-3). Bone loss is defined either as "horizontal" or "angular". If bone loss has progressed at similar rates in the dentition, the crestal contour of the remaining bone in the radiograph is even and defined as being "horizontal". In contrast, angular bony defects are the result of bone loss that developed at different rates around teeth/tooth surfaces and, hence, that type is defined as being "vertical" or "angular".

In a histological section, periodontitis is characterized by the presence of an inflammatory cell infiltrate within a 1–2 mm wide zone of the gingival connec-

tive tissue adjacent to the biofilm on the tooth (Fig. 26-4). Within the infiltrated area there is a pronounced loss of collagen. In more advanced forms of periodontitis, marked loss of connective tissue attachment to the root and apical downgrowth of the dentogingival epithelium along the root are important characteristics.

Results from clinical and animal research have demonstrated that chronic and aggressive forms of periodontal disease:

1. Affect individuals with various susceptibility at different rates (Löe *et al.* 1986)
2. Affect different parts of the dentition to a varying degree (Papapanou *et al.* 1988)
3. Are site specific in nature for a given area (Socransky *et al.* 1984)
4. Are sometimes progressive in character and, if left untreated, may result in tooth loss (Löe *et al.* 1986)
5. Can be arrested following proper therapy (Rosling *et al.* 2001).

For effective treatment planning, the location, topography, and extent of periodontal lesions must be recognized in all parts of the dentition. It is, therefore, mandatory to examine all sites of all teeth for the presence or absence of periodontal lesions. This, in turn, means that single-rooted teeth will have to be examined at least at four sites (e.g. mesial, buccal, distal, and oral) and multi-rooted teeth at least at six sites (e.g. mesio-buccal, buccal, disto-buccal, disto-oral, oral, and mesio-oral) with special attention to the furcation areas.

Since periodontitis includes inflammatory alterations of the gingiva and a progressive loss of periodontal attachment and alveolar bone, the comprehensive examination must include assessments describing such pathologic alterations. Figure 26-1 illustrates the clinical status of a 59-year-old patient diagnosed with advanced generalized chronic periodontitis. The examination procedures used to assess the location and extension of periodontal disease will be demonstrated by using this case as an example.

The gingiva

Clinical signs of gingivitis include changes in color and texture of the soft marginal gingival tissue and bleeding on probing.

Various index systems have been developed to describe gingivitis in epidemiologic and clinical research. They are discussed in Chapter 7. Even though the composition of the inflammatory infiltrate can only be identified in histologic sections, the correct clinical diagnosis for inflamed gingival tissue is made on the basis of the tendency to bleed on probing. The symptom "bleeding on probing" (BoP) to the bottom of the gingival sulcus/pocket is associ-

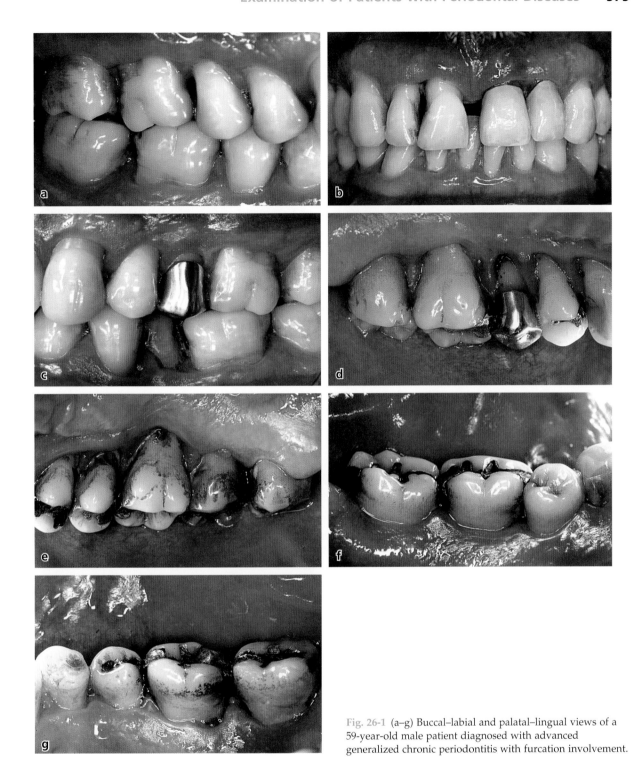

Fig. 26-1 (a–g) Buccal–labial and palatal–lingual views of a 59-year-old male patient diagnosed with advanced generalized chronic periodontitis with furcation involvement.

ated with the presence of an inflammatory cell infiltrate. The occurrence of such bleeding, especially in repeated examinations, is indicative for disease progression (Lang *et al.* 1986), although the predictive value of this single parameter remains rather low (i.e. 30%). On the other hand, the absence of bleeding on probing yields a high negative predictive value (i.e. 98.5%) and, hence, is an important indicator of periodontal stability (Lang *et al.* 1990; Joss *et al.* 1994).

Since trauma to the tissues provoked by probing should be avoided to assess the true vascular permeability changes associated with inflammation, a probing pressure of 0.25 N should be applied for assessing "bleeding on probing" (Lang *et al.* 1991; Karayiannis *et al.* 1992). The identification of the apical extent of the gingival lesion is made in conjunction with pocket probing depth (PPD) measurements. In sites where "shallow" pockets are present, inflammatory lesions in the overt portion of the gingiva are distinguished by probing in the superficial marginal tissue. When the infiltrate is in sites with attachment loss, the inflammatory lesion in the

apical part of the pocket must be identified by probing to the bottom of the deepened pocket.

Bleeding on probing (BoP)

A periodontal probe is inserted to the "bottom" of the gingival/periodontal pocket applying light force and is moved gently along the tooth (root) surface (Fig. 26-5). If bleeding is provoked by this instrumentation upon retrieval of the probe, the site examined is considered "bleeding on probing" (BoP)-positive and, hence, inflamed.

Figure 26-6 illustrates the chart used to identify BoP-positive sites in a dichotomous way at the initial examination. Each tooth in the chart is represented and each tooth surface is indicated by a triangle. The inner segments represent the palatal/lingual gingival units, the outer segments the buccal/labial units and the remaining fields the two approximal gingival units. The fields of the chart corresponding to the

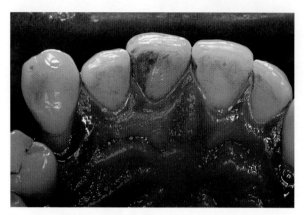

Fig. 26-2 Buccal migration of tooth 13 as a sign of advanced periodontitis.

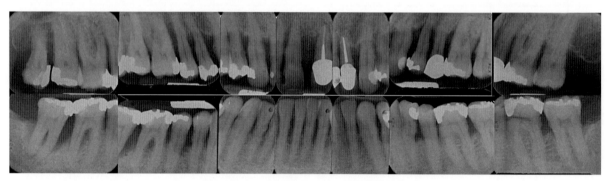

Fig. 26-3 Periapical radiographs of the patient presented in Fig. 26-1.

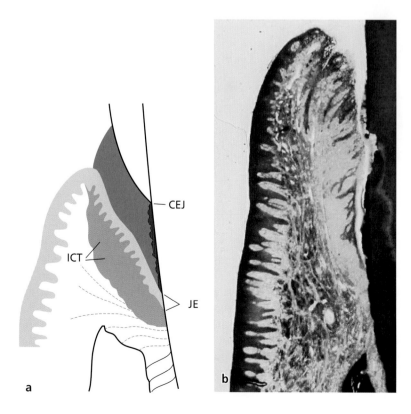

Fig. 26-4 Schematic drawing (a) and histologic section (b) illustrating the characteristics of periodontal disease. Note the zone of infiltrated connective tissue (ICT) lateral to the junctional epithelium (JE). CEJ = cemento-enamel junction; JE = junctional epithelium.

inflamed gingival units are marked in red. The mean BoP score (i.e. gingivitis) is given as a percentage. In the present example, 104 out of a total number of 116 gingival units bled on probing, amounting to a BoP percentage of 89%. This method of charting not only serves as a means of documenting areas of health and disease in the dentition but similar charting during the course of therapy or maintenance will disclose sites which become healthy or remain inflamed. The topographical pattern will also identify sites with consistent or repeated BoP at various observation periods.

The periodontal ligament and the root cementum

In order to evaluate the amount of tissue lost in periodontitis and also to identify the apical extension of the inflammatory lesion, the following parameters should be recorded:

1. Probing pocket depth (PPD)
2. Probing attachment level (PAL)
3. Furcation involvement (FI)
4. Tooth mobility (TM).

Assessment of probing pocket depth

The probing depth, i.e. the distance from the gingival margin to the bottom of the gingival sulcus/pocket, is measured to the nearest millimeter by means of a graduated periodontal probe with a standardized tip diameter of approximately 0.4–0.5 mm (Fig. 26-7). The pocket depth should be assessed at each surface

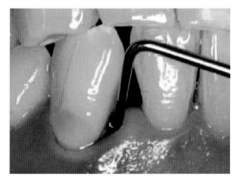

Fig. 26-5 Probing pocket depth (PPD) in conjunction with bleeding on probing (BoP). A graduated periodontal probe is inserted to the "bottom" of the gingival/periodontal pocket applying light force and is moved gently along the tooth (root) surface.

of all teeth in the dentition. In the periodontal chart (Fig. 26-8), PPD <4 mm are indicated in black figures, while deeper PPD (i.e. ≥4 mm) are marked in red. This allows an immediate evaluation of diseased sites (i.e. red figures) both from an extent and severity point of view. The chart may be used for case presentation and discussion with the patient.

Results from pocket depth measurements will only give proper information regarding the extent of loss of probing attachment in rare situations (when the gingival margin coincides with the cemento-enamel junction, CEJ). For example, an inflammatory edema may cause swelling of the free gingiva resulting in coronal displacement of the gingival margin without a concomitant migration of the dentogingival epithelium to a level apical to the CEJ. In such a situation, a pocket depth exceeding 3–4 mm represents a "pseudopocket". In other situations, an obvious loss of periodontal attachment may have occurred without a concomitant increase of probing pocket depth. A situation of this kind is illustrated in Fig. 26-9, where multiple recessions of the gingiva can be seen. Hence, the assessment of the probing depth in relation to the CEJ is an indispensable parameter for the evaluation of the periodontal condition (i.e. PAL).

Assessment of probing attachment level

PAL may be assessed to the nearest millimeter by means of a graduated probe and expressed as the distance in millimeters from the CEJ to the bottom of the probeable gingival/periodontal pocket. The clinical assessment requires the measurement of the distance from the free gingival margin (FGM) to the CEJ for each tooth surface. After this recording, PAL may be calculated from the periodontal chart (i.e. PPD – distance CEJ to FGM). In cases with gingival recession, the distance FGM–CEJ turns negative and, hence, will be added to the PPD to determine PAL.

Errors inherent in periodontal probing

The distances recorded in a periodontal examination using a periodontal probe have generally been assumed to represent a fairly accurate estimate of the PPD or PAL at a given site. In other words, the tip of the periodontal probe has been assumed to identify the level of the most apical cells of the dentogingival (junctional epithelium) epithelium. Results from research, however, indicated that this is seldom the

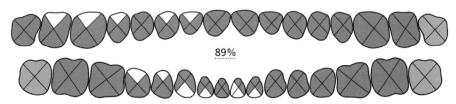

89%

Fig. 26-6 Chart used to identify BoP-positive sites in a dichotomous way at the initial examination and during maintenance care.

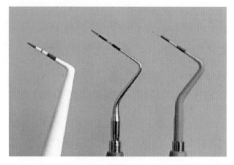

Fig. 26-7 Examples of graduated periodontal probes with a standardized tip diameter of approximately 0.4–0.5 mm.

case (Saglie *et al.* 1975; Listgarten *et al.* 1976; Armitage *et al.* 1977; Ezis & Burgett 1978; Spray *et al.* 1978; Robinson & Vitek 1979; van der Velden 1979; Magnusson & Listgarten 1980; Polson *et al.* 1980). A variety of factors influencing measurements made with periodontal probes include: (1) the thickness of the probe used, (2) angulation and positioning of the probe due to anatomic features such as the contour of the tooth surface, (3) the graduation scale of the periodontal probe, (4) the pressure applied on the instrument during probing, and (5) the degree of

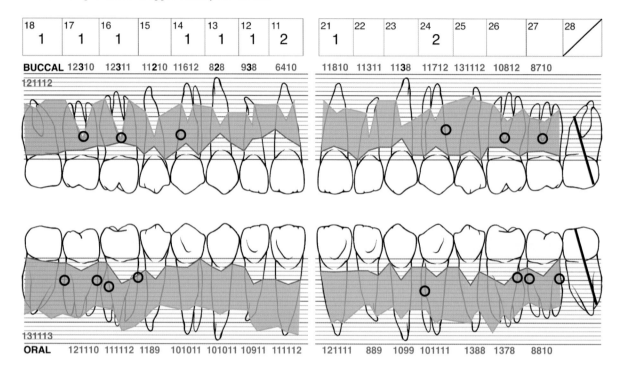

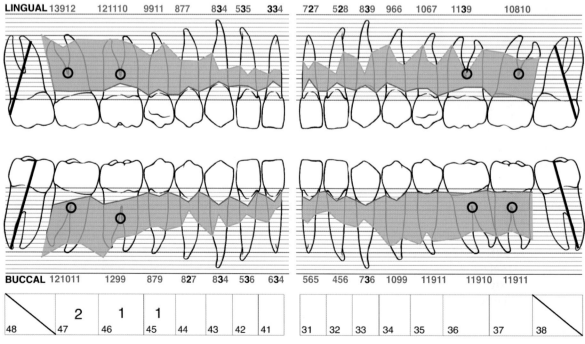

Fig. 26-8 Periodontal chart indicating PPD <4 mm in black figures and PPD ≥4 mm in red figures. This allows an immediate evaluation of diseased sites (i.e. red figures) both from an extent and severity point of view.

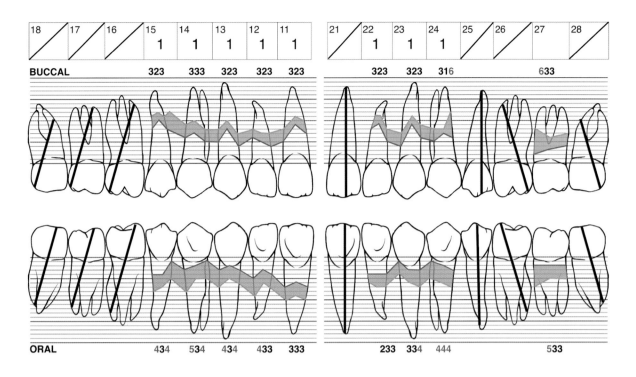

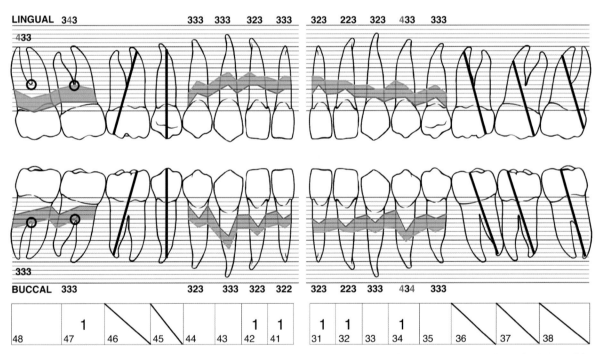

Fig. 26-9 Periodontal attachment loss has occurred without a concomitant increase of probing pocket depth. Multiple buccal/labial as well as palatal/lingual gingival recessions can be seen.

inflammatory cell infiltration in the soft tissue and accompanying loss of collagen. Therefore, a distinction should be made between the histologic and the clinical PPD to differentiate between the depth of the actual anatomic defect and the measurement recorded by the probe (Listgarten 1980).

Measurement errors depending on factors such as the thickness of the probe, the contour of the tooth surface, incorrect angulation, and the graduation scale of the probe can be reduced or avoided by the selection of a standardized instrument and careful

management of the examination procedure. More difficult to avoid, however, are errors resulting from variations in probing force and the extent of inflammatory alterations of the periodontal tissues. As a rule, the greater the probing pressure applied, the deeper the penetration of the probe into the tissue. In this context, it should be realized that in investigations designed to disclose the pressure (force) used by different clinicians, the probing pressure was found to range from 0.03–1.3 N (Gabathuler & Hassell 1971; Hassell *et al.* 1973), and also, to differ by as

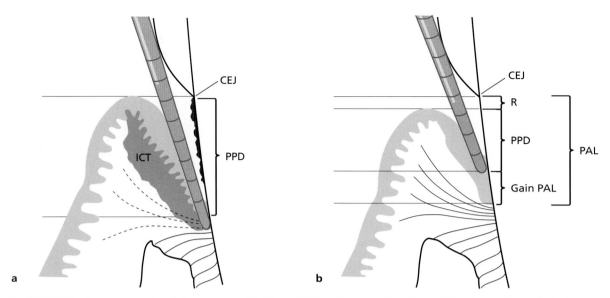

Fig. 26-10 (a) In the presence of an inflammatory cell infiltrate (ICT) in the connective tissue of the gingiva, the periodontal probe penetrates apically to the bottom of the histologic pocket. (b) Following successful periodontal therapy, the swelling is reduced and the connective tissue cell infiltrate is replaced by collagen. The periodontal probe fails to reach the apical part of the dentogingival epithelium. CEJ = cemento-enamel junction; PPD = probing pocket depth; PAL = probing attachment level; R = recession; Gain PAL = recorded false gain of attachment ("clinical attachment").

much as 2:1 for the same dentist from one examination to another. In order to exclude measurement errors related to the effect of variations in probing pressure, so-called pressure-sensitive probes have been developed. Such probes will enable the examiner to probe with a predetermined pressure (van der Velden & de Vries 1978; Vitek *et al.* 1979; Polson *et al.* 1980). However, over- and underestimation of the "true" PPD or PAL may also occur when this type of probing device is employed (Armitage *et al.* 1977; Robinson & Vitek 1979; Polson *et al.* 1980). Thus, when the connective tissue subjacent to the pocket epithelium is infiltrated by inflammatory cells (Fig. 26-10), the periodontal probe will most certainly penetrate beyond the apical termination of the dentogingival epithelium. This results in an overestimation of the "true" depth of the pocket. Conversely, when the inflammatory infiltrate decreases in size following successful periodontal treatment, and a concomitant deposition of new collagen occurs within the previously inflamed tissue area, the dentogingival tissue will become more resistant to penetration by the probe. The probe may now fail to reach the apical termination of the epithelium using the same probing pressure. This, in turn, results in an underestimation of the "true" PPD or PAL. The magnitude of the difference between the probing measurement and the histologic "true" pocket depth (Fig. 26-10) may range from fractions of a millimeter to a couple of millimeters (Listgarten 1980).

From this discussion it should be understood that reductions in PPD following periodontal treatment and/or gain of PAL, assessed by periodontal probing, do not necessarily indicate the formation of a new connective tissue attachment at the bottom of the previous lesion. Rather, such a change may merely represent a resolution of the inflammatory process and may thus occur without an accompanying histologic gain of attachment (Fig. 26-10). In this context it should be realized that the terms "probing pocket depth" (PPD) and "probing attachment level" (PAL) have replaced the previously used terms "pocket depth" and "gain and loss of attachment". Likewise, PAL is used in conjunction with "gain" and/or "loss" to indicate that changes in PAL have been assessed by clinical probing.

Current knowledge of the histopathology of periodontal lesions and healing thereof has thus resulted in an altered concept regarding the validity of periodontal probing. However, despite difficulties in interpreting the significance of PPD and PAL measurements, such determinations still give the clinician a useful estimate of the degree of disease involvement, and particularly so, when the information obtained is related to other findings of the examination procedure such as BoP and changes in alveolar bone height.

In recent years, periodontal probing procedures have been standardized to the extent that automated probing systems such as, e.g. the Florida Probe™, have been developed, yielding periodontal charts with PPD, PAL, BoP, furcation involvement (FI) and tooth mobility (TM) at one glance (Gibbs *et al.* 1988). Also, repeated examinations allow the comparison of parameters, and, hence, an assessment of the healing process (Fig. 26-11).

Assessment of furcation involvement

In the progression of periodontitis around multirooted teeth, the destructive process may involve the supporting structures of the furcation area (Fig.

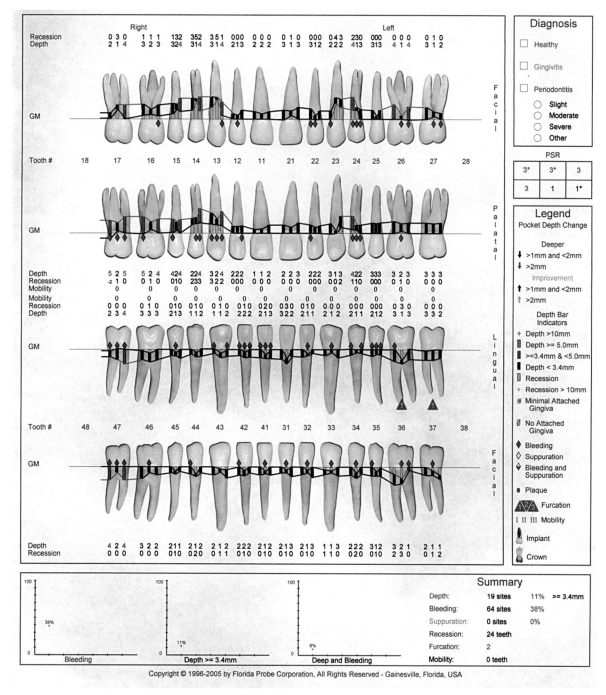

Fig. 26-11 Periodontal chart using an automated probing system (Florida Probe™). Reproduced with permission, © Copyright 1996–2005 Florida Probe Corporation.

26-12). In order to plan treatment for such involvement, a detailed and precise identification of the presence and extension of periodontal tissue breakdown within the furcation area is of importance for proper diagnosis.

Furcation involvement is assessed from all the entrances of possible periodontal lesions of multirooted teeth, i.e. buccal and/or lingual entrances of the mandibular molars. Maxillary molars and premolars are examined from the buccal, disto-palatal, and mesio-palatal entrances. Owing to the position of the first maxillary molars within the alveolar process, the furcation between the mesio-buccal and the palatal

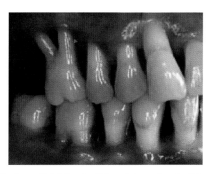

Fig. 26-12 Superficial (tooth 46) and deep (tooth 16) periodontal tissue destruction in the buccal furcation areas.

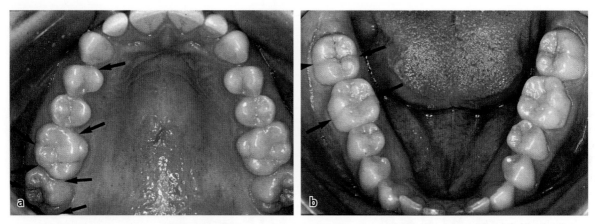

Fig. 26-13 (a,b) Anatomic locations for the assessment of furcation involvement (FI) in the maxilla and in the mandible.

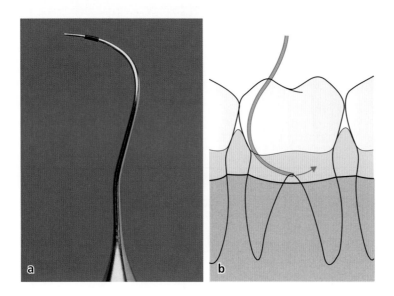

Fig. 26-14 (a,b) Furcation involvement (FI) is explored using a curved periodontal probe graduated at 3 mm (Nabers furcation probe).

roots is best explored from the palatal aspect (Fig. 26-13).

Furcation involvement is explored using a curved periodontal probe graduated at 3 mm (Nabers furcation probe) (Fig. 26-14). Depending on the penetration depth, the FI is classified as "superficial" or "deep":

- Horizontal probing depth ≤3 mm from one or two entrances is classified as a degree I FI.
- Horizontal probing depth >3 mm in at the most one furcation entrance and/or in combination with a degree I FI is classified as degree II FI.
- Horizontal probing depth >3 mm in two or more furcation entrances usually represents a "through-and-through" destruction of the supporting tissues in the furcation and is classified as degree III FI.

The FI degree is presented in the periodontal chart (Fig. 26-15) together with a description of which tooth surface the involvement has been identified on. A detailed discussion regarding the management

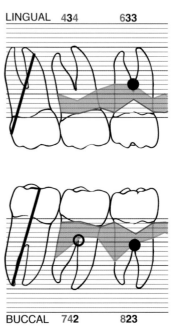

Fig. 26-15 The FI degree is illustrated in the periodontal chart. Open circles represent a superficial FI (i.e horizontal probe penetration ≤3 mm) whereas filled black circles represent a deep FI (i.e. horizontal probe penetration >3 mm).

of furcation-involved teeth is presented in Chapter 39.

Assessment of tooth mobility

The continuous loss of the supporting tissues during periodontal disease progression may result in increased tooth mobility. However, trauma from occlusion may also lead to increased tooth mobility. Therefore, the reason for increased tooth mobility as being the result of a widened periodontal ligament or a reduced height of the supporting tissues or a combination thereof should be elaborated. Increased tooth mobility may be classified according to Miller (1950).

- Degree 0: "physiological" mobility measured at the crown level. The tooth is mobile within the alveolus to approximately 0.1–0.2 mm in a horizontal direction.
- Degree 1: increased mobility of the crown of the tooth to at the most 1 mm in a horizontal direction.
- Degree 2: visually increased mobility of the crown of the tooth exceeding 1 mm in a horizontal direction.
- Degree 3: severe mobility of the crown of the tooth both in horizontal and vertical directions impinging on the function of the tooth.

It must be understood that plaque-associated periodontal disease is not the only cause of increased tooth mobility. For instance, overloading of teeth and trauma may result in tooth hypermobility. Increased tooth mobility can frequently also be observed in conjunction with periapical lesions or immediately following periodontal surgery. From a therapeutic point of view it is important, therefore, to assess not only the degree of increased tooth mobility but also the cause of the observed hypermobility (see Chapters 14 and 57).

All data collected in conjunction with measurements of PPD, PAL, as well as from the assessments of FI and tooth mobility are included in the periodontal chart (Fig. 26-8). The various teeth in this chart are denoted according to the two-digit system adopted by the FDI in 1970.

The alveolar bone

The height of the alveolar bone and the outline of the bony crest are examined in radiographs (Fig. 26-3). Radiographs provide information on the height and configuration of the interproximal alveolar bone. Obscuring structures such as roots of the teeth often make it difficult to identify the outline of the buccal and lingual alveolar bony crest. Analysis of radiographs must, therefore, be combined with a detailed evaluation of the periodontal chart in order to come

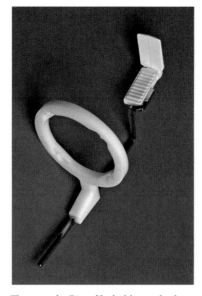

Fig. 26-16 The use of a Rinn filmholder and a long-cone paralleling technique yield reproducible radiographs.

up with a correct estimate concerning "horizontal" and "angular" bony defects.

As opposed to the periodontal chart that represents a sensitive diagnostic estimate of the lesions, the radiographic analysis is a specific diagnostic test yielding few false-negative results and, hence, is confirmatory to the periodontal chart (Lang & Hill 1977).

To enable meaningful comparative analysis, a radiographic technique should be used which yields reproducible radiographs. In this context, a long-cone paralleling technique (Updegrave 1951) is recommended (Fig. 26-16).

Diagnosis of periodontal lesions

Based on the information regarding the condition of the various periodontal structures (i.e. the gingiva, the periodontal ligament, and the alveolar bone) which has been obtained through the comprehensive examination presented above, a classification of the patient as well as a diagnosis for each tooth regarding the periodontal conditions may be given (Table 26-1). Four different tooth-based diagnoses may be used:

- *Gingivitis.* This diagnosis is applied to teeth displaying bleeding on probing. The sulcus depth usually remains at levels of 1–3 mm irrespective of the level of clinical attachment. "Pseudopockets" may be present in cases of slightly increased probing depth without concomitant attachment and alveolar bone loss and presence/absence of bleeding on probing. The diagnosis of gingivitis usually characterizes lesions confined to the gingival margin.
- *Parodontitis superficialis* (mild–moderate periodontitis). Gingivitis in combination with attachment loss is termed "periodontitis". If the PPD does not exceed 6 mm, a diagnosis of mild–moderate

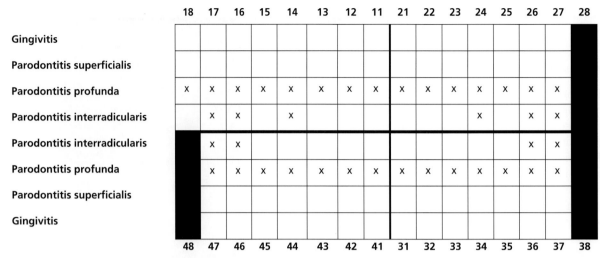

Fig. 26-17 Chart of the individual tooth diagnosis of the patient presented in Fig. 26-1.

Table 26-1 The diagnosis of the periodontal tissue conditions around each tooth in the dentition is given using main criteria (i.e. periodontal chart and radiographic analysis) and additional criteria (i.e. bleeding on probing)

Diagnosis	Main criteria	Additional criteria
Gingivitis	Bleeding on probing (BoP) No loss of PAL and alveolar bone PPD ≤3 mm Pseudopockets	
Parodontitis superficialis	PPD ≤5 mm, irrespective of the morphology of the periodontal lesion Angular and/or horizontal alveolar bone loss	Bleeding on probing (BoP)
Parodontitis profunda	PPD ≥6 mm, irrespective of the morphology of the periodontal lesion Angular and/or horizontal alveolar bone loss	Bleeding on probing (BoP)
Parodontitis interradicularis	Horizontal PPD ≤3 mm: superficial FI Horizontal PPD >3 mm: deep FI	Bleeding on probing (BoP)

periodontitis is given irrespective of the morphology of periodontal lesions. This diagnosis may, therefore, be applied to teeth with "horizontal" loss of supporting tissues, representing suprabony lesions, and/or to teeth with "angular" or "vertical" loss of supporting tissues, representing infrabony lesions. "Infrabony" lesions include "intrabony one-, two- and three-wall defects" as well as "craters" between two adjacent teeth.
• *Parodontitis profunda* (advanced periodontitis). If the PPD does exceeds 6 mm, a diagnosis of

advanced periodontitis is given irrespective of the morphology of periodontal lesions. As for mild–moderate periodontitis, angular as well as horizontal alveolar bone loss are included in this diagnosis. The distinction between mild–moderate and advanced periodontitis is only based on increased PPD.
• *Parodontitis interradicularis* (periodontitis in the furcation area). Adjunctive diagnoses may be attributed to multi-rooted teeth with FI (see above): superficial FI if horizontal PPD ≤3 mm (parodontitis interradicularis superficialis) and deep FI for horizontal PPD >3 mm (parodontitis interradicularis profunda).

In the presence of necrotizing and/or ulcerative lesions, these terms may be added to tooth-related diagnoses of both gingivitis and periodontitis (Chapter 20). Acute lesions including gingival and periodontal abscesses are diagnosed as indicated in Chapter 22.

The various teeth of the patient whose clinical status is shown in Fig. 26-1, the radiographs in Fig. 26-3 and the periodontal chart in Fig. 26-8 have received the diagnoses described in Fig. 26-17.

Oral hygiene status

In conjunction with the examination of the periodontal tissues, the patient's oral hygiene practices must also be evaluated. Absence or presence of plaque on each tooth surface in the dentition is recorded in a dichotomous manner (O'Leary et al. 1972). The bacterial deposits may be stained with a disclosing solution to facilitate their detection. The presence of plaque is marked in appropriate fields in the plaque chart shown in Fig. 26-18. The mean plaque score for the dentition is given as a percentage in correspondence with the system used for BoP (Fig. 26-6).

Alterations with respect to the presence of plaque and gingival inflammation are illustrated in a simple

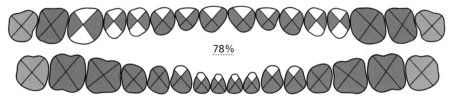

Fig. 26-18 The presence of bacterial deposits is marked in the appropriate fields in the plaque chart.

way by the repeated use of the combined BoP (Fig. 26-6) and plaque (Fig. 26-18) charts during the course of treatment. Repeated plaque recordings alone (Fig. 26-18) are predominantly indicated during the initial phase of periodontal therapy (i.e. infection control) and are used for improving self-performed plaque control. Repeated BoP charts alone (Fig. 26-6), on the other hand, are predominantly recommended during maintenance care.

Additional dental examinations

In addition to the assessment of plaque, retentive factors for plaque, such as supra- and subgingival calculus and defective margins of dental restorations, should also be identified. Furthermore, the assessment of tooth sensitivity is essential for comprehensive treatment planning. Sensitivity to percussion may indicate acute changes in pulp vitality and lead to emergency treatment prior to systematic periodontal therapy. It is obvious that a complete examination and assessment of the patient will have to include the search for carious lesions both clinically as well as radiographically.

Screening for functional disturbances may be performed using a short (i.e. 1/2 minute) test according to Shore (1963). In this test, harmonious function of the jaws with simultaneous palpation of the temporomandibular joints during opening, closing, and excursive movements is verified. Maximal mouth opening is assessed and finally, the lodge of the lateral pterygoid muscles is palpated for muscle tenderness. Further morphologic characteristics of the dentition as well as occlusal and articulating contacts may be identified.

Conclusion

The methods described above for the examination of patients with respect to periodontal disease provide a thorough analysis of the presence, extent and severity of the disease in the dentition. The classification of the patient and the correct diagnosis for each individual tooth should form the basis for a pretherapeutic prognosis and the treatment planning of the individual patient (see Chapter 31).

References

Armitage, G.C., Svanberg, G.K. & Löe, H. (1977). Microscopic evaluation of clinical measurements of connective tissue attachment level. *Journal of Clinical Periodontology* **4**, 173–190.

Ezis, I. & Burgett, F. (1978). Probing related to attachment levels on recently erupted teeth. *Journal of Dental Research* **57**, Spec Issue A 307, Abstract No. 932.

Gabathuler, H. & Hassell, T. (1971). A pressure sensitive periodontal probe. *Helvetica Odontologica Acta* **15**, 114–117.

Gibbs, C.H., Hirschfeld, J.W., Lee, J.G., Low, S.B., Magnusson, I., Thousand, R.R., Yerneni, P. & Clark, W.B. (1988). Description and clinical evaluation of a new computerized periodontal probe – the Florida probe. *Journal of Clinical Periodontology* **15**, 137–144.

Hassell, T.M., Germann, M.A. & Saxer, U.P. (1973). Periodontal probing: investigator discrepancies and correlations between probing force and recorded depth. *Helvetica Odontologica Acta* **17**, 38–42.

Joss, A., Adler, R. & Lang, N.P. (1994). Bleeding on probing. A parameter for monitoring periodontal conditions in clinical practice. *Journal of Clinical Periodontology* **21**, 402–408.

Karayiannis, A., Lang, N.P., Joss, A. & Nyman, S. (1992). Bleeding on probing as it relates to probing pressure and gingival health in patients with a reduced but healthy periodontium. A clinical study. *Journal of Clinical Periodontology* **19**, 471–475.

Kinane, D.F., Peterson, M. & Stathoupoulou, P.G. (2006). Environmental and other modifying factors of the periodontal diseases. *Periodontology 2000* **40**, 107–119.

Lang, N.P., Adler, R., Joss, A. & Nyman, S. (1990). Absence of bleeding on probing. An indicator of periodontal stability. *Journal of Clinical Periodontology* **17**, 714–721.

Lang, N.P. & Hill, R.W. (1977). Radiographs in periodontics. *Journal of Clinical Periodontology* **4**, 16–28.

Lang, N.P., Joss, A., Orsanic, T., Gusberti, F.A. & Siegrist, B.E. (1986) Bleeding on probing. A predictor for the progression of periodontal disease? *Journal of Clinical Periodontology* **13**, 590–596.

Lang, N.P., Nyman, S., Senn, C. & Joss, A. (1991). Bleeding on probing as it relates to probing pressure and gingival health. *Journal of Clinical Periodontology* **18**, 257–261.

Listgarten, M.A. (1980). Periodontal probing: What does it mean? *Journal of Clinical Periodontology* **7**, 165–176.

Listgarten, M.A., Mao, R. & Robinson, P.J. (1976). Periodontal probing and the relationship of the probe tip to periodontal tissues. *Journal of Periodontology* **47**, 511–513.

Löe, H., Anerud, Å., Boysen, H. & Morrison, E. (1986). Natural history of periodontal disease in man. Rapid, moderate and no loss of attachment in Sri Lankan laborers 14 to 46 years of age. *Journal of Clinical Periodontology* **13**, 431–445.

Magnusson, I. & Listgarten, M.A. (1980). Histological evaluation of probing depth following periodontal treatment. *Journal of Clinical Periodontology* **7**, 26–31.

Miller, S.C. (1950) *Textbook of Periodontia*, 3rd edn. Philadelphia: The Blakeston Co., p. 125.

O'Leary, T.J., Drake, R.B. & Naylor, J.E. (1972). The plaque control record. *Journal of Periodontology* **43**, 38.

Papapanou, P.N., Wennström, J.L. & Gröndahl, K. (1988). Periodontal status in relation to age and tooth type. A cross-sectional radiographic study. *Journal of Clinical Periodontology* **15**, 469–478.

Polson, A.M., Caton, J.G., Yeaple, R.N. & Zander, H.A. (1980). Histological determination of probe tip penetration into gingival sulcus of humans using an electronic pressure-sensitive probe. *Journal of Clinical Periodontology* **7**, 479–488.

Robinson, P.J. & Vitek, R.M. (1979). The relationship between gingival inflammation and resistance to probe penetration. *Journal of Periodontal Research* **14**, 239–243.

Rosling, B., Serino, G., Hellström, M.K., Socransky, S.S. & Lindhe, J. (2001). Longitudinal periodontal tissue alterations during supportive therapy. Findings from subjects with normal and high susceptibility to periodontal disease. *Journal of Clinical Periodontology* **28**, 241–249.

Saglie, R., Johansen, J.R. & Flötra, L. (1975). The zone of completely and partially destructed periodontal fibers in pathological pockets. *Journal of Clinical Periodontology* **2**, 198–202.

Shore, N.A. (1963). Recognition and recording of symptoms of temporomandibular joint dysfunction. *Journal of the American Dental Association* **66**, 19–23.

Socransky, S.S., Haffajee, A.D., Goodson, J.M. & Lindhe, J. (1984). New concepts of destructive periodontal disease. *Journal of Clinical Periodontology* **11**, 21–32.

Spray, J.R., Garnick, J.J., Doles, L.R. & Klawitter, J.J. (1978). Microscopic demonstration of the position of periodontal probes. *Journal of Periodontology* **49**, 148–152.

Updegrave, W.J. (1951). The paralleling extension-cone technique in intraoral dental radiography. *Oral Surgery, Oral Medicine and Oral Pathology* **4**, 1250–1261.

van der Velden, U. (1979). Probing force and the relationship of the probe tip to the periodontal tissues. *Journal of Clinical Periodontology* **6**, 106–114.

van der Velden, U. & de Vries, J.H. (1978). Introduction of a new periodontal probe: the pressure probe. *Journal of Clinical Periodontology* **5**, 188–197.

Vitek, R.M., Robinson, P.J. & Lautenschlager, E.P. (1979). Development of a force-controlled periodontal instrument. *Journal of Periodontal Research* **14**, 93–94.

Chapter 27

Examination of the Candidate for Implant Therapy

Hans-Peter Weber, Daniel Buser, and Urs C. Belser

Dental implants in periodontally compromised patients, 587
Patient history, 590
  Chief complaint and expectations, 590
  Social and family history, 590
  Dental history, 590
  Motivation and compliance, 591
  Habits, 591
  Medical history and medications, 591

Local examination, 591
  Extraoral, 591
  General intraoral examination, 592
  Radiographic examination, 592
  Implant-specific intraoral examination, 592
Patient-specific risk assessment, 597
  Risk assessment for sites without esthetic implications, 597
  Risk assessment for sites with esthetic implications, 597

Dental implants in periodontally compromised patients

Modern comprehensive dental care for patients with periodontally compromised dentitions has to include the consideration of dental implants. Since the initial description of osseointegration experimentally (Branemark *et al.* 1969; Schroeder *et al.* 1976, 1981), scientific evidence has been established through human clinical studies that dental implants will serve as long-term predictable anchors for fixed and removable prostheses in fully and partially edentulous patients and that patient satisfaction with dental implant therapy is high (Adell *et al.* 1990; Fritz 1996; Buser *et al.* 1997; Lindh *et al.* 1998; Moy *et al.* 2005; Pjetursson *et al.* 2005). Furthermore, substantial scientific and clinical evidence has become available to help the understanding of factors enhancing or compromising treatment success with regard to esthetic concerns (Belser *et al.* 2004a,b; Buser *et al.* 2004, 2006; Higginbottom *et al.* 2004; Martin *et al.* 2006). Overall, the pool of information on contributing factors enhancing or compromising treatment success with dental implants continues to grow and is becoming more and more valuable despite its diversity and scientific inconsistency. This is possible through a focused interpretation of the published information via systematic reviews.

The decision whether to use remaining natural teeth as abutments for conventional fixed prostheses or to add dental implants for the replacement of diseased natural teeth is influenced by a number of factors, such as location in the dental arches, strategic value and treatment prognosis for such teeth, subjective and objective need for tooth replacement, dimensions of the alveolar process, esthetic impact, as well as access for treatment. Indications for dental implants in the periodontally compromised dentition include the replacement of single or multiple "hopeless" or missing teeth within or as distal extensions to partially dentate maxillary and mandibular arches (Fig. 27-1).

In the edentulous jaw, implants supporting fixed or removable prostheses will more frequently be inserted in the anterior regions where there are more favorable alveolar bone dimensions and quality. In partially edentulous patients, implants are more likely indicated in posterior regions with less favorable anatomic conditions. The volume of the alveolar process may be substantially reduced, especially in dentitions where teeth have been lost due to periodontal disease (Fig. 27-2). This introduces a number of concerns related to the longevity of implant anchorage, function, and esthetics.

In the posterior areas of the jaw, such concerns may primarily be of biomechanical nature due to the resulting unfavorable "crown–root ratios" in the region of the greatest masticatory forces. Treatment alternatives include the use of multiple short implants splinted together with the fixed partial denture they support (Fig. 27-3), external or internal sinus floor elevation (Fig. 27-4), vertical ridge augmentation with various bone grafting techniques or distraction osteogenesis, nerve repositioning, distal extension

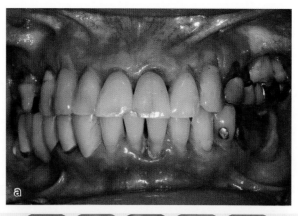

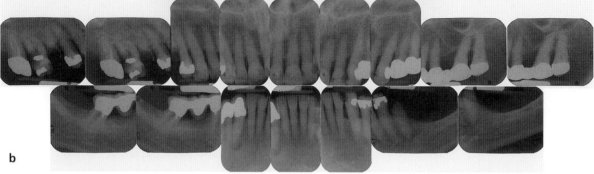

Fig. 27-1 (a) Intraoral image of a 77-year-old female patient with multiple dental problems including severe adult periodontitis after several years of neglect. At the initial examination on 12/6/06, the patient states that she does not want removable prostheses and asks for dental implants to replace the teeth, which may require extraction. (b) Full-mouth set of periapical radiographs of the same patient.

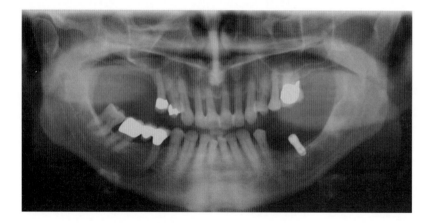

Fig. 27-2 Typical example of patient with reduced alveolar bone volume in the posterior areas of the upper right and lower left quadrant due to preceding severe periodontal bone loss. The lower left quadrant reveals a failed *alio loco* attempt for implant restoration of the lower left quadrant. According to the patient, one of the two short implants originally placed failed shortly after delivery of the fixed partial denture.

fixed prostheses anchored on remaining natural teeth or premolar occlusion without replacement of the failed molars (shortened dental arch concept) (Fig. 27-5).

Prior to the availability of dental implants and bone augmentation techniques for the replacement of posterior teeth lost to periodontal disease, cantilevered fixed partial dentures were a widely used alternative to extend dental arches distally where indicated and to spare the patient from removable partial dentures (Nyman and Lindhe 1976). Whereas this type of periodontal prosthesis performed admirably when designed and maintained properly (Fig. 27-5), the biological and biomechanical risks associated with such reconstructions have been shown to be consid-

erable (Hammerle *et al.* 2000; Pjetursson *et al.* 2004). In the patient with advanced *generalized* periodontal disease and a lack of sufficient posterior bone volume for dental implants, the extraction of the remaining compromised anterior dentition for the purpose of placing implants in combination with cantilevered full-arch prostheses as originally described by Brånemark *et al.* (1985) may prognostically be the most favorable treatment approach (Adell *et al.* 1990).

This generally supportive evidence for implant therapy has to be weighed against the long-term performance of dental implants in patients with a history of periodontal disease. This issue has recently received increased attention in the peer-reviewed dental literature (Ellegaard *et al.* 1997; Baelum &

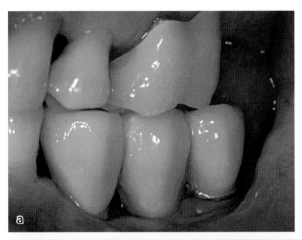

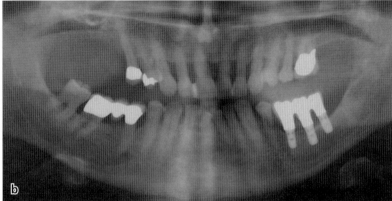

Fig. 27-3 (a) Intraoral clinical image of the same patient after prosthodontic reconstruction of the lower left quadrant with three short implants and a three-unit fixed partial denture. Note the resulting extensive crown heights. (b) Panoramic radiographic image of the implant restoration in the lower left quadrant using three 6 mm long implants. Five-year follow-up. The patient decided to wait with any prosthodontic treatment of the upper right quadrant, where a vertical ridge augmentation combined with external sinus elevation is required.

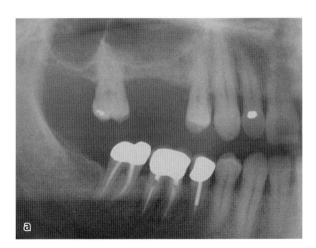

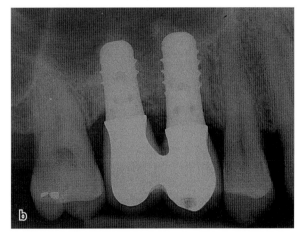

Fig. 27-4 (a) Reduced alveolar bone height in area of second premolar and first molar in the upper right quadrant. Teeth lost due to endodontic complications and periodontal disease combined. (b) Area restored with implant-supported, splinted restorations after internal sinus augmentation procedure at time of implant placement. Four-year follow-up.

Ellegaard 2004). Whereas after 5 years of function no difference was observed between implants in patients free of periodontal disease versus those with disease, a somewhat increased risk for peri-implantitis with bone loss and subsequent implant failure was found for certain implants after 10 years of follow-up. Despite this finding, the authors concluded that dental implants remain a good treatment alternative for patients with periodontal disease. In this context, the outcome with implants placed in sinus grafts in periodontitis patients was not different from subjects free of periodontal disease (Ellegaard *et al.* 2006).

A potential correlation of interleukin-1 (IL-1) gene polymorphism and susceptibility to severe periodontal disease has been reported by Kornman *et al.* (1997). Furthermore, the risk associated with IL-1 polymorphism, smoking and peri-implant bone loss was assessed in a study by Feloutzis *et al.* (2003). The results suggested that in heavy cigarette smokers, the presence of a functionally significant IL-1 gene complex polymorphism is associated with an increased risk for peri-implant bone loss following prosthetic reconstruction and during the supportive periodontal care phase of the treatment. More

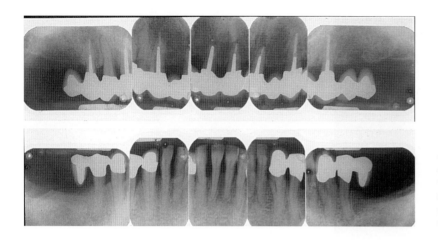

Fig. 27-5 Radiographic documentation of periodontal prostheses with distal cantilevers in all four quadrants as used prior to the availability of dental implants. The patient tolerated the shortened dental arches without difficulty.

recently, Laine *et al.* (2006) found that IL-1 gene polymorphism is associated with peri-implantitis (odds ratio = 2.6!). The authors conclude that this has to be considered a long-term risk factor for implant therapy.

In the anterior region, the loss of periodontal hard and soft tissues and the subsequent 'lengthening' of teeth brings along esthetic concerns, which can become complex, especially in patients with high expectations and smile lines as will be discussed later in this chapter. It is important to envision such problems and analyze local conditions carefully at the time of examination so that expected outcomes can be appropriately discussed with the patient prior to the initiation of therapy.

Patient history

Implant therapy is part of a comprehensive treatment plan. This is especially true for patients with a history of periodontal disease and tooth loss. An understanding of the patient's needs, social and economic background, general medical condition, etc., is a prerequisite for successful therapy. In order to expedite history taking, the patient should fill out a health questionnaire prior to the initial examination visit. As discussed in Chapter 26, such questionnaires are best constructed in a way that the professional immediately realizes compromising factors that may modify the treatment plan and may have to be discussed in detail with the patient during the initial visit or may require medical consultations to enable proper treatment planning. The assessment of the patient's history should include (1) chief complaint and expectations, (2) social and family history, (3) dental history, (4) motivation and compliance (e.g. oral hygiene), (5) habits (smoking, recreational drugs, bruxism), and (6) medical history and medications.

Chief complaint and expectations

To facilitate a successful treatment outcome, it is of critical importance to recognize and understand the patient's needs and desires for treatment. Patients usually have specific desires and expectations regarding treatment procedures and results. These may not be in tune with the attainable outcome projected by the clinician after assessment of the specific clinical situation. Optimal individual treatment results may only be achieved if the patient's demands are in balance with the objective evaluation of the condition and the projected treatment outcomes. Therefore, the patient's expectations have to be taken seriously and must be incorporated in the evaluation. A clear understanding of the patient's views is essential, especially in regard to dentofacial esthetics. Esthetic compromises need to be made often when implant restorations are performed in the periodontally compromised dentition because of the loss of hard and soft tissues. If a patient has been referred for specific treatment, the extent of the desired treatment has to be defined and the referring dentist informed of the intentions for treatment and the expectations regarding outcomes.

Social and family history

Before assessing the clinical condition in detail, it is helpful to interview the patient on her/his professional and social environment and on his/her priorities in life, especially when extensive, time-consuming, and costly dental treatment is envisioned as it is often the case with dental implant treatment. Likewise, a family history may reveal important clues with respect to time and cause of tooth loss, systemic or local diseases such as aggressive forms of periodontitis or other genetic predispositions, habits, compliance, and other behavioral aspects.

Dental history

It is important that previous dental care, including prophylaxis and maintenance, is explored with the patient if not stated by a referring dentist. As described in Chapter 26, information regarding cause of tooth loss, signs and symptoms of periodontitis noted by the patient such as migration and increasing mobility of teeth, bleeding gums, food impaction, and difficulties in chewing have to be explored in this context. Patient comfort with regard to function and esthetics and the subjective need for tooth replacement is assessed at this time.

Motivation and compliance

In this part of the communication, an assessment is made of the patient's interest and motivation for extended and costly therapy. The patient's view on oral health, her/his last visit to a dentist and/or hygienist, frequency and regularity of visits to the dentist, and detailed information on home care procedures are helpful pieces of information in this regard.

Habits

Cigarette smoking has been shown to be a risk factor for implant failure (Bain & Moy 1993; Chuang *et al.* 2002; McDermott *et al.* 2003). In the patient with (severe) periodontal disease, smoking has to be of even greater concern when combined with IL-1 gene polymorphism as discussed earlier in this chapter (Feloutzis *et al.* 2003; Laine *et al.* 2006). The patient's smoking status including details on exposure time and quantity should be assessed as part of a comprehensive examination of the implant candidate. Furthermore, testing for IL-1 gene polymorphism is strongly recommended. In this context, the importance of smoking counseling cannot be overestimated. Further aspects of smoking cessation programs are presented in Chapter 33.

Whereas the scientific evidence for a correlation of bruxism and implant failure is lacking, prosthetic complications, such as fractures of the veneering material, appear to be more frequent. Reports in the literature support the value of including precautionary measures in the implant treatment plan such as the use of implants of sufficient length and diameter, splinting of multiple implants, and use of retrievable restorations and occlusal guards. Whereas early recognition of bruxism or clenching is beneficial for appropriate treatment planning (Lobbezoo *et al.* 2006), it often cannot be diagnosed at the outset of treatment.

Medical history and medications

A thorough review of the patient's medical history is important. Certain medical conditions may contraindicate dental implant therapy. Any condition which has the potential to negatively affect wound healing has to be considered at least a conditional contraindication. This includes chemotherapy and radiation therapy for the treatment of cancers, bisphosphonate therapy, antimetabolic therapy for the treatment of arthritis, uncontrolled diabetes, seriously impaired cardiovascular function, bleeding disorders including medication-induced anticoagulation, active drug addiction including alcohol, and

heavy smoking. Patients with psychiatric conditions may not be good candidates for implant therapy. Such conditions are often difficult to identify at time of initial examination. If identified, these patients should be thoroughly examined by medical specialists before they are accepted for implant treatment (Hollender *et al.* 2003).

In light of the increasing need for medications in the aging population, an accurate assessment has to be made of the patient's prescribed and over-the-counter medications with their potential interactions and effects on therapeutic procedures. Most frequent in this context are anticoagulants, such as coumadin and aspirin. Also the need for antibiotic prophylaxis for dental surgical procedures should be recognized. Recently, the occurrence of osteonecrosis of the jaw in patients on current long-term bisphosphonate therapy or a history thereof has been described. The occurrence of osteonecrosis has primarily been observed after oral surgical procedures in patients on long-term intravenous bisphosphonate therapy as used in the treatment of cancers, but has also been observed in patients taking oral drugs of this kind (Marx *et al.* 2005). According to the American Dental Association (online member information), the risk for osteonecrosis translates into about seven cases per year for every million people taking oral bisphosphonates. In the most recent article addressing this issue, Mortensen *et al.* (2007) conclude that the increasing number of reports about bisphosphonate-associated osteomyelitis and the difficulty in treating these patients require further investigation to identify those patients who are at increased risk. Also, the optimal and safe duration of treatment with bisphosphonates remains to be determined. Due to the existing uncertainty in this area, recognition of patients on bisphosphonate therapy, communication with the treating physician(s), and a risk:benefit assessment have to be made for such patients who are being considered for implant therapy.

In summary, while most of this medical information can be extracted from a health questionnaire as mentioned earlier (see example in Chapter 26), it is important for the clinician to ask specific questions related to the patient's answers in the questionnaire to clarify their potential impact on treatment with dental implants. In many instances it will be necessary to contact the patient's physician for detailed information relevant to the planned treatment. Further aspects are presented in Chapters 30 and 33.

Local examination

Extraoral

An extraoral examination should form part of any initial patient examination. The clinician should look for asymmetries, lesions or swellings of the head and

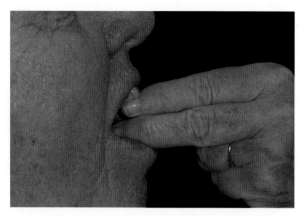

Fig. 27-6 Examination of patient's mouth-opening ability. The width of at least two of the patient's fingers placed vertically between upper and lower incisors is necessary to allow proper access for implant placement in posterior sites.

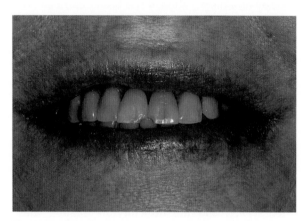

Fig. 27-7 Smile characteristics of patient introduced in Fig. 27-1.

neck areas. Observation of function and palpation of the head and neck musculature and temporomandibular joints are performed. Assessment of the opening amplitude of the mandible is especially important, since instrumentation involved with dental implant therapy requires that the patient is able to open sufficiently wide (Fig. 27-6). This is also the perfect time to take note of esthetic characteristics such as smile line, lip line, gingival line, and facial and dental midline (Fig. 27-7).

General intraoral examination

The general intraoral examination includes the assessment of the condition of soft and hard tissues of the oral cavity. This also entails a careful cancer screening. Soft or hard tissue lesions will most likely require treatment prior to the placement of dental implants. Pathological soft tissue conditions include herpetic stomatitis, candidiasis, prosthesis-induced stomatitis, tumors, hyperplasia, etc. Hard tissue pathologies, which most likely require treatment prior to implant therapy, include tooth impactions, bone cysts, root fragments, residual infections in the alveolar bone, e.g. caused by failed endodontic treatment, or tumors.

Dental hard tissues are equally carefully examined to determine the need for restorative treatment in the remaining dentition, most importantly those teeth directly adjacent to edentulous spaces. The need for restoration of the latter may influence the treatment plan in terms of choosing a conventional fixed partial denture over an implant-supported restoration to replace a missing tooth. Pathologies such as caries, fractures, attrition, abrasion, abfraction, tooth mobility, or tooth misalignment are noted. Existing restorations are recorded and deficiencies such as open margins, open contacts, or fractures identified. Testing for vitality of teeth, especially of those adjacent to potential implant sites, will point to possible endodontic pathologies, which should be treated prior to implant placement. The examination of periodontal tissues including the assessment of the patient's oral hygiene is described in detail in Chapter 26.

Finally, static and dynamic aspects of the patient's occlusion are determined, including the adequacy of the patient's vertical dimension of occlusion, maxillomandibular relationship (angle classification), overbite, overjet, stability in habitual occlusion, centric relation, slide in centric, and lateral and anterior excursive contacts (canine guidance, group function, anterior guidance).

Radiographic examination

The initial patient evaluation will include a radiographic survey. For the implant candidate with a history of periodontal disease and, hence, comprehensive treatment needs, a full-mouth set of periapical radiographs is needed to supplement the intraoral examination (Fig. 27-1b). A panoramic view will often be required as well, to reveal structures apical to the remaining teeth such as the infra-alveolar nerve canal, the mental foramina, the floor of the maxillary and nasal sinuses, and pathologic findings in the jaws (Fig. 27-8). Minimal radiographic bone height requirements for implant placement depend on a number of factors such as recommended implant length for a single implant restoration, single vs. multiple adjacent implants, jaw location, and ease and predictability of ridge augmentation in that location. For detailed planning of implant placement, additional radiographs such as occlusal views, cephalometric images, conventional or computer tomograms may be indicated. Implant-specific radiographic studies and their indications are described in Chapter 28, and treatment planning details are discussed in Chapter 32.

Implant-specific intraoral examination

Sites without esthetic implications

An implant-specific intraoral examination, emphasizing the local characteristics of potential implant

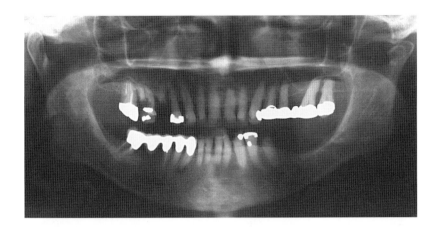

Fig. 27-8 Panoramic radiograph supporting the full-mouth radiographs shown in Fig. 27-1b.

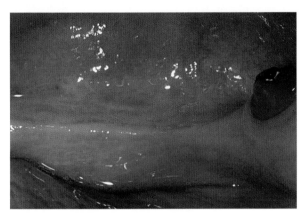

Fig. 27-9 Examination of alveolar ridge in lower left edentulous area. The ridge appears narrow in the area of the missing second premolar. Further radiographic information (lateral tomograms, computer tomograms) are recommended if dental implants are being considered.

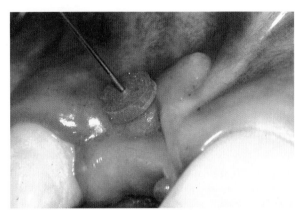

Fig. 27-10 Area of local soft tissue hyperplasia. Bone mapping is applied to explore the soft tissue thickness and the location of the underlying bone.

sites, is important. Different locations in the oral cavity have varying requirements in this regard, primarily due to differing esthetic impacts of implant treatment. They are, therefore, addressed separately in this text.

Although esthetic concerns are overall of lesser importance in mandibular and posterior maxillary sites, the evaluation of the condition of the local mucosa needs to be part of the examination in these areas as well. The clinical width and height of the alveolar process in potential implant areas is examined (Fig. 27-9). At the same time, pathologic changes are noted including mucosal hyperplasia or hypertrophy (Fig. 27-10). Probing of the local tissues may be indicated to assess tissue thickness and confirm the presence of sufficient alveolar bone. This can be done with a bone mapping procedure using a fine needle or explorer after local anesthesia has been applied (Fig. 27-10).

Besides the above, local assessment of sites with low esthetic impact consists primarily of a three-dimensional space assessment and evaluation of the condition of the adjacent teeth and their surrounding hard and soft tissues. A detailed and accurate space assessment is often difficult intraorally. Thus, it is

strongly recommended to obtain diagnostic impressions and adequate bite records to produce articulator-mounted casts, on which these critical diagnostic steps can be properly performed, including a diagnostic tooth set-up or wax-up. This is especially important when multiple teeth need to be replaced (Fig. 27-11).

From a comprehensive restorative point of view, edentulous spaces to be restored with implant restorations should ideally have the mesio-distal width of the natural tooth (teeth) that would normally be there. In the patient with a history of periodontal disease, tooth movements occur frequently and space assessment becomes important. Orthodontic pretreatment may be desirable or even required (Fig. 27-12).

From the perspective of implant placement, a mesio-distal width of 7 mm will allow the insertion of a regular-platform or regular-neck implant (3.75–5 mm). For spaces only 5–6 mm wide, narrow-platform or narrow-neck implants of approximately 3.5 mm diameter are available. For single-tooth spaces larger than 7 mm, wide-platform or wide-neck implants with a platform diameter of 6–7 mm may be the choice.

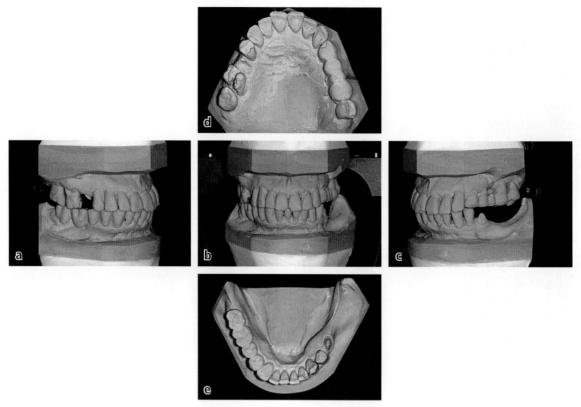

Fig. 27-11 Mounted diagnostic casts of patient introduced in Fig. 27-1: (a) right lateral view; (b) frontal view; (c) left lateral view; (d) maxillary occlusal view; (e) mandibular occlusal view.

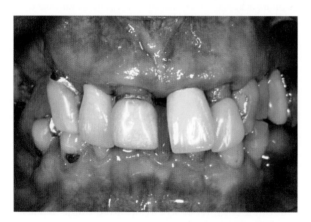

Fig. 27-12 Patient with severe periodontitis and resulting tooth movement in addition to pre-existing malocclusion.

It is important to note that wide-neck or -platform implants generally will also have a wider screw diameter. Thus, sufficient buccal–lingual bone width for the placement of a wider diameter implant is important so as to avoid perforation of the alveolar bone buccal or lingual to the implant. The bucco-lingual width of the alveolar process at an implant site is assessed either by bone mapping or cross-sectional radiographs (see Chapter 28).

A minimum vertical distance from the crestal mucosa of the potential implant site(s) to the opposing dentition is needed for implant restorations. This space requirement may vary depending on the design of the restoration, including the choice of abutments. As a general guideline, a vertical distance of at least 4 mm from the top of the mucosa to the opposing tooth (teeth) is required for straightforward implant placement and restoration. In the patient with tooth loss due to periodontal disease, this usually does not pose a problem. In contrast, due to concomitant bone loss, the distance is generally greater than the original height of a natural tooth (teeth) so that the potential esthetic and biomechanical impacts of the resulting overlong implant restoration have to be taken in consideration as documented earlier (Fig. 27-3).

Sites with esthetic implications

Definition of the problem
In the specific context of implant therapy in the *periodontally* compromised dentition with esthetic implications, which is primarily the anterior (maxillary) dentition, the local, implant-related examination will have to focus particularly on the esthetic consequences of periodontal disease in this area of the jaw. The most common visible sequels of generalized periodontal disease which may have a direct impact on esthetic appearance, depending on the patient's smile line, comprise (over-)long clinical crowns and flattening of the originally scalloped course of the gingival line, including loss of papillary tissue

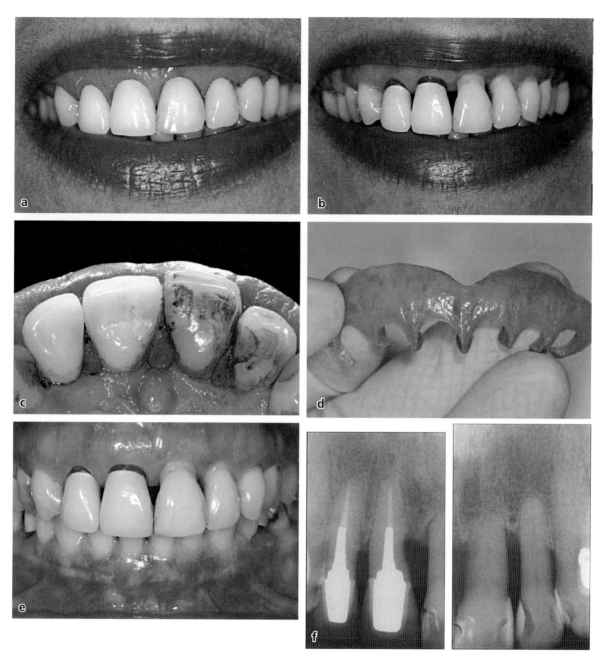

Fig. 27-13 (a) Frontal view of a 60-year-old female patient. During unforced smiling the transition between the clinical crowns and the artificial gingival epithesis is completely exposed. (b) The view without gingival epithesis displays long clinical crowns and open embrasures, both affecting the esthetic appearance. (c) The occlusal close-up view of the maxillary incisor region highlights the anchorage mechanism of the epithesis in the region of the open embrasures. (d) The gingival epithesis made of pink silicone is characterized by its regular scalloped occlusal course, compensating for the missing interproximal soft tissue. (e) The clinical view in centric occlusal reveals an average inter-arch relationship, but an altered length-to-width ratio of the clinical crowns of the four maxillary incisors as a consequence of periodontal tissue loss. (f) The corresponding radiographs document the advanced interproximal bone loss, indicating in particular that tooth #21 cannot be maintained.

leading to unsightly, "black interdental triangles". This is particularly pronounced in patients with an originally "*scalloped thin*" *gingival morphotype*, in contrast to a rather "*flat thick*" *phenotype* (Seibert & Lindhe 1989; Olsson & Lindhe 1991; Olsson *et al.* 1993). Not infrequently, vertical and/or lateral migration of teeth may also have occurred which, in turn, can significantly affect esthetic parameters. Furthermore, in case of more localized periodontal disease and loss of attachment, abrupt changes in vertical

tissue height between neighboring teeth can be present.

The resulting major shortcomings from an esthetic point of view mainly consist of an altered length-to-width ratio of the involved clinical crowns (*long teeth syndrome*) on the one hand and of interdental spaces that are not completely filled-out with gingival tissue on the other hand (Fig. 27-13). The latter may not only affect esthetics, but also lead to food retention and phonetic disturbances. As a consequence, reconstructive measures generally, and in implant therapy in particular, have not only to aim at a predictable and long-lasting functional rehabilitation, but need also to re-establish harmony from an esthetics and phonetics perspective. In general, fixed prosthodontic measures have somewhat limited potential of correcting length-to-width discrepancies of clinical crowns and to diminish open inter-proximal embrasures. Furthermore, the clinician should be aware of the additional specific limitations associated with current implant therapy (as described in Chapter 53), particularly when it comes to esthetic parameters, and therefore include this notion while proceeding to the local examination. In this context, the importance of assessing the height of the patient's smile line and his individual treatment expectations, should be once more underlined.

In the scope of this chapter and specifically addressing the local, pre-implant examination, two distinct clinical conditions can be theoretically encountered:

- One or several elements (teeth) of the anterior maxillary segment are periodontally compromised to such an extent (degree) that they can not be maintained and thus require replacement.
- One or several elements (teeth) of the anterior maxillary segment have already been lost due to periodontal disease.

This distinction is of importance, as the removal of a tooth consistently leads to horizontal and vertical tissue loss which includes soft and underlying bone tissue and which has been reported to vary between 2 and 3 mm vertically (Kois 1996; Araujo & Lindhe 2005; Araujo et al. 2005, 2006). This means that in the case of teeth still being present, but considered *irrational to treat*, an additional esthetic aggravation has to be expected. In this context, the beneficial potential of a slow orthodontic *"forced eruption"* procedure prior to tooth extraction, has to be mentioned (Salama & Salama 1993). Furthermore, as described in more detail in Chapter 53, one has to keep in mind that single-tooth replacement is significantly more predictable when it comes to long-term esthetic treatment outcome, than multiple adjacent implant restorations in the anterior maxilla (Belser et al. 2004a,b; Buser et al. 2004, 2006; Higginbottom et al. 2004). Clearly, single-tooth implant restorations benefit from tissue support provided by the adjacent natural teeth. As a consequence, the currently recommended *extraction strategy* for this area of the jaw should try to avoid, whenever feasible, ending up with *two-unit* tooth gaps. In other terms, one should either aim for *single-tooth gaps* or, if this is not possible, for *more extended edentulous segments* (three or more missing adjacent teeth). The latter concept, on the one hand, permits one to replace part of the missing teeth with pontics and thus benefit from their inherent superior esthetics (eventually

Table 27-1 Elements of the local, implant-specific examination of the periodontally compromised dentition in the esthetic zone

- Patient's smile line (high, medium, low)
- Periodontal examination (including gingival index, plaque index, probing pocket depth, clinical attachment level, bleeding on probing, width of the keratinized mucosa, gingival recessions, tooth mobility, tooth migrations)
- Inter-proximal bone height (as assessed on radiographs)
- Bone anatomy of the existing and/or anticipated (in case of inevitable tooth extractions) edentulous ridge
- Soft tissue anatomy (course of the gingival line in relation to the cemento-enamel junction of existing teeth and/or the osseous ridge)
- Gingival phenotype ("flat thick" vs. "scalloped thin")
- Shape of anatomic tooth crowns ("square" vs. "triangular")
- Length-to-width ratio of clinical crowns
- Overbite, overjet, malposition of teeth, occlusal parafunctions (wear facets, bruxism)
- Restorative/endodontic status of remaining teeth
- Width of existing and/or prospective edentulous spaces (single-tooth vs. multiple-unit gaps; identification of edentulous spaces that do not correspond to the volume of the respective missing teeth)

enhanced by connective tissue grafting procedures), and, on the other hand, to avoid adjacent implant restorations.

Clinical and radiographic examination

A structured comprehensive examination of the periodontally compromised anterior maxillary dentition (Table 27-1) should logically start with the assessment of the height of the patient's smile line. This will immediately indicate if the major esthetic shortcomings associated with an implant rehabilitation under such conditions, i.e. *long clinical crowns and open embrasures*, will become visible during unforced smiling. The examination will then focus on the detailed periodontal status, aiming at determining the prognosis of each individual unit of the respective dentition from a primarily periodontal perspective. As it is anticipated in the scope of this chapter that either one or several teeth cannot be maintained for periodontal reasons, or that one or several teeth have already been lost due to periodontal disease, the examination will have to assess whether implant therapy represents the adequate treatment solution or not. This means that additional parameters, directly related to implant therapy, have to be included in the examination process. These parameters comprise the localization of interproximal bone height assessed on radiographs, the bone anatomy of the existing or prospective (after additional tooth extractions) edentulous ridge, the course of the gingival (mucosal) line in relation to the cemento-enamel junction, as well as the width of the edentulous spaces. Furthermore, the general shape of the anatomic crowns (square or triangular) and the length-to-width ratio of the clinical crowns have to be assessed. Finally, the restorative and endodontic status of the remaining teeth and the overall occlusal conditions such as overbite, overjet, and the presence of occlusal parafunctions (wear facets, bruxism) have to be registered. In other words, all additional information which refers directly to implant therapy (e.g. bone volume) is a prerequisite for the decision-making process, to determine if implant therapy is feasible under these specific circumstances.

Patient-specific risk assessment

Summarizing the above mentioned aspects of a comprehensive preoperative examination, an individual risk profile is recommended for every candidate for implant therapy. Two different risk assessment forms are routinely used by the authors when examining potential implant patients, one for implant sites without esthetic priority, generally those in the mandible or in the posterior maxilla depending on the patient's smile profile, and a more detailed version for sites where esthetic aspects play a dominant role, primarily those in the (anterior) maxilla.

Risk assessment for sites without esthetic implications

The risk assessment in partially edentulous patients without or with low objective and subjective esthetic concerns is less complex. It should include the patient's health status, periodontal disease susceptibility, smoking history, interleukin-1 phenotype, history of bruxism, patient compliance including oral hygiene, and presence and type of alveolar bone deficiencies at potential implants sites (Table 27-2). In most patients, it takes less than 5 minutes to complete the proposed risk assessment form. Utilizing the obtained information, each implant candidate is categorized as low, medium or high risk. In patients

with a 'high risk' mark in multiple areas, the appropriateness of implant therapy must be questioned. For example, heavy smokers with advanced or refractory periodontal disease and a positive IL-1 test have to be considered overall high risk when extended bone augmentation procedures are needed to enable sufficient bony implant anchorage. It is important to discuss the individual risk situation with the patient prior to therapy and obtain the patient's consent based on the given circumstances.

Risk assessment for sites with esthetic implications

Risk assessment for implant sites with esthetic importance is much more detailed and complex. The risk assessment form contains additional surgical and prosthetic parameters, which are critical for an esthetic treatment outcome (Table 27-3). These parameters have been outlined in detail by Martin *et al.* (2006) in the first ITI Treatment Guide. In periodontally compromised patients, clinicians are often confronted with medium- to high-risk situations, since vertical bone and soft tissue deficiencies are a frequent clinical finding.

Conclusion

Modern comprehensive dental care for patients with a periodontally compromised dentition has to include the consideration of dental implants. Implant-assisted replacement of teeth that are missing or need to be extracted due to periodontal disease is an overall predictable treatment alternative in this type patient. A meticulous comprehensive examination of implant candidates is crucial and should include a patient and indication-specific risk assessment to achieve favorable short- and long-term treatment outcomes with regard to function and esthetics.

Table 27-2 Risk assessment for patients/sites without esthetic treatment implications

	Low risk	Medium risk	High risk
Health status (see Medical history and medications)	Normal wound healing		Conditions with potential for impaired wound healing
Periodontal disease susceptibility	Gingivitis	Mild to moderate chronic periodontitis	Severe or refractory periodontitis
Smoking	Non-smoking	<10 cigarettes per day	≥10 cigarettes per day
IL-1 gene phenotype	Negative		Positive
Bruxism	No		Yes
Compliance including oral hygiene	Good	Fair	Poor
Bone deficiency at implant site	None	Horizontal deficiency	Vertical deficiency

Table 27-3 Risk assessment for patients/sites with esthetic treatment implications

	Low risk	Medium risk	High risk
Health status (see Medical history and medications)	Normal wound healing		Conditions with potential for impaired wound healing
Periodontal disease susceptibility	Gingivitis	Mild to moderate chronic periodontitis	Severe or refractory periodontitis
Smoking	Non-smoking	<10 cigarettes per day	≥10 cigarettes per day
IL-1 gene phenotype	Negative		Positive
Bruxism	No		Yes
Patient's esthetic demand	Low	Medium	High
Lip line	Low	Medium	High
Gingival biotype	Thick, low scalloped	Medium thick, medium scalloped	Thin, highly scalloped
Shape of tooth crown	Rectangular		Triangular
Bone level at adjacent teeth	≤5 mm to contact point	5.5–6.5 mm to contact point	≥7 mm to contact point
Local infection at implant site	None	Chronic	Acute
Restorative status of neighboring teeth	Virgin		Restored
Width of edentulous space	One tooth ≥7 mm* One tooth ≥5.5 mm**	One tooth <7 mm* One tooth <5.5 mm**	Two teeth and more
Soft tissue anatomy	Intact soft tissues		Soft tissue defect
Bone deficiency at implant site	No bone deficiency	Horizontal bone deficiency	Vertical bone deficiency

* For regular neck/regular platform implants.
** For narrow neck/narrow platform implants.

References

Adell, R., Ericsson B., Lekholm, U, Brånemark P.-I. & Jemt, T.A. (1990). A long-term follow-up study of osseointegrated implants in the treatment of totally edentulous jaws. *International Journal of Oral and Maxillofacial Implants* **5**, 347–359.

Araujo, M.G. & Lindhe, J. (2005). Dimensional ridge alterations following tooth extraction. An experimental study in the dog. *Journal of Clinical Periodontology* **32**, 645–652.

Araujo, M.G., Sukekava, F., Wennstrom, J.L. & Lindhe, J. (2005). Ridge alterations following implant placement in fresh extraction sockets: an experimental study in the dog. *Journal of Clinical Periodontology* **32**, 212–218.

Araujo, M.G., Sukekava, F., Wennstrom, J.L. & Lindhe, J. (2006). Tissue modeling following implant placement in fresh extraction sockets. *Clinical Oral Implants Research* **17**, 615–624.

Baelum, V. & Ellegaard, B. (2004). Implant survival in periodontally compromised patients. *Journal of Periodontology* **75**, 1404–1412.

Bain, C.A. & Moy, P.K. (1993). The association between the failure of dental implants and cigarette smoking. *International Journal of Oral and Maxillofacial Implants* **8**, 609–615.

Belser, U.C., Schmid, B., Higginbottom, F. & Buser, D. (2004a). Outcome analysis of implant restorations located in the anterior maxilla: a review of the recent literature. *International Journal of Oral and Maxillofacial Implants* **19** (Suppl), 30–42.

Belser, U., Buser, D. & Higginbottom, F. (2004b). Consensus statements and recommended clinical procedures regarding esthetics in implant dentistry. *International Journal of Oral and Maxillofacial Implants* **19** (Suppl), 73–74.

Bragger, U., Karoussis, I., Persson, R., Pjetursson, B., Salvi, G. & Lang, N. (2005). Technical and biological complications/failures with single crowns and fixed partial dentures on implants: a 10-year prospective cohort study. *Clinical Oral Implants Research* **16**, 326–324.

Brånemark, P.-I., Adell, R., Breine, U., Hansson, B.O., Lindstrom, J. & Ohlsson, A. (1969). Intraosseous anchorage of dental prostheses. I. Experimental studies. *Scandinavian Journal of Plastic and Reconstructive Surgery* **3**, 81–100.

Brånemark, P.I., Zarb G.A. & Albrektsson, T. (1985). *Tissue-Integrated Prostheses: Osseointegration in Clinical Dentistry*. Chicago: Quintessence Publishing Co.

Buser, D., Mericske-Stern, R., Bernard, J.P., Behneke, A., Behneke, N., Hirt, H.P., Belser, U.C. & Lang, N.P. (1997). Long-term evaluation of non-submerged ITI implants. Part 1: 8-year life table analysis of a prospective multi-center study with 2359 implants. *Clinical Oral Implants Research* **8**, 161–72.

Buser, D., Martin, W. & Belser, U.C. (2004). Optimizing esthetics for implant restorations in the anterior maxilla: anatomic and surgical considerations. *International Journal of Oral and Maxillofacial Implants* **19** (Suppl), 43–61.

Buser, D., Martin, W. & Belser, U.C. (2006). Surgical considerations with regard to single-tooth replacements in the esthetic zone: standard procedure in sites without bone deficiencies. *ITI Treatment Guide* (Vol. 1), pp. 26–37.

Chuang, S.K., Wei, L.J., Douglass, C.W. & Dodson, T.B. (2002). Risk factors for dental implant failure: a strategy for the analysis of clustered failure-time observations. *Journal of Dental Research* **81**, 572–577.

Ellegaard, B., Baelum V. & Karring T. (1997). Implant therapy in periodontally compromised patients. *Clinical Oral Implants Research* **8**, 180–188.

Ellegaard, B., Baelum V. & Kølsen-Petersen J. (2006). Nongrafted sinus implants in periodontally compromised patients: a time-to-event analysis. *Clinical Oral Implants Research* **17**, 156–164.

Feloutzis, A., Lang, N.P., Tonetti, M.S., Burgin, W., Brägger, U., Buser, D., Duff, G.W. & Kornman, K.S. (2003). L-1 gene polymorphism and smoking as risk factors for peri-implant bone loss in a well-maintained population. *Clinical Oral Implants Research* **14**, 10–17.

Fritz, M. (1996). Implant therapy II. *Annals of Periodontology* **1**, 796–815.

Hammerle, C.H., Ungerer M.C., Fantoni, P.C., Bragger, U., Burgin, W. & Lang, N.P. (2000). Long-term analysis of biologic and technical aspects of fixed partial dentures with cantilevers. *International Journal of Prosthodontics* **13**, 409–415.

Higginbottom, F., Belser, U.C., Jones J.D. & Keith, S.E. (2004). Prosthetic management of implants in the esthetic zone. *International Journal of Oral and Maxillofacial Implants* **19** (Suppl), 62–72.

Hollender, L.G., Arcuri M.R., & Lang, B.R. (2003). Diagnosis and treatment planning. In: *Osseointegration in Dentistry. An Overview*. Chicago, Quintessence Publishing, pp. 19–29.

Iacono, V.J. (2000). Dental implants in periodontal therapy. *Journal of Periodontology* **71**, 1934–1942.

Kois, J.C. (1996). The restorative-periodontal interface: biological parameters. *Periodontology 2000* **11**, 29–38.

Kornman, K., Crane, A., Wang, H.Y., di Giovine, F.S., Newman. M.G., Pirk, F.W., Wilson. T.G. Jr., Higginbottom, F.L. & Duff, G.W. (1997). The interleukin-1 genotype as a severity factor in adult periodontal disease. *Journal of Clinical Periodontology* **24**, 72–77.

Laine, M.L., Leonhardt, A., Roos-Jansaker, A.M., Pena, A.S., van Winkelhoff, A.J., Winkel, E.G. & Renvert, S. (2006). IL-1RN gene polymorphism is associated with peri-implantitis. *Clinical Oral Implants Research* **17**, 380–385.

Lindh, T., Gunne, J. Tillberg, A. & Molin, M. (1998). A meta-analysis of implants in partial edentulism. *Clinical Oral Implants Research* **9**, 80–90.

Lobbezoo, F., Van Der Zaag, J. & Naeije, M. (2006). Bruxism: its multiple causes and its effects on dental implants – an updated review. *Journal of Oral Rehabilitation* **33**, 293–300.

Marx, R.E., Sawatari, Y., Fortin, M. & Broumand, V. (2005). Bisphosphonate-induced exposed bone (osteonecrosis/osteopetrosis) of the jaws: risk factors, recognition, prevention, and treatment. *Journal of Oral and Maxillofacial Surgery* **63**, 1567–1575.

Martin, W., Morton, D. & Buser, D. (2006). Pre-operative analysis and prosthetic treatment planning in esthetic implant dentistry. In: Buser, D., Belser, U.C. & Wismeijer, D., eds. *ITI Treatment Guide. Implant Therapy in the Esthetic Zone –*

Single Tooth Replacements. Chicago: Quintessence Publishing Co., Volume 1; pp. 9–24.

McDermott, N.E., Chuang, S.K., Woo, V.V. & Dodson, T.B. (2003). Complications of dental implants: identification, frequency, and associated risk factors. *International Journal of Oral and Maxillofacial Implants* **18**, 848–855.

Melo, M.D. & Obeid, G. (2005). Osteonecrosis of the jaws in patients with a history of receiving bisphosphonate therapy: strategies for prevention and early recognition. *Journal of the American Dental Association* **136**, 1675–1681.

Moy, P.K., Medina, D., Shetty, V. & Aghaloo, T.L. (2005). Dental implant failure rates and associated risk factors. *International Journal of Oral and Maxillofacial Implants* **20**, 569–577.

Mortensen, M., Lawson, W. & Montazem, A. (2007). Osteonecrosis of the jaw associated with bisphosphonate use: presentation of seven cases and literature review. *Laryngoscope* **117**, 30–34.

Nyman, S. & Lindhe, J. (1976). Prosthetic rehabilitation of patients with advanced periodontal disease. *Journal of Clinical Periodontology* **3**, 135–147.

Olsson, M. & Lindhe, J. (1991). Periodontal characteristics in individuals with varying form of the upper central incisors. *Journal of Clinical Periodontology* **18**, 78–82.

Olsson, M., Lindhe, J. & Marinello, C.P. (1993). On the relationship between crown form and clinical features of the gingival in adolescents. *Journal of Clinical Periodontology* **20**, 570–577.

Pjeturrson, B.E., Karoussis, I., Burgin, W., Bragger, U. & Lang, N.P. (2005). Patients' satisfaction following implant therapy. A 10-year prospective cohort study. *Clinical Oral Implants Research* **16**, 185–193.

Pjeturrson, B.E., Tan K., Lang, N.P., Bragger, U., Egger, M. & Zwahlen, M. (2004). A systematic review of the survival and complication rates of fixed partial dentures (FPDs) after an observation period of at least 5 years. *Clinical Oral Implants Research* **15**, 667–676.

Salama, H. & Salama, M. (1993). The role of orthodontic extrusive modeling in the enhancement of soft and hard tissue profiles prior to implant placement: a systematic approach to the management of extraction site defects. *International Journal of Periodontics and Restorative Dentistry* **13**, 312–334.

Schroeder, A., Pohler, O. & Sutter, F. (1976). Tissue reaction to an implant of a titanium hollow cylinder with a titanium surface spray layer. *Schweizerische Monatsschrift für Zahnheilkunde* **86**, 713–27.

Schroeder, A., van der Zypen, E., Stich, H. & Sutter, F. (1981). The reactions of bone, connective tissue, and epithelium to endosteal implants with titanium-sprayed surfaces. *Journal of Maxillofacial Surgery* **9**, 15–25.

Seibert, J. & Lindhe, J. (1989). Esthetics and periodontal therapy. In: Lindhe, J., ed. *Textbook of Clinical Periodontology*, 2nd edn. Copenhagen: Munksgaard, pp. 477–514.

Wallace, S.S. & Froum S.J. (2003). Effect of maxillary sinus augmentation on the survival of endosseous dental implants. *Annals of Periodontology* **8**, 328–343.

Chapter 28

Radiographic Examination of the Implant Patient

Hans-Göran Gröndahl and Kerstin Gröndahl

Introduction, 600
Radiographic examination for implant planning purposes – general aspects, 601
  The clinical vs. the radiologic examination, 601
  What is the necessary radiographic information?, 601
  Radiographic methods for obtaining the information required for implant planning, 603

Radiographic examination for implant planning purposes – upper jaw examination, 607
Radiographic examination for implant planning purposes – lower jaw examination, 610
Radiographic monitoring of implant treatment, 614
  Radiation detectors for intraoral radiography, 618
Image-guided surgery, 621

Introduction

In 1965, Brånemark installed the first dental implants made of titanium in the mandible of a 35-year-old male who, due to a cleft palate and loss of most of his teeth, could neither speak nor eat properly (Brånemark *et al.* 2005). The era of osseointegration, as a means to restore oral function compromised as a result of missing teeth, had begun.

The foundation for the use of titanium as the metal of choice for prostheses placed in the bone was laid many years earlier. In 1940, Bothe, Beaton and Davenport published the results of a study in which they had inserted pegs of different metals, among them titanium, in cat femurs. They found that "... the response to titanium was as good as, if not better, than that to the non-corrosive alloys in that there was more tendency for the bone to fuse with it". In 1951, Leventhal inserted screws made of titanium into the femurs of rats. He describes that "At the end of six weeks, the screws were slightly tighter than when originally put in; at twelve weeks the screws were more difficult to remove; and at the end of sixteen weeks, the screws were so tight that in one specimen the femur was fractured when an attempt was made to remove the screw". He continues: "In the past, the use of some prostheses has not become popular because it has been felt that these would remain separate from the bone and eventually loosen. Since titanium adheres to bone, it may prove to be an ideal metal for such prostheses".

Brånemark realized that screw-shaped titanium implants placed in the human jawbone could serve as substitutes for teeth that had been lost or never developed. In 1977, results from a 10-year study period were published (Brånemark *et al.* 1977) that demonstrated the clinical usefulness of what would become known as osseointegrated implants.

In the beginning of the osseointegration era limited numbers of people, and practically only those with no teeth left, were treated with dental implants. Gradually the indications were widened until partially edentulous and the patient missing just a single tooth also became candidates for implant treatment. From having been a treatment modality offered by a small number of specialists, it has emerged as a treatment mode provided by more and more dentists worldwide. It seems to grow exponentially and many more years probably remain before the vertex of its diffusion curve has been reached (Fig. 28-1a).

From a radiological point of view this must give us pause because it means that more people will undergo more extensive radiographic examination than people who receive conventional prosthetic treatment do. Consequently, we must try to use radiographic methods that do not unnecessarily increase the radiation burden to the population whilst providing us with all the information that is necessary for successful long-term treatment results.

In this chapter we will show how radiographic examinations for implant treatment purposes can be made so that they yield all necessary information at a reasonable cost both in terms of radiation dosage and economical resources. We will, in other words, adhere to the very important principle in radiography, the ALARA principle. This states that all radiographic information should be obtained with radiation doses that are As Low As Reasonably

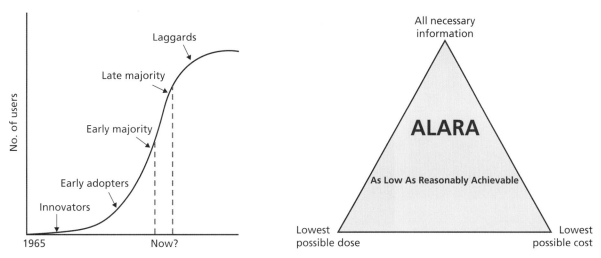

Fig. 28-1 (a, b) With the increasing use of implant treatment, it becomes increasingly important to adhere to the ALARA principle and keep radiation doses and monetary costs as low as possible.

Achievable. This principle may well be broadened so that it is also understood as stating that the monetary costs should be as low as reasonably achievable (Fig. 28-1b).

Radiographic examination for implant planning purposes – general aspects

The clinical vs. the radiologic examination

Too often a distinction is made between the clinical and the radiographic examination. The latter depends on the former and a meticulous clinical examination, including a thorough patient history, is the foundation upon which any radiologic examination must be based. Without it one can neither decide whether radiographic information is necessary, nor where and how it must be sought. The clinical examiner, whether or not he or she plans to make the radiographic examination her/himself, or refer the patient to a radiologist, thereby plays a decisive role when it comes to keeping radiation doses as low as reasonably achievable whilst obtaining the radiographic information that is necessary for a successful treatment planning. According to the International Commission on Radiation Protection, ICRP 60 (1991) all radiographic examinations should be justified and optimized. It is the clinical need of radiographic information that can make the radiographic examination justified. It is then the responsibility of the person, who will plan and perform the latter, to make certain that it will be made optimally.

What is the necessary radiographic information?

Before any radiographic technique can be chosen for any type of clinical problem one needs to clarify what radiographic information that is needed to enable a proper diagnosis and treatment plan. As regards the prospective implant patient, the necessary radiographic information is that which allows the clinician to determine:

- Whether implant treatment is the treatment option that offers the best long-term prognosis
- Whether pathological conditions are present in the jaws or remaining teeth that must be taken into account before implant treatment can be contemplated
- Where and how implants can be placed so that they have the best possibilities to become integrated with the surrounding bone and the associated crown/bridge can come into best clinical use
- How to place the implant(s) so that the surgical procedure becomes as safe as possible and the risk for post-operative failures as small as possible

A pre-operative radiographic examination is essential for all implant patients but how much of the jawbones that need to be examined and in what way will vary from patient to patient. Therefore, different radiographic techniques have to be used for different patients.

The pre-operative radiographic examination has several roles to play in respect to the clinician's needs. More specifically, the clinician needs to know the height of the bone that can be used for implant placement. One must then bear in mind that the bone height that can be used for implant placement is not necessarily the same as the total bone height (Fig. 28-2). The bone must also preferably be of a width which allows the implant to be surrounded by bone around its entire circumference. It is not only the available height that is of interest. When planning for implants to be placed adjacent to teeth or other implants one should try to ensure that they do not become positioned too close to each other (Fig. 28-3). Hence, the horizontal dimension of a potential implant site also needs to be assessed. When an

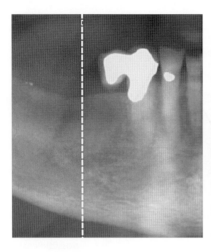
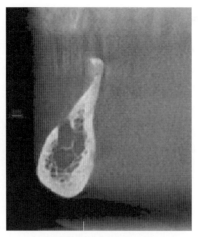

Fig. 28-2 An apparent height, as seen in the cropped panoramic image to the left, does not necessarily correspond to a bone volume useful for implant placement, as revealed by a tomogram (right image) representing a layer indicated by the dotted line.

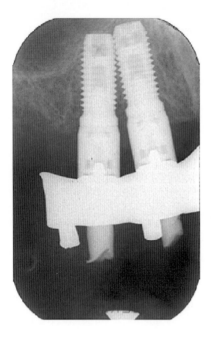
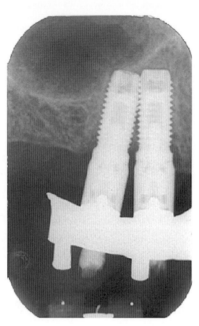

Fig. 28-3 Two implants placed very close to each other. A control radiograph taken 1 year after bridge connection (on right) demonstrates, by the thin radiolucent lines around the implants, that they have not become integrated with the surrounding bone.

implant will be placed adjacent to a tooth one should make certain that it does not become inserted too close to the tooth. Should this happen there is an increased risk of bone loss at the adjacent tooth or implant at least in the immediate period after implant surgery (Esposito *et al.* 1993; Andersson *et al.* 1995; Cardaropoli *et al.* 2003).

It is of great importance that the implant can be placed so that it will remain stable during the healing phase. The marginal bone crest may be used as a supporting bone cuff and a bony border in which the "apical" part of the implant can be placed will render some support. This can also be provided by the lingual and/or buccal cortical bone plate(s). The lower borders of the nasal cavity and the maxillary sinuses can give support to an implant (Fig. 28-4), but the upper border of the mandibular canal must not be used as anchorage of the implant tip (Worthington 2004).

A crucial aspect is that which concerns the location of anatomic structures that must not be damaged during implant surgery. In the lower jaw the mandibular canal, with its nerve bundle and blood vessels, is the most important. In the upper jaw placement of

the implants so that they come in conflict with the nasopalatine canals should be avoided.

To make the placing of the implant(s) as safe a procedure as possible the radiographic examination must also enable a description of the outer contours of the jawbones so that, for example, tilting of the alveolar bone as well as the presence and depth of bony fossae will be observed and accounted for.

From the above it can be concluded that it is important to evaluate different aspects of the bone in which one intends to place an implant and that accurate and precise measurements of different distances are essential.

The pre-operative radiographic examination serves more purposes than those described above. When implants are to be placed in jaws with remaining teeth, the condition of those and their surrounding bone must be thoroughly evaluated. Inflammatory lesions in the vicinity of an implant site may compromise the implant treatment result. Careful assessment of the remaining teeth may also lead to the choice of an alternative treatment modality. The pre-operative radiographic examination thus serves to:

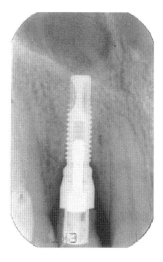
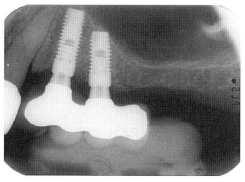

Fig. 28-4 The lower border of the nasal cavity and the maxillary sinus can provide support to an implant.

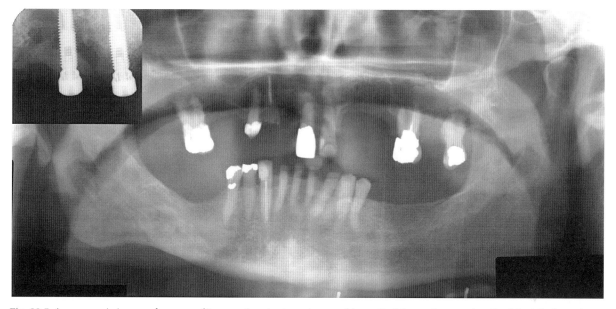

Fig. 28-5 A panoramic image of poor quality can give rise to serious problems. In this one it was not noticed that the bone in the upper right anterior region was not suitable for implant placement. Nevertheless, implants were placed (see inlay in upper left corner), soon to be lost.

- Ascertain that implant treatment is an appropriate treatment given the condition of the remaining teeth
- Make certain that bone height and width are sufficient for implant placement
- Provide measurements so that implants can be inserted without damaging neighboring structures
- Make implant insertion a safe procedure.

Needless to say, none of these objectives can be obtained without a radiographic examination of the best possible quality.

Radiographic methods for obtaining the information required for implant planning

In this chapter we will not discuss the examination of totally edentulous patients, only of those who have lost one or several teeth in jaws where some teeth still remain. As already mentioned one must then take into account the conditions of the remaining teeth in order not to jeopardize the implant treatment. A comprehensive examination, clinical as well as radiologic, of the dentition should therefore be made prior to a decision about where and how to insert implants. Depending upon the result of the clinical examination, the primary radiographic examination can be made with a combination of panoramic and intraoral radiography or by one or the other. One should not hesitate to take intraoral radiographs in regions where the panoramic radiograph has not been able to provide a clear view of the anatomic structures.

An adage well worth remembering, when determining whether an image is good enough for diagnosis and treatment planning, is that optimal diagnostic quality is only present when all diagnostically important structures are clearly visualized. Figure 28-5 illustrates a case when a panoramic radiograph was considered of good enough quality to be used for implant planning purposes. However, implants were lost, even before being subjected to

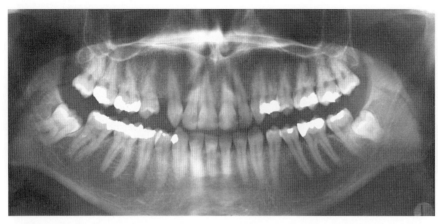
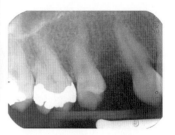

Fig. 28-6 Horizontal distortions are common in panoramic radiographs, especially in the upper premolar area, and give a false impression of available horizontal bone dimensions. Compare the distance between the second premolar and the cuspid in the two images.

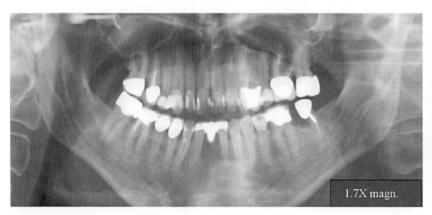
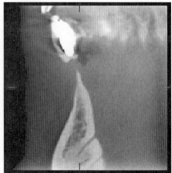

1.7X magn.

Fig. 28-7 The panoramic radiograph does not provide information about the width of the alveolar bone. A sagittal tomographic image reveals the true conditions in the lower anterior region.

occlusal loads, due to the poor bone conditions in the region that could have been observed had a better pre-operative radiographic examination been made.

Intraoral radiography should be performed according to the paralleling technique and radiographs taken so that there will be some overlapping between adjacent image fields. Most teeth will then be seen from two different angulations allowing for a better appreciation of the location of different structures.

Panoramic radiography may seem easy to perform but is a technique where many mistakes are made, not least in patient positioning. Panoramic radiographs taken on incorrectly positioned patients may provide a severely distorted view of the patient's jaws (Tronje 1982). This can cause large overlapping of neighboring teeth that can prevent a proper diagnosis. In regions where teeth are present the distortions are evident due to the overlapping of tooth surfaces (Fig. 28-6). In edentulous areas, however, distortions may not be that apparent which can lead to misjudgement of distances within the jaws. The panoramic technique can be used to provide a quick estimate of the bone height. A tomographic examination needs to be carried out in many cases to determine whether it is sufficient for implant placement (Fig. 28-7). The magnification in panoramic images varies between different types of panoramic machines. Some units also permit various types of radiographic images to be taken, that differ in magnification. It is thus important that one makes certain what magnification is indicated in the image to be evaluated.

Tomography can be used to obtain cross-sectional images, that is, images that are perpendicular to the curvature of the jawbones in the intended implant site. This is the best way in which to assess the width of the jawbone, and thereby the height available for implant placement, as well as other important aspects of the jawbone anatomy. Equipment for tomographic examinations shows much more variation than does that for panoramic and intraoral radiography. Widely different imaging principles are used resulting in different types of images.

The implant treatment spectrum varies from the single implant case to that where large parts of the facial skeleton are missing, and making an implant-anchored facial prosthesis necessary. Ideally, a clinic for oral and maxillofacial radiology is therefore equipped with a spectrum of X-ray machines for tomography capable of satisfying different demands

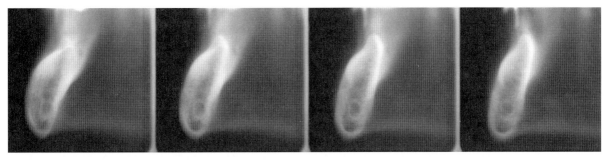

Fig. 28-8 Conventional spiral tomography of the lower jaw. Contiguous, 4 mm wide slices with the most anterior one taken in the region of the mental foramen (image to far right) that serves as an anatomic landmark.

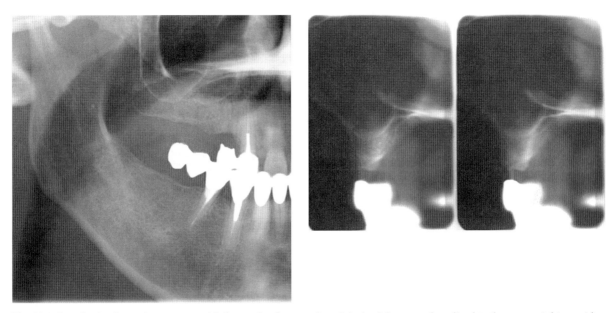

Fig. 28-9 By selecting just a few tomographic layers the dose can be minimized. Images taken distal to the upper right cuspid (see cropped) panoramic image.

and providing high-quality tomographic examinations. There is a difference between what different machines are best suited for. Three main groups of tomographic techniques are used for pre-implant tomography: motion (conventional) tomography, computed tomography (CT), and digital volume tomography (DVT), also known as cone beam CT. This is not the place to present these techniques in any detail but a little will be said about each of them as it relates to the examination of the implant patient.

Conventional tomography as applied for dental purposes underwent a profound development in the end of the 1980s when tomographic X-ray machines dedicated for the examination of the jawbones entered the market. Units such as the Scanora (Soredex Co, Helsinki, Finland) later to be followed by Cranex Tome from the same company meant that, most of the time, a comprehensive pre-implant examination of the patient could be made in the same unit and with the patient in the same position (Gröndahl *et al*. 1996, 2003). From a panoramic image one determines where in the jaw(s) one needs information that can only be found in cross-sectional, tomographic images.

The tomographic examination of the selected region is then accomplished by means of a synchronized, spiral, movement of the X-ray tube and the detector (film or image plate) permitting image layers of 2–4 mm width to be obtained containing a minimum of spurious contours from adjacent structures.

One to four images of contiguous tomographic layers can be taken during the same examination, that is, without changing patient position or detector. They will then appear on the same film, or within the same digital image frame (Fig. 28-8). By selecting just a few layers to be exposed, radiation doses can be minimized (Fig. 28-9).

By means of multimodality units, conventional spiral tomography provides the possibility of tomographic examinations of limited regions selected from a panoramic view of the entire jaw or a part of it. It has the advantage of being done with a small unit that can also be used for many other radiographic examinations of the oromaxillofacial regions. Spiral tomography can be made with film or image plates but not with CCD or CMOS solid-state detectors: these are not yet available for use with the dental multimodality-type of X-ray machines.

Computed tomography is widely used for pre-implant tomography, often because other techniques are not available (Ekestubbe *et al.* 1997). In the overwhelming majority of cases a stack of axial tomographic layer images is first taken. The height of the stack should be such that it covers a distance from just outside the marginal bone crest down to and including the base of the mandible or, for the upper jaw, up to and including the hard palate. In the upper jaw the slices should be parallel to the hard palate, in the lower jaw to the base of the mandible (Fig. 28-10). The information in the axial slices can be used for image reformatting so that cross-sectional views of the jawbone will be displayed (Fig. 28-11). These are perpendicular to a curve corresponding to the shape of the jaw as seen in a representative axial view.

Computed tomography is easily performed but can also be associated with high radiation doses (Dula *et al.* 1996, 1997; Frederiksen *et al.* 1995; BouSerhal *et al.* 2001). Doses can, however, be significantly reduced by adhering to so-called low-dose protocols which are well suited for studies where the primary interest lies in examining bony structures (Ekestubbe *et al.* 1996, 1999). When using computed tomography it is also important that the height of the examined volume is kept as small as possible. Computed tomography is not ideal for tomographic examinations of partially dentate patients. This is because the volume of diagnostic interest, even when the height of the exposed volume is small, constitutes only a small fraction of the latter. Exposing as small a volume as diagnostically feasible is one of the best ways of adhering to the ALARA principle. Should several edentulous regions within the same jaw need to be tomographically examined, computed tomography may be justified (Buser *et al.* 2002).

Digital volume tomography (DVT) is becoming exceedingly popular as a tool for maxillofacial imaging not least for pre-implant planning purposes. With the midpoint of the region of interest as a centre, the X-ray tube moves along the periphery of a circle, on the other side of which is positioned the detector. During this movement a cone-shaped X-ray beam, the diameter of which differs between different types of equipment, exposes the region of interest either continuously or in short bursts. From the X-ray detector a signal is sent to a computer where the electronic signal is converted into a digital one. Based on this information images can be reconstructed so that layer images (axial, sagittal, and coronal) of the exposed volume will appear on the screen. It is possible to travel in either direction within the volume so that the entire volume can be easily searched. Many DVT units make it possible to display curved layers of varying width so that something similar to a conventional panoramic view, although with thinner layer thickness, is obtained.

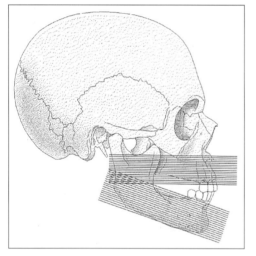

Fig. 28-10 Orientation of the axial tomographic slices differs between jaws. The height of the stack should be kept to a minimum.

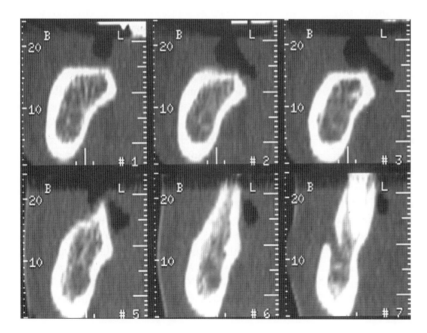

Fig. 28-11 Some reformatted cross-sectional images from the right side of the mandible.

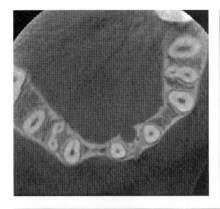
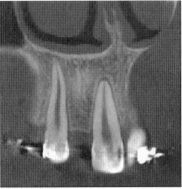
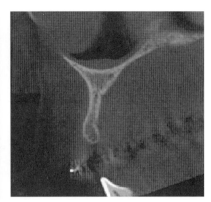
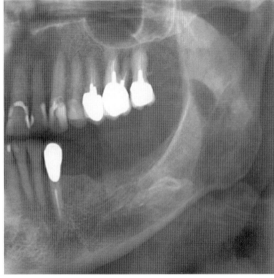
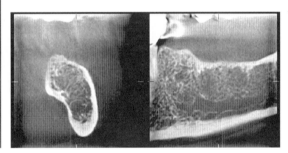

Fig. 28-12 Images (except the panoramic view) taken with 3DX Accuitomo DVT unit (J. Morita Co., Kyoto, Japan). The upper row images show the conditions in the right upper lateral incisor region. In the lower row the coronal and the sagittal tomographic images show the mandibular canal that is barely visible in the panoramic image.

Equipment for digital volume tomography comes in many different shapes (Frederiksen 2004), and they vary with regard to size of the volume that can be examined, geometric resolution, ease of use etc. They also differ as regards the radiation dose to the patient due to, above all, differences in volume size, resolution, and type of detector (Ludlow *et al.* 2006). Digital volume tomography could very well become the technique with which most partially dentate patients in need of implant treatment will be examined. The examination is easily done and radiation doses can be kept low, especially when machines that permit different sized volumes are used. An excellent way of reducing radiation dose is to expose the smallest possible volume. An advantage with digital volume tomography is its applicability in many areas of clinical dentistry. Figures 28-12 and 28-13 provide examples of images taken with DVT units.

Realizing that far from everybody has access to a wide spectrum of X-ray machines we will present various types of commonly seen cases. We will describe how they can be radiographically examined by means of different techniques but not include the totally edentulous patient or the patient in need of facial prosthetic constructions.

Radiographic examination for implant planning purposes – upper jaw examination

Depending upon where in the upper jaw implant treatment is to be planned one must take different anatomic factors into account. A common denominator is of course that the width and height of the bone must be evaluated. The available height depends on the bucco-palatal width of the bone because, ideally, the implant should be covered by bone both on its buccal and palatal aspects. The length of implants that can be used thus depends on the distance between the inferior border of the nasal cavity, or the maxillary sinus, and that part of the alveolar bone where it is sufficiently wide for implant placement (Fig. 28-14). When implants are to be placed in the vicinity of the midline one must evaluate the width of the incisive foramen and the nasopalatine canal. One must assess the height and width of the alveolar bone on the buccal and distal side of these structures to determine whether and where an implant can be placed (Fig. 28-15).

In the upper frontal region it is not uncommon for a single tooth be missing as a result of previous

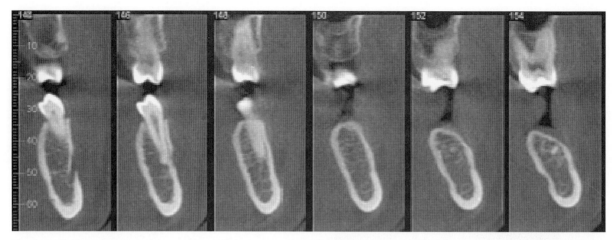

Fig. 28-13 Lower jaw tomography performed by i-CAT cone beam CT machine (Imaging Sciences International, Hatfield, PA, USA). Courtesy of Dr. Allan Farman, University of Louisville, Kentucky, USA.

Fig. 28-14 The height of the bone available for implant placement depends on its width. It may therefore be less than the height as it appears in e.g. intraoral or panoramic radiographs.

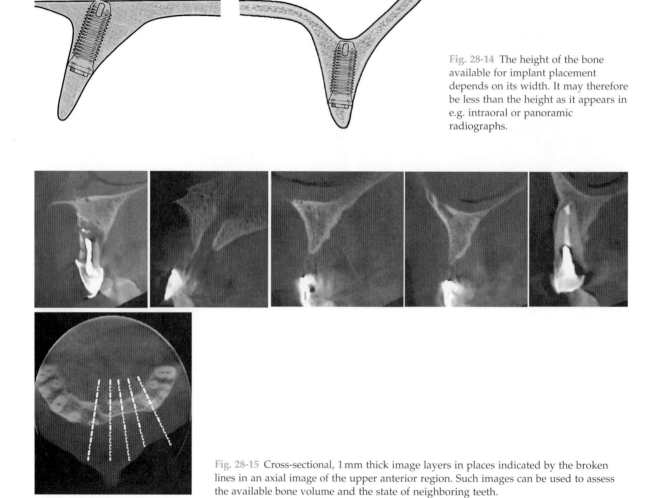

Fig. 28-15 Cross-sectional, 1 mm thick image layers in places indicated by the broken lines in an axial image of the upper anterior region. Such images can be used to assess the available bone volume and the state of neighboring teeth.

trauma. In these cases the radiographic examination can be done in a simple, yet comprehensive, way by one or two intraoral radiographs and a single tomographic image (Fig. 28-16).

Should the available bone lack the dimensions needed for the placement of an implant, the patient may be willing to accept that bone augmentation is performed to provide for sufficient height and width of the bone. In the latter case tomographic images will be of help when determining exactly where the bone is of less than sufficient width or height and the extent to which it needs to be augmented. Tomographic images can also be used to observe the results after healing (Figs. 28-17 and 28-18).

In areas where teeth have been extracted and it is uncertain how much of the alveolus has become

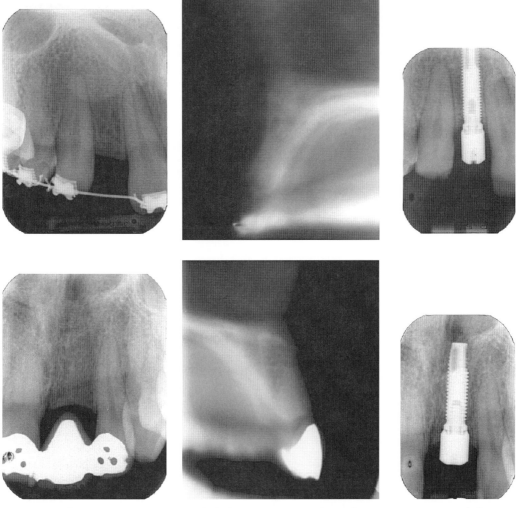

Fig. 28-16 Two cases of missing upper incisors in which the pre-operative radiographic examination was made by intraoral radiographs and conventional spiral tomography. In the lower row case an implant could be placed buccal to the nasopalatine canal.

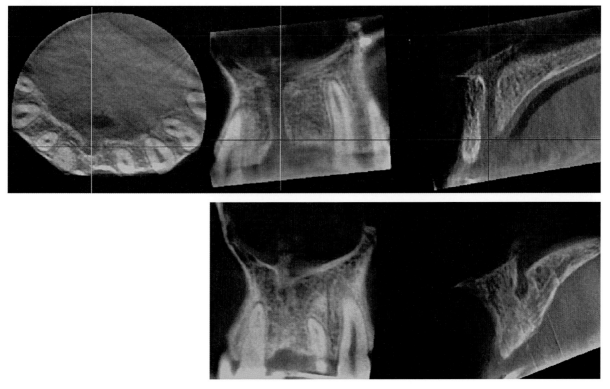

Fig. 28-17 Pre-operative (upper row) and post-operative images of a patient in whom a bone substitute was placed both buccally and in the nasopalatine canal to enable insertion of an implant in an optimal position.

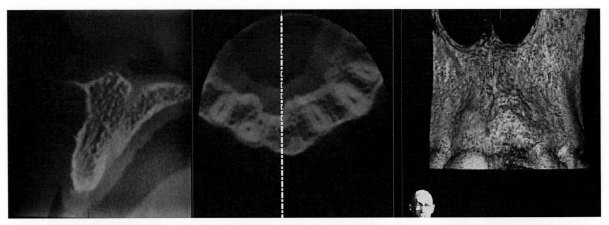

Fig. 28-18 A sagittal (left) and an axial tomographic image (middle) after a bone substitute has been placed on the buccal surface. The dotted line indicates the position of the sagittal slice. To the right is a three-dimensional image reconstructed from the volume data.

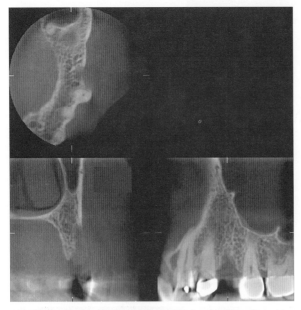

Fig. 28-19 Digital volume tomography in the upper first premolar area. Notice the lack of complete bone filling of the extraction socket and the relation of the alveolar bone to the nasal and maxillary sinus cavity.

filled with new bone, digital volume tomography is a helpful tool. This is illustrated in Fig. 28-19, where it is also apparent how well this technique is able to demonstrate the conditions anterior and inferior to the frontal border of the maxillary sinus.

In some patients in whom the available bone height below the maxillary sinus is too small one can occasionally find bone suitable for implant placement on the palatal side of the sinus. Tomography must be performed so that this can be determined (Fig. 28-20).

In the posterior parts of the upper jaw the maxillary sinus may extend so far down into the alveolar bone that there is not enough bone available in which to insert an implant. By entering the sinus through a buccal window, bone substitutes can be placed under the mucosal lining. Digital volume tomography is an ideal method to evaluate how the bone substitute is positioned and its relation to the adjacent bone (Fig. 28-21).

When implants are intended to be placed in more than one region, the use of computed tomography may be justified (Buser *et al*. 2002) provided that low-dose protocols are applied (Rustemeyer *et al*. 2004). A panoramic radiograph and, when remaining teeth are not well displayed in it, complementary intraoral radiographs are nevertheless important. Figure 28-22 describes how the results of such an examination can look. From the stack of axial images a representative image is chosen in which the curvature of the jaw is drawn. A dedicated computer program then makes new tomographic images at chosen distances. These images describe layers that are perpendicular to the curve and in which measurements of bone height and width can be made.

Computed tomography is mostly performed in medical radiology departments and images considered relevant for the purpose are sent to the clinician. Sometimes these are limited to the axial image describing the curvature of the jaw and the reconstructed cross-sectional images. We recommend that the referring dentist should also receive the scout image and the stack of axial images. In the scout image it is possible to see what reference plane that was used and, if needed, make the appropriate adjustment of the measurements taken in the cross-sectional views. In the axial images one may be able to pick up information about the remaining teeth not displayed in the panoramic or intraoral radiographs (Huumonen *et al*. 2006).

Radiographic examination for implant planning purposes – lower jaw examination

In the lower jaw there is a distinction between implant placement in the region anterior to the mental foramina and in regions posterior to the foramina. The height of the anterior region is usually well preserved

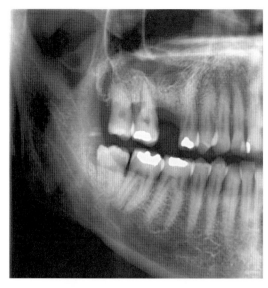
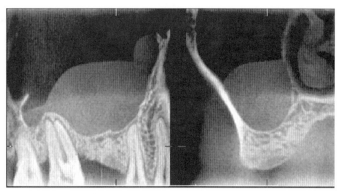

Fig. 28-20 From the panoramic image (left) it is not possible to determine that bone for implant placement is available on the palatal side of the maxillary sinus, as is clearly seen in the tomographic image (right). Notice the soft tissue swelling in the sinus.

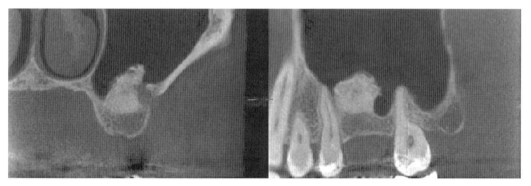

Fig. 28-21 A coronal and a sagittal tomographic layer of the lower part of the maxillary sinus in which a bone substitute has been placed.

if teeth have not been missing for a long time. This is rarely the case in the partially dentate patient. Its width, however, may be a limiting factor. One can get an indication that the alveolar bone is thinner than normal from periapical radiographs or from panoramic images, provided that the anterior region is well reproduced. This is often the case when one can see vertically running radiolucent structures corresponding to the blood vessel canals in the inner walls of the cortex. They become visible when the bone is thin or has fewer and thinner bone trabeculae than normal. In such cases a tomographic examination may be advisable so that one can determine beforehand whether a thin upper ridge will be removed or a bone augmentation procedure applied.

When implants are to be placed posterior to the mental foramina one must not only take into account the factors one had to consider in the frontal regions. One must also be able to identify the path of the mandibular canal and accurately assess the distance between the upper level of the alveolar bone, where it is sufficiently wide, to the upper border of the

canal. To do this before surgery requires that tomography is performed, so that the jawbone anatomy can be evaluated in image layers that correspond to cross sections of the mandible. Estimating this distance in panoramic radiographs, as many seem to do (Worthington 2004), requires so many assumptions of unknown variables that mistakes can easily be made (Fig. 28-23). These can result in temporary or permanent damage to the inferior alveolar nerve. These problems "are more frequent than expected" (Worthington 2004). We are convinced that careful presurgical planning, including the use of tomography, will keep the incidence of nerve damage to an absolute minimum.

The entire distance from where sufficient width of the mandible is found to the upper border of the mandibular canal cannot be used for implant surgery. One reason is that the drill used for preparing the implant site will go deeper than the implant itself. Another is that one cannot always measure distances in radiographs with absolute accuracy and precision. Therefore, prudent clinicians make use of at least a 2 mm safety zone between the upper border of the

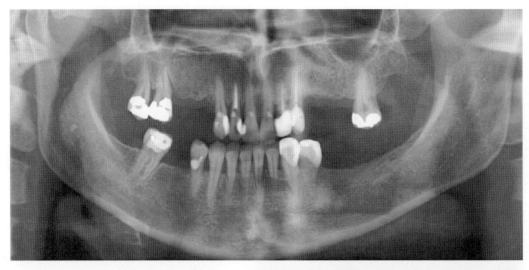

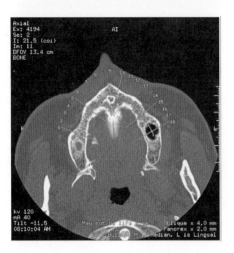 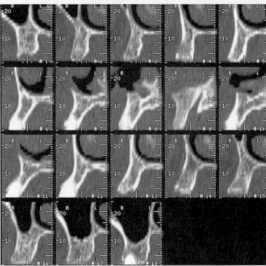

Fig. 28-22 Computed tomography of the upper jaw where implants are planned to be installed on both sides. To the lower right are cross-sectional views from one side to the other, perpendicular to the curve seen in the axial view to the left.

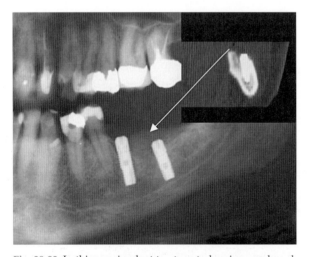

Fig. 28-23 In this case implant treatment planning was based on a panoramic radiograph only. One of the implants was placed with its tip into the mandibular canal as seen in a subsequent CT image. The positioning of the implant into the canal may have been caused by a misinterpretation of the panoramic radiograph. It is the lingual part of the upper alveolar bone that gives rise to the upper contour in the panoramic image.

mandibular canal, as seen in the radiograph, and the planned level of the tip of the implant (Fig. 28-24).

Among other factors that must be considered in the planning process is the outer shape of the mandible. Both concavities and the lingual tilt differ in extension between patients and between different parts of the jaw (Figs. 28-25 and 28-26). Accidental penetration of the lingual wall of the mandible can more easily occur under those conditions than when they are not present. Severing of arteries in the underlying soft tissues can cause severe, even fatal, bleeding (Darriba & Mendonca-Caridad 1977; Niamtu 2001).

Sometimes the mandibular canal, before it ends at the mental foramen, continues a little bit in an anterior direction before going upwards and distally toward the foramen making a so-called anterior loop (Arzouman *et al.* 1993). Therefore it is recommended not to place an implant immediately anterior to the foramen. In other cases there can be a relatively wide anterior continuation of the canal, as indicated by Fig. 28-27. It is then recommended that a radiographic

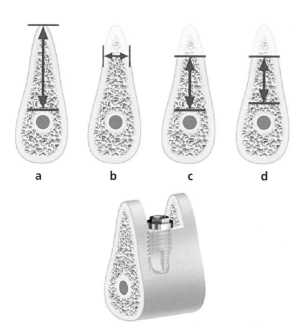

Fig. 28-24 How measurements can be made in tomographic images to ensure that the tip of the implant will not enter the mandibular canal. (a) Measure the entire height from the upper border of the canal to the marginal bone crest. (This value can be used as a reference during surgery.) (b) Assess where the bone is wide enough for the implant. (c) Measure from this level to the canal. (d) Subtract 2 mm from the latter value. From Gröndahl *et al.* (2003).

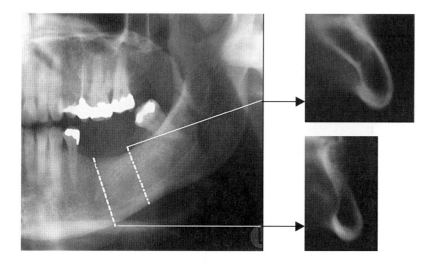

Fig. 28-25 Lingual concavity and a small bucco-lingual width just distal to the mental foramen and a different shape and width in a more distal position.

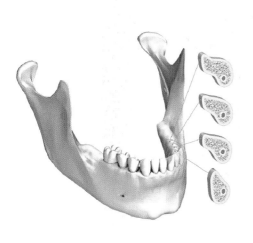

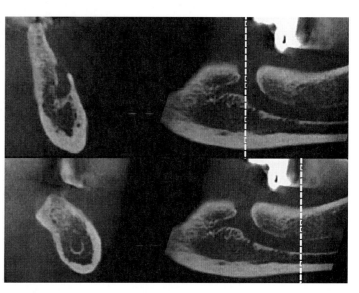

Fig. 28-26 The shape and angulation of the mandibular jawbone can be very different just a short distance apart. The dotted lines in the sagittal tomograms indicate the positions of the cross-sectional tomographic layers. This information can only be obtained pre-operatively by means of tomography.

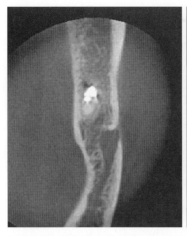 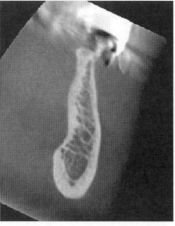 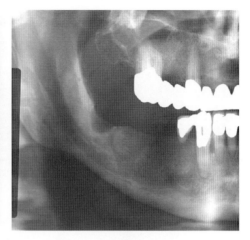

Fig. 28-27 An anterior continuation of the mandibular canal from the mental foramen as seen in tomographic images (same patient as in Fig. 28-26) and as it may appear in a panoramic view (different patient).

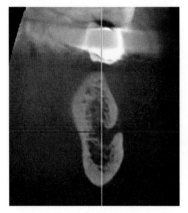 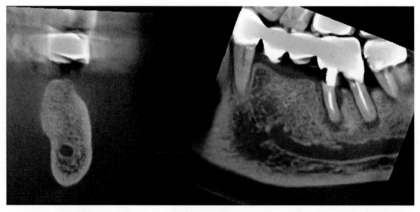

Fig. 28-28 Large local differences in bone density and architecture. The much denser bone in the most distal tomographic layer most probably is due to the inflammatory conditions at the adjacent molar.

evaluation is performed to determine its position relative to potential implant positions.

This is not the place to discuss factors related to general health that may have an influence on bone structure and architecture. In can be noted however, that in tomographic images, given that their resolution is sufficiently high, the cancellous bone pattern in intended implant sites can be studied and the thickness of the cortical bone evaluated. Local factors can contribute to local variations in bone density. In Fig. 28-28 large differences in bone density can be seen in tomographic images less than 1 cm apart. The higher density in the more distal region is most likely a reaction to the inflammatory conditions seen at an adjacent tooth.

Radiographic monitoring of implant treatment

Meticulous planning of the implant treatment together with gentle surgical technique for the insertion of the implants make immediate post-operative radiographic examination superfluous unless something unexpected occurs during surgery. Under normal conditions, however, there is simply nothing,

apart from the expected, to be found. Should the patient experience symptoms before the first post-operative radiographic examination is scheduled, one should of course not hesitate in taking radiographs if information from them is considered essential for a proper diagnosis.

The radiographs in Fig. 28-29 are from a patient who presented with severe pain very soon after implants were inserted. The images show unevenly demarcated radiolucent areas around the implants, especially the most distally and the most mesially placed. This is a strong indication of bone infection. In addition, the most mesially placed implant appears to have its tip in close proximity to the anterior loop of the mandibular canal. This is confirmed by a tomographic examination. The affected implants were removed and the symptoms soon subsided.

When implants are inserted in dense bone heat necrosis can occur around the "apical" part of the implants, particularly when the implants are long and effective cooling during their insertion has not been applied. Usually this is accompanied by pain. In the radiograph one can see a radiolucent area surrounding the apical part of the implant. A radiolucent area just beneath the apical part and caused by

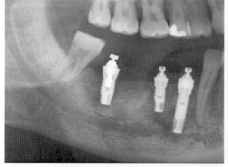
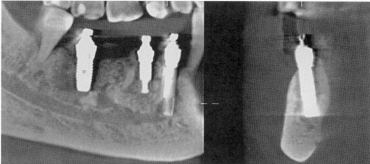
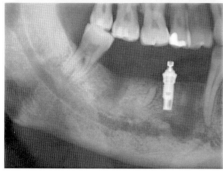

Fig. 28-29 A scanogram (upper left image) indicates an inflammatory reaction around the most distal and the most mesial implant and that the tip of the latter may interfere with the anterior loop of the mandibular canal. This is confirmed by the tomographic examination (upper right images) and after removal of the two implants, the symptoms disappeared.

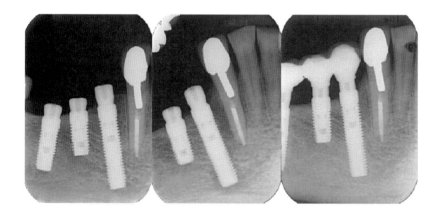

Fig. 28-30 Soon after implant insertion the patient presented with slight pain. A radiograph (left image) was interpreted as showing normal conditions. Two weeks later the pain had increased in intensity and a radiolucency could now be seen around the tip of the most mesial implant (middle image). The right image, taken some months later shows completely normal conditions.

the drill should not be confused with the radiolucency that is a result of heat necrosis. Heat necrosis is most commonly seen in the lower jaw (Fig. 28-30).

Often it is not possible to take radiographs of implants using standard intraoral techniques. One either has to take radiographs more from below or use panoramic radiography or, better yet, so-called scanograms (Fig. 28-31).

Implants that have not been correctly placed in the bone may cause symptoms as well. Should an intraoral examination fail to show the cause of the problem a tomographic examination may be needed (Fig. 28-32). It should preferably be performed with digital volume tomography, as it is less prone to cause artifacts from the implants than computed tomography.

Depending upon the implant system used there may or may not be a need for a radiographic examination when abutments are placed. To examine

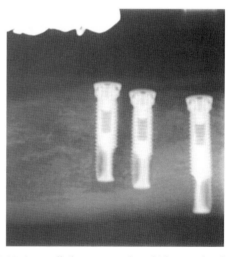

Fig. 28-31 A so-called scanogram by which even deeply seated implants can be displayed in their entirety.

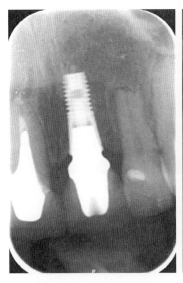
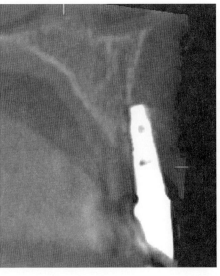

Fig. 28-32 An intraoral radiograph (left) failed to reveal the cause of the problem in a patient with pain in the region of a newly placed implant A DVT image demonstrated that most of the implant was not placed in the bone.

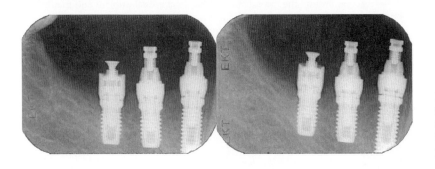

Fig. 28-33 Small gaps between abutment and implant pillar (most mesial implant) may go unnoticed in radiographs taken with less than perfect geometry (left image).

whether abutments are correctly positioned on top of the implant pillar the X-rays need to pass at right angles to the implant. If not, gaps between the abutment and implant pillar may go unnoticed and uncorrected for (Fig. 28-33). The occlusal load will then not be optimally distributed which can later cause component fractures. Marginal bone loss has also been attributed to gaps between the abutment and the implant pillar (Hermann *et al.* 2001; King *et al.* 2002).

Reference radiographs, with which later radiographs can be compared to monitor the interaction between implant and bone, are preferably taken when crowns or bridges are placed. Little can come out of such comparisons if the quality of the radiographs is not high. It must be possible to notice small marginal bone level differences over time as well as the condition of the bone–implant interface. This requires radiographs to be taken with the X-rays being directed perpendicular to the longitudinal axis of the implant and the surface of the detector. When threaded implants are used the radiographic appearance of the threads provides useful information about the irradiation geometry used and how to change it should it not be correct to start with. One must be able to get a clear picture of the inner parts of the threads on either side of the implant (Fig. 28-34).

Intraoral radiography is the method of choice for monitoring of implant treatment. Irradiation geometry and exposure can be individualized for different implants or group of implants. Panoramic radiogra-

phy cannot provide the same detailed information and should be reserved for the few cases when intraoral radiography cannot be tolerated. A better alternative can be used by those who have access to multimodality units able to provide multiple exposures of selected small areas using slightly different irradiation geometry.

With high-quality intraoral radiography it is possible to follow the course of events in the marginal and peri-implant bone over time. A fairly typical course of events for lower jaw implants, from abutment placement via bridge installation to a 5-year follow-up examination, can be seen in Fig. 28-35. With well trained and motivated personnel it is possible to get high-quality and comparable radiographs over long periods of time even without going to the effort of using particular film-holding devices. The images in Fig. 28-36 are taken over a 5-year period by different radiographers.

High-quality radiographs make it possible to detect, observe, and quantify bone level changes over time. In the majority of patients the bone level remains at the position it had after the post-surgical remodeling over as long periods that it has been hitherto possible to cover in longitudinal studies (Adell *et al.* 1990; Snauwert *et al.* 2000; Ekelund *et al.* 2003). In other patients one can find loss of bone at the marginal bone crest that affects all implants or, more often, one or a few. It is important to detect those so that the cause of the bone loss can be identified (Figs. 28-37 and 28-38).

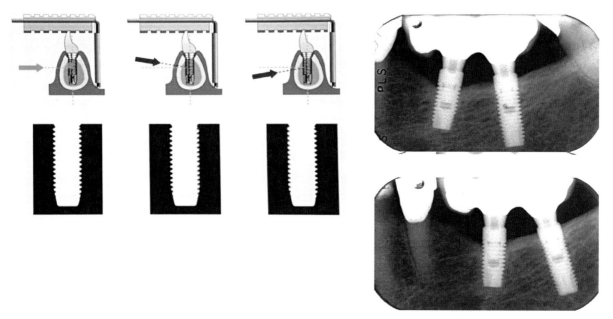

Fig. 28-34 The appearance of the threads of an implant provides useful information about how to change the direction of the X-ray beam so that it can become directed perpendicular to the implant. From Gröndahl *et al.* (1996).

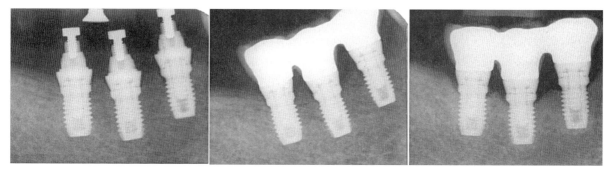

Fig. 28-35 From abutment connection via bridge installation to a 5-year follow-up examination.

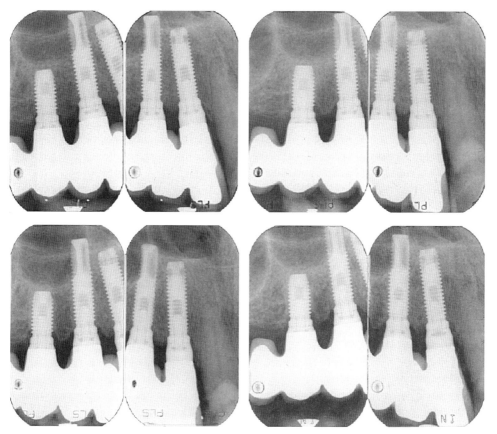

Fig. 28-36 Intraoral radiographs taken with a free-hand technique and by different radiographers at bridge installation (upper left corner) and at follow-up examinations (1, 3, and 5 years later) demonstrate excellent possibilities of monitoring the post-operative course of events.

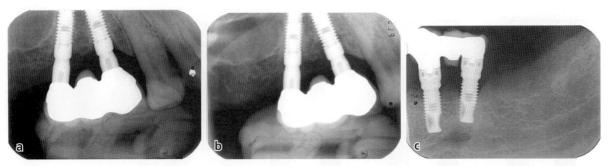

Fig. 28-37 In radiograph (b), the mesial implant has marginal bone loss that was not evident a year before. In radiograph (c), the most distal implant has marginal bone loss involving about a third of the implant length.

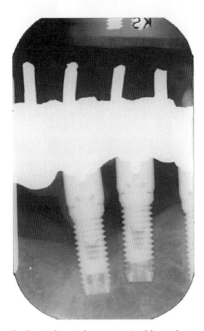

Fig. 28-38 Both implants show marginal bone loss exceeding one third of the implant length. The implant to the right is also surrounded by a thin radiolucent zone. This indicates that the implant is not osseointegrated. At a clinical examination it was found to be mobile and consequently removed.

In high-quality radiographs it is possible to identify implants that are not osseointegrated with an accuracy that is on a par with what one can find when radiography is used for other dental diagnostic purposes (Sundén *et al.* 1995; Gröndahl & Lekholm 1997). Since the first radiographic signs are very subtle, as seen in the radiographs in Fig. 28-39, it is very helpful if one is able to compare radiographs with ones taken previously. Most implants that have not become integrated are found during the first year after bridge installation, or even before that. This stresses the importance that radiographs taken at abutment connection and at bridge installation are of the highest possible quality. Radiographs should be of a quality so that it is possible to evaluate not only the conditions in the surrounding bone and the marginal bone level but also the conditions of all the technical implant components. Such conditions are,

for example, fractures of the centre screw or of the implant pillar itself and gaps between abutment and implant pillar, or between bridgework and abutment (Figs. 28-40, 28-41 and 28-42).

Radiation detectors for intraoral radiography

Although a correctly exposed and optimally processed film, in our opinion, provides the best quality images for implant monitoring we have to accept that digital imaging techniques are gaining wider and wider acceptance among dentists. There are some advantages of digital images over film-based ones, in that they can be subjected to image processing algorithms that can enhance their diagnostic quality and adapt them to various diagnostic tasks (Analoui 2001a,b). This can of course be of value when the diagnostic tasks are so varied as they are in implant monitoring when one must be able to evaluate both thin marginal bone and the metal components of the implant construction.

As we have pointed out several times in this chapter the irradiation geometry is essential when implants are to be monitored. The X-rays should come perpendicular to the longitudinal axis of the implant and to the detector plane. Therefore one must have a digital detector that can be placed in the mouth, and relative to the implants, as easily as can film. When the X-ray beam has passed through a jaw in which implants have been inserted, the transmitted radiation consists of a wide spectrum of X-rays of different intensity. Thus, the detector has to be able to respond to a wide range of exposure differences; its exposure latitude must be wide. Image plate systems possess a wider exposure latitude than most solid-state systems (Farman & Farman 2005). With solid-state systems it is therefore easier that thin bone structures become over-exposed and not visible in the radiograph (Fig. 28-43). For this reason, and because image plates are as easy to use as films, we have chosen image plate systems for implant monitoring purposes. Image plates are, however, not without problems. They can easily get scratched if not handled with extreme care.

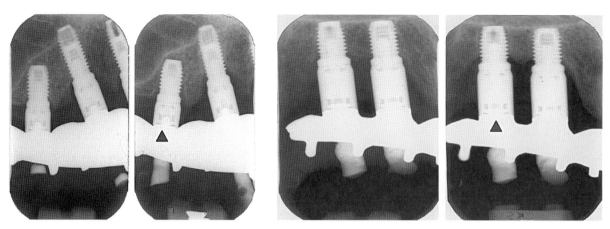

Fig. 28-39 Notice the very subtle sign, a thin radiolucent zone around the implants, indicating that the implants marked by arrows are not osseointegrated. Comparison of the radiographs with those taken earlier, the ones to the left in each image pair, makes the detection of subtle signs much easier.

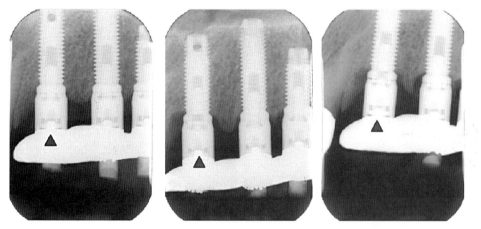

Fig. 28-40 In the implant marked by an arrow normal conditions were found at bridge installation (left image). One year later, a fracture of the centre screw went unnoticed (middle image) resulting in a gap between abutment and implant pillar seen in an image taken another year later. Notice that the irradiation geometry was not optimal at the second occasion.

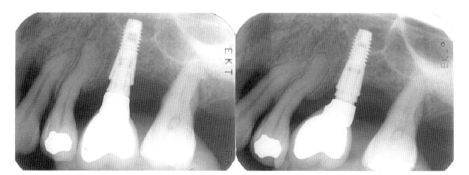

Fig. 28-41 In this case the conical abutment was not correctly placed (left image). After correction for this, the crown was remade but a later control then found a gap between crown and abutment. Notice the difference in marginal bone height on the distal side.

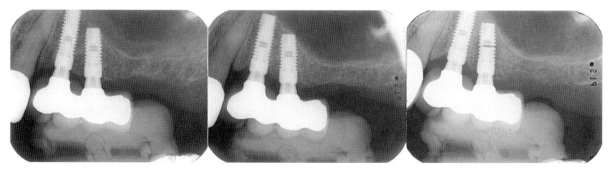

Fig. 28-42 Fracture of the implant pillar seen in radiographs taken 2 years after bridge installation. Neither the image from the latter occasion, nor the one taken at a 1-year control examination show any sign of fracture. Notice the inflammatory reaction along both sides of the implant.

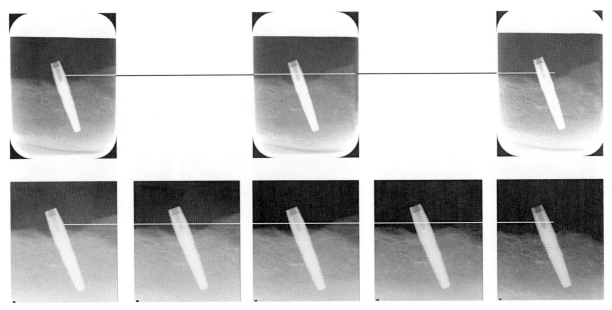

Fig. 28-43 Images taken with an image plate system, exposure times: 0.25 sec, 0.40 sec and 0.63 sec (upper row) and a CMOS system, exposure times: 0.25 sec, 0.32 sec, 0.40 sec, 0.50 sec and 0.63 sec (lower row). In the upper images the marginal bone is seen at the same level. In the lower ones it seems lower with increasing exposure. Compare with the horizontal reference line.

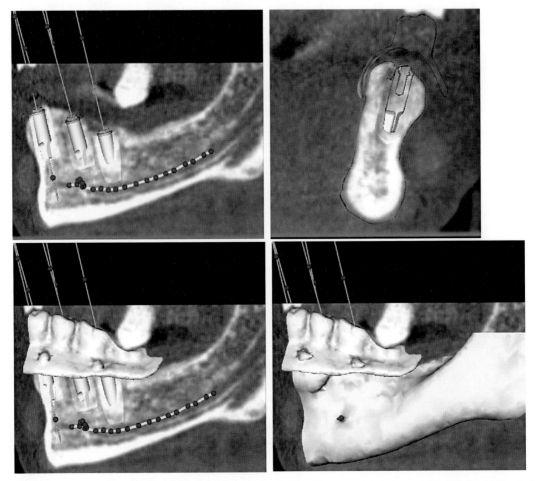

Fig. 28-44 Images describing the use of a system for surgical planning and image-guided surgery. Courtesy of Matts Andersson and Andreas Pettersson, Nobel Biocare, Göteborg, Sweden.

Image-guided surgery

Due to the three-dimensional information offered by computed tomography and digital volume tomography it is possible to use those techniques to play a more direct role in the surgical placement of the implants (BouSerhal 2001; Guerrero 2005). The exact placement and angulation of implants are determined by means of the radiographs. Guiding templates are then constructed and applied during surgery so that the implants will be positioned as intended, so-called image-guided surgery. It is also possible to build up images in which the result of the treatment, with specific implants and the final pros-

thesis "in place". Development in this area is rapid with implant companies, manufacturers of radiographic equipment, and software companies all working to develop and refine these techniques. For that reason we will do no more than mention the possibility and show just a few images that can shed some light on how these techniques can be used (Fig. 28-44). We strongly recommend that radiographic techniques that limit the radiation dose to the patient as much as possible are used. We also recommend that a careful scrutiny for diagnostic purposes is made of all radiographs before they are used for surgical implant planning and guiding.

References

Adell, R., Eriksson, B., Lekholm, U., Brånemark, P-I. & Jemt, T. (1990). A long-term follow-up study of osseointegrated implants in the treatment of totally edentulous jaws. *International Journal of Oral and Maxillofacial Implants* **10**, 303–311.

Analoui, M. (2001a). Radiographic digital image enhancement. Part I: Spatial domain techniques. *Dentomaxillofacial Radiology* **30**, 1–9.

Analoui, M. (2001b). Radiographic digital image enhancement. Part II: Transform domain techniques. *Dentomaxillofacial Radiology* **30**, 56–77.

Andersson, B., Ödman, P., Lindvall, A-M. & Lithner, B. (1995). Single-tooth restorations on osseointegrated implants. Results and experiences from a prospective study after 2–3 years. *International Journal of Oral and Maxillofacial Implants* **10**, 702–711.

Arzouman, M., Otis, L., Kipnis, V. & Levine, D. (1993). Observations of the anterior loop of the inferior alveolar canal. *International Journal of Oral and Maxillofacial Implants* **8**, 295–300.

Bothe, R.T., Beaton, L.E. & Davenport, H.A. (1940). Reaction of bone to multiple metallic implants. *Surgery, Gynecology and Obstetrics* **71**, 598–602.

BouSerhal, C. (2001). The applicability of different radiographic techniques for the preoperative planning of oral implant placement. Dissertation. Leuven: Katholieke Universiteit Leuven.

BouSerhal, C., Jacobs, R., Gijbels, F., Bosmans, H., Hermans, R., Quirynen, M. & van Steenberghe D. (2001). Adsorbed doses from spiral CT and conventional spiral tomography: a phantom vs. cadaver study. *Clinical Oral Implants Research* **12**, 473–478.

Brånemark, P-I., Gröndahl, K. & Brånemark, B. (2005). How human applications began. Why osseointegration would work and how it did in the first patients treated. Basic facts and philosophical thoughts. In: Chien, S., Gröndahl, H-G. & Robinson, K., eds. *The Osseointegration Book*. Berlin: Quintessenz Verlags-GmbH, pp. 19–114.

Brånemark, P-I., Hansson, B.O., Adell, R. Breine, U., Lindström, J., Hallén, O. & Öhman, A. (1977). Osseointegrated implants in the treatment of the edentulous jaw. Experience from a 10-year period. *Scandinavian Journal of Plastic and Reconstructive Surgery* **11**, Suppl 16.

Buser, D., Dula, K., Gröndahl, K., Harris, D., Jacobs, R., Lekholm, U., Nakielny, R., van Steenberghe, D. & van der Stelt, P. (2002). E.A.O. Guidelines for the use of Diagnostic Imaging in Implant Dentistry: A consensus workshop organized by the European Association for Osseointegration in Trinity College Dublin. *Clinical Oral Implants Research* **13**, 576–580.

Cardaropoli, G., Wennström, J.L. & Lekholm, U. (2003). Peri-implant bone alterations in relation to inter-unit distances. A 3-year retrospective study. *Clinical Oral Implants Research* **14**, 430–436.

Darriba, M.A. & Mendonca-Caridad, J.J. (1997). Profuse bleeding and life-threatening airway obstruction after placement of mandibular dental implants. *Journal of Oral Maxillofacial Surgery* **55**, 1328–1330.

Dula, K., Mini, R., Lambrecht, J.T., van der Stelt, P.F., Schneeberger, P., Clemens, G., Sanderink, H. & Buser, D. (1997). Hypothetical mortality risk associated with spiral tomography of the maxilla and mandible prior to endosseous implant treatment. *European Journal of Oral Sciences* **105**, 123–129.

Dula, K., Mini, R. & van der Stelt, P.F. (1996). Hypothetical mortality risk associated with spiral computed tomography of the maxilla and mandible. *European Journal of Oral Sciences* **104**, 503–510.

Ekelund, J-A., Lindqvist, L.W., Carlsson, G.E. & Jemt, T. (2003). Implant treatment in the edentulous mandible: a prospective study on Brånemark system implants over more than 20 years. *International Journal of Prosthodontics* **16**, 602–608.

Ekestubbe, A., Gröndahl, K., Ekholm, S., Johansson, P.E. & Gröndahl, H-G. (1996). Low-dose tomographic techniques for dental implant planning. *International Journal of Oral and Maxillofacial Implants* **5**, 650–659.

Ekestubbe, A., Gröndahl, K. & Gröndahl, H-G. (1997). The use of tomography for dental implant planning. *Dentomaxillofacial Radiology* **26**, 206–213.

Ekestubbe, A., Gröndahl, K. & Gröndahl, H-G. (1999). Quality of preimplant low-dose tomography. *Oral Surgery, Oral Medicine, Oral Pathology, Oral Radiology, and Endodontics* **88**, 738–744.

Esposito, M., Ekestubbe, A. & Gröndahl, K. (1993). Radiological evaluation of marginal bone loss at tooth surfaces facing single Brånemark implants. *Clinical Oral Implants Research* **4**, 151–157.

Farman, G. & Farman, T.T. (2005). A comparison of 18 different x-ray detectors currently used in dentistry. *Oral Surgery, Oral Medicine, Oral Pathology, Oral Radiology, and Endodontics* **99**, 485–489.

Frederiksen, N.L. (2004). Specialized radiographic techniques. In: White, S.C. & Pharoah, M.J., eds. *Oral Radiology: Principles and Interpretation*, 5th edn. St. Louis, Missouri: Mosby, pp. 245–264.

Frederiksen, N.L., Benson, B.W. & Solokowski, T.W. (1995). Effective dose and risk assessment from computed tomography of the maxillofacial complex. *Dentomaxillofacial Radiology* **24**, 55–58.

Gröndahl, K., Ekestubbe, A. & Gröndahl, H-G. (1996). *Radiography in Oral Endosseous Prosthetics*. Göteborg: Nobel Biocare.

Gröndahl, K. & Lekholm, U. (1997). The predictive value of radiographic diagnosis of implant instability. *International Journal of Oral and Maxillofacial Implants* **12**, 59–64.

Gröndahl, H-G., Ekestubbe, A. & Gröndahl, K. (2003). *Cranex Tome & Digora PCT*. Raisio: Newprint Oy.

Guerrero, M.E. (2005). The use of cone beam CT for oral implant planning and transfer to surgical field. Dissertation. Leuven: Katholieke Universiteit Leuven.

Hermann, J.S., Schoolfield, J.D., Schenk, R.K., Buser, D. & Cochran, D.L. (2001). Influence of the size of the microgap on crestal bone changes around titanum implants. A histometric evaluation of unloaded non-submerged implants in the canine mandible. *Journal of Periodontology* **72**, 1372–1383.

Huumonen, S., Kvist, T., Gröndahl, K. & Molander, A. (2006). Diagnostic value of computed tomography in re-treatment of root fillings in maxillary molars. *International Endodontic Journal* **39**, 827–833.

ICRP 60 (1991). Recommendations of the International Commission on Radiation Protection, ICRP Publication 60. *Annals of the ICRP* **21**, 1–201.

King, G.N., Hermann, J.S., Schoolfield, J.D., Buser, D. & Cochran, DL. (2002). Influence of the size of the microgap on crestal bone levels in non-submerged dental implants: a radiographic study in the canine mandible. *Journal of Periodontology* **73**, 1111–1117.

Leventhal, G.S. (1951). Titanium, a metal for surgery. *Journal of Bone and Joint Surgery* **2**, 473–474.

Ludlow, J.B., Davies-Ludlow, L.E., Brooks, S.L. & Howerton, W.B. (2006). Dosimetry of 3 CBCT devices for oral and maxillofacial radiology: CB Mercuray, NewTom 3G and i-CAT. *Dentomaxillofacial Radiology* **35**, 219–226.

Niamtu, J., III (2001). Near-fatal airway obstruction after routine implant placement. *Oral Surgery, Oral Medicine, Oral Pathology, Oral Radiology, Endodontics* **92**, 597–600.

Rustemeyer, P., Streubuhr, U. & Suttmoeller, J. (2004). Low-dose dental computed tomography: significant dose reduction without loss of image quality. *Acta Radiologica* **45**, 847–853.

Snauwaert, K., Duyck, J., van Steenberghe, D., Quirynen, M. & Naert, I. (2000). Time dependent failure rate and marginal bone loss of implant supported prostheses: a 15-year follow-up study. *Clinical Oral Implants Research* **4**, 13–20.

Sundén, S., Gröndahl, K. & Gröndahl H-G. (1995). Accuracy and precision in the radiographic diagnosis of clinical instability in Brånemark dental implants. *Clinical Oral Implants Research* **6**, 220–226.

Tronje, G. (1982). Image distortion in rotational panoramic radiography. *Dentomaxillofacial Radiology* Suppl 3.

Worthington, P. (2004). Injury to the inferior alveolar nerve during implant placement: A formula for protection of the patient and clinician. *International Journal of Oral and Maxillofacial Implants* **19**, 731–734.

Chapter 29

Examination of Patients with Implant-Supported Restorations

Urs Brägger

Identification of the presence of implants and implant systems, 623
  Screening, 623
  Implant pass, 623
  Questionnaire for new patients, 625
  Anamnestic information from patients on maintenance, 625
  The development of implant recognition software, 625
Clinical inspection and examination, 625
  Characteristics of implant-supported restorations, 625
  Characteristics of prosthetic components and components of implant systems, 626
Technical failures/complications, 626
Function, 628
  Functional analysis, 628
  Articulation, phonetics, 628

Implant, 628
  Clinical test of mobility, 629
  Electronic tools to assess the quality of osseointegration, 629
  Bacterial deposits, 629
Soft tissues, 629
  Mucosa, 629
  Palpation/sensitivity, 629
  Recession, pocket probing depth, probing attachment level, bleeding on probing, 629
Esthetics, 630
  Papillae, interdental space and type of mucosa, 630
  Condition of adjacent teeth, 631
  Color shades, 632

Identification of the presence of implants and implant systems

Screening

With the growing use of dental implants, the number of patients with implant-supported restorations seeking dental care will soon affect most dentists on a regular basis (Österberg *et al.* 2000; Berge 2000; Zitzmann & Hagmann 2007). Cohorts with fixed or removable implant-supported restorations demonstrated considerable amounts of technical and biological failures and complications over 5- and 10-year observation periods (Berglund *et al.* 2002; Pjetursson *et al.* 2004; Brägger *et al.* 2005; Widbom *et al.* 2005; Fransson *et al.* 2005; Roos-Jansaker *et al.* 2006). In the coming decades, the profession will be challenged to prevent, diagnose, and treat technical and biological problems of implant-supported restorations. Screening of all new patients, identification of the implants, and assessment of the condition of the implants, the restoration, and the surrounding structures are therefore mandatory. Aspects related to general health, smoking, etc, which may affect the quality of implant integration and function, are discussed in Chapters 27 and 30.

Implant pass

Information gathered by means of questionnaires can often be incorrect or incomplete. After a few years, patients may not be aware of how many implants were placed or even where exactly they are located. In addition, patients cannot be expected to remember and list brand names, names of biomaterials or complex interventions.

Several professional associations and manufacturers of implant systems have therefore developed an implant pass for patients (Fig. 29-1). All implant-related information can be filled out on the pass, avoiding the loss of important data. Furthermore, tracking of components back to their origin is possible applying the corresponding lot numbers in the patient chart as well as in an implant pass. Patients with implant-supported restorations would benefit from this document whenever a dental service needs to be provided, including emergency situations, maintenance, repairs or even a new restoration. Just a simple tightening of a screw-retained implant-supported prosthesis might be tedious if the dental team is unable to identify the components and if no corresponding screwdriver is available.

CERTIFICATE FOR DENTAL IMPLANTS
This certificate is issued to patients who have received dental implants.
This certificate gives information about the implant type, implant localisation and suprastructure components.
The patient is advised to show this document at any dental examination or treatment.
This certificate must be updated at any surgical or prosthodontic treatment.

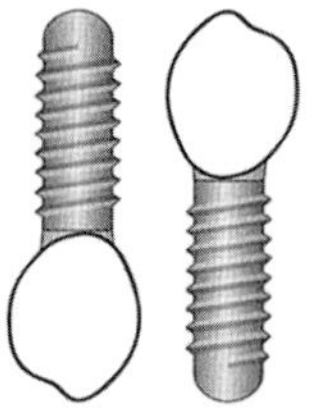

Single Crowns 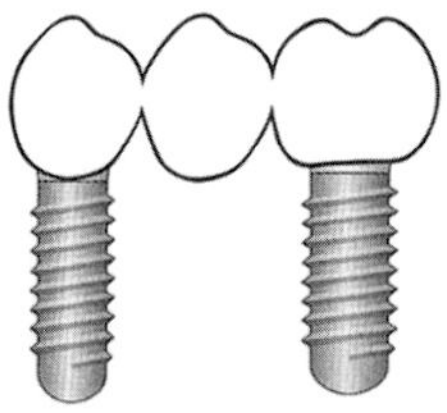   Bridge

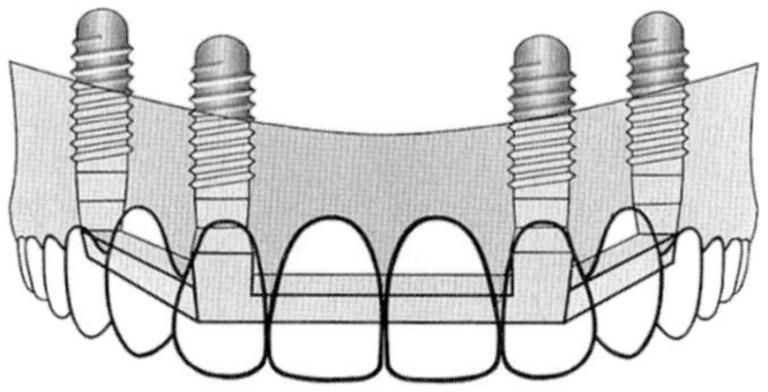

Bar Device

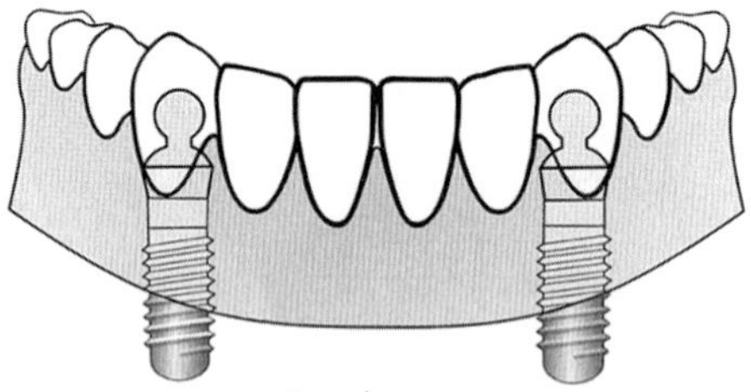

Overdenture

Name _____

First name _____

Date of birth _____

Street _____

Postal code/city _____

date	implant localisation	implant type, length, diameter	abutment type	supraconstruction			dentist/city	visum
				type*	screwed: occlusal access temporary or definitive	cemented: temporary or definitive		

*bridges: please indicate if segmented or not

Fig. 29-1 Proposal for an implant pass developed by the Swiss Society of Implantology. Copyright © Schweizerische Gesellschaft für orale Implantologie.

Questionnaire for new patients

The most straightforward way to obtain information on the presence of implants and implant-supported restorations in new patients is to ask questions related to any past implant experiences. The following comprehensive list of questions can be added to currently used questionnaires in educational programs, clinics, and private practices:

- Do you carry an implant pass?
- Did your dentist ever place implants into your jaw bones (name, address of the dentist, surgeon)?
- How many implants were placed?
- When were these implants placed (if remembered)? (How old were you when implants were placed?)
- Where are they located?
- Why were these implants placed or what were the reasons for the loss of teeth?
- Do you wear a prosthesis/crown supported by an implant (name of the dentist, prosthodontist, technician)?
- Did you have enough bone to have the implant placed?
- Were there additional treatments performed before implants could be placed?
- Did the surgeon perform a bone augmentation, sinus lift procedure?
- What was the brand name of the implants (if remembered)?
- Were bone graft particles used (if remembered)?
- What was the brand name of the biomaterials used (if remembered)?
- Have you ever experienced failures/complications with the implants?
- Have you ever experienced failures/complications with the prostheses/crowns?
- How often has this occurred?
- Are you satisfied with the way you can function with the implant-supported prosthesis/crown?
- Are you satisfied with the esthetic situation?
- Did you have to pay for the implants and prosthesis or was there insurance involved?
- How do you clean the neck portion of the implant/abutment?
- How do you clean the prosthesis/crowns?
- Do you use any special aids/disinfectants to carry out the cleaning?
- Does the mucosa/do the gums around your implant bleed?
- Do you notice a bad taste coming from underneath the prosthesis/crown?
- Is your implant mobile?
- Have you recently noticed a change with the implant-supported restorations?

Anamnestic information from patients on maintenance

Before starting to examine the oral conditions at maintenance visits, questions related to implant-supported restorations should include:

- Have you noticed a change with your implant-supported restorations?
- Are your implants stable?
- Do the gums around your implant(s) bleed?
- Are you able to clean the area around the neck portion of the implant(s) easily?
- Do you still have enough cleaning aids/disinfectants to perform daily plaque control?

In addition, general questions related to patient's satisfaction with the implant-supported reconstruction should be part of a quality management concept (Vermylen *et al.* 2003; Pjetursson *et al.* 2005).

The development of implant recognition software

Sahiwal *et al.* (2002a,b,c) collected implants from more than 50 manufacturers and divided them into threaded and non-threaded, as well as tapered and non-tapered categories. Radiographs were then taken at different angulations. Using tables and flow charts, test implants could be correctly identified in radiographs taken within ±10 degrees, according to their identifying features.

A very recent method to assist in identifying unknown implant systems applies an implant recognition software (IRS) (Michelinakis *et al.* 2006). The internet was searched for implant manufacturing companies worldwide in all languages. Relevant information on the implant designs was collected. A program was devised using key design factors for the identification of specific implants. The search revealed 87 implant manufacturers with 231 different designs. A valuable adjunct to the identification of implant systems was thus introduced for both general dental practice use and forensic identification.

Clinical inspection and examination

Characteristics of implant-supported restorations

Following the conventional extraoral and intraoral examination, the distribution of implants in the dental arch is marked in a dental record. A detailed description of the implant-borne restoration, the prosthetic components, and the components of the respective implant system may include material and design aspects.

- Restorations:
  - Crown
  - FDP, number of units
  - Extension prosthesis
  - Telescopic restoration
  - Removable partial denture
  - Bar device
  - Overdenture

- ° Defect prosthesis
- ° Other
- Material of:
  - ° Veneer
  - ° Framework
  - ° Denture teeth
- Fixation:
  - ° Cemented
  - ° Removable by the patient/dentist
  - ° Screw retained: transocclusal, transversal, access closed, access free, type of screw head, component of what system
  - ° Friction
  - ° Via attachments
  - ° Connection to teeth: one piece, detachable, attachments
  - ° Material.

Characteristics of prosthetic components and components of implant systems

- Prosthetic components:
  - ° Telescopic or conus crowns
  - ° Bar device
  - ° Riders
  - ° Matrices, patrices
  - ° Mesostructures
  - ° Individualized components
  - ° Material
- Components of implant systems:
  - ° Abutments for cementation
  - ° Abutments for transocclusal screw retention
  - ° Abutments for transversal screw retention
  - ° Angulated abutment
  - ° Anchors: ball anchor, magnets, locator system
  - ° Mesostructures
  - ° Material
  - ° CAD/CAM components
- Connection of abutments to the implants:
  - ° Localization of microgaps
  - ° How many gaps
  - ° Platform
  - ° Internal, external
  - ° Morse taper, butt joint
  - ° Geometry
  - ° Abutment screw: access free, closed, type of screwhead, components of what system.

Technical failures/complications

Until the first European Workshop on evidence-based reconstructive dentistry, held in Hünigen, Switzerland, 4–7 November 2006, there was no generally accepted definition for success and survival for reconstructions. Zöllner and Belser (2007) therefore suggested the following definitions:

- Success of abutment-reconstruction complex ("reconstruction"): survival without any biologic and/or technical complication

- Survival of abutment-reconstruction complex ("reconstruction"):
  - ° On abutment level: abutment is still *in situ*
  - ° On reconstruction level: reconstruction remaining *in situ* with or without modification
  - ° Alternatively: reconstruction remaining *in situ* in its original extension with or without modification.

In addition, factors regarded as biological or technical failures were listed but not further defined:

- Biological complications of abutment-reconstruction complex ("reconstruction"):
  - ° Natural abutment tooth: caries, loss of sensitivity, apical periodontitis, periodontitis
  - ° Implant: peri-implant diseases, implant mobility, loss of sensitivity of adjacent tooth
- Technical complications of abutment-reconstruction complex ("reconstruction"):
  - ° Tooth supported reconstruction: loss of retention, fracture of abutment, fracture of framework, fracture of veneering material
  - ° Implant supported reconstruction: loss of retention/screw loosening/abutment loosening, loss of access hole restoration, fracture of implant, fracture of abutment, screws, fracture of framework, fracture of veneering material.

While describing the above-mentioned detailed characteristics of the implant-supported restorations, any defects and irregular observations are marked.

The suprastructures are inspected for signs of loosening, loss of retention, loss of friction, wear, attrition, fractures of frame work, of denture teeth, of porcelain, of veneers, discolorations, bacterial deposits, precision or misfit at margins, cement rests (Figs. 29-2 and 29-3).

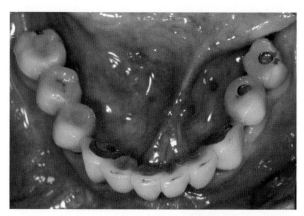

Fig. 29-2 Fractures of porcelain veneer at the distal aspects 35 and 46 as well as a porcelain chip off at 33. The patient was restored with three screw-retained porcelain fused to metal FDPs (I46 × I44/I43xxxxI33/I35I35). Three repairs within 3 years were needed. In the opposing jaw, the patient still had all his natural teeth. At night the patient wears an occlusal protective splint on an irregular basis.

The torque of occlusal screws can be checked where corresponding equipment is available. Obviously, loose screw-retained suprastructures are removed for further inspection, cleaning and retightening. Stable fixed restorations do not need to be disassembled if there were no complications reported

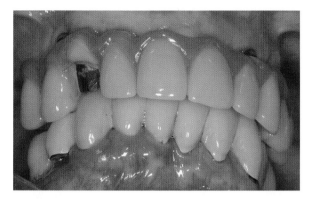

Fig. 29-3 Fracture of the denture tooth 13 as well as part of the veneer from a screw-retained extension prosthesis on five implants. In the lower jaw, the patient was restored with a fixed partial denture with bilateral distal extensions. The prosthesis could be removed and repaired.

by the patient and if the clinical examination did not reveal any technical problems.

Defective screw heads might complicate the removal of the suprastructure since screw drivers might not catch anymore. Occlusal screws that were tightened together with cementation might as well be very difficult to be removed with the regular instruments. In such cases, repair sets are needed to remove defective screws in a controllable standardized manner (Fig. 29-4). Repair sets might also be very helpful in cases with fractured abutment screws that are completely blocked in the implant (Luterbacher *et al.* 2000a) (Fig. 29-5). Abutments are also checked for their torque, the presence of bacterial deposits, corrosion products, cement rests, fractures, and deformations.

If replacement of a component is needed, the corresponding brand name and ordering number should be identified; a task that can be very tedious in the light of numerous implant producers and, in addition, a long list of copycat products (Jokstad *et al.* 2003).

Some manufacturers of implant components offer a complaint system to protect their customers from

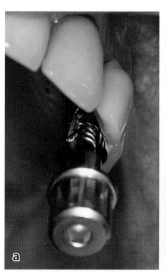
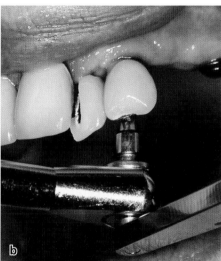

Fig. 29-4 (a) Removal of a screw-retained FDP using a screwdriver was impossible since the head of the occlusal screw was completely worn down due to attrition. The components of the repair set developed for the Straumann Dental Implant System® include an extraction bolt which can be tightened into a hole prepared with drills into the head of the occlusal screw. (b) Applying sufficient torque, the segmented part of the FDP is being removed together with the occlusal screw, the abutment, and the abutment screw. The implant was then used again for the support and fixation of a new extension prosthesis shown in Fig. 29-3.

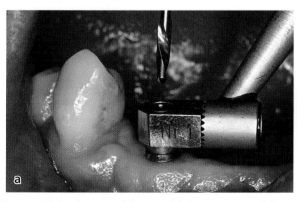
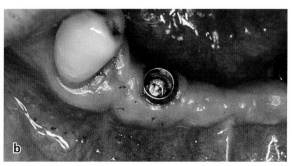

Fig. 29-5 (a) Application of the assembled components of the repair system developed for the Straumann Dental Implant System® for the removal of fractured abutment screws. The conical insert at the end of the handle secures the centered guidance of the drill. (b) After counter-clockwise drilling with ample cooling, the fractured portion of the abutment screw is removed. The threads are then recut by hand instruments with conical and cylindrical configurations.

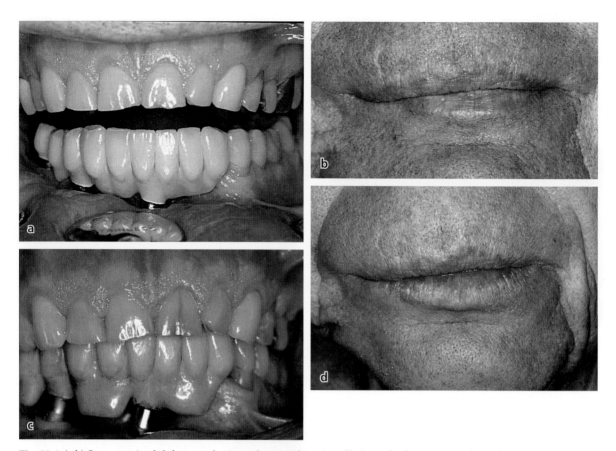

Fig. 29-6 (a,b) Screw-retained defect prosthesis on three implants in a fibula graft after excision of a malignant tumor. Function and phonetics are acceptable considering the severity of the defect. (c,d) After 5 years, some of the grafted bone has been resorbed. The soft tissues receded, leaving a large space underneath the pontics. Articulation and phonetics became more and more difficult. In addition, loss of saliva during speaking became intolerable. The FDP was removed and reshaped to fill out the missing soft tissues.

undue costs arising because of a potential error in production. Forms are completed with all the relevant information related to the loss of implants or a damaged component of the respective implant system. The defective components are sent in and exposed to a metallurgic evaluation and other tests. If the components were applied for the correct indications and a possible production error has been confirmed, the manufacturer will replace components and may even help to finance part of a new restoration as decided case by case.

If the abutment was individualized, it may also be impossible to just replace the component and use the existing suprastructure. In such cases, a new impression at the implant level will be needed to replace the abutment; a remake of the entire restoration may be necessary.

Function

Functional analysis

A functional analysis of the dentition with fixed and/or removable dental prostheses on implants needs to be carried out according to standard protocols in prosthodontics and includes parameters

assessing articulation, occlusion, phonetics, denture stability, etc.

Articulation, phonetics

Disturbed articulation after placement of implant supported restorations may be very difficult to assess without the use of objective parameters (Fig 29-6). Heydecke *et al.* (2004) recorded test words articulated by 30 patients having adjusted to different implant-supported maxillary restorations for 2 months. Lay judges were asked to rate the quality of the articulation. This within-subjects crossover trial demonstrated that overdentures with or without palate enabled patients to produce better speech quality than with fixed prostheses on the implants.

Implant

Cases with removable implant-borne restorations allow direct access for clinical inspection and examination of the implant components and the peri-implant soft tissue conditions. Cemented or screw-retained crowns or fixed dental prostheses may complicate the access for visual inspection and probing.

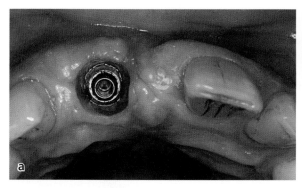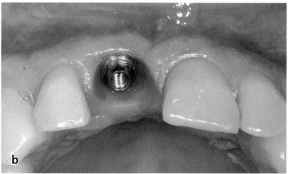

Fig. 29-7 (a) After removal of a screw-retained crown on an octa abutment, the amount of submucosal biofilm was impressive (3 years after placement of the crown). The epithetical lining of the emergence profile was ulcerated which led to bleeding after removal of the crown. (b) In a similar case, there were no obvious bacterial deposits detectable. The peri-implant soft tissues appeared epithelialized with few signs of inflammation.

Clinical test of mobility

Presence or absence of mobility is checked manually/digitally or with the help of instruments trying to move the implants. A perceived mobility of the restoration *per se* does not necessarily mean that the implant is loose. The connection suprastructure/abutment and/or abutment/implant might be loose leading to the mobility. Implant mobility can only be confirmed after disassembling all the components.

In the case of a multi-unit fixed restoration, the absence of mobility does not necessarily mean that the implants are all well integrated. Actual mobility might be obscured by the splinting effect.

Electronic tools to assess the quality of osseointegration

Resonance frequency analyses and Periotest® readings were part of numerous study protocols to quantitate the stability of implants. Changes in the readings were interpreted to reflect biological processes such as bone apposition, bone remodeling, bone maturation or, in a negative sense, deterioriation of the firmness of the bone to implant connection. Recent evidence from the literature was condensed to the following consensus statements (Hobkirk & Wiskott 2006): stability may be confirmed by performing repeated Periotest® measurements of the same implant over time. Increases of these measurements, however, became evident, when the implants are clinically obviously loose. Implants with high implant stability quotient (ISQ) values during maintenance appear to stay firmly integrated, while decreasing ISQ values may be indicative of developing instability. For both biomechanical testing methods, however, the lack of normative values and the wide range of reported values for stable implants and potentially failing implants would not justify their routine clinical use.

Bacterial deposits

The amount and distribution of visual bacterial deposits are evaluated at the emerging portion of the implant-borne restorations (implant neck, abutment, mesostructures, patrices) (Fig. 29-7). A *yes* or *no* for presence of bacterial deposits may be noted or marked in a scheme. In clinical studies, a gradual index such as the mPl (by Mombelli *et al.* 1987) has often been used.

Soft tissues

Mucosa

The inspection of the soft tissues will include the detection and description of visual signs of infection and/or other pathologic conditions, such as swelling, edema, redness, irregular keratinization, tattoos, pigmentation, hyperplasia, ulceration, soft tissue dehiscencies, or fistula. All soft tissues of the oral cavity, not only the peri-implant tissues, need to be examined (Fig. 29-8).

Palpation/sensitivity

Palpation at the buccal aspects of the implants may assist in the detection of loose implants (osseo-disintegration). Palpation furthermore reveals pus, swelling and pain, and the exudation of grafting particles. During palpation and sensitivity testing any morbidity due to, for example, grafting procedures (Clavero & Lundgren 2003) or side effects of implant placement, e.g. close to the mandibular nerve, may be detected.

Recession, pocket probing depth, probing attachment level, bleeding on probing

Measuring the localization of the margin of the mucosa in relation to a fixed reference point such as the connection suprastructure/abutment, abutment/

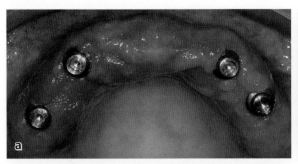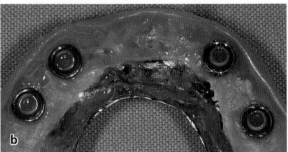

Fig. 29-8 (a) This 55-year-old female patient is wearing a palate free overdenture. Signs of denture stomatitis are an alarming signal to reinforce plaque control using chlorhexidine gel and rinses. (b) The base of the overdenture as well as the locator® matrices appear to be kept clean.

implant, suprastructure/implant, suprastructure/mesostructure as well as the pocket probing depth (PPD) reflects the anatomic situation after implant placement and reconstructive rehabilitation. Clinical parameters assessed by means of probing were first described around the neck of a one-piece transmucosal implant and included the distance between the implant shoulder and the mucosal margin (DIM), and the pocket probing depth (PPD). By adding PPD and DIM, the probing attachment level was calculated (PAL) (Buser et al. 1990).

Applying similar force, the insertion depth of a periodontal probe is usually deeper at implants compared to contralateral natural teeth. In addition, it seems to be easier to provoke bleeding after probing at implants compared to teeth (Brägger et al. 1997; Karoussis et al. 2004). Repeated probing using similar direction, localization, force, and the same references reveals stable conditions or increasing probing depths and/or increasing recession as signs of continuous loss of tissue or osseointegration.

With increasing PPD, the accuracy of repeated probing will decrease (Christensen et al. 1997). Precise readings of tissue destruction in deeper lesions are hindered by blocked access for probing and the lack of a continuous smooth surface to guide the probe tip apically. This occurs mostly at screw threads no longer covered by bone or horizontal steps between implants and abutments (Mombelli et al. 1997).

Similarly to periodontal disease, the absence of bleeding on probing (BoP) may reflect a stable condition, while repeated BoP may be indicative of a higher chance to develop tissue disintegration. Clinical and microbiological tests for monitoring tissue conditions during supportive periodontal therapy were performed in 19 patients, and the results indicated statistically significant better diagnostic characteristics of both tests at implants compared to teeth. The inclusion of an additional microbiologic test significantly enhanced the diagnostic characteristics of BoP alone at teeth as well as at implants (Luterbacher et al. 2000b).

Increased PPD combined with BoP and/or pus secretion may indicate various stages of mucositis or peri-implantitis.

According to one of the proposed concepts for the prevention and treatment of mucositis and peri-implantitis (cumulative interceptive supportive therapy), a cascade of anti-infective and corrective treatment modalities is applied depending on the severity of the findings (Lang et al. 2000). The treatment decisions are based on the clinical findings described above. In case of a suspected peri-implantitis, radiographic evaluation may be required to visualize bone levels or changes in bone levels in relation to reference points. If antibiotics are considered, information on the microbiologic composition of plaque samples as well as resistance testing will assist in decision making.

Esthetics

Papillae, interdental space and type of mucosa

A comprehensive assessment and documentation of the soft tissue condition may be of importance, especially for fixed restorations in esthetically critical areas (Fig. 29-9). The appearance of papillae and interdental spaces can be evaluated objectively using various indices, possibly including metric measurement (Jemt 1997). When linear measurements and stable reference points were used, valuable parameters for the long-term observation of changes in the papilla characteristics could be obtained (Jemt & Lekholm 2005). This also required that no changes to the crown contour were made (Klinge & Meyle 2006).

Some factors, such as the thickness of the peri-implant soft tissues, the amount of the available keratinized mucosa, the space between implants or between teeth and implants, and the underlying bone levels, may influence the esthetic appearance of the papilla/interdental space complex (Tarnow et al. 2000; Choquet et al. 2001; Gastaldo et al. 2004; Lee et al. 2005). In some cohorts reformation of papillae was also described (Jemt 1997; Chang et al. 1999). Metallic markers can be used to indicate the tip of the papilla in a radiograph in order to assess the distance between the underlying bone level and a papilla (Tarnow et al.

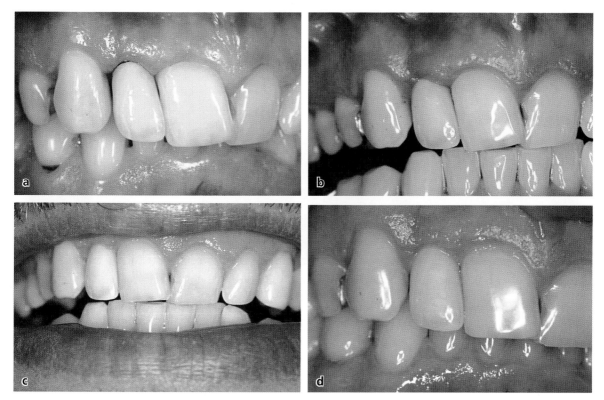

Fig. 29-9 A porcelain fused to metal crown was cemented on an implant of the Straumann Dental Implant System®. The clinical slides document the situation after cementation and after 1, 5, and 10 years. After 1 year, soft tissue seems to cover the implant shoulder and fill the interdental space: a result that was completely maintained over 5 and 10 years.

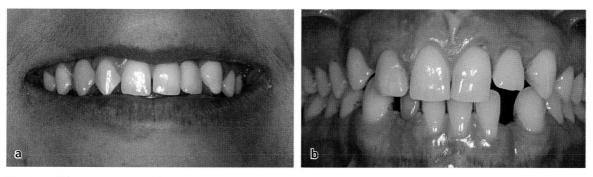

Fig. 29-10 Fifteen years ago, implants were sometimes not correctly placed to fulfill today's esthetic expectations. As a disappointing result, implant margins as well as the implant body were shining through the thin mucosa of this 20-year-old female patient. Due to the continuous eruption of the neighboring teeth, soft tissues now cover the dark implants. The crowns on I13 and I22, however, are no longer in occlusion.

1992). Assessment of the width of the keratinized mucosa can be facilitated by staining the lining non-keratinized mucosa with Schiller's (IKI) solution (Fasske & Morgenroth 1958; Brägger *et al.* 1997).

Condition of adjacent teeth

Implants placed too closely to adjacent teeth might lead to unfavorable periodontal conditions. In some studies, alveolar bone loss was observed if distances were chosen below a minimum distance (Krennmair *et al.* 2003). Adjacent teeth might have been damaged while preparing the implant bed. Delayed loss of sensitivity (vitality) may lead to endodontic interventions.

Long-term vertical changes of anterior maxillary teeth adjacent to implants in 14 young and 14 mature adults were measured in radiographs. In both groups, the tooth eruption process resulted in considerable changes ranging between 0.1 mm and 1.65 mm and 0.12 mm to 1.86 mm (Bernard *et al.* 2004) after an average observation period of about 4 years.

The lack of an implant eruption may result in the formation of steps related to adjacent teeth, incisal edges, etc. Occlusal contacts may still be present, however, due to the different eruption in the opposing jaw; step formation can also be observed (Zachrisson 2006) (Fig. 29-10).

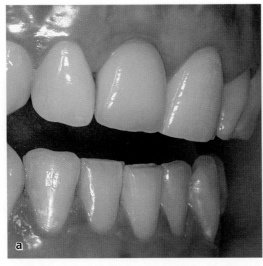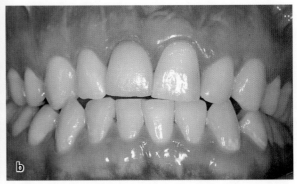

Fig. 29-11 In this 25-year-old female patient, a full ceramic crown and mesostructure were placed on an implant of the Straumann Dental Implant System®. After only 3 years, a step appeared in relation to the adjacent incisal edges. In addition, the color shade of the full ceramic crown appears to be too dark due to the fact that the patient had been bleaching her teeth.

Color shades

For a complete documentation of implant-supported restoration, a set of intraoral images of the area of interest may be desirable. In addition, an assessment of color shades based on visual or digital/electronic measurements are helpful. Of special concern are changes in color shade due to aging or bleaching of the adjacent natural teeth leading to noticeable unpleasant shade differences (Fig. 29-11).

Receding margins of the peri-implant mucosa result in visible implant components, potentially interfering with esthetics in visible zones. Even white ceramic components may result in an esthetically unfavorable situation if color matching over a wider range is not possible (Zachrisson 2006). Coverage of recessions or enlargement of the thickness of the mucosa can technically be achieved by means of free mucosa transplants. The predictability and the long-term success of such interventions remains to be assessed.

References

Berge, T.I. (2000). Public awareness, information sources and evaluation of oral implant treatment in Norway. *Clinical Oral Implants Research* 11, 401–408.

Berglund, T., Persson, L. & Klinge, B. (2002). A systematic review of the incidence of biological and technical complications in implant dentistry reported in prospective longitudinal studies of at least 5 years. *Journal of Clinical Periodontology* 29 (Suppl 3), 197–212.

Bernard, J.P., Schatz, J.P., Christou, P., Belser, U. & Kiliaridis, S. (2004). Long-term vertical changes of the anterior maxillary teeth adjacent to single implants in young and mature adults. A retrospective study. *Journal of Clinical Periodontology* 31, 1024–1028.

Brägger, U., Bürgin, W., Hämmerle, C.H.F. & Lang, N.P. (1997). Associations between clinical parameters assessed around implants and teeth. *Clinical Oral Implants Research* 8, 412–421.

Brägger, U., Karoussis, I., Persson, R., Pjetursson, B., Salvi, G. & Lang, N. (2005). Technical and biological complications/failures with single crowns and fixed partial dentures on implants: a 10-year prospective cohort study. *Clinical Oral Implants Research* 16, 326–334.

Buser, D., Weber, H.P. & Lang, N.P. (1990). Tissue integration of non-submerged implants. 1-year results of a prospective study with 100 ITI hollowcylinder and hollowscrew implants. *Clinical Oral Implants Research* 1, 33–40.

Chang, M., Ödman, P.A., Wennström, J.L. & Andersson, B. (1999). Implant supported single-tooth replacements com-

pared to contralateral neutral teeth. Crown and soft tissue dimensions. *Clinical Oral Implants Research* 10, 185–194.

Choquet, V., Hermans, M., Adriaenssens, P., Daelemans, P., Tarnow, D.P. & Malevez, C. (2001). Clinical and radiographic evaluation of the papilla level adjacent to single-tooth dental implants. A retrospective study in the maxillary anterior region. *Journal of Periodontology* 72, 1364–1371.

Christensen, M.M., Joss, A. & Lang, N.P. (1997). Reproducibility of automated periodontal probing around teeth and osseointegrated oral implants. *Clinical Oral Implants Research* 8, 455–464.

Clavero, J. & Lundgren, S. (2003). Ramus or chin grafts for maxillary sinus inlay and local onlay augmentation: comparison of donor site morbidity and complications. *Clinical Implant Dentistry and Related Research* 5, 154–160.

Fasske, E. & Morgenroth, K. (1958). Glycogen content in carcinoma of the oral cavity. *Zeitschrift für Krebsforschung* 62, 375–382.

Fransson, C., Lekholm, U., Jemt, T. & Berglundh, T. (2005). Prevalence of subjects with progressive bone loss at implants. *Clinical Oral Implants Research* 16, 440–446.

Gastaldo, J.F., Cury, P.R. & Sendyk, W.R. (2004). Effect of the vertical and horizontal distances between adjacent implants and between a tooth and an implant on the incidence of interproximal papilla. *Journal of Periodontology* 75, 1242–1246.

Heydecke, G., McFarland, D.H., Feine, J.S. & Lund, J.P. (2004). Speech with maxillary implant prostheses: ratings of articulation. *Journal of Dental Research* **83**, 236–240.

Hobkirk, J.A. & Wiskott, H.W.A. (2006). Biochemical aspects of oral implants. Consensus report of Working Group 1. *Clinical Oral Implants Research* **17** (Suppl 2), 52–54.

Jemt, T. & Lekholm, U. (2005). Single implants and buccal bone grafts in the anterior maxilla: measurements of buccal crestal contours in a 6-year prospective clinical study. *Clinical Implant Dentistry and Related Research* **7**, 127–135.

Jemt, T. (1997). Regeneration of gingival papillae after single-implant treatment. *International Journal of Periodontics and Restorative Dentistry* **17**, 326–333.

Jokstad, A., Brägger, U., Brunski, J.B., Carr, A.B., Naert, I. & Wennerberg, A. (2003). Quality of dental implants. *International Dental Journal* **53**, 409–443.

Karoussis, I.K., Müller, S., Salvi, G.E., Heitz-Mayfield, L.J., Brägger, U. and Lang, N.P. (2004). Association between periodontal and peri-implant conditions: a 10-year prospective study. *Clinical Oral Implants Research* **15**, 1–7.

Klinge, B. & Meyle, J. (2006). Soft-tissue integration of implants. Consensus report of Working Group 1. *Clinical Oral Implants Research* **17** (Suppl 2), 93–96.

Krennmair, G., Piehslinger, E. & Wagner, H. (2003). Status of teeth adjacent to single-tooth implants. *International Journal of Prosthodontics* **16**, 524–528.

Lang, N.P., Wilson, T.G. & Corbet, E.F. (2000). Biological complications with dental implants: their prevention, diagnosis and treatment. *Clinical Oral Implants Research* **11** (Suppl 1), 146–155.

Lee, D.W., Par, K.H. & Moon, I.S. (2005). Dimension of keratinized mucosa and the interproximal papilla between adjacent implants. *Journal of Periodontology* **76**, 1856–1860.

Luterbacher, S., Fourmousis, I., Lang, N.P. & Brägger, U. (2000a). Fractured prosthetic abutments in osseointegrated implants: a technical complication to cope with. *Clinical Oral Implants Research* **11**, 163–170.

Luterbacher, S., Mayfield, L., Brägger, U. & Lang, N.P. (2000b). Diagnostic characteristics of clinical and microbiological tests for monitoring periodontal and peri-implant mucosal tissue conditions during supportive periodontal therapy (SPT). *Clinical Oral Implants Research* **11**, 521–529.

Michelinakis, G., Sharrock, A. & Barclay, C.W. (2006). Identification of dental implants through the use of Implant Recognition Software (IRS). *International Dental Journal* **65**, 203–208.

Mombelli, A., Mühle, T., Brägger, U., Lang, N.P. & Bürgin, W.B. (1997). Comparison of periodontal and peri-implant probing by depth-force pattern analysis. *Clinical Oral Implants Research* **8**, 448–454.

Mombelli, A., Van Oosten, M.A.C., Schürch, E. & Lang, N.P. (1987). The microbiota associated with successful or failing osseointegrated titanium implants. *Oral Microbiology and Immunology* **2**, 145–151.

Österberg, T., Carlsson, G.E. & Sundh, V. (2000). Trends and prognoses of dental status in the Swedish population: Analysis based on interviews in 1975 to 1997 by Statistics Sweden. *Acta Odontologica Scandinavica* **58**, 177–182.

Pjetursson, B.E., Karoussis, I., Bürgin, W., Brägger, U. & Lang, N.P. (2005). Patients' satisfaction following implant therapy. A 10-year prospective cohort study. *Clinical Oral Implants Research* **16**, 185–193.

Pjetursson, B.E., Tan, K., Lang, N.P., Brägger, U., Egger, M. & Zwahlen, M. (2004). A systematic review of the survival and complication rates of fixed partial dentures (FPDs) after an observation period of at least 5 years. Implant supported FPDs. *Clinical Oral Implants Research* **15**, 625–642.

Roos-Jansaker, A.M., Lindahl, C., Renvert, H. & Renvert, S. (2006). Nine- to fourteen-year follow-up of implant treatment. Part II: presence of peri-implant lesions. *Journal of Clinical Periodontology* **33**, 290–295.

Sahiwal, I.G., Woody, R.D., Benson, B.W. & Guillen, G.E. (2002a). Macro design morphology of endosseous dental implants. *Journal of Prosthetic Dentistry* **87**, 543–551.

Sahiwal, I.G., Woody, R.D., Benson, B.W. & Guillen, G.E. (2002c). Radiographic identification of threaded endosseous dental implants. *Journal of Prosthetic Dentistry* **87**, 563–577.

Sahiwal, I.G., Woody, R.D., Benson, B.W. & Guillen, G.E. (2002b). Radiographic identification of nonthreaded endosseous dental implants. *Journal of Prosthetic Dentistry* **87**, 552–562.

Tarnow, D.P., Cho, S.C. & Wallace, S.S. (2000). The effect of inter-implant distance on the height of inter-implant bone crest. *Journal of Periodontology* **71**, 546–549.

Tarnow, D.P., Magner, A.W. & Fletcher, P. (1992). The effect of the distance from the contact point to the crest of bone on the presence or absence of the interproximal dental papilla. *Journal of Periodontology* **63**, 995–996.

Vermylen, K., Collaert, B., Linden, U., Bjorn, A.L. & De Bruyn, H. (2003). Patient satisfaction and quality of single-tooth restorations. *Clinical Oral Implants Research* **14**, 119–124.

Widbom, C., Soderfeldt, B. & Kronstrom, M. (2005). A retrospective evaluation of treatments with implant-supported maxillary overdentures. *Clinical Implant Dentistry and Related Research* **7**, 166–172.

Zachrisson, B.U. (2006). Single implant-supported crowns in the anterior maxilla – potential esthetic long-term (>5 years) problems. *World Journal of Orthodontics* **7**, 306–312.

Zitzmann, N.U., Hagmann, E. & Weiger, R. (2007). What is the prevalence of various types of dental restorations in Europe? *Clinical Oral Implants Research* **18** (Suppl 3), 20–33.

Zöllner, A. & Belser, U. (2007). Factors influencing survival of reconstructions. Consensus report of Working Group 2. *Clinical Oral Implants Research* **18** (Suppl 3), 114–116.

Chapter 30

Risk Assessment of the Implant Patient

Gary C. Armitage and Tord Lundgren

Principles of risk assessment, 634
  Clinical information required for risk assessment, 636
  Technical procedures to help minimize risk, 636
Local risk factors and conditions, 637
  Presence of ongoing oral infections, 637
Systemic risk factors, 639
  Age, 639
  Smoking, 640
  Medication history, 640
  Immunosuppression, 642
  History of radiation therapy to the jaws, 642
  Diabetes mellitus, 642
  Metabolic bone disease, 643

Connective tissue and autoimmune disorders, 643
Xerostomia, 644
Hematologic and lymphoreticular disorders, 644
Genetic traits and disorders, 644
Importance of behavioral considerations in risk
  assessment, 645
  Dental history of compliance behaviors, 645
  Substance use/abuse, 645
  Psychiatric/psychological issues, 645
  Lack of understanding or communication, 645
  Patient's expectations, 646
Interest and commitment to post-treatment care and
  maintenance program, 646

In the past few decades the widespread availability and successful use of dental implants have greatly expanded the treatment options for replacement of missing teeth. Data from numerous follow-up studies of the retention rates of implants indicate that well over 90% of the fixtures are functional for 5–10 years after insertion (Lindh *et al.* 1998; Berglundh *et al.* 2002; Weng *et al.* 2003; Fugazzotto *et al.* 2004; Pjetursson *et al.* 2004; Romeo *et al.* 2004). It is clear, however, that some implants fail. In addition, the risk for implant failures and complications is not evenly distributed among all people in a given population since implant problems tend to cluster in certain subsets of patients (Weyant & Burt 1993). There are many possible reasons for failure but it is generally acknowledged that biological, mechanical, or behavioral causes can be important. In general, any factor that increases the risk of developing periodontitis also increases the risk of implant failure. Therefore, in clinical practice it is essential that practitioners understand the possible reasons for implant failures so these threats to implant survival can be minimized. Risk assessment for endosseous implants is an evolving field and it is essential that clinicians have a working knowledge of the current literature dealing with risk factors for the development of implant complications and failure. Without this knowledge an intelligent assessment of risk cannot be conducted.

Principles of risk assessment

Risk assessment is the deliberate and thoughtful evaluation of all circumstances that can affect the outcome of a therapeutic intervention. In the case of dental implants the assessment is intended to identify variables that increase the risk of complications leading to implant loss. In many cases, early identification of these variables makes it possible to avoid or eliminate them. At the very least, knowledge of the risk-altering variables allows the clinician to discuss with the patient circumstances that might affect implant survival. Risk assessment should be performed: (1) before placement of implants (designed to avoid high failure rates by identifying suitable candidates for implant treatment), (2) during the phase of implant placement and osseointegration (designed to identify and avoid technical issues that can affect implant survival), (3) during the phase of implant maintenance (designed to minimize failure by heading off problems), and (4) after an implant has failed and been removed. This "post-mortem" analysis tries to identify the causes of failure and incorporates the experience into future risk-assessment analyses of other patients.

In the literature the therapeutic outcomes of implant placement are usually described in terms of the fixture's survival, success, or its failure. A detailed

Table 30-1 Criteria for implant success, as suggested by Albrektsson *et al.* (1986)

1. That an individual, unattached implant is immobile when tested clinically

2. That a radiograph does not demonstrate any evidence of peri-implant radiolucency

3. That vertical bone loss be less than 0.2 mm annually following the implant's first year of service

4. That individual implant performance be characterized by an absence of persistent and/or irreversible signs and symptoms such as pain, infections, neuropathies, paresthesia, or violation of the mandibular canal

5. That, in the context of the above, a successful rate of 85% at the end of a 5-year observation period and 80% at the end of a 10-year period be a minimum criterion for success

Table 30-2 Potential risk factors for peri-implantitis and implant failure that should be considered in the risk-assessment process

Local risk factors
Presence of ongoing (or incompletely treated) oral infections
　Periodontal infections
　Oral hygiene
　Probing depths around remaining teeth (deep pockets are
　　habitats or reservoirs of microorganisms that can lead to
　　implant failure)
　Endodontic infections
Parafunctional habits (e.g. bruxism, clenching, grinding)
Dentoalveolar conditions
　Ridge anatomy (e.g. width, height)
　Bone quality
　Existing prosthetic restorations in region
Maxillary sinus location

Systemic risk factors
Age
Smoking
Medication history
　Bisphosphonate therapy
　Phenytoin, calcium-channel antagonists
　Cancer chemotherapy
　Anticoagulants
　Immunosuppressive agents (e.g. corticosteroids)
Immunosuppression
　HIV infection/AIDS
History of radiation therapy to the jaws
Diabetes mellitus
Bone disorders
　Osteoporosis
Connective tissue and autoimmune disorders
　Scleroderma
　Lupus erythematosus
Xerostomia
　Sjögren syndrome
Hematological and lymphoreticular disorders
　Neutrophil defects or insufficiency
　Aplastic anemia
Genetic traits and disorders
　Polymorphisms (e.g. proinflammatory genotype)
　Down syndrome
　Papillon-Lefèvre syndrome
　Crohn's disease
　Ectodermal dysplasia
　Vitamin D-resistant rickets

Behavioral risk factors
History of poor compliance
Substance use/abuse
Psychiatric/psychological issues
Lack of understanding or communication

discussion of these terms has been reviewed by others and will not be repeated here (Mombelli 1994; Esposito *et al.* 1998a). Criteria for these outcomes have not been consistently used in the literature. Success is often difficult to define since it implies that a large number of criteria have been met, such as stability, functionality, little or no change in bone support, radiographic evidence of osseointegration, absence of infection, lack of paresthesia, comfort, acceptable esthetics, and overall patient satisfaction. However, the criteria for "success" as presented by Albrektsson *et al.* (1986) over 20 years ago are still useful (Table 30-1).

Many authors simply use the outcome of implant "survival" which implies that at least some criteria for overall success have been met. An implant can, of course, survive and meet all of the criteria for success except those dealing with patient satisfaction. If the patient regards the implant as a failure, it is a failure since a major criterion for success has not been met (i.e. patient satisfaction). Since implant failure is often the end result of a gradual accumulation of unwanted events, most studies use surrogates for failure such as the development of implant mobility, abscess formation, and loss of function. Therefore in many papers, failure is defined as the appearance of failure-associated complications such as the development of peri-implantitis.

There are very few *absolute* or unequivocal contraindications to the placement of dental implants. Depending on a number of patient-centered circumstances, dental implants can be considered even in individuals who are at an elevated risk for implant failure. Like most situations in clinical practice, the potential benefits of an intervention need to be weighed against the morbidity of potential adverse outcomes.

A *risk factor* is an environmental, behavioral, or biological factor that, if present directly increases the probability of a disease (or adverse event) occurring and, if absent or removed, reduces that probability. Risk factors are part of the causal chain, or expose the host to the causal chain (Genco *et al.* 1996). In the case of risk assessment for implant failure, risk factors can be broadly categorized as local, systemic, or behavioral factors (Table 30-2). In general, risk factors for implant failure make outcomes of implant treatment less predictable. A *risk indicator* is a probable risk factor that has not been confirmed by carefully conducted longitudinal studies. A *risk predictor* is a characteristic that is associated with an elevated risk for a disease (or adverse event), but may not be part of the causal chain (Genco *et al*. 1996). In the case of dental implants, a good risk predictor might be a documented history of the failure of previously inserted implants. In the risk assessment process for multifactorial conditions, such as implant failure, it is important to remember that the presence of several risk factors is required to result in implant loss. One or two risk factors are rarely sufficient to cause implant failure.

Clinical information required for risk assessment

The process of risk assessment begins with taking thorough medical/dental histories and conducting a complete examination of the prospective candidate for dental implants. Details of these procedures are discussed in Chapters 27–29 and will not be repeated here. However, items that are required for risk assessment include anything that helps identify individuals who might be at an increased risk of implant complications and failure.

A comprehensive evaluation of the patient should contain a review of past dental history including earlier periodontal treatment, reasons for tooth loss, how extraction sockets were treated at the time of extraction, history of increased susceptibility to infection, and awareness of parafunctional habits such as clenching and grinding. It should also include an evaluation of the patient's socioeconomic status and willingness to adjust to an often long treatment process. Dissatisfaction with earlier dental treatment may indicate an increased risk for complications during implant therapy.

The comprehensive medical history should include past and present medications and any substance use or abuse. A standard medical history form filled out and signed by the patient is an efficient way to collect basic information. This should always be followed by a verbal interview to explore in more depth any potential medical risks of implant therapy. If any uncertainties remain regarding the patient's health after the interview, a written medical consultation should be obtained from the patient's physician.

Components of a complete examination

A complete intraoral examination should be performed to determine the feasibility of placing implants in desired locations. This examination includes oral hygiene status, periodontal status, jaw relationships, occlusion, signs of bruxism, temporomandibular joint conditions, endodontic lesions, status of existing restorations, presence of non-restored caries, crown–root ratio, interocclusal space, available space for implants, ridge morphology, soft and hard tissue conditions, phonetics, and prosthetic restorability.

An appropriate radiographic evaluation of the quality and quantity of available bone is required in order to determine the optimal site(s) for implant placement. Assessments from periapical radiographs, panoramic projections, and tomographic cross-sectional imaging can individually or in combination be helpful diagnostic tools. It is important to understand that accurate estimations of bone height and width cannot be made without a comprehensive clinical examination followed by cross-sectional tomographic images. A comprehensive radiographic evaluation minimizes the risk of injuring vital anatomic structures during the surgical procedure and is also helpful in determining which cases require bone augmentation surgery before implants can be placed. A custom-made stent with radiopaque markers worn by the patient during the radiographic imaging can help locate the proper position for implant placement and also help in evaluation of the relationship between the planned implant location and available bone.

An evaluation of the quality and quantity of peri-implant soft tissues at the proposed implant site will help determine how closely this tissue will mimic the appearance of gingival tissue once the implant has been inserted. The presence of keratinized mucosa around a dental implant is an important part of an esthetically successful dental implant. It is important to evaluate the patient's perception of esthetics prior to implant placement. This is especially true in situations with compromised hard and soft tissues where esthetics can be a real challenge. Diagnostic casts and intraoral photographs can be helpful in evaluating potential esthetic outcomes as well as in the overall treatment-planning process. In general, to minimize the risk of implant complications and failure, any diseases of the soft or hard oral tissues should be treated before implant therapy.

Technical procedures to help minimize risk

Minimizing post-surgical infection

Post-operative infections increase the risk of early implant failure. It is important to perform implant surgeries with a strict hygiene protocol to minimize bacterial contamination of the surgical site. Although the incidence of post-operative infection associated with implant placement is only about 1% (Powell *et al*. 2005), some clinicians attempt to reduce this risk by prescribing pre-operative systemic antibiotics (Dent *et al*. 1997; Laskin *et al*. 2000). However, the value of pre-operative antimicrobial treatment has not been established in randomized placebo-controlled clinical trials (Lawler *et al*. 2005). In addition, the results of several case–control studies indicate that there is no advantage in using antibiotics in conjunction with implant placement (Gynther *et al*. 1998; Morris *et al*. 2004; Powell *et al*. 2005).

Minimizing tissue damage

Surgical techniques that are designed to avoid unnecessary tissue damage should be used whenever possible. Thermal damage to bone can be caused during the drilling sequence if dull drills are used or if osteotomy is performed without using enough liquid coolant. It is important to follow the manufacturer's guidelines and change the drills in the surgical kit accordingly.

Achieving early stability of implant

An important goal of the osteotomy is to prepare a site for the implant that will allow good stability of the implant during the healing process (Sennerby *et al.* 1992). Post-insertion stability lowers the risk of implant complications or failure. The presence of good-quality bone with a sufficient amount of cortical bone at the implant site is desirable to achieve this objective. In situations where there are less than optimal bone conditions (i.e. thin cortex, low trabecular density), increased initial stability can still be established by using implants with rough surfaces, parallel walls, and optimal height and width. In a study of implants placed in rabbit tibias it was found that good initial stability could be achieved by bicortical placement of an implant that engages two cortical layers of bone (Ivanoff *et al.* 1996). However, the same authors found that in a 15-year retrospective study in humans, bicortically anchored implants failed nearly four times more often than the monocortical ones (Ivanoff *et al.* 2000). They speculated that the overambitious fixation of the bicortical anchorage increased the likelihood of implant fractures that accounted for 80% of the failures in the study.

Avoiding anatomic structures

Anatomic structures that are at risk of serious collateral or accidental damage during the placement of implants include: nerves, blood vessels, floor of the mouth, nasal cavity, maxillary sinuses, and adjacent teeth. The risks to these structures can be minimized by careful assessment of radiographs and meticulous treatment planning. It is important to remember that the drills used for osteotomies penetrate further than the depth indicators on the drills. In certain situations radiographic indicator methods should be performed during surgery to help determine direction of the implant and its proximity to vital structures.

For implants that are to be placed in the mandible, the distance from the edentulous alveolar crest to the upper border of the inferior alveolar canal should be assessed from cross-sectional tomographic radiographs. The safety zone between the tip of the implant and the border of the canal should be at least 1–2 mm. Patients with compromised vertical bone dimension can sometimes be treated by placing multiple shorter implants of optimal width followed by splinting the prosthetic crowns together during the restorative phase of therapy.

The position of the mental foramen should be identified and located when implant surgeries in the premolar and molar areas of the mandible are performed. In some situations a loop of the nerve can be found to extend mesially. In one report the anterior loop of the mental neurovascular bundle extended mesially from 1.1–3.3 mm and a safety zone of 4 mm was recommended to avoid damaging the nerve during implant placement (Kuzmanovic *et al.* 2003). When placing an implant in the anterior part of the maxilla the size and location of the incisive papilla need to be determined. In addition, it must be established if there is enough bone in the area to place an implant or if the area needs to be grafted.

Anatomic concavities are frequently found on the lingual side of the mandible. It is important to avoid perforating the lingual plate during preparation of the implant site since perforations in this location can result in extensive and even life-threatening bleeding (Bruggenkate *et al.* 1993). A safe way of performing surgery in this area is to reflect a lingual flap at least to a level corresponding to the length of the implant to be placed. If this precaution is taken, any perforation that might occur is detected before any extensive damage and serious bleeding occur.

Some of the challenges of treating the partially edentulous patient are related to biological and functional differences between teeth and implants. If these differences are ignored there is an increased risk for complications. For example, in cases where there are compromised hard and soft tissues a few implants may not be able to withstand heavy occlusal forces associated with extensive posterior reconstructions (Albrektsson *et al.* 1988). Differences in morphology between implants and teeth can present another challenge. In the anterior part of the mouth an implant should blend in with the neighboring natural teeth. To accomplish this, an implant with the correct diameter must be selected and then placed in the optimal position in order to mimic a tooth esthetically and functionally.

After tooth extractions in the maxillary anterior region the alveolar ridge resorbs in a palatal direction. This will affect the position in which the anterior implants need to be placed since the relation of the implants to the lip and opposing dentition is critically important for a successful outcome (Jansen & Weisgold 1995). Where to place anterior implants in patients with a high smile line and thin periodontal tissues should be carefully evaluated to achieve acceptable esthetic and functional results.

Local risk factors and conditions

Presence of ongoing oral infections

There are abundant data showing that poor oral hygiene and microbial biofilms are important etiologic factors leading to the development of peri-implant infections and implant loss (Mombelli *et al.* 1987; Jepsen *et al.* 1996; Salcetti *et al.* 1997; Esposito *et al.* 1998a,b; Lindquist *et al.* 1988; Listgarten & Lai 1999; van Winkelhoff *et al.* 2000; Heydenrijk *et al.* 2002; Quirynen & Teughels 2003; Fugazzotto *et al.* 2004). Therefore any risk assessment for implant survival should include an evaluation of the patient's ability to perform oral hygiene procedures (Salvi & Lang 2004).

Periodontitis

There are several reasons to believe that untreated or incompletely treated periodontitis increases the risk for implant failure. First, there are case reports that suggest an association (Malmstrom *et al.* 1990; Fardal *et al.* 1999). Second, a similar subgingival microbiota has been found in pockets around teeth and implants with similar probing depths (Papaioannou *et al.* 1996; Sbordone *et al.* 1999; Hultin *et al.* 2000; Agerbaek *et al.* 2006). Third, evidence exists that periodontal pockets might serve as reservoirs of pathogens (Apse *et al.* 1989; Quirynen & Listgarten 1990; Papaioannou *et al.* 1996) that hypothetically can be transmitted from teeth to implants (Quirynen *et al.* 1996; Sumida *et al.* 2002).

Studies dealing with the microbiota of failing or failed implants clearly indicate the presence of multiple periodontal pathogens (Table 30-3). However, one of the striking features of the microbiota associated with implant failures is its extensive diversity. It would be naïve to assume that infections around implants are due to a narrow range of microorganisms. A more realistic view is that peri-implant infections are caused by a consortium of multiple

Table 30-3 Components of the subgingival microbiota frequently (≥10%) detected around failed or failing implants

Elevated microbial component	Reference	Elevated microbial component	Reference
Spirochetes	Hultin *et al.* 2000	*Aggregatibacter*	Alcoforado *et al.* 1991
	Listgarten & Lai 1999	*actinomycetemcomitans*[†]	Hultin *et al.* 2000
	Mombelli *et al.* 1987		Leonhardt *et al.* 1999
	Quirynen & Listgarten 1990		Rutar *et al.* 2001
	Rosenberg *et al.* 1991		Van Winkelhoff & Wolf
Fusobacterium spp.	Alcoforado *et al.* 1991		2000
	Laine *et al.* 2005	*Tannerella forsythia*[§]	Hultin *et al.* 2000
	Listgarten & Lai 1999		Listgarten & Lai 1999
	Malmstrom *et al.* 1990	*Campylobacter rectus*	Alcoforado *et al.* 1991
	Mombelli *et al.* 1987		Listgarten & Lai 1999
	Rams *et al.* 1991		Malmstrom *et al.* 1990
	Rosenberg *et al.* 1991	*Eikenella corrodens*	Listgarten & Lai 1999
	Salcetti *et al.* 1997		Malmstrom *et al.* 1990
Micromonas micros[*]	Alcoforado *et al.* 1991	*Actinomyces* spp.	Laine *et al.* 2005
	Laine *et al.* 2005	*Streptococcus anginosus* (milleri) group	Laine *et al.* 2005
	Listgarten & Lai 1999	*Streptococcus sanguinis*	Fardal *et al.* 1999
	Rosenberg *et al.* 1991	*Streptococcus oralis*	Fardal *et al.* 1999
	Salcetti *et al.* 1997	*Capnocytophaga* spp.	Fardal *et al.* 1999
Peptostreptococcus prevotii	Rams *et al.* 1991	Enteric rods	Alcoforado *et al.* 1991
Porphyromonas gingivalis	Hultin *et al.* 2000		Leonhardt *et al.* 1999
	Leonhardt *et al.* 1999		Listgarten & Lai 1999
	Listgarten & Lai 1999		Rams *et al.* 1991
	Rutar *et al.* 2001		Rosenberg *et al.* 1991
	Van Winkelhoff *et al.* 2000	*Escherichia coli*	Leonhardt *et al.* 1999
Prevotella intermedia	Alcoforado *et al.* 1991	Enterococci	Rams *et al.* 1991
	Hultin *et al.* 2000	Yeasts (*Candida* spp.)	Alcoforado *et al.* 1991
	Laine *et al.* 2005		Laine *et al.* 2005
	Leonhardt *et al.* 1999		Leonhardt *et al.* 1999
	Listgarten & Lai 1999		Rosenberg *et al.* 1991
	Mombelli *et al.* 1987	*Klebsiella* spp.	Leonhardt *et al.* 1999
Prevotella nigrescens	Laine *et al.* 2005	Pseudomonads	Alcoforado *et al.* 1991
	Leonhardt *et al.* 1999		Rams *et al.* 1991
	Listgarten & Lai 1999	*Staphylococcus* spp.	Alcoforado *et al.* 1991
	Salcetti *et al.* 1997		Leonhardt *et al.* 1999
			Rams *et al.* 1990, 1991
			Rosenberg *et al.* 1991

[*] Formerly *Peptostreptococcus micros*.
[†] Formerly *Actinobacillus actinomycetemcomitans*.
[§] Formerly *Bacteroides forsythus* and *Tannerella forsythensis*.

microorganisms living on the implant surface in a biofilm. Contrary to the view of some (Heydenrijk *et al.* 2002), peri-implant infections are not simply caused by Gram-negative anaerobic bacteria. Certainly this group of bacteria is important, but yeasts and Gram-positive bacteria such as *Micromonas micros* and *Staphylococcus* species are often implicated in peri-implant infections (Table 30-3). Furthermore, in the implant literature the methods used to examine subgingival biofilms have primarily relied on microscopic (morphologic), cultural, and DNA probe analyses to characterize the microbiota. Culture-independent molecular analyses (e.g. studies of 16S ribosomal RNA gene sequences) have not been used to characterize the microbiota associated with implant failures. Application of such techniques to the subgingival microbiota associated with periodontitis has revealed the existence of a more diverse and complex microbial community than can be detected by conventional methods (Paster *et al.* 2001; Brinig *et al.* 2003; Lepp *et al.* 2004). In the case of periodontitis it is estimated that only about 50% of the subgingival flora can be characterized using conventional methods (Wilson *et al.* 1997) and therefore culture-independent analyses are required to get a more complete picture. This will probably also be true of the peri-implant subgingival microbiota once culture-independent molecular methods of analyses are applied to this ecosystem. Based on the documented diversity of the microbiota associated with failing implants, it is unlikely that testing for the presence of a small number of suspect bacteria for risk assessment purposes would have any clinical value.

Subgingival sites are micro-ecosystems that are preferentially colonized by oral bacteria well adapted to thriving in such environments. Indeed, subgingival sites are the natural or preferred habitat of a diverse group of oral microorganisms. In an interesting study of 15 patients, Devides and Franco (2006) sampled mucosa-associated biofilms of edentulous sites with paper points and analyzed the specimens using polymerase chain reaction (PCR) methods to detect certain periodontal pathogens. At the edentulous sites *Aggregatibacter actinomycetemcomitans* was detected in 13.3% of subjects, *Prevotella intermedia* was detected in 46.7% of subjects, and *Porphyromonas gingivalis* was not detected. Six months after placement of endosteal implants at the same sites, subgingival plaque samples taken from around the implants were positive for *A. actinomycetemcomitans* in 73.3% of subjects, *Pr. intermedia* in 53.3% of subjects, and *P. gingivalis* in 53.3% of subjects. None of the implants showed any clinical signs of either failure or peri-implantitis. These results indicate that healthy subgingival sites around implants are readily colonized by periodontal pathogens without any concomitant development of clinically detectable disease. The mere presence of PCR-detected pathogens is not a valid surrogate for peri-implant disease.

It is important to remember that the microbiota adjacent to failing implants will differ depending on the cause of the failure. For example, Rosenberg *et al.* (1991) demonstrated that the microbiota associated with implants failing because of traumatic loads was different to that found around implants failing because of infection.

There are several reports that the survival rate of implants is decreased when the patient has a history of periodontitis (Hardt *et al.* 2001; Evian *et al.* 2004; Karoussis *et al.* 2004; Wagenberg & Froum 2006). One implication of these observations is that patients who have had periodontitis might also be more susceptible to peri-implant infections. However, this is clearly not always the case since it has also been demonstrated that periodontally compromised patients who have lost a considerable amount of alveolar bone can be successfully treated with dental implants (Nevins & Langer 1995; Ellegaard *et al.* 1997; Sbordone *et al.* 1999). Since there is no clear-cut consensus in the literature on this topic, in risk-assessment discussions with patients it is a good idea to emphasize that based on their history of periodontitis they might be at an increased risk of developing peri-implantitis and therefore should be extra diligent in adhering to a rigorous post-insertion implant maintenance program.

Endodontic infections

The presence of untreated or insufficiently treated endodontic infections adjacent to the site of implant placement can adversely affect the outcome (Sussman & Moss 1993; Shaffer *et al.* 1998). There are numerous reports of retrograde peri-implantitis in which it is hypothesized that a periapical infection on a tooth spreads to an adjacent implant (Ayangco & Sheridan 2001; Chaffee *et al.* 2001; Jalbout & Tarnow 2001; Quirynen *et al.* 2005b). However, successful retention of implants has been reported when implants were inserted immediately after extraction of endodontically infected teeth (Villa & Rangert 2005).

Based on the strength of existing data discussed above, it is highly recommended that any existing periodontal or endodontic infections should be controlled before dental implants are placed. Although the presence of ongoing oral infections does not guarantee that implants will fail, such infections appear to increase the risk of failure. Finally, since it has been documented that some peri-implant infections may be associated with *Candida* spp. (Table 30-3) it is probably wise to control and treat any existing candidiasis before implants are inserted.

Systemic risk factors

Age

In adult patients, age is usually not considered an important risk factor for implant loss. Indeed, most longitudinal studies of survival rates of implants include some subjects who are well over 75 years of age (Dao *et al.* 1993; Hutton *et al.* 1995; Nevins & Langer 1995; Davarpanah *et al.* 2002; Becktor *et al.* 2004; Fugazzotto *et al.* 2004; Karoussis *et al.* 2004; Fransson *et al.* 2005; Herrmann *et al.* 2005; Quirynen *et al.* 2005a; Mundt *et al.* 2006; Wagenberg & Froum 2006). An upper age limit is usually not listed as an exclusion criterion in such studies. It is clear that implants can be quite successful when placed in patients who are in their eighth and ninth decades of life. Several reports indicate that there is not a statistically significant relationship between age of the patient and implant failure (Dao *et al.* 1993; Hutton *et al.* 1995; Bryant & Zarb 1999; Fransson *et al.* 2005; Herrmann *et al.* 2005; Mundt *et al.* 2006; Wagenberg & Froum 2006). However, a thorough risk-assessment process involves evaluation of multiple possible risk factors. It is possible that there may have been some selection bias in the above studies since some older patients might have been excluded for medical reasons. Older individuals included in the above studies may be atypical in that they were healthy enough to be good candidates for implant placement.

In one retrospective study of the success of 4680 dental implants placed by a single surgeon over a 21-year period in 1140 patients, it was reported that increasing age was strongly associated with implant failure (Moy *et al.* 2005). A univariate analysis of the data indicated that compared to patients younger than 40 years (n = 181), patients in the 60–79-years age group (n = 499) had a significantly higher risk of implant failure (relative risk = 2.24; $P < 0.05$). However, in a multivariate analysis of the data from the entire study population, age was not a significant predictor of implant failure (Moy *et al.* 2005).

At the other end of the spectrum, a potential problem associated with the placement of dental implants in still-growing children and adolescents is the possibility of interfering with growth patterns of the jaws (Op Heij *et al.* 2003). Osseointegrated implants in growing jaws behave like ankylosed teeth in that they do not erupt and the surrounding alveolar housing remains underdeveloped. Dental implants can be a superb service to young people who have lost teeth due to trauma or have congenitally missing permanent teeth. However, because of the potential deleterious effects of implants on growing jaws it is highly recommended that implants not be placed until craniofacial growth has ceased or is almost complete (Thilander *et al.* 2001).

Smoking

Based on data generated by several follow-up studies of implant survival, cigarette smoking is often identified as a statistically significant risk factor for implant failure (Bain & Moy 1993; Lindquist *et al.* 1997; Wilson & Nunn 1999; Feloutzis *et al.* 2003; Gruica *et al.* 2004;

Karoussis *et al.* 2004; Levin *et al.* 2004; Galindo-Moreno *et al.* 2005; Moy *et al.* 2005; Nitzan *et al.* 2005; Mundt *et al.* 2006). In addition, smoking has been associated with increased post-operative complications after sinus-lift operations and placement of onlay bone grafts (Levin *et al.* 2004).

Smoking is now generally accepted as an important modifiable risk factor for the development and progression of periodontitis (Johnson & Hill 2004). The reasons that smokers are more susceptible to both periodontitis and peri-implantitis are complex, but usually involve impairment of innate and adaptive immune responses (Kinane & Chestnutt 2000; Johnson & Hill 2004) and interference with wound healing (Johnson & Hill 2004; Labriola *et al.* 2005). Smoking is such a strong risk factor for implant failure that some clinicians highly recommend smoking-cessation protocols as part of the treatment plan for implant patients (Bain 1996; Johnson & Hill 2004).

Nevertheless, it should be emphasized that smoking is not an absolute contraindication for the placement of dental implants. Indeed, there are reports indicating that smoking did not adversely affect the rate of implant survival (Peleg *et al.* 2006; Wagenberg & Froum 2006). For multifactorial problems such as peri-implantitis and implant failure, the presence of one risk factor alone is usually insufficient to cause the adverse outcome.

Medication history

Bisphosphonates

Bisphosphonates are a widely prescribed class of drugs used for the treatment of osteoporosis and to reduce the bone-lytic effects of certain malignancies such as multiple myeloma and metastatic breast cancer (Woo *et al.* 2006). These pyrophosphate drugs are potent inhibitors of osteoclast activity that also have anti-angiogenic effects. The drugs have a high affinity for hydroxyapatite and are rapidly incorporated into all parts of the skeleton and have a very long half-life (i.e. decades). Relative potencies of the agents depend on their formulation (Table 30-4). An uncommon complication associated with the use of bisphosphonates is the increased risk of developing osteochemonecrosis or osteonecrosis of the jaws (ONJ) (Ruggiero *et al.* 2004; Marx *et al.* 2005; Braun & Iacono 2006). The vast majority of cases of ONJ occur in cancer patients who have received high-potency aminobisphosphonates (e.g. zoledronate, pamidronate) given intravenously to decrease the osteolytic effects of multiple myeloma or malignancies that have metastasized to bone (e.g. breast or prostate cancer).

Of major concern to the prospective implant patient who has been taking an oral bisphosphonate for osteoporosis is the possible risk of developing ONJ after implant placement. Oral bisphosphonates

Table 30-4 Relative potency for inhibition of osteoclast activity of various bisphosphonates, adapted from Braun & Iacono (2006)

Drug	Manufacturer	Potency factor
Etidronate (Didronel®)	Procter & Gamble	1
Tiludronate (Skelid®)	Sanofi	10
Clodronate (Bonefos®)	Schering	10
Clodronate (Loron®)	Roche	10
Neridronate (Nerixia®)	Abiogen	100
Pamidronate (Aredia®)	Novartis	100
Alendronate (Fosamax®)	Merck	500
Ibandronate (Bondronat®)	Roche	1 000
Risedronate (Actonel®)	Procter & Gamble	2 000
Zoledronate (Zometa®)	Novartis	10 000

have been reported to be associated with implant failure (Starck & Epker 1995) and ONJ (Ruggiero *et al*. 2004; Marx *et al*. 2005). Although rare, the risk is real. Since bisphosphonates tightly bind to hydroxyapatite and have a very long half-life, it is likely that the length of time a patient has been taking oral bisphosphonates is important in determining the level of risk. Since oral bisphosphonates slowly accumulate in bone with time, an osteoporosis patient who has been taking the drug for 1 year is at a lower risk of developing ONJ or implant failure than someone who has been on the drug for many years. In general, it is not recommended that implants be placed in patients who have been on the drug for more than 3 years. It has been suggested by some that prolonged use of bisphosphonates is a contraindication to implant placement (Scully *et al*. 2006).

It is important to remember that bone-remodeling processes are severely inhibited in patients who have been chronically taking oral bisphosphonates for osteoporosis. Because of this such patients are poor candidates for bone-grafting procedures and sinus-lift operations. Therefore, many ridge-augmentation procedures that often make implant placement possible are ill advised in these individuals.

Drug-influenced gingival enlargement

It is well known that one of the side effects of phenytoin, calcium-channel antagonists, and cyclosporin is gingival enlargement in about 25–50% of the individuals who take one or more of these drugs (Peñarrocha-Diago *et al*. 1990; Hassell & Hefti 1991). Gingival enlargement has also been reported around dental implants in individuals taking either phenytoin (Chee & Jansen 1994) or a calcium-channel antagonist (Silverstein *et al*. 1995). When there is significant gingival enlargement around teeth or implants, oral hygiene and maintenance procedures

can become quite difficult. Therefore, medications associated with gingival enlargement should be considered in the overall risk assessment prior to implant placement.

Cancer chemotherapy

Oral cancer patients are frequently candidates for the placement of endosteal dental implants since prostheses designed to replace missing portions of the jaws need to be anchored to implants. Since antimitotic drugs used as chemotherapy for cancer might affect wound healing and suppress certain components of the immune system, it is important to know if these drugs interfere with osseointegration and success of dental implants. In a retrospective study, implant success was compared in 16 oral cancer patients who had no chemotherapy with the success in 20 patients who received postsurgical adjuvant chemotherapy with either cis- or carboplatin and 5-fluorouracil (Kovács 2001). It was found that these drugs did not have any detrimental effects on the survival and success of implants placed in the mandible.

It has also been reported that some cancer patients who received cytotoxic antineoplastic drugs experienced infections around existing transmucosal or endosteal dental implants (Karr *et al*. 1992). Therefore, it is important to recognize that many anticancer drugs suppress or kill cells necessary for optimal innate and adaptive immunity. Patients who are receiving cancer chemotherapy should have thorough periodontal and implant maintenance care to minimize the development of adverse events.

Anticoagulants

Patients who have blood-coagulation disorders or are taking high doses of anticoagulants are at an elevated risk of experiencing post-operative bleeding problems after implant surgery. Some patients with coagulation disorders may be at an elevated risk of implant failure (van Steenberghe *et al*. 2003) whereas other patients who chronically take oral anticoagulants can safely receive dental implants (Weischer *et al*. 2005). Patients who are on continuous oral anticoagulant therapy (e.g. coumarin derivatives) to reduce the risk of thromboembolic events and require dental implants for optimal restorative care should be evaluated on a case-by-case basis. Most of these patients can safely continue their warfarin or other anticoagulant therapy when they have their dental implant surgery (Wahl 1998, 2000). In such patients, local bleeding after the placement of dental implants can usually be well controlled by conventional hemostatic methods. The risk of developing life-threatening bleeding or bleeding that cannot be controlled using local measures following placement of dental implants is so low that there is no need to stop oral anticoagulant therapy (Beirne 2005).

Therapeutic levels of an anticoagulant drug such as warfarin are measured by the international normalized ratio (INR) which is the patient's prothrombin time (PT) divided by the mean normal PT for the laboratory (i.e. PTR). The PTR is then adjusted for the reagents used to arrive at a standardized INR value that will be comparable anywhere in the world. A higher INR reflects a higher level of anticoagulation with an attendant increased risk of hemorrhage (Herman *et al.* 1997). Although there are insufficient data to draw any evidence-based conclusions, placement of single implants is regarded as safe when the INR target values are 2.0–2.4 (Herman *et al.* 1997).

Immunosuppressive agents

Any medication that interferes with wound healing or suppresses components of innate and adaptive immunity can theoretically increase the risk of implant failure. Corticosteroids are a good example. They are potent anti-inflammatory agents that are widely used for the management of a wide variety of ailments. These drugs can interfere with wound healing by blocking key inflammatory events needed for satisfactory repair. In addition, through their immunosuppressive effects on lymphocytes, they can increase the rate of post-operative infections. In general, these undesirable effects are greatest in patients who take high doses of the drugs for long periods of time.

Immunosuppression

In the early years of the AIDS epidemic placement of dental implants was ill advised since affected patients developed major life-threatening oral infections. With the advent of effective HAART (highly active anti-retroviral therapy) regimens, most HIV-positive patients who take their medications live for many years without developing severe opportunistic infections. There have been no controlled studies dealing with the risk of dental implant failures in HIV-positive individuals. However, several case reports suggest that placement of dental implants in HIV-positive patients is not associated with elevated failure rates (Rajnay & Hochstetter 1998; Baron *et al.* 2004; Shetty & Achong 2005; Achong *et al.* 2006). Low T-helper (CD4) cell counts (i.e. <200/μL) do not appear to predict increased susceptibility to intraoral wound infections or elevated failure rates of dental implants (Achong *et al.* 2006). Although more studies are needed, it appears that it is safe to place dental implants if the patient's HIV disease is under medical control.

History of radiation therapy to the jaws

Patients who have received radiation (i.e. absorbed dose of ≥60 Gy) to the head and neck as part of the treatment for malignancies are at an increased risk of developing osteoradionecrosis (ORN). Most cases of this complication of cancer treatment are triggered by the extraction of teeth or other oral surgery procedures such as insertion of implants. Implant failure rates of up to 40% have been reported in patients who have had a history of radiation therapy (Granström *et al.* 1993, 1999; Beumer *et al.* 1995; Esposito *et al.* 1998a,b; Lindquist *et al.* 1988). At one time it was believed that ORN was due to vascular derangement and hypoxia of bone cells caused by the tissue-damaging effects of radiation (Teng & Futran 2005). Based on this hypothesis, it has been recommended that oral surgical procedures in patients at risk of ORN be performed in conjunction with hyperbaric oxygen (HBO) therapy. Indeed, Granström *et al.* (1999) reported that use of HBO therapy improved implant survival rates. However, the value of HBO therapy for the management of ORN has been called into question partly based on a placebo-controlled, randomized clinical trial (Annane *et al.* 2004) and other reports showing no advantage to HBO interventions (Maier *et al.* 2000; Gal *et al.* 2003). In addition, a systematic review by Coulthard *et al.* (2003) indicated that there is no high-quality evidence that HBO therapy improves implant survival in irradiated patients.

It is now believed that the pathogenesis of ONR is much more complex than a simple hypoxia-related phenomenon related to poor vascularity of irradiated tissues. Current evidence supports the view that ONR is a fibroatrophic process (Teng & Futran 2005). From the perspective of risk-assessment procedures for implant placement, patients who have a history of irradiation to the jaws should be considered at high risk for implant failure and HBO interventions will probably not lower that risk.

Diabetes mellitus

Although there is a slight tendency for more failures of implants in a diabetic compared to a non-diabetic population, the increased risk is not substantial in patients who are under good metabolic control (Shernoff *et al.* 1994; Kapur *et al.* 1998; Balshi & Wolfinger 1999; Fiorellini *et al.* 2000; Morris *et al.* 2000; Olson *et al.* 2000). In the general population the 5-year overall success rate for implants is approximately 95% (Buser *et al.* 1997; Weber *et al.* 2000; Davarpanah *et al.* 2002; Fugazzotto 2005), whereas in a diabetic population the rate is approximately 86% (Fiorellini *et al.* 2000).

Diabetics under suboptimal metabolic control often experience wound-healing difficulties and have an increased susceptibility to infections due to a variety of problems associated with immune dysfunctions (Geerlings & Hoepelman 1999). In the risk evaluation of diabetics it is important to establish the level of metabolic control of the disease. A useful test to determine the level of control over the last 90 days is a blood test for glycosylated hemoglobin (HbA_{1c}). This is a test for the percentage of hemoglobin to which glucose is bound. Normal values for a non-diabetic or a diabetic under good metabolic control are HbA$_{1c}$ <6–6.5% and fasting blood glucose <6.1 mmol/L (110 mg/dL). Diabetics with HbA$_{1c}$ values of ≥8% are under poor control and have an elevated risk of encountering wound healing problems and infection if dental implants are placed.

Metabolic bone disease

Osteoporosis

Osteoporosis is a complex group of systemic skeletal conditions characterized by low bone mass and microarchitectural deterioration of bone tissue. Osteoporotic bone is fragile and has an increased susceptibility to fracture. Primary osteoporosis is a common condition and is diagnosed when other disorders known to cause osteoporosis are not present. Secondary osteoporosis is diagnosed when the condition is related to, or occurs as a consequence of, osteoporosis-inducing circumstances. These might include diet (e.g. starvation, calcium deficiency), congenital conditions (e.g. hypophosphatasia, osteogenesis imperfecta), drugs (e.g. alcohol abuse, glucocorticoids), endocrine disorders (e.g. Cushing's syndrome), and certain systemic diseases (e.g. diabetes mellitus, rheumatoid arthritis). Osteoporosis is assessed using bone densitometry in which a patient's bone mass or bone mineral density (BMD) is determined. BMD refers to grams of bone mineral per square centimeter of bone cross-section and is expressed in units of g/cm^2.

There are multiple case reports that conclude that osteoporosis alone is not a significant risk factor for implant failure (Dao *et al.* 1993; Friberg 1994; Fujimoto *et al.* 1996; Friberg *et al.* 2001). Implants placed in individuals with osteoporosis appear to successfully osseointegrate and can be retained for years. However, in cases of secondary osteoporosis there are often accompanying illnesses or conditions that increase the risk of implant failure (e.g. poorly controlled diabetes mellitus, corticosteroid medications). Therefore, in the risk-evaluation process the presence of osteoporosis should alert the clinician to the possible presence of osteoporosis-associated circumstances that are known to increase the risk of implant failure.

In the implant literature the concept of "poor bone quality" was introduced by Lekholm and Zarb (1985). This is something quite different to osteoporosis. Poor bone quality refers to the subjective appraisal of the presence and amount of compact and trabecular bone as visualized in radiographs. The radiographic appraisal of bone quality is reassessed during explorative drilling at the fixture-preparation site. The assessment system uses the following four groups:

- Type 1 = almost the entire jaw is comprised of homogenous compact bone

- Type 2 = a thick layer of compact bone surrounds a core of dense trabecular bone
- Type 3 = a thin layer of cortical bone surrounds a core of dense trabecular bone of favorable strength
- Type 4 = a thin layer of cortical bone surrounds a core of low density trabecular bone.

The system has serious reproducibility problems that limit its usefulness in the risk-assessment process. Nevertheless, there are reports indicating that jaw bone quality is significantly related to implant failure especially when there is type 4 bone (Jaffin & Berman 1991; Hutton *et al.* 1995; Herrmann *et al.* 2005).

Connective tissue and autoimmune disorders

Scleroderma

Systemic sclerososis or scleroderma is a chronic autoimmune disease that targets the skin, lungs, heart, gastrointestinal tract, kidneys, and musculoskeletal system. The disease is characterized by widespread tissue fibrosis, endothelial dysfunction of small blood vessels, and formation of auto-antibodies against a number of tissue components. The skin loses much of its flexibility and becomes leatherlike. Patients often experience stiffening of the finger joints making it almost impossible to grasp items such as a toothbrush and other oral hygiene devices. The lips become so stiff and taut that opening the mouth is restricted to only a few centimeters. As a result of these access problems, all types of dental care (i.e. self-administered and professionally delivered) become extraordinarily difficult. The overall effect is long-standing poor oral hygiene leading to the inevitable loss of multiple teeth due to caries and periodontal disease.

There are no well controlled studies on the success rates of dental implants in patients with scleroderma. However, there are some case reports showing that patients with this disease can have implants successfully placed and maintained for several years (Jensen & Sindet-Pedersen 1990; Patel *et al.* 1998; Hodgson *et al.* 2006). If the decision is made to place dental implants in patients with scleroderma, it is critical that a rigorous maintenance program be incorporated into the treatment plan.

Systemic lupus erythematosus

Systemic lupus erythematosus (SLE) is an autoimmune disease that affects many organ systems, with the joints, kidneys, heart, and lungs being the most commonly affected. It is well established that SLE patients have increased susceptibility to many opportunistic infections (Zandman-Goddard & Shoenfeld 2003; Bosch *et al.* 2006). The reasons for this increased susceptibility are not well understood but SLE-associated abnormalities of both humoral and cellular immunological responses and use of immunosuppressive therapy (e.g. corticosteroids) are undoubtedly important. If implants are absolutely required for a patient with SLE, it should be emphasized that bacteremias from oral surgery procedures increase the risk of developing infections of SLE-affected joints. In such cases it is recommended that antibiotic coverage be considered to minimize this potential problem (Fitzgerald *et al*. 2003). There are no well controlled studies, or even a well documented case series, of the success rates of implants placed in patients with SLE.

Xerostomia

Xerostomia or dry mouth can be caused by a wide range of factors, including certain medications, aging, and damage to salivary glands (Beikler & Flemmig 2003). Sjögren syndrome (SS) is a group of autoimmune diseases that may be limited to lacrimal and salivary glands leading to xerostomia and keratoconjunctivitis (primary SS). In secondary SS the xerostomia and keratoconjunctivitis occur along with a number of connective tissue disorders such as rheumatoid arthritis and scleroderma. One of the main oral problems associated with SS is severe xerostomia that often leads to severe dental caries, burning sensations of the oral mucosa, oral candidiasis, and difficulty in swallowing. In many cases all of the teeth are lost because of rampant root and coronal caries. Patients with severe xerostomia find wearing artificial dentures to be a difficult and very unpleasant experience because of the lack of lubrication ordinarily supplied by saliva. Based on a few case reports it appears that dental implants can be successfully used in patients with SS (Payne *et al*. 1997; Isidor *et al*. 1999; Binon 2005). However, since SS often accompanies other conditions that increase the risk of implant failure (e.g. scleroderma, lupus erythematosus), it is important that implant candidates with SS be carefully evaluated for numerous other risk factors that might be present.

Hematologic and lymphoreticular disorders

A number of hematologic and lymphoreticular disorders carry with them an increased susceptibility to periodontitis and other infections (Kinane 1999). Among these disorders are: agranulocytosis, acquired neutropenias, cyclic neutropenias, leukocyte adherence deficiency, and aplastic anemia (e.g. Fanconi's syndrome). Since patients with these diseases frequently lose teeth early in life they often have extensive prosthetic needs that can be met by the placement of dental implants. In the risk-assessment process prior to implant placement the major concern to be considered is the increased susceptibility to infec-

tions that could occur around any implants that might be placed. There are no well controlled studies of the success rates of implants placed in patients with these disorders. However, implants can be placed if the patient's disease is under control or in remission and a rigorous post-insertion implant maintenance program is an integral part of the overall treatment plan.

Genetic traits and disorders

Polymorphisms (IL-1 and MMP)

Polymorphisms are small variations in base-pair components of DNA that occur with a frequency of approximately 1–2% in the general population (Kornman & Newman 2000). These small variations in genes are biologically normal and do not cause disease. However, gene polymorphisms can affect in subtle ways how different people respond to environmental challenges. Within the context of risk assessment for implant failure, they affect how people respond to a microbial challenge and how efficiently their wounds heal.

Polymorphisms in the interleukin-1 (IL-1) gene cluster on chromosome 2q 13 have been associated with a hyper-responsive inflammatory reaction to a microbial challenge. A specific composite genotype of *IL-1A* and *IL-1B* polymorphisms, consisting of allele 2 of both IL-1A −889 (or the concordant +4845) and *IL-1B* +3954 has been associated with an increased risk of severe chronic periodontitis in non-smokers (Kornman *et al*. 1997). Several investigators have attempted to determine if this composite IL-1 genotype can serve as a risk factor for complications associated with implants such as bone loss or their eventual failure (Wilson & Nunn 1999; Rogers *et al*. 2002; Feloutzis *et al*. 2003; Gruica *et al*. 2004; Jansson *et al*. 2005). All of these reports found that being positive for the composite IL-1 genotype was not associated with an increased risk of bone loss or other implant-related problems. However, in some populations there appears to be a synergistic effect between a positive IL-1 genotype and smoking that puts dental implants at a higher risk of developing peri-implant bone loss (Feloutzis *et al*. 2003; Gruica *et al*. 2004).

Matrix metalloproteinases (MMPs) are a family of at least 15 zinc-dependent endopeptidases that function extracellularly. They are important in both normal and pathologic remodeling of tissues and differ in some of their substrate specificities. For example, MMP-1 is an interstitial collagenase capable of cleaving collagen types I, II, III, VII, and X. While another enzyme called MMP-9 or gelatinase B cleaves collagen types IV, V, VII, and XIV. In a pilot study of 46 patients it was found that a polymorphism in the promoter region of the *MMP-1* gene was associated with early implant failure, whereas a polymorphism in the promoter region of the *MMP-9* gene had no relationship with implant loss (Santos *et al.* 2004). Further studies in this general area are warranted since a validated genetic risk factor for implant failure would have immense clinical utility.

Genetic disorders

A number of genetic disorders such as those associated with chromosomal defects (e.g. Down syndrome) or those transmitted as Mendelian traits (e.g. Papillon-Lefèvre syndrome) often lead to tooth loss due to increased susceptibility to infections. An important question in the restorative care of these individuals is, will the increased susceptibility to periodontal infections also increase the risk of implant failure? In the risk-evaluation process it is probably best to assume that the answer to this question is "yes". However, with good post-operative and effective long-term maintenance care, implants can be successfully placed and retained in high-risk patients. For example, Papillon-Lefèvre syndrome is due to loss-of-function mutations in the cathepsin C gene that impairs innate immune responses (Toomes *et al.* 1999). Even in patients with this genetic disorder dental implants can be successful (Ullbro *et al.* 2000).

Importance of behavioral considerations in risk assessment

In the examination and evaluation of a candidate for dental implants, one of the most difficult tasks is to analyze the behavioral aspects of risk assessment. This area has not been well studied and falls within the realm of the art, rather than the science, of clinical practice. Important behavioral issues that need to be assessed include compliance history, substance use/abuse habits, psychiatric/psychological issues, practitioner–patient communications, and expectations of the patient.

Dental history of compliance behaviors

Long-term success of dental implants requires that the patient is able and willing to comply with the recommended post-insertion maintenance procedures required for long-term survival and success of implants. Since poor oral hygiene is a documented risk factor associated with failure of implants, it is critically important that patients understand this and are taught the skills necessary to perform plaque removal on a daily basis (Mombelli *et al.* 1987; Lindquist *et al.* 1988; Jepsen *et al.* 1996; Salcetti *et al.* 1997; Esposito *et al.* 1998a,b; Listgarten & Lai 1999; van Winkelhoff *et al.* 2000; Heydenrijk *et al.* 2002; Fugazzotto *et al.* 2004; Quirynen & Teughels 2003).

The teaching of oral hygiene is not a trivial task and often requires a considerable investment of time over multiple visits. In addition, since patient-performed oral hygiene does not adequately remove or disrupt dental plaque biofilms at subgingival locations, periodic maintenance visits are needed so the oral healthcare provider can deliver this care. It is recommended that these visits be at 3-month intervals until it can be established that a less intense schedule is sufficient. The patient's compliance with the recommended maintenance schedule is a major key to long-term success.

Substance use/abuse

Cigarette smoking as a risk factor for peri-implantitis and implant loss has been discussed earlier in this chapter. Smoking is a well documented risk factor that has both local and systemic effects on implant success. In addition, smoking is a powerful addiction with many complex behavioral components. In the consultation visit with the patient it is important that the clinician explain that smoking can contribute to complications after implant insertion. Referral to experts who conduct smoking-cessation programs is often helpful.

Patients who have addictions to alcohol and drugs are usually poor candidates for dental implants. Since the success of implant therapy requires a considerable amount of patient cooperation at all stages of care, individuals with substance-abuse problems should receive prosthetic care that does not depend on implants.

Psychiatric/psychological issues

In general, patients who have severe mental health problems or exhibit psychotic behavior are not good candidates for dental implants. As in the case of individuals with substance-abuse problems, the cooperation needed for successful implant therapy is missing. However, people with medically controlled mental health problems, such as depression, can be successfully treated with implants. In cases where there is uncertainty regarding how well the problem is under medical control, a consultation with the patient's physician is advisable.

Lack of understanding or communication

Most practitioners explain to their patients what the proposed dental care involves. However, in many cases patients do not understand what has been explained to them. It is important that the practitioner determine if the information they tried to convey was understood. One of the best ways to do this is to convey the information in easily understood (non-technical) language and in small increments. A common mistake is to rapidly present too much information. It is highly recommended that the patient be encouraged to give some feedback showing that they actually understand what they have been told. Patients who understand what is being done are usually quite cooperative and this cooperation leads to the increased probability of successful therapeutic outcomes.

Patient's expectations

It is important to remember that the practitioner's and patient's perspectives may be somewhat different regarding the primary criteria used to measure implant success. From the patient's point of view the successful implant should be esthetically acceptable, comfortable, low-cost, and functional. Practitioners usually discuss implant success in terms of extent of osseointegration, level of alveolar bone, probing depths, and stability. Although the two sets of criteria are not in conflict, they emphasize different things. During the consultation visit, before any care is delivered, the practitioner should discuss, using patient-centered outcomes, what can be expected from placement of the implant.

A final comprehensive treatment plan should be presented to the patient that includes all recommended dental therapy and alternative treatment options. The patient should also be informed about the sequencing of the clinical procedures, risks and costs involved, and the anticipated total treatment time. This discussion between practitioner and patient is critically important in lowering the overall risk of treatment problems. Patients who understand what will be done, and why, are more likely to cooperate with the recommended treatment.

Interest and commitment to post-treatment care and maintenance program

As discussed above, daily self-care (oral hygiene) and adherence to a maintenance-recall schedule is absolutely required for long-term success. This is best discussed and conveyed to the patient at the consultation visit. Long-term success of both periodontal and implant therapy depends on an effective partnership between the patient and practitioner. Many patients play a passive role when it comes to oral care. They place themselves in the hands of the therapist and expect most of the care to be done for them. An effective way to reduce the risk of implant complications and failure is to stress the importance of the patient's role as an active participant in the overall therapeutic program.

Summary and conclusions

A key part of implant therapy is the risk-assessment process in which an attempt is made to identify variables that increase the risk of complications leading to implant failure. In many cases, early identification of these variables makes it possible to avoid or eliminate them, thereby increasing the chances of long-term implant survival. Risk factors for implant failure are environmental, biologic, or behavioral factors that are part of the causal chain leading to implant complications. For multifactorial problems, such as peri-implantitis and implant failure, the presence of one risk factor alone is usually insufficient to cause the adverse outcome. It is the combination of multiple risk factors that has clinical importance.

To minimize the risk of implant complications clinicians can use a number of technical procedures, such as adhering to a strict hygienic surgical protocol, performing the osteotomies with sharp drills, achieving early implant stability, and avoiding damage to vital anatomic structures during surgery. Since ongoing oral infections can lead to implant complications it is highly recommended that any endodontic, periodontal, and other oral infections be treated prior to implant placement. Conventional microbiologic methods have revealed that a large number of microorganisms are associated with peri-implant infections. Because of this microbial diversity, it is unlikely that testing for the presence of a small number of suspect bacteria for risk-assessment purposes will have any clinical value. Existing evidence does not support the routine use of pre-operative systemic antibiotics in implant therapy.

Most of the systemic risk factors for implant complications are those that increase the patient's susceptibility to infections or those that interfere with wound healing. Particularly important risk factors that suppress or alter neutrophil function are cigarette smoking, poor metabolic control of diabetes mellitus, and certain hematologic disorders. Factors that can significantly suppress adaptive immune functions are chronic use of corticosteroid medications and the presence of systemic lupus erythematosus. Important risk factors that can interfere with healing around implants are long-term use of bisphosphonates, history of radiation therapy to the jaws, and poor metabolic control of diabetes mellitus.

An effective risk-assessment process includes thorough medical and dental histories, a complete clinical examination, and an appropriate radiographic survey. Important behavioral issues that need to be assessed include compliance history, substance use/abuse habits, psychiatric/psychologic issues, effectiveness of practitioner–patient communication, and expectations of the patient. Depending on a number of circumstances, dental implants can be considered even in individuals who are at an elevated risk for implant complications. Risk assessment of the implant patient is a critically important preamble to treatment planning and if properly done can minimize the complications associated with endosseous implants.

References

Achong, R.M, Shetty, K., Arribas, A., & Block, M.S. (2006). Implants in HIV-positive patients: 3 case reports. *Journal of Oral & Maxillofacial Surgery* **64**, 1199–1203.

Agerbaek, M.R., Lang, N.P. & Persson, G.R. (2006). Comparisons of bacterial patterns present at implant and tooth sites in subjects on supportive periodontal therapy. I. Impact of clinical variables, gender and smoking. *Clinical Oral Implants Research* **17**, 18–24.

Albrektsson, T., Zarb, G., Worthington, P. & Eriksson, A.R. (1986). The long-term efficacy of currently used dental implants: A review and proposed criteria for success. *International Journal of Oral & Maxillofacial Implants* **1**, 11–25.

Albrektsson, T., Dahl, E., Enbom, L., Engevall, S., Enquist, B., Eriksson, A.R., Feldmann, G., Freiberg, N., Glantz, P.-O., Kjellman, O., Kristersson, L., Kvint, S., Köndell, P.-Å., Palmquist, J., Werndahl, L. & Åstrand, P. (1988). Osseointegrated oral implants. A Swedish multicenter study of 8139 consecutively inserted Nobelpharma implants. *Journal of Periodontology* **59**, 287–296.

Alcoforado, G.A., Rams, T.E., Feik, D. & Slots, J. (1991). Microbial aspects of failing osseointegrated dental implants in humans. *Journal de Parodontologie* **10**, 11–18.

Annane, D., Depondt, J., Aubert, P., Villart, M., Géhanno, P., Gajdos, P. & Chevret, S. (2004). Hyperbaric oxygen therapy for radionecrosis of the jaw: A randomized, placebo-controlled, double-blind trial from the ORN96 study group. *Journal of Clinical Oncology* **22**, 4893–4900.

Apse, P., Ellen, R.P., Overall, C.M. & Zarb, G.A. (1989). Microbiota and crevicular fluid collagenase activity in the osseointegrated dental implant sulcus: A comparison of sites in edentulous and partially edentulous patients. *Journal of Periodontal Research* **24**, 96–105.

Ayangco, L. & Sheridan, P.J. (2001). Development and treatment of retrograde peri-implantitis involving a site with a history of failed endodontic and apicoectomy procedures: A series of reports. *International Journal of Oral & Maxillofacial Implants* **16**, 412–417.

Bain, C.A. & Moy, P.K. (1993). The association between the failure of dental implants and cigarette smoking. *International Journal of Oral & Maxillofacial Implants* **8**, 609–615.

Bain, C.A. (1996). Smoking and implant failure – Benefits of a smoking cessation protocol. *International Journal of Oral & Maxillofacial Implants* **11**, 756–759.

Balshi, T.J. & Wolfinger, G.J. (1999). Dental implants in the diabetic patient: a retrospective study. *Implant Dentistry* **8**, 355–359.

Baron, M., Gritsch, F, Hansy, A.-M. & Haas, R. (2004). Implants in an HIV-positive patient: A case report. *International Journal of Oral & Maxillofacial Implants* **19**, 425–430.

Becktor, J.P., Isaksson, S. & Sennerby, L. (2004). Survival analysis of endosseous implants in grafted and nongrafted edentulous maxillae. *International Journal of Oral & Maxillofacial Implants* **19**, 107–115.

Beikler, T. & Flemmig, T.F. (2003). Implants in the medically compromised patient. *Critical Reviews in Oral Biology & Medicine* **14**, 305–316.

Beirne, O.R. (2005). Evidence to continue oral anticoagulant therapy for ambulatory oral surgery. *Journal of Oral & Maxillofacial Surgery* **63**, 540–545.

Berglundh, T., Persson, L. & Klinge, B. (2002). A systematic review of the incidence of biological and technical complications in implant dentistry reported in prospective longitudinal studies of at least 5 years. *Journal of Clinical Periodontology* **29** (Suppl 3), 197–212.

Beumer, J., Roumanas, E. & Nishimura, R. (1995). Advances in osseointegrated implants for dental and facial rehabilitation following major head and neck surgery. *Seminars in Surgical Oncology* **11**, 200–207.

Binon, P.P. (2005). Thirteen-year follow-up of a mandibular implant-supported fixed complete denture in a patient with Sjogren's syndrome: A clinical report. *Journal of Prosthetic Dentistry* **94**, 409–413.

Bosch, X., Guilabert, A., Pallarés, L., Cervera, R., Ramos-Casals, M., Bové, A. Ingelmo, M. & Font, J. (2006). Infections in systemic lupus erythematosus: a prospective and controlled study of 110 patients. *Lupus* **15**, 584–589.

Braun, E. & Iacono, V.J. (2006). Bisphosphonates: case report of nonsurgical periodontal therapy and osteochemonecrosis. *International Journal of Periodontics & Restorative Dentistry* **26**, 315–319.

Brinig, M.M., Lepp, P.W., Ouverney, C.C., Armitage, G.C. & Relman, D.A. (2003). Prevalence and disease association of bacteria of division TM7 in human subgingival plaque. *Applied & Environmental Microbiology* **69**, 1687–1694.

Bruggenkate, C.M., Krekeler, G., Kraaijenhagen, H.A., Foitzik, C., Nat, P. & Oosterbeek, H.S. (1993). Hemorrhage of the floor of the mouth resulting from lingual perforation during implant placement: a clinical report. *International Journal of Oral & Maxillofacial Implants* **8**, 329–334.

Bryant, S.R. & Zarb, G.A. (1998). Osseointegration of oral implants in older and younger adults. *International Journal of Oral & Maxillofacial Implants* **13**, 492–499.

Buser, D., Mericske-Stern, R., Bernard, J.P., Behneke, A., Behneke, N., Hirt, H.P., Belser, U.C. & Lang, N.P. (1997). Long-term evaluation of non-submerged ITI implants. Part 1: 8-year life table analysis of a prospective multi-center study with 2359 implants. *Clinical Oral Implants Research* **8**, 161–172.

Chaffee, N.R., Lowden, K., Tiffee, J.C. & Cooper, L.F. (2001). Periapical abscess formation and resolution adjacent to dental implants: A clinical report. *Journal of Prosthetic Dentistry* **85**, 109–112.

Chee, W.W.L. & Jansen, C.E. (1994). Phenytoin hyperplasia occurring in relation to titanium implants: A clinical report. *International Journal of Oral & Maxillofacial Implants* **9**, 107–109.

Coulthard, P., Esposito, M., Worthington, H.V. & Jokstad, A. (2003). Therapeutic use of hyperbaric oxygen for irradiated dental implant patients: A systematic review. *Journal of Dental Education* **67**, 64–68.

Dao, T.T.T., Anderson, J.D. & Zarb, G.A. (1993). Is osteoporosis a risk factor for osseointegration of dental implants? *International Journal of Oral & Maxillofacial Implants* **8**, 137–144.

Davarpanah, M., Martinez, H., Etienne, D., Zabalegui, I., Mattout, P. Chiche, F. & Michel, J.-F. (2002). A prospective multicenter evaluation of 1,583 3i implants: 1- to 5-year data. *International Journal of Oral & Maxillofacial Implants* **17**, 820–828.

Dent, C.D., Olson, J.W., Farish, S.E., Bellome, J., Casino, A.J., Morris, H.F. & Ochi, S. (1997). The influence of preoperative antibiotics on success of endosseous implants up to and including stage II surgery: a study of 2,641 implants. *Journal of Oral & Maxillofacial Surgery* **55** (Suppl 5), 19–24.

Devides, S.L. & Franco, A.T.M. (2006). Evaluation of peri-implant microbiota using polymerase chain reaction in completely edentulous patients before and after placement of implant-supported prostheses submitted to immediate load. *International Journal of Oral & Maxillofacial Implants* **21**, 262–269.

Ellegaard, B., Baelum, V. & Karring, T. (1997). Implant therapy in periodontally compromised patients. *Clinical Oral Implants Research* **8**, 180–188.

Esposito, M., Hirsch, J.-M., Lekholm, U. & Thomsen, P. (1998a). Biological factors contributing to failures of osseointegrated oral implants. I. Success criteria and epidemiology. *European Journal of Oral Sciences* **106**, 527–551.

Esposito, M., Hirsch, J.-M., Lekholm, U. & Thomsen, P. (1998b). Biological factors contributing to failures of osseointegrated oral implants. II. Etiopathogenesis. *European Journal of Oral Sciences* **106**, 721–764.

Evian, C.I., Emling, R., Rosenberg, E.S., Waasdorp, J.A., Halpern, W., Shah, S. & Garcia, M. (2004). Retrospective analysis of implant survival and the influence of periodontal disease and immediate placement on long-term results. *International Journal of Oral & Maxillofacial Implants* **19**, 393–398.

Fardal, Ø., Johannessen, A.C. & Olsen, I. (1999). Severe, rapidly progressing peri-implantitis. *Journal of Clinical Periodontology* **26**, 313–317.

Feloutzis, A., Lang, N.P., Tonetti, M.S., Bürgin, W., Brägger, U., Buser, D., Duff, G.W. & Kornman, K.S. (2003). IL-1 gene polymorphism and smoking as risk factors for peri-implant bone loss in a well-maintained population. *Clinical Oral Implants Research* **14**, 10–17.

Fiorellini, J.P., Chen, P.K., Nevins, M. & Nevins, M.L. (2000). A retrospective study of dental implants in diabetic patients. *International Journal of Periodontics & Restorative Dentistry* **20**, 367–373.

Fitzgerald, R.E. Jr., Jacobsen, J.J., Luck, J.V. Jr., Nelson, C.L., Nelson, J.P., Osman, D.R. & Pallasch, T.J. (2003). Antibiotic prophylaxis for dental patients with total joint replacements. *Journal of the American Dental Association* **134**, 895–899.

Fransson, C., Lekholm, U., Jemt, T. & Berglundh, T. (2005). Prevalence of subjects with progressive bone loss at implants. *Clinical Oral Implants Research* **16**, 440–446.

Friberg, B. (1994). Treatment with dental implants in patients with severe osteoporosis: a case report. *International Journal of Periodontics & Restorative Dentistry* **14**, 349–353.

Friberg, B., Ekestubbe, A., Mellström, D. & Sennerby, L. (2001). Brånemark implants and osteoporosis: a clinical exploratory study. *Clinical Implant Dentistry & Related Research* **3**, 50–56.

Fugazzotto, P.A., Vlassis, J. & Butler, B. (2004). ITI implant use in private practice: Clinical results with 5,526 implants followed up to 72+ months in function. *International Journal of Oral & Maxillofacial Implants* **19**, 408–412.

Fugazzotto, P.A. (2005). Success and failure rates of osseointegrated implants in function in regenerated bone for 72 to 133 months. *International Journal of Oral & Maxillofacial Implants* **20**, 77–83.

Fujimoto, T., Niimi, A., Nakai, H. & Ueda, M. (1996). Osseointegrated implants in a patient with osteoporosis: A case report. *International Journal of Oral & Maxillofacial Implants* **11**, 539–542.

Gal, T.J., Yueh, B. & Futran, N.D. (2003). Influence of prior hyperbaric oxygen therapy in complications following microvascular reconstruction for advanced osteoradionecrosis. *Archives of Otolaryngology – Head & Neck Surgery* **129**, 72–76.

Galindo-Moreno, P., Fauri, M., Ávila-Ortiz, G., Fernández-Barbero, J.E., Cabrera-León, A. & Sánchez-Fernández, E. (2005). Influence of alcohol and tobacco habits on peri-implant marginal bone loss: a prospective study. *Clinical Oral Implants Research* **16**, 579–586.

Genco, R.J., Jeffcoat, M., Caton, J., Papapanou, P., Armitage, G., Grossi, S., Johnson, N., Lamster, I., Lang, N., Robertson, P. & Sanz, M. (1996). Consensus report. Periodontal diseases: Epidemiology and diagnosis. *Annals of Periodontology* **1**, 216–222.

Geerlings, S.E. & Hoepelman, A.I.M. (1999). Immune dysfunction in patients with diabetes mellitus (DM). *FEMS Immunology & Medical Microbiology* **26**, 259–265.

Granström, G., Tjellström, A., Brånemark, P.-I. & Fornander, J. (1993). Bone-anchored reconstruction of the irradiated head and neck cancer patient. *Otolaryngology – Head & Neck Surgery* **108**, 334–343.

Granström, G., Tjellström, A. & Brånemark, P.-I. (1999). Osseointegrated implants in irradiated bone: A case-controlled study using adjunctive hyperbaric oxygen therapy. *Journal of Oral & Maxillofacial Surgery* **57**, 493–499.

Gruica, B., Wang, H.-Y., Lang, N.P. & Buser, D. (2004). Impact of IL-1 genotype and smoking status on the prognosis of osseointegrated implants. *Clinical Oral Implants Research* **15**, 393–400.

Gynther, G.W., Köndell, P.Å., Moberg, L.-E. & Heimdahl, A. (1998). Dental implant installation without antibiotic prophylaxis. *Oral Surgery Oral Medicine Oral Pathology Oral Radiology & Endodontics* **85**, 509–511.

Hardt, C.R.E., Gröndahl, K., Lekholm, U. & Wennström, J.L. (2002). Outcome of implant therapy in relation to experienced loss of periodontal bone support. A retrospective 5-year study. *Clinical Oral Implants Research* **13**, 488–494.

Hassell, T.M. & Hefti, A.F. (1991). Drug-induced gingival overgrowth: Old problem, new problem. *Critical Reviews in Oral Biology & Medicine* **2**, 103–137.

Herman, W.W., Konzelman, J.L. Jr. & Sutley, S.H. (1997). Current perspectives on dental patients receiving coumarin anticoagulant therapy. *Journal of the American Dental Association* **128**, 327–335.

Herrmann, I., Lekholm, U., Holm, S. & Kultje, C. (2005). Evaluation of patient and implant characteristics as potential prognostic factors for oral implant failures. *International Journal of Oral & Maxillofacial Implants* **20**, 220–230.

Heydenrijk, K., Meijer, H.J.A., van der Reijden, W.A., Raghoebar, G.M., Vissink, A. & Stegenga, B. (2002). Microbiota around root-form endosseous implants: A review of the literature. *International Journal of Oral & Maxillofacial Implants* **17**, 829–838.

Hodgson, T.A., Lewis, N., Darbar, U., Welfare, R.D., Boulter, A. & Porter, S.R. (2006). The short-term efficacy of osseointegrated implants in patients with non-malignant oral mucosal disease: a case series. *Oral Diseases* **12** (s1), 11.

Hultin, M., Gustafsson, A. & Klinge, B. (2000). Long-term evaluation of osseointegrated dental implants in the treatment of partly edentulous patients. *Journal of Clinical Periodontology* **27**, 128–133.

Hutton, J.F., Heath, M.R., Chai, J.Y., Harnett, J., Jemt, T., Johns, R.B., McKenna, S., McNamara, D.C., van Steenberghe, D., Taylor, R., Watson, R.M. & Herrmann, I. (1995). Factors related to success and failure rates at 3-year follow-up in a multicenter study of overdentures supported by Brånemark implants. *International Journal of Oral & Maxillofacial Implants* **10**, 33–42.

Isidor, F., Brøndum, K., Hansen, H.J., Jensen, J. & Sindet-Pedersen, S. (1999). Outcome of treatment with implant-retained dental prostheses in patients with Sjögren syndrome. *International Journal of Oral & Maxillofacial Implants* **14**, 736–743.

Ivanoff, C.-J., Sennerby, L. & Lekholm, U. (1996). Influence of mono- and bicortical anchorage on the integration of titanium implants. A study in the rabbit tibia. *International Journal of Oral and Maxillofacial Surgery* **25**, 229–235.

Ivanoff, C.-J., Gröndahl, K., Bergström, C., Lekhom, U. & Brånemark, P.-I. (2000). Influence of bicortical or monocortical anchorage on maxillary implant stability: A 15-year retrospective study of Brånemark system implants. *International Journal of Oral & Maxillofacial Implants* 15, 103–110.

Jaffin, R.A. & Berman, C.L. (1991). The excessive loss of Branemark fixtures in type IV bone: A 5-year analysis. *Journal of Periodontology* **62**, 2–4.

Jalbout, Z.N. & Tarnow, D.P. (2001). The implant periapical lesion: Four case reports and review of the literature. *Practical Procedures & Aesthetic Dentistry* **13**, 107–112.

Jansen, C.E. & Weisgold, A. (1995). Presurgical planning for the anterior single-tooth implant restoration. *Compendium of Continuing Education in Dentistry* **8**, 746, 748–752, 754.

Jansson, H., Hamberg, K., De Bruyn, H. & Bratthall, G. (2005). Clinical consequences of IL-1 genotype on early implant failures in patients undergoing periodontal maintenance care. *Clinical Implant Dentistry & Related Research* **7**, 51–59.

Jensen, J. & Sindet-Pedersen, S. (1990). Osseointegrated implants for prosthetic reconstruction in a patient with scleroderma: report of a case. *Journal of Oral & Maxillofacial Surgery* **48**, 739–741.

Jepsen, S., Rühling, A., Jepsen, K., Ohlenbusch, B. & Albers, H.-K. (1996). Progressive peri-implantitis. Incidence and prediction of peri-implant attachment loss. *Clinical Oral Implants Research* **7**, 133–142.

Johnson, G.K. & Hill, M. (2004). Cigarette smoking and the periodontal patient. *Journal of Periodontology* **75**, 196–209.

Kapur, K.K., Garrett, N.R., Hamada, M.O., Roumanas, E.D., Freymiller, E., Han, T., Diener, R.M., Levin, S. & Ida, R. (1998). A randomized clinical trial comparing the efficacy of mandibular implant-supported overdentures and conventional dentures in diabetic patients. Part I: Methodology and clinical outcomes. *Journal of Prosthetic Dentistry* **79**, 555–569.

Karoussis, J.K., Müller, S., Salvi, G.E., Heitz-Mayfield, L.J.A., Brägger, U. & Lang, N.P. (2004). Association between peri-odontal and peri-implant conditions: a 10-year prospective study. *Clinical Oral Implants Research* **15**, 1–7.

Karr, R.A., Kramer, D.C. & Toth, B.B. (1992). Dental implants and chemotherapy complications. *Journal of Prosthetic Dentistry* **67**, 683–687.

Kinane, D. (1999). Blood and lymphoreticular disorders. *Periodontology 2000* **21**, 84–93.

Kinane, D.F. & Chestnutt, I.G. (2000). Smoking and periodontal disease. *Critical Reviews in Oral Biology & Medicine* **11**, 356–365.

Kornman, K.S., Crane, A., Wang, H.-Y., di Giovine, F.S., Newman, M.G., Pirk, F.W., Wilson, T.G. Jr., Higginbottom, F.L. & Duff, G.W. (1997). The interleukin-1 genotype as a severity factor in adult periodontal disease. *Journal of Clinical Periodontology* **24**, 72–77.

Kornman, K.S. & Newman, M.G. (2000). Role of genetics in assessment, risk, and management of adult periodontitis. In: Rose, L.F., Genco, R.J., Mealey, B.L., Cohen, D.W., eds. *Periodontal Medicine*. Hamilton: B.C. Decker, pp. 45–62.

Kovács, A.F. (2001). Influence of chemotherapy on endosteal implant survival and success in oral cancer patients. *International Journal of Oral & Maxillofacial Surgery* **30**, 144–147.

Kuzmanovic, D.V., Payne, A.G.T., Kieser, J.A. & Dias, G.J. (2003). Anterior loop of the mental nerve: a morphological and radiographic study. *Clinical Oral Implants Research* **14**, 464–471.

Labriola, A., Needleman, I. & Moles, D.R. (2005). Systematic review of the effect of smoking on nonsurgical periodontal therapy. *Periodontology 2000* **37**, 124–137.

Laine, P., Salo, A., Kontio, R., Ylijoki, S., Lindqvist, C. & Suuronen, R. (2005). Failed dental implants – clinical, radio-logical and bacteriological findings in 17 patients. *Journal of Cranio-Maxillofacial Surgery* **33**, 212–217.

Laskin, D.M., Dent, C.D., Morris, H.F., Ochi, S. & Olson, J.W. (2000). The influence of preoperative antibiotics on success of endosseous implants at 36 months. *Annals of Periodontology* **5**, 166–174.

Lawler, B., Sambrook, P.J. & Goss, A.N. (2005). Antibiotic pro-phylaxis for dentoalveolar surgery: is it indicated? *Australian Dental Journal* **50** (Suppl 2), S54-S59.

Lekholm, U. & Zarb, G.A. (1985). Patient selection and prepara-tion. In: Brånemark, P.-I., Zarb, G.A., Albrektsson, T., eds. *Tissue-Integrated Prostheses. Osseointegration in Clinical Dentistry*. Chicago: Quintessence Publishing, pp. 199–209.

Leonhardt, Å., Renvert, S. & Dahlén, G. (1999). Microbial find-ings at failing implants. *Clinical Oral Implants Research* **10**, 3339–345.

Lepp, P.W., Brinig, M.M., Ouverney, C.C., Palm, K., Armitage, G.C. & Relman, D.A. (2004). Methanogenic *Archaea* and human periodontal disease. *Proceedings of the National Academy of Sciences, USA* **101**, 6176–6181.

Levin, L., Herzberg, R., Dolev, E. & Schwartz-Arad, D. (2004). Smoking and complications of onlay bone grafts and sinus lift operations. *International Journal of Oral & Maxillofacial Implants* **19**, 369–373.

Lindh, T., Gunne, J. & Molin, M. (1998). A meta-analysis of implants in partial edentulism. *Clinical Oral Implants Research* **9**, 80–90.

Lindquist, L.W., Rockler, B. & Carlsson, G.E. (1988). Bone resorption around fixtures in edentulous patients treated with mandibular fixed tissue-integrated prostheses. *Journal of Prosthetic Dentistry* **59**, 59–63.

Lindquist, L.W., Carlsson, G.E. & Jemt, T. (1997). Association between marginal bone loss around osseointegrated man-dibular implants and smoking habits: A 10-year follow-up study. *Journal of Dental Research* **76**, 1667–1674.

Listgarten, M.A. & Lai, C.-H. (1999). Comparative microbio-logical characteristics of failing implants and periodontally diseased teeth. *Journal of Periodontology* **70**, 431–437.

Maier, A., Gaggl, A., Klemen, H., Santler, G., Anegg, U., Fell, B., Kärcher, H., Smolle-Jüttner, F.M. & Friehs, G.B. (2000). Review of severe osteoradionecrosis treated by surgery alone or surgery with postoperative hyperbaric oxygen-ation. *British Journal of Oral & Maxillofacial Surgery* **38**, 173–176.

Malmstrom, H.S., Fritz, M.E., Timmis, D.P. & Van Dyke, T.E. (1990). Osseo-integrated implant treatment of a patient with rapidly progressive periodontitis. A case report. *Journal of Periodontology* **61**, 300–304.

Marx, R.E., Sawatari, Y., Fortin, M. & Broumand, V. (2005). Bisphosphonate-induced exposed bone (osteonecrosis/osteopetrosis) of the jaws: Risk factors, recognition, preven-tion, and treatment. *Journal of Oral & Maxillofacial Surgery* **63**, 1567–1575.

Mombelli, A., Van Oosten, M.A.C., Schürch, E. & Lang, N.P. (1987). The microbiota associated with successful or failing osseointegrated titanium implants. *Oral Microbiology & Immunology* **2**, 145–151.

Mombelli, A., Buser, D. & Lang, N.P. (1988). Colonization of osseointegrated titanium implants in edentulous patients. Early results. *Oral Microbiology & Immunology* **3**, 113–120.

Mombelli, A. (1994). Criteria for success. Monitoring. In: Lang, N.P. & Karring, T., eds. *Proceedings of the 1st European Work-shop on Periodontology*. London: Quintessence Publishing Co., Ltd., pp. 317–325.

Morris, H.F., Ochi, S. & Winkler, S. (2000). Implant survival in patients with type 2 diabetes: Placement to 36 months. *Annals of Periodontology* **5**, 157–165.

Morris, H.F., Ochi, S., Plezia, R., Gilbert, H., Dent, C.D., Pikul-ski, J. & Lambert, P.M. (2004). AICRG, Part III: The influence of antibiotic use on the survival of a new implant design. *Journal of Oral Implantology* **30**, 144–151.

Moy, P.K., Medina, D., Shetty, V. & Aghaloo, T.L. (2005). Dental implant failure rates and associated risk factors. *Interna-tional Journal of Oral & Maxillofacial Implants* **20**, 569–577.

Mundt, T., Mack, F., Schwahn, C. & Biffar, R. (2006). Private practice results of screw-type tapered implants: Survival and evaluation of risk factors. *International Journal of Oral & Maxillofacial Implants* **21**, 607–614.

Nevins, M. & Langer, B. (1995). The successful use of osseoin-tegrated implants for the treatment of the recalcitrant peri-odontal patient. *Journal of Periodontology* **66**, 150–157.

Nitzan, D., Mamlider, A., Levin, L. & Schwartz-Arad, D. (2005). Impact of smoking on marginal bone loss. *International Journal of Oral & Maxillofacial Implants* **20**, 605–609.

Olson, J.W., Shernoff, A.F., Tarlow, J.L., Colwell, J.A., Scheetz, J.P. & Bingham, S.F. (2000). Dental endosseous implant assessments in a type 2 diabetic population: A prospective study. *International Journal of Oral Maxillofacial Implants* **15**, 811–818.

Op Heij, D.G., Opdebeeck, H., van Steenberghe, D. & Quirynen, M. (2003). Age as compromising factor for implant insertion. *Periodontology 2000* **33**, 172–184.

Papaioannou, W., Quirynen, M. & van Steenberghe, D. (1996). The influence of periodontitis on the subgingival flora around implants in partially edentulous patients. *Clinical Oral Implants Research* **7**, 405–409.

Paster, B.J., Boches, S.K., Galvin, J.L., Ericson, R.E., Lau, C.N., Levanos, V.A., Sahasrabudhe, A. & Dewhirst, F.E. (2001). Bacterial diversity in human subgingival plaque. *Journal of Bacteriology* **183**, 3770–3783.

Patel, K., Welfare, R. & Coonar, H.S. (1998). The provision of dental implants and a fixed prosthesis in the treatment of a patient with scleroderma: A clinical report. *Journal of Prosthetic Dentistry* **79**, 611–612.

Payne, A.G.T., Lownie, J.F. & Van der Linden, W.J. (1997). Implant-supported prostheses in patients with Sjögren's syndrome: A clinical report on three patients. *International Journal of Oral & Maxillofacial Implants* **12**, 679–685.

Peleg, M., Garg, A.K. & Mazor, Z. (2006). Healing in smokers versus nonsmokers: Survival rates for sinus floor augmentation with simultaneous implant placement. *International Journal of Oral & Maxillofacial Implants* **21**, 551–559.

Peñarrocha-Diago, M., Bagán-Sebastián, J.V. & Vera-Sempere, F. (1990). Diphenylhydantoin-induced gingival overgrowth in man: A clinico-pathological study. *Journal of Periodontology* **61**, 571–574.

Pjetursson, B.E., Tan, K., Lang, N.P., Brägger, U., Egger, M. & Zwahlen, M. (2004). A systematic review of the survival and complication rates of fixed partial dentures (FPDs) after an observation period of at least 5 years. I. Implant-supported FPDs. *Clinical Oral Implants Research* **15**, 625–642.

Powell, C.A., Mealey, B.L., Deas, D.E., McDonnell, H.T. & Moritz, A.J. (2005). Post-surgical infections: Prevalence associated with various periodontal surgical procedures. *Journal of Periodontology* **76**, 329–333.

Quirynen, M. & Listgarten, M.A. (1990). The distribution of bacterial morphotypes around natural teeth and titanium implants ad modum Brånemark. *Clinical Oral Implants Research* **1**, 8–12.

Quirynen, M., Papaioannou, W. & van Steenberghe, D. (1996). Intraoral transmission and the colonization of oral hard surfaces. *Journal of Periodontology* **67**, 986–993.

Quirynen, M. & Teughels, W. (2003). Microbiologically compromised patients and impact on oral implants. *Periodontology 2000* **33**, 119–123.

Quirynen, M., Alsaadi, G., Pauwels, M., Haffajee, A., van Steenberghe, D. & Naert, I. (2005a). Microbiological and clinical outcomes and patient satisfaction for two treatment options in the edentulous lower jaw after 10 years of function. *Clinical Oral Implants Research* **16**, 277–287.

Quirynen, M., Vogels, R., Alsaadi, G., Naert, I., Jacobs, R. & van Steenberghe, D. (2005b). Predisposing conditions for retrograde peri-implantitis, and treatment suggestions. *Clinical Oral Implants Research* **16**, 599–608.

Rajnay, Z.W. & Hochstetter, R.L. (1998). Immediate placement of an endosseous root-form implant in an HIV-positive patient: Report of a case. *Journal of Periodontology* **69**, 1167–1171.

Rams, T.E., Feik, D. & Slots, J. (1990). Staphylococci in human periodontal diseases. *Oral Microbiology & Immunology* **5**, 29–32.

Rams, T.E., Roberts, T.W., Feik, D., Molzan, A.K. & Slots, J. (1991). Clinical and microbiological findings on newly inserted hydroxyapatite-coated and pure titanium human dental implants. *Clinical Oral Implants Research* **2**, 121–127.

Rogers, M.A., Figliomeni, L., Baluchova, K., Tan, A.E.S., Davies, G., Henry, P.J. & Price, P. (2002). Do interleukin-1 polymorphisms predict the development of periodontitis or the success of dental implants? *Journal of Periodontal Research* **37**, 37–41.

Romeo, E., Lops, D., Margutti E., Ghisolfi. M., Chiapasco, M. & Vogel, G. (2004). Long-term survival and success of oral implants in the treatment of full and partial arches: A 7-year prospective study with the ITI dental implant system. *International Journal of Oral & Maxillofacial Implants* **19**, 247–259.

Rosenberg, E.S., Torosian, J.P. & Slots, J. (1991). Microbial differences in 2 clinically distinct types of failures of osseointegrated implants. *Clinical Oral Implants Research* **2**, 135–144.

Ruggiero, S.L., Mehrotra, B., Rosenberg, T.J. & Engroff, S.L. (2004). Osteonecrosis of the jaws associated with the use of bisphosphonates: A review of 63 cases. *Journal of Oral & Maxillofacial Surgery* **62**, 527–534.

Rutar, A., Lang, N.P., Buser, D., Bürgin, W. & Mombelli, A. (2001). Retrospective assessment of clinical and microbiological factors affecting periimplant tissue conditions. *Clinical Oral Implants Research* **12**, 189–195.

Salcetti, J.M., Moriarty, J.D., Cooper, L.F., Smith F.W., Collins, J.G., Socransky, S.S. & Offenbacher, S. (1997). The clinical, microbial, and host response characteristics of the failing implant. *International Journal of Oral & Maxillofacial Implants* **12**, 32–42.

Salvi, G.E. & Lang, N.P. (2004). Diagnostic parameters for monitoring implant conditions. *International Journal of Oral & Maxillofacial Implants* **19** (Suppl), 116–127.

Santos, M.C.L., Campos, M.I.G., Souza, A.P., Trevilatto, P.C. & Line, S.R.P. (2004). Analysis of MMP-1 and MMP-9 promoter polymorphisms in early osseointegrated implant failure. *International Journal of Oral & Maxillofacial Implants* **19**, 38–43.

Sbordone, L., Barone, A., Ciaglia, R.N., Ramaglia, L. & Iacono, V.J. (1999). Longitudinal study of dental implants in a periodontally compromised population. *Journal of Periodontology* **70**, 1322–1329.

Scully, C., Madrid, C. & Bagan, J. (2006). Dental endosseous implants in patients on bisphosphonate therapy. *Implant Dentistry* **15**, 212–218.

Sennerby, L., Thomsen, P. & Ericson, L.E. (1992). A morphometric and biomechanic comparison of titanium implants inserted in rabbit cortical and cancellous bone. *International Journal of Oral and Maxillofacial Surgery* **7**, 62–71.

Shaffer, M.D., Juruaz, D.A. & Haggerty, P.C. (1998). The effect of periradicular endodontic pathosis on the apical region of adjacent implants. *Oral Surgery Oral Medicine Oral Pathology Oral Radiology & Endodontics* **86**, 578–581.

Shernoff, A.F., Colwell, J.A. & Bingham, S.F. (1994). Implants for type II diabetic patients: interim report. VA implants in diabetes study group. *Implant Dentistry* **3**, 183–185.

Shetty, K. & Achong, R. (2005). Dental implants in the HIV-positive patient – Case report and review of the literature. *General Dentistry* **53**, 434–437.

Silverstein, L.H., Koch, J.P., Lefkove, M.D., Garnick, J.J., Singh, B. & Steflik, D.E. (1995). Nifedipine-induced gingival enlargement around dental implants: a clinical report. *Journal of Oral Implantology* **21**, 116–120.

Starck, W.J. & Epker, B.N. (1995). Failure of osseointegrated dental implants after diphosphonate therapy for osteoporosis: A case report. *International Journal of Oral & Maxillofacial Implants* **10**, 74–78.

Sumida, S., Ishihara, K., Kishi, M. & Okuda, K. (2002). Transmission of periodontal disease-associated bacteria from teeth to osseointegrated implant regions. *International Journal of Oral & Maxillofacial Implants* **17**, 696–702.

Sussman, H.I. & Moss, S.S. (1993). Localized osteomyelitis secondary to endodontic-implant pathosis. A case report. *Journal of Periodontology* **64**, 306–310.

Teng, M.S. & Futran, N.D. (2005). Osteoradionecrosis of the mandible. *Current Opinion in Otolaryngology & Head and Neck Surgery* **13**, 217–221.

Thilander, B., Ödman, J. & Lekholm U. (2001). Orthodontic aspects of the use of oral implants in adolescents: a 10-year follow-up study. *European Journal of Orthodontics* **23**, 715–731.

Toomes, C., James, J., Wood, A.J., Wu, C.L., McCormick, D., Lench, N., Hewitt, C., Moynihan, L., Roberts, E., Woods, C.G., Markham, A., Wong, M., Widmer, R., Ghaffar, K.A., Pemberton, M., Hussein, I.R., Temtamy, S.A., Davis, R., Read, A.P., Sloan, P., Dixon, M.J. & Thakker, N.S. (1999). Loss-of-function mutations in the cathepsin C gene result in periodontal disease and palmoplantar keratosis. *Nature Genetics* **23**, 421–424.

Ullbro, C., Crossner, C.-G., Lundgren, T., Stålblad, P.-Å. & Renvert, S. (2000). Osseointegrated implants in a patients with Papillon-Lefèvre syndrome. A 4$\frac{1}{2}$-year follow-up. *Journal of Clinical Periodontology* **27**, 951–954.

Van Steenberghe, D., Quirynen, M., Molly, L. & Jacobs, R. (2003). Impact of systemic diseases and medication on osseointegration. *Periodontology 2000* **33**, 163–171.

Van Winkelhoff, A.J., Goené, R.J., Benschop, C. & Folmer, T. (2000). Early colonization of dental implants by putative periodontal pathogens in partially edentulous patients. *Clinical Oral Implants Research* **11**, 511–520.

Van Winkelhoff, A.J. & Wolf, J.W.A. (2000). *Actinobacillus actinomycetemcomitans*-associated peri-implantitis in an edentulous patient. A case report. *Journal of Clinical Periodontology* **27**, 531–535.

Villa, R. & Rangert, B. (2005). Early loading of interforaminal implants immediately installed after extraction of teeth presenting endodontic and periodontal lesions. *Clinical Implant Dentistry & Related Research* **7** (Suppl 1), S28–S35.

Wagenberg, B. & Froum, S.J. (2006). A retrospective study of 1,925 consecutively placed immediate implants from 1988 to 2004. *International Journal of Oral & Maxillofacial Implants* **21**, 71–80.

Wahl, M.J. (1998). Dental surgery in anticoagulated patients. *Archives of Internal Medicine* **158**, 1610–1616.

Wahl, M.J. (2000). Myths of dental surgery in patients receiving anticoagulant therapy. *Journal of the American Dental Association* **131**, 77–81.

Weber, H.P., Crohin, C.C. & Fiorellini, J.P. (2000). A 5-year prospective clinical and radiographic study of non-submerged dental implants. *Clinical Oral Implants Research* **11**, 144–153.

Weischer, T., Kandt, M. & Reidick, T. (2005). Immediate loading of mandibular implants in compromised patients: Preliminary results. *International Journal of Periodontics & Restorative Dentistry* **25**, 501–507.

Weng, D., Jacobson, Z., Tarnow, D., Hürzeler, M.B., Faehn, O., Sanavi, F., Barkvoll, P. & Stach, R.M. (2003). A prospective multicenter clinical trial of 3i machined-surface implants: Results after 6 years of follow-up. *International Journal of Oral & Maxillofacial Implants* **18**, 417–423.

Weyant, R.J. & Burt, B.A. (1993). An assessment of survival rates and within-patient clustering of failures for endosseous oral implants. *Journal of Dental Research* **73**, 2–8.

Wilson, M.J., Weightman, A.J. & Wade, W.G. (1997). Applications of molecular biology in the characterisation of uncultured microorganisms associated with human disease. *Reviews in Medical Microbiology* **8**, 91–101.

Wilson, T.G. Jr. & Nunn, M. (1999). The relationship between the interleukin-1 periodontal genotype and implant loss. Initial data. *Journal of Periodontology* **70**, 724–729.

Woo, S.-B., Hellstein, J.W. & Kalmar, J.R. (2006). Systematic review: Bisphosphonates and osteonecrosis of the jaws. *Annals of Internal Medicine* **144**, 753–761.

Zandman-Goddard, G. & Shoenfeld, Y. (2003). SLE and infections. *Clinical Reviews in Allergy & Immunology* **25**, 29–40.

Part 10: Treatment Planning Protocols

31 Treatment Planning of Patients with Periodontal Diseases, 655
Giovanni E. Salvi, Jan Lindhe, and Niklaus P. Lang

32 Treatment Planning for Implant Therapy in the Periodontally Compromised
Patient, 675
Jan L. Wennström and Niklaus P. Lang

33 Systemic Phase of Therapy, 687
Niklaus P. Lang and Hans-Rudolf Baur

Chapter 31

Treatment Planning of Patients with Periodontal Diseases

Giovanni E. Salvi, Jan Lindhe, and Niklaus P. Lang

Screening for periodontal disease, 656
  Basic periodontal examination, 656
Diagnosis, 657
Treatment planning, 658
  Initial treatment plan, 658

Pre-therapeutic single tooth prognosis, 660
Case presentation, 660
Case report, 667
  Patient S.K. (male, 35 years old), 667

Caries and periodontal diseases represent opportunistic infections associated with biofilm formation on the surfaces of teeth. Factors such as bacterial specificity and pathogenicity as well as the disposition of the individual for disease, e.g. local and general resistance, may influence the onset, the rate of progression, and clinical characteristics of plaque-associated dental disorders. Findings from animal experiments and longitudinal studies in humans, however, have demonstrated that treatment, including the elimination or the control of the biofilm infection and the introduction of careful plaque control measures, in most, if not all, cases results in dental and periodontal health. Even if health cannot always be achieved and maintained, the arrest of disease progression following treatment must be the goal of modern dental care.

The treatment of patients affected by caries and periodontal disease, including symptoms of associated pathologic conditions such as pulpitis, periapical periodontitis, marginal abscesses, tooth migration, etc., may from a didactic point of view be divided into four different phases:

1. Systemic phase of therapy including smoking counseling
2. Initial (or hygiene) phase of periodontal therapy, i.e. cause-related therapy
3. Corrective phase of therapy, i.e. additional measures such as periodontal surgery, and/or endodontic therapy, implant surgery, restorative, orthodontic and/or prosthetic treatment
4. Maintenance phase (care), i.e. supportive periodontal therapy (SPT).

Treatment goals

In every patient diagnosed with periodontitis, a treatment strategy, including the elimination of the opportunistic infection, must be defined and followed. This treatment strategy must also define the clinical outcome parameters to be reached through therapy. Such clinical parameters include:

- Reduction or resolution of gingivitis (bleeding on probing; BoP). A patient full mouth mean BoP ≤25% should be reached.
- Reduction in probing pocket depth (PPD). No residual pockets with PPD >5 mm should be present.
- Elimination of (through-and-through) open furcations in multi-rooted teeth. Initial furcation involvement should not exceed 3 mm.
- Absence of pain.
- Individually satisfactory esthetics and function.

In this context it must be emphasized that risk factors for periodontitis that can be controlled must be addressed as well. The three main risk factors for chronic periodontitis are (1) improper plaque control, (2) cigarette smoking, and (3) uncontrolled diabetes mellitus (Kinane *et al.* 2006).

Systemic phase

The goal of this phase is to eliminate or decrease the influence of systemic conditions on the outcomes of therapy and to protect the patient and the dental care providers against infectious hazards. Contact with a physician or specialist should enable appropriate preventive measures to be taken, if necessary. Efforts must be undertaken to stimulate a smoker to enroll in a smoking cessation program. Additional aspects are discussed in Chapter 33.

Initial (hygiene) phase

This phase represents the cause-related therapy. The objective of this phase is the achievement of clean and infection-free conditions in the oral cavity through complete removal of all soft and hard deposits and their retentive factors. Furthermore, this phase should aim at motivating the patient to perform optimal plaque control. The initial phase of periodontal therapy is concluded by re-evaluation and planning of both additional and supportive therapies.

Corrective phase (additional therapeutic measures)

This phase addresses the sequelae of the oportunistic infections and includes therapeutic measures, such as periodontal and implant surgery, endodontic therapy, restorative and/or prosthetic treatment. The amount of corrective therapy required and the selection of the type of restorative and prosthetic therapy can be determined only when the degree of success of the cause-related therapy can be properly evaluated. The patient's willingness and ability to cooperate in the overall therapy must determine the type of corrective treatment. If this cooperation is inadequate, it may not be worth initiating treatment procedures: permanent improvement of oral health, function and esthetics may therefore not be achieved. The validity of this statement can be exemplified by the results of studies aimed at assessing the relative value of different types of surgical methods in the treatment of periodontal disease. A number of clinical trials (Lindhe & Nyman 1975; Nyman *et al.* 1975, 1977; Rosling *et al.* 1976a,b; Nyman & Lindhe 1979) have demonstrated that gingivectomy and flap procedures performed in patients with proper plaque control levels often result in gain of alveolar bone and clinical attachment, while surgery in plaque-contaminated dentitions may cause additional destruction of the periodontium.

Maintenance phase (supportive periodontal therapy)

The aim of this treatment is the prevention of re-infection and disease recurrence. For each individual patient a recall system must be designed that includes (1) assessment of deepened sites with bleeding on probing, (2) instrumentation of such sites, and (3) fluoride application for the prevention of dental caries. In addition, this treatment involves the regular control of prosthetic restorations incorporated during the corrective phase of therapy. Tooth sensitivity testing should be applied to abutment teeth as loss of vitality is a frequently encountered complication (Bergenholtz & Nyman 1984; Lang *et al.* 2004; Lulic *et al.* 2007). Based upon the individual caries activity, bitewing radiographs should be incorporated into SPT at regular intervals.

Screening for periodontal disease

A patient seeking dental care is usually screened for the presence of carious lesions by means of clinical and radiographic tools. Likewise, it is imperative that such a patient is screened for the presence of periodontitis as well, using a procedure termed the basic periodontal examination (BPE) (or periodontal screening record; PSR).

Basic periodontal examination

The goal of the BPE is to screen the periodontal conditions of a new patient and to facilitate treatment planning. BPE scoring will allow the therapist to identify:

- A patient with reasonably healthy periodontal conditions, but in need of long-term preventive measures
- A patient with periodontitis and in need of periodontal therapy.

In the BPE the screening of each tooth or implant is evaluated. For this purpose, the use of a thin graduated periodontal probe is recommended. At least two sites per tooth/implant (i.e. mesio-buccal and disto-buccal) should be probed using a light force (i.e. 0.2 N). Each dentate sextant within the dentition is given a BPE code or score, whereby the *highest* individual site score is used.

BPE system code

- Code 0 = probing pocket depth (PPD) ≤3 mm, BoP negative, no calculus or overhanging fillings (Fig. 31-1a)
- Code 1 = PPD ≤3 mm, BoP positive, no calculus or overhanging fillings (Fig. 31-1b)
- Code 2 = PPD ≤3 mm, BoP positive, presence of supra- and/or subgingival calculus and/or overhanging fillings (Fig. 31-1c)
- Code 3 = PPD >3 mm but ≤5 mm, BoP positive (Fig. 31-1d)
- Code 4 = PPD >5 mm (Fig. 31-1e).

If an examiner identifies a single site with a PPD >5 mm within a sextant, the sextant will receive a code of 4, and no further assessments are needed in this particular sextant. Patients with sextants given codes of 0, 1 or 2 belong to the relatively periodontally healthy category. A patient exhibiting a sextant with codes of 3 or 4 must undergo a more comprehensive periodontal examination (for details see Chapter 26).

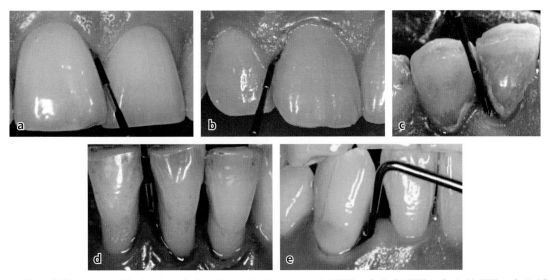

Fig. 31-1 Clinical illustration of the basic periodontal examination scores. (a) BPE code 0. (b) BPE code 1. (c) BPE code 2. (d) BPE code 3. (e) BPE code 4.

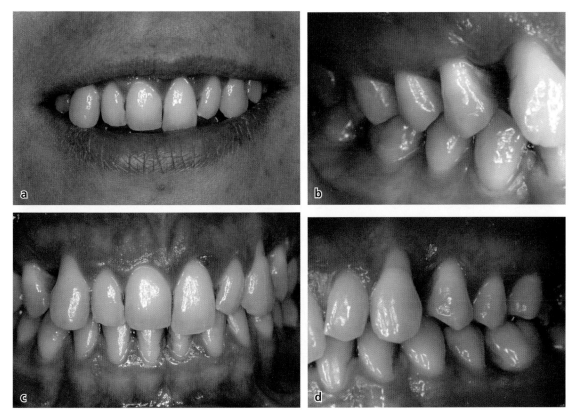

Fig. 31-2 (a–d) Clinical status of a 27-year-old female patient (S.B.) diagnosed with generalized aggressive periodontitis with furcation involvement.

The aim of the following text is to explain the overall objectives of the treatment planning of patients with BPE codes of 3 and 4 undergoing a comprehensive diagnostic process.

Diagnosis

The basis for the treatment planning described in this chapter is established by the clinical data collected from the patient's examination (see Chapter 26). This patient (Ms. S.B., 27 years of age) was sys-

temically healthy and a non-smoker. She was examined with respect to her periodontal conditions, i.e. gingival sites displaying signs of *bleeding on probing* were identified, *probing pocket depths* were measured, the *periodontal attachment level* was calculated, *furcation involvements* were graded, *tooth mobility* was assessed, and the radiographs were analyzed to determine the *height* and *outline* of the *alveolar bone crest*.

The clinical characteristics of the dentition of this patient are shown in Fig. 31-2. The periodontal chart

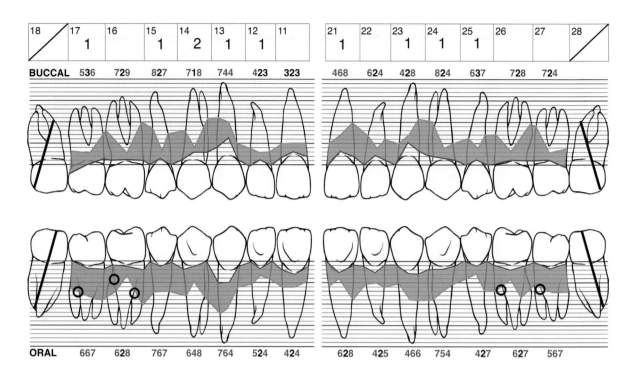

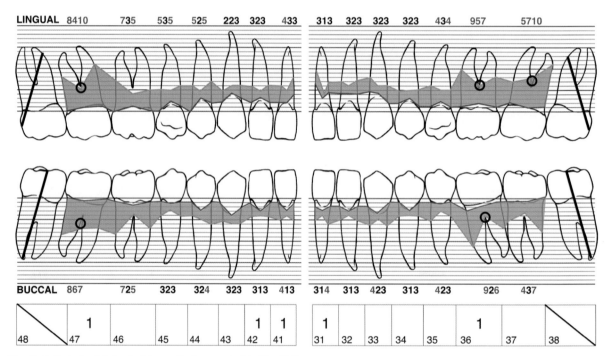

Fig. 31-3 Periodontal chart of the patient presented in Fig. 31-2.

and the radiographs are presented in Figs. 31-3 and 31-4, respectively. Based on these findings, each tooth in the dentition was given a diagnosis (Fig. 31-5) and a pre-therapeutic prognosis (Fig. 31-6). In addition to the examination of the periodontal condition, detailed assessments of primary pland recurrent caries were made for all tooth surfaces in the dentition. Furthermore, the patient was examined with respect to endodontic and occlusal problems as well as temporomandibular joint dysfunction.

Treatment planning

Initial treatment plan

Provided that the patient's examination has been completed (see Chapter 26) and a diagnosis of all pathologic conditions has been made, an initial treatment plan can been established. At this early stage in the management of a patient, it is, in most instances,

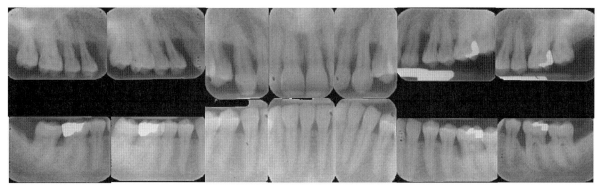

Fig. 31-4 Radiographs of the patient presented in Fig. 31-2.

	18	17	16	15	14	13	12	11	21	22	23	24	25	26	27	28
Gingivitis																
Parodontitis superficialis							X	X								
Parodontitis profunda		X	X	X	X	X			X	X	X	X	X	X	X	
Parodontitis interradicularis		X	X											X	X	
Parodontitis interradicularis		X	X											X	X	
Parodontitis profunda		X	X											X	X	
Parodontitis superficialis			X	X			X	X		X		X				
Gingivitis					X	X			X		X					
	48	47	46	45	44	43	42	41	31	32	33	34	35	36	37	38

Fig. 31-5 Single tooth diagnosis of the patient presented in Fig. 31-2.

	18	17	16	15	14	13	12	11	21	22	23	24	25	26	27	28
Irrational to treat																
Doubtful (unsecure)		X	X	X	X						X	X		X	X	
Good (secure)						X	X	X	X				X			
Good (secure)			X	X	X	X	X	X	X	X	X	X	X			
Doubtful (unsecure)		X	X											X	X	
Irrational to treat																
	48	47	46	45	44	43	42	41	31	32	33	34	35	36	37	38

Fig. 31-6 Pre-therapeutic single tooth prognosis of the patient presented in Fig. 31-2.

impossible to make definite decisions regarding all aspects of the treatment sequence, because:

1. *The degree of success of initial therapy is unknown.* The re-evaluation after initial, cause-related therapy forms the basis for the selection of means for additional therapy. The degree of disease elimination that can be reached depends on the outcome of subgingival instrumentation, but also on the patient's ability and willingness to exercise proper plaque control and to adopt adequate dietary habits.

2. *The patient's "subjective" need for additional (periodontal and/or restorative) therapy is unknown.* When the dentist has completed the examination of the patient and an inventory has been made regarding periodontal disease, caries, pulpal disease, and temporomandibular joint disorders, the observations are presented to the patient (i.e. "the case presentation"). During the case presentation

session it is important to find out if the patient's subjective need for dental therapy coincides with the dentist's professional appreciation of the type and amount of therapy that is required. It is important that the dentist understands that the main objective of dental therapy, besides *elimination of pain*, is *to satisfy the patient's demands regarding chewing function (comfort) and esthetics*, demands that certainly vary considerably from one individual to another.

3. *The result of some treatment steps cannot be predicted.* In patients exhibiting advanced forms of caries and periodontal disease it is often impossible to anticipate whether or not all teeth that are present at the initial examination can be successfully treated, or to predict the result of certain parts of the intended therapy. In other words, critical and difficult parts of the treatment must be performed first, and the outcome of this treatment must be evaluated before all aspects of the definitive corrective treatment can be properly anticipated and described.

Pre-therapeutic single tooth prognosis

Based on the results of the comprehensive examination, including assessments of periodontitis, caries, tooth sensitivity, and the resulting diagnosis, as well as considering the patient's needs regarding esthetics and function, a pre-therapeutic prognosis for each individual tooth (root) is made. Three major questions are addressed:

1. Which tooth/root has a *"good"* (secure) prognosis?
2. Which tooth/root is *"irrational-to-treat"*?
3. Which tooth/root has a *"doubtful"* (unsecure) prognosis?

Teeth with a *good* prognosis will require relatively simple therapy and may be regarded as secure abutments for function.

Teeth that are considered "irrational-to-treat" should be extracted during initial, cause-related therapy. Such teeth may be identified on the basis of the following criteria:

- Periodontal:
  ○ Recurrent periodontal abscesses
  ○ Combined periodontal–endodontic lesions
  ○ Attachment loss to the apex
- Endodontal:
  ○ Root perforation in the apical half of the root
- Dental:
  ○ Vertical fracture of the root
  ○ Oblique fracture in the middle third of the root
  ○ Caries lesions that extend into the root canal
- Functional:
  ○ Third molars without antagonists and with periodontitis/caries.

Teeth with a *doubtful* prognosis are usually in need of comprehensive therapy and must be brought into the category of teeth with a *good* prognosis by means of additional therapy. Such teeth may be identified on the basis of the following criteria:

- Periodontal:
  ○ Furcation involvement
  ○ Angular (i.e. vertical) bony defects
  ○ "Horizontal" bone loss involving more than two thirds of the root
- Endodontal:
  ○ Incomplete root canal therapy
  ○ Periapical pathology
  ○ Presence of voluminous posts/screws
- Dental:
  ○ Extensive root caries.

Case presentation

The "case presentation" is an essential component of the initial treatment plan and must include a description for the patient of different therapeutic goals and the modalities by which these may be reached. At the case presentation for Ms. S.B. the following treatment plan was described:

- The teeth in the dentition from 12 to 22 and from 45 to 35 will probably not confront the dentist with any major therapeutic challenges. For the remaining teeth in the dentition, however, the treatment plan may involve several additional measures.

Expected benefits inherent to a certain treatment plan versus obvious disadvantages should always be explained to and discussed with the patient. His/her attitude to the alternatives presented must guide the dentist in the design of the overall treatment plan.

Based on the pre-therapeutic single tooth prognosis (Fig. 31-6), the following detailed treatment plan was presented to the patient.

Systemic phase

Owing to the fact that the patient was systemically healthy and a non-smoker, no medical examination and smoking cessation counseling were required.

Initial phase (cause-related therapy)

The treatment was initiated and included the following measures to eliminate or control the bacterial infection:

1. *Motivation* of the patient and *instruction* in oral hygiene measures with subsequent check-ups and re-instruction
2. *Scaling and root planing* under local anesthesia in combination with removal of plaque-retentive factors

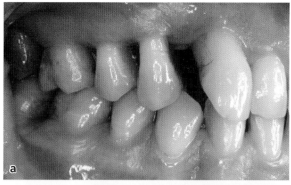

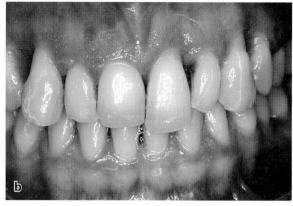

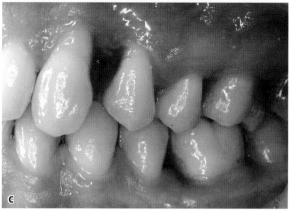

Fig. 31-7 (a–c) Clinical front and lateral views of the patient presented in Fig. 31-2 at re-evaluation after initial periodontal therapy.

3. *Excavation and restoration* of carious lesions (16 and 26)
4. *Endodontic treatment* of tooth 46.

Re-evaluation after initial phase

The initial phase of therapy is completed with a thorough analysis of the results obtained with respect to the elimination or degree of control of the dental infections. This implies that a re-evaluation of the patient's periodontal conditions and caries activity must be performed. The results of this re-evaluation (Figs. 31-7 and 31-8) form the basis for the selection, if necessary, of additional corrective measures to be performed in the phase of definitive treatment (i.e. corrective phase). In order to provide time for the tissues to heal, the re-evaluation should be performed no earlier than 6–8 weeks following the last session of instrumentation.

Planning of the corrective phase (i.e. additional definitive therapy)

If the results from the re-evaluation, made 6–8 weeks after the termination of the initial treatment phase, show that periodontal disease and caries have been brought under control, the additional treatment may be carried out. The main goal of this phase is to correct the sequelae caused by oral infections (i.e. periodontal disease and caries). The following procedures may be performed:

- *Additional endodontic treatment with/without post-and-core build-ups*

- *Periodontal surgery.* The type (i.e. open-flap debridement, regenerative or resective surgery) and extent of surgical treatment should be based on probing depth measurements, degree of furcation involvement and BoP score assessed at re-evaluation. Periodontal surgery is often confined to those areas of the dentition where the inflammatory lesions were not resolved by root instrumentation and in areas with angular bony defects or in furcation-involved molars.
- *Installation of oral implants.* In regions of the dentition where tooth abutments are missing, implant therapy for esthetic and functional reasons may be considered. It is essential to realize that implant therapy must be initiated once all dental infections are under control, i.e. after successful periodontal therapy.
- *Definitive restorative and prosthetic treatment* including fixed or removable dental prostheses.

Corrective phase (additional therapy)

After initial therapy the patient (Ms. S.B.) exhibited low plaque and gingivitis scores (i.e. 5–10%) and no active carious lesions. The corrective phase therefore included the following components:

1. *Periodontal surgery* (i.e. open-flap debridement) in the maxillary left and right quadrants as well as in the mandibular molar regions (Fig. 31-9)
2. *Guided tissue regeneration* (GTR) for tooth 36
3. *Re-evaluation* after periodontal surgery (Figs. 31-10 and 31-11)

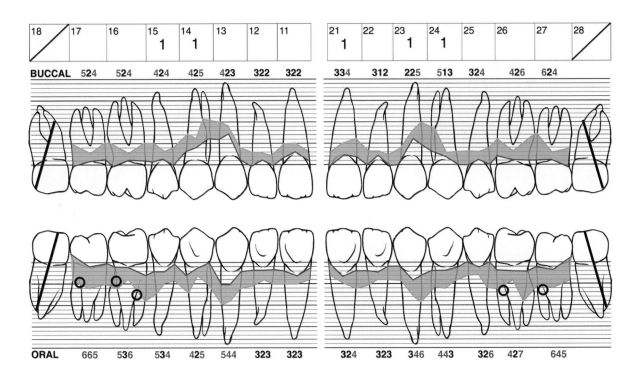

18	17	16	15	14	13	12	11
			1	1			

BUCCAL 524 524 424 425 423 322 322

ORAL 665 536 534 425 544 323 323

21	22	23	24	25	26	27	28
1		1	1				

BUCCAL 334 312 225 513 324 426 624

ORAL 324 323 346 443 326 427 645

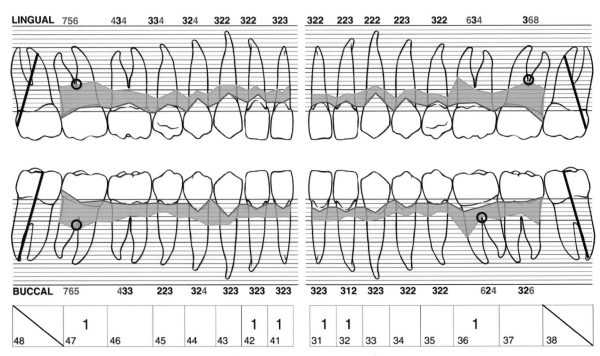

LINGUAL 756 434 334 324 322 322 323

BUCCAL 765 433 223 324 323 323 323

LINGUAL 322 223 222 223 322 634 368

BUCCAL 323 312 323 322 322 624 326

48	47	46	45	44	43	42	41
	1					1	1

31	32	33	34	35	36	37	38
1	1				1		

Fig. 31-8 Periodontal chart of the patient presented in Fig. 31-2 at re-evaluation after initial periodontal therapy.

4. *Orthodontic therapy* in the maxillary front area (Fig. 31-12)
5. *Restorative therapy* in the maxillary front area for esthetic reasons (Fig. 31-13).

Re-evaluation after corrective phase

The corrective phase of therapy is completed with a thorough analysis of the results obtained with respect to the elimination of the sequelae of periodontal tissue destruction (Figs. 31-14, 31-15 and 31-16). This implies that a re-evaluation of the patient's periodon-

tal and peri-implant conditions must be performed. The results of this re-evaluation form the basis for the assessment of the residual periodontal risk. The outcomes of the periodontal risk assessment (PRA), in turn, will determine the recall frequency of the patient during maintenance phase.

Maintenance phase (care)

Following completion of cause-related therapy, the patient must be enrolled in a recall system aiming at

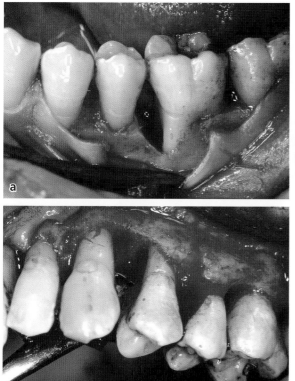
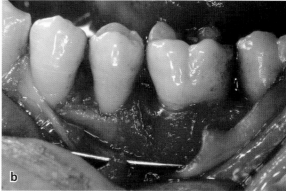
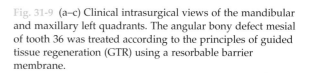

Fig. 31-9 (a–c) Clinical intrasurgical views of the mandibular and maxillary left quadrants. The angular bony defect mesial of tooth 36 was treated according to the principles of guided tissue regeneration (GTR) using a resorbable barrier membrane.

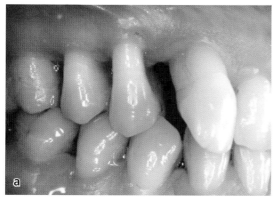
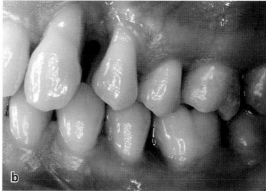

Fig. 31-10 (a,b) Clinical lateral views of the patient presented in Fig. 31-2 at re-evaluation after periodontal surgery.

preventing the recurrence of oral infections (i.e. periodontitis, caries, and peri-implantitis). Supportive periodontal therapy (SPT) should be scheduled at the re-evaluation after initial therapy and independently of the need for additional therapy. The time interval between the recall appointments should be based on a periodontal risk assessment established at the re-evaluation after the corrective phase. It is well established that self-performed plaque control combined with regular maintenance care visits following active periodontal treatment represents an effective means of controlling gingivitis and periodontitis and limiting tooth mortality over a 30-year period (Axelsson *et al.* 2004). It is important to emphasize, however, that the recall program must be designed to meet the individual needs of the patient. According to a PRA performed after completion of active therapy, some patients should be recalled every 3 months, while

others may have to be checked only once a year (Lang & Tonetti 2003).

At the various recall visits the following procedures should be carried out:

1. Update of the medical and smoking history
2. Soft tissue examination as cancer screening
3. Recording of the full-mouth PPD ≥5 mm with concomitant BoP
4. Re-instrumentation of bleeding sites with PPD ≥5 mm
5. Polishing and fluoridation for the prevention of dental caries.

The patient (Ms. S.B.), presented to describe the guiding principles of treatment planning, was recalled twice during the first 6 months after active treatment (i.e. every 3 months) and subsequently only once every 6 months based on the individual PRA.

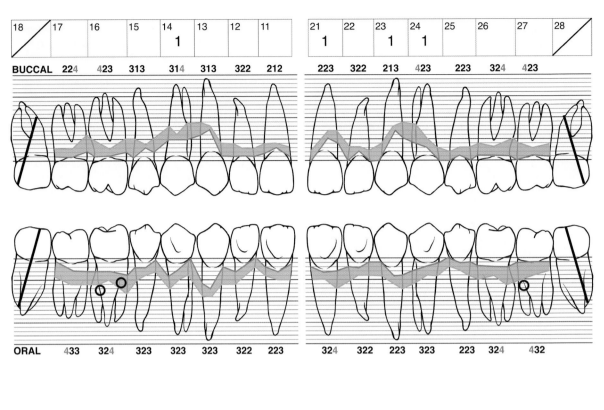

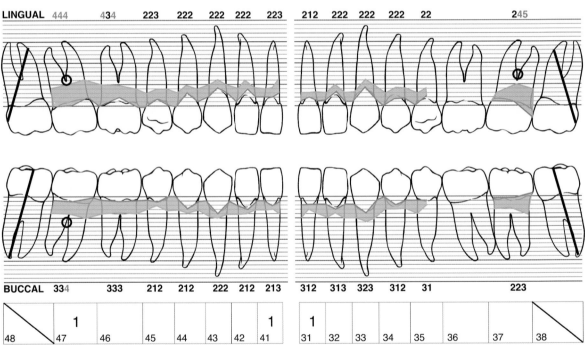

Fig. 31-11 Periodontal chart of the patient presented in Fig. 31-2 at re-evaluation after periodontal surgery.

Concluding remarks

The overall treatment plan and the sequence of the different treatment procedures used in this case were selected for presentation in order to illustrate the following principle: *in patients exhibiting a generalized advanced breakdown of the periodontal tissues, but with an intact number of teeth, considerable efforts should be made to maintain all teeth*. Extraction of a single tooth in such a dentition will frequently also call for the extraction of several others for "prosthetic reasons". The end result of such an approach thus includes a prosthetic rehabilitation that, if the treatment planning had been properly done, would have been unnecessary.

The large variety of treatment problems that different patients present may obviously require deviations from the sequence of treatment phases (i.e. systemic phase, initial cause-related therapy, corrective therapy, and maintenance care) discussed above.

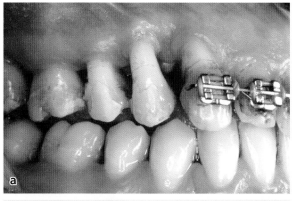
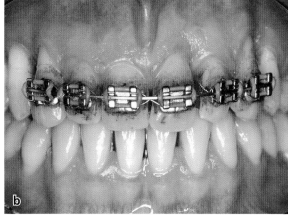
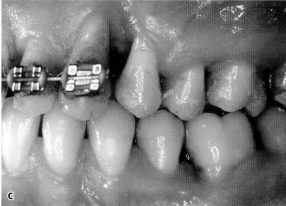

Fig. 31-12 (a–c) Clinical front and lateral views of the patient presented in Fig. 31-2 during orthodontic therapy of the maxillary front teeth.

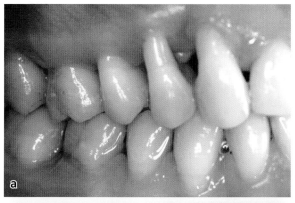
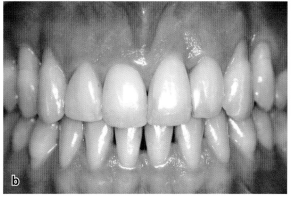
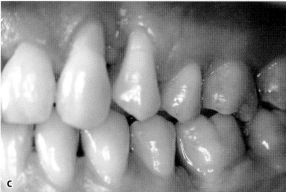

Fig. 31-13 (a–c) Clinical front and lateral views of the patient presented in Fig. 31-2 at the final re-evaluation. To improve the esthetic outcome, the maxillary front teeth were restored with composite fillings.

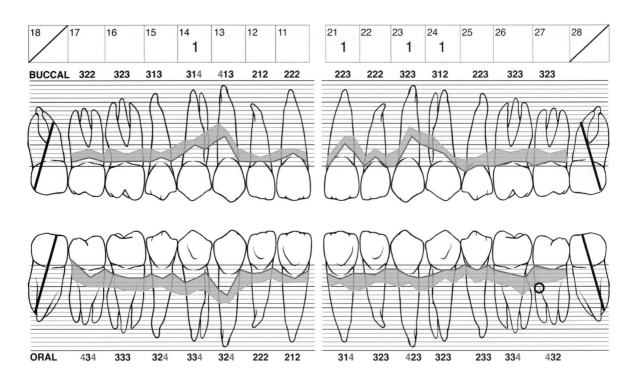

18	17	16	15	14	13	12	11
				1			

21	22	23	24	25	26	27	28
1		1	1				

BUCCAL 322 323 313 314 413 212 222   223 222 323 312 223 323 323

ORAL 434 333 324 334 324 222 212   314 323 423 323 233 334 432

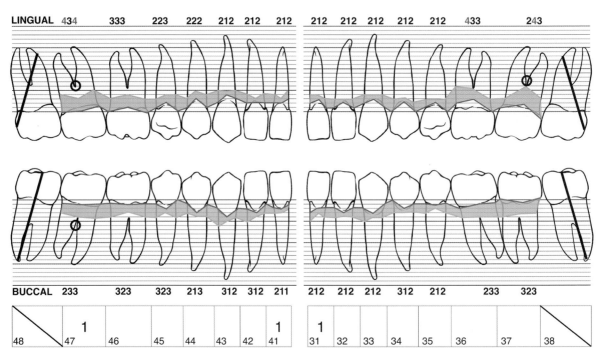

LINGUAL 434 333 223 222 212 212 212   212 212 212 212 212 433 243

BUCCAL 233 323 323 213 312 312 211   212 212 212 312 212 233 323

48	47	46	45	44	43	42	41
	1						1

31	32	33	34	35	36	37	38
1							

Fig. 31-14 Periodontal chart of the patient presented in Fig. 31-2 at the final re-evaluation.

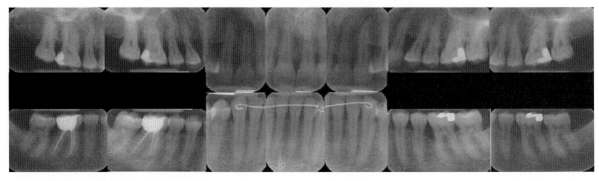

Fig. 31-15 Radiographs of the patient presented in Fig. 31-2 at the final re-evaluation.

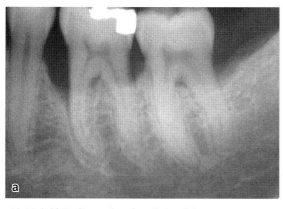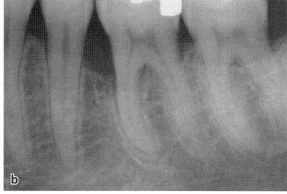

Fig. 31-16 (a,b) Radiographs of tooth 36 of the patient presented in Fig. 31-2 before and after regenerative periodontal therapy according to the principles of GTR.

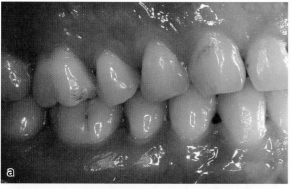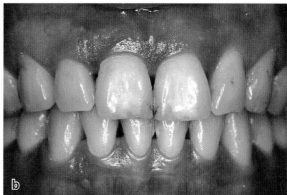

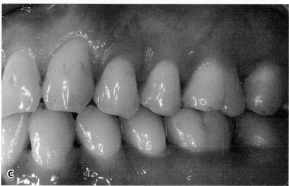

Fig. 31-17 (a–c) Clinical front and lateral views of patient S.K. at initial examination.

Such deviations may be accepted as long as the fundamental principles characterizing the treatment phases are understood.

Case report

A patient will be presented below together with a brief description of his specific dental problems and the treatment delivered in order to demonstrate the rationale behind such treatment phases.

Patient S.K. (male, 35 years old)

Initial examination

The chief complaint of the patient was the slightly increased mobility of tooth 21. The periodontal con-

ditions (i.e. probing pocket depths, furcation involvements, tooth mobility, and periapical radiographs) from the initial examination are shown in Figs. 31-17, 31-18, and 31-19.

The data obtained from the initial examination disclosed the presence of an advanced destruction of the supporting tissues in most parts of the dentition (Fig. 31-18) and the presence of several angular bony defects (Fig. 31-19). The full-mouth plaque score (FMPS) and full-mouth bleeding score (FMBS) were 32% and 86%, respectively. The patient was systemically healthy and a former smoker.

Diagnosis

The patient was diagnosed with generalized chronic periodontitis with furcation involvement.

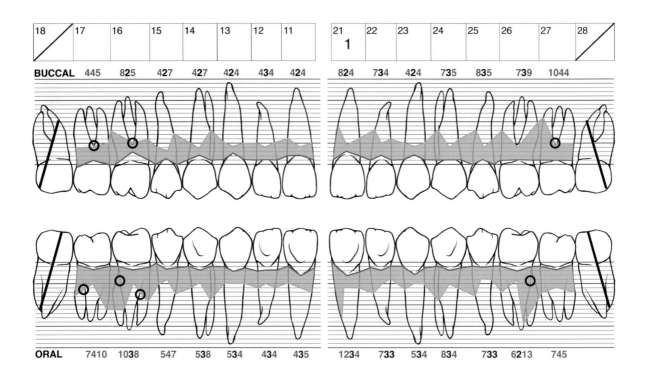

18	17	16	15	14	13	12	11	21	22	23	24	25	26	27	28
								1							

BUCCAL	445	825	427	427	424	434	424	824	734	424	735	835	739	1044

ORAL	7410	1038	547	538	534	434	435	1234	733	534	834	733	6213	745

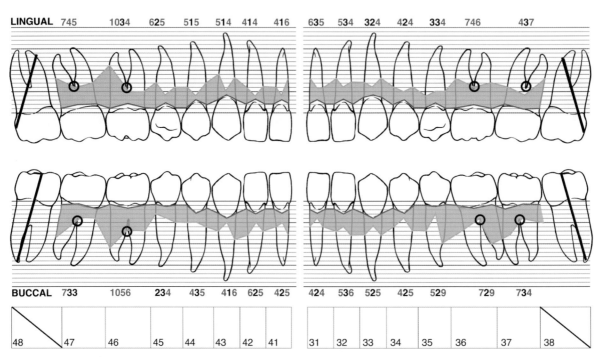

LINGUAL	745	1034	625	515	514	414	416	635	534	324	424	334	746	437

BUCCAL	733	1056	234	435	416	625	425	424	536	525	425	529	729	734

48	47	46	45	44	43	42	41	31	32	33	34	35	36	37	38

Fig. 31-18 Periodontal chart of the patient presented in Fig. 31-17.

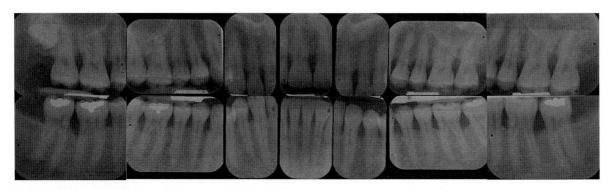

Fig. 31-19 Radiographs of the patient presented in Fig. 31-17.

Etiology

The supra- and subgingival bacterial deposits were identified as the main etiologic factors. Past cigarette smoking was considered a modifying factor.

Pre-therapeutic single tooth prognosis

Teeth 28, 38, and 48 were missing. Tooth 18 was impacted and considered irrational-to-treat. Teeth 13, 12, 11, and 23 in the maxilla and from 45 to 35 in the mandible were classified as secure. A doubtful prognosis was assigned to 17, 16, 15, 14, 21, 22, 24, 25, 26, and 27 in the maxilla and to 36, 37, 46, and 47 in the mandible (Fig. 31-20).

Treatment planning

In the treatment planning of this young patient, it seemed reasonable to anticipate the retention of all teeth of his periodontally compromised dentition. The prerequisites for a good long-term prognosis after therapy included (1) optimal self-performed plaque control, (2) proper healing of the periodontal tissues following non-surgical and surgical therapy, and (3) a carefully monitored maintenance care program. As stated above, tooth 21 displayed increased mobility. This mobility, however, did not disturb the chewing comfort of the patient.

In such a young patient, extensive efforts were made to treat inflammatory periodontal disease pro-

	18	17	16	15	14	13	12	11	21	22	23	24	25	26	27	28
Irrational to treat	X															
Doubtful (unsecure)		X	X	X	X				X	X		X	X	X	X	
Good (secure)						X	X	X			X					
Good (secure)			X	X	X	X	X	X	X	X	X	X	X			
Doubtful (unsecure)		X	X											X	X	
Irrational to treat																
	48	47	46	45	44	43	42	41	31	32	33	34	35	36	37	38

Fig. 31-20 Pre-therapeutic single tooth prognosis of the patient presented in Fig. 31-17.

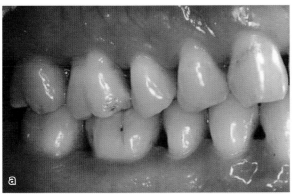

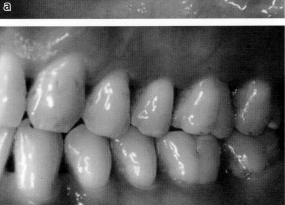

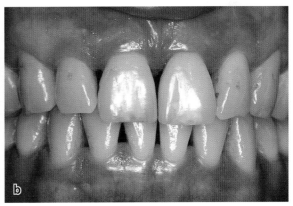

Fig. 31-21 (a–c) Clinical front and lateral views of the patient presented in Fig. 31-17 at re-evaluation after initial therapy.

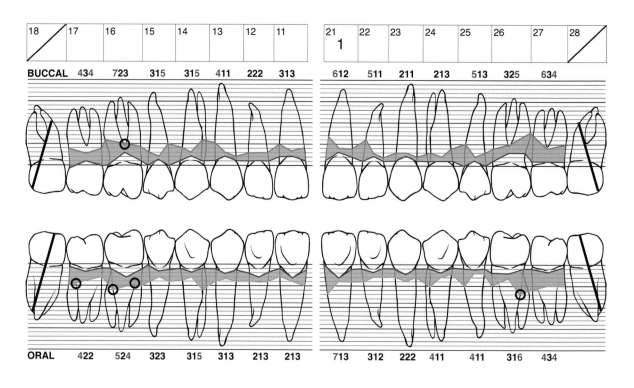

18	17	16	15	14	13	12	11

21	22	23	24	25	26	27	28
1							

BUCCAL 434   723   315   315   411   222   313

BUCCAL 612   511   211   213   513   325   634

ORAL 422   524   323   315   313   213   213

ORAL 713   312   222   411   411   316   434

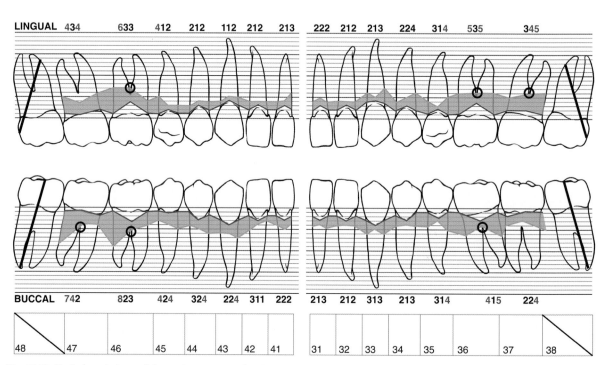

LINGUAL 434   633   412   212   112   212   213

LINGUAL 222   212   213   224   314   535   345

BUCCAL 742   823   424   324   224   311   222

BUCCAL 213   212   313   213   314   415   224

48	47	46	45	44	43	42	41

31	32	33	34	35	36	37	38

Fig. 31-22 Periodontal chart of the patient presented in Fig. 31-17 at re-evaluation after initial therapy.

perly in the entire dentition, in order to avoid tooth extraction and subsequent prosthetic rehabilitation.

Treatment

Subsequent to initial examination, the patient was given a detailed "case presentation" and information regarding alternative goals of and prerequisites for the overall treatment. This information included a description of the role of dental biofilms in the etiol-

ogy of periodontal disease and the significance of optimal plaque control for a successful outcome of therapy. A treatment program was subsequently planned which aimed at maintaining all teeth. The overall treatment was performed in the sequence described below.

Initial cause-related therapy

The patient was counseled not to start smoking again. After thorough motivation, the patient was instructed

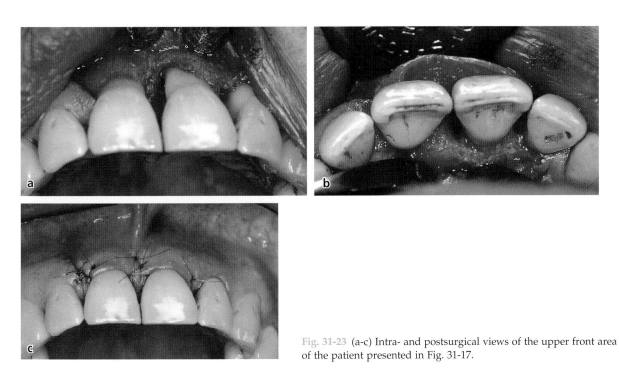

Fig. 31-23 (a-c) Intra- and postsurgical views of the upper front area of the patient presented in Fig. 31-17.

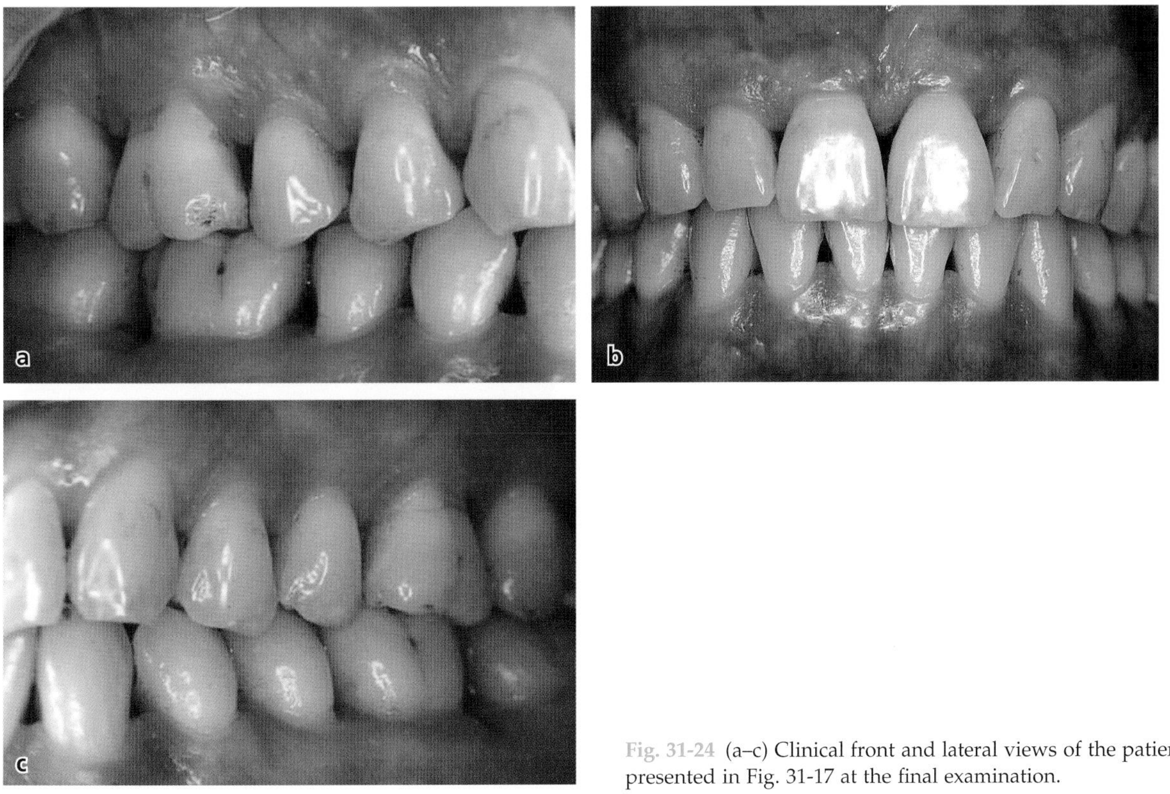

Fig. 31-24 (a–c) Clinical front and lateral views of the patient presented in Fig. 31-17 at the final examination.

in the toothbrushing technique according to Bass and in the use of interdental brushes. Scaling and root planing of all teeth were performed under local anesthesia. The front and lateral views as well as the periodontal chart at re-evaluation after initial therapy are presented in Figs. 31-21 and 31-22, respectively.

Additional therapy
The need for additional therapy was based on the re-evaluation after initial therapy (Fig. 31-22). Periodontal surgery in conjunction with regenerative procedures was deemed necessary in all quadrants. During access flap surgery in the first quadrant extending from 13 to 17, tooth 18 was extracted.

Between the upper front teeth 11 and 21, the modified papilla preservation technique (Cortellini *et al.* 1995) was incorporated in the surgical procedure to gain access to the angular bony defect of tooth 21 (Fig. 31-23). In this area, the application of enamel matrix derivatives (i.e. Emdogain®) aimed at regenerating the lost periodontal tissues on the mesial aspect of 21.

In the third quadrant, the surgical access flap extended from 35 to 37. In the fourth quadrant, flap surgery in conjunction with the simplified papilla preservation technique (Cortellini *et al.* 1999) was used to gain access to the angular bony defect on the distal aspect of 46. In this area, the application of enamel matrix derivatives (i.e. Emdogain®) aimed at regenerating the lost periodontal tissues. Six months after completion of the corrective phase (Fig. 31-24), a re-evaluation of the periodontal conditions (Fig. 31-25), including radiographs (Figs. 31-26 and 31-27) followed by a PRA, were performed.

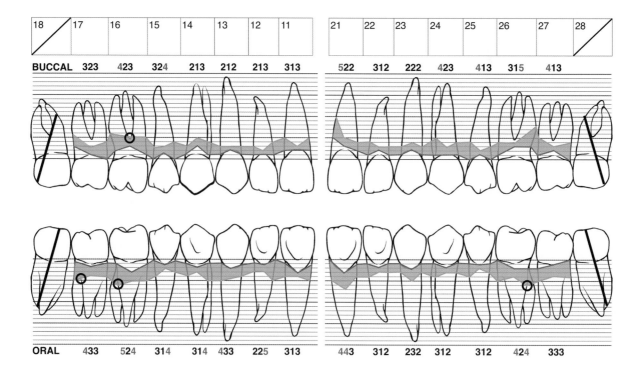

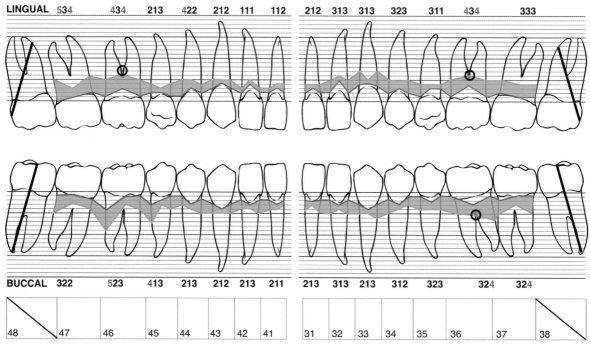

Fig. 31-25 Periodontal chart of the patient presented in Fig. 31-17 at the final examination.

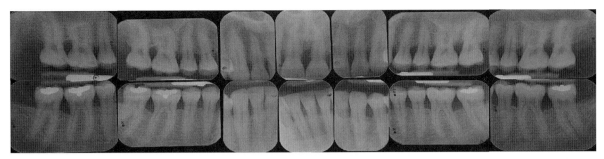

Fig. 31-26 Radiographs of the patient presented in Fig. 31-17 at the final examination.

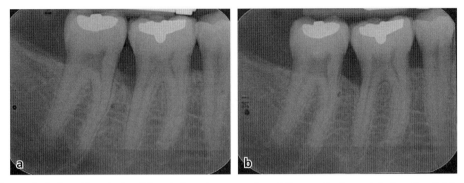

Fig. 31-27 Radiographs before (a) and after (b) periodontal regeneration of the angular bony defect on the distal aspect of tooth 46.

Supportive periodontal therapy

After completion of initial and corrective therapy, the patient was recalled for maintenance care every 3 months. During recall appointments, sites bleeding on probing and with a PPD ≥5 mm were re-instru-mented. If necessary, the patient was remotivated and re-instructed in oral hygiene procedures. Fluoride was regularly applied in order to prevent the onset of dental caries.

References

Axelsson, P., Nyström, B. & Lindhe, J. (2004). The long-term effect of a plaque control program on tooth mortality, caries and periodontal disease in adults. Results after 30 years of maintenance. *Journal of Clinical Periodontology* **31**, 749–757.

Bergenholtz, G. & Nyman, S. (1984). Endodontic complications following periodontal and prosthetic treatment of patients with advanced periodontal disease. *Journal of Periodontology* **55**, 63–68.

Cortellini, P., Pini-Prato, G.P. & Tonetti, M.S. (1995). The modified papilla preservation technique. A new surgical approach for interproximal regenerative procedures. *Journal of Periodontology* **66**, 261–266.

Cortellini, P., Pini-Prato, G.P. & Tonetti, M.S. (1999). The simplified papilla preservation flap. A novel surgical approach for the management of soft tissues in regenerative procedures. *International Journal of Periodontics and Restorative Dentistry* **19**, 589–599.

Kinane, D.F., Peterson, M. & Stathoupoulou, P.G. (2006). Environmental and other modifying factors of the periodontal diseases. *Periodontology 2000* **40**, 107–119.

Lang, N.P., Pjetursson, B.E., Tan, K., Brägger, U., Egger, M. & Zwahlen, M. (2004). A systematic review of the survival and complication rates of fixed partial dentures (FPDs) after an observation period of at least 5 years. II. Combined tooth-implant supported FPDs. *Clinical Oral Implants Research* **15**, 643–653.

Lang, N.P. & Tonetti, M.S. (2003). Periodontal risk assessment (PRA) for patients in supportive periodontal therapy (SPT). *Oral Health and Preventive Dentistry* **1**, 7–16.

Lindhe, J. & Nyman, S. (1975). The effect of plaque control and surgical pocket elimination on the establishment and maintenance of periodontal health. A longitudinal study of periodontal therapy in cases of advanced disease. *Journal of Clinical Periodontology* **2**, 67–79.

Lulic, M., Brägger, U., Lang, N.P., Zwahlen, M. & Salvi, G.E. (2007). Ante's (1926) law revisited. A systematic review on survival rates and complications of fixed dental prostheses (FDPs) on severely reduced periodontal tissue support. *Clinical Oral Implants Research* **18** (Suppl 3), 63–72.

Nyman, S. & Lindhe, J. (1979). A longitudinal study of combined periodontal and prosthetic treatment of patients with advanced periodontal disease. *Journal of Periodontology* **50**, 163–169.

Nyman, S., Lindhe, J. & Rosling, B. (1977). Periodontal surgery in plaque-infected dentitions. *Journal of Clinical Periodontology* **4**, 240–249.

Nyman, S., Rosling, B. & Lindhe, J. (1975). Effect of professional tooth cleaning on healing after periodontal surgery. *Journal of Clinical Periodontology* **2**, 80–86.

Rosling, B., Nyman, S. & Lindhe, J. (1976a). The effect of systematic plaque control on bone regeneration in infrabony pockets. *Journal of Clinical Periodontology* **3**, 38–53.

Rosling, B., Nyman, S., Lindhe, J. & Jern, B. (1976b). The healing potential of the periodontal tissues following different techniques of periodontal surgery in plaque-free dentitions. A 2-year clinical study. *Journal of Clinical Periodontology* **3**, 233–250.

Chapter 32

Treatment Planning for Implant Therapy in the Periodontally Compromised Patient

Jan L. Wennström and Niklaus P. Lang

Prognosis of implant therapy in the periodontally compromised patient, 675
Strategies in treatment planning, 676
Treatment decisions – case reports, 676
  Posterior segments, 676

Tooth versus implant, 679
Aggressive periodontitis, 680
Furcation problems, 682
Single-tooth problem in the esthetic zone, 683

The use of dental implants for replacement of missing teeth is a viable option in the rehabilitation of the periodontally compromised patient, and certainly the availability of this treatment option may also influence our decisions regarding the preservation of teeth with varying degrees of periodontal tissue destruction.

Prognosis of implant therapy in the periodontally compromised patient

Global data on survival rates of dental implants indicate a rather low incidence of implant loss. The question is, however, whether the long-term prognosis for implants is better than that for teeth. In a systematic review by Berglundh et al. (2002), including 16 studies reporting data on implant-supporting fixed partial dentures (FPDs), the overall 5-year failure rate was calculated as about 5%. In the few studies that included a follow-up of 10 years the figure for implant loss was about 10%. It should be noted, however, that these studies did not specifically address the prognosis of implant therapy in periodontally compromised patients. Hardt et al. (2002) reported from a 5-year study that 8% of the implants were lost in patients who at time of implant placement presented advanced loss of periodontal support at their natural teeth. The corresponding figure in patients without periodontal tissue destruction was only 3% (Table 32-1). In the periodontally compromised patients most of the

Table 32-1 Proportion (%) of implants lost in relation to experience of destructive periodontal disease

Authors	Follow-up (years)	No history of destructive periodontal disease (%)	History of destructive periodontal disease (%)
Hardt et al. (2002)	5	3.3	8.0
Karoussis et al. (2003)	10	3.5	9.5

implants that were lost were so-called late failures. Furthermore, after 5 years 64% of the periodontally compromised patients showed a mean bone loss at the implants of >2 mm compared to only 24% among the non-compromised patients. Karoussis et al. (2003) found a failure rate of 10% after 10 years in patients that had been treated for periodontitis before implant placement, compared to 4% in patients who had received implant therapy because of tooth loss for reasons other than periodontal disease. The data reported above indicate that there is an increased risk for implant failure in individuals susceptible to periodontitis.

A question of concern in relation to treatment decisions in a periodontally compromised patient is whether the failure rate of implants is different from that of teeth. In order to give an answer to this

Table 32-2 Proportion (%) of teeth lost in patients treated for advanced destructive periodontal disease and maintained in supportive care programs

Authors	Mean follow-up (years)	Percentage of teeth lost	Percentage of teeth lost per 10 years
Lindhe & Nyman (1984)	14	2.3	1.6
Yi et al. (1995)	15	8	5
Rosling et al. (2001)	12	1.9	1.6
König et al. (2002)	12	3.1	2.6
Karoussis et al. (2004)	10	5	5

question we have to know the incidence of tooth loss in periodontally treated patients. Based on data from studies involving patients that have been treated for advanced periodontal disease and thereafter been provided with regular supportive periodontal therapy (SPT), the average incidence of tooth loss during a 10-year period can be estimated to be between 2 and 5% (Table 32-2). These figures, in comparison with the data for implant loss presented above, indicate that the prognosis for long-term survival of implants is not better than that of properly treated periodontitis-affected teeth. Furthermore, evidence is accumulating that suggests that longitudinal bone loss at implants is positively correlated with periodontal disease susceptibility and that implant therapy in the periodontally compromised patient may not be as successful as the global data for implant therapy in general has indicated.

Strategies in treatment planning

A comprehensive clinical and radiographic examination forms the basis for the treatment planning of the periodontally compromised patient. In relation to implant therapy, careful risk assessments should also be made (see Chapter 30) and additional radiographic examinations may be required (see Chapter 28). The goal of the treatment is to satisfy the patient's demands regarding chewing comfort and esthetics, with a favorable long-term prognosis of the restoration. The use of implants as a means to restore chewing function and esthetics in the periodontitis-susceptible patient has to be carefully evaluated in relation to the patient's standard of infection control. In partially dentate patients with remaining periodontal lesions, implants are rapidly colonized by periodontal pathogens, which indicates that periodontal pockets may act as reservoirs for microbial colonization of implants (see Chapter 10). Since there is no evidence that the host response to the microbial challenge is altered when a tooth is substituted with

an implant, it should be anticipated that a periodontitis-susceptible individual with improper infection control will face similar risk for disease-induced bone loss at implants and teeth.

Elimination of periodontitis lesions before implant placement and the establishment of a high standard of infection control are consequently decisive factors for the success of implant therapy. Regular recalls for supportive care should be scheduled after the completion of the therapy (see Chapter 59). Provided such a treatment program is adhered to, the long-term success of implant therapy in the periodontally compromised patient may not deviate from that in a non-susceptible patient (Baelum & Ellegaard 2004; Wennström et al. 2004).

Treatment decisions – case reports

Posterior segments

In the periodontally compromised patient the posterior segments of the dentition are usually those that are most severely affected by the disease and tooth loss. Figure 32-1 shows the clinical and radiographic status of a 53-year-old male following the completion of basic periodontal therapy for the establishment of infection control. Following periodontal treatment, the patient, originally diagnosed with severe chronic periodontitis, demonstrated a high standard of self-performed infection control and all lesions in the periodontal tissues have now been resolved. Because of the severity of the periodontal destruction, remaining teeth posterior to the canines in the maxilla as well as one remaining mandibular molar had to be removed. Hence, the dentition is markedly reduced, not only with regard to the number of teeth but also in terms of the amount of remaining periodontal support. From a chewing comfort point of view the patient is in need of prosthetic rehabilitation, particularly in the posterior segments of the maxilla. The treatment options available include (1) a removable prosthesis or (2) implant-supported FPDs. Considering that the remaining teeth show slightly increased mobility, the treatment alternative involving implant-supported FPDs seems most appropriate. In addition, the patient would if possible prefer to have fixed prosthetic reconstructions.

Clinical and radiographic evaluation of the posterior jaw segments of the maxilla revealed that two implants might be placed in quadrant 1 between the canine and the anterior border of the maxillary sinus, while the dimension of the bone inferior of the sinus was judged inadequate for placement of implants (Fig. 32-1b,c). If the implant in position 15 was placed along the anterior wall of the sinus cavity and was angulated slightly distally, space might be available to insert a pontic between the two implants and to provide the patient with a three-unit FPD. In the quadrant 2, the bone dimensions were more

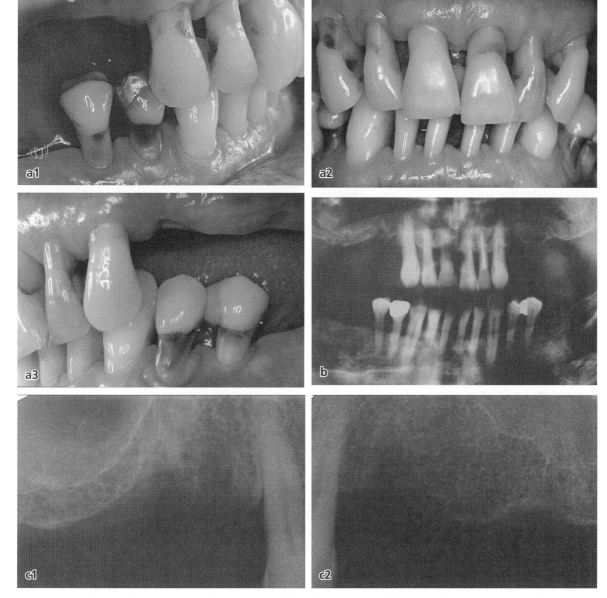

Fig. 32-1 (a–c) A 53-year-old male patient (H.L.) with periodontally compromised dentition. Clinical and radiographic status after periodontal treatment and establishment of infection control.

favorable and it was judged feasible to install three implants. Hence, by providing the patient with two three-unit implant-supported FPDs in the posterior segments of the maxilla a premolar occlusion could be established. The patient considered this treatment solution to be satisfactory with regard to his demands for improved chewing function. He had no requests for improved esthetics in the anterior segments, most likely because of a low lip line and because he only exposed the incisial half of the crown when smiling.

Figure 32-1d–f shows the outcome of the restorative treatment. In order to further improve the patient's chewing comfort a single implant was inserted in the left side of the mandible, after the second premolar had been tilted mesially. After completion of the restorative treatment the patient was enrolled in a maintenance care program, including

recalls once every 6 months to secure a high standard of infection control and to provide preventive means to reduce the risk for development of root caries. The 10-year follow-up status (Fig. 32-1g–h) reveals healthy marginal tissues and no loss of supporting structures, neither at the implants nor at the teeth. The standard of self-performed infection control has been excellent throughout the follow-up period.

In conclusion: The treatment outcome in this case clearly illustrates that the periodontitis-susceptible patient can be successfully treated with the use of implants and without signs of peri-implant bone loss over time, provided proper infection control is established and maintained. The recall visits for supportive therapy must include careful evaluation of both the periodontal and the peri-implant tissues for detection of signs of pathology, and proper decisions regarding indicated treatment (see Chapter 59).

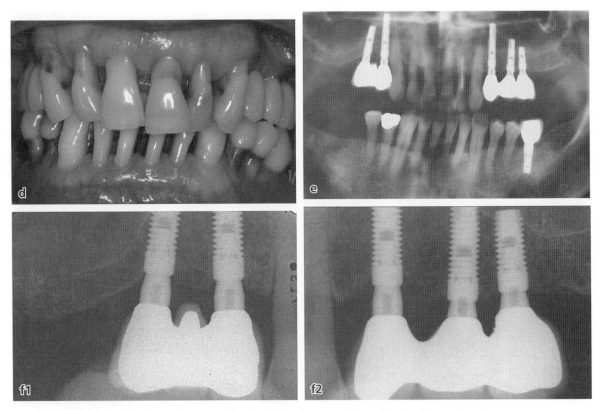

Fig. 32-1 (d–f) Clinical and radiographic status of patient H.L. after completion of the implant treatment.

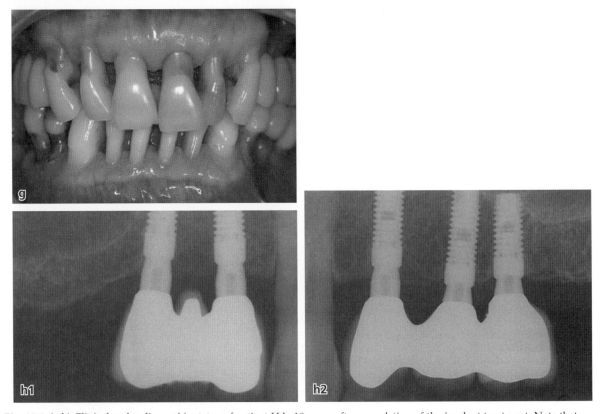

Fig. 32-1 (g,h) Clinical and radiographic status of patient H.L. 10 years after completion of the implant treatment. Note that there is no loss of bone support at the implants.

Tooth versus implant

Our treatment decisions regarding implant therapy or advanced periodontal therapy often relate to a single tooth. Figure 32-2(a,b) illustrates such a case. A 67-year-old woman presents with a localized advanced periodontal lesion at an abutment tooth in a three-unit FPD. The FPD is about 15 years old and the patient has no esthetic or functional complaints with regard to the FPD. Tooth 15 has a 10 mm deep pocket at the mesial aspect. The pocket is associated with a wide angular bone defect, and the tooth is positioned with its root in close proximity to the anterior wall of the maxillary sinus. If the tooth is extracted one may anticipate a marked remodeling of the ridge in the area, and the amount of bone available in the region might become insufficient for

implant placement to support a new FPD, unless sinus elevation and bone grafting procedures are performed.

The question in the treatment planning with regard to tooth 15 is whether there is a reasonable chance to save 15 and maintain the FPD with periodontal therapy, or should the tooth be extracted and implants placed to support a new FPD? Considering the great functional value of the tooth, it was decided to perform flap elevation and to evaluate the potential for tissue regeneration. Following debridement (Fig. 32-2c), it was observed that the defect was wide and had the morphology of a combined one-/two-/three-wall defect. A regenerative approach (application of enamel matrix proteins; see Chapter 43) was selected. The healing resulted in 6 mm gain in clinical attachment level and radiographic bone fill. The amount of

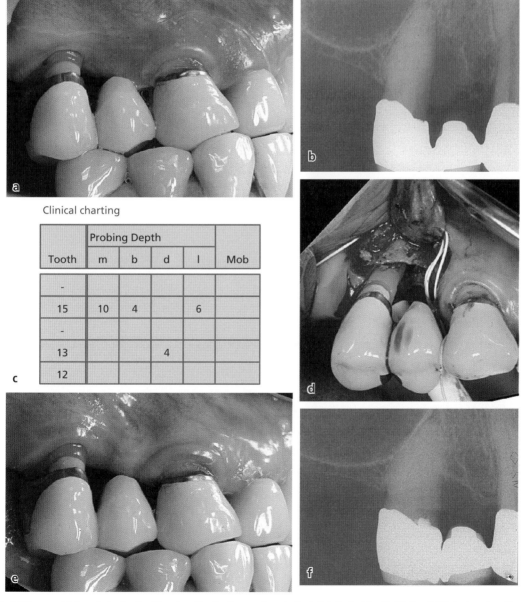

Clinical charting

Tooth	Probing Depth				Mob
	m	b	d	l	
-					
15	10	4		6	
-					
13			4		
12					

Fig. 32-2 A 67-year-old female patient with a localized advanced periodontal defect at tooth 15. (a–c) Clinical and radiographic status at the initial examination. (d) Flap elevated and the morphology of the defect can be determined as a wide combined one-/two-/three-wall defect. (e,f) Clinical and radiographic status 6 years after active treatment. Courtesy of Dr. G. Heden, Sweden.

soft tissue recession was minimal as seen from the 6-year follow-up documentation (Fig. 32-2d, e).

In conclusion, considering that implant therapy in this case most likely would have required sinus elevation and bone grafting to satisfy the patient's demands for esthetics and chewing function, the maintenance of 15 through proper periodontal therapy was of great benefit for the patient.

Aggressive periodontitis

Figure 32-3 shows a 22-year-old female patient diagnosed as a case of aggressive periodontitis. The first molar in the maxillary right quadrant and in the mandibular left quadrant have already been lost due to advanced periodontal destruction. The patient is asking for prosthetic replacement of the missing

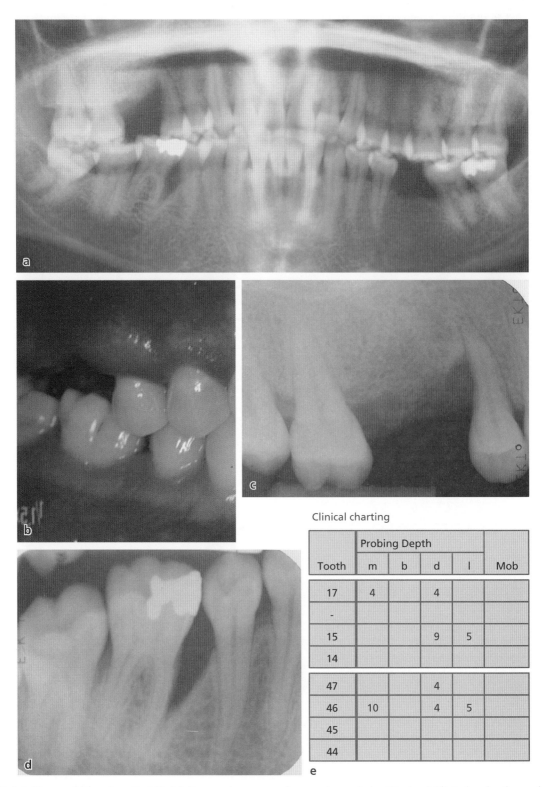

Clinical charting

Tooth	Probing Depth				Mob
	m	b	d	l	
17	4		4		
-					
15			9	5	
14					
47			4		
46	10		4	5	
45					
44					

Fig. 32-3 A 22-year-old female patient (A.A.) diagnosed as a case of Aggressive periodontitis. (a–e) Clinical and radiographic status at the initial examination. Localized advanced periodontal lesions are diagnosed at teeth 15 and 46. (f) Radiographic view after periodontal and implant treatment. (g–j) Clinical and radiographic status 12 years after active treatment.

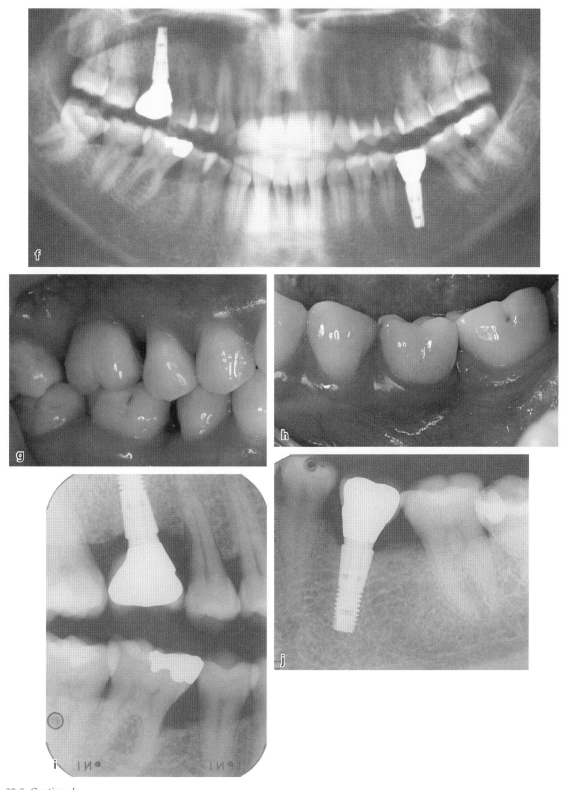

Fig. 32-3 *Continued*

teeth. The clinical examination also disclosed the presence of deep angular defects at the first molar in the mandibular right quadrant and at the second premolar in the maxillary right quadrant. It seems reasonable to plan for implant-supported restorations to replace the missing 16 and 36. The more difficult question, however, is related to the treatment of the periodontally compromised 15 and 46 (Fig. 32-3c,d).

Is it possible to successfully eliminate the periodontal lesions at 15 and 46 with a good long-term prognosis for the teeth? Or should the teeth be removed and replaced with implant-supported restorations? For tooth 15 extraction may be seen as a rational decision since implant therapy is planned in the region of 16. However, from an esthetic perspective it would be preferable to maintain 15 because the crown is intact and there is no loss of attachment or soft tissue height at the mesial aspect of the tooth (Fig. 32-3b).

Patients with aggressive periodontitis can be successfully treated, and this is well documented in the literature. Further, by applying a regenerative method in the surgical treatment of deep angular defects like those at 15 and 46, the chance of attachment gain of a magnitude of >4 mm is markedly increased (Giannobile *et al.* 2003; Murphy & Gunsolley 2003). Hence, the treatment decisions made in this case were to first establish proper infection control and then to apply a regenerative surgical approach (guided tissue regeneration) in the periodontal treatment of the lesions at 15 and 46.

Evaluation of the periodontal healing revealed closure of the pockets and *de novo* bone tissue formation. Single implant-supported restorations were subsequently performed to restore for the loss of teeth 16 and 36 (Fig. 32-3e). After completion of the active treatment the patient was assigned to a supportive care program with recall appointments once every 6 months. Fig. 32-3f–i illustrates the outcome

at 12 years post treatment. The regained height of the periodontal tissue support at 15 and 46 following the active treatment was maintained over the years, and optimal bone height is seen around the single implants. The good long-term prognosis in this case is attributed to a high quality of infection control and careful monitoring during the maintenance period.

Furcation problems

Even if the goal of the treatment of patients with periodontitis should be to preserve the teeth, there may be situations when this goal seems less meaningful in relation to the patient's need for prosthetic rehabilitation. Such a situation is illustrated in Fig. 32-4(a–d). The patient is missing the two premolars in the first quadrant and the molars present with advanced periodontal destruction and through-and-through furcation involvement (grade III). The patient requests a fixed restoration to substitute for the missing premolars. A possible treatment solution following periodontal therapy could include root sepa-

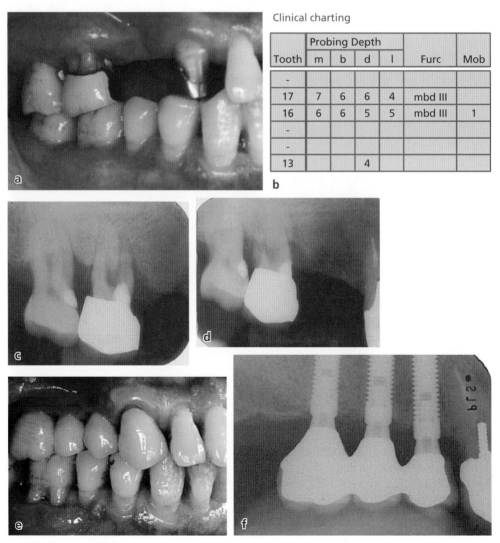

Clinical charting

Tooth	Probing Depth				Furc	Mob
	m	b	d	l		
-						
17	7	6	6	4	mbd III	
16	6	6	5	5	mbd III	1
-						
-						
13			4			

Fig. 32-4 A 52-year-old male patient with advanced periodontal destruction at remaining molars in the maxillary right quadrant. (a–d) Clinical and radiographic status at the initial examination. (e,f) Clinical and radiographic status 2 years after active treatment.

ration of the molars, after proper endodontic therapy, and the maintenance of, for example, the palatal roots of the molars to be used as posterior abutments in a fixed tooth-supported prosthesis 17 . . . 13. However, advanced inter-radicular periodontal destruction was identified by furcation probing, indicating that the palatal roots might not have enough remaining periodontal support in order to provide functional stability of a straight FPD (17 . . . 13). The clinical and radiographic examination reveals that the alveolar process in the premolar–molar region has proper dimensions for implant placement. An alternative treatment solution to satisfy the patient's demands for improved function and esthetics could therefore include implant placement to support a FPD.

The decision made in this case was to extract the two molars and, following proper periodontal treatment of the remaining dentition and establishment of adequate infection control, provide the patient with a three-unit implant-supported FPD and a single-crown restoration on tooth 13 (Fig. 32-4e,f). After completion of active treatment this patient was enrolled in a maintenance care program including recall appointments once every 4 months.

Single-tooth problem in the esthetic zone

Figure 32-5(a–e) illustrates the maxillary front tooth region of a 45-year-old female patient diagnosed with generalized chronic periodontitis. The right central incisor has severe periodontal destruction with probing pocket depths of 10–11 mm and obvious signs of inflammation at its distal and palatal surfaces. The tooth responded positively to sensibility testing. Interdental black triangles can be seen in the entire anterior tooth region because of approximal loss of periodontal attachment and soft tissue recession. Based on the results of the comprehensive examination, tooth 11 was judged to have a questionable prognosis, whereas it would be possible to resolve the periodontal lesions at the other anterior teeth by non-surgical means and improved self-performed infection control. Since the patient had a high lip line, potential recession of the soft tissue margins as a consequence of the treatment was a factor that had to be considered, particularly in relation to the treatment decision for the severely affected right central incisor. By regenerative therapy it might be possible to maintain the tooth, but will the treatment result in acceptable esthetics? The fact that the defect had a wide extension (buccally–lingually) and that the adjacent teeth presented with approximal attachment loss indicated that there was an obvious risk for loss of tissue height during healing following a surgical intervention. An alternative treatment approach could include the extraction of tooth 11 and to perform installation of a single implant. This alternative solution would also offer the possibility of correcting the position of the crown of 11. In discussing the different treatment alternatives and their con-

sequences with the patient, it was apparent that she preferred to have the position of the tooth corrected as part of the treatment. Hence, based on the careful analysis of the esthetic problems associated with the treatment of the tooth, the decision made was to extract the tooth and make an implant-supported restoration. By the use of the crown together with a portion of the root as a pontic, support to the surrounding soft tissues during initial healing of the extraction socket was provided (Fig. 32-5f).

Evaluation of the outcome of the cause-related phase of therapy, which included oral hygiene instructions, plaque control evaluations, and full-mouth pocket/root debridement, disclosed no remaining pathologically deepened pockets in the front tooth region (Fig. 32-5g). The radiographic evaluation of the extraction site 2 months after the removal of 11 (Fig. 32-5h) showed a preserved bone height at the neighboring approximal tooth sites and gain of bone in the extraction socket. Clinically only minor changes had taken place in the position of the soft tissue margin at the extraction site. A single implant was installed and after 3 months the prosthetic therapy was completed.

Following the completion of the active treatment, the patient was scheduled for supportive care every 6 months. Figure 32-5(i–k) shows the clinical and radiographic status at the 1-year follow-up examination. The position of the soft tissue margin is located at a similar level at the implant-supported crown and the contralateral incisor. Compared to the pre-treatment conditions (Fig. 32-5a), only minimal changes in the position of the soft tissue margins at the implant-borne restoration are evident. Overall some recession of the soft tissue margin has occurred as a consequence of the establishment of healthy marginal tissues.

In conclusion: Although it may be possible to maintain a tooth with severe local periodontal destruction by regenerative periodontal surgery, soft tissue recession as a consequence of the treatment may render the treatment outcome unsatisfactory from an esthetic perspective. Selection of a treatment approach involving tooth extraction and implant therapy instead of periodontal therapy should be based on a careful evaluation of the potential of the various treatment approaches to satisfy the patient's demands for esthetics.

Conclusions

- The prognosis for the properly treated periodontitis-affected tooth is at least as good as that for the implant.
- An increased risk of failure of implant therapy has been reported for periodontitis-susceptible patients.
- Proper infection control is a critical factor for the long-term success of implant therapy in the periodontally compromised patient.

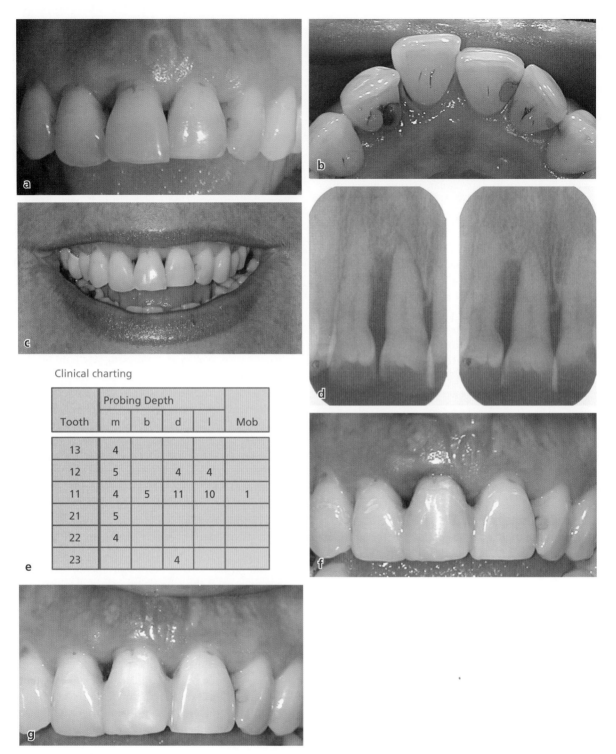

Clinical charting

Tooth	Probing Depth				Mob
	m	b	d	l	
13	4				
12	5		4	4	
11	4	5	11	10	1
21	5				
22	4				
23			4		

Fig. 32-5 A 45-year-old female patient with generalized chronic periodontitis. (a–e) Clinical and radiographic status of the maxillary anterior teeth at the initial examination. The right central incisor has severe periodontal destruction with probing pocket depths of 10–11 mm. (f) Tooth 11 was extracted and the tooth was reshaped and fixed to the neighboring teeth to support the soft tissues during the initial healing of the extraction socket. (g,h) Clinical and radiographic status 2 months post extraction when the implant placement surgery was performed. (i–k) Clinical and radiographic status 1 year after completion of the periodontal and implant treatment.

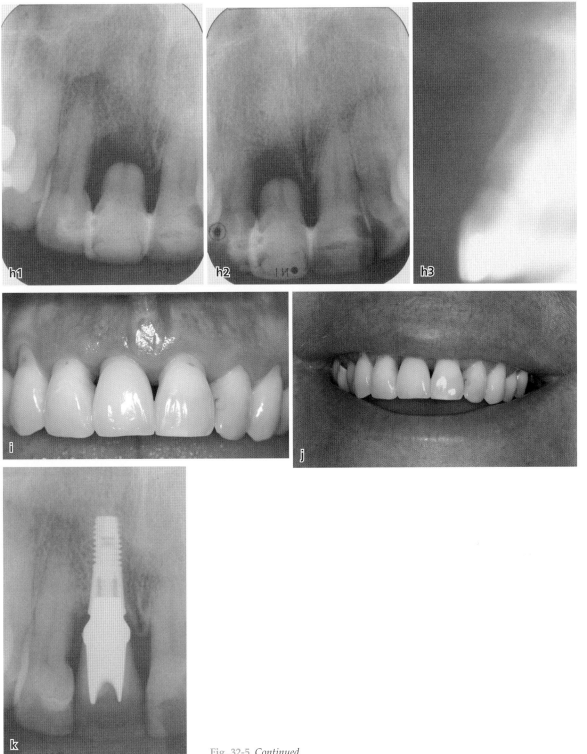

Fig. 32-5 *Continued*

References

Baelum, V. & Ellegaard, B. (2004). Implant survival in perio-dontally compromised patients. *Journal of Periodontology* **75**, 1404–1412.

Berglund, T., Persson, L. & Klinge, B. (2002). A systematic review of the incidence of biological and technical compli-cations in implant dentistry reported in prospective longi-tudinal studies of at least 5 years. *Journal of Clinical Periodontology* **29** (Suppl 3), 197–212.

Giannobile, W.V., Al-Shammari, K.F. & Sarment, D.P. (2003). Matrix molecules and growth factors as indicators of per-iodontal disease activity. *Periodontology 2000* **31**, 125–134.

Hardt, C.R.E., Gröndahl, K., Lekholm, U. & Wennström, J.L. (2002). Outcome of implant therapy in relation to experi-enced loss of periodontal bone support. A retrospec-tive 5-year study. *Clinical Oral Implants Research* **13**, 488–494.

Karoussis, I.K., Salvi, G.E., Heitz-Mayfield, L.J.A., Hämmerle, C.H.F. & Lang, N.P. (2003). Long-term implant prognosis in patients with and without a history of chronic periodontitis: a 10-year prospective cohort study of the ITI® Dental Implant System. *Clinical Oral Implants Research* **14**, 329–339.

Karoussis, I.K., Müller, S., Salvi, G.E., Heitz-Mayfield, L.J.A., Brägger, U. & Lang, N.P. (2004). Association between periodontal and peri-implant conditions: a 10-year prospective study. *Clinical Oral Implants Research* **15**, 1–7.

König, J., Plagmann, H.C., Ruuhling, A. & Kocher, T. (2002). Tooth loss and pocket probing depths in compliant periodontally treated patients: a retrospective analysis. *Journal of Clinical Periodontology* **29**, 1092–1100.

Lindhe, J. & Nyman, S. (1984). Long-term maintenance of patients treated for advanced periodontal disease. *Journal of Clinical Periodontology* **11**, 504–514.

Murphy K.G. & Gunsolley, J.C. (2003). Guided tissue regeneration for the treatment of periodontal intrabony and furcation defects. A systematic review. *Annals of Periodontology* **8**, 266–302.

Rosling, B., Serino, G., Hellström, M.K., Socransky, S.S. & Lindhe, J. (2001). Longitudinal periodontal tissue alterations during supportive therapy. Findings from subjects with normal and high susceptibility to periodontal disease. *Journal of Clinical Periodontology* **28**, 241–249.

Wennström, J.L., Ekestubbe, A., Gröndahl, K., Karlsson, S. & Lindhe, J. (2004). Oral rehabilitation with implant-supported fixed partial dentures in periodontitis-susceptible subjects. A 5-year prospective study. *Journal of Clinical Periodontology* **31**, 713–724.

Yi, S.W., Ericsson, I., Carlsson, G.E. & Wennström, J.L. (1995). Long-term follow-up of cross-arch fixed partial dentures in patients with advanced periodontal destruction. Evaluation of the supporting tissues. *Acta Odontologica Scandinavica* **53**, 242–248.

Chapter 33

Systemic Phase of Therapy

Niklaus P. Lang and Hans-Rudolf Baur

Introduction, 687
Protection of the dental team and other patients against infectious
  diseases, 687
Protection of the patient's health, 688
Prevention of complications, 688
  Infection, specifically bacterial endocarditis, 688
  Bleeding, 689

Cardiovascular incidents, 690
  Allergic reactions and drug interactions, 690
Systemic diseases, disorders or conditions influencing pathogenesis
  and healing potential, 690
Control of anxiety and pain, 690
Smoking counseling, 691

Introduction

The systemic phase of periodontal therapy should be concerned with general health implications of periodontal diseases and periodontal treatment. While the former aspects are described in Chapters 12, 13, 16, and 21, the latter aspects are presented in this chapter.

The systemic phase of periodontal therapy is designed to protect the patient against unforeseen systemic reactions, to prevent complications affecting the general health of the patient and to protect the health care providers from (predominantly infectious) hazards in conjunction with the treatment of risk patients.

In order to adequately plan the systemic phase, results from a health questionnaire (Chapter 26) filled in by the patient in the waiting area, the family and social history, the general medical and, in particular, the smoking history have to be evaluated. Also, any extra- and intraoral findings pertinent to the patient's systemic health have to be considered.

The systemic phase of periodontal therapy encompasses:

- Precautions for protecting the general health of the dental team and other patients against infectious and contagious diseases
- Protection against potentially harmful systemic effects of routine therapy
- Making allowances for systemic diseases or disorders that may influence the etiology of the patient's periodontal conditions, the healing potential, and the systemic response to therapy
- Controlling anxiety and low pain threshold
- Risk assessment and considerations of systemic supportive therapy

- Smoking counseling and instituting tobacco use cessation programs.

Protection of the dental team and other patients against infectious diseases

As a rule, routine periodontal therapy should be postponed in a patient with an active contagious state of a disease until the patient has received adequate medical treatment. Given the fact that patients may not always be aware of such a state or that all manifestations of disease may have abated, but the patient may still be carrier of infectious agents, routine dental treatment should be carried out under special precautions against transmission of the most serious diseases being transmitted orally. These include infectious hepatitis (Levin et al. 1974), HIV infection, and venereal diseases (Chue 1975). Hygiene in the dental office, therefore, has to address the most contagious level of infective agents, the hepatitis virus, and cope with the prevention of the transmission of these infections. As a minimal precaution, the wearing of rubber gloves and mouth masks is strongly recommended for all dental therapy in all patients. Also protective glasses for both the therapist and the patient should be worn during procedures generating aerosols.

Herpes simplex virus (Nahmias & Roizman 1973) and tuberculosis are other infectious diseases with a high transmission potential. Special precautions should be observed in patients with a recent history (2–3 years) of infectious hepatitis, although the dental team may be vaccinated against hepatitis. If the medical history and the oral examination reveal that the patient may have overt or hidden systemic disease, she/he should be referred for medical examination prior to enrolling the patient into comprehensive periodontal therapy.

Protection of the patient's health

A number of systemic conditions may affect treatment planning, although there may be no direct relevance in the pathogenesis and healing potential of periodontal lesions. Since over 50% of all patients over 40 years of age may have systemic conditions or take medications affecting periodontal therapy, these aspects have to be carefully appraised prior to instituting therapy.

For patients with life-threatening systemic conditions, such as coronary insufficiency or hypertensive heart disease, the patient's physician should be consulted about appropriate patient management and whether treatment should be performed in a hospital or clinic rather than a private practice setting. If the dental office is considered to be the adequate environment for treating these patients, short appointments should be planned and treatment performed with complete pain control using local anesthesia without any or with minimal vasoconstrictive drugs.

Prevention of complications

The complications most commonly encountered in the dental office are:

- Infection
- Bleeding
- Cardiovascular incidents
- Allergic reactions.

These may be prevented if appropriate precautions are taken. Hence, gaining awareness of possible complications from a medical history is an important step for treatment planning and total patient care.

Infection, specifically bacterial endocarditis

Patients with cardiac disease or disorders involving the endocardium are susceptible to endocarditis as a result of blood-borne infection. Such conditions include rheumatic heart disease, congenital valvular heart defects, aortic valvular diseases, and collagen diseases involving the endocardium. In addition, patients wearing prosthetic heart appliances belong to this risk group.

The major procedures thought to be the cause of bacterial endocarditis are extractions and scaling and/or root planing leading to significant bleeding and possible bacteremia (Durack 1995). Hence, it is not surprising that national societies have issued guidelines for antibiotic prophylaxis against bacterial endocarditis (USA: Dajani *et al.* 1997; UK: Gould *et al.*

2006; FDI, 1987). The common belief is that a bacteremia occurs only when dental procedures cause bleeding and does not occur when there is no bleeding. Hence, procedures such as extractions, root instrumentation, and periodontal and implant surgical procedures would require antibiotic prophylaxis, while for example the placement of fillings does not. This hypothesis was addressed in a study in children in which 14 various dentogingival manipulative procedures were evaluated (Roberts *et al.* 1997). It was clearly demonstrated that no relationship existed between the existence of bleeding and bacteremia. However, the number of oral organisms isolated from the blood where bleeding was present was statistically significantly higher than when there was no bleeding. It was concluded that the cumulative exposure to bacteremia is significantly greater from "everyday" procedures, when compared to dental procedures and hence, the cause of bacterial endocarditis may be attributable to such cumulative everyday exposures that are often thousands to millions of times greater than that occurring following surgical procedures, such as extractions of teeth (Roberts 1999).

Antibiotic prophylaxis to prevent bacterial endocarditis is predominantly based on anecdotal and circumstantial evidence suggesting a causal association between various procedures and bacteremia (Baltch *et al.* 1982). A case study, however, did not identify a link between endocarditis and dental treatment (Guntheroth 1984; Strom *et al.* 1998). Moreover, accumulating evidence suggests that bacteremia may easily be produced, e.g. by toothbrushing or chewing, rather than by single procedures causing bleeding. Hence, endocarditis causation has shifted from procedure-related bacteremia to cumulative or "everyday" bacteremia (Gould *et al.* 2006).

Indeed, a recent systematic review of the Cochrane Collaboration (Oliver *et al.* 2004) concluded that there was no conclusive evidence to support the use of prophylactic penicillin to prevent bacterial endocarditis in invasive dental procedures. This review did not find any randomized controlled clinical trials, any controlled clinical trials or any cohort studies. From a total of three case–control studies (Imperiale & Horowitz 1990; Van der Meer *et al.* 1992; Lacassin *et al.* 1995), only one study (Van der Meer *et al.* 1992) complied with the inclusion criteria. Details of 349 individuals who developed definite native-valve endocarditis in the Netherlands within a 2-year period were collected. Controls had not been diagnosed with endocarditis, but had one of the cardiac conditions and were outpatients of one of five hospitals. Controls were matched for age and had undergone dental procedure within 180 days of their interview. No significant protective effect of antibiotic prophylaxis was seen against endocarditis.

It has to be realized, however, that clinicians feel bound by guidelines and medico-legal considerations to provide antibiotic prophylaxis rather than by the best scientific evidence available. Ethically, practitio-

Table 33-1 Recommendations of the British Society for Antimicrobial Chemotherapy (BSAC) for prophylaxis of bacterial endocarditis

Population	Age			Timing of dose before procedure
	>10 years	≥5 to <10 years	<5 years	
General	Amoxicillin 3 g *per os*	Amoxicillin 1.5 g *per os*	Amoxicillin 750 mg *per os*	1 hour
Allergic to penicillin	Clindamycin 600 mg *per os*	Clindamycin 300 mg *per os*	Clindamycin 150 mg *per os*	1 hour
Allergic to penicillin and unable to swallow capsules	Azithromycin 500 mg *per os*	Azithromycin 300 mg *per os*	Azithromycin 200 mg *per os*	1 hour

From Gould *et al.* (2006).
Where a course of treatment involves several visits, the antibiotic regimen should alternate between amoxicillin and clindamycin.
Pre-operative mouth rinse with chlorhexidine gluconate 0.2% (10 ml for 1 minute).

Table 33-2 British Society for Antimicrobial Chemotherapy (BSAC) Prevention of Infective Endocarditis Guidelines Information for Patients and Parents February 2006

A BSAC group of experts has spent a lot of time carefully looking at whether dental treatment procedures are a possible cause of infective endocarditis (IE) (sometimes called bacterial endocarditis (BE)), which is infection of the heart valve.

After a very detailed analysis of all the available evidence they have concluded that there is no evidence that dental treatment procedures increase the risk of these infections.

Therefore, it is recommended that the current practice of giving patients antibiotics before dental treatment be stopped for all patients with cardiac abnormalities, except for those who have a history of healed IE, prosthetic heart valves and surgically constructed conduits.

The main reasons for this are the lack of any supporting evidence that dental treatment leads to IE and the increasing worry that administration of antibiotics may lead to other serious complications such as anaphylaxis (severe allergy) or antibiotic resistance.

The advice from the BSAC is that patients should concentrate on achieving and keeping a high standard of oral and dental health, as this does reduce the risk of endocarditis. Help for this will be provided by your Dental Professional.

British Society for Antimicrobial Chemotherapy (BSAC), 2 February 2006

ners need to discuss the potential benefits and harms of antibiotic prophylaxis with the patients and their cardiologists before the decision is made about administration (Oliver *et al.* 2004). Considering the change in paradigms regarding bacterial endocarditis, a task force of the British Society for Antimicrobial Chemotherapy has recently published new guidelines (Gould *et al.* 2006) (Table 33-1). According to these, the practice of giving patients antibiotics is reserved for those patients with a history of healed bacterial endocarditis, prosthetic heart valves, and surgically constructed conduits, while patients with cardiac abnormalities should no longer receive antibiotic prophylaxis before dental procedures. A patient information form has also been published (Table 33-2).

Bleeding

Due consideration must be given to patient on anticoagulant medication or patients on preventive anticoagulant drugs such as salicylates. For the first group of patients, a consultation with the patient's physician is indispensable. Especially prior to periodontal or implant surgical procedures, temporary adjustment of the intake of anticoagulant medication may have to be initiated in cooperation with the phy-

sician. Careful planning and timing of these procedures is mandatory.

Preventive anticoagulant therapy does not generally create problems for routine dental therapy, including surgical procedures, although consultation with the patient's physician still is advisable.

Individuals with known cirrhosis of the liver, or even patients with high alcohol consumption over many years without diagnosed cirrhosis, are at a potential risk for bleeding complications during periodontal and/or implant surgery, as their clotting mechanisms may be affected (Nichols *et al.* 1974). Again, medical consultation is recommended prior to periodontal treatment of such patients.

Extra precautions against bleeding should be taken when treating patients with any kind of blood dyscrasia or hemophilia. Following mandatory consultation with the patient's physician, it is recommended to render treatment in small segments (only a few teeth being instrumented at each visit) and to apply periodontal dressings over the treated area, even if the treatment only consisted of root instrumentation. With systematic periodontal treatment and institution of efficacious oral hygiene measures, the annoying symptom of oral bleeding can often be controlled irrespective of the patient's bleeding disorder.

Cardiovascular incidents

Cardiac patients are often treated with anticoagulants and, hence, may develop bleeding problems (as indicated above), especially if given drugs (e.g. aspirin, indomethacin, sulfonamide, tetracycline) that interact with coagulation. Other cardiovascular drugs (antihypertensive, anti-arrhythmic, diuretic) are often used in these patients which may increase the danger of hypotensive episodes during dental treatment.

Stress associated with dental procedures may precipitate anginal pain or congestive heart failure in patients with cardiovascular disease. Therefore, every effort should be made to keep procedures short and control anxiety and pain in this patient population.

Allergic reactions and drug interactions

Full knowledge of the patient's known allergies and the medications administered is essential before any drug is prescribed, administered or used during treatment. The most common allergic reactions encountered in the dental office are allergies to some local anesthetics (Novocain®), penicillins, sulfa derivatives, and disinfectants, such as iodine. In case of known allergies, such drugs have to be avoided. A consultation with the patient's physician is advisable to discuss the possible administration of replacement drugs.

Many patients – over 90% over the age of 60 years – regularly take medications for various systemic conditions, special attention has to be devoted to possible drug interactions, especially in the elderly. Drugs prescribed as part of periodontal therapy or used during treatment may interfere with the effectiveness of drugs the patient is already taking or create hazardous or synergistic action with such drugs. Hence, no new drugs should be prescribed without fully understanding their possible interaction with drugs already in use. Dentists should never change an existing drug therapy without prior discussion and preferably written consent of the physician.

Many patients regularly take tranquilizers and antidepressant drugs that have the potential for summation and synergistic effects with drugs that may be used during periodontal therapy. Moreover, the interaction with and potentiation of these drugs with alcohol should be discussed with the patient.

Systemic diseases, disorders or conditions influencing pathogenesis and healing potential

All possible attempts should be made to alleviate the effects of systemic diseases, such as blood disorders and diabetes mellitus, as much as possible before definitive periodontal treatment is initiated. However,

cause-related therapy may easily be carried out and generally results in remarkable success even during active stages of these systemic conditions. How far the treatment plan should progress with respect to pocket reduction and/or regenerative procedures depends on the seriousness of the patient's systemic involvement and likewise, to a great extent, on the potential threat to the patient's health from incomplete periodontal therapy.

Diabetes control, as an example, may be facilitated by successful control of the periodontal infection (Grossi *et al.* 1997; Genco *et al.* 2005). Thus, periodontal treatment may have a beneficial effect on the systemic health of the patient (see Chapter 21). Palliative treatment of advanced periodontitis with furcation involvement and residual deep pockets that cannot be reduced should not be undertaken for such patients. Rather the involved teeth with repeated abscesses and pus formation should be extracted if needed to accomplish infection control.

Clinical experience indicates that the healing response of the periodontal tissues is as good in diabetic as in non-diabetic patients provided that the diabetes is fairly well controlled. However, juvenile diabetics may have angiopathic changes associated with a lowered resistance to infection that may require the use of antibiotics following periodontal or implant surgery. With controlled diabetes, premedication with antibiotics is not indicated. Hypoglycemia may become aggravated by the stress of periodontal surgery and, hence, precautions have to be taken to avoid hypoglycemic reactions in such patients.

Patients taking therapeutic doses of cortisone over a long period of time may yield considerable metabolic effects with systemic manifestations of a reduced rate of fibroblastic activity and hence, a lowered resistance to infection during wound healing. Nevertheless, such patients can be treated successfully by regular cause-related therapy with no significant delay in healing. The use of antibiotics is not recommended for these patients, unless there is a serious infectious condition in the mouth associated with the development of fever.

Control of anxiety and pain

Many patients interested in maintaining a healthy dentition do not regularly seek dental care because of anxiety and apprehension related to such treatment. Since modern dentistry offers a variety of effective means for controlling pain and apprehension, patients should no longer suffer from dental treatment. During history taking and the oral examination, the patient's profile regarding anxiety and pain thresholds should be explored.

Prior to therapy, it may be advisable to premedicate an apprehensive patient using diazepams (Benzodiazepine, Valium®, 2–5 mg) to be taken the night before, in the morning and half an hour before an extensive and/or surgical procedure. Painless dental care can be achieved by carefully applying local anesthetics.

Post-operative analgesic medication, such as non-steroidal anti-inflammatory drugs (NSAIDs) with analgesic and antipyretic properties are recommended. Diclofenac potassium, the active ingredient of Voltaren® Rapide, inhibits prostaglandin synthesis by interfering with the action of prostaglandin synthetase. Following any kind of periodontal and implant surgery, 50 mg twice daily of Voltaren® Rapide is administered for 3 days. In addition, further adjunctive pain killers (Mefenaminic acid, e.g. Ponstan®, 500 mg not more than every 6–8 hours) may be prescribed depending on the individual patient's need and pain threshold.

Favorable personality interactions between the patient, the therapist, and the entire office staff may contribute to the control of anxiety, but may require more time and consideration than that allocated to the routine patient.

Smoking counseling

Cigarette smoking constitutes the second most important risk factor in the etiology and pathogenesis of periodontal diseases after poor oral hygiene standards. A careful assessment of the patient's smoking history is therefore indispensable. Depending on the duration of the exposure to tobacco smoking, daily consumption, and the patient's periodontal status, smoking counseling has to be undertaken as one of the primary measures. In all patients that smoke, the contributory role of tobacco consumption to the pathogenesis of periodontitis has to be addressed. Depending on the patient's response, smoking cessation programs may be instituted. Short-term interventions lasting 3–5 minutes using motivational interviewing techniques (Chapter 34) may be included during the initial phase of periodontal therapy. If a heavy smoker is ready to quit the habit, professional cessation programs may be the appropriate measures to take. Smoking counseling is further discussed in Chapter 34.

Conclusions

The goals of the systemic phase of periodontal therapy are to appraise the aspects that may require protection of both the dental team and the systemic health of the patient. Infection control in the dental office plays a central role. Protecting the patient against presumptive complications, such as infection, especially bacterial endocarditis, bleeding, cardiovascular incidences, and allergies, requires in-depth knowledge of the patient's medical history and oral examination.

Bacterial endocarditis prophylaxis is nowadays reserved for those patients with a history of a healed bacterial endocarditis, prosthetic heart valves or surgically constructed conduits, while the use of antibiotics before dental treatment is not necessary for patients with cardiac abnormalities. Patients with systemic diseases such as diabetes mellitus or cardiovascular diseases usually are treated with a number of medications that may interact with drugs prescribed during periodontal therapy. Precautions should be taken, and consultation with the patient's physician prior to systematic periodontal therapy is recommended.

It has to be realized that periodontal treatment may have a beneficial effect on the systemic health of the patient as well. Glycemic control may be facilitated in diabetics if proper periodontal therapy is rendered.

Finally, smoking counseling is part of modern periodontal treatment owing to the fact that, after inadequate oral hygiene standards, cigarette smoking constitutes the second most important risk factor for periodontitis.

References

Baltch, A.L., Schaffer, C., Hammer, M.C., Sutphen, N.T., Smith, R.P., Conroy, J. & Shayegani, M. (1982). Bacteraemia following dental cleaning in patients with and without penicillin prophylaxis. *American Heart Journal* **104**, 1335–1339.

Chue, P.W.Y. (1975). Gonorrhoea – its natural history, oral manifestations diagnosis, treatment and prevention. *Journal of the American Dental Association* **90**, 1297–1301.

Dajani, A.S., Taubert, K.A., Wilson, W., Bolger, A.F., Bayer, A., Ferrieri, P., Gewitz, M.H., Shulman, S.T., Nouri, S., Newburger, J.W., Hutto, C., Pallasch, T.J., Gage, T.W., Levison, M.E., Peter, G. & Zuccaro, G. Jr. (1997). Prevention of bacterial endocarditis. Recommendations by the American Heart Association. *Journal of the American Medical Association* **227**, 1794–1801.

Durack, D.T. (1995). Prevention of infective endocarditis. *New England Journal of Medicine* **332**, 38–44.

Federation Dentaire Internationale (1987). Guideline for antibiotic prophylaxis of infective endocarditis for dental patients with cardiovascular disease. *International Dental Journal* **37**, 235–236.

Genco, R.J., Grossi, S.G., Ho, A., Nishimura, F. & Murayama, Y. (2005). A proposed model linking inflammation to obesity, diabetes, and periodontal infections. *Journal of Periodontology* **76** (Suppl), 2075–2084.

Gould, F.K., Elliott, T.S.J., Foweraker, J., Fulford, M., Perry, J.D., Roberts, G.J., Sandoe, J.A.T. & Watkin, R.W. (2006). Guidelines of the prevention of endocarditis: report of the Working Party of the British Society of Antimicrobial Chemotherapy. *Journal of Antimicrobial Chemotherapy* **57**, 1035–1042.

Grossi, S.G., Skrepcinski, F.B., DeCaro, T., Robertson, D.C., Ho, A.W., Dunford, R.G. & Genco, R.J. (1997) Treatment of periodontal disease in diabetics reduces glycated hemoglobin. *Journal of Periodontology* **68**, 713–719.

Guntheroth, W. (1984). How important are dental procedures as a cause of infective endocarditis? *American Journal of Cardiology* **54**, 797–801.

Imperiale, T.F. & Horowitz, R.I. (1990). Does prophylaxis prevent post dental infective endocarditis? A controlled evaluation of protective efficacy. *American Journal of Medicine* **88**, 131–136.

Lacassin, F., Hoen, B., Leport, C., Selton-Suty, C., Delahaye F., Goulet, V., Etienne, J. & Briancon, S. (1995). Procedures associated with infective endocarditis in adults – a case control study. *European Heart Journal* **16**, 1968–1974.

Levin, M.L., Maddrey, W.C., Wands, J.R. & Mendeloff, A.L. (1974). Hepatitis B transmission by dentists. *Journal of the American Medical Association* **228**, 1139–1140.

Nahmias, A.J. & Roizman, B. (1973). Infection with herpes simplex viruses 1 and 2. Parts I, II, III. *New England Journal of Medicine* **289**, 667–674, 719–725, 781–789.

Nichols, C., Roller, N.W., Garfunkel, A. & Ship, I.I. (1974). Gingival bleeding: the only sign in a case of fibrinolysis. *Oral Surgery, Oral Medicine, Oral Pathology* **38**, 681–690.

Oliver, R., Roberts G.J. & Hooper, J. (2004). Penicillins for the prophylaxis of bacterial endocarditis in dentistry (Review). *The Cochrane Database of Systematic Reviews*. Issue 2. Art. No.: CD003813.pub2. DOI: 10.1002/14651858.CD003813.pub2. New York: John Wiley & Sons Ltd, 1–20.

Roberts, G.J., Holzel, H., Sury, M.R.J., Simmons, N.A., Gardner, P. & Longhurst, P. (1997). Dental bacteraemia in children. *Pediatric Cardiology* **18**, 24–27.

Roberts, G.J. (1999). Dentists are innocent! "Everyday" bacteraemia is the real culprit: a review and assessment of the evidence that dental surgical procedures are a principal cause of bacterial endocarditis in children. *Pediatric Cardiology* **20**, 317–325.

Strom, B.L., Abrutyn, E., Berlin, J.A., *et al.* (1998). Dental and cardiac risk factors for infective endocarditis. A population based, case-control study. *Annals of Internal Medicine* **129**, 761–769.

Van der Meer, J.T.M., van Wijk, W., Thompson, J., Valkenburg, H.A. & Michel, M.F. (1992). Efficacy of antibiotic prophylaxis for the prevention of native-valve endocarditis. *Lancet* **339**, 135–139.

Part 11: Initial Periodontal Therapy (Infection Control)

34 Motivational Interviewing, 695
    Christoph A. Ramseier, Delwyn Catley, Susan Krigel, and Robert A. Bagramian

35 Mechanical Supragingival Plaque Control, 705
    Fridus Van der Weijden, José J. Echeverría, Mariano Sanz, and Jan Lindhe

36 Chemical Supragingival Plaque Control, 734
    Martin Addy and John Moran

37 Non-surgical Therapy, 766
    Noel Claffey and Ioannis Polyzois

Part III: Initial Periodontal Therapy (Infection Control)

Chapter 34

Motivational Interviewing

Christoph A. Ramseier, Delwyn Catley, Susan Krigel, and Robert A. Bagramian

The importance of behavioral change counseling in
    periodontal care, 695
Development of motivational interviewing, 696
    History of motivational interviewing, 697
    What is motivational interviewing?, 697
Evidence for motivational interviewing, 697
Implementation of motivational interviewing into the periodontal
    treatment plan, 698

Key principles of motivational interviewing, 698
Basic communication skills, 698
Giving advice, 700
Case examples for oral hygiene motivation, 700
    Oral hygiene motivation 1, 700
    Oral hygiene motivation 2, 701
Case example for tobacco use cessation, 702

The importance of behavioral change counseling in periodontal care

Periodontal health is supported by appropriate behaviors such as regularly self-performed plaque control, avoidance of tobacco, and consumption of a healthy diet. Inadequate oral hygiene, tobacco use, and uncontrolled diet in type 2 diabetes mellitus, on the other hand, are shown to have a destructive impact on periodontal tissues. The prevention and control of periodontal disease needs to be addressed on both the population and the individual level. Efficient public health approaches consider the entire population and focus on health issues that present the largest burden within a community. The dental community involved with oral health care should gain an understanding of the health effects of inappropriate behaviors in order to successfully target prevention and disease control. As a consequence, services for primary and secondary prevention on an individual level oriented towards the change of inappropriate behavior become a professional responsibility for all oral health care providers.

Data from epidemiologic studies consistently reveal the prevalence of periodontal disease in more than 50% of the adult population (Albandar *et al.* 1999; Albandar 2002). In addition to the causal relationship with dental biofilms, a positive association with tobacco use has been documented (Bergstrom 1989; Haber *et al.* 1993; Tomar & Asma 2000). Tobacco use contributes to the global burden of public health with almost one third of the adult population using various forms of tobacco and an increasing number of annual deaths from tobacco-related diseases. Moreover, dietary excess has been shown to significantly impact chronic diseases including obesity, cardiovascular diseases, type 2 diabetes, cancer, osteoporosis, and oral diseases (Petersen 2003).

There is growing evidence that the patient's individual behavior is seen to be influential or even critical for the success of periodontal therapy; since the results of periodontal therapy appear to be limited in patients who especially lack appropriate behavior. In a recent literature review by Ramseier (2005) it was shown that second to plaque control, smoking cessation was the most important measure for the management of chronic periodontitis. Therefore, it appears to be reasonable in clinical concepts for periodontal care to (1) include assessments of patient behavior, and (2) if necessary apply effective behavior change counseling methods.

Traditional periodontal care includes the instruction of proper oral hygiene methods. In practice, as an example, a demonstration of a suitable toothbrushing method is given to the patient, followed by recommendations of both the frequency and the time spent per brushing. Past and recent studies on the effectiveness of oral hygiene instructions consistently revealed that the patient adherence to a proper daily oral hygiene regime generally remains poor (Johansson *et al.* 1984; Schuz *et al.* 2006). The reinforcement of oral hygiene habits through additional appointments can compensate somewhat for the ineffectiveness of one-time or repeated oral hygiene instructions. However, due to weak patient adherence, visits for supportive periodontal care are often cancelled, resulting in a lack of professional maintenance care and the potential recurrence of periodontal disease (Wilson *et al.* 1984; Demetriou *et al.* 1995; Schuz *et al.* 2006).

Unfortunately, many health education approaches seem to be inefficient in accomplishing long-term change, potentially leading to frustration of both the patient and the clinician. The following hypothetical dialogue between a clinician (Dr) and a patient (P) illustrates how using a directive advice-oriented method for behavior change counseling can lead to an unproductive conversation and little likelihood of change by the patient:

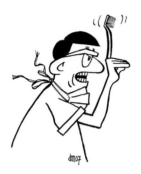

Dr   Are you flossing regularly?
P   Yes, but not as often as I should.
Dr   I strongly recommend that you floss every day. There are serious consequences if you don't floss frequently enough.
P   I know I should do it more often, but . . .
Dr   It is really important!
P   I know . . . . . . but I don't have the time!

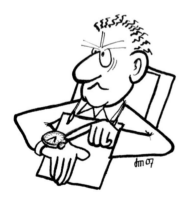

Since the clinician doesn't offer the patient a chance to discuss the reasons to floss as well as the patient's perceived barriers to flossing, the conversation reaches an impasse and behavior change will be unlikely. In certain cases, the patient may even be blamed for poor compliance and further oral health education may be seen to be pointless.

There is a shortage of evidence in both the dental and behavioral literature on effective methods for behavior counseling in periodontal care, in particular regarding:

- Individual oral hygiene instructions for optimal oral hygiene

- Effective tobacco use prevention and cessation counseling to help abstain from tobacco
- Appropriate dietary counseling for a healthy diet.

In order to get reliably effective outcomes in periodontal care, it may be necessary to apply different behavior change counseling methods for each individual behavior. According to the best available evidence for oral hygiene instructions, the repeated demonstration of a cleaning device may be applied, while for tobacco use cessation, in addition to pharmacotherapy, the method of the five As (ask, advise, assess, assist, arrange) may be used (Fiore 2000). Additionally, type 2 diabetic patients or patients with a high carbohydrate diet may be referred to nutritionists for dietary counseling. From a practical point of view, however, it may be complicated and even discouraging to approach the periodontal patient with a variety of different methods targeting the same purpose: establishing appropriate behavior to improve the outcomes of both periodontal therapy and long-term supportive periodontal care.

Hence, aiming for simplicity, it may be preferable to apply one single method for behavior change counseling in periodontal care that is shown to be effective in both primary and secondary prevention of oral diseases. This method should be:

- Based on the best available evidence
- Applicable to oral hygiene behavior, tobacco use prevention and cessation, and dietary counseling
- Suitable for implementation by the dental practice team in a cost-effective way.

Development of motivational interviewing

As discussed, health *education* efforts provided by practitioners are frequently ineffective in changing patient behavior. Considerable behavioral research suggests that the root of this common problem can be traced back to a false assumption inherent in the health education approach. Specifically, that behavior change is simply a function of a patient having the requisite knowledge or understanding, and that it is up to the practitioner to provide the relevant information. Motivational interviewing (MI), in contrast, is based on a different assumption of human behavior change. It assumes that the knowledge is insufficient to bring about behavior change and that, instead, sustained behavior change is much more likely when change is connected to something the individual values. In other words, motivation is elicited "from within the patient" rather than externally imposed upon the patient by a practitioner. In MI, the assumption is that individuals have "within them" their own reasons for changing and that the role of the practitioner is to elicit and reinforce these reasons.

MI originated in the field of addictive behavior but has increasingly been applied to a wide variety of other behavior change problems, including health behaviors such as tobacco use and diet and exercise (Burke *et al.* 2004; Hettema *et al.* 2005). MI principles and methods have also been specifically adapted for brief interventions in medical settings (Butler *et al.* 1999; Rollnick *et al.* 1999) and have recently been tested in a dental setting (Weinstein *et al.* 2006).

History of motivational interviewing

William Richard Miller, the originator of MI, developed the method in response to his observations regarding the treatment of patients with alcohol problems in the 1970s. The standard approach to the treatment of alcoholic patients was confrontational, and failure of treatment was attributed either to "denial", seen as a personality deficit on the part of the client, or the failure of the client to engage with the program (Miller 1983). In contrast, he observed that the research literature suggested that positive outcomes were mostly related to a strong bond or "therapeutic alliance" between the counselor and the patient. Miller began to test his empathy-centered treatments on problem drinkers and found that change was occurring more quickly than with traditional methods (Moyers 2004). This brief treatment which used the *therapeutic alliance* and *empathy* to engender the client's inherent motivation to change was first described in an article by Miller in Behavioural Psychotherapy (1983). Subsequently Miller met Stephen Rollnick, the co-founder of the MI method, who had been concentrating on ambivalence, or the extent to which the client envisioned the pros and cons of changing. Miller and Rollnick began to explore the use of language during MI, concentrating on the elicitation of client "change talk" to promote behavior change. In 1991, Miller and Rollnick published the first edition of *"Motivational Interviewing: Preparing People to Change Addictive Behaviors"* in which they provided a detailed description of the approach. Since then there has been an explosion in the research and application of MI with many researchers addressing the applicability of the method to addressing health behavior change (Resnicow *et al.* 2002).

What is motivational interviewing?

MI has been defined as "a client-centered, directive method for enhancing intrinsic motivation to change by exploring and resolving ambivalence" (Miller & Rollnick 2002). The client-centered element refers to the emphasis that is placed on understanding and working from the perspective of the patient and their view of what it means to make a behavior change. For example, rather than a clinician simply telling a patient about the benefits of quitting smoking (from the practitioner perspective), the practitioner invites the patient to describe *his or her own view* of the advantages and disadvantages of quitting continuing to smoke. Although the patient's perspective is central, because MI is also directive, the practitioner takes deliberate steps to facilitate a particular behavioral outcome. For example, without ignoring patient concerns about changing, the practitioner selectively reinforces and encourages elaboration of any patient statements that are oriented toward the possibility or benefits of making a change. By eliciting and elaborating upon the patient's own reasons for change the motivation for change that is fostered is intrinsic or internal, rather than externally imposed. This approach rests on the assumption that individuals are almost always ambivalent about changing their behavior (i.e., it is almost always the case that individuals can identify both pros and cons of changing). MI practitioners therefore attempt to enhance intrinsic reasons for change by facilitating an exploration and resolution of the patient's underlying ambivalence.

Evidence for motivational interviewing

Because MI was initially developed for the treatment of addictive behavior, particularly alcohol addiction, the bulk of empirical studies has been conducted in this area. Nevertheless, the explosion in the application (Hettema *et al.* 2005) of MI to other areas of behavior change has been sufficient that there are now four published meta-analyses (Burke *et al.* 2003, 2004; Hettema *et al.* 2005; Rubak *et al.* 2005), the more recent of which include more than 70 clinical trials. Generally, the meta-analyses indicate that MI-based interventions are at least equivalent to other active treatments and superior to no-treatment or placebo controls for problems involving addictive behavior (drugs, alcohol, and gambling), adoption of water purification/safety technology, diet and exercise, and treatment engagement, retention, and adherence. Effect sizes are on average in the small to medium range but are highly variable (Hettema *et al.* 2005). Of particular relevance to dental settings where only brief counseling is feasible, is that MI-based interventions are just as efficacious as alternative active interventions despite involving significantly less contact time, suggesting that MI may be a particularly efficient method of counseling (Burke *et al.* 2004). Rubak *et al.* (2005) report that in brief encounters of 15 minutes, 64% of studies showed an effect. In addition, when the intervention was delivered by physicians an effect was observed in approximately 80% of studies suggesting that it is feasible for professionals who are not counseling experts to deliver effectively MI in brief encounters.

Studies of MI for tobacco use cessation are also of particular relevance. Although fewer studies were available, the meta-analyses cited above did not find

MI to be efficacious for smoking cessation. Nevertheless, most of the smoking cessation studies can be criticized for various reasons, including not having procedures to ensure and document fidelity to MI principles by the interventionists (Colby *et al.* 1998; Butler *et al.* 1999; Stotts *et al.* 2002; Wakefield *et al.* 2004), testing the intervention with smokers who are already motivated to quit which may be counterproductive (Smith *et al.* 2001; Ahluwalia *et al.* 2006), and not providing sufficient guidance on *how* to quit once participants were motivated by MI (Butler *et al.* 1999; Okuyemi *et al.* 2007). On the positive side, these studies also show that MI leads to significantly more quit attempts (Wakefield *et al.* 2004; Borrelli *et al.* 2005); greater reductions in smoking level (Borrelli *et al.* 2005); greater advances in readiness to quit (Butler *et al.* 1999); greater self-reported abstinence in the previous 24 hours (Butler *et al.* 1999); and a lower rate of increased smoking among pregnant women who were smoking early in pregnancy (Tappin *et al.* 2005). Importantly, a recent study (published subsequent to the meta-analyses) of primary care patients has shown that three 20-minute sessions of MI delivered by family physicians can increase smoking cessation more than five-fold compared to brief advice (Soria *et al.* 2006). This study addressed many of the limitations of prior studies by recruiting a large proportion of smokers not necessarily ready to quit, and incorporating procedures to ensure fidelity to MI principles.

Another particularly relevant target behavior for oral health is dietary habits. As indicated, meta-analyses have found significant effects of MI for changing diet. Specifically, these studies have documented changes due to MI in overall dietary intake (Mhurchu *et al.* 1998), fat intake (Mhurchu *et al.* 1998; Bowen *et al.* 2002), carbohydrate consumption (Mhurchu *et al.* 1998), cholesterol intake (Mhurchu *et al.* 1998), body mass index (BMI) (Mhurchu *et al.* 1998), weight (Woollard *et al.* 1995), salt intake (Woollard *et al.* 1995), alcohol consumption (Woollard *et al.* 1995), and consumption of fruits and vegetables (Resnicow *et al.* 2001; Richards *et al.* 2006).

At the time of writing, there was only one published study focused on oral health. This study examined the effect of using MI compared to traditional health education for motivating 240 mothers of young children with high risk for developing dental caries to use dietary and non-dietary behaviors for caries prevention (Weinstein *et al.* 2004, 2006). An MI session and six follow-up phone calls over a year in addition to an educational pamphlet and video was more effective than the pamphlet and video alone in preventing new dental caries among the children after 2 years. This result is consistent with the results of the meta-analyses that have found MI to be efficacious for dietary change (Burke *et al.* 2003; Hettema *et al.* 2005).

In summary, there is generally a wealth of support for MI as an effective method of counseling for behav-ior change. MI has also been shown to be relatively efficient and has been successfully delivered by medical practitioners. In areas of specific relevance to oral health practitioners, MI has either already been shown to be efficacious or offers significant promise. Given the extraordinary explosion in the application of MI we anticipate that it will not be long before there will be many more studies specific to dental settings.

Implementation of motivational interviewing into the periodontal treatment plan

Key principles of motivational interviewing

Although MI methods and techniques provide a wealth of guidance of what to do and what not to do when counseling patients, Miller and Rollnick have emphasized that to be an effective MI practitioner it is more important to embody the underlying philosophy than to be able to apply the collection of techniques. They have identified four general principles that capture the underlying philosophy of the method. First, a practitioner should *express empathy* for the patient's behavior change dilemma. In other words, the practitioner should communicate acceptance of the patient's perspective, providing and *expressing* full acknowledgement of the patient's feelings and concerns. The second principle is to *develop discrepancy* between the patient's current behavior and how they would ideally like to behave to be consistent with their broader goals and values. For example, the goal of being strong or responsible, or a good spouse or parent, can often be linked to being healthy and suggest the need for improved health behaviors. The third principle is to *roll with resistance*. When patients argue against change there is a strong tendency to fall into the trap of providing counter arguments. As a result the patient expends all of their energy arguing against change which is precisely the opposite of what is desired, perhaps making them even less likely to change. MI practitioners therefore avoid arguing and instead use MI methods to "roll with resistance". The fourth principle is to *support self-efficacy* or the patient's confidence in their ability to make a change. Patients are unlikely to succeed in making a change even if they are motivated, when they don't know how or don't believe they can. MI practitioners therefore make efforts to enhance their patients' confidence through such means as expressing their belief in the patient's ability to change or pointing out past successes or steps in the right direction.

Basic communication skills

Implementing MI in a dental setting requires consideration of how to ensure the collaborative and

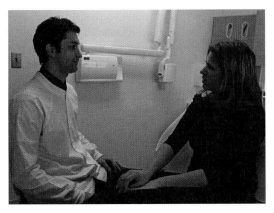

Fig. 34-1 Appropriate position for a conversation: the clinician is facing the patient on the same seating level.

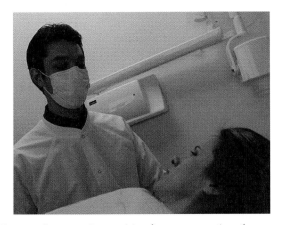

Fig. 34-2 Inappropriate position for a conversation: the clinician is wearing a face mask and is at a higher level than the supine patient.

empathic spirit of the method. Even such basic matters as how the patient and practitioner are seated can contribute to the patient feeling like they are truly being invited to engage in a dialogue as a partner (Fig. 34-1), rather than feeling they are simply to be the recipient of expert advice (Fig. 34-2).

There are four primary activities for the beginning stages of a brief MI session. These can be summarized with the acronym OARS, for **o**pen-ended questions, **a**ffirm the patient, **r**eflect, and **s**ummarize.

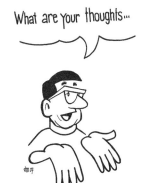

- *Ask open-ended questions.* Approaching the patient with multiple closed-ended questions (question

that will be answered with "yes" or "no") sets the patient's role to be a rather passive one. In contrast, open-ended questions invite thought, collaboration, and effort on the part of the patient. Example: "How do you feel about your smoking?"

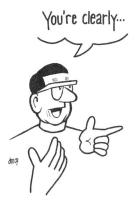

- *Affirm the patient.* It is human nature to presume a negative attitude, particularly when one's own behavior is coming under scrutiny. Acknowledging the patient's strengths and appreciation of his or her honesty will decrease defensiveness, increase openness, and the likelihood of change. Example: "You're telling me clearly why you're not very concerned about your toothbrushing and I appreciate that honesty."

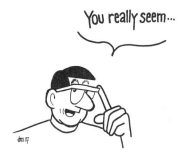

- *Reflect what the patient is communicating.* Reflection is the primary way to demonstrate empathy (ability to understand another person's perspective). Appropriate reflection includes the genuine effort to understand the patient's perspective. It (1) captures the underlying meaning of the patient's words, (2) is concise, (3) is spoken as an observation or a comment, and (4) conveys understanding rather than judgment. Example: "You really seem to have lost hope that you can ever really quit smoking."

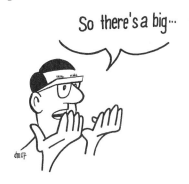

- *Summarize*. Summarizing the patient demonstrates interest, organizes the interview, and gets things back on track if necessary. It involves the compilation of the patient's thoughts on change mentioned during the counseling. Example: "So there's a big part of you that doesn't feel ready to change right now. You really enjoy smoking, but you have been a little worried by the way some people react when they find out that you smoke. Is that about right?"

Giving advice

Although we have highlighted the distinction between advice-oriented health education and MI in this chapter, it is important to recognize that at times it is appropriate to provide information to address patient's questions, misapprehensions, or lack of knowledge. The Motivational Interviewing Skill Code (Moyers *et al.* 2003), which is used to assess practitioner's adherence to principles of MI distinguishes between giving advice *without* permission, which is proscribed, and giving advice *with* permission, which is consistent with MI principles. In essence, it is consistent with MI to provide information when the patient is willing and interested in receiving it. Practitioners commonly err by providing advice too soon in an encounter with a patient, resulting in patients perceiving the practitioner as having an agenda that they are trying to "push". In contrast, it is common in MI practice to find that the process of eliciting the patient's perspective reveals gaps in knowledge, questions and concerns, and misapprehensions that the patient would appreciate receiving more information about. The practitioner can then provide particularly relevant information that is much more likely to be well received. Rollnick *et al.* (1999) have outlined a three-step process that serves as a useful framework for providing advice in an MI consistent style:

- Step 1: *elicit* the patient's readiness and interest in hearing the information. For example a practitioner might say to a patient "I have some information related to (that topic) that you may be interested in. Would you be interested in hearing more about that?"
- Step 2: *provide* the information in as neutral a fashion as possible. For example, a practitioner might say "Research indicates that. . . ." or "Many of my patients tell me that . . ." This allows factual information to be presented in a manner that supports the patient's autonomy.
- Step 3: *elicit* the patient's reaction to the information presented. Following up will often facilitate the patient to integrate the new information in a way that brings about a new perspective and increases motivation to change. Alternatively, following up may reveal further gaps in knowledge or misunderstandings that can be addressed. If a

patient "rejects" the information it is important not to get into a debate. It is generally better to simply acknowledge the patient's perspective with statements such as "This information doesn't fit with your experience" or "This information doesn't seem relevant to your situation" and then move on to a more productive area of conversation.

Case examples for oral hygiene motivation

Oral hygiene motivation 1

Using the following case example, MI is demonstrated in a dialogue for oral hygiene motivation between a periodontist (Dr) and a patient (P) diagnosed with chronic periodontitis at the beginning of periodontal therapy.

Dr   Would you mind if we talk about methods to improve your oral hygiene during and after your gum treatment?

P   No, I don't mind.

Dr   Good. Let me know a little bit about how you usually clean your teeth.

P   I usually brush once or twice a day.

Dr   So you brush your teeth regularly. What are you using when you clean your teeth?

P   I use a toothbrush and toothpaste.

Dr   Very good. Could you let me know how you use your toothbrush?

P   I brush all upper and lower teeth on the outside and the inside as I was shown a long time ago.

Dr   And how do you feel about brushing your teeth that way?

P   I generally feel quite good about it. But since I have been told I have gum disease, I'm wondering if I haven't been brushing enough?

Dr   So you have been making efforts to keeping your teeth clean but you're worried that maybe you haven't been brushing enough.
It can be difficult to get to all the areas of your teeth and gums to remove the plaque that causes gum disease. I have some information related to prevention of gum disease that you might be interested in. Would you like to hear about it?

P   Yes.

Dr   The chronic gum or periodontal disease you are diagnosed with was caused by bacterial plaque attached to your teeth over time. Plaque has to be entirely removed from all the tooth surfaces on a daily basis in order to prevent and control this disease.
How confident are you that you were cleaning all the surfaces on a regular basis?

P   Not very, although I thought that I was doing enough.

Dr Well actually, research indicates that using a toothbrush alone is not sufficient to clean between the teeth. In order to clean these areas, an interdental device is needed such as a dental floss, a toothpick, or an interdental brush. Are you using any one of these devices?

P Yes, I've tried using dental floss.

Dr How did you find the use of dental floss?

P I had some trouble getting to some of the spaces between my teeth. In other areas, the floss used to rip up too, so I quit using it.

Dr I am sorry to hear that you had trouble using the dental floss. The floss can rip up at the edges of dental fillings or crowns. In spaces with extensive tartar built-up, the gap between your teeth may even be blocked out with tartar. Are you using anything else for cleaning?

P Yes, I use a toothpick whenever I have something stuck between my teeth.

Dr So in addition to your regular brushing with toothpaste you are also using a toothpick from time to time to clean your teeth?

P That's right.

Dr Good. During gum treatment, fillings and crowns with rough edges will be smoothed over and tartar can be removed which should make it easier to use things like dental floss or a toothpick between your teeth. Thinking of a 10-point scale where 0 is not at all important and 10 is extremely important, how important is it to you to floss or use a toothpick every day to clean the gaps between your teeth?

P Probably a 7.

Dr That sounds quite important. What makes this so important to you?

P I want to do everything needed to keep my teeth. However, I am not quite sure if I will be able to keep doing it over time.

Dr So you are quite motivated now because you want to look after your teeth, but you are worried about the long term. If you were to use the same 10-point scale to rate how confident you are that you can do it over the long-term, where would rate yourself?

P I would be at a 6.

Dr That sounds fairly confident. What gives you that level of confidence?

P Well, taking care of my teeth and gums is part of my routine already so this would just need to be added to it. But it does take extra effort, so it's a matter of realizing that it's really that important for my gums.

Dr So the fact that it can be part of your existing routine will help. But perhaps I can help you remain motivated in the long run by showing you at your follow-up visits the benefits you are achieving with your treatment by doing it regularly. How do you think that might help you to stick with it over time?

P Well, yes I think that would probably help a lot to see or learn from you that it really is making a difference to the success of my treatment.

Dr Great! So let me summarize what we have discussed. You plan to keep brushing on a regular basis with toothbrush and toothpaste and you will start to use a device for cleaning the gaps between your teeth after the issues with the rough filling and crown margins have been resolved. Then, each time you visit we'll see how you are progressing with your cleaning at home and see if we need to find any other ways to help. Does that sound like it would work for you?

P Yes, that sounds like it would work.

Oral hygiene motivation 2

In this second case example dialogue, MI is used in a conversation about oral hygiene at a visit for supportive periodontal therapy (SPT).

Dr From looking at your plaque index, I noticed today that compared to your visit 3 months ago there is more plaque around the areas between your teeth. I was wondering if you could tell me a little bit about how you find the cleaning between your teeth.

P Oh . . . I guess that I don't do it as often as I should. I barely have time now to do it every day, you know.

Dr I understand. It takes time to clean all the areas between your teeth, you are right. May I ask you a few questions about your current oral hygiene habits so I could understand your situation better?

P Sure you can.

Dr Good. So what do you use to clean your teeth currently?

P I am using an electric toothbrush and the interdental brushes you showed me.

Dr OK. How often do you use these?

P I use the electric toothbrush every day and I use the interdental brushes from time to time.

Dr So you are using the toothbrush on a regular basis, but only occasionally using the interdental brushes. What is prompting you when you do decide to use the interdental brushes?

P Well, sometimes I just feel guilty that I haven't been using them and sometimes I can see the tartar on my teeth and am reminded to use them again.

Dr So you sometimes worry that you are not using them enough and sometimes you can see on your teeth that you are not using them enough.

P Right, I suppose I should be doing better.

Dr Well let me ask you this. If you had to rate how important it is for you to use the interdental brushes every day on a scale from 0 to 10, 0 being not important at all and 10 being very important, where would you place yourself?

P I guess the use of these brushes is pretty important. I'd say an 8.

Dr Well that sounds very motivated. What makes it that important for you?

P Well I don't want to have a lot of problems with my teeth – I hate having fillings and of course I don't want to lose any teeth in the long run.

Dr So avoiding pain and discomfort and keeping your teeth is important to you. So how confident are you that you can use the brushes on a daily basis? Where would you rate yourself on that 0 to 10 scale?

P As I said, I know that I should use them more often, but finding the time is hard and I even just forget sometimes. I'd give it a 3.

Dr Using them daily seems quite hard for you. Out of curiosity, though, it seems you do have a little bit of confidence in doing this – may I ask you why a 3 instead of a 0 or a 1?

P Well, I just think that I would use them more often if they would become a part of my routine tooth cleaning, you know? I used to have toothpicks on my dinner table too and so I used them whenever I saw them sitting there. I could think about putting my interdental brushes on my sink next to my toothbrush. So I would be reminded to use them after brushing my teeth with the electric toothbrush.

Dr That sounds like a really good plan. Can you see any problems with doing that?

P No, not really. Once I have that reminder in place it's just a matter of staying committed to doing it.

Dr Very good. So if I can summarize, it sounds like you feel quite motivated to use the interdental brushes everyday, and that you think that if you put your interdental brushes on your sink next to your electric toothbrush that would help you remember to actually do it.

P Yes, that's right.

Dr Well does that sound like something you want to do?

P Yes, I'll do that tonight.

Case example for tobacco use cessation

A brief intervention for tobacco use cessation using MI is presented in a clinical case example dialogue between a periodontist (Dr) and a patient (P) at the beginning of periodontal therapy.

Dr According to your tobacco use history, you are currently smoking cigarettes. May I ask you a few questions about your smoking?

P Yes.

Dr Tell me how you feel about your smoking.

P Well I know I should quit. I know it's not good for my health. But I don't want to quit right now.

Dr So you don't feel that you want to quit right now, but you do have some concern about the health effects.

P Yes.

Dr Well, tell me more about what concerns you?

P Well, mainly that I would get lung cancer or something.

Dr So you worry a bit about getting cancer because of smoking. Is there anything else that you don't like about smoking?

P Well if I quit my clothes would stop smelling.

Dr So the smell of tobacco smoke is something you would like to be rid of?

P Yes, but I've smoked for many years, you know and I tried to quit once before.

Dr So even though you would like to be a non-smoker for health and other reasons you haven't had much success quitting.

P Yes, and right now I'm enjoying smoking so there's not much motivation to try.

Dr Well it sounds like even though you have some important reasons to quit, you're not very confident you could succeed and you don't feel ready to take on this challenge right now. I wonder if it would be OK for us to talk about this again next time to see where you are with it and whether I could help?

P Yes that sounds fine.

Conclusion

Chronic damaging behaviors not only affect general and oral health that individuals face but also impact the burden of disease on a community level. Hence, the services for primary and secondary prevention on an individual level oriented towards the change of inappropriate behavior become a professional responsibility for all oral health care providers. Motivational interviewing, encouraging the modification of all common risk factors for periodontal diseases such as insufficient oral hygiene, tobacco use, unhealthy dietary habits, and alcohol abuse, appears to be suitable for implementation into the periodontal treatment plan.

Acknowledgment

We are grateful to Dr. Dieter Müller, Bremgarten, Berne, Switzerland, for providing the cartoons of this chapter.

References

Ahluwalia, J.S., Okuyemi, K., Nollen, N., Choi, W.S., Kaur, H., Pulvers, K. & Mayo, M.S. (2006). The effects of nicotine gum and counseling among African American light smokers: a 2 × 2 factorial design. *Addiction* **101**, 883–891.

Albandar, J.M. (2002). Periodontal diseases in North America. *Periodontology 2000* **29**, 31–69.

Albandar, J.M., Brunelle, J.A. & Kingman, A. (1999). Destructive periodontal disease in adults 30 years of age and older in the United States, 1988–1994. *Journal of Periodontology* **70**, 13–29.

Bergstrom, J. (1989). Cigarette smoking as risk factor in chronic periodontal disease. *Community Dentistry and Oral Epidemiology* **17**, 245–247.

Borrelli, B., Novak, S., Hecht, J., Emmons, K., Papandonatos, G. & Abrams, D. (2005). Home health care nurses as a new channel for smoking cessation treatment: outcomes from project CARES (Community-nurse Assisted Research and Education on Smoking). *Preventive Medicine* **41**, 815–821.

Bowen, D., Ehret, C., Pedersen, M., Snetselaar, L., Johnson, M., Tinker, L., Hollinger, D., Ilona, L., Bland, K., Sivertsen, D., Ocke, D., Staats, L. & Beedoe, J.W. (2002). Results of an adjunct dietary intervention program in the Women's Health Initiative. *Journal of the American Diet Association* **102**, 1631–1637.

Burke, B.L., Arkowitz, H. & Menchola, M. (2003). The efficacy of motivational interviewing: a meta-analysis of controlled clinical trials. *Journal of Consulting and Clinical Psychology* **71**, 843–861.

Burke, B.L., Dunn, C.W., Atkins, D.C. & Phelps, J.S. (2004). The emerging evidence base for motivational interviewing: A meta-analytic and qualitative inquiry. *Journal of Cognitive Psychotherapy* **18**, 309–322.

Butler, C.C., Rollnick, S., Cohen, D., Bachmann, M., Russell, I. & Stott, N. (1999). Motivational consulting versus brief advice for smokers in general practice: a randomized trial. *British Journal of General Practice* **49**, 611–616.

Colby, S.M., Monti, P.M., Barnett, N.P., Rohsenow, D.J., Weissman, K., Spirito, A., Woolard, R.H. & Lewander, W.J. (1998). Brief motivational interviewing in a hospital setting for adolescent smoking: a preliminary study. *Journal of Consulting and Clinical Psychology* **66**, 574–578.

Demetriou, N., Tsami-Pandi, A. & Parashis, A. (1995). Compliance with supportive periodontal treatment in private periodontal practice. A 14-year retrospective study. *Journal of Periodontology* **66**, 145–149.

Fiore, M.C. (2000). US public health service clinical practice guideline: treating tobacco use and dependence. *Respiratory Care* **45**, 1200–1262.

Haber, J., Wattles, J., Crowley, M., Mandell, R., Joshipura, K. & Kent, R.L. (1993). Evidence for cigarette smoking as a major risk factor for periodontitis. *Journal of Periodontology* **64**, 16–23.

Hettema, J., Steele, J. & Miller, W.R. (2005). Motivational interviewing. *Annual Review of Clinical Psychology* **1**, 91–111.

Johansson, L.A., Oster, B. & Hamp, S.E. (1984). Evaluation of cause-related periodontal therapy and compliance with maintenance care recommendations. *Journal of Clinical Periodontology* **11**, 689–699.

Mhurchu, C.N., Margetts, B.M. & Speller, V. (1998). Randomized clinical trial comparing the effectiveness of two dietary interventions for patients with hyperlipidaemia. *Clinical Science* **95**, 479–487.

Miller, W.R. (1983). Motivational interviewing with problem drinkers. *Behavioural Psychotherapy* **11**, 147–172.

Miller, W.R. & Rollnick, S. (2002). *Motivational Interviewing: Preparing People for Change*, 2nd edn. New York: The Guillford Press.

Moyers, T.B. (2004). History and happenstance: how motivational interviewing got its start. *Journal of Cognitive Psychotherapy* **18**, 291–298.

Moyers, T.B., Martin, T., Catley, D., Harris, K. & Ahluwalia, J.S. (2003). Assessing the integrity of motivational interviewing interventions: Reliability of the motivational interviewing skills code. *Behavioural Cognitive Psychotherapy* **31**, 177–184.

Okuyemi, K.S., James, A.S., Mayo, M.S., Nollen, N., Catley, D., Choi, W.S. & Ahluwalia, J.S. (2007). Pathways to health: a cluster randomized trial of nicotine gum and motivational interviewing for smoking cessation in low-income housing. *Health Education & Behavior: the official publication of the Society for Public Health Education* **34**, 43–54.

Petersen, P.E. (2003). The World Oral Health Report 2003: continuous improvement of oral health in the 21st century – the approach of the WHO Global Oral Health Programme. *Community Dentistry and Oral Epidemiology* **31** (Suppl 1), 3–23.

Ramseier, C.A. (2005). Potential impact of subject-based risk factor control on periodontitis. *Journal of Clinical Periodontology* **32** (Suppl 6), 283–290.

Resnicow, K., Jackson, A., Wang, T., De, A.K., McCarty, F., Dudley, W.N. & Baranowski, T. (2001). A motivational interviewing intervention to increase fruit and vegetable intake through Black churches: results of the Eat for Life trial. *American Journal of Public Health* **91**, 1686–1693.

Resnicow, K., DiIorio, C., Soet, J.E., Ernst, D., Borrelli, B. & Hecht, J. (2002). Motivational interviewing in health promotion: it sounds like something is changing. *Health Psychology: official journal of the Division of Health Psychology, American Psychological Association* **21**, 444–451.

Richards, A., Kattelmann, K.K. & Ren, C. (2006). Motivating 18- to 24-year-olds to increase their fruit and vegetable consumption. *Journal of the American Diet Association* **106**, 1405–1411.

Rollnick, S., Mason, P. & Butler, C.C. (1999). *Health Behavior Change: A Guide for Practitioners*. Edinburgh: Churchill Livingstone.

Rubak, S., Sandbaek, A., Lauritzen, T. & Christensen, B. (2005). Motivational interviewing: a systematic review and meta-analysis. *British Journal of General Practice* **55**, 305–312.

Schuz, B., Sniehotta, F.F., Wiedemann, A. & Seemann, R. (2006). Adherence to a daily flossing regimen in university students: effects of planning when, where, how and what to do in the face of barriers. *Journal of Clinical Periodontology* **33**, 612–619.

Smith, S.S., Jorenby, D.E., Fiore, M.C., Anderson, J.E., Mielke, M.M., Beach, K.E., Piasecki, T.M. & Baker, T.B. (2001). Strike while the iron is hot: can stepped-care treatments resurrect relapsing smokers? *Journal of Consulting and Clinical Psychology* **69**, 429–439.

Soria, R., Legido, A., Escolano, C., Lopez Yeste, A. & Montoya, J. (2006). A randomised controlled trial of motivational interviewing for smoking cessation. *British Journal of General Practice* **56**, 768–774.

Stotts, A.L., Diclemente, C.C. & Dolan-Mullen, P. (2002). One-to-one: a motivational intervention for resistant pregnant smokers. *Addictive Behaviors* **27**, 275–292.

Tappin, D.M., Lumsden, M.A., Gilmour, W.H., Crawford, F., McIntyre, D., Stone, D.H., Webber, R., MacIndoe, S. & Mohammed, E. (2005). Randomised controlled trial of home based motivational interviewing by midwives to help pregnant smokers quit or cut down. *Brittish Medical Journal* **331**, 373–377.

Tomar, S.L. & Asma, S. (2000). Smoking-attributable periodontitis in the United States: findings from NHANES III. National Health and Nutrition Examination Survey. *Journal of Periodontology* **71**, 743–751.

Wakefield, M., Olver, I., Whitford, H. & Rosenfeld, E. (2004). Motivational interviewing as a smoking cessation intervention for patients with cancer: randomized controlled trial. *Nursing Research* **53**, 396–405.

Weinstein, P., Harrison, R. & Benton, T. (2004). Motivating parents to prevent caries in their young children: one-year findings. *Journal of the American Dental Association* **135**, 731–738.

Weinstein, P., Harrison, R. & Benton, T. (2006). Motivating mothers to prevent caries: confirming the beneficial effect of counseling. *Journal of the American Dental Association* **137**, 789–793.

Wilson, T.G., Jr., Glover, M.E., Schoen, J., Baus, C. & Jacobs, T. (1984). Compliance with maintenance therapy in a private periodontal practice. *Journal of Periodontology* **55**, 468–473.

Woollard, J., Beilin, L., Lord, T., Puddey, I., MacAdam, D. & Rouse, I. (1995). A controlled trial of nurse counselling on lifestyle change for hypertensives treated in general practice: preliminary results. *Clinical and Experimental Pharmacology and Physiology* **22**, 466–468.

Chapter 35

Mechanical Supragingival Plaque Control

Fridus Van der Weijden, José J. Echeverría, Mariano Sanz, and Jan Lindhe

Importance of supragingival plaque removal, 705
Self-performed plaque control, 706
  Brushing, 706
  Interdental cleaning, 714

Adjunctive aids, 717
Side effects, 718
Importance of instruction and motivation in mechanical
  plaque control, 719

Importance of supragingival plaque removal

Dental plaque is a bacterial biofilm that is not easily removed from the surface of teeth. Biofilms consist of complex communities of bacterial species that reside on tooth surfaces or soft tissues. It has been estimated that between 400 and 1000 species may, at some time, colonize oral biofilms. In these microbial communities, there are observable associations between specific bacteria due in part to synergistic or antagonistic relationships and in part to the nature of the available surfaces for colonization or nutrient availability (Chapter 9). The products of biofilm bacteria are known to initiate a chain of reactions leading to host protection but also to tissue destruction (Chapter 11).

The dental biofilm is a complex configuration leading many to speculate that traditional plaque indices are inadequate because they fail to evaluate qualitative features. Furthermore, the term *plaque* is not precise. Plaque may be supragingival or subgingival and may be adherent or non-adherent to tooth or tissue. In addition the microbial composition of plaque varies from person to person and from site to site within the same mouth (Thomas 2004).

Supragingival plaque is exposed to saliva and to the natural self-cleansing mechanisms existing in the oral cavity. Friction through mastication may have a limiting effect on occlusal and incisal extensions of plaque. However, in most populations natural cleaning of the human dentition appears unimportant (Löe 2000). Therefore, in order to maintain oral health, regular personal plaque removal measures must be undertaken. The most widespread means of actively removing plaque at home is toothbrushing. There is substantial evidence which shows that plaque and gingivitis/periodontitis can be controlled most reliably through toothbrushing supported by other mechanical cleansing procedures. Thus, evidence stemming from large cohort studies demonstrated that high standards of oral hygiene will ensure the stability of periodontal tissue support (Hujoel *et al.* 1998; Axelsson *et al.* 2004).

As meaningful as oral hygiene measures are for disease prevention, they are relatively ineffective when used *alone* for treatment of moderate and severe forms of periodontitis (Loos *et al.* 1988; Lindhe *et al.* 1989). On the other hand, without an adequate level of oral hygiene in periodontitis-susceptible subjects, periodontal health tends to deteriorate once periodontitis is established and further loss of attachment may occur (Lindhe & Nyman 1984).

Meticulous, self-performed plaque removal measures can modify both the quantity and composition of subgingival plaque (Dahlén *et al.* 1992). The Socransky group (Haffajee 2001) confirmed this finding and reported that a permanent optimal supragingival plaque control regimen can alter the composition of the pocket microbiota and lower the percentage of periodontopathic bacteria.

At present both primary prevention of gingivitis and primary and secondary prevention of periodontitis are based on the achievement of sufficient plaque removal. Almost 50 years of experimental research, clinical trials in different geographical and social settings, have confirmed that effective removal of dental plaque is essential to dental and periodontal health (Löe 2000). The concept of the primary prevention of gingivitis derives from the assumption that gingivitis is the precursor of periodontitis and that maintenance of a healthy gingiva will prevent periodontitis.

Consequently, preventing gingivitis could have a major impact on expenditure for periodontal care (Baehni & Takeuchi 2003). Primary prevention of periodontal diseases includes educational interventions on periodontal diseases and related risk factors as well as regular self-performed plaque removal and professional mechanical removal of plaque and calculus. Optimal oral hygiene requires appropriate motivation of the patient, adequate tools, and professional oral hygiene instruction.

Self-performed plaque control

Personal oral hygiene refers to the effort of the patient to remove supragingival plaque. Procedures used to remove supragingival plaque are as old as recorded history. The earliest record of the chewstick which has been considered the primitive toothbrush dates back in the Chinese literature to about 1600 BC (Carranza & Shklar 2003). In his writings, Hippocrates (460–377 BC) included commentaries on the importance of removing deposits from the tooth surfaces. The observation that self-performed plaque removal is one of the foundations of periodontal health was clearly described by Antonie van Leeuwenhoek in 1683, who wrote (Carranza & Shklar 2003):

"Tis my wont of a morning to rub my teeth with salt and then swill my mouth out with water; and often, after eating, to clean my back teeth with a toothpick, as well as rubbing them hard with a cloth; wherefore my teeth, back and front, remain as clean and white as falleth to the lot of few men of my years, **and my gums never start bleeding**."

The Chinese are given credit for developing the first bristle toothbrush which was introduced in the Western world in the sixteenth century. Currently, toothbrushes of various kinds are important aids for mechanical plaque removal. Furthermore, a fluoridated dentifrice is an integral component of daily home care. The use of toothbrush and dentifrices is almost universal. The use of interdental cleaning devices, mouthrinses, and other oral hygiene aids is less well documented, but available evidence tends to suggest that only a small percentage of the population use such additional measures on a regular basis (Bakdash 1995).

There is an increasing public awareness of the value of good oral health practices. This fact is proven by a recorded increase in both public spending on oral hygiene products (over $3.2 billion a year in the US) and industry spending on consumer-related advertising (over $272 million a year in the US) (Bakdash 1995).

Brushing

Different cleaning devices have been used in different cultures (toothbrushes, chewing sticks, chewing sponges, etc.). Toothbrushing is currently the most commonly used measure in oral hygiene practice. Toothbrushing alone, however, does not provide adequate interdental cleaning since a toothbrush may only reach the facial, oral, and occlusal tooth surfaces. It was suggested (Frandsen 1986) that the outcome of toothbrushing is dependent on: (1) the design of the brush, (2) the skill of the individual using the brush, and (3) the frequency and (4) duration of brushing.

Dental professionals must become familiar with the variety in shapes, sizes, textures, and other characteristics of available toothbrushes in order to provide their patients with proper advice. From the numerous products present on the market only a few should be selected for the individual patient. It is important that the dental care provider understands the advantages and disadvantages of the various toothbrushes (and other aids) to provide the patient with proper information during the oral hygiene instruction session.

For the most part, studies that have compared the effectiveness of different manual brushes have found relatively little difference among designs (see below). It is quite possible that a given patient may obtain better results with one particular toothbrush than with another. Providing oral hygiene information should therefore be tailored to the individual.

Motivation

Oral hygiene education is essential in primary prevention of gingivitis. Improvement in a patient's oral hygiene is often accomplished through cooperative interaction between the patient and the dental professional. The role of the patient is to seek education regarding efficient self-performed plaque removal and accept regular check-ups to ensure a high level of oral hygiene. The patient must be interested in maintaining the health of the tissues, interested in a proposed treatment plan, and motivated to participate. Without compliance, which has been described as the degree to which a patient follows a regimen prescribed by a dental professional, a good treatment outcome will not be achieved. In this context it should be realized that compliance with treatment recommendations is generally poor, particularly in patients with chronic diseases in which the risk of complications is not immediate or life threatening. Also compliance with oral hygiene recommendations is generally poor (Thomas 2004).

So, however effective any toothbrushing method is, it will only be of any real value if the patient is prepared to use the technique on a regular basis (Warren & Chater 1996a). Merely the patient's positive attitude to treatment may have a positive long-term effect on her/his tooth cleaning efforts. Thus, well motivated patients who are compliant with professional advice and instruction are likely to achieve and sustain ideal levels of plaque control.

There is an increasing public awareness of the value of personal oral hygiene. Good oral hygiene should form an integral part of overall health practices, such as regular exercise, stress management, diet and weight control, smoking cessation, and moderation in alcohol consumption. If the clinician can establish the link between oral health and general health for the patient, this individual may be more willing to establish proper oral hygiene measures as part of her/his lifestyle.

The issue of changing a patient's lifestyle is the more difficult part of motivational sessions (Chapter 34). The principles of brushing and flossing are easy to learn. Integrating them into one's daily routine is far more difficult. This can form a source of frustration for the clinician who has provided a patient with information about the necessity of personal oral hygiene measures.

Toothbrush (see Procedure 1)

It is believed that the first toothbrush made of hog's bristles was mentioned in the early Chinese literature. In 1698 Cornelis van Solingen, a doctor from The Hague, published a book in which he presented the first illustration of a toothbrush in Europe (Fig. 35-1). Nylon filaments were introduced in 1938 since complications of World War II prevented the Chinese export of wild boar bristles. Nearly all current toothbrushes are made exclusively of synthetic materials (Wilkins, 1999). Such nylon filaments and plastic handle are easy to manufacture, and therefore more affordable. This has made toothbrushing a common practice in most societies.

During toothbrushing the removal of dental plaque is achieved primarily through direct contact between the filaments of the toothbrush and the surfaces of teeth and soft tissues. At the European Workshop on Mechanical Plaque Control, it was agreed that the features of an ideal manual toothbrush should include (Egelberg & Claffey 1998):

1. Handle size appropriate to user age and dexterity so that the brush can easily and efficiently be manipulated
2. Head size appropriate to the size of the individual patient's requirements
3. Use of end-rounded nylon or polyester filaments not larger than 0.23 mm (0.009 inches) in diameter
4. Use of soft filament configurations as defined by the acceptable international industry standards (ISO)
5. Filament patterns which enhance plaque removal in the approximal spaces and along the gum line.

Additional characteristics could be: inexpensive, durable, impervious to moisture, and easily cleaned.

Modern toothbrushes have filament patterns designed to enhance plaque removal from hard-to-reach areas of the dentition, in particular from proximal areas. Cross-placed filaments, crimped, and tapered filaments are the most recent improvements. Such designs are based on the premise that the majority of subjects in any population use a simple horizontal brushing action. In order to improve patient comfort brush head shape, filament shape, and placement of filaments into the handles also have been subject to change over time. Multiple tufts of filaments, sometimes angled in different directions, are currently used (Jepsen 1998). Thus, when the head of the toothbrush is located horizontal to the tooth surface, there are filaments angled in the direction of the approximal tooth surfaces. Toothbrushes with this design facilitate more plaque removal in such difficult-to-reach areas when compared with flat-headed brushes (Cugini & Warren 2006).

Double- and triple-headed toothbrushes have been proposed in order to reach lingual surfaces more easily, especially in molar areas, which are normally the tooth surfaces hardest to reach with a regular toothbrush. Although some studies have indicated that the use of such multi-headed toothbrushes may improve plaque control in lingual areas (Agerholm 1991; Yankell *et al*. 1996), their use is not widespread.

Where handles used to be straight and flat, nowadays round and curved handles are more common. Today, a modern toothbrush has a handle size that is appropriate to the hand size of the prospective user, and much emphasis has been placed on new ergonomic designs (Löe 2002). Several studies have investigated differences in plaque removal between brushes with different handle design. In such studies brushes with long and contoured handles appeared to remove more plaque than brushes with traditional handles (Saxer & Yankell 1997).

When brushes with hard, soft, multi-tufted, and space-tufted filaments were compared, no significant clinical differences were found with respect to plaque removal. It is worth considering that most of such

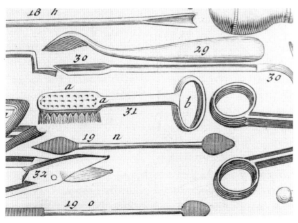

Fig. 35-1 Illustration of a toothbrush and tongue scraper from the book of Cornelis van Solingen with special thanks to the University Museum of Dentistry in Utrecht, The Netherlands.

toothbrush studies involved highly motivated participants such as dental students, who do not represent the general population. Most studies on manual brushes are 'single-use' tests. Although such short-term trials may be useful as pilot experiments, they need to be supplemented with studies of longer duration. Numerous manual toothbrushes are available on the market. There is still, however, insufficient evidence that one specific toothbrush design is superior to another. In 1994, two well performed clinical trials which assessed the efficacy of two toothbrushes came to entirely different conclusions (Grossman et al. 1994; Sharma et al. 1994). In the one trial toothbrush A was more effective than brush B while in the other trial brush B was superior to brush A. The trial which proved that brush A was most effective was sponsored by the manufacturer of brush A. The finances of the other trial which proved that brush B was more effective came from the manufacturer of brush B. As with many other aspects of oral hygiene aids, there is insufficient information to make evidence-based recommendations. Thus, in absence of this evidence, the best toothbrush continues to be the one that is (properly) used by the patient (Cancro & Fischman 1995; Jepsen 1998).

Efficacy of toothbrushing

The enthusiastic use of the toothbrush is not synonymous with a high standard of oral hygiene. Adults, despite their apparent efforts, appear not to be as effective in their plaque removal as might be expected. Most individuals only remove about 50% of plaque by toothbrushing (Jepsen 1998). De la Rosa and co-workers (1979) studied the pattern of plaque accumulation and removal with daily toothbrushing during a 28-day period following a dental prophylaxis. On average about 60% of the plaque was left after the self-performed brushing. Morris et al. (2001) reported on the 1998 UK Adult Dental Health survey and observed that the mean proportion of teeth with plaque deposits was 30% in the 25–34-year age group and 44% in those aged 65 years and above. At the Academic Centre for Dentistry Amsterdam (ACTA) a study was conducted which assessed the efficacy of a single 1-minute brushing exercise in subjects adhering to their customary brushing method (Van der Weijden et al. 1998a). It was observed that after 1 minute of brushing, approximately 39% of the plaque had been removed. The results of the studies described above indicate that most subjects are not effective brushers and that they probably live with large amounts of plaque on their teeth, even though they brush once every day.

Methods of toothbrushing

There is no single oral hygiene method that is correct for all patients. The morphology of the dentition (crowding, spacing, gingival phenotype etc.), the type and severity of the periodontal tissue destruction, as well as the patient's own manual dexterity

determine what kind of hygiene aids and cleaning techniques are to be recommended. It should also be realized that during the course of periodontitis therapy, the techniques may have to be changed or adapted to the morphologic situation (longer teeth, open interdental spaces, exposed dentin).

The ideal brushing technique is the one that allows complete plaque removal in the least possible time, without causing any damage to the tissues (Hansen & Gjermo 1971). Different toothbrushing methods have been recommended over time, but also been abandoned. Such methods can be classified based on the position and motion of the brush.

Horizontal brushing is probably the most commonly used toothbrushing method. It is most frequently used by individuals who never had instruction in oral hygiene techniques. Despite the efforts of the dental profession to instruct patients to adopt other more efficient brushing techniques, most individuals use horizontal brushing since it is simple. The head of the brush is positioned perpendicular to the tooth surface and then a horizontal back and forth movement is applied. The occlusal, lingual, and palatal surfaces of the teeth are brushed with open mouth. In order to reduce pressure of the cheek on the brush head the vestibular surfaces are cleaned with the mouth closed.

Vertical brushing (Leonard (1939) technique) is similar to the horizontal brushing technique, but the movement is applied in vertical direction using up and down strokes.

Circular brushing (Fones (1934) method): with the teeth closed the brush is placed inside the cheek and a fast circular motion is applied that extends from the maxillary gingiva to the mandibular gingiva using light pressure. Back and forth strokes are used on the lingual and palatal tooth surfaces. The *scrubbing method* includes a combination of horizontal, vertical, and circular strokes.

Sulcular brushing (Bass (1948) technique): this method emphasizes cleaning of the area directly beneath the gingival margin. The head of the brush is positioned in an oblique direction towards the apex. Filament tips are directed into the sulcus at approximately 45° to the long axis of the tooth. The brush is moved in a back and forth direction using short strokes without disengaging the tips of the filaments from the sulci. On the lingual surfaces in the anterior tooth regions the brush head is kept in the vertical direction. The Bass technique is widely accepted as an effective method for removing plaque not only at the gingival margin, but also subgingivally. A few studies have been carried out on teeth affected with periodontal disease and scheduled for extraction, where the gingival margin was marked with a groove and the depth of subgingival cleaning was measured. These studies showed that with the use of this brushing method the plaque removal could reach a depth of approximately 1 mm subgingivally (Waerhaug 1981a).

Vibratory technique (Stillman (1932) method): as originally described by Stillman the method was designed for massage and stimulation of the gingiva as well as for cleaning the cervical areas of the teeth. The head of the brush is positioned in an oblique direction toward the apex, with the filaments placed partly in the gingival margin and partly on the tooth surface. Light pressure together with a vibratory (slight rotary) movement is then applied to the handle, while the filament tips are maintained in position on the tooth surface.

Vibratory technique (Charters (1948) method): this method was originally developed to increase cleansing effectiveness and gingival stimulation in the interproximal areas. It uses a reverse position of the brushhead as compared to the Stillman technique. The head of the brush is positioned in an oblique direction with the filament tips directed towards the occlusal or incisal surfaces. Light pressure is used to flex the filaments and gently force the tips into the interproximal embrassures. A vibratory (slight rotary) movement is then applied to the handle while the filament tips are maintained in position on the tooth surface. This method is particularly effective in cases with receded interdental papillae because the filament tips can easily penetrate the interdental space (Fig. 35-2).

Roll technique: the head of the brush is positioned in an oblique direction toward the apex of the teeth, with the filaments placed partly in the gingival margin and partly on the tooth surface. The sides of the filaments are pressed lightly against the gingiva. Next the head of the brush is rolled over the gingiva and tooth in occlusal direction.

Modified Bass/Stillman technique: the Bass and Stillman methods were designed to concentrate on the cervical portion of the teeth and adjacent gingival tissues. Each of these methods can be modified to add a roll stroke. The brush is positioned similarly to the Bass/Stillman technique. After activation of the brushhead in a back and forth direction, the head of the brush is rolled over the gingiva and tooth in occlusal direction making it possible for some of the filaments to reach interdentally.

In the 1970s several investigators compared various methods of brushing. Because of varying experimental conditions the outcomes of such studies are difficult to compare. To date no methods of toothbrushing have been shown to be clearly superior to others. As early as 1986, Frandsen commented on this issue by stating: "Researchers have realized that improvement in oral hygiene is not as dependent upon the development of better brushing methods as upon improved performance by the persons using any one of the accepted methods." Therefore, since no particular toothbrushing method has been found to be clearly superior to another, there is no reason to introduce a specific toothbrushing technique in each new periodontal patient. In most cases, small changes in the patient's own method of toothbrushing will suffice, always bearing in mind that more important than the selection of a certain method of

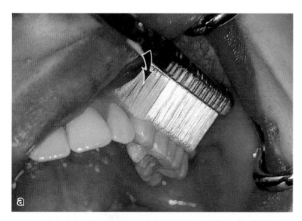
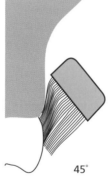
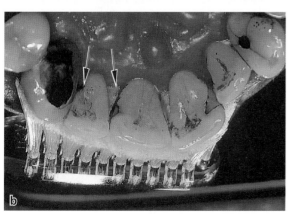

Fig. 35-2 (a) The Charters method of toothbrushing. The head of the toothbrush is placed in the left maxilla. Note the angulation of the bristles against the buccal tooth surfaces. The bristles are forced into the interproximal areas. (b) The palatal aspect of the incisor region in the maxilla illustrating the penetration of the bristles through the interproximal spaces (arrows).

toothbrushing is the willingness and thoroughness on the part of the patients to effectively clean their teeth. Implementation of the toothbrushing methods described above must be made according to patient´s needs. For example, since the Bass method has been associated with gingival recession (O'Leary 1980), it would be hardly indicated in individuals with energetic toothbrushing habits who have a thin gingival biotype.

Frequency of toothbrushing

There is no consensus as to the optimum frequency of toothbrushing. How often and how much plaque has to be removed in order to prevent dental disease from developing is not known. The majority of individuals, including periodontal patients, are usually not able to remove dental plaque completely as a result of daily brushing. However complete plaque removal does not seem to be necessary. A proper level of oral hygiene theoretically is the extent of plaque removal that prevents gingivitis/periodontal disease and tooth decay in the individual patient. Prevention of gingival inflammation is important because the inflammatory condition of soft tissues also favors plaque accumulation (Ramberg et al. 1994; Rowshani et al. 2004).

Results in cross-sectional studies have been equivocal when the self-reported frequency of tooth cleaning has been related to caries and periodontal disease. Disease appears to be more related to quality of cleaning than to its frequency (Bjertness 1991). Kressin and co-workers (2003) evaluated the effect of oral hygiene practices on tooth retention in a longitudinal study with a 26-year follow-up. They observed that consistent brushing (at least once a day) resulted in a 49% reduction of the risk of tooth loss compared to a lack of consistent oral hygiene habits.

If plaque is allowed to accumulate freely in the dentogingival region, subclinical signs of gingival inflammation (gingival fluid) appear within 4 days (Egelberg 1964). The minimum frequency of tooth cleaning to reverse experimentally induced gingivitis is once every day or every second day. Bosman and Powell (1977) induced experimental gingivitis in a group of students. The signs of gingival inflammation persisted in those students who removed plaque only every third or fifth day. In groups who properly cleaned their teeth once a day or every second day, the gingivae healed within 7–10 days.

Based on the observation that the onset of gingivitis appears to be more related to the maturation and age of the plaque than to its amount, the minimum frequency needed to prevent the development of gingivitis has been investigated in a prospective study. Dental students and young dental faculty members with healthy periodontal conditions were assigned to study groups with different cleaning frequencies over periods of 4–6 weeks. The results showed that that students who thoroughly removed plaque once daily or even every second day, did not develop clinical signs of gingival inflammation over a 6-week period. This tooth cleaning included the use of interproximal aids (dental floss and woodsticks) as well as the toothbrush (Lang et al. 1973). Caution should be excercised in extrapolating the results obtained from studies including dentally aware subjects to the average patient.

From a practical standpoint, it is generally recommended that patients brush their teeth at least twice daily, not only to remove plaque but also to apply fluoride through the use of dentifrice in order to prevent caries. This advice is also conceivable based on reasons of practibility and feeling of oral freshness. For most patients, it may be desirable to perform all necessary procedures (e.g. brushing and interdental cleaning) at the same time and in the same manner each day. Unfortunately, with subjects who live busy, stressful lives, this may be difficult to achive (Thomas 2004). Despite the fact that most individuals claim to brush their teeth at least twice a day, it is clear from both epidemiologic and clinical studies that mechanical oral hygiene procedures as performed by most subjects are insufficient to control supragingival plaque formation and to prevent gingivitis and more severe forms of periodontal disease (Sheiham & Netuveli 2002).

Brushing duration

Patients usually believe that they spend more time on toothbrushing than they actually do (Saxer et al. 1998). The least time spent on brushing was observed in a study carried out on English schoolchildren; in the 13 years age group, the children spent approximately 33 seconds on brushing (Macgregor & Rugg-Gunn 1985). About one third of the studies that were reviewed reported an average brushing time of less than 56 seconds whereas two thirds of the studies reported a brushing time of ≥56 seconds and <70 seconds. One investigation which used dental students as study population reported an average of 90 seconds (Ayer et al. 1965). The best estimate of actual manual brushing time seems to range between 30 and 60 seconds (Van der Weijden et al. 1993).

In reviewing the literature for studies that addressed the question whether in adult patients the duration of toothbrushing is correlated with efficacy of plaque removal five studies were identified. Three of these evaluated the use of electric toothbrushes (Van der Weijden et al. 1996a; McCracken et al. 2003, 2005). One study compared a manual toothbrush with an electric toothbrush (Preber et al. 1991), while one study included only manual toothbrushes (Hawkins et al. 1986). Results from all five studies indicate that duration of brushing is consistently correlated with the amount of plaque that is removed. In one study, toothbrushing was delivered by a dentist/dental hygienist. This study compared the effect of brushing time on plaque removal using manual and electric toothbrushes utilizing five different brushing times (30, 60, 120, 180, and 360 seconds).

This study showed that 2 minutes of electric toothbrushing can be as effective as 6 minutes of manual toothbrushing. The authors furthermore observed that at 2 minutes an optimum in plaque-removing efficacy was reached with both a manual and electric toothbrushes (Van der Weijden *et al.* 1993). Based on these observations the duration of toothbrushing should also be stressed during the toothbrushing instruction session.

Brushing filaments

Most current toothbrushes have nylon filaments. The degree of hardness and stiffness of a toothbrush depends on the filament characteristics, such as material, diameter, and length. Also the density of filaments in a tuft influences stiffness, since each filament gives support to the adjacent fiaments and each tuft gives support to adjacent tufts. Toothbrushes with thinner filaments are softer while thicker filament diameters are stiffer and less flexible. This increased stiffness will prevent the filament ends from bending back during brushing, avoiding the potential risk of damaging the gums. However, the filament must be sufficiently stiff so that during brushing enough pressure is exerted to allow proper plaque removal. Consider that a rod represents a filament of a toothbrush. Whilst brushing, a vertical upward load is exerted, which in turn exerts an effect of the same order of magnitude on the oral mucosa. The force of the brush, acting on the individual filament, is thus always as great as the load exercised by the filament on the mucosa. If the load is increased then the load on the mucosa increases to the same extent. Consequently the risk of soft tissue damage increases in that the filament's tip can penetrate into the mucosa. However, elastic rods demonstrate a peculiarity in their behavior. They suddenly fold back laterally when a certain limit load is reached. When folding back, the rod suddenly gives way elastically (without breaking) and the load on the oral mucosa diminishes abruptly. A load higher than this fold-back limit can thus not be transferred to the mucosa by the rod, via its tip. Tapered filaments (Fig. 35-3) have endings with the

shape of an extreme rotational ellipsoid instead of a hemisphere. This is suggested to give the filaments very soft endings combined with a good stability of the filament corpus. Curved filaments may be more flexible and less stiff than straight filaments of equal length and diameter.

As late as 1967, most people were buying hard brushes (Fanning & Henning 1967). The shift in preference to soft brushes of specific design paralleled the change that occurred in oral health care when calculus was the prime etiologic agent in periodontal disease (Mandell 1990). The concentration on plaque, especially in the crevicular area and the attention to intrasulcular brushing strongly influenced the change from hard to soft filaments, primarily because of the concern of trauma to the gingival tissues (Niemi *et al.* 1984). The cleaning performance of a toothbrush is influenced by its degree of hardness. The toothbrush must not be too hard, to avoid damaging the gums when positioning the toothbrush. The harder the toothbrush filaments are the greater is risk of gingival abrasion (Khocht *et al.* 1993). But there is no point in using a brush with very thin filaments that merely strokes across the tooth and, as a result of the lack of load, no longer cleans the tooth surface.

Filament end-rounding

The end of a toothbrush filament can be cut bluntly or rounded. End-rounding has become increasingly common in the manufacturing process to reduce gingival abrasion (Fig. 35-4). The logic that smooth filament tips would cause less trauma than filament tips with sharp edges or jagged projections has been validated with both animal and clinical studies (Breitenmoser *et al.* 1979). Danser *et al.* (1998) evaluated two types of end-rounding, and saw an effect of end-rounding on the incidence of abrasion. The form to which the ends were rounded, however, had no effect on the level of plaque removal.

Toothbrush wear and replacement

It is generally recommended that toothbrushes be replaced before the first signs of the filaments

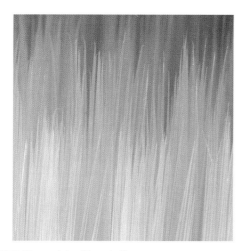

Fig. 35-3 Tapered toothbrush filaments.

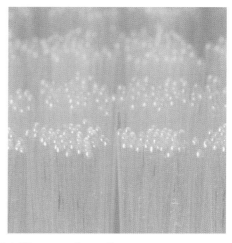

Fig. 35-4 Filament end-rounding.

becoming worn. The useful life of an average tooth-brush has been estimated to be 2–3 months. Not all patients take this advice, and evidence indicates that the average age at which a toothbrush is replaced ranges from 2.5–6 months (Bergström 1973). Common sense would suggest that a worn toothbrush with splayed or frayed filaments loses resilience and is less likely to be as effective in removing plaque than a new brush. This is why dental professionals often recommend that toothbrushes are used for a maximum of 3 months before they are they are replaced. Whilst this advice would seem reasonable, there is little actual clinical proof that this recommendation is correct. Because of variability in subjects' brushing techniques and the force applied to the teeth whilst brushing, the degree of wear varies significantly from subject to subject. It is also likely that different brushes, made from various materials, would exhibit differences in longevity. Some commercially available brushes have filaments that change color after a certain amount of use. This serves as a reminder to the patients that it is time to replace the brush.

Kreifeldt and co-workers (1980) showed that new brushes were more efficient in removing dental plaque than old brushes. They examined worn tooth-brushes and observed that, as a result of wear, the filaments showed a taper, proceeding from the insertion to the free end. For example filaments were seen which tapered from 0.28 mm at one end to 0.020–0.015 mm at the free end. They concluded that among other wear factors, tapering contributed the most to loss of effectiveness. Their explanation for this observation was that as the tapering will result in a reduction of filament diameter, the brush will become softer and remove less plaque.

Since many patients use a brush for periods significantly longer than the recommended time of 3 months, it is important to know whether excessive wear is of clinical relevance. Several studies have examined this question but there is inconclusive evidence about the relationship between toothbrush wear and plaque removal. Studies with laboratory-worn toothbrushes reported that such used tooth-brushes had inferior plaque removal efficacy as compared to new brushes (Kreifeldt et al. 1980; Warren et al. 2002). However, artificially worn tooth-brushes may not mimic the characteristics of a naturally worn brush. In a laboratory study of the wear of toothbrushes, wear will inevitably be highly uniform and not reflect the variation in wear seen in normal toothbrush use. Most studies in which naturally worn toothbrushes were used reported no statistically significant decrease in reduction of whole-mouth plaque scores after brushing when compared to using new toothbrushes (Daly et al. 1996; Sforza et al. 2000; Tan & Daly 2002; Conforti et al. 2003; Van Palenstein Helderman et al. 2006). From this brief review of the literature it may be concluded that in contrast to what is generally thought, the wear status of a toothbrush might be less critical for maintaining good plaque control.

Electric toothbrushes (see Procedure 2)

In well motivated and properly instructed individuals who are willing to invest the necessary time and effort, mechanical measures, using traditional tooth-brushes and adjunctive manual (interdental) devices, are effective in removing plaque. Maintaining a dentition close to plaque-free is, however, not easy. The electric toothbrush represents an advance that has the potential to both enhance plaque removal and patient motivation. Electric toothbrushes were introduced to the market more than 50 years ago. The first toothbrush powered by electricity was developed by Bemann & Woog in Switzerland and was introduced in the United States in 1960 as the Broxodent. In 1961 a cordless rechargeable model was introduced by General Electric (Darby & Walsh 2003). Studies of the use of these early electric tootbrushes showed that there was no difference in plaque removal when compared with a manual toothbrush and they had mixed effects on gingivitis. The consensus of the research reports on toothbrushing of the World Workshop in Periodontics in 1966 states: "in non-dentally oriented persons, in persons not high motivated to oral health care, or in those who have difficulty in mastering suitable hand brushing technique the use of an electric brush with its standard movements may result in more frequent and better cleansing of the teeth".

Since the 1980s, tremendous advances have been made in the technology of electrically powered tooth-brushes. Various electric toothbrushes have been developed to improve the efficiency of plaque removal using increased filament velocity, brush stroke frequency, and various filament patterns and motions. Where old electric toothbrushes were using a combination of horizontal and vertical movements mimicking closely the back-and-forth motion of the traditional brushing methods, the more recent designs apply rotary motion or oscillating/rotating motion with pulsation, or have brush heads which move at high frequencies.

After reviewing many of the published reports over the past decades, it may be concluded that certain newer types of rechargeable electric tooth-brushes have become more effective in removing supragingival plaque and controlling gingivitis. It is also clear that the effectiveness of particularly the low-cost battery-operated brushes are not well documented. To some extent, power brushes have overcome the limitations of the manual dexterity and skill of the user. Modern design features appear to be responsible for this (Fig. 35-5). These newer designed toothbrushes remove plaque in a shorter time than a standard manual brush (Van der Weijden et al. 1993, 1996a). The new generation of electric brushes have better plaque removal efficacy and gingival inflammation control in the approximal tooth surfaces

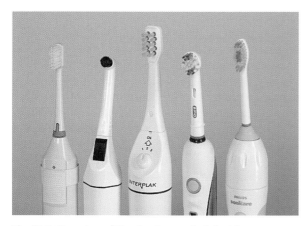

Fig. 35-5 Overview of the development of electric toothbrushes from brushes mimicking a manual toothbrush to high-frequency brushhead movement. From left to right: the Braun D3®, Rotadent®, Interplak®, Braun/Oral-B Triumph®, Sonicare Elite®.

(Egelberg & Claffey 1998). This superiority was clearly demonstrated in a study carried out on extracted teeth (Rapley & Killoy 1994). The electric toothbrush should not be considered a substitute for a specific interdental cleaning method, such as flossing, but it may offer advantages in terms of an overall approach to improved oral hygiene.

Two independent systematic reviews confirmed that oscillating rotating toothbrushes have superior efficacy over manual toothbrushes in reducing plaque and gingivitis (Sicilia *et al.* 2002; Robinson *et al.* 2005). Toothbrushes with this mode of action reduced plaque by 7% and gingival bleeding by 17% when compared with manual brushes (Robinson *et al.* 2005).

One electric toothbrush that has consistently been shown to be more effective than a manual toothbrush, both with respect to plaque removal and improvement of the gingival condition, is the original Braun Oral-B Plaque Remover (D7) (Warren & Chater 1996b). This toothbrush features a small round brush head that makes rotating and oscillating movements at a speed of 2800 oscillating rotations per minute. A further development of this brush, the Braun Oral-B Ultra Plaque Remover (D9) maintained the oscillating rotating action but at an increased speed (3600 rotations per minute). A clinical study with the D9 demonstrated equivalence in safety and a trend towards greater plaque removal when compared with the D7 (Van der Weijden *et al.* 1996b). Newer developments in the oscillating rotating brush technology add the additional high-frequency vibrations in the direction of the bristles creating three-dimensional movements during brushing. This modification was developed to enhance penetration and removal of plaque from approximal spaces of the dentition. Studies have shown the three-dimensional movements carried out by the brush are safe to use and more efficient regarding plaque removal (Danser *et al.* 1998).

Another approach in this technology was the development of sonic toothbrushes that have a high frequency of filament movement in excess of approximately 30 000 strokes per minute. Two recently introduced sonic toothbrushes are the Oral-B Sonic Complete® (SC; Oral-B Laboratories, Boston, MA, USA) rechargeable toothbrush with a side-to-side filament operating at 260 Hz, and the Philips Sonicare® Elite (SE; Philips Oral Healthcare, Snoqualmie, WA, US) based on a different technology, with a side-to-side motion also operating at a frequency of 260 Hz. Some clinical studies have shown sonic technology to be comparable or more effective than a manual toothbrush in removing plaque and reducing gingival inflammation (Johnson & McInnes 1994; Tritten & Armitage 1996; Zimmer *et al.* 2000; Moritis *et al.* 2002). Two studies using the same experimental gingivitis model compared an earlier Sonicare device and the Oral-B oscillating rotating toothbrush. In both studies the oscillating rotating brush was more effective in improving the level of gingival health (Putt *et al.* 2001; Van der Weijden *et al.* 2002a,b). This confirmed the findings of an earlier 6-week crossover study (Isaacs *et al.* 1998) where improvement in gingival condition was 8.6% greater with the oscillating rotating brush. Rosema and co-workers (2005) compared the Sonicare Elite to the Oral-B Professional Care 7000 and again found the oscillating rotating pulsation brush to be more effective. On the other hand, Tritten & Armitage (1996) compared the Sonicare advance to a traditional manual toothbrush in a 12-week parallel group study and concluded that both brushes were equally effective in reducing gingival inflammation.

Modern power toothbrushes are known to enhance long-term compliance. In a study involving periodontitis patients with persistent poor compliance, Hellstadius and co-workers (1993) found that switching from a manual to a power toothbrush reduced plaque levels and that the reduced levels were maintained over a period of between 12 and 36 months. The power brush significantly improved compliance, and patients expressed a positive attitude to the new brush. In a survey carried out in Germany most dentists stated that the time their patients spent on toothbrushing was too small (Warren 1998). Approximately half of the dentists stated that they recommend their patients to use a power toothbrush, and the vast majority of the dentists believed that changing to a power toothbrush would improve the condition of their patients' teeth and gums. Findings from a recent US practice-based study, involving a large number of subjects who switched from a manual toothbrush to the Braun Oral-B Ultra Plaque Remover (D9), confirmed the findings from the German study (Warren *et al.* 2000).

Electrically active (ionic) toothbrush

Several toothbrushes have been marketed over the years, which are designed to send a small imperceptible electronic current through the brush head, presumedly to enhance the efficacy of the brush in plaque elimination. The electrons should reduce the H⁺ ions from the organic acid in the plaque which may result in a decomposition of the bacterial plaque (Hoover *et al.* 1992). The first record of a charged toothbrush, the "Dr. Scott's Electric Toothbrush" was found in the February 1886 issue of Harper's weekly magazine. The handle of Dr. Scott's toothbrush was purportedly "charged with an electromagnetic current which acts without any shock, immediately upon the nerves and tissues of the teeth and gums . . . arresting decay . . . and restoring the natural whiteness of the enamel."

Short-term clinical studies with the use of these kinds of brushes documented a beneficial effect in terms of plaque reduction and gingivitis resolution (Hoover *et al.* 1992; Weiger 1998). Hotta and Aono (1992) studied an electrically active manual toothbrush that was designed with a piezo-electric element in the handle. This brush generates a voltage potential corresponding to the bending motion of the handle as the teeth are brushed. In this study no difference in the amount of remaining plaque after brushing was observed between the placebo and the electrically active brush. Other toothbrushes, which have a claimed 'electrochemical' effect on dental plaque, have a semiconductor of TiO_2 incorporated in the brush handle. In the presence of light, saturated low energy electrons in the wet semiconductor are transformed into high-energy electrons. An electron current of approximately 10 nA was measured to run from the semiconductor to the tooth (Weiger 1988).

Interdental cleaning

There is confusion in the literature with respect to the definitions of approximal, interproximal, interdental, and proximal sites. Commonly used indices are not suitable for assessing interdental plaque (directly under the contact area), and thereby limit interpretation of interdental plaque removal. The European Workshop on Mechanical Plaque Control in 1999 proposed the following definitions: *approximal* (proximal) areas are the visible spaces between teeth that are not under the contact area. In health these areas are small, although they may increase after periodontal attachment loss. The terms *interproximal* and *interdental* may be used interchangeably and refer to the area under and related to the contact point.

As stated above, the toothbrush does not reach the approximal surfaces of teeth as efficiently as it does for the facial, lingual, and ooclusal aspects nor does it reach into the interproximal area between adjacent teeth. Therefore measures for interdental plaque control should be selected to complement plaque control by toothbrushing (Lang *et al.* 1977; Hugoson & Koch 1979).

The interdental gingiva fills the embrasure between two teeth apical to their contact point. This is a 'shel-

tered' area, difficult to access, when teeth are in normal position. In populations that use a toothbrush, the interproximal surfaces of the molars and premolars are the predominant sites of residual plaque. The removal of plaque from these surfaces remains a valid objective, since in patients susceptible to periodontal diseases, gingivitis and periodontitis are usually more pronounced in this interdental area than on oral or facial aspects (Löe 1979). Dental caries also occurs more frequently in the interdental region than on oral or facial smooth surfaces. A fundamental principle of prevention is that the effect is greatest where the risk of disease is greatest. Therefore, interdental plaque removal, which cannot be achieved with the toothbrush, is of critical importance for most patients. A number of interdental cleaning methods have been developed, ranging from floss to the more recently introduced electrically powered cleaning aids. Flossing is the most universally applicable method, since it may be used effectively in nearly all clinical situations. However, not all interdental cleaning devices suit all patients or all types of dentitions. Factors such as the contour and consistency of gingival tissues, the size of the interproximal embrasure, tooth position and alignment, and the ability and motivation of the patient should be taken into consideration when recommending an interdental cleaning method. The most appropriate interdental hygiene aids must be selected for each individual patient. The selection made from the numerous commercially available devices is dependent for the most part on the size and shape of the interdental space as well as on the morphology of the proximal tooth surface. In subjects with normal gingival contours and embrasures, dental floss or tape should be recommended. At sites where soft tissue recession has become pronounced, flossing becomes progressively less effective. Then an alternative method (either woodsticks or interdental brushes) should be recommended. A review on interdental cleaning methods (Warren & Chater 1996a) concluded that all conventional devices are effective, but each method should be suited to a particular patient but also to a particular situation in the mouth (Table 35-1).

The use of dental floss, interproximal brushes, and woodsticks may also induce soft tissue damage. In most cases, however, this damage is limited to acute lesions, such as lacerations and gingival erosions (Gillette & Van House 1980). Gingival bleeding during interdental cleaning can be a result of trauma or an indication of inflammation. Patients must be aware that bleeding *per se* is not a sign that interdental cleaning should be avoided but more likely an indicator of inflammation that needs to be treated.

Dental floss and tape (see Procedure 3)

Of all the methods used for removing interproximal plaque, dental flossing is the most frequently recom-

Table 35-1 Interdental cleaning methods recommended for particular situations in the mouth

Situation	Interdental cleaning method
Intact interdental papillae; narrow interdental space	Dental floss or small woodstick
Moderate papillary recession; slightly open interdental space	Dental floss, woodstick or small interdental brush
Complete loss of papilla; wide open interdental space	Interdental brush
Wide embrassure space; diastema, extraction diastema, furcation or posterior surface of most distal molar, root concavities or grooves	Single-tufted/end-tufted brush or gauze strip

mended technique. Levi Spear Parmly, a dentist based in New Orleans, is credited as being the inventor of modern dental floss. As early as 1815 Parmly recommended teeth flossing with a piece of silk thread. Clinical studies clearly show that, when toothbrushing is used together with flossing, more plaque is removed from the proximal surfaces than by toothbrushing alone (Reitman *et al*. 1980; Kinane *et al*. 1992). Dental floss and tape – a type of broader dental floss – are most useful where the interdental papillae completely fill the embrasure space. When properly used, flossing effectively removes up to 80% of proximal plaque. Even subgingival plaque can be removed, since dental floss can be introduced 2–3.5 mm below the tip of the papilla (Waerhaug 1981b). Several types of floss (waxed, unwaxed) are available. Studies have shown no difference in the effectiveness of unwaxed versus waxed dental floss. Unwaxed dental floss is generally recommended for patients with normal tooth contacts because it slides through the contact area easily. It is the thinnest type of floss available, yet when it separates during use it covers a larger surface area of the tooth than waxed floss. Waxed floss is recommended for patients with tight proximal tooth contacts. *Ease of use* is the most important factor that influences whether patients will use floss on a daily basis. Recently, powered flossing devices have been introduced. In comparison with manual flossing no differences have been found in terms of plaque removal and gingivitis reduction, although patients preferred flossing with the automated device (Gordon *et al*. 1996).

Frequent reinstruction and reinforcement in the use of floss are necessary because flossing is a difficult skill to master. Flossing is also time-consuming. When a patient is unwilling to use dental floss alternative interdental hygiene aids should be recommended even if these are less efficient. If a patient finds a particular method or device more appealing to use, long-term compliance becomes an achievable

goal. Although it is clear that flossing, when properly used, removes plaque in a very efficient manner, there is no evidence that flossing in adult patients with preserved interproximal periodontal tissues should be routinely indicated (Burt & Eklund 1999).

To facilitate flossing a special floss holder may be used. The holder may be re-used and is normally made of plastic material, durable, lightweight, and easily cleaned. Research reveals that reductions in bacterial plaque biofilm and gingivitis are equivalent with either the use of a hand flossing or flossholder. A Swedish national dental survey showed that approximately 46% of adults use woodsticks sporadically and only 12% use woodsticks daily. On the other hand, dental floss is used occasionally by 12% of adults and daily by only 2%. In other words, adults use woodsticks as an oral hygiene aid four to six times more frequently than dental floss (Axelsson 1994).

Woodsticks (see Procedure 4)

Picking our teeth may well be one of humanity's oldest habits and the toothpick one of the earliest tools. The evolution of the primitive toothpick took a second pathway in the more acquisitive societies. It became part of a personal care kit along with a depilatory tweezer and a ear wax scoop (Mandel 1990). In 1872, Silas Noble and J.P. Cooley patented the first toothpick-manufacturing machine.

The key difference between a toothpick and a woodstick (wooden stimulator/cleaner) relates to the triangular (wedge-like) design. Woodsticks should not be confused with toothpicks which are simply meant for removing food debris after a meal (Warren & Chater 1996a). Woodsticks are inserted interdentally with the base of the triangle resting on the gingival side. The tip should point occlusally or incisally and the triangles against the adjacent tooth surfaces. Triangular wedge-like woodsticks have been found to be superior in plaque removal when compared with round or rectangluar woodsticks since they fit the interdental area more snugly (Bergenholtz *et al*. 1980; Mandel 1990). Woodsticks are usually made of soft wood to prevent injury to the gingiva. The tapered form makes it possible for the patient to angle the woodstick interdentally and even clean the lingually localized interdental surfaces. Unlike floss they can be used on the concave surfaces of the tooth root. Some are hand held, while others are designed to be mounted in a handle, which helps gain access to the interdental areas in the posterior region of the mouth (Axelsson 2004).

The wood can store fluoride crystals both on the surface and in the porosities. These crystals readily dissolve when the woodstick is moistened with saliva (Axelsson 2004). During use the soft wood may become splayed. As soon as the first signs of splaying are evident the woodstick should be discarded. As stated above most patients prefer to use woodsticks for the removal of interdental plaque. Woodsticks have the advantage that they are easy to use, and can be used throughout the day without the need for special facilities such as a bathroom or a mirror. Woodsticks may also be used in primary prevention, even in cases of poor manual dexterity, including posterior areas. To use woodsticks there must be sufficient interdental space available and in these cases woodsticks are an excellent substitute to dental floss. Although woodsticks have a good cleansing capacity in the center part of the interproximal surfaces of teeth in contact, their effect is reduced on the lingual side of these surfaces. The woodstick is somewhat difficult to use in the far posterior regions of the jaws because of the lack of accessibility and since the triangular cross section must pass into the embrassure space at a specific angle (Bassiouny & Grant 1981).

When used in healthy dentitions, woodsticks may depress the gingival margin and clean the toothsurface up to 2–3 mm subgingivally (Morch & Waerhaug 1956). Long-term use may cause a permanent loss of the papilla and opening of the embrasure which may have important esthetic implications in the anterior dentition. Woodsticks can clearly be recommended in patients with open interdental spaces as secondary prevention for periodontal diseases.

A review of the literature for studies that have addressed the question whether woodsticks used as adjunct to toothbrushing in adult patients have an effect on plaque and periodontal inflammation identified eight publications. In only one study a significant reduction in plaque scores was reported as result of the use of woodsticks (Schmid *et al.* 1976). In three studies the use of woodsticks resulted in reduction of gingival bleeding (Anaise 1976; Bassiouny & Grant 1981; Bouwsma *et al.* 1992).

Interdental brushes (see Procedure 5)

Interdental brushes were introduced in the 1960s as an alternative to woodsticks. They are effective in the removal of plaque from the proximal tooth surfaces (Bergenholtz & Olsson 1984). The interdental brush consists of soft nylon filaments twisted into a fine stainless steel wire. This 'metal' wire can prove uncomfortable for patients with sensitive root surfaces. For such patients the use of plastic-coated metal wires may be recommended. The support wire is continuous or inserted into a metal/plastic handle. Interdental brushes are manufactured in different sizes and forms The most common forms are cylindrical or conical/tapered (like a Christmas tree). The length of the bristles in cross section should be tailored to the interdental space. Appropriate interdental brushes are currently available for the smallest to the largest interdental space (Fig. 35-6). Although unconfirmed with scientific documentation, it is believed that the most effcient cleaning is achieved if the brush selected is slightly larger than the embrasure space. The brush is inserted obliquely into the

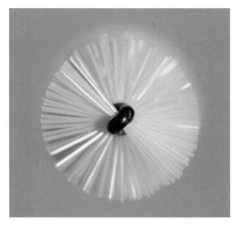

Fig. 35-6 With interdental brushes the diameter of the metal wire core is a detemining factor with respect to access. A close fit of the brushing filaments influences the cleaning ability.

interdental space, from an apical direction. Cleaning is performed with a back-and-forth motion. The interdental brush is the aid of choice when root surfaces with concavities or grooves have been exposed. The interdental brush is also the most suitable cleaning device in "through-and-through" furcation defects. Like woodsticks, interdental brushes are easy to use, although they may have some drawbacks, including the fact that different types may be needed to fit differently sized open interproximal spaces. When not properly used, interdental brushes may elicit dentin hypersensitivity. In order to minimize the risk of hard tissue abrasion interdental brushes should be used without dentifrice except in special cases and then only short-term. They can also be regularly used as a carrier to apply fluoride or antimicrobial agents, e.g. chlorhexidine gel into the interdental space to prevent caries or the recolonization of residual pockets. The brush should be discarded when the filaments become loose or deformed.

Interdental brushes represent the ideal interdental cleaning tool, especially for periodontitis patients. Waerhaug (1976) showed that individuals who habitually used an interdental brush were able to maintain supragingival proximal surfaces free of plaque and to remove some subgingival plaque below the gingival margin. In a more recent study in patients with moderate to severe periodontitis Christou and co-workers (1998) showed the interdental brush to be more effective than dental floss in the removal of plaque and in promoting pocket reduction. Patients reported that the use of interdental brushes was easier than the use of dental floss. This is in agreement with previous studies (e.g. Wolffe 1976). Also the perception of efficacy was better for the interdental brushes. Significantly less patients reported problems with the use of interdental brushes. Even if efficacy of interdental brushes were not better than that of floss, the long-term use of interdental brushes might be more easily implemented in a patient's routine than that of floss.

Single-tufted/end-tufted brush (see Procedure 6)

Single-tufted brushes are designed with smaller brush heads that have a small group of tufts or a single tuft. The tuft may be 3–6 mm in diameter and can be flat or tapered. The handle can be straight or contra-angled. Angulated handles permit easier access to lingual and palatal aspects. The filaments are directed into the area to be cleaned and activated with a rotating motion. Single-tufted toothbrushes are designed to improve access to distal surfaces of posterior molars, tipped, rotated or displaced teeth, to clean around and under fixed partial dentures, pontic, orthodontic appliances, or precission attachment, and to clean teeth affected by gingival recession and irregular gingival margin or furcation involvement.

Adjunctive aids

Dental water jet

The dental water jet was introduced in 1962. This device, also called an oral irrigator, has been demonstrated to be safe and effective. Oral irrigation has been a source of controversy within the field of periodontology. The daily use of oral irrigation has been shown to reduce dental plaque, calculus, gingivitis, bleeding, probing depth, periodontal pathogens, and host inflammatory mediators (Cutler *et al*. 2000). The strongest and most consistent evidence for the benefit of daily use of a dental water jet is the ability of the device to reduce gingivitis and bleeding. It has been reported that a pulsating stream of water is better than a continuous flow. The pulsating, hydrodynamic forces produced by irrigators can rinse away food debris from interdental spaces and plaque-retentive areas. Irrigation is not, however, a monotherapy but an adjunct designed to supplement or enhance other home care methods (brushing and flossing) intended for mechanical plaque removal (Hugoson 1978; Cutler *et al*. 2000).

Irrigation devices may be used with water or with disinfective ingredients (Lang & Raber 1982). In a study by Flemmig and co-workers (1990) it was observed that the addition of water irrigation to regular oral hygiene reduced bleeding on probing by 50% over a 6-month timeframe. The use of chlorhexidine in suboptimum concentrations (e.g. 0.06%) led to improved plaque inhibition and had an anti-inflammatory effect (Lang & Räber 1982; Flemmig *et al*. 1990). The success of pulsating irrigators with regular tips is limited in the subgingival area, and in periodontal pockets (Wennström *et al*. 1987). With specially designed tips (PikPocket: Waterpik Technologies, Inc.; Newport Beach, CA, USA), the pulsat-

ing stream of fluid may penetrate more deeply into the pocket areas (Cobb *et al*. 1988).

Tongue cleaners (see Procedure 7)

The dorsum of the tongue, with its papillary structure and furrows, harbors a great number of microorganisms (Chapter 60). It forms a unique ecologic oral site with a large surface area (Danser *et al*. 2003). The tongue is said to act as a reservoir which permits the accumulation and stagnation of bacteria and food residues (Outhouse *et al*. 2006). The tongue bacteria may serve as a source of bacterial dissemination to other parts of the oral cavity, e.g. the tooth surfaces and may contribute to dental plaque formation. Therefore, tongue brushing has been advocated as part of daily home oral hygiene together with toothbrushing and flossing (Christen & Swanson 1978). Tongue brushing has also been advocated as a component of the so-called "full-mouth disinfection" approach in the treatment of periodontitis, with the aim of reducing possible reservoirs of pathogenic bacteria (Quirynen *et al*. 2000).

Regular tongue cleaning has been used since ancient times and is still used by natives of Africa, Arabic countries, India, and South America. Many ancient religions emphasized cleanliness of the entire mouth, including the tongue. Indian people's daily ritual of oral hygiene was not only confined to brushing of the teeth but also the tongue was scraped and the mouth was rinsed with concoctions of betel leaves, cardamom, camphor or other herbs.

A large variety of tongue cleaners is commercially available. A modern tongue-scraping instrument may consist of a long strip of plastic ribbon. This is held in both hands and bent so that the edge can be pulled down over the dorsal surface of the tongue. Brushing also appears to be an easy method of cleaning the tongue providing that the gagging reflex can be controlled. In a recent systematic review it was concluded that scrapers or cleaners are more effective than toothbrushes for tongue cleaning (Outhouse *et al*. 2006). Patients should be informed that it is most important to clean the posterior portion of the tongue dorsum.

Tongue cleaning is a simple and fast procedure that helps to remove microorganisms and debris from the tongue. When tongue cleaning is practiced on a daily basis, the process becomes easier. Eventually, the patient may indeed feel "unclean" when tongue debris is not removed on a regular basis. In a study by Gross and co-workers (1975) the test group was instructed to brush their tongues as an adjunct to their normal oral hygiene measures. The members of a control group were not instructed to clean the tongue. A reduction in the presence of tongue coating was found of 40% in the test group as compared to the control group.

Some studies have shown that tongue brushing in combination with other methods of oral hygiene is an effective method in reducing the formation of dental plaque. In contrast, Badersten and co-workers (1975) found no difference in *de novo* plaque accumulation between a 4-day period of tongue brushing and a 4-day period of no oral hygiene procedures. The authors suggested that the majority of the important plaque-forming bacteria might not originate from the tongue. Another reason for not finding an effect of tongue brushing on plaque formation may be that brushing of the posterior part of the dorsum of the tongue is difficult due to inaccesibility and discomfort.

Dentifrices

The use of a toothbrush is usually combined with a dentifrice (sold as *toothpaste*) with the purpose of facilitating plaque removal and applying agents to the tooth surfaces for therapeutic or preventive reasons (Chapter 36). In 1824, a dentist named Peabody was the first person to add soap to toothpaste. John Harris first added chalk as an ingredient to toothpaste in the 1850s. Colgate mass-produced the first toothpaste in a jar. In 1892, Dr. Washington Sheffield of Connecticut manufactured toothpaste into a collapsible tube. The traditional role of dentifrice is primarily cosmetic, in aiding the cleaning of teeth and producing fresh breath. It also makes toothbrushing more pleasant.

The studies by de la Rosa and co-workers (1979) and Stean and Forward (1980) validated the use of dentifrice since they found that there was a reduction in plaque growth after brushing with a dentifrice as opposed to brushing with water. In the course of the years many dentifrice formulations were tested and became well established because of their anti-plaque and/or anti-gingivitis properties. For additional information see Chapter 36.

Foam brushes, swabs or tooth towelettes

Tooth towelettes are being marketed as a method of plaque removal when toothbrushing is not possible. Their use is not meant to replace a daily toothbrushing regimen. Recently the I-Brush® has been introduced. This swab is mounted on the index finger of the brushing hand. It uses the agility and sensitivity of the finger. Consequently it could permit a better control over the finger pressure because the finger can actually feel the tooth and gingival surfaces and help positioning the brush for more effective scrubbing. During a 3-week clinical trial, no adverse effects were found. The results show that the finger brush removed less plaque than a regular manual toothbrush. In particular approximal plaque reduction was poor in comparison with the manual toothbrush. Based on these results, it is concluded that there is no beneficial effect of the finger brush in comparison with a regular manual toothbrush (Graveland *et al.* 2004).

Foam brushes resemble a disposable soft sponge on a stick and have been dispensed to hospital patients for intraoral cleansing and refreshing as early as the 1970s. They are particularly used for oral care in medically compromised and immunocompromised patients, to reduce the risk of oral and systemic infection (Pearson & Hutton 2002). Lefkoff and co-workers (1995) studied the effectiveness of such a disposable foam brush on plaque. In this study the regular manual toothbrush was found to be significantly more effective in retarding the accumulation of plaque from a plaque-free baseline on both facial and lingual surfaces. The foam brush did, however, show some plaque-preventive capabilities by maintaining plaque formation below 2 mm at the cervical margin of the tooth. Nevertheless, according to most authors, foam brushes should not be considered as a substitute for a regular toothbrush. In a study by Ransier and co-workers (1995) foam brushes were saturated with a chlorhexidine solution. They found the foam brush which had been soaked in chlorhexidine to be as effective as a regular toothbrush in controlling plaque and gingivitis levels. Therefore, if a toothbrush cannot be used in hospitalized patients, an alternative may be the use of chlorhexidine applied with a foam brush.

Side effects

Brushing force

Studies have shown brushing force with powered toothbrushes to be lower than that of a manual toothbrush (Van der Weijden *et al.* 1996c). This appears to be a consistent finding. There is an approximately 1.0 N difference between manual and powered toothbrushes. Recently McCracken and co-workers (2003) observed, in a range from 0.75–3.0 N, that the improvement in plaque removal, using a power toothbrush with forces in excess of 1.5 N was negligible. In a feedback study a professional brusher was asked to brush at 1.0 N, 1.5 N, 2.0 N, 2.5 N, and 3.0 N, during which the efficacy in relation of brushing force to brushing was determined. An increase in efficacy was observed with raising brushing force from 1.0 N to 3.0 N (Van der Weijden *et al.* 1996c). Hasegawa and co-workers (1992) evaluated the effect of different toothbrushing forces on plaque reduction by brushing with 100 g intervals on a scale from 100–500 g. The results of their study corroborate the findings of earlier studies that with increasing force more plaque is removed. In addition they observed that 300 g seems to be the most effective brushing force when using a manual toothbrush for both children and adults. Forces exceeding 300 g caused pain and gingival bleeding in the test patients. As shown in a manual brushing study in which efficacy was plotted against brushing force the relationship between force and efficacy appears not to be linear (Van der Weijden *et al.* 1998a). Using this particular manual toothbrush a positive correlation between efficacy and force up to 4.0 N was found. The more force was used, the more effective was the plaque removal. However efficacy was reduced when forces above 4.0 N were used. Indeed there appeared to be a negative correlation. The hypothesis is that this negative correlation had to do with distortion of the brushing filaments. Above 4.0 N the brushing was no longer performed with the tip of the filament, but due to bending, with its side. This indicates that brushing force is not the sole factor which determines efficacy. Other factors such as action of the brush, size of the brushhead, brushing time, and manual dexterity may be of greater importance.

Excessive brushing force has been mentioned as a factor which is partly responsible for the origin of toothbrush trauma (gingival abrasion). In response to patients that use excessive force, manual and electric toothbrush manufacturers have introduced toothbrush designs, which can limit the amount of force used and thus reduce the chance of damage to soft and hard tissues. However there is no linear correlation between brushing force and abrasion. Mierau and Spindler (1989) performed a quantitative assessment of habit patterns of toothbrushing in 28 subjects and nine sessions. Least variations within each individual were observed with regard to brushing force. Brushing force ranged from 1.0–7.4 N between individuals. They did not observe any (visual) lesions from brushing in those individuals using a brushing force <2 N. If the brushing force was >2 N, co-factors such as brushing time, brushing method, and frequency of brushing appeared to be associated with acute brushing lesions. Burgett & Ash (1974) argued that the potential detrimental effect of brushing is related to the force applied at a particular point, i.e. pressure. it must be recognized that the head of a manual brush is larger than the head of the electric brush. Since the forces are given as a total of the force over the entire brush it may be that the unit pressure was less for the manual than for the electric brushes. They observed no difference in pressure between a soft manual (11.32 g/mm^2) and an electric toothbrush (11.29 g/mm^2). These data which show that the pressure for the electric and the manual brush are similar are also in agreement with findings presented by Van der Weijden and co-workers (1996c).

Toothbrush abrasion

Since various mechanical products are used in personal control of supragingival plaque, the possibility exists that some deleterious effects may appear as a consequence of these oral hygiene practices (Echeverría 1998). It has already been known for a long time that toothbrushing may have some unwanted effects on the gingiva and hard tooth tissues (Kitchin 1941). Trauma to hard tissues leads to cervical abrasion of the tooth surface. These lesions have been associated with toothbrush stiffness, the method of brushing, and brushing frequency. Cervical tooth abrasion has a multifactorial etiology, but in most cases it is the consequence of toothbrushing due to an excessive pressure of the brush and an excessive number of

toothbrushing episodes/time. Both situations are probably linked to personality traits (*compulsive brushers*). Tooth wear has also been associated with toothbrush characteristics, especially related to the finishing and hardness of the filaments (Fishman 1997). It has been stated that hard tissue damage is mainly caused by the abrasives in the dentifrice, whereas lesions of the gingival tissues are caused by the toothbrush (Axelsson *et al.* 1997; Meyers *et al.* 2000).

In many instances, *tooth abrasion* is found in combination with *gingival recession*. Whereas gingival recession is associated with different etiologic/risk factors, e.g. periodontal inflammation, smoking, gingival biotype or repeated periodontal instrumentation, inadequate toothbrushing is probably the most significant one (Björn *et al.* 1981). Clinical experience does support the idea that, with improper use, toothbrushing can cause superficial damage to the gingival tissues. Patients with good oral hygiene have been found to have more gingival recession and more dental abrasion than those with poor oral hygiene. Unfortunately there are few studies in the dental literature concerning gingival lesions resulting from toothbrushing. Thus, to what extent oral hygiene procedures may traumatize the gingival tissues is not clear. Gingival abrasions as a result of brushing are often reversible localized superficial lesions. It is unlikely that gingival abrasion is induced by a single factor. One factor which has already been mentioned to be related to gingival abrasion is brushing force. In the literature, other factors have been suggested such as brushing method (e.g. Bass method), abusive toothbrush use, manual or powered toothbrushing, toothbrush grip, brush head shape, stiffness of filaments, end-rounding of toothbrush filaments, and toothbrushing frequency (Van der Weijden & Danser 2000).

Interestingly, there has been little debate on the role of dentifrice in the abrasion of soft tissues. This is somewhat surprising when abrasion of dental hard tissues is almost entirely a function of dentifrice. Detergents in dentifrice, agitated over a mucosal surface, could enhance the removal of the protective salivary glycoprotein layer and exert cytotoxic action on the overlying epithelial cells (Addy & Hunter 2003). No statistically significant difference in the incidence of gingival abrasion was found between brushing with dentifrice or without dentifrice (Versteeg *et al.* 2005) (Fig. 35-7).

Importance of instruction and motivation in mechanical plaque control

A fundamental principle for all preventive action is that the effect is greatest where the risk of development of disease is greatest. Needs-related instruction in oral hygiene should therefore intensify mechanical plaque removal on those individual teeth and surfaces that are at risk. A prerequisite for establishing needs-related toothcleaning habits is a well

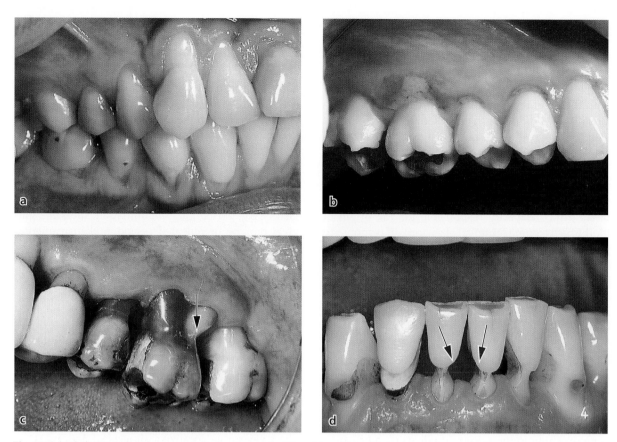

Fig. 35-7 (a) Soft tissue damage as a result of extensive toothbrushing. Note gingival recession on the buccal gingival surface of tooth 13. (b) Note multiple ulcerations of the buccal gingival margin in the right maxilla. (c,d) Hard tissue damage has resulted after extensive use of interdental brushes.

motivated, well informed, and well instructed patient (Axelsson 2004). Mechanical plaque control demands active participation of the individual subject, and therefore the establishment of proper oral home care habits is a process that involves and depends on behavioral changes to a great extent. When implementing behavioral changes, dental professionals should try to ensure that the patient recognizes his/ her oral health status and the role of his/her personal oral hygiene procedures in the prevention of caries and periodontal diseases. The patient should be informed about the casual relationship that led to the disease process and should be encouraged to take responsibility for his/her own oral health. The dental team has numerous possibilities to demonstrate soft tissue alterations elicited by inflammation to the patient, and the responsible etiologic factors. Most commonly, as with sports coaching, a one-to-one professional–patient approach should be employed.

Many patients spend too little time brushing or they brush haphazardly. The importance of thorough plaque removal should be stressed. Toothbrushing instruction for a patient involves teaching what, when, where, and how. In addition, instruction should also involve a description of specific toothbrushing methods, the grasp of the brush, the sequence and amount of brushing, the areas of limited access, supplementary brushing for occlusal surfaces and the tongue. The possible detrimental effects from improper toothbrushing and variations for special condition are described (Wilkins 1999). The design of toothbrushes or a specific toothbrushing method are of secondary importance to the skills of the individual in using the brush (Frandsen 1986). The simplest, least time-consuming procedures that will effectively remove bacterial plaque and maintain oral health should be recommended. If a patient prefers a specific oral hygiene strategy the clinician can evaluate this and modify the technique to maximize effectiveness, rather than changing it. Although it is necessary to give all patients honest feedback on their plaque removal efforts, it is also important to reward a positive performance and not entertain unrealistic expectations, so that the patient will not dread each maintenance visit.

Oral hygiene instruction should also include components such as self-assessment, self-examination, self-monitoring, and self-instruction. With this purpose, several devices and chemical agents have been used in order to make dental plaque more evident to the patient. The interested patient can be informed and motivated, for example, through use of disclosing agents to visualize plaque at the gingival margin or in the interdental spaces. Disclosing agents are chemical compounds such as erythrosine, fuchsin or a fluorescein-containing dye that stains dental plaque and thus makes it fully evident to the patient, either with regular or ultraviolet light. Erythrosine

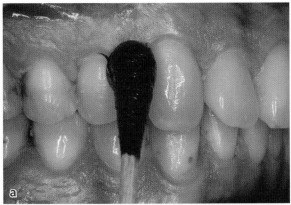
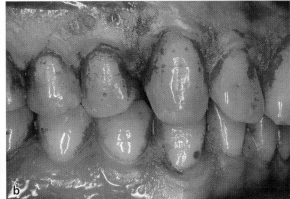
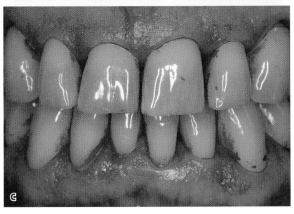

Fig. 35-8 (a) Disclosing solution is often used to identify plaque. (b) Note remaining plaque on the buccal tooth surfaces after staining. (c) After self-performed tooth cleaning, remaining plaque can be identified by the patient following rinsing with a disclosing solution.

has already been used for many years and has received an FDA approval (Arnim 1963) (Fig. 35-8).

When applied immediately before toothbrushing, the patient can identify the amount of plaque formed after the last toothbrushing episode, thus receiving an immediate feedback about his/her cleaning performance. This procedure is useful during the early phase of plaque control. Later on, the disclosing agent should be applied after toothbrushing, which allows the patient to identify those areas needing additional cleaning efforts. Disclosing solution is available in either liquid or tablet form. The liquid may offer some advantages in that the operator can ensure that all surfaces are adequately covered. The red disclosing solution remains in the mouth for some time and may temporarily stain the lips and gingiva.

Disclosing of plaque in the patient's mouth is usually not enough to establish good oral hygiene habits, however. Other factors might influence the individual to modify or determine his or her behavior. These factors may be more or less beyond the control of the dental personnel (such as social and personal factors, environmental setting, and past dental experiences) or may lie within the control of dental personnel (such as conditions of treatment, instruction, and education of the patient). All of these should be considered in the design of an individualized oral hygiene program.

A variety of methods can be used to deliver advice and instruction. The effect of various oral hygiene instruction programs, administered individually or in groups, has been evaluated in a number of clinical studies. These studies have evaluated whether instruction given during one visit only is similar to step-by-step instruction provided during several visits, or whether the use of pamphlets or video tapes is superior to self-instruction manuals and to personal instruction given by a dental professional. In a study by Renton-Harper and co-workers (1999) an instructional video for an oscillating rotating electric toothbrush was evaluated. The subjects that followed the instructional video benefited significantly and considerably in terms of plaque removal compared to subjects receiving only written instructions. Different types and amounts of feedback to the patients using disclosed plaque scores and phase contrast demonstrations have also been investigated. These studies have usually reported similar improvements in plaque and gingivitis scores, irrespective of the mode of instruction. However, these results should be interpreted with caution since the subjects participating in these studies were examined at regular intervals, and therefore it is difficult to separate the effect of repeated examinations from the effect of the instructions (Renvert & Glavind 1998).

If oral hygiene motivation, information, and instruction are combined with professional tooth cleaning the effect in terms of reduction of plaque levels and levels of gingival inflammation may persist even after 6 months. A recent systematic review concluded, based on studies ≥6 months of duration, that a single oral hygiene instruction, describing the use of a mechanical toothbrush, in addition to a single professional "oral prophylaxis" provided at baseline, had a significant, albeit small, positive effect on the reduction of gingivitis (Van der Weijden & Hioe 2005).

Rylander and Lindhe (1997) have recommended that oral hygiene instruction be given during a series of visits allowing the possibility of giving the patient immediate feedback and reinforcing the patient in his/her home care activities. The protocol below is based on the one used in several clinical trials by Lindhe and Nyman (1975), Rosling and co-workers (1976), and Lindhe and co-workers (1982), where the role of plaque control in preventing and arresting periodontal diseases was clearly proven.

First session

1. Apply a plaque-disclosing solution to the teeth and, with aid of a hand mirror, demonstrate all sites with plaque to the patient (Fig. 35-8b). The plaque score should be recorded using a plaque control record (Fig. 35-9).
2. Ask the patient to clean the teeth using his/her traditional technique. With the aid of a hand mirror, demonstrate the results of the toothbrushing to the patient, again identifying all sites with plaque (Fig. 35-8c).
3. Without changing the technique, ask the patient to clean the surfaces with plaque.

Depending on the plaque remaining after this second toothbrushing, the dental professional should either improve the technique or introduce an alterna-

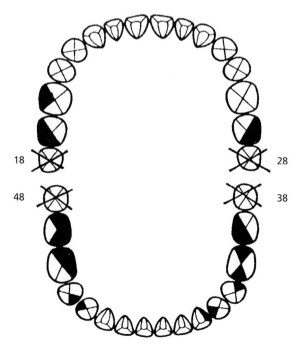

Fig. 35-9 A chart illustrating the teeth and tooth surfaces in the maxilla and mandible. The distribution of tooth surfaces with dental plaque (shadowed areas) is identified. In this case the plaque score is 17%.

tive system of toothbrushing. In order not to overload the patient with too much information during the first session, the use of adjunctive devices for interproximal cleaning can be introduced or improved in the second session.

Second session

1. A few days after the previous session, the disclosing solution is again applied. The results, in terms of plaque deposits, are identified in the mouth, recorded in the plaque control record, and discussed with the patient.
2. The patient is then invited to clean the teeth, according to the directions previously given in the first session, until all staining is removed. In many cases, toothbrushing instructions will need to be reinforced. Reinforcement and positive recognition should be given to the patient at the same time.

If necessary, the use of interproximal cleaning aids can now be introduced or improved.

Third and following sessions

1. One or two weeks later the same procedure used in the second session is repeated. However, the efficacy of self-performed plaque control should be evaluated and presented to the patient at each appointment. This repeated instruction, supervision, and evaluation aims to reinforce the necessary behavioral changes.

The long-term result of oral hygiene instruction is dependent on behavioral changes. Patients may fail to comply with given instructions for many reasons, ranging from unwillingness to perform oral self-care, poor understanding, lack of motivation, poor dental health beliefs, and unfavorable dental health values, to stressful life events or low socioeconomic status. Although the use of behavior-modification techniques may offer an advantage over traditional instruction techniques, there is limited research in this area to clarify the relationship between health beliefs and compliance.

Conclusion

- Oral hygiene instruction should be tailored to each individual patient on the basis of his/her personal needs and other factors.
- The patient should be involved in the instructional process.
- An individualized maintenance program should follow the basic oral hygiene instruction.

All the illustrations for the following procedures are used with permission from *Paro Praktijk Utrecht*.

Procedure 1: Instruction for Manual Toothbrush

It is of utmost importance that in addition to using the correct toothpaste and also brushing for at least 2 minutes to brush the teeth in a set sequence. This prevents missing out certain areas. Areas untouched by the brush allow plaque to continue to grow. Try to choose a brush with medium or soft bristles and a small head.

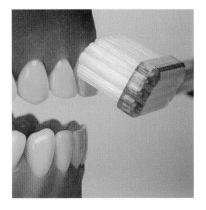

Instruction
- Hold the brush firmly and place the bristles at an angle against the edge of your gums (use a 45° angle). Take care to ensure that the bristles are in contact with a small part of the gum margin.
- Place the brush against the molar or tooth at the back of the mouth and make short back and forth scrubbing movements. Brush from the back to the front of the mouth and try to overlap the strokes. Do not brush more than two teeth simultaneously. Always start at the back and work slowly forwards.
- Always hold the brush head horizontal when cleaning the outside surfaces of the teeth. It is easier to hold the head vertically when brushing the inside surfaces of the top and bottom teeth.
- Avoid too much pressure and fast movements and be aware of feeling contact with the gum margin. Also avoid brushing too vigorously thereby preventing damage to the gums.

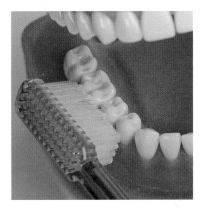

When cleaning the teeth keep using the same sequence of brushing. For example, inside of bottom jaw left (15 seconds) inside right (15 seconds). Then left on the outside (15 seconds), followed by right on the outside (15 seconds). Repeat the same sequence in the top jaw. Finally, brush the chewing surfaces with small scrubbing movements. Replace the brush when the bristles start to splay.

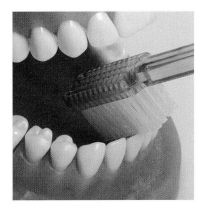

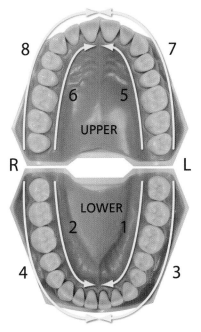

Procedure 2: Instruction for the Electric Toothbrush

The importance of using a set sequence of brushing movements is also applicable when using an electric toothbrush. The question as to whether an electric brush is better than a manual one has been asked many times. Both allow to one achieve a high level of oral hygiene. However research has shown that electric toothbrushes are more efficient and many people report that they are easier to use.

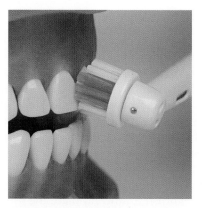

Instruction
- Place the brush firmly on the hand piece. Grip the brush in the palm so that the bristles of the head are somewhat angled toward the gums (at an angle of approximately 70°). Try to allow the longer bristles to penetrate between the teeth and take care that the bristles contact your gums.
- Switch on the brush and place the head on the last tooth in the mouth (check the angle) and move the head gradually (in about 2 seconds) from the back to the front of this tooth.
- Try to follow the contour of both the tooth and the gums. Place the brush head on the next tooth and repeat this process.
- Allow the electric toothbrush to do the work. It is not necessary to press hard or make brushing movements.
- Use a timer! Many brushes will give some form of signal after 30 seconds (the apparatus stops for a moment). This is the point at which to move on to a new part of the mouth.

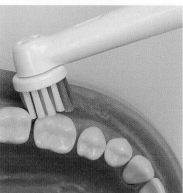

Remember to thoroughly clean the brush and its head when finished.

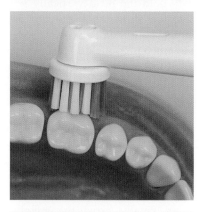

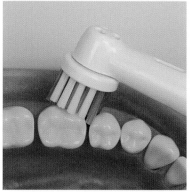

Procedure 3: Use of Dental Floss

The use of dental floss has become part of oral care in addition to correct, more frequent and longer tooth brushing. Floss can be purchased in a variety of thicknesses and types and with or without a layer of wax. If there is sufficient space between the front and back teeth is it advisable to use the somewhat thicker tape than the thinner floss.

Instruction
- Take approximately 40 cm of floss and wind the ends loosely around the middle finger. Allow for 10 cm between the middle fingers. Then hold the floss between the thumb and first finger so that about 3 cm remains between the thumbs.
- Using a sawing movement, allow the tightly stretched piece of floss to pass between the front and back teeth. This may be difficult where teeth are so close that the space between them is limited. Avoid allowing the floss to slip so fast between the teeth that the gums become damaged.
- Stretch the floss around one of the teeth and carefully allow it to pass just under the gum, once again with a sawing movement.
- Draw the floss up to the contact point with a sawing movement and then repeat the process on the other tooth bordering the space filled with gum tissue.
- Remove the floss from between the teeth, once again with a sawing movement and repeat this process for all the other spaces in the mouth.
- Use a clean piece of floss for each separate space by unwinding part of it from around one middle finger whilst winding it around the other middle finger.

Do not worry if at first your gums bleed slightly. This will stop after using the floss a number of times. Don't give up!

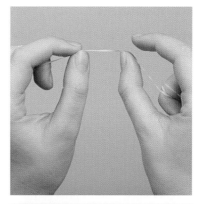
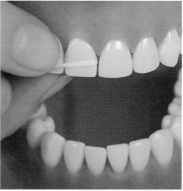
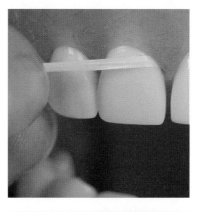
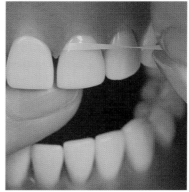

Procedure 4: Woodsticks

Most adults have sufficient space available between the incisors and molars to allow woodsticks to be used. These come in differing thicknesses and are made from wood and have a triangular cross section, mimicking the shape of the space between the teeth. Woodsticks can only be used once and are ideal when you have a few spare moments – for example when sitting in a traffic queue!

Instruction
- Hold the woodstick firmly between the thumb and first finger about halfway along its length. When possible place the other fingers for support on the chin. Moisten the tip of the woodstick by sucking on the point of it, thus making it softer and more flexible.
- Place the flat side of the woodstick (i.e. not the sharp side) against the gum. In the upper jaw the flat surface will face upwards and in the lower jaw downwards.
- Push the woodstick firmly from the outer side of the space into it until it becomes just wedged. Then pull it back slightly and push it back once again, using a light sawing motion at right angles to the outer surfaces of the teeth. Light pressure can also be applied simultaneously to the gums. Repeat this a few times, angling the woodstick so as to contact the surfaces of the teeth enclosing the space.
- When using a woodstick between the premolars and molars, close the mouth slightly to reduce tension in the cheeks making the movements easier.

With this method, all spaces between the teeth throughout the mouth can be cleaned. Should the woodstick prick the surface of the gums with the point, angle it a little differently – in the upper jaw the point will face downwards and in the lower jaw upwards. Do not be concerned if your gums bleed a little at first – this will disappear after using the woodsticks repeatedly for a period of time.

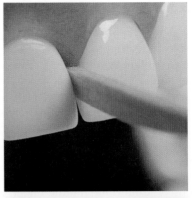

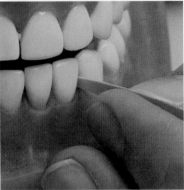

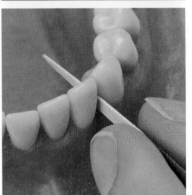

Procedure 5: Interproximal Brushes

Interdental brushes are purchasable in a variety of sizes varying from small to very large. It is of importance to choose the correct diameter of the bristle part of the brush. The size of the space between the teeth determines the size of the diameter of the bristles on the brush. It is often necessary to use different size of brush within one mouth for optimal cleansing. In order to effectively remove dental plaque there should be a slight degree of resistance when the brush is moved back and forth between the teeth.

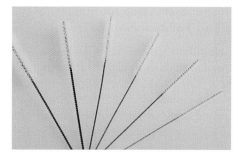

Instruction
- Always use the interdental brush *without* toothpaste
- Hold the interdental brush between the thumb and first finger just behind the bristles. Support can be achieved when necessary by placing your other fingers on your chin. Push, from the outer side of the space, the interdental brush carefully between the teeth, taking care that the brush remains at right angles to the teeth.
- Avoid scraping the centre (metal spiral part) of the brush against the teeth.
- Slide the brush in and out of the space using the full length of the bristle part of the brush. This will remove the dental plaque.
- The area of contact between the brush and the teeth can be somewhat increased by using differing angles of insertion.
- Slight pressure of the brush against the gums should be used as this will allow the bristles to penetrate a little underneath the gum margin.
- By slightly closing the mouth it will be easier to manipulate the brush as the tension in the cheeks is lessened. It may also be of help to slightly bend the brush to ease insertion.
- Cleanse all areas between the teeth where an interdental brush will fit. Rinse the interdental brushes thoroughly after use and allow them to dry out. It is often a good idea to combine the use if interdental brushes and woodsticks.

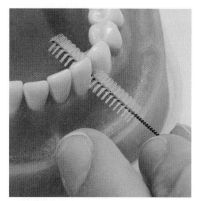

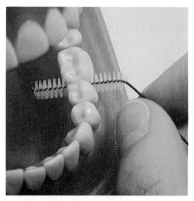

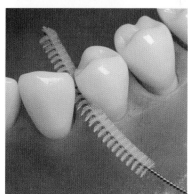

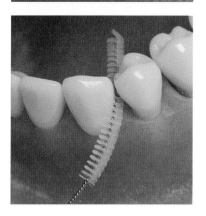

Procedure 6: Instruction for Single-Tufted/End-Tufted Brush

The single-tufted toothbrush is a small brush with a small, single tuft of short bristles attached to the end. The end-tufted brush has a number of small tufts attached in a similar manner. These brushes are ideal for cleansing areas of the dentition which cannot be reached with other oral hygiene aids. For example a lone standing tooth, the back surface of the last molar or tooth in the arch, wires and locks of orthodontic braces, grooves or the entrance to areas where roots split apart.

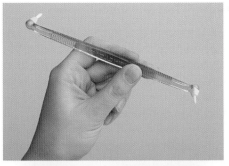

Instruction
- Hold the single-tufted brush in the same way as a pen. This prevents too much force being applied to the gums.
- Place the single-tufted brush at an angle directed toward the gums (about 45°) – this allows the bristles to reach just under the gum margin.
- Use small, rotational pencil movements.
- The bristles of the brush will then rotate under and along the gum margin. The brush should then be slowly moved along the tooth surface to cover all areas.

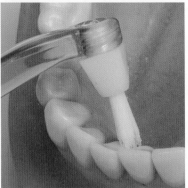

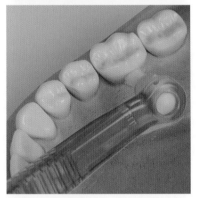

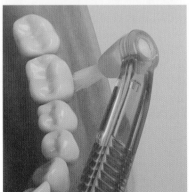

Procedure 7: Use of Tongue Cleaners

Tongue cleaning is a useful addition to the daily oral hygiene routine. Many bacteria can be found within the grooves on the back of the tongue which can cause bad breath. By brushing or scraping the tongue this problem can be markedly helped or prevented entirely. One of the problems associated with tongue cleaning is that it can stimulate a gag reflex, especially when first using this procedure. This occurs more frequently with brushing than when using a scraper. Some people find it less of a problem if they clean their tongue in the evening.

Instruction
- There are various types of tongue cleaners: the most effective seems to be one having the form of a loop.
- Extend the tongue as far as possible out of your mouth.
- Breathe calmly through your nose.
- Place the tongue cleaner as far as possible on the back of the tongue and press lightly with it so that the tongue becomes flattened.
- Ensure full contact of the tongue cleaner with the tongue.
- Pull the tongue cleaner slowly forward.
- Clean the middle part of the tongue first using the raised edge on one side of the instrument.
- Use the smooth surface of the tongue cleaner on the sides of the tongue.
- Repeat these scraping movements a number of times.
- Rinse the mouth several times.

Remember to clean the tongue cleaner thoroughly after use.

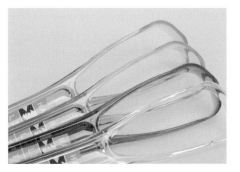

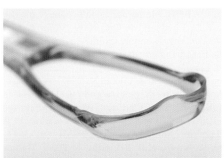

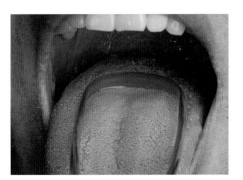

References

Addy, M. & Hunter, M.L. (2003). Can toothbrushing damage your health? Effects on oral and dental tissues. *International Dental Journal* **53** (Suppl 3), 177–186.

Agerholm, D.M. (1991). A clinical trial to evaluate plaque removal with a double-headed toothbrush. *British Dental Journal* **170**, 411–413.

Anaise, J.Z. (1976). Plaque removing effect of dental floss and toothpicks in children 12–13 years of age. *Community Dentistry and Oral Epidemiology* **4**, 137–139.

Arnim, S.S. (1963). The use of disclosing agents for measuring the tooth cleanliness. *Journal of Periodontology* **34**, 227–245.

Axelsson, P. (1994). Mechanical plaque control In: Lang, N.P. & Karring, T., eds. *Proceedings of the 1st European Workshop on Periodontology.* London: Quintessence, pp. 219–243.

Axelsson, P. (2004). *Preventive Materials, Methods and Programs.* Vol 4. London: Quintessence, pp. 37–102.

Axelsson, P., Kocher, T. & Vivien, N. (1997). Adverse effects of toothpastes on teeth, gingiva and bucal mucosa. In: Lang, N.P., Karring, T. & Lindhe, J. eds. *Proceedings of the 2nd European Workshop on Periodontology. Chemicals in Periodontics.* London: Quintessence, pp. 259–261.

Axelsson, P., Nyström, B. & Lindhe, J. (2004). The long-term effect of a plaque control program on tooth mortality, caries and periodontal disease in adults. Results after 30 years of maintenance. *Journal of Clinical Periodontology* **31**, 749–757

Ayer, W.A., Habgood, T.E., Deulofeu, V. & Juliani, H.R. (1965). A survey of the oral hygiene practices of dental students. *New York State Dental Journal* **31**, 106–112.

Badersten, A., Egelberg, J., Jonsson, G. & Kroneng, M. (1975). Effect of tongue brushing on formation of dental plaque. *Journal of Periodontology* **46**, 625–627.

Baehni, P.C. & Takeuchi, Y. (2003). Anti-plaque agents in the prevention of biofilm-associated oral diseases. *Oral Diseases* **1**, 23–29.

Bakdash, B. (1995). Current patterns of oral hygiene product use and practices. *Periodontology 2000* **8**, 11–14.

Bass, C.C. (1948). The optimum characteristics of toothbrushes for personal oral hygiene. *Dental Items of Interest* **70**, 696.

Bassiouny, M.A. & Grant, A.A. (1981). Oral hygiene for the partially edentulous. *Journal of Periodontology* **52**, 214–218.

Bergenholtz, A., Bjorne, A., Glantz, P.O. & Vikstrom, B. (1980). Plaque removal by various triangular toothpicks. *Journal of Clinical Periodontology* **7**, 121–128.

Bergenholtz, A., Bjorne, A. & Vikstrom, B. (1974). The plaque-removing ability of some common interdental aids. An intra-individual study. *Journal of Clinical Periodontology* **1**, 160–165.

Bergenholtz, A. & Olsson, A. (1984). Efficacy of plaque-removal using interdental brushes and waxed dental floss. *Scandinavian Journal of Dental Research* **92**, 198–203.

Bergström, J. (1973). Wear and hygiene status of toothbrushes in relation to some social background factors. *Swedish Dental Journal* **66**, 383–391.

Bjertness, E. (1991). The importance of oral hygiene on variation in dental caries in adults. *Acta Odontologica Scandinavica* **49**, 97–102.

Björn, A.L., Andersson, U. & Olsson, A. (1981). Gingival recession in 15-year-old pupils. *Swedish Dental Journal* **5**, 141–146.

Bosman, C.W. & Powell, R.N. (1977). The reversal of localized experimental gingivitis. A comparison between mechanical toothbrushing procedures and a 0.2% chlorhexidine mouthrinse. *Journal of Clinical Periodontology* **4**, 161–172.

Bouwsma, O.J., Yost, K.G. & Baron, H.J. (1992). Comparison of a chlorhexidine rinse and a wooden interdental cleaner in reducing interdental gingivitis. *American Journal of Dentistry* **5**, 143–146.

Breitenmoser, J., Mormann, W. & Muhlemann, H.R. (1979). Damaging effects of toothbrush bristle end form on gingiva. *Journal of Periodontology* **50**, 212–216.

Burgett, F.G. & Ash, M.M. (1974). Comparative study of the pressure of brushing with three types of toothbrushes. *Journal of Periodontology* **45**, 410–413.

Burt, B.A. & Eklund, S.A. (1999). Prevention of periodontal diseases. In: Burt, B.A. & Eklund, S.A., eds. *Dentistry, Dental Practice and the Community.* Philadelphia: W.B. Saunders Company, pp. 358–370.

Cancro, L.P. & Fischman, S.L. (1995). The expected effect on oral health of dental plaque control through mechanical removal. *Periodontology 2000* **8**, 60–74.

Carranza, F. & Shklar, G. (2003). Ancient India and China. In: *History of Periodontology.* London: Quintessence, pp. 9–13.

Charters, W.J. (1948). Home care of the mouth. I. Proper home care of the mouth. *Journal of Periodontology* **19**, 136.

Christen, A.G. & Swanson, B.Z. Jr. (1978). Oral hygiene: a history of tongue scraping and brushing. *Journal of the American Dental Association* **96**, 215–219.

Christou, V., Timmerman, M.F., van der Velden, U. & Van der Weijden, G.A. (1998). Comparison of different approaches of interdental oral hygiene: interdental brushes versus dental floss. *Journal of Periodontology* **69**, 759–764.

Conforti, N.J., Cordero, R.E., Liebman, J., Bowman, J.P., Putt, M.S., Kuebler, D.S., Davidson, K.R., Cugini, M. & Warren, P.R. (2003). An investigation into the effect of three months' clinical wear on toothbrush efficacy: results from two independent studies. *Journal of Clinical Dentistry* **14**, 29–33.

Cobb, C.M., Rodgers, R.L. & Killoy, W.J. (1988). Ultrastructural examination of human periodontal pockets following the use of an oral irrigation device in vivo. *Journal of Periodontology* **59**, 155–163.

Cronin, M.J., Dembling, W.Z., Low, M.A., Jacobs, D.M. & Weber, D.A. (2000). A comparative clinical investigation of a novel toothbrush designed to enhance plaque removal efficacy. *American Journal of Dentistry* **13** (special issue), 21–26.

Cugini, M. & Warren, P.R. (2006). The Oral-B CrossAction manual toothbrush: a 5-year literature review. *Journal of the Canadian Dental Association* **72**, 323.

Cutler, C.W., Stanford, T.W., Abraham, C., Cederberg, R.A., Boardman, T.J. & Ross, C. (2000). Clinical benefits of oral irrigation for periodontitis are related to reduction of proinflammatory cytokine levels and plaque. *Journal of Clinical Periodontology* **27**, 134–143.

Dahlén, G., Lindhe, J., Sato, K., Hanamura, H. & Okamoto, H. (1992). The effect of supragingival plaque control on the subgingival microbiota in subjects with periodontal disease. *Journal of Clinical Periodontology* **19**, 802–809.

Daly, C.G., Chapple C.C. & Cameron, A.C. (1996). Effect of toothbrush wear on plaque control. *Journal of Clinical Periodontology* **23**, 45–49.

Danser, M.M., Timmerman, M.F., Ijzerman, Y., van der Velden, U., Warren, P.R. & Van der Weijden, G.A. (1998) A comparison of electric toothbrushes in their potential to cause gingival abrasion of oral soft tissues. *American Journal of Dentistry* **11**, S35–S39.

Danser, M.M., Mantilla Gómez, S. & Van der Weijden, G.A. (2003). Tongue coating and tongue brushing: a literature review. *International Journal of Dental Hygiene* **1**, 151–158.

Darby, M.L. & Walsh, M.M. (2003). Mechanical plaque control: Toothbrushes and toothbrushing. In: *Dental Hygiene: Theory and Practice,* 2nd edn. St Louis: Saunders, pp. 348–384.

Davies, R.M., Ellwood, R.P. & Davies, G.M. (2004). The effectiveness of a toothpaste containing Triclosan and polyvinylmethyl ether maleic acid copolymer in improving plaque control and gingival health: a systematic review. *Journal of Clinical Periodontology* **31**, 1029–1033.

De la Rosa, M., Zacarias Guerra, J., Johnston, D.A. & Radike, A.W. (1979). Plaque growth and removal with daily toothbrushing. *Journal of Periodontology* **50**, 660–664.

Echeverría, J.J. (1998). Managing the use of oral hygiene aids to prevent damage: Effects and sequelae of the incorrect use of mechanical plaque removal devices. In: Lang, N.P., Attström, R. & Löe, H., eds. *Proceedings of the European Workshop on Mechanical Plaque Control.* London: Quintessence, pp. 268–278.

Egelberg, J. (1964). Gingival exudates measurements for evaluation of inflammatory changes of the gingivae. *Odontologisk Revy* **15**, 381–398.

Egelberg, J. & Claffey, N. (1998). Role of mechanical dental plaque removal in prevention and therapy of caries and periodontal diseases. Consensus Report of Group B. In: Lang, N.P., Attström, R. & Löe, H., eds. *Proceedings of the European Workshop on Mechanical Plaque Control.* London: Quintessence, pp. 169–172.

Fanning, E.A. & Henning, F.R. (1967). Toothbrush design and its relation to oral health. *Australian Dental Journal* **12**, 464–467.

Fishman, S.L. (1997). The history of oral hygiene products: How far have we come in 6000 years? *Periodontology 2000* **15**, 7–14.

Flemmig, T.F., Newman, M.G., Doherty, F.M., Grossman, E., Meckel, A.H. & Bakdash, M.B. (1990). Supragingival irrigation with 0.06% chlorhexidine in naturally occurring gingivitis. I. 6-month clinical observations. *Journal of Periodontology* **61**, 112–117.

Fones, A.C., ed. (1934). *Mouth Hygiene,* 4th edn. Philadelphia: Lea & Febiger, pp. 299–306.

Frandsen, A. (1986). Mechanical oral hygiene practices. In: Löe, H. & Kleinman, D.V., eds. *Dental Plaque Control Measures and Oral Hygiene Practices.* Oxford, Washington DC: IRL Press, pp. 93–116.

Gaffar, A., Afflito, J., Nabi, N., Herles, S., Kruger, I. & Olsen, S. (1994). Recent advances in plaque, gingivitis, tartar and caries prevention technology. *International Dental Journal* **44** (suppl 1), 63–70.

Gillette, W.B. & Van House, R.L. (1980). III effects of improper oral hygiene procedure. *Journal of the American Dental Association* **101**, 476–80.

Gordon, J.M., Frascella, J.A. & Reardon, R.C. (1996). A clinical study of the safety and efficacy of a novel electric interdental cleaning device. *Journal of Clinical Dentistry* **7**, 70–73.

Graveland, M.P., Rosema, N.A., Timmerman, M.F. & Van der Weijden, G.A. (2004). The plaque-removing efficacy of a finger brush (I-Brush®). *Journal of Clinical Periodontology* **31**, 1084–1087.

Gross, A., Barnes, G.P. & Lyon, T.C. (1975). Effects of tongue brushing on tongue coating and dental plaque scores. *Journal of Dental Research* **54**, 1236.

Grossman, E., Dembling, W. & Walley, D.R. (1994). Two long-term clinical studies comparing the plaque removal and gingivitis reduction efficacy of the Oral-B advantage plaque remover to five manual toothbrushes. *Journal of Clinical Dentistry* **5**, 46–53.

Haffajee, A.D., Smith, C., Torresyap, G., Thompson, M., Guerrero, D. & Socransky, S.S. (2001). Efficacy of manual and powered toothbrushes (II). Effect on microbiological parameters. *Journal of Clinical Periodontology* **28**, 947–54.

Hansen, F. & Gjermo, P. (1971). The plaque-removal effect of four toothbrushing methods. *Scandinavian Journal of Dental Research* **79**, 502–506.

Hawkins, B.F., Kohout, F.J., Lainson, P.A. & Heckert, A. (1986). Duration of toothbrushing for effective plaque control. *Quintessence International* **17**, 361–365.

Hasegawa, K., Machida, Y., Matsuzaki, K. & Ichinohe, S. (1992). The most effective toothbrushing force. *Pediatric Dental Journal* **2**, 139–143.

Hellstadius, K., Asman, B. & Gustafsson, A. (1993). Improved maintenance of plaque control by electrical toothbrushing in periodontitis patients with low compliance. *Journal of Clinical Periodontology* **20**, 235–237.

Hoover, J.N., Singer, D.L., Pahwa, P. & Komiyama, K. (1992). Clinical evaluation of a light energy conversion toothbrush. *Journal of Clinical Periodontology* **19**, 434–436.

Hotta, M. & Aono, M. (1992). A clinical study on the control of dental plaque using an electronic toothbrush with piezo-electric element. *Clinical Preventive Dentistry* **14**, 16–18.

Hugoson, A. (1978) Effect of the Water-Pik® device on plaque accumulation and development of gingivitis. *Journal of Clinical Periodontology* **5**, 95–104.

Hugoson, A. & Koch, G. (1979). Oral health in 1000 individuals aged 3–70 years in the Community of Jönköping, Sweden. *Swedish Dental Journal* **3**, 69–87.

Hujoel, P.P., Löe, H., Ånerud, Å., Boysen, H. & Leroux, B.G. (1998). Forty-five-year tooth survival probabilities among men in Oslo, Norway. *Journal of Dental Reasearch* **77**, 2020–2027.

Isaacs, R.L., Beiswanger, B.B., Rosenfield, S.T., Crawford, J.L., Mau, M.S., Eckert, G.J. & Warren, P.R. (1998). A crossover clinical investigation of the safety and efficacy of a new oscillating/rotating electric toothbrush and a high frequency electric toothbrush. *American Journal of Dentistry* **11**, 7–12.

Jepsen, S. (1998). The role of manual toothbrushes in effective plaque control: advantages and limitations. In: Lang, N.P., Attström, R. & Löe, H., eds. *Proceedings of the European Workshop on Mechanical Plaque Control.* London: Quintessence, pp. 121–137.

Johnson, B. D. & McInnes, C. (1994). Clinical evaluation of the efficacy and safety of a new sonic toothbrush. *Journal of Periodontology* **65**, 692–697.

Khocht, A., Simon, G., Person, P. & Denepitiya, J.L. (1993). Gingival recession in relation to history of hard toothbrush use. *Journal of Periodontology* **64**, 900–905.

Kinane, D. F., Jenkins, W.M. & Paterson, A.J. (1992). Comparative efficacy of the standard flossing procedure and a new floss applicator in reducing interproximal bleeding: a short-term study. *Journal of Periodontology* **63**, 757–760.

Kitchin, P. (1941). The prevalence of tooth root exposure and the relation of the extent of such exposure to the degree of abrasion in different age classes. *Journal of Dental Research* **20**, 565–581.

Kreifeldt, J., Hill, P.H. & Calisti, L.J. (1980). A systematic study of the plaque-removal efficiency of worn toothbrushes. *Journal of Dental Research* **59**, 2047–2055.

Kressin, N.R., Boehmer, U., Nunn, M.E. & Spiro, A., 3rd (2003). Increased preventive practices lead to greater tooth retention. *Journal of Dental Research* **82**, 223–227.

Kuusela, S., Honkala, E., Kannas, L., Tynjala, J. & Wold, B. (1997). Oral hygiene habits of 11 year-olds in 22 European countries and Canada in 1993–1994. *Journal of Dental Research* **76**, 1602–1609.

Lang, N.P., Cumming, B.R. & Löe, H. (1973). Toothbrushing frequency as it relates to plaque development and gingival health. *Journal of Periodontology* **44**, 396–405.

Lang, N.P., Cummings, B.R. & Löe, H.A. (1977). Oral hygiene and gingival health in Danish dental students and faculty. *Community Dentistry and Oral Epidemiology* **5**, 237–242.

Lang, N.P. & Räber, K. (1982). Use of oral irrigators as vehicle for the application of antimicrobial agents in chemical plaque control. *Journal of Clinical Periodontology* **8**, 177–188.

Lefkoff, M.H., Beck, F.M. & Horton, J.E. (1995). The effectiveness of a disposable tooth cleansing device on plaque. *Journal of Periodontology* **66**, 218–221.

Leonard, H.J. (1939). Conservative treatment of periodontoclasia. *Journal of the American Dental Association* **26**, 1308.

Lindhe, J. & Nyman, S. (1975). The effect of plaque control and surgical pocket elimination on the establishment and maintenance of periodontal health. A longitudinal study of periodontal therapy in cases of advanced disease. *Journal of Clinical Periodontology* **2**, 67–69.

Lindhe, J. & Nyman, S. (1984). Long-term maintenance of patients treated for advanced periodontal disease. *Journal of Clinical Periodontology* **11**, 504–514.

Lindhe, J., Okamoto H., Yoneyama, T., Haffajee, A. & Socransky, S.S. (1989). Longitudinal changes in periodontal disease in untreated subjects. *Journal of Clinical Periodontology* **16**, 662–670.

Lindhe, J., Westfeld, E., Nyman, S., Socransky, S.S., Heijl, L. & Bratthall, G. (1982). Healing following surgical/non-surgical treatment of periodontal disease. A clinical study. *Journal of Clinical Periodontology* **9**, 115–128.

Löe, H. (1979). Mechanical and chemical control of dental plaque. *Journal of Clinical Periodontology* **6**, 32–36.

Löe, H. (2000). Oral hygiene in the prevention of caries and periodontal disease. *International Dental Journal* **50**, 129–139.

Löe, H. (2002). Half a century of plaque removal. What's next? Millennium Lecture EuroPerio 2000. London: The Parthenon Publishing Group.

Löe, H., Theilade, E. & Jensen, S.B. (1965). Experimental gingivitis in man. *Journal of Periodontology* **36**, 177–187.

Loos, B., Claffey, N. & Crigger, M. (1988). Effects of oral hygiene measures on clinical and microbiological parameters of periodontal disease. *Journal of Clinical Periodontology* **15**, 211–216.

MacGregor, I.D. & Rugg-Gunn, A.J. (1985). Toothbrushing duration in 60 uninstructed young adults. *Community Dental Oral Epidemiology* **13**, 121–122.

Mandel, I.D. (1990). Why pick on teeth? *Journal of the American Dental Association* **121**, 129–132.

McCracken, G.I., Janssen, J., Swan, M., Steen, N., de Jager, M. & Heasman, P.A. (2003). Effect of brushing force and time on plaque removal using a powered toothbrush. *Journal of Clinical Periodontology* **30**, 409–413.

McCracken, G.I., Steen, N., Preshaw P.M., Heasman, L., Stacey, F. & Heasman, P.A. (2005). The crossover design to evaluate the efficacy of plaque removal in tooth-brushing studies. *Journal of Clinical Periodontology* **32**, 1157–1162.

Meyers, I.A., McQueen, M.J., Harbrow, D. & Seymour, G.J. (2000). The surface effect of dentifrices. *Australian Dental Journal* **45**, 118–124.

Mierau, H.D. & Spindler, T. (1984). Beitrag zur Ätiologie der Gingivarezessionen. *Deutsche Zahnärztliche Zeitschrift* **39**, 634–639.

Morch, T. & Waerhaug, J. (1956). Quantitative evaluation of the effect of toothbrushing and toothpicking. *Journal of Periodontology* **27**, 183–190.

Moritis, K., Delaurenti, M., Johnson, M.R., Berg, J. & Boghosian, A.A. (2002). Comparison of the Sonicare Elite and a manual toothbrush in the evaluation of plaque reduction. *American Journal of Dentistry* **15**, 23B-25B.

Morris, A.J., Steele, J. & White, D.A. (2001). The oral cleanliness and periodontal health of UK adults in 1998. *British Dental Journal* **191**, 186–192.

Mulry, C.A., Dellerman, P.A., Ludwa, R.J., White, D.J. & Wild, J.E. (1992). A comparison of the end-rounding of nylon bristles in commercial toothbrushes: Crest Complete® and Oral-B®. *Journal of Clinical Dentistry* **3**, 47–50.

Niemi, M.L., Sandholm, L. & Ainamo, J. (1984). Frequency of gingival lesions after standardized brushing related to stiffness of toothbrush and abrasiveness of dentifrice. *Journal of Clinical Periodontology* **11**, 254–261.

Outhouse, T.L., Al-Alawi, R., Fedorowicz, Z. & Keenan, J.V. (2006). Tongue scraping for treating halitosis. *Cochrane Database Systemetic Review* **1**, CD005519.

O'Leary, T.J. (1980). Plaque control. In: Shanley, D., ed. *Efficacy of Treatment Procedures in Periodontology*. Chicago: Quintessence, pp. 41–52.

Pearson, L.S. & Hutton, J.L. (2002). A controlled trial to compare the ability of foam swabs and toothbrushes to remove dental plaque. *Journal of Advanced Nursing* **39**, 480–489.

Putt, M.S., Milleman, J.L., Davidson, K.R., Kleber, C.J. & Cugini, M.A. (2001). A split-mouth comparison of a three-dimensional-action electric toothbrush and a high-frequency electric toothbrush for reducing plaque and gingivitis. *Journal of International Academic Periodontology* **3**, 95–103.

Preber, H., Ylipää, V., Bergstrom, J. & Ryden, H. (1991). A comparative study of plaque removing efficiency using rotary electric and manual toothbrushes. *Swedish Dental Journal* **15**, 229–234.

Quirynen, M., Mongardini, C., De Soete, M., Pauwels, M., Coucke, W., Van Eldere, J. & Van Steenberghe, D (2000). The role of chlorhexidine in the one-stage full-mouth disinfection treatment of patients with advanced adult periodontitis. *Journal of Clinical Periodontology* **27**, 578–589.

Ramberg, P., Lindhe, J., Dahlen, G. & Volpe, A.R. (1994). The influence of gingival inflammation on de novo plaque formation. *Journal of Clinical Periodontology* **21**, 51–56.

Ransier, A., Epstein, J.B., Lunn, R. & Spinelli, J. (1995). A combined analysis of a toothbrush, foam brush, and a chlorhexidine-soaked foam brush in maintaining oral hygiene. *Cancer Nursing* **18**, 393–396.

Rapley, J.W. & Killoy, W.J. (1994). Subgingival and interproximal plaque removal using a counter-rotational electric toothbrush and a manual toothbrush. *Quintessence International* **25**, 39–42.

Reitman, W.R., Whiteley, R.T. & Robertson, P.B. (1980). Proximal surface cleaning by dental floss. *Clinical Preventive Dentistry* **2**, 7–10.

Renton-Harper, P., Addy, M., Warren, P. & Newcombe, R.G. (1999). Comparison of video and written instructions for plaque removal by an oscillating/rotating/reciprocating electric toothbrush. *Journal of Clinical Periodontology* **26**, 752–756.

Renvert, S. & Glavind, L. (1998). Individualized instruction and compliance in oral hygiene practices: recommendations and means of delivery. In: Lang, N.P., Attström, R. & Löe, H., eds. *Proceedings of the European Workshop on Mechanical Plaque Control*. London: Quintessence, pp. 300–309.

Robinson, P.G., Deacon, S.A., Deery, C., Heanue, M., Walmsley, A.D., Worthington, H.V., Glenny, A.M. & Shaw, W.C. (2005). Manual versus powered toothbrushing for oral health. *Cochrane Database Systemetic Review* **1**, CD002281.

Rosema, N.A.M., Timmerman, M.F., Piscaer, M., Strate, J., Warren, P. R., Van der Velden, U. & Van der Weijden, G.A. (2005). An oscillating/pulsating electric toothbrush versus a high frequency electric toothbrush in the treatment of gingivitis. *Journal of Dentistry* **33S1**, 29–36.

Rosling, B., Nyman, S. & Lindhe, J. (1976). The effect of systematic plaque control on bone regeneration in infrabony pockets. *Journal of Clinical Periodontology* **3**, 38–53.

Rowshani, B., Timmerman, M.F. & van der Velden, U. (2004). Plaque development in relation to the periodontal condition and bacterial load of the saliva. *Journal of Clinical Periodontology* **31**, 214–218.

Rylander, H. & Lindhe, J. (1997). Cause-related periodontal therapy. In: Lindhe, J., Karring, T. & Lang, N.P., eds. *Clinical Periodontology and Implant Dentistry*. Copenhagen: Munksgaard, pp. 438–447.

Saxer, U.P., Barbakow, J. & Yankell, S.L. (1998). New studies on estimated and actual toothbrushing times and dentifrice use. *Journal of Clinical Dentistry* **9**, 49–51.

Saxer, U.P. & Yankel, S.L. (1997). Impact of improved toothbrushes on dental diseases I. *Quintessence International* **28**, 513–525.

Schmid, M.O., Balmelli, O.P. & Saxer, U.P. (1976). Plaque removing effect of a toothbrush, dental floss and a toothpick. *Journal of Clinical Periodontology* **3**, 157–165.

Sforza, N.M., Rimondini, L., di Menna, F. & Camorali, C. (2000). Plaque removal by worn toothbrush. *Journal of Clinical Periodontology* **27**, 212–216.

Sharma, N.C., Galustians, J., McCool, J.J., Rustogi, K.N. & Volpe, A.R. (1994). The clinical effect on plaque and gingivitis over three month's use of four complex-design manual toothbrushes. *Journal of Clinical Dentistry* **5**, 114–118.

Sharma, N.C., Galustians, J., Rustogi, K.N., Petrone, M., Volpe, A.R., Korn, L.R. & Petrone, D. (1992). Comparative plaque removal efficacy of three toothbrushes in two independent clinical studies. *Journal of Clinical Dentistry* **3** (suppl C), 13–20.

Sharma, N.C., Qaqish, J.G., Galustians, H.J., King, D.W., Low, M.A., Jacobs, D.M. & Weber, D.A. (2000). An advanced toothbrush with improved plaque removal efficacy. *American Journal of Dentistry* **13** (spec. no), 15A-19A.

Sheiham, A. & Netuveli, G.S. (2002). Periodontal diseases in Europe. *Periodontology 2000* **29**, 104–121.

Sicilia, A., Arregui, I., Gallego, M., Cabezas, B. & Cuesta, S. (2002). A systematic review of powered v.s. manual tooth-brushes in periodontal cause-related therapy. *Journal of Clinical Periodontology* **29**, 39–54.

Singh, S.M. & Deasy, M.J. (1993). Clinical plaque removal performance of two manual toothbrushes. *Journal of Clinical Dentistry* **4** (suppl D), 13–16.

Stean, H. & Forward, G.C. (1980). Measurement of plaque growth following toothbrushing. *Community Dentistry and Oral Epidemiololgy* **8**, 420–423.

Stillman, P.R. (1932). A philosophy of treatment of periodontal disease. *Dental Digest* **38**, 315–322.

Tan, E. & Daly, C. (2002). Comparison of new and 3-month-old toothbrushes in plaque removal. *Journal of Clinical Periodontology* **29**, 645–650.

Thomas, M.V. (2004). Oral physiotherapy. In: Rose, L.F., Mealey, B.L., Genco, R.J. & Cohen, W., eds. *Periodontics, Medicine, Surgery and Implants*. St Louis, USA: Mosby, pp. 214–236.

Tritten, C.B. & Armitage, G.C. (1996). Comparison of a sonic and a manual toothbrush for efficacy in supragingival plaque removal and reduction of gingivitis. *Journal of Clinical Periodontology* **23**, 641–648.

Van der Weijden, G.A. & Danser, M.M. (2000). Toothbrushes: benefits versus effects on hard and soft tissues. In: Addy, M., Emberry, G., Edgar, W.M. & Orchardson, R., eds. *Tooth Wear and Sensitivity*. London: Martin Dunitz Ltd., pp. 217–248.

Van der Weijden, G.A. &, Hioe, K.P.A. (2005). Systematic review of the effectiveness of self-performed mechanical plaque removal in adults with gingivitis using a manual toothbrush. *Journal of Clinical Periodontology* **32**, 214–228.

Van der Weijden, G.A., Timmerman, M.F., Danser, M.M. & van der Velden, U. (1998a). Relationship between the plaque removal efficacy of a manual toothbrush and brushing force. *Journal of Clinical Periodontology* **25**, 413–416.

Van der Weijden, G.A., Timmerman, M.F., Danser, M.M. & van der Velden, U. (1998b). The role of electric tooth-brushes: advantages and limitations. In: Lang, N.P., Attström, R. & Löe, H., eds. *Proceedings of the European Workshop on Mechanical Plaque Control*. Berlin: Quintessence, pp. 138–155.

Van der Weijden, G.A., Timmerman, M.F., Nijboer, A., Lie, M.A. & van der Velden, U. (1993). A comparative study of electric toothbrushes for the effectiveness of plaque removal in relation to toothbrushing duration. *Journal of Clinical Periodontology* **20**, 476–481.

Van der Weijden, G.A., Timmerman M.F., Piscaer, M., IJzerman, Y. & van der Velden, U. (2002). A clinical comparison of three powered toothbrushes. *Journal of Clinical Periodontology* **29**, 1042–1047.

Van der Weijden, G.A., Timmerman, M.F., Piscaer, M., Snoek, C.M., van der Velden, U. & Galgut, P.N. (2002). The effectiveness of an electrically active toothbrush in the removal of overnight plaque and treatment of gingivitis. *Journal of Clinical Periodontology* **29**, 699–704.

Van der Weijden, G.A., Timmerman, M.F., Reijerse, E., Mantel, M.S. & van der Velden, U. (1995). The effectiveness of an electronic toothbrush in the removal of established plaque and treatment of gingivitis. *Journal of Clinical Periodontology* **22**, 179–182.

Van der Weijden, G.A., Timmerman, M.F., Reijerse, E., Snoek, C.M. & van der Velden, U. (1996b). Comparison of an oscil-lating/rotating electric toothbrush and a 'sonic' toothbrush in plaque removing ability. A professional toothbrushing and supervised brushing study. *Journal of Clinical Periodontology* **23**, 407–411.

Van der Weijden, G.A., Timmerman, M.F., Reijerse, E., Snoek, C.M. & van der Velden, U. (1996c). Toothbrushing force in relation to plaque removal. *Journal of Clinical Periodontology* **23**, 724–729.

Van der Weijden, G.A., Timmerman, M.F., Snoek, C.M., Reijerse, E. & van der Velden, U. (1996a). Toothbrushing duration and plaque removal efficacy of electric tooth-brushes. *American Journal of Dentistry* **9**, 31–36.

Van Palenstein Helderman, W.H., Kyaing, M.M., Aung, M.T., Soe, W., Rosema, N.A., Van der Weijden, G.A. & van 't Hof, M.A. (2006). Plaque removal by young children using old and new toothbrushes. *Journal of Dental Research* **85**, 1138–1142.

Van Swol, R.L., Van Scotter, D.E., Pucher, J.J. & Dentino, A.R. (1996). Clinical evaluation of an ionic toothbrush in the removal of established plaque and reduction of gingivitis. *Quintessence International* **27**, 389–394.

Versteeg, P.A., Timmerman M.F., Piscaer. M., van der Velden, U. & Van der Weijden, G.A. (2005). Brushing with and without dentifrice on gingival abrasion. *Journal of Clinical Periodontology* **32**, 158–162.

Waerhaug, J. (1976). The interdental brush and its place in operative and crown and bridge dentistry. *Journal of Oral Rehabilitation* **3**, 107–113.

Waerhaug, J. (1981a). Effect of toothbrushing on subgingival plaque formation. *Journal of Periodontology* **52**, 30–34.

Waerhaug, J. (1981b). Healing of the dento-epithelial junction following the use of dental floss. *Journal of Clinical Periodontology* **8**, 144–150.

Warren, P.R. (1998). Electric toothbrush use – Attitudes and experience among dental practitioners in Germany. *American Journal of Dentistry* **11**, S3–S6.

Warren, P.R. & Chater, B.V. (1996a). An overview of established interdental cleaning methods. *Journal of Clinical Dentistry* **7** (Spec. No. 3), 65–69.

Warren, P.R. & Chater, B. (1996b). The role of the electric toothbrush in the control of plaque and gingivitis: a review of 5 years clinical experience with the Braun Oral-B Plaque Remover (D7). *American Journal Dentistry* **9**, 5–11.

Warren, P.R., Jacobs, D., Low, M.A., Chater, B.V. & King, D.W. (2002). A clinical investigation into the effect of toothbrush wear on efficacy. *Journal of Clinical Dentistry* **13**, 119–124.

Warren, P.R., Ray, T.S., Cugini, M. & Chater, B.V. (2000). A practice-based study of a power toothbrush: assessment of effectiveness and acceptance. *Journal of the American Dental Association* **13**, 389–394.

Weiger, R. (1988). Die "Denta-Solar"-klinische untersuchung einer neuen zahnbürste mit intergriertem halbleiter aus TiO_2. *Oralprophylaxe* **10**, 79–83.

Wennstrom, J.L., Heijl, L., Dahlen, G. & Grondahl, K. (1987). Periodic subgingival antimicrobial irrigation of periodontal pockets (I). Clinical observations. *Journal of Clinical Periodontology* **14**, 541–550.

Wilkins, E.M. (1999). Oral Infection control: toothbrushes and toothbrushing In: *Clinical Practice of the Dental Hygienist*. Philadelphia: Lippincott Williams & Wilkins, pp. 350–369.

Wolffe, G.N. (1976). An evaluation of proximal surface cleansing agents. *Journal of Clinical Periodontology* **3**, 148–156.

Yankell, S.L., Emling, R.C. & Pérez, B. (1996). A six-month clinical evaluation of the Dentrust toothbrush. *Journal of Clinical Dentistry* **7**, 106–109.

Zimmer, S., Fosca, M. & Roulet, J.F. (2000) Clinical study of the effectiveness of two sonic toothbrushes. *Journal of Clinical Dentistry* **11**, 24–27.

Chapter 36

Chemical Supragingival Plaque Control

Martin Addy and John Moran

Classification and terminology of agents, 734
The concept of chemical supragingival plaque control, 735
 Supragingival plaque control, 736
 Chemical supragingival plaque control, 737
 Rationale for chemical supragingival plaque control, 738
 Approaches to chemical supragingival plaque control, 739
 Vehicles for the delivery of chemical agents, 740
Chemical plaque control agents, 742
 Systemic antimicrobials including antibiotics, 743
 Enzymes, 744
 Bisbiguanide antiseptics, 744
 Quaternary ammonium compounds, 744
 Phenols and essential oils, 745
 Natural products, 745
 Fluorides, 746
 Metal salts, 746

Oxygenating agents, 746
Detergents, 746
Amine alcohols, 746
Salifluor, 747
Acidified sodium chlorite, 747
Other antiseptics, 747
Chlorhexidine, 748
 Toxicology, safety, and side effects, 748
 Chlorhexidine staining, 749
 Mechanism of action, 750
 Chlorhexidine products, 750
 Clinical uses of chlorhexidine, 751
Evaluation of chemical agents and products, 754
 Studies *in vitro*, 755
 Study methods *in vitro*, 755
 Clinical trial design considerations, 757

This chapter will consider the past and present status and success of chemical supragingival plaque control in the prevention of gingivitis and thereby the occurrence or recurrence of chronic periodontal diseases. Chlorhexidine, arguably the most studied agent, will be used to consider the possible applications of chemical plaque control in periodontal practice.

Classification and terminology of agents

Agents that could inhibit the development or maturation of supragingival plaque have been classified according to possible mechanisms of action (for review see Addy & Moran 1997): (1) anti-adhesive; (2) antimicrobial; (3) plaque removal; and (4) anti-pathogenic. The majority of agents used to control supragingival plaque are contained in "oral hygiene" products and available to the general public either directly "over the counter" or following recommendation/prescription by a dental or medical professional. Manufacturers of these products and, for that matter, published literature use a variety of terms to describe the action of these chemical agents, often interchangeably, which has tended to cause confusion. In an attempt to clarify the various descriptive

terms used the European Federation of Periodontology in the 1996 European Workshop on Periodontology recommended definitions for the terminology employed for agents in chemical supragingival plaque control (Lang & Newman, 1997) as follows:

- Antimicrobial agents: chemicals that have a bacteriostatic or bactericidal effect *in vitro* that alone cannot be extrapolated to a proven efficacy *in vivo* against plaque.
- Plaque reducing/inhibitory agents: chemicals that have only been shown to reduce the quantity and/or affect the quality of plaque, which may or may not be sufficient to influence gingivitis and/or caries.
- Antiplaque agents: chemicals that have an effect on plaque sufficient to benefit gingivitis and/or caries (Addy *et al.* 1983).
- Antigingivitis agents: chemicals which reduce gingival inflammation without necessarily influencing bacterial plaque (includes anti-inflammatory agents).

The classification, terminology, and definitions are presented here because of their fundamental importance to understanding the concept of chemical supragingival plaque control. They will be considered in greater detail however under the headings of "Approaches to chemical supragingival plaque control" and "Evaluation of chemical agents and products" and, particularly for the latter, in respect of implied and inferred claims made by manufacturers.

The concept of chemical supragingival plaque control

Epidemiologic studies revealed a peculiarly high correlation between supragingival plaque levels and chronic gingivitis (Ash *et al.* 1964), and clinical research (Löe *et al.* 1965) led to the proof that plaque was the primary etiologic factor in gingival inflammation. Subgingival plaque, derived from supragingival plaque, is also intimately associated with the advancing lesions of chronic periodontal diseases. On the basis that plaque-induced gingivitis always precedes the occurrence and recurrence of periodontitis (Lindhe 1986; Löe 1986), the mainstay of primary and secondary prevention of periodontal diseases is the control of supragingival plaque (for review see Hancock 1996). Periodontal diseases appear to occur when a pathogenic microbial plaque acts on a susceptible host (for review see Haffajee & Socransky 1994). What constitutes a pathogenic subgingival plaque has been, and continues to be, a much researched area in periodontology. In the 1996 World Workshop on Periodontology a small number of bacteria were confirmed as true pathogens with a longer list considered as putative pathogens (for reviews see Zambon 1996). Much has been learned in the intervening decade, not the least of which is the bacterial diversity of subgingival plaque in health and disease, highlighted in a number of reviews (for review see Socransky & Haffajee 2005). The possibility that viruses may be involved has also been postulated (for review see Slots 2003). If the latter postulate becomes proven an extension of the classification of chemical agents, to include antiviral, will be necessary. Interestingly, and alluded to later in this chapter, some of the antimicrobial agents used in chemical plaque control do have antiviral activity.

Susceptibility to periodontal disease is less well understood and, at this time, certainly difficult to predict and quantify, although risk factors have been identified including genetic markers (for reviews see Kinane *et al.* 2005) (see Chapters 11 and 18). The relationship of plaque levels to pathogenicity and susceptibility is also poorly understood and therefore, for any one individual, what constitutes a satisfactory level of oral hygiene cannot be stated. This aside, there is evidence which demonstrates that improving oral hygiene and gingival health, over several decades, noted in developed countries (Hugoson *et al.* 1998a), has been associated with a decreasing incidence of periodontal disease (Hugoson *et al.* 1998b). Additionally, long-term follow-up of treated periodontal disease patients has shown that success is dependent on maintaining plaque levels compatible with gingival health (Axelsson & Lindhe 1981). Supragingival plaque control is thus fundamental to the prevention and management of periodontal diseases and, with appropriate advice and instruction from professionals, is primarily the responsibility of the individual.

It could be argued that the heavy reliance on mechanical methods to prevent what are microbially associated diseases is outdated. Very few hygiene practices against microorganisms used by humans on themselves, in the home, at the workplace or in the environment rely on mechanical methods alone and some methods are only chemical. The contrary argument must be that the prevention of periodontitis, through the control of gingivitis, would require the discovery of a safe and effective agent. Also, such a preventive agent would have to be applied from an early age to a large proportion of all populations, many of whom would have low or no susceptibility to periodontal disease (for review see Papapanou 1994).

These discussions aside, chemical preventive agents, aimed at the microbial plaque, have been a feature of periodontal disease management for almost a century (for review see Fischman 1997). The consensus appears to be that the use of preventive agents should be as adjuncts and not replacements for the more conventional and accepted effective mechanical methods and only then when these appear partially or totally ineffective alone.

Mechanical tooth cleaning through toothbrushing with toothpaste is arguably the most common and potentially effective form of oral hygiene practiced by peoples in developed countries (for reviews see Frandsen 1986; Jepsen 1998); although, *per capita* in the world, wood sticks are probably more commonly used. Interdental cleaning is a secondary adjunct and would seem particularly important in individuals who, through the presence of disease, can be retrospectively assessed as susceptible (for reviews see Hancock 1996; Kinane 1998). Unfortunately, it is a fact of life that a significant proportion of all individuals fail to practice a high enough standard of plaque removal such that gingivitis is highly prevalent and from an early age (Lavstedt *et al.* 1982; Addy *et al.* 1986). This, presumably, arises either or both from a failure to comply with the recommendation to regularly clean teeth or lack of dexterity with tooth cleaning habits (Frandsen 1986). Certainly, many individuals remove only around half of the plaque from their teeth even when brushing for 2 minutes (de la Rosa *et al.* 1979). Presumably this occurs because certain tooth surfaces receive little or no attention during the brushing cycle (Rugg-Gunn & MacGregor 1978; MacGregor & Rugg-Gunn 1979). The adjunctive use of chemicals would therefore appear a way of overcoming deficiencies in mechanical tooth cleaning habits as practiced by many individuals.

Supragingival plaque control

The formation of plaque on a tooth surface is a dynamic and ordered process, commencing with the attachment of primary plaque-forming bacteria. The attachment of these organisms appears essential for initiating the sequence of attachment of other organisms such that, with time, the mass and complexity of the plaque increases (see Chapter 8). Left undisturbed, supragingival plaque reaches a quantitative and qualitative level of bacterial complexity that is incompatible with gingival health, and gingivitis ensues. Even though, as yet, the microbiology of gingivitis is poorly understood, the sequencing of plaque formation highlights how interventions may prevent the development of gingivitis. Thus, any method of plaque control, which prevents plaque achieving the critical point where gingival health deteriorates, will stop gingivitis. Unfortunately, the lack of knowledge of bacterial specificity for gingivitis does not allow targeting or the control of particular organisms except for perhaps the primary plaque formers. Plaque inhibition has, therefore, targeted plaque formation at particular points – bacterial attachment, bacterial proliferation, and plaque maturation – and these will be discussed in more detail in the later section "Approaches to chemical supragingival plaque control".

The mainstay of supragingival plaque control has been regular plaque removal using mechanical methods which, in developed countries, means the toothbrush, manual or electric, and in less well developed countries the use of wood or chewing sticks (for review see Frandsen 1986, Hancock 1996). These devices primarily access smooth surface plaque and not interdental deposits. Interdental cleaning devices include wood sticks, floss, tape, interdental brushes, and, more recently, electric interdental devices (for reviews see Egelberg & Claffey 1998; Kinane 1998). Regular mechanical tooth cleaning is directed towards maintaining a level of plaque, quantitatively and/or qualitatively, which is compatible with gingival health, and not rendering the tooth surface bacteria free. Theoretically, mechanical cleaning of teeth could prevent caries but workshops have concluded that tooth brushing *per se* and interdental cleaning as performed by the individual do not prevent caries (for review see Frandsen 1986). Clearly, but outside the scope of this chapter, the toothbrush and other mechanical devices do provide a vehicle whereby anticaries agents, such as fluoride, can be delivered to the tooth surface. Under the conditions of clinical experimentation, tooth cleaning performed once every 2 days was shown to prevent gingivitis (Lang et al. 1973). The professional recommendation however, has been to brush twice per day, for which there is evidence of a benefit to gingival health over less frequent cleaning with no additional benefit for more frequent brushing (for review see Frandsen 1986). Indeed, recommendations to increase the fre-quency of brushing more than twice daily may result in more damage to hard and soft tissues (for review see Addy & Hunter 2003). The duration of brushing is somewhat controversial given that most surveys or studies reveal an average brushing time of 60 seconds or less (Rugg-Gunn & MacGregor 1978; MacGregor & Rugg-Gunn 1979). It is worth noting that one study showed less than 50% plaque removal after 2 minutes' brushing (de la Rosa et al. 1979). This perhaps highlights that many individuals spend little or no time during the brushing cycle at some tooth surfaces, notably lingually (Rugg-Gunn & MacGregor 1978; MacGregor & Rugg-Gunn 1979).

Oral hygiene, oral hygiene instruction, and the effect of supragingival plaque control alone on subgingival plaque and therefore periodontal disease is the subject of other chapters. Nevertheless, some further comments on mechanical tooth cleaning are pertinent in this chapter, particularly in respect of comparative efficacy of devices. The manual toothbrush as known today, man-made filaments in a plastic head, was invented as recently as the 1930s. Evidence for such devices dates back to China, approximately 1000 years ago, re-emerging in the 1800s in Europe, but too expensive for common usage (for reviews see Fischman 1997). Numerous changes in manual toothbrush design have occurred, particularly recently, and similarly numerous claims have been made for the efficacy of individual designs. Despite this, researchers, workshop reports, and consensus views have repeatedly concluded that there is no best design of manual toothbrush nor an optimal method of tooth cleaning: the major variable being the person using the brush (for reviews see Frandsen 1986; Jepsen 1998). Limited evidence is available comparing the modern toothbrush with chewing sticks but what is available suggests similar efficacy (Norton & Addy 1989), perhaps not surprisingly if indeed the user is the important factor. Interdental cleaning is considered important particularly for those individuals who are known to be susceptible to or have periodontal disease (for reviews see Egelberg & Claffey 1998; Kinane 1998). Here again, there is little evidence supporting one interdental cleaning method over another, leaving patients and professionals to hold subjectively related preferences (for review see Kinane 1998). Electric toothbrushes of the counter-rotation type found prominence for a short time in the 1960s and 1970s but were unreliable and proven of no greater efficacy over manual brushes, except for handicapped individuals (for reviews see Frandsen 1986). More recently, ranges of new electric brushes have appeared with a variety of head, tuft, and filament actions. For these, consensus reports conclude that there is evidence for greater efficacy over manual brushes particularly when professional advice in their use is provided (for reviews see Hancock 1996; Egelberg & Claffey 1998; van der Weijden et al. 1998). More recently, a Cochrane systematic review concluded that only oscillating rotating electric toothbrushes could be proven significantly more effective than manual toothbrushes in reducing plaque and gingivitis (Heanue *et al.* 2004). Despite this, there is no clear evidence that any one electric design or head motion is superior and, again, the user appears the major variable. As with manual brushes advice and instruction in the use of electric brushes can result in very high levels of plaque control (Renton Harper *et al.* 2001). Given the speed of head movement for electric versus manual brushes, there must be concerns over potential harmful effect to hard and soft tissues. In this respect, Phaneuf and co-workers (1962) hypothesized that electric brushes would produce the same or less harm, postulating that the users would apply less force. Many years later the application of less pressure to electric compared to manual brushes was proven (for review see van der Weijden *et al.* 1998). Overall, therefore, it has been concluded that the benefits of normal tooth-brushing alone and as a vehicle for toothpaste with a variety of active ingredients far outweigh the potential for harm to hard and soft tissues (for review see Addy & Hunter 2003).

Chemical supragingival plaque control

History of oral hygiene products

The terminology "oral hygiene products" is recent but there is evidence dating back at least 6000 years that formulations and recipes existed to benefit oral and dental health (for reviews see Fischman 1997). This includes the written Ebers Papyrus 1500 BC containing recipes for tooth powders and mouth rinses dating back to 4000 BC. A considerable number of formulations can be attributed to the writer and scientist Hippocrates (circa 480 BC). By today's standards the early formulations appear strange if not disgusting but they were not always without logic. Thus, bodies or body parts of animals perceived to have good or continuously erupting teeth were used in the belief that they would impart health and strength to the teeth of the user. Hippocrates, for example, recommended the head of one hare and three whole mice, after taking out the intestines of two, mixing the powder derived from burning the animals with greasy wool, honey, aniseeds, myrrh, and white wine. This early toothpaste was to be rubbed on the teeth frequently.

Mouth rinses similarly contained ingredients which would have had some stimulating effect on salivary flow, breath odor masking and antimicrobial actions, albeit not necessarily formulated with all these activities in mind. Alcohol-based mouth rinses were particularly popular with the Romans and included white wine and beer. Urine, as a mouth rinse, appeared to be popular with many peoples and over many centuries. There even appeared differences in opinion, with the Cantabri and other peoples of Spain preferring stale urine, whereas Fauchard

(1690–1761) in France recommended fresh urine. The Arab nations were purported to prefer children's urine and the Romans to prefer Arab urine. Anecdotal reports suggest the use of urine as a mouth rinse to this very day with individuals rinsing with their own urine. There could, indeed, be benefits to oral health from rinsing with urine by virtue of the urea content; however this has never been evaluated, and given today's Guidelines for Good Clinical Practice, it is unlikely that study protocols would receive ethical approval.

Throughout the centuries, most tooth powders, toothpastes, and mouth rinses appear to have been formulated for cosmetic reasons including tooth cleaning and breath freshening rather than the control of dental and periodontal diseases. Many formulations contained very abrasive ingredients and/or acidic substances. However, ingredients with antimicrobial properties were used, perhaps not intentionally, and included arsenic and herbal materials. Herbal extracts are, perhaps, increasingly being used in toothpastes and mouth rinses, although there are little data to support efficacy for gingivitis and none for caries. Many agents prescribed well into the twentieth century, usually as rinses, had the potential to cause local damage to tissues, if not systemic toxicity, including aromatic sulfuric acid, mercuric perchloride, carbolic acid, and formaldehyde (Dilling & Hallam 1936).

Perhaps the biggest change to toothpastes came with the chemoparasitic theory of tooth decay of W.D. Miller in 1890. The theory that organic acids were produced by oral bacteria acting on fermentable carbohydrates in contact with enamel led to both the introduction of agents into toothpaste which might influence this process, and the production of alkaline products. Shortly after, and at the beginning of the twentieth century, various potassium and sodium salts were added to toothpaste as a therapy for periodontal disease. The first half of the twentieth century saw numerous claims for toothpastes for oral health benefits, including tooth decay and periodontal disease. For example, with the early recognition that periodontal diseases were associated with microorganisms, emetin hydrochloride was added to toothpaste to treat possible amoebic infections. Perhaps with the exception of the well known essential oil mouth rinse marketed at the end of the nineteenth century, the addition of antimicrobial and/or antiseptic agents to toothpastes and mouth rinses is a relatively recent practice by manufacturers. During the nineteenth and twentieth centuries, toothpastes also became less abrasive. Interestingly, the importance of a level of abrasivity in toothpastes to the prevention of extrinsic dental stain became apparent when one manufacturer marketed a non-abrasive liquid dentifrice. The unsightly brown tooth staining that developed in many users resulted in the early removal of this product from the marketplace. Standard organizations, notably the British Standards

Institute (BSI) and the International Standards Organisation (ISO), have written standards for toothpaste (BS5136:1981, ISO11609:1995). The ISO standard for toothpaste is, at this time, under review although, as for the original standard, it is safety rather than efficacy, which is the key issue. Toxicity and abrasivity (see later under Vehicles) are important sections of the toothpaste standard although evaluations for fluoride availability are likely to feature in the next finalized toothpaste standard. An ISO standard for mouth rinses is also under preparation where the hard tissue safety issue of low pH mouth rinses is under consideration. Throughout the ages, and until relatively recently, scientific evaluations of agents and formulations for gum health were not performed and claims for efficacy appear based on anecdotal reports at best. Indeed, given the nature of many ingredients and the recipes recommended in the past for oral hygiene benefits, it is unlikely that efficacy will ever be tested. In the 6000 years history of oral hygiene products, scientific evaluation must be seen as an extremely recent event: an observation which can, of course, be applied to almost all aspects of chemoprevention and chemotherapy of human diseases. Indeed, perhaps the first ever, double-blind, randomized cross-over design clinical trial in dentistry was less than 50 years ago (Cooke & Armitage 1960).

Rationale for chemical supragingival plaque control

The epidemiologic data and clinical research (Ash et al. 1964; Löe et al. 1965) directly associating plaque with gingivitis perhaps, unfortunately, led to a rather simplistic view that regular tooth cleaning would prevent gingivitis and thereby periodontal disease. Theoretically correct, this concept did not appear to consider the multiplicity of factors which influence the ability of individuals to clean their teeth sufficiently well to prevent disease, not the least of which are those factors which affect individual compliance with advice, and dexterity in performing such tasks. The need for research into those psychosocial factors which might influence attitude to and performance in oral hygiene, was stated in a workshop report on plaque control and oral hygiene practices (Frandsen 1986) but appears not to have been heeded to this day. Moreover, and as described in other chapters, epidemiologic data suggest that not all individuals are particularly susceptible to periodontal disease. The most severe disease is accounted for by a relatively small proportion of any population and then by only a proportion of sites in their dentition (Baelum et al. 1986). Even accepting that a considerable proportion of middle-aged adults will have one or more sites in the dentition with moderate periodontal disease, this will be of the chronic type and a minimal threat to the longevity of their dentition (Papapanou 1994) (see Chapter 7). The prevention of chronic peri-odontal diseases, through improved oral hygiene practices, will therefore be grossly over-prescribed as the early identification of susceptible individuals is impossible at present.

Host susceptibility is described retrospectively in the already diseased individual but, even here, an explanation for their susceptibility, except for a few risk factors, cannot be made. These risk factors include smoking, diabetes, and polymorph defects, and possibly stress (for review see Chapters 11 and 12). Genetic markers for periodontal disease have been identified but, at present, appear to be applied retrospectively rather than prospectively (Kornman et al. 1997; Kinane et al. 2005) and the value to early onset disease has been questioned (Hodge et al. 2001).

One definition of periodontal disease is chronic gingivitis with loss of attachment. This is a particularly useful definition, since not only does it describe the pathogenic processes occurring but also alludes to the approach to prevent, treat or prevent recurrence of the disease. Therefore prevention through supragingival plaque control still remains the mainstay of controling gingivitis and therefore the occurrence or recurrence of periodontitis. The importance of oral hygiene to outcome and long-term success of therapy for periodontal disease is hampered by the frequent ineffectiveness of mechanical cleaning of specific sites using a toothbrush, and the limited or lack of use of interdental cleaning by many individuals. Despite the encouraging improvements in oral hygiene, gingivitis and, to some extent, periodontitis in developed countries, gingival inflammation is still highly prevalent (see Chapter 7). Taken with the microbial etiology of both gingivitis and periodontitis, this supports the concept of employing agents to control plaque which require minimal compliance and skill in their use. This is the concept that underlies chemical supragingival plaque control, but as with oral hygiene instruction in mechanical methods, it will have to be vastly over-prescribed if periodontal disease prevention is to be achieved in susceptible individuals. Chemical supragingival plaque control has thus been the subject of extensive research using scientific methodologies for 40 years. The question to be addressed here is whether a chemical or chemicals have been discovered and proven efficacious in, firstly, the prevention of gingivitis and, secondly, periodontitis.

Conclusions

- Gingivitis and periodontitis are highly prevalent diseases and prevention of occurrence or recurrence is dependent on supragingival plaque control.
- Tooth cleaning is largely influenced by the compliance and dexterity of the individual and little by design features of oral hygiene appliances and aids.

- The concept of chemical plaque control may be justified as a means of overcoming inadequacies of mechanical cleaning.
- Gingivitis is highly prevalent and from a young age in all populations, but the proportion of individuals susceptible to tooth loss through periodontal disease is small.
- Prediction of susceptibility to periodontal disease from an early age is at present impossible.
- Mechanical and/or chemical supragingival plaque control measures for prevention of periodontitis will have to be greatly over-prescribed.
- In those individuals with chronic periodontal disease, and therefore considered susceptible, a daily form of interdental cleaning must be essential to long-term treatment success.

Approaches to chemical supragingival plaque control

The well ordered and dynamic process of plaque formation is summarized in Fig. 36-1. It is apparent that this process can be interrupted, interfered with, reversed or modified at several points and before the plaque mass and/or complexity reach a level whereby gingival health deteriorates. Mechanical cleaning aims to regularly remove sufficient microorganisms to leave a "healthy plaque" present, which cannot induce gingival inflammation. Chemical agents, on the other hand, could influence plaque quantitatively and qualitatively via a number of processes and these are summarized in Fig. 36-1. The action of the chemicals could fit into four categories:

1. Antiadhesive
2. Antimicrobial
3. Plaque removal
4. Antipathogenic.

Antiadhesive agents

Antiadhesive agents would act at the pellicle surface to prevent the initial attachment of the primary plaque-forming bacteria. Such antiadhesive agents would probably have to be totally preventive in their effects, acting most effectively on an initially clean

tooth surface. Antiadhesive agents do exist and are used in industry, domestically, and in the environment. Such chemicals prevent the attachment and development of a variety of biofilms and are usually described as antifouling agents. Unfortunately the chemicals found in such applications are either too toxic for oral use or ineffective against dental bacteria plaques. Nevertheless, the concept of antiadhesives continues to attract research interest (for review see Wade & Slayne 1997). To date, effective formulations or products with antiadhesive properties are not available to the general public, although the amine alcohol, delmopinol, which appears to interfere with bacterial matrix formation and therefore fits somewhere between the concepts of antiadhesion and plaque removal, has been shown effective against plaque and gingivitis (Collaert *et al.* 1992; Claydon *et al.* 1996). Were antiadhesive agents to be discovered, a secondary benefit of extrinsic stain prevention of teeth may be expected.

Antimicrobial agents

The bacterial nature of dental plaque, not surprisingly, attracted interest in prevention of plaque formation through the use of antimicrobial agents. Antimicrobial agents could inhibit plaque formation through one of two mechanisms alone or combined. The first would be the inhibition of bacterial proliferation and would be directed, as with antiadhesive agents, at the primary plaque-forming bacteria. Antimicrobial agents therefore could exert their effects either at the pellicle-coated tooth surface before the primary plaque formers attach or after attachment but before division of these bacteria. This plaque inhibitory effect would be bacteriostatic in type, with the result that the lack of bacterial proliferation would not allow attachment of subsequent bacterial types on to the primary plaque-forming bacteria. The second effect could be bactericidal, whereby the antimicrobial agent destroys all of the microorganisms either attaching or already attached to the tooth surface. Many antimicrobial agents exist which could produce this effect; however, as will be discussed, to be effective in inhibiting plaque, the bactericidal effect would have to be absolute and/or persistent.

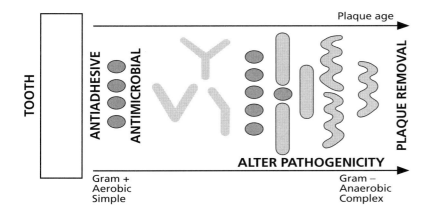

Fig. 36-1 Bacterial succession plaque formation. There is increasing mass and bacterial complexity as plaque bacteria attach and proliferate. Ideal sites of action for chemicals which might influence plaque accumulation are shown. Acknowledgment to Dr. William Wade for permission to publish this diagram.

If not, other bacteria within the oral environment would colonize the tooth surface immediately following the loss of the bactericidal effect and the biofilm would be re-established. For the most part biofilms in themselves are fairly resistant to total bactericidal effects of antimicrobial agents and, thus far, there does not appear to have been any agent discovered which effectively would sterilize the tooth surface after each application. If such an agent were found it could, of course, have potentially dangerous implications for the oral cavity since it would almost certainly destroy most of the commensal bacteria which normally colonize the oral cavity. This would open up the potential for exogenous microorganisms, with dangerous pathogenic potential, colonizing the oral cavity. In the event, it is probable that antimicrobial agents exert both a bactericidal effect followed by a bacteriostatic action of variable duration. The bactericidal effect will occur when the antimicrobial agent is at high concentration within the oral cavity and usually this will represent the time when the formulation is actually within the oral cavity. This bactericidal effect would be expected to be lost very soon after expectoration.

As will be discussed in respect of chlorhexidine, it is almost certainly the persistence of the bacteriostatic action of antimicrobial agents which accounts for their plaque-inhibitory activity. Calculations by Stralfors (1961) indicated that plaque inhibition through a bactericidal effect would require the immediate killing of 99.9% of the oral bacteria to effect a plaque-inhibitory action of significant duration. Antimicrobial agents for plaque inhibition, to date, are the only agents that have found common usage in oral hygiene products. The efficacy of these agents and products varies at the extremes (for reviews see Addy 1986; Kornman 1986; Mandel 1988; Addy *et al.* 1994; Addy & Renton-Harper 1996; Rolla *et al.* 1997; Eley 1999).

Plaque removal agents

The idea of employing a chemical agent which would act in an identical manner to a toothbrush and remove bacteria from the tooth surface, is an attractive proposition. Such an agent, contained in a mouth rinse, would be expected to reach all tooth surfaces and thereby be totally effective. For this reason, the idea of chemical plaque removal agents has attracted the terminology of "the chemical toothbrush". As with antiadhesives, there are agents, such as the hypochlorites, which might be expected to remove bacterial deposits and are commonly employed within the domestic environment. Again, such chemicals would likely be toxic were they to be applied within the oral cavity. Perhaps, the nearest success was with enzymes, directed at both pellicle, e.g. proteases, or bacterial matrices, e.g. dextranase and mutanase (for review see Kornman 1986). Again, as will be discussed, these enzymes, albeit potentially effective,

lacked substantivity within the oral cavity and had local side effects.

Antipathogenic agents

It is theoretically possible that an agent could have an effect on plaque microorganisms, which might inhibit the expression of their pathogenicity without necessarily destroying the microorganisms. In some respects antimicrobial agents, which exert a bacteriostatic effect, achieve such results. At present the understanding of the pathogenesis of gingivitis is so poor that this approach has received no attention. Were our knowledge on the microbial etiology of gingivitis to improve, there exists the possibility of an alternative, but related, approach: the introduction into the oral cavity of organisms which have been modified to remove their pathogenic potential to the gingival tissues. This is not a new concept and was an approach experimented with to replace pathogenic staphylococci within the nasal cavities of surgeons with the idea of reducing the potential for wound infection caused by the operator. At present such an approach within the oral cavity for either gingivitis or caries is perhaps within the realms of science fiction.

Conclusions

- At present most antiplaque agents are antimicrobial and prevent the bacterial proliferation phase of plaque development.
- Plaque formation could be controlled by antiadhesive or plaque removal agents, but these are not, as yet, available or safe for oral use.
- Alteration of bacterial plaque pathogenicity through chemical agents or bacterial modification would require a greater understanding of the bacterial etiology of gingivitis.

Vehicles for the delivery of chemical agents

The carriage of chemical agents into the mouth for supragingival plaque control has involved a small but varied range of vehicles (for reviews see Addy 1994; Cummins 1997).

Toothpaste

By virtue of common usage the ideal vehicle for the carriage of plaque-control agents is toothpaste. A number of ingredients go to make up toothpaste and each has a role in either influencing the consistency and stability of the product or its function (for review see Forward *et al.* 1997).

The major ingredients may be classified under the following headings:

1. *Abrasives*, such as silica, alumina, dicalcium phosphate, and calcium carbonate either alone, or more usually today, in combination. Abrasives affect

the consistency of the toothpaste and assist in the control of extrinsic dental staining. The range of abrasivity of toothpaste against dental hard tissues is defined in the BSI and ISO toothpaste standards (presently under review) in an attempt to minimize tooth wear from normal toothbrushing with toothpaste. Dentine abrasion is of prime importance as the majority of abrasives used in toothpastes produce little or no wear to enamel: non-hydrated alumina being the exception. Also, toothpaste detergents produce wear to dentine (Moore & Addy 2005). Abrasivity is calculated by relating the wear of dentine (enamel) by toothpaste to a standard formulation: the relative dentine abrasivity (RDA) value (relative enamel abrasivity (REA)). For the BSI standard a calcium carbonate based abrasive formulation is used whereas for the ISO standard it is calcium pyrophosphate based. The wear of dentine, measured directly by profilometry or release of P^{52}, by the standard is considered as 100. Toothpastes, according to the two standards, can be up to twice the standard for BSI (RDA range 0–200) and two and a half times for ISO (RDA range 0–250).

2. *Detergents*: the most common detergent used in toothpaste is sodium lauryl sulfate, which imparts the foaming and "feel" properties to the product. Additionally, detergents may help dissolve active ingredients and the anionic detergent sodium lauryl sulfate has both antimicrobial and plaque inhibitory properties (Jenkins *et al.* 1991a,b). Certain toothpaste products cannot employ anionic detergents as they interact with cationic substances that may be added to the product, such as chlorhexidine, or polyvalent metal salts, such as strontium, used in the treatment of dentine hypersensitivity.
3. *Thickeners*, such as silica and gums, primarily influence the viscosity of the product.
4. *Sweeteners*, including saccharine.
5. *Humectants*, notably glycerine and sorbitol to prevent drying out of the paste once the tube has been opened.
6. *Flavors*, of which there are many but mint or peppermint are popular in the western world although rarely found in toothpaste in the Indian subcontinent where herbal flavors are more popular.
7. *Actives*, notably fluorides for caries prevention; for plaque control triclosan and stannous fluoride and, to a lesser extent, chlorhexidine have been the most studied examples. Other actives relate to different aspects of oral care including anticalculus agents (pyrophosphates), whitening agents (polyphosphates), and desensitizing agents (strontium and potassium salts).

As stated, the addition of cationic antiseptics to toothpastes is difficult but chlorhexidine has been formulated into toothpastes and shown to be effective (Yates *et al.* 1993; Sanz *et al.* 1994), although

few products have reached or lasted in the marketplace.

Mouth rinses

Despite the ideal nature of the toothpaste vehicle, most chemical plaque-control agents have been evaluated and later formulated in the mouth rinse vehicle. Mouth rinses vary in their constituents but are usually considerably less complex than toothpastes. They can be simple aqueous solutions, but the need for products, purchased by the general public, to be stable and acceptable in taste usually requires the addition of flavoring, coloring, and preservatives such as sodium benzoate. Anionic detergents are included in some products but, again, cannot be formulated with cationic antiseptics such as cetylpyridinium chloride or chlorhexidine (Barkvoll *et al.* 1989). Ethyl alcohol is commonly used both to stabilize certain active ingredients and to improve the shelf-life of the product. Several concerns, not always well substantiated, have been expressed over alcohol-containing mouth rinses (for review see Eley 1999). The possible association of alcohol intake with oropharyngeal cancer, has been extended to include alcohol-containing mouth rinses. Whether these concerns are scientifically valid has not been established and separating out the well established role of smoking in these cancers is difficult, if not impossible, as is other sources of alcohol. Also, since at present there seems little support for the long-term use of mouth rinses for gingival health benefits, when mouth rinses are correctly prescribed the risk from contained alcohol is probably minuscule. This, however, does not obviate the possible risk from self-prescription, the chronic use of mouth rinses, or the ingestion of alcoholic mouth rinses by children. In the latter case, toxicity has been reported. Additionally, alcohol may adversely affect the physical properties of some esthetic restoration materials. Sensibly the prescription or recommendation of alcohol-containing mouth rinses would seem inappropriate to known alcoholics or to those individuals whose religion or culture forbids the intake of alcohol. The proportion of alcohol is usually less than 10% but some rinses have in excess of 20% alcohol. Some manufacturers are now producing alcohol-free mouth rinses.

Spray

Spray delivery of chemical plaque-control agents has attracted both research interest and the development of products by some manufacturers in some countries. Sprays have the advantage of focusing delivery on the required site. The dose is clearly reduced and for antiseptics such as chlorhexidine this has taste advantages. When correctly applied, chlorhexidine sprays were as effective as mouth rinses for plaque inhibition, although there was no reduction in staining (Francis *et al.* 1987a; Kalaga *et al.* 1989a). Chlorhexidine sprays were found particularly useful for plaque

Irrigators

Irrigators were designed to spray water, under pressure, around the teeth. As such they only removed debris, with little effect on plaque deposits (for review see Frandsen 1986). Antiseptics and other chemical plaque-control agents, such as chlorhexidine, have been added to the reservoir of such devices. A variety of dilutions of chlorhexidine has been employed to good effect (Lang & Raber 1981) but again with the incumbent local side effects of this agent.

Chewing gum

Over a relatively short period there has been interest in employing chewing gum to deliver a variety of agents for oral health benefits. Also, there appear to be significant benefits to dental health through the use of sugar-free chewing gum. Unfortunately, chewing gums alone appear to have little in the way of plaque-control benefits particularly at sites prone to gingivitis (Hanham & Addy 2001). They can reduce occlusal plaque deposits (Addy et al. 1998), but whether this is directly relevant to the prevention of fissure caries has not been proven, indeed is unlikely. Nonetheless, the vehicle has been used to deliver chemical agents such as chlorhexidine and, when used as an adjunct to normal toothbrushing, reduced plaque and gingivitis levels have been shown (Ainamo & Etemadzadeh 1987; Smith et al. 1996).

Varnishes

Varnishes have been employed to deliver antiseptics including chlorhexidine, but the purpose has been to prevent root caries rather than as a reservoir for plaque control throughout the mouth.

Conclusions

- Many vehicles may be used to deliver antiplaque agents but most information relates to mouth rinses and toothpaste.
- Toothpaste appears the most practical and cost-effective method for chemical plaque control for most individuals.
- In formulating antiplaque agents into toothpaste, potential inactivation by other ingredients must be considered.
- Minority groups, such as the handicapped, may benefit from other delivery systems.

Chemical plaque control agents

Over a period of nearly four decades there has been quite intense interest in the use of chemical agents to control supragingival plaque and thereby gingivitis. The number and variation of chemical agents evaluated are quite large but most have antiseptic or anti-

microbial actions and success has been extremely variable. It is important to emphasize that formulations based on antimicrobial agents provide a considerably greater preventive than therapeutic action. The most effective agents inhibit the development of plaque and gingivitis but are limited or slow to affect established plaque and gingivitis. Were they available, antiadhesive agents would similarly be expected to provide preventive rather than therapeutic effects. Plaque removal agents, on the other hand, would almost certainly provide both preventive and therapeutic actions. Chemical plaque-control agents have been the subject of many detailed reviews since 1980 (Hull 1980; Addy 1986; Kornman 1986; Mandel 1988; Gjermo 1989; Addy et al. 1994; Heasman & Seymour 1994; Jackson 1997; Eley 1999). Based on knowledge derived from chlorhexidine (for review see Jones 1997), the most effective plaque-inhibitory agents in the antiseptic or antimicrobial group are those showing persistence of action in the mouth measured in hours. Such persistence of action, sometimes termed substantivity (Kornman 1986), appears dependent on several factors:

1. Adsorption and prolonged retention on oral surfaces including, importantly, pellicle-coated teeth
2. Maintenance of antimicrobial activity once adsorbed primarily through a bacteriostatic action against the primary plaque-forming bacteria
3. Minimal or slow neutralization of antimicrobial activity within the oral environment or slow desorption from surfaces.

The latter concepts will be discussed later under chlorhexidine.

Antimicrobial activity of antiseptics in vitro is not a reliable predictor of plaque-inhibitory activity in vivo (Gjermo et al. 1970, 1973). Early studies on a number of antiseptics revealed similar antimicrobial profiles but a large variation in clinical effects. For example, compared to chlorhexidine, the cationic quaternary ammonium compound, cetylpyridinium chloride, has a similar antimicrobial profile in vitro (Gjermo et al. 1970, 1973; Roberts & Addy 1981) and is initially adsorbed in the mouth to a considerably greater extent (Bonesvoll & Gjermo 1978). The persistence of action of cetylpyridinium chloride is, however, much shorter than chlorhexidine (Schiott et al. 1970; Roberts & Addy, 1981), and plaque inhibition is considerably less (for review see Mandel 1988). Several reasons may explain these apparent anomalies, including poor retention of cetylpyridinium chloride within the oral cavity (Bonesvoll & Gjermo 1978), reduced activity once adsorbed, and neutralization in the oral environment (Moran & Addy 1984), or a combination of these factors. Attempts to improve efficacy of cetylpyridinium chloride can, of course, include increasing the frequency of use, but this is likely to incur compliance problems and side effects (Bonesvoll & Gjermo 1978). Alternatively,

Table 36-1 Groups of agents used in the control of dental plaque and/or gingivitis

Group	Example of agents	Action	Used now/product
Antibiotics	Penicillin Vancomycin Kanamycin Niddamycin Spiromycin	Antimicrobial	No
Enzymes	Protease Lipase Nuclease Dextranase Mutanase	Plaque removal	No
	*Glucose oxidase *Amyloglucosidase	Antimicrobial	*Yes Toothpaste
Bisbiguanide antiseptics	*Chlorhexidine Alexidine Octenidine	Antimicrobial	*Yes Mouthrinse Spray Gel Toothpaste Chewing gum Varnish
Quaternary ammonium compounds	*Cetylpyridinium chloride *Benzalconium chloride	Antimicrobial	*Yes Mouthrinse
Phenols and essential oils	*Thymol *Hexylresorcinol *Ecalyptol *Triclosan+	*Antimicrobial +Anti-inflammatory	*Yes Mouthrinse Toothpaste
Natural products	*Sanguinarine	Antimicrobial	No
Fluorides	(*)Sodium fluoride (*)Sodium monofluoro-phosphate *Stannous fluoride+ +Amine fluoride	*Antimicrobial () minimal + ?	+*Yes Toothpaste Mouthrinse +Gel
Metal salts	*Tin+ *Zinc Copper	Antimicrobial	*Yes Toothpaste Mouthrinse +Gel
Oxygenating agents	*Hydrogen peroxide *Sodium peroxyborate *Sodium peroxycarbonate	Antimicrobial ? plaque removal	*Yes Mouthrinse
Detergents	*Sodium lauryl sulfate	Antimicrobial ? plaque removal	*Yes Toothpaste Mouthrinse
Amine alcohols	Octapinol Delmopinol	Plaque matrix Inhibition	No Yes Toothpaste Mouthrinse
Salicylanide	Salifluor	Antimicrobial and anti-inflammatory	No

substantivity could be improved by combining anti-microbials or using agents to increase the retention of antimicrobials (Gaffar *et al.* 1992). Individual groups of compounds, together with the specific agents within the group, are listed in Table 36-1 and discussed below.

Systemic antimicrobials including antibiotics
(For reviews see Addy 1986; Kornman 1986)

Despite evidence for efficacy in preventing caries and gingivitis or resolving gingivitis, the opinion today is that systemic antimicrobials should not be used either topically or systemically as preventive agents against these diseases. The risk-to-benefit ratio is high and even systemic antimicrobial use in the treatment of adult periodontitis is open to debate (for reviews see Slots & Rams 1990; Addy & Martin 2003) (see Chapter 42). Thus, systemic antimicrobials have their own specific side effects not all of which can be avoided by topical application. Perhaps of greatest importance is the development of bacterial resistance within human populations, for example methicillin-resistant *Staphylococcus aureus* (MRSA), which causes serious and life-threatening wound infections, particularly within hospitalized patients.

Enzymes
(For reviews see Addy 1986)

Enzymes fall into two groups. Those in the first group are not truly antimicrobial agents but more plaque removal agents in that they have the potential to disrupt the early plaque matrix, thereby dislodging bacteria from the tooth surface. In the late 1960s and early 1970s enzymes such as dextranase, mutanase and various proteases were thought to be a major breakthrough in dental plaque control that might prevent the development of both caries and gingivitis. Such agents, unfortunately, had poor substantivity and were not without unpleasant local side effects, notably mucosal erosion. The second group of enzymes employed glucose oxidase and amyloglucosidase to enhance the host defense mechanism. The aim was to catalyse the conversion of endogenous and exogenous thiocyanate to hypothiocyanite via the salivary lactoperoxydase system. Hypothiocyanite produces inhibitory effects upon oral bacteria, particularly streptococci, by interfering with their metabolism. This approach is a theoretical possibility and the chemical processes can be produced in the laboratory. A toothpaste product containing the enzymes and thiocyanate was produced but equivocal results for benefits to gingivitis were obtained and there are no convincing long-term studies of efficacy.

Bisbiguanide antiseptics
(For reviews see Addy 1986; Addy *et al.* 1994; Kornman 1986; Gjermo 1989; Jones 1997; Eley 1999)

Chlorhexidine is thus far the most studied and effective antiseptic for plaque inhibition and the prevention of gingivitis. Consequent upon the original publication (Löe & Schiott 1970), chlorhexidine arguably represents the nearest that research has come to identifying a chemical agent that could be used as a replacement for, rather than an adjunct to, mechanical oral hygiene practices. Other bisbiguanides such as alexidine and octenidine have less or similar activity, respectively, to chlorhexidine but bring with

them no improvement in local side effects and have less toxicity data available. Chlorhexidine has thus remained the only bisbiguanide used in a number of vehicles and available in commercial products. In view of the importance of this antiseptic within preventive dentistry, a separate section later in the chapter will be devoted to considering its activity and usage in the mouth.

Quaternary ammonium compounds
(For reviews see Mandel 1988; Eley 1999)

Benzalconium chloride and, more particularly, cetylpyridinium chloride are the most studied of this family of antiseptics. Cetylpyridinium chloride is used in a wide variety of antiseptic mouth rinse products, usually at a concentration of 0.05%. At oral pH these antiseptics are monocationic and adsorb readily and quantitatively, to a greater extent, than chlorhexidine to oral surfaces (Bonesvoll & Gjermo 1978). The substantivity of cetylpyridinium chloride however appears to be only 3–5 hours (Roberts & Addy 1981) due either to loss of activity once adsorbed or rapid desorption. Cetylpyridinium chloride in mouth rinses has some chemical plaque-inhibitory action but evidence for gingivitis benefits is equivocal, particularly when formulations are used alongside toothbrushing with toothpaste. Home use studies, given the large number of rinse products containing this antiseptic, are surprisingly few. Those available, with one exception, failed to demonstrate any adjunctive benefits to toothbrushing with toothpaste. The one exception (Allen *et al.* 1998) was peculiar in that there was a lack of the expected Hawthorne effect in the control group (see section "Evaluation of chemical agents and products" later in this chapter) and the plaque reduction in the active group, 28%, was as great as seen in no brushing chemical plaque inhibition studies. As will be discussed, it is not unusual to find chemicals that provide modest, even moderate, plaque inhibition in no brushing studies but fail to show effects in adjunctive home use studies. This occurs because the range over which to show a benefit of the chemical is limited by the mechanical oral hygiene practices of the study subjects. Additionally, the plaque-inhibitory properties of cetylpyridinium chloride are reduced by toothpaste used before or after the rinse (Sheen *et al.* 2001, 2003). This may explain why a pre-brushing cetylpyridinium mouth rinse offered no adjunctive benefit to mechanical plaque control (Moran & Addy 1991). The efficacy of cetylpyridinium chloride can be increased by doubling the frequency of rinsing to four times per day (Bonsvoll & Gjermo 1978), but this increases local side effects, including tooth staining, and would probably affect compliance. Mouth rinses combining cetylpyridinium chloride with chlorhexidine are available and compare well with established chlorhexidine products (Quirynen *et al.* 2001, 2005). Whether the cetylpyridinium chloride actually contributes to the activity of the chlorhexidine cannot be assessed. A slow-release system and lozenges have been used to deliver cetylpyridinium chloride but provided no greater plaque inhibition than the cetylpyridinium mouth rinse and significantly less than a chlorhexidine rinse (Vandekerchove *et al.* 1995). Interestingly, in this study, the lozenges produced the most dental staining. There is limited information on quaternary ammonium compounds in toothpastes and very few products are available.

Phenols and essential oils

(For reviews see Mandel 1988; Jackson 1997; Eley 1999)

Phenols and essential oils have been used in mouth rinses and lozenges for many years. One mouth rinse formulation dates back more than 100 years and, although not as efficacious as chlorhexidine, has antiplaque activity supported by a number of short- and long-term home use studies. This mouth rinse product may reduce gingivitis via both a plaque-inhibitory action and an anti-inflammatory action possibly due to an anti-oxidative activity (Firalti *et al.* 1994). The data from home use studies led the American Dental Association to accept the product as an aid to home oral hygiene measures (for review see Eley 1999). When compared directly with chlorhexidine one 6-month study has demonstrated equivalent effects on plaque and gingivitis but without the inherent side effects of chlorhexidine (Charles *et al.* 2004). Nevertheless, the pH of the product is low (pH 4.3) and has been shown *in vitro* and *in situ* to cause erosion of dentine and enamel respectively, albeit to a considerably less degree than orange juice (Addy *et al.* 1991; Pontefract *et al.* 2001). Combining essential oils with cetylpyridinium chloride has been attempted and with promising results from initial studies (Hunter *et al.* 1994).

The non-ionic antimicrobial triclosan, a trichlora-2-hydroxy phenyl ether, is usually considered to belong to the phenol group and has been widely used over many years in a number of medicated products including antiperspirants and soaps. More recently, it has been formulated into toothpaste and mouth rinses and, for the former, has accumulated an impressive amount of literature, some of which is conflicting. In simple solutions, at relatively high concentrations (0.2%) and dose (20 mg twice per day), triclosan has moderate plaque-inhibitory action and antimicrobial substantivity of around 5 hours (Jenkins *et al.* 1991a,b). The dose response against plaque of triclosan alone is relatively flat (Jenkins *et al.* 1993), although significantly greater benefits are obtained at 20 mg doses twice daily compared to 10 mg doses. In terms of plaque inhibition, a 0.1% triclosan concentration (10 mg dose twice per day) was considerably less effective than a 0.01% chlorhexidine mouth rinse (1 mg twice per day) (Jenkins *et al.* 1994).

The activity of triclosan appears to be enhanced by the addition of zinc citrate or the co-polymer, polyvinylmethyl ether maleic acid (for review see Gaffar *et al.* 1992). The co-polymer appears to enhance the retention of triclosan whereas the zinc is thought to increase the antimicrobial activity. Only triclosan toothpastes with the co-polymer or zinc citrate have shown antiplaque activity in long-term home use studies (for review see Jackson 1997). Some home use studies showed little or no effect for one or other of the products on plaque alone, gingivitis alone or both compared to the control paste or conventional fluoride toothpaste (Palomo *et al.* 1994; Kanchanakamol *et al.* 1995; Renvert & Birkhed 1995; Binney *et al.* 1996; Owens *et al.* 1997a). Triclosan toothpastes appear to provide greater gingivitis benefits in some studies than plaque reductions and this could be explained by a possible anti-inflammatory action for this agent (Barkvoll & Rolla 1994).

More recently, long-term studies have suggested that triclosan-containing toothpaste can reduce the progress of periodontitis, although the effects have been considered small (Rosling *et al.* 1997; Ellwood *et al.* 1998). Mouth rinses containing triclosan and the co-polymer are available, with some evidence of adjunctive benefits to oral hygiene and gingival health when used alongside normal tooth cleaning (Worthington *et al.* 1993). This latter study was again interesting with, unusually, no clear Hawthorne effect in the control group. Other studies on the plaque inhibitory properties of a triclosan/co-polymer mouth rinse showed effects significantly less than those of an essential oil mouth rinse product (Moran *et al.* 1997).

Natural products

(For review see Mandel 1988; Eley 1999)

Herb and plant extracts have been used in oral hygiene products for many years if not centuries. Unfortunately, there are few data available and such toothpaste products provide no greater benefits to oral hygiene and gingival health than do conventional fluoride toothpaste (Moran *et al.* 1991). The plant extract sanguinarine has been used in a number of formulations. Zinc salts are also incorporated, which makes it difficult to evaluate the efficacy of sanguinarine alone. Even when it is combined with zinc, however, data are equivocal for benefits (Moran *et al.* 1988, 1992a; Quirynen *et al.* 1990). Some positive findings were reported for the combined use of sanguinarine/zinc toothpaste and mouth rinses (Kopczyk *et al.* 1991), but the benefit-to-cost ratio must be low. Importantly and very recently, sanguinarine-containing mouth rinses have been shown to increase the likelihood of oral precancerous lesions almost ten-fold even after cessation of mouth rinse use. The manufacturer of the most well known product has replaced sanguinarine in the mouth rinses with an alternative agent. More recently, tea tree oil has been suggested to be of value when topically delivered with positive effects at reducing gingival inflammation (Sookoulis & Hirsch 2004) but as yet no conclusive evidence for effects on plaque accumulation.

Fluorides

The caries-preventive benefits for a number of fluoride salts are well established but the fluoride ion has no effect against the development of plaque and gingivitis. Amine fluoride and stannous fluoride provide some plaque-inhibitory activity, particularly when combined; however, the effects appear to be derived from the non-fluoride portion of the molecules. A mouth rinse product containing amine fluoride and stannous fluoride is available and there is some evidence from home use studies of efficacy against plaque and gingivitis (Brecx et al. 1990, 1992), but less so than chlorhexidine.

Metal salts
(For reviews see Addy et al. 1994; Jackson 1997)

Antimicrobial actions including plaque inhibition by metal salts have been appreciated for many years, with most research interest centered on copper, tin, and zinc. Results have been somewhat contradictory but appear dependent on the metal salt used, its concentration, and frequency of use. Essentially, polyvalent metal salts alone are effective plaque inhibitors at relatively high concentration when taste and toxicity problems may arise. Stannous fluoride is an exception but is difficult to formulate into oral hygiene products because of stability problems, with hydrolysis occurring in the presence of water. Stable anhydrous gel and toothpaste products are available with evidence of efficacy against plaque and gingivitis (Beiswanger et al. 1995; Perlich et al. 1995). Stannous pyrophosphate at 1% has been added to some stannous fluoride toothpaste to good effect (Svatun 1978). Indeed, it appears that the concentration of available stannous ions is the most significant factor in determining efficacy (Addy et al. 1997). Dental staining, however, occurs with stannous formulations and appears to occur by the same mechanism as for chlorhexidine and other cationic antiseptics, involving interaction with dietary chromogens (for reviews see Addy & Moran 1995; Watts & Addy 2001). Combining metal salts with other antiseptics produces added plaque and gingivitis inhibitory effects, for example zinc and hexetidine (Saxer & Muhlemann 1983) and, as already described, zinc and triclosan. Copper also causes dental staining but is not available in oral hygiene products. Zinc, at low concentration, has no side effects and is used in a number of toothpastes and mouth rinses; however, alone it has little effect on plaque (Addy et al. 1980) except at higher concentrations. Zinc salts nevertheless, may be of value at reducing volatile sulfur compounds associated with oral malodor (Rosing et al. 2002).

Oxygenating agents
(For review see Addy et al. 1994)

Oxygenating agents have been used as disinfectants in various disciplines of dentistry, including endodontics and periodontics. Hydrogen peroxide has been employed for supragingival plaque control and more recently has become important as bleach in tooth whitening. Similarly, peroxyborate may be used in the treatment of acute ulcerative gingivitis (Wade et al. 1966). Products containing peroxyborate and peroxycarbonate were, until recently, available in Britain and Europe with evidence of antimicrobial and plaque-inhibitory activity (Moran et al. 1995). There are little data from long-term home use studies and such evaluations would seem warranted before conclusions about true antiplaque activity can be drawn.

Detergents

Detergents, such as sodium lauryl sulfate, are common ingredients in toothpaste and mouth rinse products. Besides other qualities and, for that matter, side effects, detergents such as sodium lauryl sulfate have antimicrobial activity (Jenkins et al. 1991b) and probably provide most of the modest plaque-inhibitory action of toothpaste (Addy et al. 1983). Alone, sodium lauryl sulfate was shown to have moderate substantivity, measured at between 5 and 7 hours, and plaque-inhibitory action similar to triclosan (Jenkins et al. 1991a,b). Detergent-only formulations are not available and no long-term evaluations have been performed.

Amine alcohols

This group of compounds does not truly fit into an antimicrobial or antiseptic category; indeed they exhibit minimal effects against microbes. Of these morpholinoethenol derivatives, octopinol was the first to be shown effective as an antiplaque agent but was withdrawn for toxicologic reasons. Delmopinol followed and at 0.1% and 0.2% in mouth rinses was shown to be effective against plaque and gingivitis in short-term no oral hygiene and long-term home use studies (Collaert et al. 1992; Moran et al. 1992b; Claydon et al. 1996; Hase et al. 1998; Lang et al. 1998). Arguably, the short-term no oral hygiene studies showed plaque inhibition closer to chlorhexidine than any other previous agent (Moran et al. 1992b). Recently, the data from eight studies from seven independent research groups in five European countries using a 0.2% delmopinol mouth rinse as an adjunct to normal oral hygiene practices were subjected to a meta-analysis. Delmopinol, one of the very few chemical plaque-control agents to be subjected to such analyses, was shown to be a significantly effective adjunct for reducing the plaque burden and severity of gingivitis (Addy *et al.* 2007). The data for gingivitis in several studies met the efficacy criteria for gingivitis reduction of the American Dental Association. The mode of action of delmopinol can be debated but appears to be an interference with plaque matrix formation, reducing the adherence of the primary plaque-forming bacteria of the successional bacteria (Simonsson *et al.* 1991a,b). If correct, delmopinol would closest fit classification as an antiadhesive agent. Side effects include tooth discoloration, transient numbness of the tongue, and burning sensations in the mouth (Claydon *et al.* 1996; Hase *et al.* 1998; Lang *et al.* 1998). Interestingly, the staining was considerably less than with chlorhexidine, rarely reported by study participants and easily removed. In these adjunctive studies discontinuations were considerably less with delmopinol than chlorhexidine. Rinses containing 0.2% delmopinol are available in some countries.

Salifluor
(For review see Eley 1999)

Salifluor, a salicylanide with both antibacterial and anti-inflammatory properties, has been studied for its effects of plaque inhibition and retardation of onset of gingivitis (Furuichi *et al.* 1996). To improve oral retention and to maximize adsorption, Gantrez (PVM/MA) has been incorporated in salifluor toothpaste and mouth rinse formulations. Perhaps surprisingly, salifluor has not been extensively evaluated, since initial 4-day plaque regrowth studies and 14-day gingivitis studies have suggested equivalent efficacy to a 0.12% chlorhexidine mouth rinse (Furuichi *et al.* 1996). In spite of this evidence to suggest the potential value of the chemical as an antiplaque agent, further long-term studies have yet to be carried out.

Acidified sodium chlorite
(For review see Yates *et al.* 1997)

This agent does not sit well with any particular group listed in Table 36-1; however, depending on the acid chosen and the conditions of the reaction between the acid and the sodium chlorite, a varied and complex range of reaction products can ensue. Under ideal conditions for antimicrobial benefits sodium chlorite is reacted with a protic acid to produce chlorous acid, which then liberates a range of higher oxidant species but contains minimal amounts of chlorine dioxide. These higher oxidant species have a broad range of antimicrobial action against bacteria, fungi, yeast, and viruses, and products are available in the US within the veterinary and food industry, both as a preventive for mastitis in cows and for the preservation of frozen poultry. Experimental mouth rinses have been tested in short-term plaque regrowth studies and salivary bacterial count investigations (Yates *et al.* 1997). Surprisingly, given that the acid and sodium chlorite are mixed immediately before rinsing, and that the duration of the chemical reaction would be limited to the rinsing time, three experimental formulations were shown to be as good as chlorhexidine against plaque regrowth and showed the same substantivity as chlorhexidine. Although not tested in longer-term studies, side effects, particularly staining and alteration of taste, would appear unlikely with the acidified sodium chlorite mouth rinses. Unfortunately, the low pH of the formulations would be expected to cause some dental erosion and this has been proven in studies *in situ* (Pontefract *et al.* 2001). Such erosion, which was found comparable to that of orange juice *in situ*, would tend to obviate the long-term continuous use of such agents. Acidified sodium chlorite mouth rinses, however, could find application in preventive dentistry similar to those to be described for chlorhexidine (see later in this chapter). The erosive effects would not, in short- to medium-term use, reach clinically significant levels. To date no commercial products are available.

Other antiseptics
(For review see Addy 1986)

A number of antiseptics/antimicrobial agents have been studied for plaque inhibition. Most have been found to have little or no effect *in vivo*; a few have been formulated in mouth rinse products including povidone iodine and hexetidine. Povidone iodine at 1% has a substantivity of only 60 minutes (Addy & Wright 1978) and lacks appreciable plaque-inhibitory activity (Addy *et al.* 1977) or action in acute infections such as acute ulcerative gingivitis (Addy & Llewelyn 1978), for which it is recommended. Povidone iodine is largely without side effects but as a rinse has potential to affect thyroid function adversely (Wray *et al.* 1978). Hexetidine, a saturated pyrimidine, at 0.1% was shown to have limited plaque-inhibitory action (Bergenholtz & Hanstrom 1974) and no evidence for antiplaque activity when used as an adjunct for oral hygiene (Chadwick *et al.* 1991). The action of hexetidine against plaque appears enhanced by zinc salts (Saxer & Muhlemann 1983) but data are derived only from short-term studies. Side effects for hexetidine include tooth staining and mucosal erosion, although both are uncommon (Bergenholtz & Hanstrom 1974). Nevertheless, mucosal erosion is markedly increased in incidence if the concentration is raised to 0.14% (Bergenholtz & Hanstrom 1974). A mouth rinse product containing 0.1% hexetidine is available in some European countries. Recent studies have shown favorable effects on plaque and gingivitis (Sharma *et al.* 2003; Ernst *et al.* 2005) and when compared to 0.1% chlorhexidine, less tendency for stain production (Ernst *et al.* 2005).

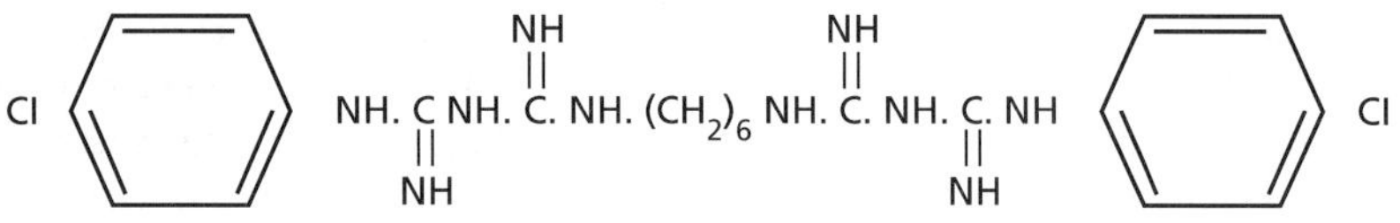

1,6–di (4–chlorophenyldiguanido) hexane

Fig. 36-2 Chlorhexidine molecule.

Conclusions

- Effective antimicrobial antiplaque agents show prolonged persistence of action in the mouth (substantivity). Chlorhexidine is the most effective antiplaque agent to date. Stannous fluoride and triclosan oral hygiene products are available with proven antiplaque activity. The long established mouth rinse, based on essential oils, has some evidence for adjunctive antiplaque activity.
- The limited information on natural products, for example herbal formulations, is not encouraging and the root extract sanguinarine has been withdrawn because of the potential to cause precancerous oral lesions.
- The amine alcohol, delmopinol, is an effective antiplaque agent and products are becoming available.
- Acidified sodium chlorite appears as effective as chlorhexidine against plaque but the acidic nature of the rinse may obviate oral hygiene products ever coming to the marketplace.
- Combinations of agents sometimes provide additive or synergistic action, but with the exception of triclosan, few products are available.

Chlorhexidine

Chlorhexidine is available in three forms, the digluconate, acetate, and hydrochloride salts. Most studies and most oral formulations and products have used the digluconate salt, which is manufactured as a 20% V/V concentrate. Digluconate and acetate salts are water soluble but hydrochloride is very sparingly soluble in water. Chlorhexidine was developed in the 1940s by Imperial Chemical Industries, England, and marketed in 1954 as an antiseptic for skin wounds. Later, the antiseptic was more widely used in medicine and surgery including obstetrics, gynecology, urology, and presurgical skin preparation for both patient and surgeon. Use in dentistry was initially for presurgical disinfection of the mouth and in endodontics. The first definitive study on chlorhexidine was performed by Löe and Schiott (1970). This study showed that rinsing for 60 seconds twice per day with 10 ml of a 0.2% (20 mg dose) chlorhexidine gluconate solution in the absence of normal tooth cleaning, inhibited plaque regrowth and the development of gingivitis. Numerous studies followed, such that chlorhexidine is one of the most investigated compounds in dentistry (for reviews see Jones 1997; Eley 1998). Chlorhexidine is a bisbiguanide antiseptic, being a symmetrical molecule consisting of four chlo-

rophenyl rings and two biguanide groups connected by a central hexamethylene bridge (Fig. 36-2). The compound is a strong base and dicationic at pH levels above 3.5, with two positive charges on either side of a hexamethylene bridge. Indeed, it is the dicationic nature of chlorhexidine, making it extremely interactive with anions, which is relevant to its efficacy, safety, local side effects, and difficulties with formulation in products.

Toxicology, safety, and side effects

The cationic nature of chlorhexidine minimizes absorption through the skin and mucosa, including from the gastrointestinal tract. Systemic toxicity from topical application or ingestion is therefore not reported, nor is there evidence of teratogenicity in the animal model. Even in intravenous infusion in animals, chlorhexidine is well tolerated and this has occurred accidentally in humans without serious consequences. Hypersensitivity reactions including anaphylaxis have been reported in fewer than 10 people in Japan and resulted from the application of non-proprietary chlorhexidine products to sites other than the mouth. There was insufficient information to confirm that the reactions were actually due to chlorhexidine. Neurosensory deafness can occur if chlorhexidine is introduced into the middle ear and the antiseptic should not be placed in the outer ear in case the eardrum is perforated. The antiseptic has a broad antimicrobial action, including a wide range of Gram-positive and Gram-negative bacteria (Wade & Addy 1989). It is also effective against some fungi and yeasts including *Candida*, and some viruses including HBV and HIV. Bacterial resistance has not been reported with long-term, oral use or evidence of super-infection by fungi, yeasts or viruses. Long-term oral use resulted in a small shift in the flora towards the less sensitive organisms but this was rapidly reversible at the end of the 2-year study (Schiott *et al.* 1976).

In oral use as a mouth rinse, chlorhexidine has been reported to have a number of local side effects (Flotra *et al.* 1971). These side effects are:

1. Brown discoloration of the teeth and some restorative materials and the dorsum of the tongue (Figs. 36-3 and 36-4).
2. Taste perturbation where the salt taste appears to be preferentially affected (Lang *et al.* 1988) to leave food and drinks with a rather bland taste.
3. Oral mucosal erosion (Fig. 36-5). This appears to be an idiosyncratic reaction and concentration

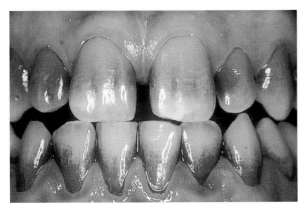

Fig. 36-3 Brown discoloration of the teeth of an individual rinsing twice a day for 3 weeks with a 0.2% chlorhexidine mouth rinse.

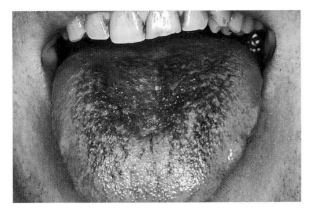

Fig. 36-4 Brown discoloration of the tongue of an individual rinsing twice a day for 2 weeks with a 0.2% chlorhexidine mouth rinse.

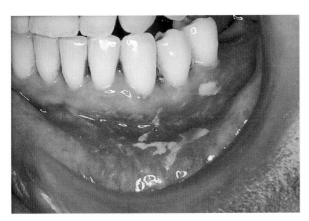

Fig. 36-5 Mucosal erosion occurring following a few days of rinsing twice a day with a 0.2% chlorhexidine mouth rinse.

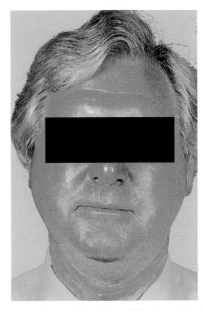

Fig. 36-6 Bilateral parotid swelling following a few days of rinsing with a 0.2% chlorhexidine mouth rinse.

proteins on to the tooth surface, thereby increasing pellicle thickness and/or precipitation of inorganic salts on to or into the pellicle layer.

Chlorhexidine also has a bitter taste, which is difficult to mask completely.

Chlorhexidine staining

The mechanisms proposed for chlorhexidine staining can be debated (Eriksen *et al*. 1985; for reviews see Addy & Moran 1995; Watts & Addy 2001) but have been proposed as:

1. Degradation of the chlorhexidine molecule to release parachloraniline
2. Catalysis of Maillard reactions
3. Protein denaturation with metal sulfide formation
4. Precipitation of anionic dietary chromogens.

Degradation of chlorhexidine to release parachloraniline appears not to occur on storage or as a result of metabolic processes. Also, alexidine, a related bisbiguanide, does not have parachloraniline groups, yet causes staining identical to that of chlorhexidine. Non-enzymatic browning reactions (Maillard reactions) catalyzed by chlorhexidine are a theoretical possibility; however, evidence is indirect, circumstantial or inconclusive (Eriksen *et al*. 1985). The theory does not consider the fact that other antiseptics and metals such as tin, iron, and copper also produce dental staining. Protein denaturation produced by chlorhexidine with the interaction of exposed sulfide radicals with metal ions is also theoretically possible but there is no direct evidence to support this concept. Again, the theory does not take into account similar staining by other antiseptics and metal ions. Laboratory and clinical studies also could

dependent. Dilution of the 0.2% formulation to 0.1%, but rinsing with the whole volume to maintain dose, usually alleviates the problem. Erosions are rarely seen with 0.12% rinse products used at 15 ml volume.
4. Unilateral or bilateral parotid swelling (Fig. 36-6). This is an extremely rare occurrence and an explanation is not available.
5. Enhanced supragingival calculus formation. This effect may be due to the precipitation of salivary

not reproduce this process (for reviews see Addy & Moran 1985; Watts & Addy 2001). Precipitation of anionic dietary chromogens by cationic antiseptics, including chlorhexidine and polyvalent metal ions as an explanation for the phenomenon of staining by these substances, is supported by a number of well controlled laboratory and clinical studies (for reviews see Addy & Moran 1995; Watts & Addy 2001). Thus, the locally bound antiseptics or metal ions on mucosa or teeth can react with polyphenols in dietary substances to produce staining. Beverages such as tea, coffee, and red wine are particularly chromogenic, but other foods and beverages will interact to produce various colored stains. These reactions between chlorhexidine and other cationic antiseptics and polyvalent metal ions with chromogenic beverages can be performed within the test tube. Interestingly, most of the precipitates formed between polyvalent metal ions and chromogens have the same color as their sulfide salts. It is for this reason that original theories considered that staining, seen in individuals exposed to these polyvalent metal ions, usually in the workplace, was due to metal sulfide formation. Again, laboratory and clinical experiments have failed to produce such interactions.

It is perhaps the staining side effect that limits long-term use of chlorhexidine in preventive dentistry (Flotra *et al.* 1971) and occurs with all correctly formulated products including gels, toothpastes, and sprays. Indeed, the staining side effect can be used to assess patient compliance in the use and activity of formulations. In the latter case laboratory and clinical studies on staining have revealed a proprietary chlorhexidine mouth rinse product to be inactive (Renton-Harper *et al.* 1995). Interestingly, this particular chlorhexidine product was reformulated in the UK to produce an active formulation (Addy *et al.* 1991), but the manufacturers maintained the original formulation within France when both laboratory and clinical studies confirmed markedly reduced potential of the product to cause staining in the laboratory, and plaque inhibition in the clinic (Renton-Harper *et al.* 1995). Recently, a chlorhexidine product with an anti-discoloration system (ADS) was launched in Europe. A clinical study purporting to show reduced staining had significant drawbacks in design and presentation (Bernadi *et al.* 2004). A laboratory study found no difference in staining potential (Addy *et al.* 2005) and a plaque regrowth study showed significantly reduced plaque inhibition for the ADS rinse (Arweiler *et al.* 2006). The old adage concerning chlorhexidine products appears to still hold true: "If it does not stain it does not work".

Mechanism of action
(For reviews see Addy 1986; Jenkins *et al.* 1988)

Chlorhexidine is a potent antibacterial substance but this alone does not explain its antiplaque action. The antiseptic binds strongly to bacterial cell membranes.

At low concentration this results in increased permeability with leakage of intracellular components including potassium. At high concentration, chlorhexidine causes precipitation of bacterial cytoplasm and cell death. In the mouth chlorhexidine readily adsorbs to surfaces including pellicle-coated teeth. Once adsorbed, and unlike some other antiseptics, chlorhexidine shows a persistent bacteriostatic action lasting in excess of 12 hours (Schiott *et al.* 1970). Radio-labelled chlorhexidine studies suggest a slow release of the antiseptic from surfaces (Bonesvoll *et al.* 1974a,b) and this was suggested to produce a prolonged antibacterial milieu in the mouth (Gjermo *et al.* 1974). The methods used, however, could not determine the activity of the chlorhexidine, which was almost certainly attached to the salivary proteins and desquamating epithelial cells and therefore unavailable for action. Consistent with the original work and conclusions (Davies *et al.* 1970), a more recent study and review suggested that plaque inhibition is derived only from the chlorhexidine adsorbed to the tooth surface (Jenkins *et al.* 1988). It is possible that the molecule attaches to pellicle by one cation leaving the other free to interact with bacteria attempting to colonize the tooth surface. This mechanism would, therefore, be similar to that associated with tooth staining. It would also explain why anionic substances, such as sodium lauryl sulfate based toothpastes, reduce the plaque inhibition of chlorhexidine if used shortly after rinses with the antiseptic (Barkvoll *et al.* 1989). Indeed, a more recent study has demonstrated that plaque inhibition by chlorhexidine mouth rinses is reduced if toothpaste is used immediately before or immediately after the rinse (Owens *et al.* 1997b). These inhibitory effects on chlorhexidine activity by substances such as toothpastes can be modeled using the chlorhexidine tea staining method, which shows reduced staining activity by the chlorhexidine solutions resulting from an interaction with toothpaste (Sheen *et al.* 2001).

Plaque inhibition by chlorhexidine mouth rinses appears to be dose related (Jenkins *et al.* 1994) such that similar effects to that seen with the more usual 10 ml, 0.2% solution (20 mg) can be achieved with high volumes of low-concentration solutions (Lang & Ramseier-Grossman 1981). It is worth noting, however, that not inconsiderable plaque inhibition is obtained with doses as low as 1–5 mg twice daily (Jenkins *et al.* 1994). Also, and relevant to the probable mechanism of action, topically applying 0.2% solutions of chlorhexidine only to the tooth surface, including by the use of sprays, produces the same level of plaque inhibition as rinsing with the full 20 mg dose (Addy & Moran 1983; Francis *et al.* 1987a; Jenkins *et al.* 1988; Kalaga *et al.* 1989a).

Chlorhexidine products

Chlorhexidine has been formulated into a number of products.

Mouth rinses

Aqueous alcohol solutions of 0.2% chlorhexidine were first made available for mouth rinse products for twice daily use in Europe in the 1970s. A 0.1% mouth rinse product also became available; however questions were raised over the activity of the 0.1% product and in some countries the efficacy of this product is less than would be expected from a 0.1% solution (Jenkins *et al.* 1989). Later, in the US, a 0.12% mouth rinse was manufactured but to maintain the almost optimum 20 mg doses derived from 10 ml of 0.2% rinses, the product was recommended as a 15 ml rinse (18 mg dose). The studies revealed equal efficacy for 0.2% and 0.12% rinses when used at appropriate similar doses (Segreto *et al.* 1986). More recently alcohol-free chlorhexidine rinses have become available, some formulated with the inclusion of 0.05% CPC. Such formulations have been shown to possess equivalent effects at inhibiting plaque and gingivitis compared to alcohol-containing chlorhexidine rinses but with better taste acceptability with the non-alcoholic rinse (Quirynen *et al.* 2001; Van Strydonck *et al.* 2005)

Gel

A 1% chlorhexidine gel product is available and can be delivered on a toothbrush or in trays. The distribution of the gel by toothbrush around the mouth appears to be poor and preparations must be delivered to all tooth surfaces to be effective (Saxen *et al.* 1976).

In trays the chlorhexidine gel was found to be particularly effective against plaque and gingivitis in handicapped individuals (Francis *et al.* 1987a). The acceptability of this tray delivery system to the recipients and the carers was found to be poor (Francis *et al.* 1987b). More recently, 0.2% and 0.12% chlorhexidine gels have become available.

Sprays

Sprays containing 0.1% and 0.2% chlorhexidine are commercially available in some countries. Studies with the 0.2% spray have revealed that small doses of approximately 1–2 mg delivered to all tooth surfaces produces similar plaque inhibition to a rinse with 0.2% mouth rinses (Kalaga *et al.* 1989a). Sprays appear particularly useful for the physically and mentally handicapped groups, being well received by individuals and their carers (Francis *et al.* 1987a,b; Kalaga *et al.* 1989b).

Toothpaste
(For review see Yates *et al.* 1993)

Chlorhexidine is difficult to formulate into toothpaste for reasons already given and early studies produced variable outcomes for benefits to plaque and gingivitis. More recently, a 1% chlorhexidine toothpaste with and without fluoride was found to be superior to the control product for the prevention of plaque and gingivitis in a 6-month home use study (Yates *et al.* 1993). Stain scores however, were markedly increased as was supragingival calculus formation, and the manufacturer did not produce a commercial product. For a short time a commercial product was available, having been shown to be efficacious for both plaque and gingivitis (Sanz *et al.* 1994). Although effective, chlorhexidine products based on toothpaste and sprays produce similar tooth staining to mouth rinses and gels; taste disturbance, mucosal erosion, and parotid swellings tend to be less or have never been reported.

Varnishes

Chlorhexidine varnishes have been used mainly for prophylaxis against root caries rather than an antiplaque depot for chlorhexidine in the mouth.

Slow-release vehicles

A chlorhexidine chip has been produced commercially for placement into periodontal pockets as an adjunct to scaling and root planning. This will be discussed in Chapter 42.

Conclusions

- Chlorhexidine to date is the proven most effective antiplaque agent, for which commercial products are available to the public.
- Chlorhexidine is free from systemic toxicity in oral use, and microbial resistance and super-infection do not occur.
- Local side effects are reported which are mainly cosmetic problems.
- The antiplaque action of chlorhexidine appears dependent on prolonged persistence of antimicrobial action in the mouth (substantivity).
- A number of vehicles for delivering chlorhexidine are available, but mouth rinses are most commonly recommended.
- Extrinsic dental staining and perturbation of taste are variably the two side effects of chlorhexidine mouth rinse usage, which limit acceptability to users and the long-term employment of this antiseptic in preventive dentistry.

Clinical uses of chlorhexidine

Despite the excellent plaque inhibitory properties of chlorhexidine, widespread and prolonged use of the agent is limited by local side effects. Moreover, because of the cationic nature of the chlorhexidine and therefore its poor penetrability, the antiseptic is of limited value in the therapy of established oral conditions including gingivitis, and is much more valuable in the preventive mode. A number of clinical uses, some well researched, have been recommended for chlorhexidine (for reviews see Gjermo 1974; Addy 1986; Addy & Renton-Harper 1996; Addy & Moran 1997; Eley 1999).

As an adjunct to oral hygiene and professional prophylaxis

Oral hygiene instruction is a key factor in the treatment plan for patients with periodontal disease and as part of the maintenance program following treatment. Adequate plaque control by periodontal patients is therefore essential to successful treatment and the prevention of recurrence of the disease. Chlorhexidine should therefore increase the improvement in gingival health through plaque control, particularly following professional prophylaxis to remove existing supra- and immediately subgingival plaque. There is, however, a potential disadvantage of using such an effective chemical plaque-control agent at this stage of the periodontal treatment plan. Thus, following oral hygiene instruction, it is normal, usually by the use of indices, to quantify the improvement in plaque control by patients so instructed and, in particular, the improvement at specific sites, which previously had been missed by individual patients. By virtue of the excellent plaque-control effects of chlorhexidine, the response to oral hygiene instruction cannot be accurately assessed since the antiseptic will overshadow any deficiencies in mechanical cleaning. Indeed, as the original research demonstrated, with chlorhexidine mouth rinse patients could maintain close to zero levels of plaque following a professional prophylaxis without using any form of mechanical oral hygiene (Löe & Schiott 1970). Nevertheless, chlorhexidine mouth rinse may be of value in maintaining oral hygiene following scaling and root planing when adequate tooth brushing may be compromised by post-treatment soreness or sensitivity.

Post oral surgery including periodontal surgery or root planing

Chlorhexidine may be used post-operatively since it offers the advantage of reducing the bacterial load in the oral cavity and preventing plaque formation at a time when mechanical cleaning may be difficult because of discomfort. In periodontal surgery, periodontal dressings have largely been replaced by the use of chlorhexidine preparations, in particular mouth rinses, since healing is improved and discomfort reduced (Newman & Addy 1978, 1982). Regimens vary but chlorhexidine should be used immediately post treatment and for periods of time until the patient can re-institute normal oral hygiene. Depending on the appointment schedule, chlorhexidine could be used throughout the treatment phase and for periods of weeks after completion of the treatment plan. If dressings are used, chlorhexidine is of limited value to the post-operative site since it does not penetrate beneath the periodontal dressings (Pluss et al. 1975). Although chlorhexidine rinses are probably used after root planing by many clinicians, evidence of therapeutic benefit has only recently been published (Faveri et al. 2006).

The idea of full-mouth disinfection using chlorhexidine both supra- and subgingivally as an adjunct to scaling and root planing has been assessed by one group in a number of papers since 1995 (for review see Quirynen et al. 2006). In the event, few adjunctive benefits could be shown (for review see Apatzidou 2006). It appeared that the more dominant factor was the time over which the non-surgical treatment plan was completed. Thus, root planing performed totally within 24 hours was more effective than root planing completed over more conventional periods of several weeks (Quirynen et al. 2006). Similar clinical research however, showed no difference between root planing completed within 24 hours compared to within several weeks (Apatzidou & Kinane 2004).

For patients with jaw fixation

Oral hygiene is particularly difficult when jaws are immobilized by such methods as intermaxillary fixation. Chlorhexidine mouth rinses have been shown markedly to reduce the bacterial load, which tends to increase during jaw immobilization, and to improve plaque control (Nash & Addy 1979). The more recent trend to use sub-dermal or sub-mucosal plates to stabilize bony fragments probably impedes oral hygiene procedures to a lesser degree, providing there are no oral mucosal lacerations. The influence of these factors on oral hygiene and therefore the role of chlorhexidine formulation has never been investigated.

For oral hygiene and gingival health benefits in the mentally and physically handicapped

Chlorhexidine has been found particularly useful in institutionalized mentally and physically handicapped groups, improving both oral hygiene and gingival health (Storhaug 1977). Spray delivery of 0.2% solutions was found particularly useful and acceptable to patients and care workers (Francis et al. 1987a,b; Kalaga et al. 1989b).

Medically compromised individuals predisposed to oral infections

A number of medical conditions predispose individuals to oral infections, notably candidiasis. Chlorhexidine is effective as an anticandidal agent but is most useful when combined with specific anticandidal drugs, such as nystatin or amphotericin B (Simonetti et al. 1988). Indications for chlorhexidine use combined with anticandidal drugs have been for the prevention of oral and systemic infections in the immunocompromised, including those with blood dyscrasias, those receiving chemotherapy and/or radiotherapy, and notably bone marrow transplant patients (Ferretti *et al.* 1987, 1988; Toth *et al.* 1990). The value of chlorhexidine appears greatest when initiated before oral or systemic complications arise. A chlorhexidine spray was also found to produce symptomatic/psychologic oral care benefits in the terminally ill (Jobbins *et al.* 1992).

High-risk caries patients

Chlorhexidine rinses or gels can reduce considerably the *Streptococcus mutans* counts in individuals who are caries prone. Additionally, and interestingly, chlorhexidine appears synergistic with sodium fluoride and combining chlorhexidine and fluoride rinses appears beneficial to such at-risk individuals (Dolles & Gjermo 1980). Sodium monofluorophosphate on the other hand, reduces the effect of chlorhexidine and probably *vice versa* (Barkvoll *et al.* 1988). A chlorhexidine rinse product with sodium fluoride has recently become available.

Recurrent oral ulceration

Several studies have shown that chlorhexidine mouth rinses and chlorhexidine gels reduce the incidence, duration, and severity of recurrent minor aphthous ulceration (for review see Hunter & Addy 1987). The mechanism of action is unclear but may relate to a reduction in contamination of ulcers by oral bacteria, thereby reducing the natural history of the ulceration. Regimens have included three times daily use of chlorhexidine products for several weeks. Interestingly, one study showed that triclosan rinses reduce the incidence of recurrent mouth ulcers (Skaare *et al.* 1996). There have been no controlled studies of chlorhexidine in the management of major aphthous ulceration or other oral erosive or ulcerative conditions, although anecdotally chlorhexidine appears ineffective. Again, this may reflect the low therapeutic potential of this and other antiseptics, and the considerable amount of proteinacious material associated with these lesions which would both tend to inactivate chlorhexidine and block access to underlying microorganisms (Roberts & Addy 1981). A similar explanation may be propounded for the failure of chlorhexidine mouth rinses in treatment of acute necrotizing ulcerative gingivitis (periodontitis) (Addy & Llewelyn 1978): further evidence for the lack of absorption into tissues and biofilms of this cationic antiseptic.

Removable and fixed orthodontic appliance wearers

Plaque control in the early stages of orthodontic appliance therapy may be compromised and chlorhexidine can be prescribed for the first 4–8 weeks. Additionally, chlorhexidine has been shown to reduce the number and severity of traumatic ulcers during the first 4 weeks of fixed orthodontic therapy (Shaw *et al.* 1984).

Denture stomatitis

Chlorhexidine has been recommended in the treatment of *Candida*-associated infections; however, in practice even applying chlorhexidine gel to the fitting surfaces of dentures produces, in many cases, slow and incomplete resolution of the condition. Again, chlorhexidine is less effective in the therapeutic mode and it is more advantageous to treat denture stomatitis with specific anticandidal drugs and then employ chlorhexidine to prevent recurrence. The denture itself can be usefully sterilized from *Candida* by soaking in chlorhexidine solutions (Olsen 1975).

Oral malodor

Rinsing with chlorhexidine as with other antiseptic mouth rinses containing CPC, triclosan, and essential oils, has been suggested to be of value in reducing halitosis. Reductions in volatile sulphur compounds and morning malodor have been noted with all these chemicals (Carvalho *et al.* 2004).

Immediate pre-operative chlorhexidine rinsing and irrigation

This technique can be used immediately prior to operative treatment, particularly when air polishing, ultrasonic scaling or high-speed instruments are to be used. Such pre-operative rinsing markedly reduces the bacterial load and contamination of the operative area, operator, and staff (Worral *et al.* 1987). Additionally, in susceptible patients, irrigation of chlorhexidine around the gingival margin reduces the incidence of bacteremia (MacFarlane *et al.* 1984). This should be seen, however, only as an adjunct to appropriate systemic antimicrobial prophylaxis. Chlorhexidine mouth rinsing now features as an adjunct to antibiotic prophylaxis in the new UK guidelines.

Subgingival irrigation

Numerous antimicrobial agents have been used as subgingival irrigants in the management and treatment of periodontal diseases (for reviews see Wennstrom 1992, 1997). Alone, irrigation with antimicrobial agents produces effects little different from using saline, and they are of short duration, suggesting that the action is a washing-out effect. Irrigation combined with root planing appears to provide no adjunctive benefits.

Conclusions

- There is a significant number of indications for the use of chlorhexidine in preventive dentistry, most of which rely on the antimicrobial properties of the antiseptic and its duration of action.

- The most valuable chemical plaque-control uses of chlorhexidine are in the short to medium term when mechanical tooth cleaning is not possible, difficult or inadequate and during which time local side effects are likely to be minimized.
- Chlorhexidine is more effective as a preventive rather than a therapeutic agent and therefore must be of questionable value as a subgingival adjunct in the treatment of periodontitis (see Chapter 42).

Evaluation of chemical agents and products

(For reviews see Addy *et al.* 1992; Addy 1995; Moss *et al.* 1995; Addy & Moran 1997)

The number and use of oral hygiene products has grown enormously in recent years and, as an example, hundreds of millions of pounds per year are spent on oral hygiene products in the UK and presumably billions worldwide. There can be no doubt that the oral hygiene industries, through their collaboration and research with the dental profession and their promotion of their products have, in no small way, contributed to the improvement in dental health seen in many countries. Claims for efficacy of oral hygiene products, however, are frequently made and it is essential that these are supported by scientific evidence. Without such evidence the profession and the public may be confused or misled. The dental profession is, however, faced with a large number of oral hygiene products supported by huge quantities of varied promotional literature and media advertising, which makes impossible, in many cases, any valid judgment or assessment of the efficacy or value of individual products to specific patient groups or the public as a whole. Even those with specialized interest, and research experience in specific aspects of oral hygiene product evaluation, must find validation, based on published literature, a daunting task. This is made all the more difficult since what constitutes proof of efficacy is not generally agreed even amongst so-called experts. Few countries of the world have central control over what evidence is required before efficacy claims can be made and there are very few guidelines suggesting requirements for proof of efficacy for oral hygiene products.

The scientific evaluation of dental products, and for that matter, preventive and therapeutic agents in medicine as a whole, is a relatively modern concept but today must be the backbone on which to base claims of efficacy. Anecdotal and case reports, uncontrolled studies and data listed as "held on file" by manufacturers, whilst interesting, should not be used as the basis for efficacy claims. Blind, randomized, controlled clinical and laboratory studies must be the methods used today to obtain data on the activity of agents, formulations, and products. Terminology and phraseology in product claims also needs to be

carefully reviewed and assessed. Perhaps the greatest area for criticism must be the implied claim by the manufacturer and/or the inferences left to be drawn, from promotional material, by the dental profession or public. A classic scenario for which there is precedence can be stated as follows: A is the cause of B, C reduces A, leaving the inference to be drawn that C can control B. Perhaps nowhere is this more apparent than in the use of agents which are known to control plaque, and therefore it can be implied, without evidence, they must control gingivitis. The now familiar claim would be "this product reduces plaque, the major cause of gum disease". Similarly, creative arithmetic is not infrequently used to give inflated impressions of efficacy. Proportional differences, rather than actual differences, are not infrequently quoted, as are percentages of percentages giving hundreds of percent improvements over another product or control, yet the actual benefit is a fraction of the scoring index used. Finally, "piggy back" claims are not uncommon, when a known active ingredient is formulated into a new product and equivalent efficacy to established products is assumed. It would seem reasonable here to repeat the definitions for the terminology for oral hygiene products, agreed at the European Workshop on Periodontology in 1996 which defined certain terms (Lang & Newman 1997):

- *Antimicrobial agents*: chemicals that have a bacteriostatic or bactericidal effect *in vitro* that alone cannot be extrapolated to a proven efficacy *in vivo* against plaque.
- *Plaque reducing/inhibitory agents*: chemicals that have only been shown to reduce the quantity and/or affect quality of plaque, which may or may not be sufficient to influence gingivitis and/or caries.
- *Antiplaque agents*: chemicals that have an effect on plaque sufficient to benefit gingivitis and/or caries.
- *Antigingivitis agents*: chemicals which reduce gingival inflammation without necessarily influencing bacterial plaque (includes anti-inflammatory agents).

Thus, the fact that antimicrobial agents such as antiseptics kill or inhibit the growth of bacteria does not necessarily mean they will be effective plaque inhibitors (Gjermo *et al.* 1970). Also, the mere incorporation of a known antiplaque agent into a formulation is not a guarantee of efficacy because inactivation by other ingredients may occur.

This section looks at methods that have been used to test oral hygiene products both in the laboratory and the clinic. No one protocol can provide all the answers, and research and development of agents into products is a step-by-step process, hopefully culminating in a body of evidence proving efficacy, beyond doubt, of a final product. Methods *in vitro* and *in vivo* will be summarized but animal testing will not be discussed except to acknowledge that the use of animals is still necessary in drug development, in understanding the mode of action of drugs and, particularly, in evaluating safety from a toxicologic point of view. The evaluation of oral hygiene products on animals, however, particularly for efficacy, must be questioned on a number of scientific and moral grounds.

Most laboratory and clinical methods have been developed to test antimicrobial agents but methodologies are available, or present ones could be modified, to study potential antiadhesive and plaque removal chemicals (for reviews see Addy *et al.* 1992; Addy 1995; Addy & Moran 1997).

Studies *in vitro*

Bacterial tests

Antimicrobial tests, including minimum inhibitory concentration (MIC), minimum bactericidal concentration (MBC), and kill curves, can be determined. These tests indicate the antibacterial activity and antimicrobial spectrum of agents and formulations against a range of oral bacteria. Continuous culture techniques can also be used but they may not provide more meaningful data. It is likely that, with technologic advances, laboratory models to accurately replicate the plaque biofilm will become available to test chemical plaque-control agents. At present, antimicrobial tests *in vitro* primarily only indicate activity, or lack of it, and they are very poor predictors *per se* of effects on plaque *in vivo*. This is because, so far, methods do not provide particularly reliable information on the substantivity of the antimicrobial agent. Nevertheless, antimicrobial tests are valuable for a variety of reasons. With few exceptions, agents without activity *in vitro* will not provide activity *in vivo*. The additive or negative effects of ingredient mixtures can be determined. The availability of active ingredients incorporated in the product can be assessed. The adverse influence of the oral environment can be modeled; for example, the influence of saliva or proteins on the antibacterial activity of agents can be tested.

Uptake measurements

One aspect of substantivity is adsorption of antimicrobials and other potential plaque-inhibitory agents on to surfaces. This can be quantified using a variety of substrates such as hydroxyapatite, dentine, enamel, acrylic, and other polymers. The influence of other factors or agents on the uptake of a particular agent can also be assessed. Such data are of interest but must be interpreted with caution since they only measure uptake, not activity once adsorbed. Nevertheless, desorption of an agent from such surfaces can be measured by a variety of analytical techniques, thereby giving some indication of both the adsorp-

tion profile and the subsequent substantivity of the agent to the substrate surface.

Other methods

Activity or availability of an ingredient in a formulation can be measured or assessed. Methods include chemical analyses; however, some methods chemically extract the agent from the formulation in its entirety and therefore do not necessarily demonstrate that it is freely available and active within the formulation. For the cationic antiseptics and polyvalent metal salts, their potential to bind dietary chromogens from beverages such as tea can be used to assess the possibility that they may cause staining *in vivo*. More usefully, the test method can be employed to determine and compare the availability of the same ingredient in different formulations. Such methods have shown considerable differences in availability of chlorhexidine and cetylpyridinium chloride in apparently similar mouth rinses (Addy *et al.* 1995). Moreover, how other oral hygiene products might interfere with the activity of chemical plaque-control agents, such as toothpaste with chlorhexidine and cetylpyridinium chloride, has given surprisingly accurate predictions of clinical outcome (Owens *et al.* 1997b; Sheen *et al.* 2001, 2003). Again, these methods give little indication of substantivity and therefore the staining method *in vitro* cannot be used to compare different agents for propensities to cause staining *in vivo*. For example, a 0.05% cetylpyridinium chloride mouth rinse produces comparable tea staining on a substrate surface to a 0.2% chlorhexidine mouth rinse, yet clinically the amount of staining reported for chlorhexidine is considerably greater than that for cetylpyridinium chloride and this can be explained by the fact that the substantivity of the former is greater than that of the latter.

Study methods *in vivo*

A considerable number of protocols have been developed to evaluate potential antiplaque agents and products. Ideally, because of the number of ingredients and more particularly formulations, a step-by-step pyramid approach is taken. Thus initially, study designs are used which permit, if necessary, the screening of relatively large numbers of agents and formulations and on relatively small numbers of subjects.

Depot studies

Retention of agents in the mouth may be measured by determining the amount expectorated versus the known dose (the buccal retention test) or by measuring plaque and saliva levels of the agent over time. Such retention assessments can be misleading because retention is only one aspect of substantivity and the measurement techniques do not provide information

Bacterial counts × 10^6

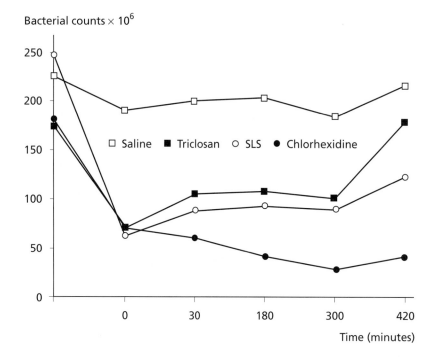

□ Saline   ■ Triclosan   ○ SLS   ● Chlorhexidine

Time (minutes)

Fig. 36-7 Salivary bacterial counts over time following mouth rinsing with chlorhexidine, saline, sodium lauryl sulfate, and triclosan. Following a single rinse with chlorhexidine, sodium lauryl sulfate, and triclosan there is an immediate large reduction in bacterial counts. This continues and persists to the 420-minute endpoint of the study for chlorhexidine (positive control) with a tendency for counts to revert towards baseline for triclosan and sodium lauryl sulfate. With saline (placebo control), there is little change in counts over time.

on the activity of the retained agents. Moreover, the buccal retention test does not distinguish drug absorption from adsorption nor determine how much is swallowed. Thus, for example, studies using radio-labeled chlorhexidine purported to demonstrate slow release from oral surfaces and this occurred over a protracted period of time (Bonesvoll *et al.* 1974a,b). However, saliva derived from subjects following rinsing with chlorhexidine only provided antimicrobial activity for up to 3 hours following rinsing (Addy & Wright 1978). This is clearly markedly less than the known substantivity or persistence of action of chlorhexidine in the mouth of at least 12 hours (Schiott *et al.* 1970). It is likely, therefore, that the initial desorption studies using a radiolabel were merely detecting chlorhexidine adsorbed to desquamating oral surfaces, particularly the mucosa.

Antimicrobial tests

For antimicrobial agents only, salivary bacterial count assessments are much more indicative of substantivity and are predictive of antiplaque action for the same agents. The method involves measuring salivary bacterial counts before, and at time points, after a single rinse with the agent (Fig. 36-7) and was first described for chlorhexidine (Schiott *et al.* 1970). In the case of toothpaste, the product can be either brushed or rinsed as an aqueous slurry (Addy *et al.* 1983; Jenkins *et al.* 1990). Agents and products produce variable reductions in counts ranging from none, as with water, to greater than 90%, as with chlorhexidine. More importantly, the duration of reduction from baseline varies from minutes to hours. Thus, povidone iodine only reduces counts for approximately 1 hour, cetylpyridinium chloride for 3 hours (Roberts & Addy 1981), whereas chlorhexidine pro-

duces such effects for over 12 hours (Schiott *et al.* 1970). Toothpastes generally show reductions in counts between 3 and 5 hours, probably largely due to contained detergents and/or specific ingredients such as triclosan (Addy *et al.* 1989).

Experimental plaque studies

Short-term plaque regrowth studies are perhaps the most commonly used clinical experiments to screen chemical oral hygiene products. They have the advantage of assessing the chemical action of the formulation divorced from the indeterminate variable of toothbrushing. Typically, plaque regrowth from a zero baseline and the influence of the test agent is recorded. Originally used for mouth rinses, the method has been modified for toothpaste by delivering the formulation in a tray applied to the teeth (Etemadzadeh *et al.* 1985) or as a slurry rinse (Addy *et al.* 1983). Studies are usually cross-over, allowing many formulations to be evaluated against suitable controls. Study periods range from 24 hours to several days, usually 4–5 days (Harrap 1974; Addy *et al.* 1983). A negative control such as water and a positive control such as chlorhexidine may be used (Fig. 36-8). These help to position the activity of the test formulations between the extremes. Also, because the results from these controls can be predicted, their use tends to confirm or otherwise the conduct of these blind, randomized study designs.

Experimental gingivitis studies

Experimental gingivitis studies (Löe & Schiott 1970) are based on the original experimental gingivitis in man protocol first used to demonstrate the direct etiologic relationship between plaque and gingivitis

Plaque Area (sq cm)

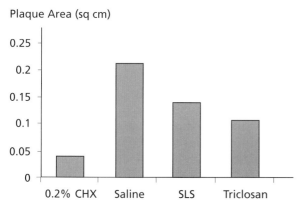

Fig. 36-8 Plaque area following the use of chlorhexidine, saline, sodium lauryl sulfate, and triclosan mouth rinses after 4-day periods. Considerable plaque inhibition was afforded by chlorhexidine (positive control) when toothcleaning was suspended. Both sodium lauryl sulfate and triclosan show significant plaque-inhibitory action compared to saline (placebo control) albeit significantly less than chlorhexidine.

Plaque Index

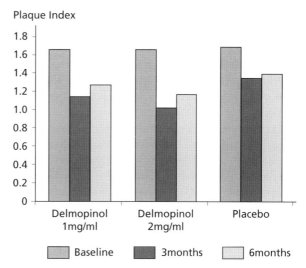

Fig. 36-9 A 6-month study of delmopinol rinses as adjuncts to oral hygiene. Significant improvements in plaque scores are seen in the delmopinol mouth rinse groups at 3 and 6 months compared to placebo. A Hawthorne effect of improved toothcleaning irrespective of the treatment is apparent in the placebo group, particularly at 3 months, although this is still present at 6 months.

(Löe *et al.* 1965). This latter original study did not return subjects to zero baseline plaque scores or gingival health, whereas most subsequent methods, to evaluate oral hygiene products, have taken this approach with baseline parameters. Study periods usually range from 12, but more particularly 19–28 days. In the absence of normal tooth cleaning, the development of plaque and gingivitis are recorded under the influence of test and control formulations. Studies may be either cross-over or parallel.

Home use studies

For chemical oral hygiene products and usually toothpastes and mouth rinses, the final evaluation requires that they are shown to be effective against plaque and, more particularly, gingivitis, when used along with normal mechanical tooth cleaning. Studies can be over days or weeks but usually, in accordance with guidelines such as those for the American Dental Association (Council of Dental Therapeutics 1985), they need to be 6 months or longer, particularly since safety needs to be assessed (Fig. 36-9). Most studies are parallel in design. Protocols have used two approaches. One is perhaps more therapeutic in concept whereby subjects have to exhibit a certain level of plaque and/or gingivitis before entry (Johansen *et al.* 1975). The other is more preventive in concept and there is a pre-study period in which subjects with gingivitis receive prophylaxis and instruction to improve their gingival health. Those satisfactorily responding are entered, and change in gingival health is monitored in the test and control groups (Stephen *et al.* 1990).

Several factors tend to confound home use studies of oral hygiene products and may mask a proven chemical antiplaque action determined from short-term plaque and experimental gingivitis studies. Most important is the so-called Hawthorne effect

where subjects knowingly involved in oral hygiene studies improve their tooth cleaning (Fig. 36-9). Secondly, baseline prophylaxes are commonly given and the influence of this on the subsequent gingivitis levels is not known. In mouth rinse studies used as adjuncts to tooth cleaning, there is the potential of interaction between toothpaste and mouth rinse, which could be additive but in most cases is more likely negative for effects on mouth rinse ingredients (Owens *et al.* 1997b; Sheen *et al.* 2001, 2003). Compliance in home use studies can also be a problem and difficult to determine accurately. In short-term studies compliance can be guaranteed through supervision but this is difficult in home use studies although was achieved, in part, in a series of delmopinol studies (for review see Addy *et al.* 2007). Finally, particularly in toothpaste studies, the control product will have some inherent plaque-inhibitory action consequent upon ingredients such as detergents (Addy *et al.* 1983). If the appropriate control products have been used in the screening plaque inhibitory and experimental gingivitis models this should not pose a problem. However, there is no doubt, and this will be discussed, that the choice of control toothpaste, used to compare an active toothpaste, could considerably influence the outcome and therefore the conclusions concerning a potential antiplaque toothpaste.

Clinical trial design considerations

Clinical trials involving human patients, subjects or healthy volunteers in many countries must now conform to the Guidelines for Good Clinical Practice (ICH 1996) including the Declaration of Helsinki (World Medical Association 1996). The Declaration of

Helsinki was introduced primarily to protect the well-being of the participants. The Guidelines for Good Clinical Practice are broadly concerned with all aspects of a clinical trial and, in particular, the ethical requirements, the design and conduct of the trial, data collection and record keeping, data analysis, and reporting of the findings. As a result, the Guidelines not only also protect the interests of the participants but of those organizing, supporting, and conducting the trials. An important additional purpose of the Guidelines is to limit the possibility of falsification of data. Requirements of ethical committees will vary locally, nationally, and internationally; however, common to all is a need for a detailed protocol covering all aspects of the clinical trial, subject or patient information, and consent. Written indemnification and/or insurance cover from the appropriate source or sources for the subjects or patients is required, although the details may vary both nationally and internationally. For example, in the UK most ethical committees would adopt the indemnification principles as set out by the Association of British Pharmaceutical Industries.

The basic requirements of a clinical trial are that it should be blind, randomized, and suitably controlled. These three aspects of clinical trial design are intimately related and are there to remove, limit or allow adjustment for possible influences that might confound the outcome of a clinical trial and thereby reduce or completely obviate the scientific value of any particular study. These three design features will be discussed individually.

Blindness

The term "blindness" is for obvious reasons not universally accepted and alternatives include "masking" or "masked". All clinical studies must be, at least, single, examiner blind. Single blindness requires that any investigator collecting data from the patients or subjects should not know the identity of the treatments used by any particular individual. Single blindness should eliminate bias in data collection. Examiner blindness, however, can be compromised to a variable degree if a particular treatment produces changes within the oral cavity, which can be perceived by the examiner. Such an example could be extrinsic staining of the teeth and/or oral mucosa by chlorhexidine formulations. The use of objective measures, which reduce or remove the requirement for subjective judgment, by the examiner, can improve the likelihood of single blindness. Unfortunately, such objective methods are not common to the recording of plaque, gingivitis, and periodontal disease parameters.

Double blindness is the ideal when neither the examiner nor subject or patient is aware of the treatment being used by the individual. Numerous factors will influence whether the subjects or patients can be maintained totally blind to their treatment(s), including whether the study is parallel or cross-over (to be discussed later), prior experience with treatments,

and the presentation, taste, and appearance of the treatments, particularly controls. Subject blindness, although ideal, is less important where the treatment outcome measures are out of the immediate control of the subject, e.g. plaque accumulation and gingivitis; assuming, that is, that lack of subject blindness does not influence compliance. Subject blindness becomes highly important where the subject is required to make a valid judgment of the effects of the treatment, for example the effects of treatments on symptoms such as pain. The term "triple blindness" is used by some investigators and relates to the blindness of the individual analyzing the data to the identity of the treatments. Thus, the data are analyzed using the treatment codes e.g. treatments A, B, and C. The identities of A, B, and C are only revealed once the statistical tests have been completed.

Randomization

The order in which treatments are received by each subject in a cross-over study, or into which treatment group subjects are placed in a parallel study, should be according to a randomized schedule. Randomization provides several important safety aspects to the study design in that firstly it is an essential part of examiner blindness. Secondly, in a cross-over study randomization should remove the potential confounding effects of the order of product use, the so-called period effects. Thirdly, the use of balanced randomization designs allows for potential carry-over effects of treatments in cross-over design studies (Newcombe *et al.* 1995). Finally, where the effects of a treatment on a disease state are to be assessed, randomization improves the chances that parallel treatment groups should be as similar as possible in baseline disease levels and, if relevant, demographic data. Randomization schedules, which use subject matching for demographic and disease status or stratification for level of disease, can be employed to improve balancing of parallel groups.

Controls

The use of appropriate control treatments is essential to the evaluation of the benefits of a particular agent or product. Without such controls, studies essentially become no more than case report data at best and anecdotal at worst, particularly when specific treatment is evaluated alone for effects on various parameters. The choice of controls, however, can vary depending on the aim of the study and the level of evaluation of an agent or product within a program of research. The choice of controls could therefore be one or more of the following:

- *Placebo control.* Here the control is a substance without any expected pharmacologic action, e.g. water. This is useful when assessing a new agent or positioning an agent or formulation between a positive or benchmark control. Placebo controls are particularly valuable where a condition or symptom may be perceived by the subject or patient to have improved, so-called placebo response, or where a condition appears to improve naturally over time, the so-called regression to the mode. Both of these phenomena are common to studies of the treatment of dentine hypersensitivity where pain is a primary outcome measure, but they are, of course, unlikely to occur in studies where the outcome measure are levels of plaque and gingivitis.

- *Minus active control (negative control)*. This type of control is commonly employed to determine whether an agent provides activity over and above its vehicle. It is particularly useful in the initial assessment of formulations such as toothpastes which have included a new active. In the later stages of development, perhaps at the product level, the use of minus active controls in home use studies is of less value since minus active controls are not normally used by the general public.
- *Bench mark control*. This term is usually used to define a control which is a commercially available product commonly used by the general public. Such controls would appear more sensible for home use studies rather than minus active products when, for example, a new toothpaste product is formulated to promote gingival health benefits. In this case it would seem reasonable to determine whether efficacy is superior to conventional fluoride toothpaste rather than the minus active toothpaste.
- *Positive control*. Positive control is an agent or formulation presently considered the most effective agent available. In this case chlorhexidine mouth rinse is arguably considered the "gold" standard antiplaque agent and is frequently used as the positive control by which to compare and position the efficacy of agents and formulations. Usually a chlorhexidine mouth rinse is used as the positive control in the early no oral hygiene study protocols.

Depending on the aims and constraints of a clinical study, more than one of the aforementioned controls may be used; for example, in the short-term studies it is not unusual to position an agent or formulation for plaque and gingivitis efficacy between a positive control, chlorhexidine, and a placebo, water.

Study groups

Study designs for oral hygiene products are usually either parallel or cross-over. Parallel group studies require that each individual uses only one of the formulations (active or control) throughout the duration of the study. Parallel designs can be used for any of the previously described oral hygiene study methods; however they are more commonly used when the study duration is protracted to weeks or months. Parallel designs require that the study groups are large in number to provide sufficient power for statis-

tical analysis. Indeed, the power of any particular study to demonstrate a statistically significant difference between treatments should be calculated prior to the study, although this may be compromised by lack of data as to the likely outcome or by difficulty in deciding the clinical relevance of any difference found. Advice from a statistician is important and group sizes can be calculated based on expected differences between test and control formulations. It must be remembered that small differences can be found statistically significant merely by using large group sizes.

Cross-over studies randomly allocate subjects to use all of the agents or formulations under test. Since each individual acts as their own control, paired statistical analytical techniques mean that the power to detect differences is markedly increased compared to parallel designs, and thereby the total study cohort of subjects can be relatively small. Furthermore, a considerable number of formulations can be compared, although this will be limited by the duration of each study period which, in itself, will have a knock-on effect on acceptability to and compliance of the subjects. Cross-over studies require a wash-out period between each treatment period and this will depend on the known, or expected, carry-over effect of a treatment or a condition into the next period. Random incomplete block designs can be used, in which each subject only uses so many of the agents under test.

The relationship between statistical significance and clinical significance is always difficult to resolve (for review see Addy & Newcombe 2005). Statistical significance is a mathematical concept which, with varying levels of probability, supports the idea that any difference between treatments is not due to chance. Clinical significance, on the other hand, is conceptual and attempts to define the benefit to the patient of any particular treatment. Unlike some branches of medicine and surgery, in periodontology, clinical significance is particularly difficult to define because the usual outcome variables are not absolute. Thus, treatment effects on plaque and/or gingivitis indices, unless approaching 100%, cannot be translated with any certainty to the initiation or progress of periodontitis and certainly not to tooth loss. Clinical significance could be:

1. *Bench mark equivalent*: when a formulation performs as well as an established formulation or product.
2. *Bench mark superior*: when a formulation performs significantly better than an established formulation.
3. *Disease related*: when a formulation has an effect on an etiologic factor such that the related signs or symptoms of the associated disease are reduced to a significantly greater extent than the control, e.g. plaque reduction which reduced gingivitis to a greater extent than control.
4. *Positive*: when a formulation produced the effect significantly greater than the most effective agent

today, e.g. the antiplaque effect is greater than chlorhexidine.

5. *Proportional superiority*: when from the outset of a study a minimum percentage improvement over the control group is set down as clinically significant.

Conclusions

- Terminology concerning oral hygiene products needs to be standardized and defined.
- Efficacy claims, which are implied, or rely on inferences to be drawn, should be avoided.
- Studies *in vitro* can provide supportive data to clinical investigations but cannot stand alone as proof of efficacy *in vivo*.
- Research and development of oral hygiene products needs to be step-by-step processed, making available a body of knowledge supporting the efficacy of a final formulation.
- Clinical proof should be largely dependent on data from blind, randomized, controlled clinical trials conducted to the Guideline for Good Clinical Practice (GCP).
- In reporting clinical trials the clinical significance of the finding should be considered.
- Statistical significance should not necessarily be taken as proof *per se* of the benefit of an oral hygiene product to the general public.
- Clinical outcome, when possible, should be evaluated against side effects and the cost–benefit ratio should be determined.
- Where possible, systematic reviews with meta-analyses need to be conducted to prove the efficacy of agents and products for the control of supragingival plaque.

References

Addy, M. (1986). Chlorhexidine compared with other locally delivered anti-microbials. A short review. *Journal of Clinical Periodontology* **13**, 957–964.

Addy, M. (1994). Local delivery of anti-microbial agents to the oral cavity. *Advanced Drug Delivery Reviews* **13**, 123–134.

Addy, M. (1995). Evaluation of clinical trials of agents and procedures to prevent caries and periodontal disease: choosing products and recommending procedures. *International Dental Journal* **45**, 185–196.

Addy, M., Dummer, P.M.H., Griffiths, G., Hicks, R., Kingdon, A. & Shaw, W.C. (1986). Prevalence of plaque, gingivitis, and caries in 11–12 year old children in South Wales. *Community Dentistry and Oral Epidemiology* **14**, 115–118.

Addy, M., Greenman, J., Renton-Harper, P., Newcombe, R.G. & Doherty, F.M. (1997). Studies on stannous fluoride toothpaste and gel 2: Effects on salivary bacterial counts and plaque re-growth *in vivo*. *Journal of Clinical Periodontology* **24**, 86–91.

Addy, M., Griffiths, C. & Isaac, R. (1977). The effect of povidone iodine on plaque and salivary bacteria. A double blind crossover trial. *Journal of Periodontology* **48**, 730–732.

Addy, M. & Hunter, M.L. (2003) Can tooth brushing damage your health? Effects on oral and dental tissues. *International Dental Journal* **53**, 177–186.

Addy, M., Jenkins, S. & Newcombe, R. (1989). Toothpastes containing 0.3% and 0.5% triclosan. II. Effects of single brushings on salivary bacterial counts. *American Journal of Dentistry* **2**, 215–220.

Addy, M. & Llewelyn, J. (1978). Use of chlorhexidine gluconate and povidone iodine mouthwashes in the treatment of acute ulcerative gingivitis. *Journal of Clinical Periodontology* **5**, 272–277.

Addy, M., Loyn, T. & Adams, D. (1991). Dentine hypersensitivity: Effects of some proprietary mouthwashes on the dentine smear layer. An S.E.M. study. *Journal of Dentistry* **19**, 148–152.

Addy, M., Mahdavi, S.A. & Loyn, T. (1995). Dietary staining *in vitro* by mouthrinses as a comparative measure of antiseptic activity and predictor of staining *in vivo*. *Journal of Dentistry* **22**, 95–99.

Addy, M. & Martin, M.V. (2003). The use of systemic antimicrobials in the treatment of periodontal disease: A dilemma. *Oral Diseases* **9** (Suppl 1), 38–44.

Addy, M. & Moran, J. (1983). Comparison of plaque accumulation after topical application and mouth rinsing with chlorhexidine gluconate. *Journal of Clinical Periodontology* **10**, 69–71.

Addy, M. & Moran, J.M. (1995). Mechanisms of stain formation on teeth, in particular associated with metal ions and antiseptics. *Advances in Dental Research* **9**, 450–456.

Addy, M. & Moran, J.M. (1997). Clinical indications for the use of chemical adjuncts to plaque control: chlorhexidine formulations. In: Addy, M. & Moran, J.M., eds. Toothpaste, mouth rinse and other topical remedies in periodontics. *Periodontology 2000* **15**, 52–54.

Addy, M., Moran, J.M. & Newcombe, R. (1991). A comparison of 0.12% and 0.1% chlorhexidine mouth-rinses in the development of plaque and gingivitis. *Clinical Preventive Dentistry* **13**, 26–29.

Addy, M., Moran, J. & Newcombe, R.G. (2007). Meta-analyses of studies of 0.2% delmopinol mouthrinse as an adjunct to gingival health and plaque control measures. *Journal of Clinical Periodontology* **34**, 58–65.

Addy, M., Moran, J. & Wade, W. (1994). Chemical plaque control in the prevention of gingivitis and periodontitis. In: Lang, N.E. & Karring, T., eds. *Proceedings of the 71st European Workshop on Periodontology*. London: Quintessence Publishing, pp. 244–257.

Addy, M., Moran, J., Wade, W. & Jenkins, S. (1992). The evaluation of toothpaste products in promoting gingival health. In: Embery, G. & Rolla, G., eds. *Clinical and Biological Aspects of Dentifrices*. Oxford: Oxford University Press, pp. 249–262.

Addy, M. & Newcombe, R.G. (2005). Statistical versus clinical significance in periodontal research and practice. *Periodontology 2000* **39**, 132–144.

Addy, M. & Renton-Harper, P. (1996). The role of antiseptics in secondary prevention. In: Lang, N.P., Karring, T. & Lindhe, J., eds. *Proceedings of the 2nd European Workshop on Periodontology, Chemicals in Periodontics*. Berlin: Quintessence, pp. 152–173.

Addy, M., Renton-Harper, P. & Myatt, G. (1998). A plaque index for occlusal surfaces and fissures: measurement of repeatability and plaque removal. *Journal of Periodontology* **25**, 164–168.

Addy, M., Richards, J. & Williams, G. (1980). Effects of a zinc citrate mouthwash on dental plaque and salivary bacteria. *Journal of Clinical Periodontology* **7**, 309–315.

Addy, M., Sharif, N. & Moran, J. (2005). A non-staining chlorhexidine mouthwash? Probably not: a study in vitro. *International Journal of Dental Hygiene* 3, 59–63.

Addy, M., Willis, L. & Moran, J. (1983). The effect of toothpaste and chlorhexidine rinses on plaque accumulation during a 4 day period. *Journal of Clinical Periodontology* 10, 89–98.

Addy, M. & Wright, R. (1978). Comparison of the *in vivo* and *in vitro* antibacterial properties of povidone iodine and chlorhexidine gluconate mouthrinses. *Journal of Clinical Periodontology* 5, 198–205.

Ainamo, J. & Etemadzadeh, H. (1987). Prevention of plaque growth with chewing gum containing chlorhexidine acetate. *Journal of Clinical Periodontology* 14, 524–527.

Allen, D.R., Davies, R., Bradshaw, B., Ellwood, R., Simone, A.J., Robinson, R., Mukerjee, C., Petrone, M.E., Chaknis, P., Volpe, A.R. & Proskin, H.M. (1998). Efficacy of a mouth rinse containing 0.05% cetylpyridinium chloride for the control of plaque and gingivitis: a 6-month clinical study in adults. *Compendium of Continuing Education in Dentistry* 19, 20–26.

Apatzidou, D.A. (2006). One stage full-mouth disinfection – Treatment of choice? *Journal of Clinical Periodontology* 33, 942–943.

Apatzidou, D. & Kinane, D. (2004). Quadrant root planing versus same day full mouth root planning 1. Clinical Findings. *Journal of Clinical Periodontology* 31, 132–140.

Arweiler, N.B., Boehnke, N., Sculean, A., Hellwig, E. & Auschill, T.M. (2006). Differences in efficacy of two commercial 0.2% chlorhexidine mouth rinse solutions: a 4-day plaque regrowth study. *Journal of Clinical Periodontology* 33, 334–339.

Ash, M., Gitlin, B.N. & Smith, N.A. (1964). Correlation between plaque and gingivitis. *Journal of Periodontology* 35, 425–429.

Axelsson, P. & Lindhe, J. (1981). Effect of controlled oral hygiene procedures on caries and periodontal disease in adults. Results after 6 yrs. *Journal of Clinical Periodontology* 8, 239–248.

Baelum, V., Fejerskov, O. & Karring, T. (1986). Oral hygiene, gingivitis and periodontal breakdown in adult Tanzanians. *Journal of Periodontal Research* 21, 221–232.

Barkvoll, P. & Rolla, C. (1994). Triclosan protects the skin against dermatitis caused by sodium lauryl sulfate exposure. *Journal of Clinical Periodontology* 21, 717–719.

Barkvoll, P., Rolla, G. & Bellagamba, S. (1988). Interaction between chlorhexidine digluconate and sodium monofluorophosphate in vitro. *Scandanavian Journal of Dental Research* 96, 30–33.

Barkvoll, P., Rolla, G. & Svendsen, A. (1989). Interaction between chlorhexidine digluconate and sodium lauryl sulphate *in vivo*. *Journal of Clinical Periodontology* 16, 593–598.

Beiswanger, B.B., Doyle, P.M., Jackson, R.D., Mallatt, M.E., Mau, M.S., Bollmer, B.W., Crisanti, M.M., Guay, C.B., Lanzalaco, A.C., Lukacovic, M.F., Majeti, S. & McClanahan, T. (1995). The clinical effect of dentifrices containing stabilised stannous fluoride on plaque formation and gingivitis, a six-month study with *ad libitum* brushing. *Journal of Clinical Dentistry* 6, 46–53.

Bergenholtz, A. & Hanstrom, L. (1974). The plaque inhibiting effect of hexetidine (Oraldene) mouthwash compared to that of chlorhexidine. *Community Dentistry and Oral Epidemiology* 2, 70–74.

Bernadi, F., Pincelli, M.R., Carloni, S., Gatto, M.R. & Montebugoli, L. (2004). Chlorhexidine with an anti discoloration system. A comparative study. *International Journal of Dental Hygiene* 2, 122–126.

Binney, A., Addy, M., Owens, J., Faulkner, J., McKeown, S. & Everatt, L. (1996). A 3-month home use study comparing the oral hygiene and gingival health benefits of triclosan and conventional fluoride toothpastes. *Journal of Clinical Periodontology* 23, 1020–1024.

Bonesvoll, P. & Gjermo, P. (1978). A comparison between chlorhexidine and some quaternary ammonium compounds with regard to retention, salivary concentration and plaque inhibiting effect in the human mouth after mouth rinses. *Archives of Oral Biology* 23, 289–294.

Bonesvoll, P., Lokken, P. & Rolla, G. (1974a). Influence of concentration, time, temperature and pH on the retention of chlorhexidine in the human oral cavity after mouth rinses. *Archives of Oral Biology* 19, 1025–1029.

Bonesvoll, P., Lokken, P., Rolla, G. & Paus, P.N. (1974b). Retention of chlorhexidine in the human oral cavity after mouth rinses. *Archives of Oral Biology* 19, 209–212.

Brecx, M., Brownstone, E., MacDonald, L., Gelskey, S. & Cheang, M. (1992). Efficacy of Listerine, Meridol and chlorhexidine mouth rinses as supplements to regular tooth-cleaning measures. *Journal of Clinical Periodontology* 19, 202–207.

Brecx, M., Netuschil, I., Reichert, B. & Schreil, C. (1990). Efficacy of Listerine, Meridol and chlorhexidine mouth rinses on plaque, gingivitis and plaque bacteria vitality. *Journal of Clinical Periodontology* 17, 292–297.

British Standards Institution (1981). Specification for Toothpastes, BS 5136.

Carvalho, M.D., Tabchoury, C.M., Cury, J.A., Toledo, S. & Nogueira-Filho, G.R. (2004). Impact of mouthrinses on morning bad breath in healthy subjects. *Journal of Clinical Periodontology* 31, 85–90.

Chadwick, B., Addy, M. & Walker, D.M. (1991). The use of a hexetidine mouthwash in the management of minor aphthous ulceration and as an adjunct to oral hygiene. *British Dental Journal* 171, 83–87.

Charles, C.H., Mostler, K.M., Bartels, L.L. & Mankodi, S.M. (2004). Comparative antiplaque and antigingivitis effectiveness of a chlorhexidine and an essential oil mouth rinse: 6-month clinical trial. *Journal of Clinical Periodontology* 31, 878–884.

Claydon, N., Hunter, L., Moran, J., Wade, W., Kelty, F., Movert, R. & Addy, M. (1996). A 6-month home-usage trial of 0.1% and 0.2% delmopinol mouthwashes. 1. Effects on plaque, gingivitis, supragingival calculus and tooth staining. *Journal of Clinical Periodontology* 23, 220–228.

Collaert, B., Attstrom, R., de Bruyn, N. & Movert, R. (1992). The effect of delmopinol rinsing on dental plaque formation and gingivitis healing. *Journal of Clinical Periodontology* 19, 274–280.

Cooke, B.E.D. & Armitage, P. (1960). Recurrent Mikulicz's aphthae treated with topical hydrocortisone hemisuccinate sodium. *British Medical Journal* 1, 764–766.

Council of Dental Therapeutics (1985). Guidelines for acceptance of chemotherapeutic products for the control of supragingival dental plaque and gingivitis. *Journal of the American Dental Association* 112, 529–532.

Cummins, D. (1997). Vehicles: how to deliver the goods. In: Addy, M. & Moran, J.M., eds. Toothpaste, mouthrinse and other topical remedies in periodontics. *Periodontology 2000* 15, 84–99.

Davies, R.M., Jensen, S.B., Schiott, C.R. & Löe, H. (1970). The effect of topical application of chlorhexidine on the bacterial colonization of the teeth and gingiva. *Journal of Periodontal Research* 5, 96–101.

de la Rosa, M.R., Guerra, J.Z., Johnson, D.A. & Radike, A.W. (1979). Plaque growth and removal with daily tooth brushing. *Journal of Periodontology* 50, 661–664.

Dilling, W.J. & Hallam, S. (1936). *Dental Materia Medica, Pharmacology and Therapeutics*, 3rd edn. London: Cassell & Company.

Dolles, O.K. & Gjermo, P. (1980). Caries increment and gingival status during two years of chlorhexidine and fluoride containing dentifrices. *Scandinavian Journal of Dental Research* 88, 22–27.

Egelberg, J. & Claffey, N. (1998). Consensus Report of Group B: Role of mechanical plaque removal in the prevention and therapy of caries and periodontal disease. In: Lang, N.P., Attstrom, R. & Loe, H., eds. *Proceedings of the European Work-*

shop on Mechanical Plaque Control. Berlin: Quintessence Publishing Company, pp. 169–172.

Eley, B.M. (1999) Antibacterial agents in the control of supragingival plaque – a review. *British Dental Journal* **186**, 286–296.

Ellwood, R.P., Worthington, H.V., Blinkhorn, A.S.B., Volpe, A.R. & Davies, R.M. (1998). Effect of a triclosan/copolymer dentifrice on the incidence of periodontal attachment loss in adolescents. *Journal of Clinical Periodontology* **25**, 363–367.

Eriksen, H.M., Nordbo, H., Kantanen, H. & Ellingsen, J.E. (1985). Chemical plaque control and extrinsic tooth discoloration. A review of possible mechanisms. *Journal of Clinical Periodontology* **12**, 345–350.

Ernst, C.P., Canbek, K., Dillenburger, A. & Willershausen, B. (2005). Clinical study on the effectiveness and side effects of hexetidine and chlorhexidine mouthrinses versus a negative control. *Quintessence International* **36**, 641–652.

Etemadzadeh, H., Ainamo, J. & Murtoma, H. (1985). Plaque growth inhibiting effects of an abrasive fluoride-chlorhexidine toothpaste and a fluoride toothpaste containing oxidative enzymes. *Journal of Clinical Periodontology* **12**, 607–616.

Faveri, M., Gursky, L.C., Ferres, M., Shibli, J.A., Salvador, S.L. & de Figueiredo, L.C. (2006). Scaling and root planing and chlorhexidine mouth rinses in the treatment of chronic periodontitis: a randomized placebo-controlled clinical trial. *Journal of Clinical Periodontology* **33**, 819–828.

Ferretti, G., Ash, R.C., Brown, A.T., Largent, B.M., Kaplan, A. & Lillich, T.T. (1987). Chlorhexidine for prophylaxis against oral infections and associated complications in patients receiving bone marrow transplants. *Journal of the American Dental Association* **114**, 461–467.

Ferretti, G., Ash, R.C., Brown, A.T., Parr, M.D., Romand, E.H. & Lillich, T.T. (1988). Control of oral mucositis and candidiasis in marrow transplantation: a prospective double blind trial of chlorhexidine digluconate oral rinse. *Bone Marrow Transplantation* **3**, 483–493.

Firalti, E., Unal, T., Onan, U. & Sandalli, P. (1994). Antioxidative activities of some chemotherapeutics: a possible mechanism of reducing inflammation. *Journal of Clinical Periodontology* **21**, 680–683.

Fischman, S. (1997). Oral hygiene products: How far have we come in 6000 years. *Periodontology 2000* **15**, 7–14.

Flotra, L., Gjermo, P., Rolla, G. & Waerhaug, J. (1971). Side effects of chlorhexidine mouthwashes. *Scandinavian Journal of Dental Research* **79**, 119–125.

Forward, G.C., James, A.H., Barnett, P. & Jackson, R.J. (1997). Gum health product formulations: what is in them and why? *Periodontology 2000* **15**, 32–39.

Francis, J.R., Addy, M. & Hunter, B. (1987b). A comparison of three delivery methods of chlorhexidine in institutionalised physically handicapped children. *Journal of Periodontology* **58**, 456–459.

Francis, J.R., Hunter, B. & Addy, M. (1987a). A comparison of three delivery methods of chlorhexidine in handicapped children. I. Effects on plaque, gingivitis and tooth staining. *Journal of Periodontology* **58**, 451–454.

Frandsen, A. (1986). Mechanical oral hygiene practices In: Löe, H. & Kleinman, D.V., eds. *Dental Plaque Control Measures and Oral Hygiene Practices*. Oxford: IRL Press, pp. 93–116.

Furuichi, Y., Ramberg, P., Lindhe, J., Nabi, N & Gaffar, A. (1996). Some effects of mouthrinses containing salifluor on de novo plaque formation and developing gingivitis. *Journal of Clinical Periodontology* **23**, 795–802.

Gaffar, A., Volpe, A. & Lindhe, J. (1992). Recent advances in plaque/gingivitis control. In: Embery, G. & Rolla, C., eds. *Clinical and Biological Aspects of Dentifrices*. Oxford: Oxford University Press, pp. 229–248.

Gjermo, P. (1974). Chlorhexidine in dental practice. *Journal of Clinical Periodontology* **1**, 143–152.

Gjermo, P. (1989). Chlorhexidine and related compounds. *Journal of Dental Research* **68**, 1602–1608.

Gjermo, P., Baastad, K.L. & Rolla, C. (1970). The plaque inhibitory capacity of 11 antibacterial compounds. *Journal of Periodontal Research* **5**, 102–109.

Gjermo, P., Bonesvoll, P. & Rolla, C. (1974). The relationship between plaque inhibiting effect and retention of chlorhexidine in the human oral cavity. *Archives of Oral Biology* **19**, 1031–1034.

Gjermo, P., Rolla, C. & Arskaug, L. (1973). Effect on dental plaque formation and some in vitro properties of 12 bisbiguanides. *Journal of Periodontal Research* **8** (Suppl 12), 81–88.

Haffajee, A.D. & Socransky, S.S. (1994). Microbial etiological agents of periodontal destruction. *Periodontology 2000* **5**, 78–111.

Hancock, E.B. (1996). Prevention. World Workshop in Periodontics. *Annals of Periodontology* **1**, 223–249.

Hanham, A. & Addy, M. (2001). The effect of chewing sugar free gum on plaque regrowth at smooth and occlusal surfaces. *Journal of Clinical Periodontology* **28**, 255–257.

Harrap, G.J. (1974). Assessment of the effect of dentifrices on the growth of dental plaque. *Journal of Clinical Periodontology* **1**, 166–174.

Hase, J.C., Attstrom, R., Edwardsson, S., Kelty, E. & Kirsch, J. (1998). 6-month use of 0.2% delmopinol hydrochloride in comparison with 0.2% chlorhexidine digluconate and placebo. (1) Effect on plaque formation and gingivitis. *Journal of Clinical Periodontology* **25**, 746–753.

Heanue, M., Deacon, S.A., Deery, C., Robinson, P.G., Walmsley, A.D., Worthington, H.V. & Shaw, W.C. (2004). Manual versus powered tooth brushing for oral health (Cochrane Review). In: the Cochrane Library, Issue 4, Chichester, UK: John Wiley & Sons, Ltd.

Heasman, P.A. & Seymour, R.A. (1994). Pharmacological control of periodontal disease. 1. Anti-plaque agents. *Journal of Dentistry* **22**, 323–326.

Hodge, P.J., Riggio, M.P. & Kinane, D.F. (2001). Failure to detect an association with IL1 genotypes in European Caucasians with generalised early onset periodontitis. *Journal of Clinical Periodontology* **28**, 430–436.

Hugoson, A., Norderyd, O., Slotte, C. & Thorstensson, H. (1998a). Oral hygiene and gingivitis in a Swedish adult population 1973, 1983, 1993. *Journal of Clinical Periodontology* **25**, 807–812.

Hugoson, A., Norderyd, O., Slotte, C. & Thorstensson, H. (1998b). Distribution of periodontal disease in a Swedish adult population 1973, 1983, 1993. *Journal of Clinical Periodontology* **25**, 542–548.

Hull, P.S. (1980). Chemical inhibition of plaque. *Journal of Clinical Periodontology* **7**, 431–442.

Hunter, L., Addy, M., Moran, J., Kohut, B., Hovliaras, C. & Newcombe, R. (1994). A study of a pre-brushing mouth rinse as an adjunct to oral hygiene. *Journal of Periodontology* **65**, 762–765.

Hunter, M.L. & Addy, M. (1987). Chlorhexidine gluconate mouthwash in the management of minor aphthous ulceration. A double-blind, placebo-controlled cross-over trial. *British Dental Journal* **162**, 106–108.

ICH (1996). Topic 6 Guidelines for Good Clinical Practice, CPMP/ICH/135/95. Geneva: International Conference on Harmonization.

ISO 11609 (1995). International Standard: Dentistry-Toothpaste-Requirements, test methods and marking. Geneva: International Standards Organization.

Jackson, R.J. (1997). Metal salts, essential oils and phenols-old or new? In: Addy, M. & Moran, J.M., eds. Toothpaste, mouth rinse and other topical remedies in periodontics. *Periodontology 2000* **15**, 63–73.

Jenkins, S., Addy, M. & Newcombe, R. (1989). Comparison of two commercially available chlorhexidine mouth rinses. II. Effects on plaque reformation, gingivitis and tooth staining. *Clinical Preventive Dentistry* **11**, 12–16.

Jenkins, S., Addy, M. & Newcombe, R. (1990). Comparative effects of toothpaste brushing and toothpaste rinsing on salivary bacterial counts. *Journal of Periodontal Research* **25**, 316–319.

Jenkins, S., Addy, M. & Newcombe, R. (1991a). Triclosan and sodium lauryl sulphate mouth rinses. II. Effects on 4-day plaque re-growth. *Journal of Clinical Periodontology* **18**, 145–148.

Jenkins, S., Addy, M. & Newcombe, R.G. (1991b). Triclosan and sodium lauryl sulphate mouthrinses. I. Effects on salivary bacterial counts. *Journal of Clinical Periodontology* **18**, 140–144.

Jenkins, S., Addy, M. & Newcombe, R.G. (1993). A dose response study of triclosan mouth rinses on plaque re-growth. *Journal of Clinical Periodontology* **20**, 609–612.

Jenkins, S., Addy, M. & Newcombe, R. (1994). Dose response of chlorhexidine against plaque and comparison with triclosan. *Journal of Clinical Periodontology* **21**, 250–255.

Jenkins, S., Addy, M. & Wade, W. (1988). The mechanism of action of chlorhexidine: a study of plaque growth on enamel inserts *in vivo*. *Journal of Clinical Periodontology* **15**, 415–424.

Jepsen, S. (1998). The role of manual toothbrushes in effective plaque control: advantages and limitations. In: Lang, N.P., Attstrom, R. & Löe, H., eds. *Proceedings of the European Workshop on Mechanical Plaque Control*. Berlin: Quintessence Verlag, pp. 121–137.

Jobbins, J., Addy, M., Bagg, J., Finlay, I., Parsons, K. & Newcombe, R. (1992). A double blind, single phase placebo controlled clinical trial of 0.2% chlorhexidine gluconate oral spray in terminally ill cancer patients. *Palliative Medicine* **6**, 299–307.

Johansen, J.R., Gjermo, P. & Eriksen, H.M. (1975). The effect of two years use of chlorhexidine containing dentifrices on plaque, gingivitis and caries. *Scandinavian Journal of Dental Research* **83**, 288–292.

Jones, C.G. (1997). Chlorhexidine: is it still the gold standard? In: Addy, M. & Moran, J.M., eds. Toothpaste, mouth rinse and other topical remedies in periodontics, *Periodontology 2000* **15**, 55–62.

Kalaga, A., Addy, M. & Hunter, B. (1989a). Comparison of chlorhexidine delivery by mouthwash and spray on plaque accumulation. *Journal of Periodontology* **60**, 127–130.

Kalaga, A., Addy, M. & Hunter, B. (1989b). The use of 0.2% chlorhexidine as an adjunct to oral health in physically and mentally handicapped adults. *Journal of Periodontology* **60**, 381–385.

Kanchanakamol, U., Umpriwan, R., Jotikasthira, N., Srisilapanan, P., Tuongratanaphan, S., Sholitkul, W. & Chat-Uthai, T. (1995). Reduction of plaque formation and gingivitis by a dentifrice containing triclosan and copolymer. *Journal of Periodontology* **66**, 109–112.

Kinane, D.F. (1998). The role of interdental cleaning in effective plaque control: need for inter-dental cleaning in primary and secondary prevention. In: Lang, N.P., Attstrom, R. & Löe, H., eds. *Proceedings of the European Workshop on Mechanical Plaque Control*. Berlin: Quintessence Publishing Company, pp. 156–168.

Kinane, D.F., Shiba, H. & Hart, T.C. (2005). The genetic basis of periodontitis. *Periodontology 2000* **39**, 91–117.

Kopczyk, R.A., Abrams, H., Brown, A.T., Matheny, J.L. & Kaplan, A.L. (1991). Clinical and microbiological effects of a sanguinarine containing mouth-rinse and dentifrice with and without fluoride during 6 months use. *Journal of Periodontology* **62**, 617–622.

Kornman, K.S. (1986). Anti-microbial agents. In: Löe, H. & Kleinman, D.V., eds. *Dental Plaque Control Measures and Oral Hygiene Practices*. Oxford: IRL Press, pp. 121–142.

Kornman, K.S., Crane, A., Wang, H.Y., di Giovine, F.S., Newman, M.G., Pirk, F.W., Wilson, T.G., Higginbottom, F.L. & Duff, G.W. (1997). The interleukin-1 genotype as a severity factor in adult periodontal disease. *Journal of Clinical Periodontology* **24**, 72–77.

Lang, N.P., Catalanotto, F.A., Knopfli, R.U. & Antczak, A.A. (1988). Quality specific taste impairment following the application of chlorhexidine gluconate mouthrinses. *Journal of Clinical Periodontology* **15**, 43–48.

Lang, N.P., Cumming, B.R. & Löe, H. (1973). Toothbrush frequency as it's related to plaque development and gingival health. *Journal of Periodontology* **44**, 396–405.

Lang, N.P., Hase, J.C., Grassi, M., Hammerle, C.H., Weigel, C., Kelty, E. & Frutig, F. (1998). Plaque formation and gingivitis after supervised mouthrinsing with 0.2% delmopinol hydrochloride, 0.2% chlorhexidine digluconate and placebo for 6 months. *Oral Diseases* **4**, 105–113.

Lang, N.P. & Newman, H.N. (1997). Consensus report of session II. In: Lang, N.P., Karring, T. & Lindhe, J., eds. *Proceedings of the 2nd European Workshop on Periodontology. Chemicals in Periodontics*. Berlin: Quintessence Verlag, pp. 192–200.

Lang, N.P. & Raber, K. (1981). Use of oral irrigators as vehicles for the application of anti-microbial agents in chemical plaque control. *Journal of Clinical Periodontology* **8**, 177–188.

Lang, N.P. & Ramseier-Grossman, I.C. (1981). Optimal dosage of chlorhexidine gluconate in chemical plaque control when delivered by an oral irrigator. *Journal of Clinical Periodontology* **8**, 189–202.

Lavstedt, S., Modeer, T. & Welander, F. (1982). Plaque and gingivitis in a group of Swedish school children with particular reference to tooth brushing habits. *Acta Odontologica Scandinavica* **40**, 307–311.

Lindhe, J. (1986). Gingivitis, General Discussion. *Journal of Clinical Periodontology* **13**, 395.

Löe, H. (1986). Progression of natural untreated periodontal disease in man. In: *Borderland Between Caries and Periodontal Disease*, 3rd edn. Geneva: Medecin et Hygiene.

Löe, H. & Schiott, C.R. (1970). The effect of mouth rinses and topical application of chlorhexidine on the development of dental plaque and gingivitis in man. *Journal of Periodontal Research* **5**, 79–83.

Löe, H., Theilade, E. & Jensen S.B. (1965). Experimental gingivitis in man. *Journal of Periodontology* **36**, 177–187.

MacFarlane, T.W., Ferguson, M.M. & Mulgrew, C.J. (1984). Post extraction bacteraemia: role of antiseptics and antibiotics. *British Dental Journal* **156**, 179–181.

MacGregor, D.M. & Rugg-Gunn, A.J. (1979). A survey of tooth brushing sequence in children and young adults. *Journal of Periodontal Research* **14**, 225–230.

Mandel, I.D. (1988). Chemotherapeutic agents for controlling plaque and gingivitis. *Journal of Clinical Periodontology* **15**, 488–496.

Moore, C. & Addy, M. (2005). Wear of dentine *in vitro* by toothpaste abrasives and detergents alone and combined. *Journal of Clinical Periodontology* **32**, 1242–1246.

Moran, J. & Addy, M. (1984). The effect of surface adsorption and staining reactions on the anti-microbial properties of some cationic antiseptic mouthwashes. *Journal of Periodontology* **55**, 278–282.

Moran, J. & Addy, M. (1991). The effects of a cetylpyridinium chloride prebrushing rinse as an adjunct to oral hygiene and gingival health. *Journal of Periodontology* **62**, 562–564.

Moran, J., Addy, M. & Newcombe, R. (1988). A clinical trial to assess the efficacy of sanguinarine mouth rinse (Veadent) compared with a chlorhexidine mouth rinse (Corsodyl). *Journal of Clinical Periodontology* **15**, 612–616.

Moran, J., Addy, M. & Newcombe, R. (1991). Comparison of a herbal toothpaste with a fluoride toothpaste on plaque and gingivitis. *Clinical Preventive Dentistry* **13**, 12–15.

Moran, J., Addy, M. & Newcombe, R.G. (1997). A 4-day plaque re-growth study comparing an essential oil mouth rinse with a triclosan mouth rinse. *Journal of Clinical Periodontology* **24**, 636–639.

Moran, J., Addy, M. & Roberts, S. (1992a). A comparison of natural product, triclosan and chlorhexidine mouthrinses on 4-day plaque re-growth. *Journal of Clinical Periodontology* **19**, 578–582.

Moran, J., Addy, M., Wade, W.G., Maynard, J.H., Roberts, S.F., Astrom, M. & Movert, R. (1992b). A comparison of delmopinol and chlorhexidine on plaque re-growth over a 4-day period and salivary bacterial counts. *Journal of Clinical Periodontology* **19**, 749–753.

Moran, J., Addy, M., Wade, W., Milsom, S., McAndrew, R. & Newcombe, R. (1995). The effect of oxidising mouth rinses compared with chlorhexidine on salivary bacterial counts and plaque re-growth. *Journal of Clinical Periodontology* **22**, 750–755.

Moss, S., Holmgren, C. & Addy, M. (1995). A reader's and writer's guide to the publication of clinical trials. *International Dental Journal* **45**, 177–184.

Nash, E.S. & Addy, M. (1979). The use of chlorhexidine gluconate mouth rinses in patients with inter-maxillary fixation. *British Journal of Oral Surgery* **17**, 251–255.

Newcombe, R.G., Addy, M. & McKeown, S. (1995). Residual effect of chlorhexidine gluconate in 4 day plaque regrowth trials and its implications for study design. *Journal of Periodontal Research* **30**, 319–324.

Newman, P.S. & Addy, M. (1978). A comparison of a periodontal dressing and chlorhexidine gluconate mouthwash after the internal bevel flap procedure. *Journal of Periodontology* **49**, 576–579.

Newman, P.S. & Addy, M. (1982). Comparison of hypertonic saline and chlorhexidine mouthrinses after the inverse bevel flap procedure. *Journal of Periodontology* **52**, 315–318.

Norton, M.R. & Addy, M. (1989). Chewing sticks versus toothbrushes in West Africa. A pilot study. *Clinical Preventive Dentistry* **11**, 11–13.

Olsen, I. (1975). Denture stomatitis. The clinical effects of chlorhexidine and Amphotericin B. *Acta Odontologica Scandinavica* **33**, 47–52.

Owens, J., Addy, M. & Faulkner, J. (1997a). An 18 week home use study comparing the oral hygiene and gingival health benefits of triclosan and fluoride toothpaste. *Journal of Clinical Periodontology* **24**, 626–631.

Owens, J., Addy, M., Faulkner, J., Lockwood, C. & Adair, R. (1997b). A short term clinical study to investigate the chemical plaque inhibitory properties of mouthrinses when used as adjuncts to toothpastes: applied to chlorhexidine. *Journal of Clinical Peridontology* **24**, 732–737.

Palomo, F., Wantland, L., Sanchez, A., Volpe, A.R., McCool, J. & DeVizio, W. (1994). The effect of three commercially available dentifrices containing triclosan on supragingival plaque formation and gingivitis: a six month clinical study. *International Dental Journal* **44**, 75–81.

Papapanou, R.N. (1994). Epidemiology and natural history of periodontal disease. In: Lang, N.P. & Karring, T., eds. *Proceedings of the 1st European Workshop on Periodontology.* London: Quintessence, pp. 23–41.

Perlich, M.A., Bacca, L.A., Bolimer, B.W., Lanzalaco, A.C., McClanahan, L.K., Sewak, L.K., Beiswanger, B.B., Eichold, W.A., Hull, J.R., Jackson, R.D. & Mau, M.S. (1995). The clinical effect of dentifrices containing stabilised stannous fluoride on plaque formation and gingivitis and gingival bleeding – a six-month study. *Journal of Clinical Dentistry* **6**, 54–58.

Phaneuf, E.A., Harrington, J.H., Dale, P.P. & Shklar, G. (1962). Automatic toothbrush: A new reciprocating action. *Journal of the American Dental Association* **65**, 12–25.

Pluss, E.M., Engelberg, P.R. & Rateitschak, K.H. (1975). Effect of chlorhexidine on plaque formation under a periodontal pack. *Journal of Clinical Periodontology* **2**, 136–142,

Pontefract, H., Hughes, J., Kemp, K., Yates, R., Newcombe, R.G. & Addy, M. (2001). The erosive effects of some mouth rinses on enamel. A study *in situ. Journal of Clinical Periodontology* **28**, 319–324.

Quirynen, M., Aventroodt, P., Peeters, W., Pauwels, M., Coucke, W. & Van Steenberge, D. (2001). Effect of different chlorhexidine formulations in mouthrinses on de novo plaque formation. *Journal of Clinical Periodontology* **28**, 1127–1136.

Quirynen, M., De Soete, M., Boschmans, G., Pauwels, M., Coucke, W., Teughels, W. & van Steenberghe, D. (2006). Benefit of one-stage full-mouth disinfection is explained by disinfection and root planing within 24 hours: a randomised controlled trial. *Journal of Clinical Periodontology* **33**, 639–647.

Quirynen, M., Marachal, M. & van Steenberghe, D. (1990). Comparative anti-plaque activity of sanguinarine and chlorhexidine in man. *Journal of Clinical Periodontology* **17**, 223–227.

Quirynen, M., Soers, C., Desnyder, M., Dekeyser, C. & Pauwels, M. (2005). A 0.05% cetyl pyridinium chloride/0.05% chlorhexidine mouth rinse during maintenance phase after initial periodontal therapy. *Journal of Clinical Periodontology* **32**, 390–400.

Renton-Harper, P.R., Milsom, S., Wade, W.G., Addy, M., Moran, J. & Newcombe, R.G. (1995). An approach to efficacy screening of mouth rinses: studies on a group of French products (II). Inhibition of salivary bacteria and plaque *in vivo. Journal of Clinical Periodontology* **22**, 723–727.

Renvert, S. & Birkhed, D. (1995). Comparison between 3 triclosan dentifrices on plaque, gingivitis and salivary microflora. *Journal of Clinical Periodontology* **22**, 63–70.

Roberts, W.R. & Addy, M. (1981). Comparison of *in vitro* and *in vivo* antibacterial properties of antiseptic mouth rinses containing chlorhexidine, alexidine, CPC and hexetidine. Relevance to mode of action. *Journal of Clinical Periodontology* **8**, 295–310.

Rolla, G., Kjaerheim, V. & Waaler, S.M. (1997). The role of antiseptics in secondary prevention. In: Lang, N.P., Karring, T. & Lindhe, J., eds. *Proceedings of the 2nd European Workshop on Periodontology, Chemicals in Periodontics.* Berlin: Quintessence, pp. 120–130.

Rosing, C.K., Jonski, G. & Rolla, G. (2002). Comparative analysis of some mouthrinses on the production of volatile sulfur-containing compounds *Acta Odontologica Scandanavica* **60**, 10–12.

Rosling, B., Wannfors, B., Volpe, A.R., Furuichi, Y., Ramberg, P. & Lindhe, J. (1997). The use of a triclosan/copolymer dentifrice may retard the progression of periodontitis. *Journal of Clinical Periodontology* **24**, 873–880.

Rugg-Gunn, A.J. & MacGregor, D.M. (1978). A survey of tooth brushing behaviour in children and young adults. *Journal of Periodontal Research* **13**, 382–388.

Sanz, M., Vallcorba, N., Fabregues, S., Muller, I. & Herkstroter, F. (1994). The effect of a dentifrice containing chlorhexidine and zinc on plaque, gingivitis, calculus and tooth staining. *Journal of Clinical Periodontology* **21**, 431–437.

Saxen, L., Niemi, M.L. & Ainamo, J. (1976). Intra-oral spread of the antimicrobial effect of a chlorhexidine gel. *Scandinavian Journal of Dental Research* **84**, 304–307.

Saxer, U.P. & Muhlemann, H. (1983). Synergistic anti-plaque effects of a zinc fluoride/hexetidine containing mouthwash. A review. *Helvetica Odontologica Acta* **27**, 1–16.

Schiott, C.R., Löe, H. & Briner, W.N. (1976). Two years use of chlorhexidine in man. 4. Effect on various medical parameters. *Journal of Periodontal Research* **11**, 158–164.

Schiott, C., Löe, H., Jensen, S.B., Kilian, M., Davies, R.M. & Glavind, K. (1970). The effect of chlorhexidine mouthrinses on the human oral flora. *Journal of Periodontal Research* **5**, 84–89.

Segreto, V.A., Collins, E.M., Beiswanger, B.B., de la Rosa, M., Isaacs, R.L., Lang, N.P., Mallet, M.E. & Meckel, A.H. (1986). A comparison of mouthwashes containing two concentrations of chlorhexidine. *Journal of Periodontal Research* **21** (Suppl 16), 23–32.

Sharma, N.C., Galustians, H.J., Qaqish, J., Charles, C.H., Vincent, J.W. & McGuire, J.A. (2003). Antiplaque and antigingivitis effectiveness of a hexetidine mouthwash. *Journal of Clinical Periodontology* **30**, 590–594.

Shaw, W.C., Addy, M., Griffiths, S. & Price, C. (1984). Chlorhexidine and traumatic ulcers in orthodontic patients. *European Journal of Orthodontics* **6**, 137–140.

Sheen, S., Eisenburger, M. & Addy, M. (2003). The effect of toothpaste on the plaque inhibitory properties of a cetylpyridinium chloride mouth rinse. *Journal of Clinical Periodontology* **30**, 255–260.

Sheen, S., Owens, J. & Addy, M. (2001). The effect of toothpaste on the propensity of chlorhexidine and cetylpyridinium chloride to produce staining *in vitro*: a possible predictor of inactivation. *Journal of Clinical Periodontology* **28**, 46–51.

Simonetti, N., D'Aurin, F.D., Strippoli, V. & Lucchetti, G. (1988). Itraconazole: increased activity of chlorhexidine. *Drugs and Experimental Clinical Research* **14**, 19–23.

Simonsson, T., Arnebrant, T. & Peterson, L. (1991a). The effect of delmopinol on the salivary pellicles, the wettability of tooth surfaces in vivo and bacterial cell surfaces in vitro. *Biofouling* **3**, 251–260.

Simonsson, T., Bondesson, H., Rundegren, J. & Edwardsson, S. (1991b). Effect of delmopinol on *in vitro* dental plaque formation, bacterial acid production and the number of microorganisms in human saliva. *Oral Microbiology and Immunology* **6**, 305–309.

Skaare, A.B., Herlofson, B.B. & Barkvoll, P. (1996). Mouthrinses containing triclosan reduce the incidence of recurrent aphthous ulcers (RAU). *Journal of Clinical Periodontology* **23**, 778–782.

Slots, J. (2003). Update on general health risk of periodontal disease. *International Dental Journal* **53** (Suppl 3), 200–207.

Slots, J. & Rams, T.E. (1990). Antibiotics in periodontal therapy: advantages and disadvantages. *Journal of Clinical Periodontology* **17**, 479–493.

Smith, A., Moran, J., Dangler, L.V., Leight, R.S. & Addy, M. (1996). The efficacy of an anti-gingivitis chewing gum. *Journal of Clinical Periodontology* **23**, 19–23.

Socransky, S.S. & Haffajee, A.D. (2005). Periodontal microbial aetiology. *Periodontology 2000* **38**, 135–197.

Sookoulis, S. & Hirsch, R. (2004). The effect of a tea tree oil-containing gel on plaque and chronic gingivitis. *Australian Dental Journal* **49**, 78–83.

Stephen, K.W., Saxton, C.A., Jones, C.L., Richie, J.A. & Morrison, T. (1990). Control of gingivitis and calculus by a zinc salt and triclosan. *Journal of Periodontology* **61**, 674–679.

Storhaug, K. (1977). Hibitane in oral disease in handicapped patients. *Journal of Clinical Periodontology* **4**, 102–107.

Stralfors, A. (1961). In: Muhlemann, H.R. & Konig, K.G., eds. *Caries Symposium*. Berne: Hans Huber, p. 154.

Svatun, B. (1978). Plaque inhibitory effect of dentifrices containing stannous fluoride. *Acta Odontologica Scandinavica* **36**, 205–210.

Toth, B.B., Martin, J.W. & Fleming, T.J. (1990). Oral complications associated with cancer therapy. A MD Anderson Cancer Center experience. *Journal of Clinical Periodontology* **17**, 508–515.

Vandekerchhove, B.N.A., Van Steenberge, D., Tricio, J., Rosenberg, D. & Ercarnanacion, M. (1995). Efficacy on supragingival plaque control of cetylpyridinium chloride in a slow-release dosage form. *Journal of Clinical Periodontology* **22**, 824–829.

Van Strydonck, D.A., Timmerman, M.F., van der Velden, U. & van der Weijden, G.A. (2005). Plaque inhibition of two commercially available chlorhexidine mouthrinses. *Journal of Clinical Periodontology* **32**, 305–309.

Van der Weijden, G.A., Timmerman, M.F., Danser, M.M. & van der Velden, U. (1998). The role of electric toothbrushes: advantages and limitations. In: Lang, N.P., Attstrom, R. & Löe, H. *Proceedings of the European Workshop on Mechanical Plaque Control*. Berlin: Quintessence Verlag, pp. 138–155.

Wade, A.B., Blake, G.C. & Mirza, K.B. (1966). Effectiveness of metronidazole in treating the acute phase of ulcerative gingivitis. *Dental Practice* **16**, 440–443.

Wade, W. & Addy, M. (1989). *In vitro* activity of a chlorhexidine containing mouth-rinse against subgingival bacteria. *Journal of Periodontology* **60**, 521–525.

Wade, W.G. & Slayne, M.A. (1997). Controlling plaque by disrupting the process of plaque formation. *Periodontology 2000* **15**, 25–31.

Watts, A. & Addy, M. (2001). Tooth discolouration and staining: A review of the literature. *British Dental Journal* **190**, 309–316.

Wennstrom, J.L. (1992). Subgingival irrigation systems for the control of oral infections. *International Dental Journal* **42**, 281–285.

Wennstrom, J.L. (1997). Rinsing, irrigation and sustained delivery. In: Lang, N.P., Karring, T. & Lindhe, J., eds. *Proceedings of the 2nd European Workshop on Periodontology, Chemicals in Periodontics*. Berlin: Quintessence, pp. 131–151.

World Medical Association (1996). *Declaration of Helsinki*. 48th World Medical Assembly, Somerset West, Republic of South Africa.

Worral, S.F., Knibbs, P.J. & Glenwright, H.D. (1987). Methods of reducing contamination of the atmosphere from use of an air polisher. *British Dental Journal* **163**, 118–119.

Worthington, H.V., Blinkhorn, A.S., Petrone, M. & Volpe, A.R. (1993). A six month clinical study of the effect of a pre-brush rinse on plaque removal and gingivitis. *British Dental Journal* **175**, 322–329.

Wray, D., Ferguson, M.M. & Geddes, D.A.M. (1978). The effect of povidone iodine mouthwash on plaque accumulation and thyroid function. *British Dental Journal* **144**, 14–16.

Yates, R., Jenkins, S., Newcombe, R.G., Wade, W.G., Moran, J. & Addy, M. (1993). A 6-month home usage trial of a 1% chlorhexidine toothpaste. 1. Effects on plaque, gingivitis, calculus and tooth staining. *Journal of Clinical Periodontology* **20**, 130–138.

Yates, R., Moran, J., Addy, M., Mullan, P.J., Wade, W. & Newcombe, R. (1997). The comparative effect of acidified sodium chlorite and chlorhexidine mouthrinses on plaque regrowth and salivary bacterial counts. *Journal of Clinical Periodontology* **24**, 603–609.

Zambon, J.J. (1996). Periodontal Diseases: Microbial factors. Proceedings of the 1996 World Workshop in Periodontics. *Annals of Periodontology* **1**, 879–925.

Chapter 37

Non-surgical Therapy

Noel Claffey and Ioannis Polyzois

Introduction, 766
Detection and removal of dental calculus, 766
Methods used for non-surgical root surface debridement, 768
  Hand instrumentation, 768
  Sonic and ultrasonic scalers, 770
  Reciprocating instruments, 770
  Ablative laser therapy, 771
  Choice of debridement method, 771
The influence of mechanical debridement on subgingival biofilms, 772

Implication of furcation involvement, 773
Pain and discomfort following non-surgical therapy, 773
Re-evaluation, 774
  Interpretation of probing measurements at re-evaluation, 774
  Average changes in measurements due to non-surgical therapy, 775
  Interpretation of longitudinal changes at individual sites, 775
Prediction of outcome and evaluation of treatment, 775
Full-mouth disinfection, 776

Introduction

It is generally accepted that the goal of the initial periodontal treatment is to restore the biological compatibility of periodontally diseased root surfaces, thus halting the process of the disease. Figure 37-1 illustrates the role and sequencing of non-surgical therapy in the management of most periodontitis patients.

Non-surgical therapy aims to eliminate both living bacteria in the microbial biofilm and calcified biofilm microorganisms from the tooth surface and adjacent soft tissues. Complete elimination of such pathogenic microorganisms is perhaps over-ambitious. However a reduction in inflammation of the periodontium due to a lesser bacterial load leads to beneficial clinical changes. In addition, non-surgical therapy aims to create an environment in which the host can more effectively prevent pathogenic microbial recolonization using personal oral hygiene methods.

This chapter outlines the various methods used in non-surgical therapy, such as hand instrumentation, ultrasonic and sonic scalers, and ablative laser therapy. Their respective merits and shortcomings and their clinical efficacy will be discussed. The chapter will attempt to identify realistic prognostic outcomes of therapy when taking into consideration factors such as different methods of instrumentation, different root surfaces, and varying degrees of periodontitis.

Re-evaluation of the initial clinical response to non-surgical therapy as well as consideration of modifiable risk factors allows the clinician to formulate an ongoing treatment plan tailored to the individual.

Detection and removal of dental calculus

Periodontitis is strongly associated with the presence of dental calculus on root surfaces. It has been suggested that the rough surface of calculus does not in itself induce inflammation but that the deleterious effect of calculus relates to its ability to provide an ideal surface for microbial colonization (Waerhaug 1952). It has also been demonstrated that epithelial adherence to subgingival calculus can occur following its disinfection with chlorhexidine (Lisgarten & Ellegaard 1973). Thus, a rationale for the removal of calculus relates to eliminating, as far as possible, surface irregularities harboring pathogenic bacteria.

Microbes giving rise to and colonizing the surface of dental calculus have been shown to produce lipopolysaccharides (LPS). These potent triggers of host response mechanisms were thought to be present within calculus and underlying cementum. For this reason it was thought necessary to remove not only calculus but also underlying cementum. However later evidence suggested that removal of tooth substance was not necessary. Ground sections of extracted periodontally involved teeth were examined. LPS was detected on cementum which had been previously exposed to the periodontal pocket. LPS also extended 1 mm into the surrounding connective tissue attachment. On no occasion was LPS seen penetrating into sub-surface cementum (Hughes & Smales 1986). These conclusions were further supported by animal and human studies which demonstrated that removal of superficial plaque on subgingival calculus resulted in the healing of periodontal lesions and the maintenance of health,

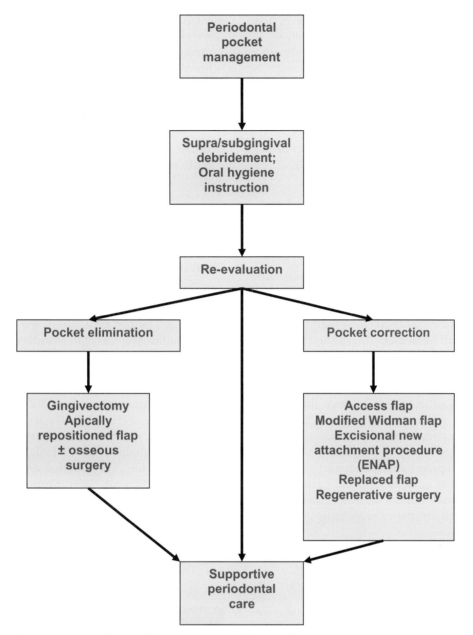

Fig. 37-1 Schematic representation of a typical treatment regimen for periodontitis patient management.

provided supragingival hygiene was meticulous (Nyman *et al*. 1986, 1988; Mombelli *et al*. 1995). From a clinical standpoint, minimizing the total volume of dental calculus present seems to be desirable. However, aggressive tooth substance removal does not seem warranted.

Factors that may influence complete calculus removal include the extent of disease, anatomic factors, the skill of the operator, and the instruments used. Waerhaug (1978) suggested that in more than 90% of cases, deposits of plaque and calculus remained in sites with pocket depths (PD) >5 mm following scaling and root planing. Similar conclusions were reported by Rabbani *et al*. (1981) and Magnusson *et al*. (1984). Brayer *et al*. (1989) investigated inter-operator variability performing non-surgical root debridement, comparing operators of two different levels of experience. It was found that the more

experienced clinician achieved a superior level of calculus removal.

Although Caffesse *et al*. (1986) found more residual calculus following non-surgical root debridement compared to root debridement as part of a surgical procedure, 50% or more of surfaces with PD >7 mm showed residual calculus irrespective of methodology. Buchanan and Robertson (1987) found more residual calculus following non-surgical treatment on molar and premolar tooth surfaces than non-molar teeth. They also demonstrated that over 60% of molar sites had residual calculus following closed root debridement. These findings may reflect increased difficulty in achieving successful root debridement in posterior areas in the mouth in addition to the more complicated anatomy of multi-rooted teeth.

Matia *et al*. (1986) noted no difference in the quality of root debridement following evaluation of ultrasonic, sonic or hand instrumentation. However none of the sites treated were totally free of calculus.

The agreement between clinicians in the detection of residual subgingival calculus has been found to be low. Furthermore microscopic studies have demonstrated that even if calculus is not detected clinically it may yet be present on a microscopic level. Nonetheless from a practical standpoint if calculus is detected clinically the site is more likely to display ongoing inflammation (Sherman *et al.* 1990).

Methods used for non-surgical root surface debridement

Scaling is a procedure which aims at the removal of plaque and calculus from the tooth surface. Depending on the location of deposits, scaling is performed by supragingival and/or subgingival instrumentation. Root planing denotes a technique of instrumentation by which the "softened cementum" is removed and the root surface is made "hard" and "smooth". However, on the basis of evidence already discussed, excessive tooth substance removal is not warranted and so perhaps the term root debridement is more appropriate. Root debridement may therefore be defined as the removal of plaque and/or calculus from the root surface without the intentional removal of tooth structure.

Non-surgical periodontal treatment may be carried out using a variety of methods including hand instruments, sonic and ultrasonic scalers reciprocating instruments, and ablative laser therapy.

Hand instrumentation

Hand instrumentation allows good tactile sensation while minimizing the risk of contaminated aerosol production. However, it tends to be more time consuming than other methods and, if aggressively performed, hand instrumentation can lead to excessive tooth substance removal. In addition, hand instrumentation is more technique sensitive and requires correct and frequent instrument sharpening.

Access to furcations and the base of deep pockets is limited compared to some machine-driven instruments which have been designed to access narrow apertures and relatively inaccessible areas (Leon *et al.* 1987; Oda & Ishikawa 1989; Dragoo *et al.* 1992; Takacs *et al.* 1993; Yukna *et al.* 1997; Kocher *et al.* 1998, 2001; Beuchat *et al.* 2001). Recently however, modified curettes with extended shanks for deep pockets and mini-bladed curettes for narrow pockets have been developed to improve efficacy of scaling and root planing in difficult areas (Singer *et al.* 1992; Landry *et al.* 1999).

Hand instruments

A hand instrument is composed of three parts: the working part (the blade), the shank, and the handle (Fig. 37-2). The cutting edges of the blade are centered over the long axis of the handle in order to give the instrument proper balance. The blade is often made of carbon steel, stainless steel or tungsten carbide.

Curettes are instruments used for both scaling and root debridement (Fig. 37-3). The working part of the curette is the spoon-shaped blade which has two curved cutting edges. The two edges are united by the rounded toe. The curettes are usually made "double-ended" with mirror-turned blades. The length and angulation of the shank as well as the dimensions of the blade differ between different brands of instruments.

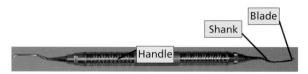

Fig. 37-2 A curette demonstrating the handle, shank, and blade.

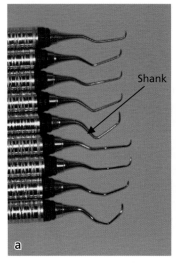
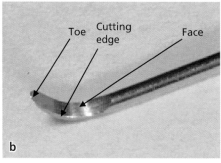

Fig. 37-3 (a) Selections of curettes with varying shank configurations to facilitate debridement of different areas of the dentition. (b) The working end of a curette demonstrating rounded toe, face, and cutting edge.

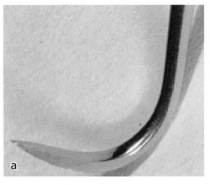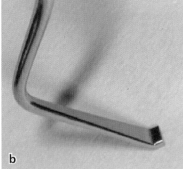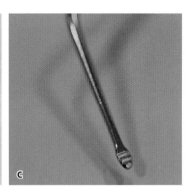

Fig. 37-4 (a) Sickle scaler. (b) Hoe. (c) File.

(a)
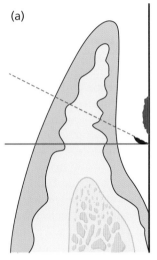

(b)
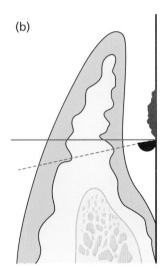

(c)
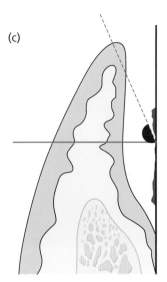

Fig. 37-5 The effect of different angulations of the cutting edge of the curette to the tooth surface. (a) Correct angle of application. (b) Too obtuse angulation resulting in ineffective calculus removal and the possibility of cratering the surface. (c) Too acute angulation resulting in ineffective calculus removal and burnishing of the calculus deposits.

The sickle is manufactured with either a curved or a straight blade which has a triangular cross section and two cutting edges. The "facial" surface between the two cutting edges is flat in the lateral direction but may be curved in the direction of its long axis. The "facial" surface converges with the two lateral surfaces of the blade. Sickles are mainly used for supragingival debridement or scaling in shallow pockets (Fig. 37-4a).

The hoe has only one cutting edge. The blade is turned at a 100° angle to the shank with the cutting edge bevelled at a 45° angle. The blade can be positioned at four different inclinations in relation to the shank: facial, lingual, distal, and mesial. The hoe is mainly used for supragingival scaling (Fig. 37-4b). Periodontal files can be useful for smoothing roots in areas of stubborn deposits (Fig. 37-4c).

Principles of curette use

Perhaps the most widely used instrument type for subgingival debridement is the curette. The angulation of the cutting edge of the curette to the tooth surface influences the efficiency of debridement. The optimal angle between the cutting edge and the tooth is approximately 80° (Fig. 37-5a). Too obtuse an angle, as shown in Fig. 37-5b, will result in cratering and consequent roughening of the root surface. Too acute an angle, as shown in Fig. 37-5c, will result in ineffective removal and burnishing of subgingival calculus deposits.

Subgingival instrumentation should preferably be performed under local anesthesia. The root surface of the diseased site is explored with a probe to identify (1) the probing depth, (2) the anatomy of the root surface (irregularities, root furrows, open furcation, etc.), and (3) the location of the calcified deposits.

The instrument is held in a modified pen grasp and the blade inserted into the periodontal pocket with the face of the blade parallel to and in light contact with the root surface. It is important that all root surface instrumentation is performed with a proper finger rest. This implies that one finger – the third or the fourth – must act as a fulcrum for the movement of the blade of the instrument. A proper finger rest serves to (1) provide a stable fulcrum, (2) permit optimal angulation of the blade, and (3) enable the use of wrist–forearm motion. The finger rest must

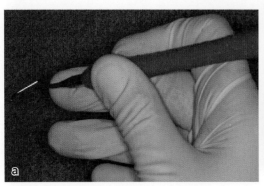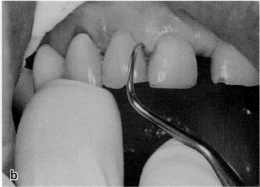

Fig. 37-6 Illustrations of (a) a modified pen grasp and (b) a finger rest in close proximity to the area of instrumentation.

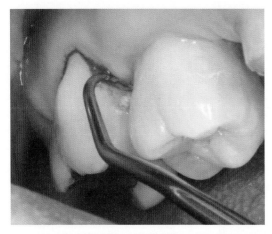

Fig. 37-7 Illustration of the shank of the curette held parallel to the long axis of the tooth during instrumentation of a posterior site.

be secured as close as possible to the site of instrumentation to facilitate controlled use of the instrument (Fig. 37-6).

After the base of the periodontal pocket has been identified with the lower edge of the blade, the instrument is turned into a proper "cutting" position: i.e. the shank is parallel to the long axis of the tooth (Fig. 37-7). The grasp of the instrument is tightened somewhat, the force between the cutting edge and the root surface is increased, and the blade is moved in a coronal direction. Strokes must be made in different directions to cover all aspects of the root surface (crosswise, back and forth) but, as stated above, strokes should always start from an apical position and be guided in a coronal direction. The probe is inserted in the pocket again and the surface of the root assessed anew for the presence of calculus.

Frequent sharpening of the cutting edge of the instrument is necessary to obtain efficient calculus removal (Fig. 37-8a). The angle between the face and the back of curettes must be maintained at approximately 70° during sharpening (Fig. 37-8b). Any greater angle will result in dulling of the cutting edge. A more acute angle results in a fragile and easily worn cutting edge.

Sonic and ultrasonic scalers

A common alternative to hand instrumention for non-surgical periodontal therapy is the use of sonic and ultrasonic scalers. Sonic scalers use air pressure to create mechanical vibration that in turn causes the instrument tip to vibrate; the frequencies of vibration ranging from 2000–6000 Hz (Gankerseer & Walmsley 1987; Shah *et al.* 1994). Ultrasonic scalers convert electrical current to mechanical energy in the form of high-frequency vibrations at the instrument tip; the vibration frequencies ranging from 18 000–45 000 Hz. There are two types of ultrasonic scalers, magnetostrictive and piezoelectric. In piezoelectric scalers the alternating electrical current causes a dimensional change in the hand piece which is transmitted to the working tip as vibrations. The pattern of vibration at the tip is primarily linear. In magnetostrictive scalers the generated electrical current produces a magnetic field in the handpiece that causes the insert to expand and contract along its length and in turn causes the insert to vibrate. The pattern of vibration at the tip is elliptical. Modified sonic and ultrasonic scaler tips, e.g. tiny, thin, periodontal probe type, and diamond coated, have been developed for use in deep pockets (Drisko *et al.* 2000).

Recently, ultrasonic instruments using a working frequency of 25 kHz and a coupling at the head of the handpiece to transfer energy indirectly to the working tip have been developed. These instruments are cooled by a water-based medium containing polishing particles of various sizes dependent on therapeutic indication. The amount of contaminated aerosol is said to be reduced compared to other ultrasonic or sonic scalers. This system has been advocated for the treatment of periodontitis and peri-implantitis, as well as minimal invasive preparation of tooth structures. This development has been shown to be equally effective as conventional methods (Sculean *et al.* 2004).

Reciprocating instruments

Few studies have been carried out to investigate the efficacy of reciprocating instruments. Results demon-

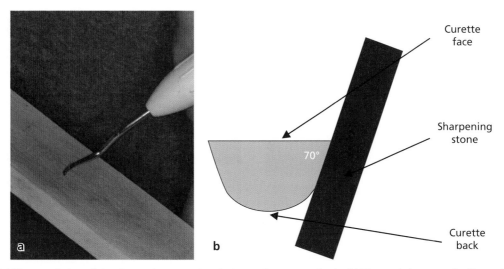

Fig. 37-8 (a) The angulation of the sharpening stone in relation to the curette shank. (b) The angle between the flat surface of the sharpening stone and the cutting edge of the curette.

strated that they produce an equivalent clinical outcome compared to hand, sonic or ultrasonic scalers. The use of reciprocating instruments is less time consuming than hand instrumentation and results in less root surface loss (Obeid *et al.* 2004; Obeid & Bercy 2005). Further evidence is awaited to support their widespread use.

Ablative laser therapy

Ablative laser therapy targets both the soft and hard tissues of the periodontium. It has bacteriocidal and detoxification effects and can remove the epithelium lining and granulation tissue within the periodontal pocket which may potentially improve healing. Considering the possibility of bacterial invasion into the soft tissues of pockets, this effect could be an important factor in the treatment of moderate to deep pockets. However, studies have shown that curettage of granulation tissues had no added benefit over scaling and root planing (Lindhe & Nyman 1985; Ramfjord *et al.* 1987). Laser therapy is capable of removing plaque and calculus with extremely low mechanical stress and no formation of a smear layer on root surfaces. In addition the use of lasers may allow access to sites that conventional mechanical instruments cannot reach.

Various types of lasers such as carbon dioxide lasers, Er:YAG lasers, and Nd:YAG lasers are currently in use. Carbon dioxide lasers, when used with relatively low energy output in a pulsed and/or defocused mode, have root conditioning, detoxification, and bacteriocidal effects on contaminated root surfaces. However, at low energy outputs they are unable to remove calculus. Er:YAG lasers are capable of effectively removing calculus from the root surface. Er:YAG laser irradiation energy is absorbed by water and organic components of the biological tissues which causes their evaporation resulting in heat generation, water vapour production, and thus an increase in internal pressure within the calculus deposits. The resulting expansion within the calculus causes its separation from the root surface.

Choice of debridement method

It has been demonstrated that hand, sonic, and ultrasonic scalers produce similar periodontal healing response with respect to probing pocket depths, bleeding on probing, and clinical attachment level (Badersten *et al.* 1981, 1984; Lindhe & Nyman 1985; Kalkwarf *et al.* 1989; Loos *et al.* 1987; Copulos *et al.* 1993; Yukna *et al.* 1997; Kocher *et al.* 2001; Obeid *et al.* 2004; Wennstrom *et al.* 2005; Christgau *et al.* 2006). With respect to time spent, several studies have shown that debridement time spent per tooth may be reduced when ultrasonic or sonic scalers used compared to hand scalers (Copulos *et al.* 1993; Boretti *et al.* 1995; Tunkel *et al.* 2002; Wennstrom *et al.* 2005; Christgau *et al.* 2006). Regarding root surface loss, sonic and ultrasonic scalers have been shown to produce less tooth surface loss compared to hand scalers (Ritz *et al.* 1991; Schmidlin *et al.* 2001).

In contrast to hand instrumentation, the use of sonic and ultrasonic scalers is less technique sensitive, requires less time to complete, and removes less root surface cementum. It has been shown to provide better access to deep pockets and furcation areas (Kocher *et al.* 1998; Beuchat *et al.* 2001). In addition the flushing action of water used in sonic and ultrasonic scalers removes, to a certain extent, debris and bacteria from the pocket area. However, tactile sensation is reduced, and there is production of contaminated aerosols (Harrel *et al.* 1998; Barnes *et al.* 1998; Rivera-Hidalgo *et al.* 1999; Timmerman *et al.* 2004). Some patients may find the vibration, sound, and water spray uncomfortable.

It has been demonstrated that the use of lasers produces results comparable to scaling and root planing (Schwarz *et al.* 2001). However, no adjunctive

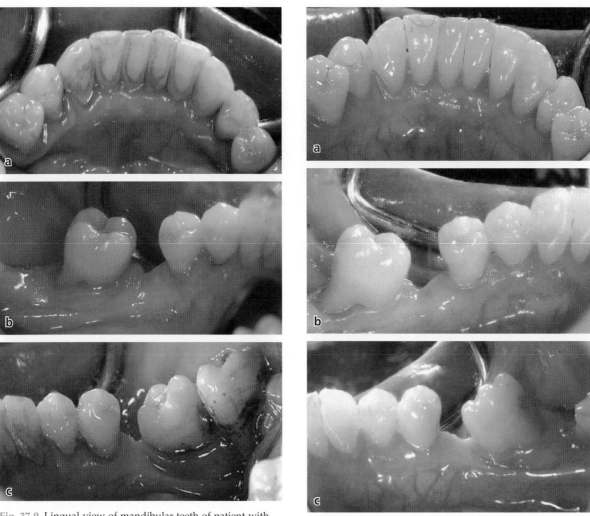

Fig. 37-9 Lingual view of mandibular teeth of patient with untreated periodontitis prior to periodontal therapy.

Fig. 37-10 Lingual view of mandibular teeth of patient 3 months following initial non-surgical therapy.

benefit of the use of lasers over scaling and root planing alone has been demonstrated (Schwarz *et al*. 2003; Ambrosini *et al*. 2005). Inadvertent irradiation and reflection from shiny metal surfaces may cause damage to patient's eyes, throat, and oral tissues other than the targeted area. In addition there is also a risk of excessive tissue destruction by direct ablation and thermal side effects. Also the high cost of the laser apparatus is a drawback for many clinicians.

Figures 37-9 and 37-10 demonstrate the effects of non-surgical therapy.

The influence of mechanical debridement on subgingival biofilms

Supra- and subgingival debridement results in the mechanical disruption of the plaque biofilm and remains the "gold standard" modality for periodontal treatment. Removal of subgingival plaque and calculus deposits through subgingival debridement exposes the cementum, root dentine, and pocket epithelium for novel colonization. Species which may

have thrived in the subgingival environment of the diseased pocket may find the new habitat less hospitable. A decreased concentration of microbial products and tissue breakdown products, and a decrease in the flow of gingival crevicular fluid, along with a more neutral subgingival biofilm pH may encourage the growth of less pathogenic bacterial species. Also a decrease in pocket depth as a result of a resolution of inflammation, decreased oedema, and a re-adaptation of apical junctional epithelium favors the recolonization of more aerobic species.

Following treatment the subgingival habitat may be repopulated by microorganisms which originate from: residual subgingival plaque deposits (Ramberg *et al*. 1994; Dahan *et al*. 2004); radicular dentinal tubules or cementum (Daly *et al*. 1982; Adriaens *et al*. 1988; Giuliana *et al*. 1997); pocket epithelium and connective tissues (Slots & Rosling 1983); supragingival plaque deposits (Magnusson *et al*. 1984; Ximenez-Fyvie *et al*. 2000); subgingival deposits of adjacent teeth and from other intraoral soft tissue sites (von Troil-Linden *et al*. 1996).

Subgingival debridement has been observed to result in a decrease in the total number of microorganisms present in subgingival sites and a shift in the relative proportion of different microbial species within the subgingival plaque biofilm. A decrease in the total bacterial count for sites of 3 mm or greater depth, from $91 \pm 11 \times 10^5$ to $23 \pm 6 \times 10^5$, has been observed immediately following subgingival debridement (Teles *et al.* 2006). Although pre-debridement subgingival microbial counts are restored in 4–7 days post debridement (Sharawy *et al.* 1966), the impact of subgingival debridement on the composition of subgingival plaque biofilms, although often transient, is more long lasting.

Subgingival debridement has been observed to result in a decrease in the mean counts and number of sites colonized by *P. gingivalis*, *A. actinomycetemcomitans*, *Pr. intermedia* (Shiloah & Patters 1994), *T. forsythia*, and *Tr. denticola* (Darby *et al.* 2005) several weeks following subgingival debridement. The persistence of *A. actinomycetemcomitans* and *P. gingivalis* following subgingival debridement is attributed to the ability of these microorganisms to invade the pocket epithelium and connective tissues (Slots & Rosling 1983; Renvert *et al.* 1990; Shiloah & Patters 1994). Haffajee *et al.* (1997) found that the only species to be significantly affected in prevalence and mean counts 3 months following non-surgical periodontal therapy were *B. forsythus*, *P. gingivalis*, and *Tr. denticola*.

An increase in the proportions of Gram-positive aerobic cocci and rods following subgingival debridement is associated with health (Cobb 2002). Haffajee *et al.* (2006) reported an increase in proportion of streptococci (including *S. gordonni*, *S. mitis*, *S. oralis*, and *S. sanguinis*) and *Actinomyces* spp., *E. corrodens*, and *G. morbillarum* post subgingival debridement.

Microorganisms do not exist in isolation in the subgingival environment, but rather as members of communities. Socransky *et al.* (1998) identified groups of organisms which were commonly found together and subdivided microorganisms into complexes accordingly. Members of the red and orange complexes are most commonly identified at sites displaying signs of periodontitis. A re-emergence of species of the red and orange complex 3–12 months post debridement may be associated with ongoing attachment loss at these sites (Haffajee *et al.* 2006).

In the absence of appropriate home care, the re-establishment of the pretreatment microflora as well as the rebound of clinical improvements due to treatment will occur in a matter of weeks (Magnusson *et al.* 1984; Loos *et al.* 1988; Sbordone *et al.* 1990). In the absence of professional maintenance an increase in the prevalence and counts of periodontopathogens is to be expected (Renvert *et al.* 1990; Shiloah & Patters 1994). Following supra- and subgingival debridement and appropriate home care the re-establishment of a pathogenic subgingival microflora and an associated rebound in clinical parameters may occur in localized sites (Beikler *et al.* 2004).

Implication of furcation involvement

Once attachment loss has progressed to the furcation area of multi-rooted teeth, patient-performed home care and professionally performed subgingival debridement become more difficult (Wylam *et al.* 1993). Microbial communities may develop relatively undisturbed in this sheltered anatomic site and increasingly anaerobic and virulent microbes may thrive.

Loos *et al.* (1988) observed that while subgingival debridement resulted in improvements in clinical and microbiologic parameters over a 1-year period post debridement, sites with furcation involvement consistently demonstrated higher microbial counts and greater proportions of suspected periodontopathogens. Generally clinical improvement was found to be less pronounced in furcation sites than in other locations (Loos *et al.* 1989). Nordland *et al.* (1987) and Claffey and Egelberg (1994) observed that the frequency of continued probing attachment loss was considerably greater in furcation-involved sites compared with all other sites. Consequently, teeth with furcation involvement may be viewed with some caution with respect to long-term prognosis.

Pain and discomfort following non-surgical therapy

It has been demonstrated that tissue trauma occurs during non-surgical periodontal therapy (Claffey *et al.* 1988). This trauma can trigger local mechano-receptors and polymodal nociceptors, the activation of which leads to the release of chemicals, such as prostaglandins, bradykinin, and histamine, and ultimately to the perception of pain in the central nervous system.

Clinical studies referring to pain experience after non-surgical therapy are limited. Quantifying pain is difficult as it cannot be measured directly. Pain perception to a similar stimulus is highly variable from individual to individual. Pain may be measured using visual analogue scales whereby the patient is asked to indicate their level of pain by a mark on a gradated scale from no pain to the most severe pain imaginable.

Pihlstrom *et al.* (1999) reported that patients experienced pain of significant duration and magnitude following scaling and root planning. Pain was reported to peak in intensity between 2 and 8 hours post therapy and on average lasted for 6 hours. Almost 25% of patients self-medicated to relieve pain after treatment.

In addition to pain resulting from soft tissue trauma, patients may also experience root sensitivity following non-surgical therapy. Good oral hygiene measures resulting in low plaque scores prior to commencement of non-surgical periodontal therapy have been shown to decrease root dentin sensitivity.

Despite this, root dentin sensitivity can be a side effect of thorough root planing. Tammaro *et al.* (2000) demonstrated only moderate increases in root dentin sensitivity in most patients with only a small portion of patients experiencing more extreme sensitivity. Patients with sensitive teeth prior to treatment had higher levels of sensitivity following treatment. Although a reduction in the intensity of root dentin sensitivity over 4 weeks was noted, the number of sensitive teeth remained unchanged.

Clinical trials have shown anxiety, depression, and stress to be related to pain perception. Kloostra *et al.* (2006) investigated these factors with regard to non-surgical as well as surgical periodontal therapy and concluded that psychosocial factors may influence pain experience and the need for medication after therapy.

In a further clinical trial concerned with patients' experience of pain during diagnosis and non-surgical treatment of periodontitis it was demonstrated that pain experience during diagnostic instrumentation correlated significantly with pain experience during root instrumentation (van Steenberghe *et al.* 2004). One third of patients took analgesic medication after non-surgical treatment. However approximately half of the total number of patients complained of gingival soreness and pain and two thirds even experienced problems while eating.

Pain during and after periodontal diagnosis and non-surgical therapy seems to be on average mild to moderate and transient in nature. Nevertheless, some patients experience significant pain during treatment. Patients' psychosocial factors such as anxiety may influence the intensity of the pain experienced. Moreover recognition of this anxiety may be the first step in the management of pain in such patients (Chung *et al.* 2003). There is some first evidence that pre-emptive analgesics (ibruprofen arginine) may have some beneficial effect and help the patient to have a much more positive experience during periodontal treatment (Ettlin *et al.* 2006).

Re-evaluation

Healing following non-surgical therapy is almost complete at 3 months. However a slower ongoing but limited healing can continue for up to 9 or more months following the treatment (Badersten *et al.* 1984). Re-evaluation is a vital stage in a periodontal treatment plan. At re-evaluation the effectiveness of treatment previously carried out is evaluated and the nature of further therapy, if needed, is established.

Measurements are made at baseline and again at 3 months as a method of evaluation of periodontal status and effectiveness of therapy. Measurements include plaque scores, bleeding on probing, suppuration on probing, probing pocket depth, recession, probing attachment level, and assessment of mobility. These are usually recorded at four to six sites around each tooth.

Interpretation of probing measurements at re-evaluation

Probing depth is defined as the distance from the gingival margin to the base of the periodontal pocket measured in millimeters using a periodontal probe. Probing attachment level change is utilized to assess events occurring at the base of the periodontal pocket. Measurements are made at different times from a fixed point, such as from a stent margin or cemento-enamel junction to the base of the pocket. It is generally accepted that any improvement in probing attachment level is not a result of connective tissue reattachment but due to a re-adaptation of the junctional epithelium at the base of the pocket (Fig. 37-11). Probing depth change is a combination of recession and the change in probing attachment level

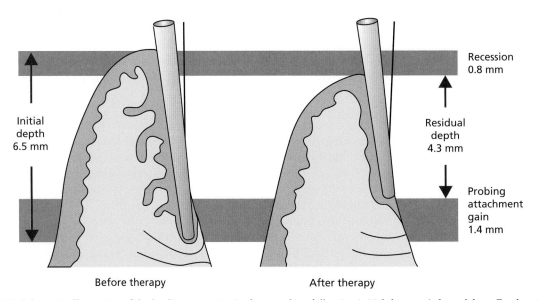

Initial depth 6.5 mm

Recession 0.8 mm

Residual depth 4.3 mm

Probing attachment gain 1.4 mm

Before therapy

After therapy

Fig. 37-11 Schematic illustration of the healing occurring in deep pockets following initial therapy (adapted from Fowler *et al.* 1982).

due to events occurring at the base of the periodontal pocket.

On average the change in pocket depth seen following treatment for deeper pockets is a combination of recession at the gingival margin due to resolution of inflammation and a tightening of the junctional epithelium at the base of the pocket. Moreover the reduced bleeding on probing scores found after treatment may reflect the increased resistance to probe penetration into the connective tissue.

Average changes in measurements due to non-surgical therapy

Tables 37-1 and 37-2 present mean changes in plaque scores, bleeding scores, probing depths, and probing attachment levels which were generally observed in studies of mean changes from baseline to re-evaluation. However the use of mean results of pooled sites can mask deterioration or improvement at individual sites.

It is important to appreciate that the extent of the initial probing depth has a marked influence on probing depth changes due to treatment. For example, for shallow pockets, non-surgical treatment results in loss of probing attachment, whereas in deep pockets there is a marked gain of probing attachment. It has been shown that there is an initial loss of probing attachment due to instrumentation trauma for pockets of all initial probing depths. However in the deeper sites this loss is reversed upon resolution of inflammation (Claffey *et al.* 1988).

Interpretation of longitudinal changes at individual sites

Difficulties arise in detecting individual sites with ongoing destruction due to the following reasons:

Table 37-1 Estimations generally observed in studies, of improvements in plaque and bleeding scores for sites of different initial probing depths after a single episode of supra- and subgingival instrumentation

Initial probing depth (mm)	Plaque	Bleeding
≤3.5	≈ 50% → 10%	≈ 55% → 15%
4–6.5	≈ 80% → 15%	≈ 80% → 25%
≥7	≈ 90% → 25%	≈ 90% → 30%

Table 37-2 Mean changes (mm) generally observed in studies in probing depth, probing attachment levels, and gingival recession after a single episode of supra- and subgingival instrumentation

Initial probing depth (mm)	Probing depth	Probing attachment level	Recession
≤3.5	0	−0.5	0.5
4–6.5	1–2	0–1	0–1
≥7	2–3	1–2	1–2

- Lack of reproducibility of probing measurements. Factors influencing the reproducibility of probing measurements include: probing force, probe tip diameter, angulation of probe, position in the mouth, probing depth itself and the inflammatory status of the tissues. A similar lack of reproducibility has been reported following recordings made by the same examiner at different time points (intra-examiner) and recordings taken by different examiners at the same time points (inter-examiner). Badersten *et al.* (1984) demonstrated that duplicate probing measurements were exactly the same in only 30–40% of cases when looking at both inter-examiner and intra-examiner reproducibility. Differences of 2 mm or more were noted in 5–7% of recordings. Therefore, such probing attachment level changes at individual sites cannot be relied upon to indicate true disease progression.
- As discussed above variations in probing attachment levels may simply reflect changes in the inflammatory status at the base of the pocket rather than true connective tissue loss or gain.

With these points in mind, in order to identify sites with ongoing connective tissue loss, probing measurements should be interpreted with caution. Various methods have been reported in the literature to address this problem. One method is to demand a high threshold of change before indicating a site as deteriorating. Others include the application of statistical methods, such as regression analysis, to a series of longitudinal measurements.

Prediction of outcome and evaluation of treatment

It would be of great benefit to the clinician to be able to predict the outcome of treatment prior to therapy and also to identify at re-evaluation the sites likely to continue to deteriorate. Prediction and evaluation must be considered both at a patient level and a site level. On a patient level, the extent of baseline bleeding scores, probing attachment loss, and probing depths have been found to relate to future probing attachment loss in untreated patients (Halazonetis *et al.* 1989; Lindhe *et al.* 1989; Haffajee *et al.* 1991). In patients treated with non-surgical therapy without the use of local anesthetic, baseline scores of attachment loss were also seen to relate to the risk of further loss of attachment (Grbic *et al.* 1991; Grbic & Lamster 1992). On a patient level, the number of sites greater then 6 mm at re-evaluation bears a direct relationship to future periodontal breakdown (Claffey & Egelberg 1995).

On a site level, bleeding on probing is, at best, a moderate predictor of future attachment loss (Badersten *et al.* 1990; Claffey *et al.* 1990). On the other hand, absence of bleeding on probing has been demonstrated as a useful indicator of health (Lang *et al.* 1990). Claffey *et al.* (1990) found that deep residual

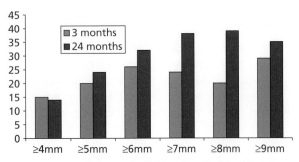

Fig. 37-12 Diagnostic predictability of residual probing depths at 3 months and 12 months following non-surgical treatment of advanced periodontitis. Diagnostic predictability is the percentage of sites with a certain feature, for instance with a deep probing depth at 3 or 6 months, which show attachment loss at a later time point.

probing depth was of limited predictive value when observed over short periods (Fig. 37-12). However, over the longer term, deep residual sites appeared to be more indicative of further attachment loss, particularly if combined with bleeding on probing. This emphasizes the need for ongoing monitoring to identify such sites and instigate appropriate intervention.

Full-mouth disinfection

Traditionally non-surgical treatment of periodontitis involves a series of appointments separated by perhaps a week or more. Each appointment typically involves root debridement of a quadrant depending on disease severity. In 1995 Quirynen *et al.* introduced the concept of total mouth disinfection as a new treatment strategy. It involved full-mouth scaling and root debridement within a 24-hour treatment period, subgingival irrigation (repeated three times within 10 minutes) with 1% chlorhexidine gel, tongue brushing with 1% chlorhexidine gel, and mouth rinsing with 0.2% chlorhexidine. This full-mouth disinfection protocol aimed to reduce the bacterial load in pockets and intraoral niches to minimize the risk of reinfection of the treated pockets from areas harboring pathogenic bacteria. Quirynen *et al.* (1995) showed that full-mouth disinfection yielded better periodontal treatment results on a short-term basis compared to conventional treatment.

Subsequent studies (Bollen *et al.* 1996, 1998; Vandekerckhove *et al.* 1996; Mongardini *et al.* 1999; Quirynen *et al.* 1999, 2000; De Soete *et al.* 2001) concluded that the full-mouth disinfection protocol resulted in clinical and microbiologic improvements comparable to the traditional technique of treatment in patients with advanced chronic periodontitis.

Many recent studies report varying degrees of efficacy of full-mouth disinfection protocol (Apatzidou & Kinane 2004). However, the full-mouth disinfection treatment approach has been promoted as a more efficient way of treating chronic periodontitis patients (Koshy *et al.* 2004; Wennstrom *et al.* 2005).

References

Adriaens, P.A., De Boever, J.A. & Loesche, W.J. (1988). Bacterial invasion in root cementum and radicular dentin of periodontally diseased teeth in humans. A reservoir of periodontopathic bacteria. *Journal of Periodontology* **59**, 222–230.

Ambrosini, P., Miller, N., Briancon, S., Gallina, S. & Penaud, J. (2005). Clinical and microbiological evaluation of the effectiveness of the Nd:Yap laser for the initial treatment of adult periodontitis. A randomized controlled study. *Journal of Clinical Periodontology* **32**, 670–676.

Apatzidou, D.A. & Kinane, D.F. (2004). Quadrant root planing versus same-day full-mouth root planing. I. Clinical findings. *Journal of Clinical Periodontology* **31**, 132–140.

Badersten, A., Nilveus, R. & Egelberg, J. (1981). Effect of non-surgical periodontal therapy 1. Moderate and advanced periodontitis. *Journal of Clinical Periodontology* **8**, 57–72.

Badersten, A., Nilveus, R. & Egelberg, J. (1984). Effect of non-surgical periodontal therapy II. *Journal of Clinical Periodontology* **11**, 63–76.

Badersten, A., Nilveus, R. & Egelberg, J. (1990). Scores of plaque, bleeding, suppuration and probing depth to predict probing attachment loss. 5 years of observation following nonsurgical periodontal therapy. *Journal of Clinical Periodontology* **17**, 102–107.

Barnes, J.B., Harrel, S.K. & Rivera Hidalgo, F. (1998). Blood contamination of the aerosols produced by in vivo use of ultrasonic scaler. *Journal of Periodontology* **69**, 434–438.

Beikler, T., Abdeen, G., Schnitzer, S., Salzer, S., Ehmke, B., Heinecke, A. & Flemmig, T.F. (2004). Microbiological shifts in intra- and extraoral habitats following mechanical periodontal therapy. *Journal of Clinical Periodontology* **31**, 777–783.

Beuchat, M., Bussliger, A., Schmidlin, P.R., Michel, B., Lehmann, B. & Lutz, F. (2001). Clinical comparison of the effectiveness of novel sonic instruments and curettes for periodontal debridement after two months. *Journal of Clinical Periodontology* **28**, 1145–1150.

Bollen, C.M., Mongardini, C., Papaioannou, W., van Steenberghe, D. & Quirynen, M. (1998). The effect of a one-stage full-mouth disinfection on different intra-oral niches. Clinical and microbiological observations. *Journal of Clinical Periodontology* **25**, 56–66.

Bollen, C.M., Vandekerckhove, B.N., Papaioannou, W., Van Eldere, J. & Quirynen, M. (1996). Full- versus partial-mouth disinfection in the treatment of periodontal infections. A pilot study: long-term microbiological observations. *Journal of Clinical Periodontology* **23**, 960–970.

Boretti, G., Zappau, U., Graf, H. & Case, D. (1995). Short term effect of phase 1 therapy on crevicular cell population: *Journal of Periodontology* **66**, 235–240.

Brayer, W.K., Mellonig, J.T., Dunlap, R.M., Marinak, K.W. & Carson, R.E. (1989). Scaling and root planing effectiveness: the effect of root surface access and operator experience. *Journal of Periodontology* **60**, 67–72.

Buchanan, S.A. & Robertson, P.B. (1987). Calculus removal by scaling/root planing with and without surgical access. *Journal of Periodontology* **58**, 159–163.

Caffesse, R.G., Sweeney, P.L. & Smith, B.A. (1986). Scaling and root planing with and without periodontal flap surgery. *Journal of Clinical Periodontology* **13**, 205–210.

Christgau, M., Männer, T., Beuer, S., Hiller, K.A. & Schmalz, G. (2006). Periodontal healing after non-surgical therapy with modified sonic scaler. *Journal of Clinical Periodontology* **33**, 749–758.

Chung, D.T., Bogle, G., Bernardini, M., Stephens, D., Riggs, M.L. & Egelberg, J.H. (2003). Pain experienced by patients during periodontal maintenance. *Journal of Periodontology* **74**, 1293–1301.

Claffey, N. & Egelberg, J. (1994). Clinical characteristics of periodontal sites with probing attachment loss following initial periodontal treatment. *Journal of Clinical Periodontology* **21**, 670–679.

Claffey, N. & Egelberg, J. (1995). Clinical indicators of probing attachment loss following initial periodontal treatment in advanced periodontitis patients. *Journal of Clinical Periodontology* **22**, 690–696.

Claffey, N., Loos, B., Gantes, B., Martin, M., Heins, P. & Egelberg, J. (1988). The relative effects of therapy and periodontal disease on loss of probing attachment after root debridement. *Journal of Clinical Periodontology* **17**, 108–114.

Claffey, N., Nylund, K., Kiger, R., Garrett, S. & Egelberg, J. (1990). Diagnostic predictability of scores of plaque, bleeding, suppuration and probing depth for probing attachment loss. 3.5 years of observation following initial periodontal therapy. *Journal of Clinical Periodontology* **17**, 108–114.

Cobb, C.M. (2002). Clinical significance of non-surgical periodontal therapy: an evidence-based perspective of scaling and root planing. *Journal of Clinical Periodontology* **29**, 6–16.

Copulos, T.A., Low, S.B., Walker, C.B., Trebilcock, Y.Y. & Hefti, A. (1993). Comparative analysis between a modified ultrasonic tip and hand instruments on clinical parameters of periodontal disease. *Journal of Periodontology* **64**, 694–700.

Dahan, M., Timmerman, M.F., van Winkelhoff, A.J. & van der Velden, U. (2004). The effect of periodontal treatment on the salivary bacterial load and early plaque formation. *Journal of Clinical Periodontology* **31**, 972–977.

Daly, C.G., Seymour, G.J., Kieser, J.B. & Corbet, E.F. (1982). Histological assessment of periodontally involved cementum. *Journal of Clinical Periodontology* **9**, 266–274.

Darby, I.B., Hodge, P.J., Riggio, M.P. & Kinane, D.F. (2005). Clinical and microbiological effect of scaling and root planing in smoker and nonsmoker chronic and aggressive periodontitis patients. *Journal of Clinical Periodontology* **32**, 200–206.

De Soete, M., Mongardini, C., Peuwels, M., Haffajee, A., Socransky, S., van Steenberghe, D. & Quirynen, M. (2001). One-stage full-mouth disinfection. Long-term microbiological results analyzed by checkerboard DNA-DNA hybridization. *Journal of Periodontology* **72**, 374–382.

Dragoo, M.R. (1992). A clinical evaluation of hand and ultrasonic instruments on subgingival debridement 1: with unmodified and modified ultrasonic inserts. *International Journal of Periodontics and Restorative Dentistry* **12**, 310–323.

Drisko, C.L., Cochran, D.L., Blieden, T., Bouwsma, O.J., Cohen, R.E., Damoulis, P., Fine, J.B., Greenstein, G., Hinrichs, J., Somerman, M.J., Iacono, V. & Genco, R.J. (2000). Research, Science and Therapy Committee of the American Accademy of Periodontology. Position paper: sonic and ultrasonic scalers in periodontics. *Journal of Periodontology* **71**, 1792–1801.

Ettlin, D.A., Ettlin, A., Bless, K., Puhan, M., Bernasconi, C., Tillmann, H.C., Palla, S. & Gallo, L.M. (2006). Ibuprofen arginine for pain control during scaling and root planing: a randomized, triple-blind trial. *Journal of Clinical Periodontology* **33**, 345–350.

Fowler, C., Garrett, S., Crigger, M. & Egelberg, J. (1982). Histologic probe position in treated and untreated human periodontal tissues. *Journal of Clinical Periodontology* **9**, 373–385.

Gankerseer, E.J. & Walmsley, A.D. (1987). Preliminary investigation into the performance of sonic scalers. *Journal of Periodontology* **58**, 780–784.

Giuliana, G., Ammatuna, P., Pizzo, G., Capone, F. & D'Angelo, M. (1997). Occurrence of invading bacteria in radicular dentin of periodontally diseased teeth: microbiological findings. *Journal of Clinical Periodontology* **24**, 478–485.

Grbic, J.T. & Lamster, I.B. (1992). Risk indicators for future clinical attachment loss in adult periodontitis. Tooth and site variable. *Journal of Periodontology* **63**, 262–329.

Grbic, J.T., Lamster, I.B., Clenti, R.S. & Fine, J.B. (1991). Risk indicators for future clinical attachment loss in adult periodontitis. *Journal of Periodontology* **63**, 322–329.

Haffajee, A.D., Cugini, M.A., Dibart, S., Smith, C., Kent, R.L. & Socransky, S.S. (1997). The effect of SRP on the clinical and microbiological parameters of periodontal diseases. *Journal of Clinical Periodontology* **24**, 324–334.

Haffajee, A.D., Socransky, S.S., Lindhe, J., Kent, R.L., Okamoto, H. & Yoneyama, T. (1991). Clinical risk indicators for periodontal attachment loss. *Journal of Clinical Periodontology* **18**, 117–125.

Haffajee, A.D., Teles, R.P. & Socransky, S.S. (2006). The effect of periodontal therapy on the composition of the subgingival microbiota. *Periodontology 2000* **42**, 219–258.

Halazonetis, T.D., Haffajee, A.D. & Socransky, S.S. (1989). Relationship of clinical parameters to attachment loss in subsets of subjects with destructive periodontal diseases. *Journal of Clinical Periodontology* **16**, 563–568.

Harrel, S.K., Barnes, J.B. & Rivera-Hidalgo, F. (1998). Aerosols and splatter contamination from the operative site during ultrasonic scaling. *Journal of the American Dental Association* **129**, 1241–1249.

Hughes, F.J. & Smales, F.C. (1986). Immunohistochemical investigation of the presence and distribution of cementum-associated lipopolysaccharides in periodontal disease. *Journal of Periodontal Research* **21**, 660–667.

Kalkwarf, K.L., Kaldal, W.B., Patil, K.D. & Molvar, M.P. (1989). Evaluation of gingival bleeding following four types of periodontal therapies. *Journal of Clinical Periodontology* **16**, 608–616.

Kloostra, P.W., Eber, R.M., Wang, H.L. & Inglehart, M.R. (2006). Surgical versus non-surgical periodontal treatment: psychosocial factors and treatment outcomes. *Journal of Periodontology* **77**, 1253–1260.

Kocher, T., Gutsche, C. & Plagmann, H.C. (1998). Instrumentation of furcation with modified sonic scaler inserts: study on manikins, Part 1. *Journal of Clinical Periodontology* **25**, 388–393.

Kocher, T., Rosin, M., Langenbeck, N. & Bernhardt, O. (2001). Subgingival polishing with a teflon-coated sonic scaler insert in comparison to conventional instruments as assessed on extracted teeth (II). Subgingival roughness. *Journal of Clinical Periodontology* **28**, 723–729.

Koshy, G., Corbet, E.F. & Ishikawa, I. (2004). A full mouth disinfection approach to nonsurgical periodontal therapy-prevention of reinfection from bacterial reservoirs. *Periodontology 2000* **36**, 166–178.

Landry, C., Long, B., Singer, D. & Senthilse Lvan, A. (1999). Comparison to conventional instruments as assessed on extracted teeth (II). Subgingival roughness. *Journal of Clinical Periodontology* **26**, 548–551.

Lang, N.P., Alder, R., Joss, A. & Nyman, S. (1990). Absence of bleeding on probing. An indicator of periodontal stability. *Journal of Clinical Periodontology* **17**, 714–721.

Leon, L.E. & Vogel, R.I.A. (1987). Comparison of the effectiveness of hand scaling and ultrasonic debridement in furcations as evaluated by different dark field microscopy. *Journal of Clinical Periodontology* **58**, 86–94.

Lindhe, J. & Nyman, S. (1985). Scaling and granulation tissue removal in periodontal therapy. *Journal of Clinical Periodontology* **12**, 374–388.

Lindhe, J., Okamoto, H., Yoneyama, T., Haffajee, A. & Socransky, S.S. (1989). Longitudinal changes in periodontal disease in untreated subjects. *Journal of Clinical Periodontology* **16**, 662–670.

Listgarten, M.A. & Ellegaard, B. (1973). Electron microscopic evidence of a cellular attachment between junctional epithelium and dental calculus. *Journal of Periodontal Research* **8**, 143–150.

Loos, B., Kiger, R. & Egelberg, J. (1987). An evaluation of basic periodontal therapy using sonic and ultrasonic scalers. *Journal of Clinical Periodontology* **14**, 29–33.

Loos, B., Claffey, N. & Egelberg, J. (1988). Clinical and microbiological effects of root debridement in periodontal furcation pockets. *Journal of Clinical Periodontology* **15**, 453–463.

Loos, B., Nylund, K., Claffey, N. & Egelberg, J. (1989). Clinical effects of root debridement in molar and non-molar teeth. A 2-year follow up. *Journal of Clinical Periodontology* **16**, 498–504.

Magnusson, I., Lindhe, J., Yoneyama, T. & Liljenberg B. (1984). Recolonization of a subgingival mcrobiota following scaling in deep pockets. *Journal of Clinical Periodontology* **11**, 193–207.

Matia, J.I., Bissada, N.F., Maybury, J.E. & Ricchetti, P. (1986). Efficiency of scaling of the molar furcation area with and without surgical access. *International Journal of Periodontics and Restorative Dentistry* **6**, 24–35.

Mombelli, A., Nyman, S., Bragger, U., Wennstrom, J. & Lang, N.P. (1995). Clinical and microbiological changes associated with an altered subgingival environment induced by periodontal pocket reduction. *Journal of Clinical Periodontology* **22**, 780–787.

Mongardini, C., van Steenberghe, D., Dekeyser, C. & Quirynen, M. (1999). One stage full- versus partial-mouth disinfection in the treatment of chronic adult or generalized early-onset periodontitis. I. Long-term clinical observations. *Journal of Clinical Periodontology* **70**, 632–645.

Nordland, P., Garrett, S., Kiger, R., Vanooteghem, R., Hutchens, L.H. & Egelberg, J. (1987). The effect of plaque control and root debridement in molar teeth. *Journal of Clinical Periodontology* **14**, 231–236.

Nyman, S., Sarhed, G., Ericsson, I., Gottlow, J. & Karring, T. (1986). Role of "diseased" root cementum in healing following treatment of periodontal disease. An experimental study in the dog. *Journal of Periodontal Research* **21**, 496–503.

Nyman, S., Westfelt, E., Sarhed, G. & Karring, T. (1988). Role of "diseased" root cementum in healing following treatment of periodontal disease. A clinical study. *Journal of Clinical Periodontology* **15**, 464–468.

Obeid, P. & Bercy, P. (2005). Loss of tooth substance during root planing with various periodontal instruments: an *in vitro* study. *Clinical Oral Investigation* **9**, 118–123.

Obeid, P.R., D'hoove, W. & Bercy, P. (2004). Comparative clinical responses related to the use of various periodontal instruments. *Journal of Clinical Periodontology* **31**, 193–199.

Oda, S. & Ishikawa, I. (1989). *In vitro* effectiveness of a newly designed ultrasonic scaler tip for furcation areas. *Journal of Periodontology* **60**, 634–639.

Pihlstrom, B.L., Hargreaves, K.M., Bouwsma, O.J., Myers, W.R., Goodale, M.B. & Doyle, M.J. (1999). Pain after periodontal scaling and root planing. *Journal of the American Dental Association* **130**, 801–807.

Quirynen, M., Bollen, C.M., Vandekerckhove, B.N., Dekeyser, C., Papaioannou, W. & Eyssen, H. (1995). Full- vs. partial-mouth disinfection in the treatment of periodontal infections: short-term clinical and microbiological observations. *Journal of Dental Research* **74**, 1459–1467.

Quirynen, M., Mongardini, C., de Soete, M., Pauwels, M., Coucke, W., van Eldere, J. & van Steenberghe, D. (2000). The role of chlorhexidine in the one-stage full-mouth disinfection treatment of patients with advanced adult periodontitis. Long-term clinical and microbiological observations. *Journal of Clinical Periodontology* **27**, 578–589.

Quirynen, M., Mongardini, C., Pauwels, M., Bollen, C.M., Van Eldere, J. & van Steenberghe, D. (1999). One stage full- versus partial-mouth disinfection in the treatment of chronic adult or generalized early-onset periodontitis. II. Long-term impact on microbial load. *Journal of Periodontology* **70**, 646–656.

Rabbani, G.M., Ash, M.M. Jr. & Caffesse, R.G. (1981). The effectiveness of subgingival scaling and root planing in calculus removal. *Journal of Periodontology* **52**, 119–123.

Ramberg, P., Lindhe, J., Dahlen, G. & Volpe, A.R. (1994). The influence of gingival inflammation on *de novo* plaque formation. *Journal of Clinical Periodontology* **21**, 51–56.

Ramfjord, S.P., Caffesse R.G., Morrison, E.C., Hill, R.W., Kerry, G.J., Appleberry, E.A., Nissle, R.R. & Stults, D.L. (1987). Four modalities of periodontal treatment compared over five years. *Journal of Periodontal Research* **22**, 222–223.

Renvert, S., Wikstrom, M., Dahlen, G., Slots J. & Egelberg, J. (1990). On the inability of root debridement and periodontal surgery to eliminate *Actinobacillus actinomycetemcomitans* from periodontal pockets. *Journal of Clinical Periodontology* **17**, 351–355.

Ritz, L., Hefti, A.F. & Rateitschak, K.H. (1991). An *in vitro* investigation on the loss of root substance in scaling with various instruments. *Journal of Clinical Periodontology* **18**, 643–647.

Rivera-Hidalgo, F., Barnes, J.B. & Harrel, S.K. (1999). Aerosols and splatter production by focused spray and standard ultrasonic inserts. *Journal of Periodontology* **70**, 473–477.

Sbordone, L., Ramaglia, L., Gulletta, E. & Iacono, V. (1990). Recolonization of the subgingival microflora after scaling and root planing in human periodontitis. *Journal of Periodontology* **61**, 579–584.

Schmidlin, P.R., Beuchat, M., Busslinger, A., Lehmann, B. & Lutz, F. (2001). Tooth substance loss resulting from mechanical, sonic and ultrasonic root instrumentation assessed by liquid scintillation. *Journal of Clinical Periodontology* **28**, 1058–1066.

Schwarz, F., Sculean, A., Berakdar, M., Georg, T., Reich, E. & Becker, J. (2003). Clinical evaluation of an Er:YAG laser combined with scaling and root planing for non-surgical periodontal treatment. A controlled, prospective clinical study. *Journal of Clinical Periodontology* **30**, 26–34.

Schwarz, F., Sculean, A., Georg, T. & Reich, E. (2001). Periodontal treatment with an Er: YAG laser compared to scaling and root planing. A controlled clinical study. *Journal of Periodontology* **72**, 361–367.

Sculean, A., Schwartz, F., Berakdurm, M., Romanos, G.E., Brecx, M., Willershausen, B. & Becker, J. (2004). Non-surgical periodontal treatment with a new ultrasonic device (Vector ultrasonic system) or hand instruments. *Journal of Clinical Periodontology* **31**, 428–433.

Shah, S., Walmsley, A.D., Chapple, I.L. & Lumley, P.J. (1994). Variability of sonic scaler tip movement. *Journal of Clinical Periodontology* **21**, 705–709.

Sharawy A.M., Sabharwal, K., Socransky, S.S. & Lobene, R.R. (1966). A quantitative study of plaque and calculus formation in normal and periodontally involved mouths. *Journal of Periodontology* **37**, 495–501.

Sherman, P.R., Hutchens, L.H. Jr. & Jewson, L.G. (1990). The effectiveness of subgingival scaling and root planing. II. Clinical responses related to residual calculus. *Journal of Periodontology* **61**, 9–15.

Shiloah, J. & Patters, M.R. (1994). DNA probe analyses of the survival of selected periodontal pathogens following scaling, root planing, and intra-pocket irrigation. *Journal of Periodontology* **65**, 568–575.

Singer, D.L., Long, A.B., Lozanoff, S. & Senthilselvan, A. (1992). Evaluation of new periodontal curettes. An *in vitro* study. *Journal of Clinical Periodontology* **19**, 549–552.

Slots, J. & Rosling, B. (1983). Suppression of the periodontopathogenic microflora in localised juvenile periodontitis by systemic tetracycline. *Journal of Clinical Periodontology* **10**, 465–486.

Socransky, S.S., Haffajee, A.D., Cugini, M.A., Smith, C. & Kent R.L. Jr. (1998). Microbial complexes in subgingival plaque. *Journal of Clinical Periodontology* **25**, 134–144.

Takacs, V.J., Lie, T., Perala, D.G. & Adams, D.F. (1993). Efficacy of 5 machining instruments in scaling of molar furcations. *Journal of Periodontology* **64**, 228–236.

Tammaro, S., Wennstrom J.L. & Bergenholtz, G. (2000). Root dentine sensitivity following non-surgical periodontal treatment. *Journal of Clinical Periodontology* **27**, 690–697.

Teles, R.P., Haffajee, A.D. & Socransky, S.S. (2006). Microbiological goals of periodontal therapy. *Periodontology 2000* **42**, 180–218.

Timmerman, M.F., Menso, L., Steinfot, J., Van Winkelhoff, A.J. & Van der Weijden, G.A. (2004). Atmospheric contamination during ultrasonic scaling. *Journal of Clinical Periodontology* **31**, 458–462.

Tunkel, J., Heinecke, A. & Flemming, T.F. (2002). Systemic review of efficiency of machine-driven and manual subgingival debridement in treatment of chronic periodontitis. *Journal of Clinical Periodontology* **29**, 72–81.

Vandekerckhove, B.N., Bollen, C.M., Dekeyser, C., Darius, P. & Quirynen, M. (1996). Full- versus partial-mouth disinfection in the treatment of periodontal infections. Long-term clinical observations of a pilot study. *Journal of Periodontology* **67**, 1251–1259.

van Steenberghe, D., Garmyn, P., Geers, L., Hendrickx, E., Marechal, M., Huizar, K., Kristofferson, A., Meyer-Rosberg, K. & Vandenhoven, G. (2004). Patients' experience of pain and discomfort during instrumentation in the diagnosis and non-surgical treatment of periodontitis. *Journal of Periodontology* **75**, 1465–1470.

von Troil-Linden, B., Saarela, M., Matto, J., Alaluusua, S., Jousimies-Somer, H. & Asikainen, S. (1996). Source of suspected periodontal pathogens re-emerging after periodontal treatment. *Journal of Clinical Periodontology* **23**, 601–617.

Waerhaug J. (1978). Healing of the dento-epithelial junction following subgingival plaque control. I. As observed in human biopsy material. *Journal of Periodontology* **49**, 1–8.

Waerhaug, J. (1952). The gingival pocket; anatomy, pathology, deepening and elimination. *Odontologisk Tidskrift* **60**, 1–186.

Wennström, J.L., Tomasi, C., Bertelle, A. & Dellagesa, E. (2005). Full mouth ultrasonic debridement versus quadrant scaling and root planing as an initial approach for treatment of chronic periodontitis. *Journal of Clinical Periodontology* **32**, 851–859.

Wylam, J.M., Mealey, B.L., Mills, M.P., Waldrop, C.T. & Moskowicz, D.C. (1993). The clinical effectiveness of open versus closed scaling and root planning on multi-rooted teeth. *Journal of Periodontology* **6**, 1023–1028.

Ximenez-Fyvie, L.A., Haffajee, A.D., Som, S., Thompson, M., Torresyap, G. & Socransky, S.S. (2000). The effect of repeated professional supragingival plaque removal on the composition of the supra- and subgingival microbiota. *Journal of Clinical Periodontology* **27**, 637–647.

Yukna, R.A., Scott, J.B., Aichelmann-Reidy, M.E., Le Blanc, D.M. & Mayer, E.T. (1997). Clinical evaluation of speed and effectiveness of subgingival calculus removal on single-rooted teeth with diamond-coated ultrasonic tips. *Journal of Periodontology* **68**, 436–442.

Part 12: Additional Therapy

38   Periodontal Surgery: Access Therapy, 783
     Jan L. Wennström, Lars Heijl, and Jan Lindhe

39   Treatment of Furcation-Involved Teeth, 823
     Gianfranco Carnevale, Roberto Pontoriero, and Jan Lindhe

40   Endodontics and Periodontics, 848
     Gunnar Bergenholtz and Gunnar Hasselgren

41   Treatment of Peri-implant Lesions, 875
     Tord Berglundh, Niklaus P. Lang, and Jan Lindhe

42   Antibiotics in Periodontal Therapy, 882
     Andrea Mombelli

Chapter 38

Periodontal Surgery: Access Therapy

Jan L. Wennström, Lars Heijl, and Jan Lindhe

Introduction, 783
Techniques in periodontal pocket surgery, 783
　Gingivectomy procedures, 784
　Flap procedures, 786
　Regenerative procedures, 793
Distal wedge procedures, 794
Osseous surgery, 795
　Osteoplasty, 796
　Ostectomy, 796
General guidelines for periodontal surgery, 797
　Objectives of surgical treatment, 797
　Indications for surgical treatment, 797
　Contraindications for periodontal surgery, 799

Local anesthesia in periodontal surgery, 800
Instruments used in periodontal surgery, 802
Selection of surgical technique, 805
Root surface instrumentation, 808
Root surface conditioning/biomodification, 808
Suturing, 808
Periodontal dressings, 811
Post-operative pain control, 812
Post-surgical care, 812
Outcome of surgical periodontal therapy, 812
　Healing following surgical pocket therapy, 812
　Clinical outcome of surgical access therapy in comparison to
　　non-surgical therapy, 814

Introduction

Since most forms of periodontal disease are plaque-associated disorders, it is obvious that surgical access therapy can only be considered as adjunctive to cause-related therapy (see Chapters 34 to 37). Therefore, the various surgical methods described below should be evaluated on the basis of their potential to facilitate removal of subgingival deposits and self-performed plaque control and thereby enhance the long-term preservation of the periodontium.

The decision concerning what type of periodontal surgery should be performed and how many sites should be included is usually made after the effect of initial cause-related measures has been evaluated. The time lapse between termination of the initial cause-related phase of therapy and this evaluation may vary from 1 to 6 months. This routine has the following advantages:

- Removal of calculus and bacterial plaque will eliminate or markedly reduce the inflammatory cell infiltrate in the gingiva (edema, hyperemia, flabby tissue consistency), thereby making assessment of the "true" gingival contours and pocket depths possible.
- Reduction of gingival inflammation makes the soft tissues more fibrous and thus firmer, which facili-

tates surgical handling of the soft tissues. The propensity for bleeding is reduced, making inspection of the surgical field easier.
- A better basis for a proper assessment of the prognosis has been established. The effectiveness of the patient's home care, which is of decisive importance for the long-term prognosis, can be properly evaluated. Lack of effective self-performed infection control will often mean that the patient should be excluded from surgical treatment.

Techniques in periodontal pocket surgery

Over the years, several different surgical techniques have been described and used in periodontal therapy. A superficial review of the literature in this area may give the reader a somewhat confusing picture of the specific objectives and indications relevant for various surgical techniques. It is a matter of historic interest that the first surgical techniques used in periodontal therapy were described as means of gaining access to diseased root surfaces. Such access could be accomplished without excision of the soft tissue pocket ("open-view operations"). Later, procedures were described by which the "diseased gingiva" was excised (gingivectomy procedures).

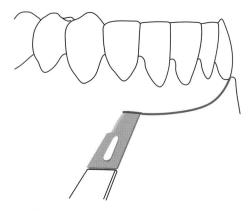

Fig. 38-1 Gingivectomy. The straight incision technique (Robicsek 1884).

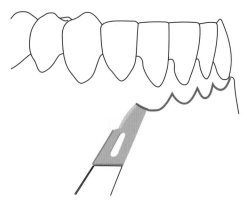

Fig. 38-2 Gingivectomy. The scalloped incision technique (Zentler 1918).

The concept that not only inflamed soft tissue but also "infected and necrotic bone" had to be eliminated called for the development of surgical techniques by which the alveolar bone could be exposed and resected (flap procedures). Other concepts such as (1) the importance of maintaining the mucogingival complex (i.e. a wide zone of gingiva) and (2) the possibility for regeneration of periodontal tissues have also prompted the introduction of "tailor-made" surgical techniques.

In the following, surgical procedures will be described which represent important steps in the development of the surgical component of periodontal therapy.

Gingivectomy procedures

The surgical approach as an alternative to subgingival scaling for pocket therapy was already recognized in the latter part of the nineteenth century, when Robicsek (1884) pioneered the so-called *gingivectomy* procedure. Gingivectomy was later defined by Grant *et al.* (1979) as being "the excision of the soft tissue wall of a pathologic periodontal pocket". The surgical procedure, which aimed at "pocket elimination", was usually combined with recontouring of the diseased gingiva to restore physiologic form.

Robicsek (1884) and, later, Zentler (1918) described the gingivectomy procedure in the following way. The line to which the gum is to be resected is determined first. Following a straight (Robicsek) (Fig. 38-1) or scalloped (Zentler) (Fig. 38-2) incision, first on the labial and then on the lingual surface of each tooth, the diseased tissue should be loosened and lifted out by means of a hook-shaped instrument. After elimination of the soft tissue, the exposed alveolar bone should be scraped. The area should then be covered with some kind of antibacterial gauze or be painted with disinfecting solutions. The result obtained should include eradication of the deepened periodontal pocket and formation of an area which can be kept clean more easily.

Technique

The gingivectomy procedure as it is employed today was described in 1951 by Goldman.

- When the dentition in the area scheduled for surgery has been properly anesthetized, the depths of the pathological pockets are identified with a conventional periodontal probe (Fig. 38-3a). At the level of the bottom of the pocket, the gingiva is pierced with the probe and a bleeding point is produced on the outer surface of the soft tissue (Fig. 38-3b). The pockets are probed and bleeding points produced at several location points around each tooth in the area. The series of bleeding points produced describes the depth of the pockets in the area scheduled for treatment and is used as a guideline for the incision.
- The primary incision (Fig. 38-4), which may be made by a scalpel (blade No. 12B or 15; Bard-Parker®) in either a Bard-Parker handle or an angulated handle (e.g. a Blake's handle), or a Kirkland knife No. 15/16, should be planned to give a thin and properly festooned margin of the remaining gingiva. Thus, in areas where the gingiva is bulky, the incision must be placed at a level more apical to the level of the bleeding points than in areas with a thin gingiva, where a less accentuated bevel is needed. The beveled incision is directed towards the base of the pocket or to a level slightly apical to the apical extension of the junctional epithelium. In areas where the interdental pockets are deeper than the buccal or lingual pockets, additional amounts of buccal and/or lingual (palatal) gingiva must be removed in order to establish a "physiologic" contour of the gingival margin. This is often accomplished by initiating the incision at a more apical level.
- Once the primary incision is completed on the buccal and lingual aspects of the teeth, the interproximal soft tissue is separated from the interdental periodontium by a secondary incision using an Orban knife (No. 1 or 2) or a Waerhaug knife (No. 1 or 2; a saw-toothed modification of the Orban knife) (Fig. 38-5).

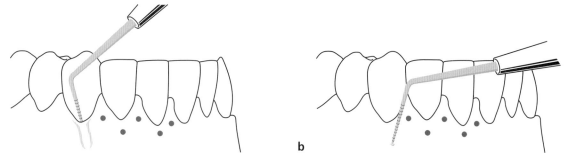

Fig. 38-3 Gingivectomy. Pocket marking. (a) An ordinary periodontal probe is used to identify the bottom of the deepened pocket. (b) When the depth of the pocket has been assessed an equivalent distance is delineated on the outer aspect of the gingiva. The tip of the probe is then turned horizontally and used to produce a bleeding point at the level of the bottom of the probeable pocket.

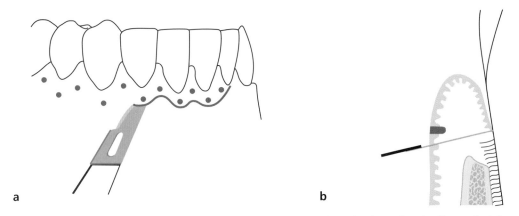

Fig. 38-4 Gingivectomy. (a) The primary incision. (b) The incision is terminated at a level apical to the "bottom" of the pocket and is angulated to give the cut surface a distinct bevel.

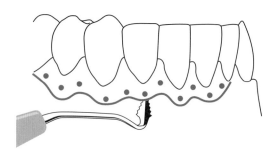

Fig. 38-5 Gingivectomy. The secondary incision through the interdental area is performed with the use of a Waerhaug knife.

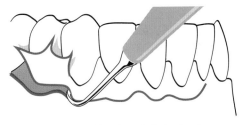

Fig. 38-6 Gingivectomy. The detached gingiva is removed with a scaler.

- The incised tissues are carefully removed by means of a curette or a scaler (Fig. 38-6). Remaining tissue tabs are removed with a curette or a pair of scissors. Pieces of gauze packs often have to be placed in the interdental areas to control bleeding. When the field of operation is properly prepared, the exposed root surfaces are carefully scaled and planed.
- Following meticulous debridement, the dentogingival regions are probed again to detect any remaining pockets (Fig. 38-7). The gingival contour is checked and, if necessary, corrected by means of knives or rotating diamond burs.
- To protect the incised area during the period of healing, the wound surface must be covered by a

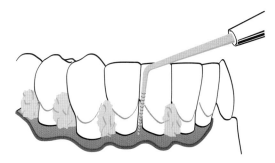

Fig. 38-7 Gingivectomy. Probing for residual pockets. Gauze packs have been placed in the interdental spaces to control bleeding.

periodontal dressing (Fig. 38-8). The dressing should be closely adapted to the buccal and lingual wound surfaces as well as to the interproximal spaces. Care should be taken not to allow the

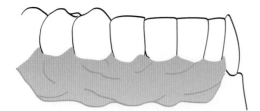

Fig. 38-8 Gingivectomy. The periodontal dressing has been applied and properly secured.

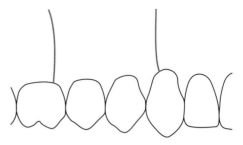

Fig. 38-9 Original Widman flap. Two releasing incisions demarcate the area scheduled for surgical therapy. A scalloped reverse bevel incision is made in the gingival margin to connect the two releasing incisions.

dressing to become too bulky, since this is not only uncomfortable for the patient, but also facilitates dislodgement of the dressing.

- The dressing should remain in position for 10–14 days. After removal of the dressing, the teeth must be cleaned and polished. The root surfaces are carefully checked and remaining calculus removed with a curette. Excessive granulation tissue is eliminated with a curette. The patient is instructed to clean properly the operated segments of the dentition, which now have a different morphology compared to the pre-operative situation.

Flap procedures

The original Widman flap

In 1918 Leonard Widman published one of the first detailed descriptions of the use of a flap procedure for pocket elimination. In his article "The operative treatment of pyorrhea alveolaris" Widman described a mucoperiosteal flap design aimed at removing the pocket epithelium and the inflamed connective tissue, thereby facilitating optimal cleaning of the root surfaces.

Technique
- Sectional releasing incisions were first made to demarcate the area scheduled for surgery (Fig. 38-9). These incisions were made from the mid-buccal gingival margins of the two peripheral teeth of the treatment area and were continued several millimeters out into the alveolar mucosa. The two releasing incisions were connected by a gingival incision, which followed the outline of the gingival margin and *separated the pocket epithelium and the inflamed connective tissue from the non-inflamed gingiva*. Similar releasing and gingival incisions, if needed, were made on the lingual aspect of the teeth.
- A mucoperiosteal flap was elevated to expose at least 2–3 mm of the marginal alveolar bone. The collar of inflamed tissue around the neck of the teeth was removed with curettes (Fig. 38-10) and the exposed root surfaces were carefully scaled. Bone recontouring was recommended in order to achieve an ideal anatomic form of the underlying alveolar bone (Fig. 38-11).

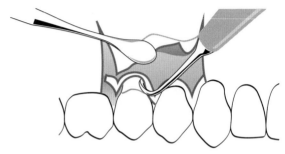

Fig. 38-10 Original Widman flap. The collar of inflamed gingival tissue is removed following the elevation of a mucoperiosteal flap.

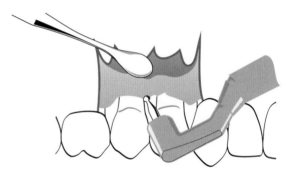

Fig. 38-11 Original Widman flap. By bone recontouring, a "physiologic" contour of the alveolar bone may be re-established.

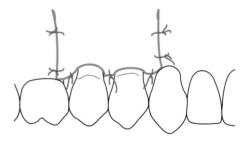

Fig. 38-12 Original Widman flap. The coronal ends of the buccal and lingual flaps are placed at the alveolar bone crest and secured in this position by interdentally placed sutures.

- Following careful debridement of the teeth in the surgical area, the buccal and lingual flaps were laid back over the alveolar bone and secured in this position with interproximal sutures (Fig. 38-12). Widman pointed out the importance of placing the soft tissue margin at the level of the alveolar bone crest, so that no pockets would remain. The surgical procedure resulted in the exposure of root surfaces. Often the interproximal areas were left without soft tissue coverage of the alveolar bone.

The main advantages of the *"original Widman flap"* procedure in comparison to the gingivectomy procedure included, according to Widman (1918):

- Less discomfort for the patient, since healing occurred by primary intention
- It was possible to re-establish a proper contour of the alveolar bone in sites with angular bony defects.

The Neumann flap

Only a few years later, Neumann (1920) suggested the use of a flap procedure, which in some respects was different from that originally described by Widman.

Technique
- According to the technique suggested by Neumann, an intracrevicular incision was made through the base of the gingival pockets and the entire gingiva (and part of the alveolar mucosa) was elevated in a mucoperiosteal flap. Sectional releasing incisions were made to demarcate the area of surgery.
- Following flap elevation, the inside of the flap was curetted to remove the pocket epithelium and the granulation tissue. The root surfaces were subsequently carefully "cleaned". Any irregularities of the alveolar bone were corrected to give the bone crest a horizontal outline.
- The flaps were then trimmed to allow both an optimal adaptation to the teeth and a proper coverage of the alveolar bone on both the buccal/lingual (palatal) and the interproximal sites. With regard to pocket elimination, Neumann (1920) pointed out the importance of removing the soft tissue pockets, i.e. replacing the flap at the crest of the alveolar bone.

The modified flap operation

In a publication from 1931 Kirkland described a surgical procedure to be used in the treatment of "periodontal pus pockets". The procedure was called the *modified flap operation*, and is basically an access flap for proper root debridement.

Technique
- In this procedure incisions were made intracrevicularly through the bottom of the pocket (Fig. 38-13) on both the labial and the lingual aspects of the interdental area. The incisions were extended in a mesial and distal direction.

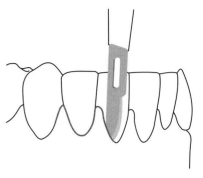

Fig. 38-13 Modified flap operation (the Kirkland flap). Intracrevicular incision.

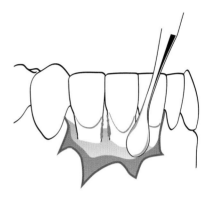

Fig. 38-14 Modified flap operation (the Kirkland flap). The gingiva is retracted to expose the "diseased" root surface.

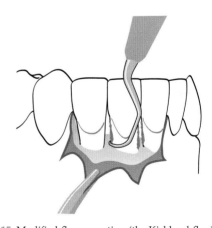

Fig. 38-15 Modified flap operation (the Kirkland flap). The exposed root surfaces are subjected to mechanical debridement.

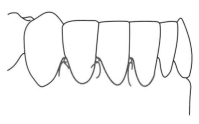

Fig. 38-16 Modified flap operation (the Kirkland flap). The flaps are replaced to their original position and sutured.

- The gingiva was retracted labially and lingually to expose the diseased root surfaces (Fig. 38-14) which were carefully debrided (Fig. 38-15). Angular bony defects were curetted.
- Following the elimination of the pocket epithelium and granulation tissue from the inner surface of the flaps, these were *replaced* to their original position and secured with interproximal sutures (Fig. 38-16). Thus, no attempt was made to reduce the pre-operative depth of the pockets.

In contrast to the *original Widman flap* as well as the *Neumann flap*, the *modified flap operation* did not include (1) extensive sacrifice of non-inflamed tissues and (2) apical displacement of the gingival margin. The method could be useful in the anterior regions of the dentition for esthetic reasons, since the root surfaces were not markedly exposed. Another advantage of the *modified flap operation* was the potential for bone regeneration in intrabony defects which frequently occurred according to Kirkland (1931).

The main objectives of the flap procedures so far described were to:

- Facilitate the debridement of the root surfaces as well as the removal of the pocket epithelium and the inflamed connective tissue
- Eliminate the deepened pockets (the *original Widman flap* and the *Neumann flap*)
- Cause a minimal amount of trauma to the periodontal tissues and discomfort to the patient.

The apically repositioned flap

In the 1950s and 1960s new surgical techniques for the removal of soft and, when indicated, hard tissue periodontal pockets were described in the literature. The importance of maintaining *an adequate zone of attached gingiva* after surgery was now emphasized. One of the first authors to describe a technique for the preservation of the gingiva following surgery was Nabers (1954). The surgical technique developed by Nabers was originally denoted "repositioning of attached gingiva" and was later modified by Ariaudo and Tyrrell (1957). In 1962 Friedman proposed the term *apically repositioned flap* to describe more appropriately the surgical technique introduced by Nabers. Friedman emphasized the fact that, at the end of the surgical procedure, the entire complex of the soft tissues (gingiva and alveolar mucosa) rather than the gingiva alone was displaced in an apical direction. Thus, rather than excising the amount of gingiva which would be in excess after osseous surgery (if performed), the whole muco-gingival complex was maintained and repositioned apically. This surgical technique was used on buccal surfaces in both upper and lower jaws and on lingual surfaces in the lower jaw, while an excisional technique had to be used on the palatal aspect of maxillary teeth where the lack of alveolar mucosa made it impossible to reposition the flap in an apical direction.

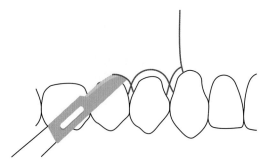

Fig. 38-17 Apically repositioned flap. Following a vertical releasing incision, the reverse bevel incision is made through the gingiva and the periosteum to separate the inflamed tissue adjacent to the tooth from the flap.

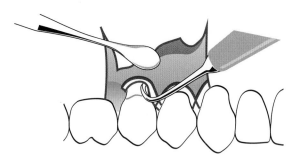

Fig. 38-18 Apically repositioned flap. A mucoperiosteal flap is raised and the tissue collar remaining around the teeth, including the pocket epithelium and the inflamed connective tissue, is removed with a currette.

Technique

According to Friedman (1962) the technique should be performed in the following way:

- A reverse bevel incision is made using a scalpel with a Bard-Parker blade (No. 12B or No. 15). How far from the buccal/lingual gingival margin the incision should be made is dependent on the pocket depth as well as the thickness and the width of the gingiva (Fig. 38-17). If pre-operatively the gingiva is thin and only a narrow zone of keratinized tissue is present, the incision should be made close to the tooth. The beveling incision should be given a scalloped outline, to ensure maximal interproximal coverage of the alveolar bone when the flap subsequently is repositioned. Vertical releasing incisions extending out into the alveolar mucosa (i.e. past the muco-gingival junction) are made at each of the end points of the reverse incision, thereby making apical repositioning of the flap possible.
- A full-thickness mucoperiosteal flap including buccal/lingual gingiva and alveolar mucosa is raised by means of a mucoperiosteal elevator. The flap has to be elevated beyond the muco-gingival line in order to be able later to reposition the soft tissue apically. The marginal collar of tissue, including pocket epithelium and granulation tissue, is removed with curettes (Fig. 38-18), and

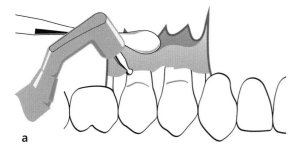
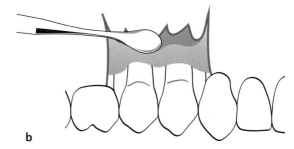

Fig. 38-19 Apically repositioned flap. Osseous surgery is performed with the use of a rotating bur (a) to recapture the physiologic contour of the alveolar bone (b).

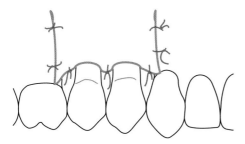

Fig. 38-20 Apically repositioned flap. The flaps are repositioned in an apical direction to the level of the recontoured alveolar bone crest and retained in this position by sutures.

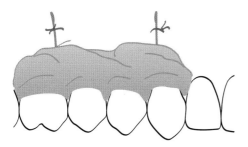

Fig. 38-21 Apically repositioned flap. A periodontal dressing is placed over the surgical area to ensure that the flaps remain in the correct position during healing.

the exposed root surfaces are carefully scaled and planed.
- The alveolar bone crest is recontoured with the objective of recapturing the normal form of the alveolar process but at a more apical level (Fig. 38-19). The osseous surgery is performed using burs and/or bone chisels.
- Following careful adjustment, the buccal/lingual flap is repositioned to the level of the newly recontoured alveolar bone crest and secured in this position (Fig. 38-20). The incisional and excisional technique used means that it is not always possible to obtain proper soft tissue coverage of the denuded interproximal alveolar bone. A periodontal dressing should therefore be applied to protect the exposed bone and to retain the soft tissue at the level of the bone crest (Fig. 38-21). After healing, an "adequate" zone of gingiva is preserved and no residual pockets should remain.

To handle periodontal pockets on the palatal aspect of the maxillary teeth, Friedman described a modification of the "apically repositioned flap", which he termed the *beveled flap*:

- In order to prepare the tissue at the gingival margin to follow the outline of the alveolar bone crest properly, a conventional mucoperiosteal flap is first resected (Fig. 38-22).
- The tooth surfaces are debrided and osseous recontouring is performed (Fig. 38-23).
- The palatal flap is subsequently replaced and the gingival margin is prepared and adjusted to the alveolar bone crest by a secondary scalloped and beveled incision (Fig. 38-24). The flap is secured in this position with interproximal sutures (Fig. 38-25).

Among a number of suggested advantages of the *apically repositioned flap* procedure, the following have been emphasized:

- Minimum pocket depth post-operatively
- If optimal soft tissue coverage of the alveolar bone is obtained, the post-surgical bone loss is minimal
- The post-operative position of the gingival margin may be controlled and the entire muco-gingival complex may be maintained.

The sacrifice of periodontal tissues by bone resection and the subsequent exposure of root surfaces (which may cause esthetic and root sensitivity problems) were regarded as the main disadvantages of this technique.

The modified Widman flap

Ramfjord and Nissle (1974) described the *modified Widman flap* technique that is also recognized as the *open flap curettage* technique. It should be noted that, while the *original Widman flap* technique included both apical displacement of the flaps and osseous recontouring (elimination of bony defects) to obtain proper pocket elimination, the *modified Widman flap* technique is not intended to meet these objectives.

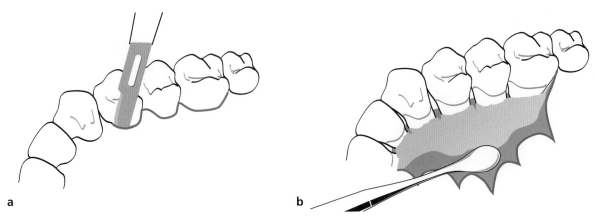

a

b

Fig. 38-22 Bevelled flap. A primary incision is made intracrevicularly through the bottom of the periodontal pocket (a) and a conventional mucoperiosteal flap is elevated (b).

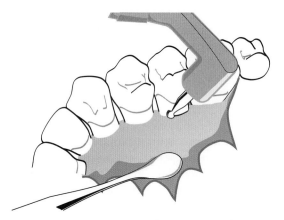

Fig. 38-23 Bevelled flap. Scaling, root planing, and osseous recontouring are performed in the surgical area.

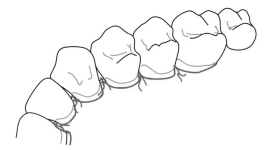

Fig. 38-25 Bevelled flap. The shortened and thinned flap is replaced over the alveolar bone and in close contact with the root surfaces.

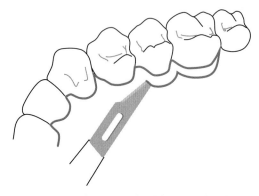

Fig. 38-24 Bevelled flap. The palatal flap is replaced and a secondary, scalloped, reverse bevel incision is made to adjust the length of the flap to the height of the remaining alveolar bone.

Technique

- According to the description by Ramfjord and Nissle (1974) the *initial incision* (Fig. 38-26), which may be performed with a Bard-Parker knife (No. 11), should be parallel to the long axis of the tooth and placed approximately 1 mm from the buccal gingival margin in order to properly separate the pocket epithelium from the flap. If the pockets on the buccal aspects of the teeth are less than 2 mm deep or if esthetic considerations are important, an intracrevicular incision may be made. Furthermore, the scalloped incision should be extended as far as possible in between the teeth, to allow maximum amounts of the interdental gingiva to be included in the flap. A similar incision technique is used on the palatal aspect. Often, however, the scalloped outline of the initial incision may be accentuated by placing the knife at a distance of 1–2 mm from the mid-palatal surface of the teeth. By extending the incision as far as possible in between the teeth, sufficient amounts of tissue can be included in the palatal flap to allow for proper coverage of the interproximal bone when the flap is sutured. Vertical releasing incisions are not usually required.
- Buccal and palatal full-thickness flaps are carefully elevated with a mucoperiosteal elevator. The flap elevation should be limited and allow only a few millimeters of the alveolar bone crest to become exposed. To facilitate the gentle separation of the collar of pocket epithelium and granulation tissue from the root surfaces, an intracrevicular incision is made around the teeth (*second incision*) to the alveolar crest (Fig. 38-27).
- A *third incision* (Fig. 38-28) made in a horizontal direction and in a position close to the surface of

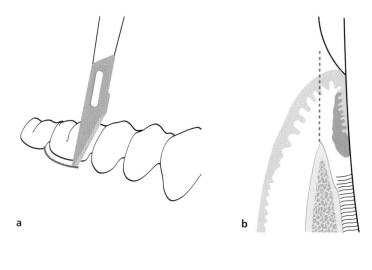

Fig. 38-26 Modified Widman flap. The initial incision is placed 0.5–1 mm from the gingival margin (a) and parallel to the long axis of the tooth (b).

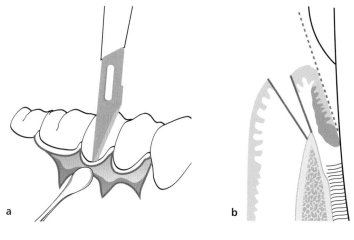

Fig. 38-27 Modified Widman flap. Following careful elevation of the flaps, a second intracrevicular incision (a) is made to the alveolar bone crest (b) to separate the tissue collar from the root surface.

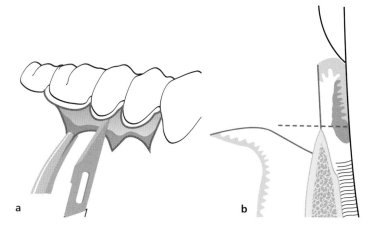

Fig. 38-28 Modified Widman flap. A third incision is made perpendicular to the root surface (a) and as close as possible to the bone crest (b), thereby separating the tissue collar from the alveolar bone.

the alveolar bone crest separates the soft tissue collar of the root surfaces from the bone.

- The pocket epithelium and the granulation tissues are removed by means of curettes. The exposed roots are carefully scaled and planed, except for a narrow area close to the alveolar bone crest in which remnants of attachment fibers may be preserved. Angular bony defects are carefully curetted.
- Following the curettage, the flaps are trimmed and adjusted to the alveolar bone to obtain complete coverage of the interproximal bone (Fig. 38-29). If this adaptation cannot be achieved by soft tissue recontouring, some bone may be removed from the outer aspects of the alveolar process in order to facilitate the all-important flap adaptation. The flaps are sutured together with individual interproximal sutures. Surgical dressing may be placed over the area to ensure close adaptation of the flaps to the alveolar bone and root surfaces. The dressing, as well as the sutures, is removed after 1 week.

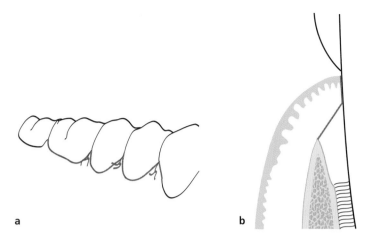

a

b

Fig. 38-29 Modified Widman flap. (a) Following proper debridement and currettage of angular bone defects, the flaps are carefully adjusted to cover the alveolar bone and sutured. (b) Complete coverage of the interdental bone as well as close adaptation of the flaps to the tooth surfaces should be accomplished.

The main advantages of the *modified Widman flap* technique in comparison to other procedures previously described are, according to Ramfjord and Nissle (1974):

- The possibility of obtaining a close adaptation of the soft tissues to the root surfaces
- The minimum of trauma to which the alveolar bone and the soft connective tissues are exposed
- Less exposure of the root surfaces, which from an esthetic point of view is an advantage in the treatment of anterior segments of the dentition.

The papilla preservation flap

In order to preserve the interdental soft tissues for maximum soft tissue coverage following surgical intervention involving treatment of proximal osseous defects, Takei *et al.* (1985) proposed a surgical approach called *papilla preservation technique*. Later, Cortellini *et al.* (1995b, 1999) described modifications of the flap design to be used in combination with regenerative procedures. For esthetic reasons, the papilla preservation technique is often utilized in the surgical treatment of anterior tooth regions.

Technique
- According to the description by Takei *et al.* (1985) the *papilla preservation flap technique* is initiated by an intra-sulcular incision at the facial and proximal aspects of the teeth without making incisions through the interdental papillae (Fig. 38-30a). Subsequently, an intra-sulcular incision is made along

the lingual/palatal aspect of the teeth with a semilunar incision made across each interdental area. The semilunar incision should dip apically at least 5 mm from the line angles of the teeth, which will allow the interdental tissue to be dissected from the lingual/palatal aspect so that it can be elevated intact with the facial flap. In situations where an osseous defect has a wide extension into the lingual/palatal area, the semilunar incision may be placed on the facial aspect of the interdental area to have the papillae included with the lingual/palatal flap.
- A curette or interproximal knife is used to free the interdental papilla carefully from the underlying hard tissue. The detached interdental tissue is pushed through the embrasure with a blunt instrument (Fig. 38-30b).
- A full-thickness flap is reflected with a periosteal elevator on both facial and lingual/palatal surfaces. The exposed root surfaces are thoroughly scaled and root planed and bone defects carefully curetted (Fig. 38-31).
- While holding the reflected flap, the margins of the flap and the interdental tissue are scraped to remove pocket epithelium and excessive granulation tissue. In anterior areas, the trimming of granulation tissue should be limited in order to maintain the maximum thickness of tissue.
- The flaps are repositioned and sutured using cross mattress sutures (Fig. 38-32). Alternatively, a direct suture of the semilunar incisions can be done as the only means of flap closure. A surgical dressing may be placed to protect the surgical

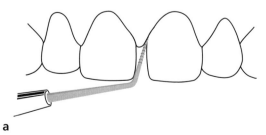

a

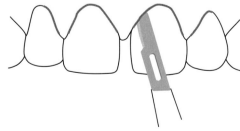

b

Fig. 38-30 Papilla preservation flap. Intracrevicular incisions are made at the facial and proximal aspects of the teeth.

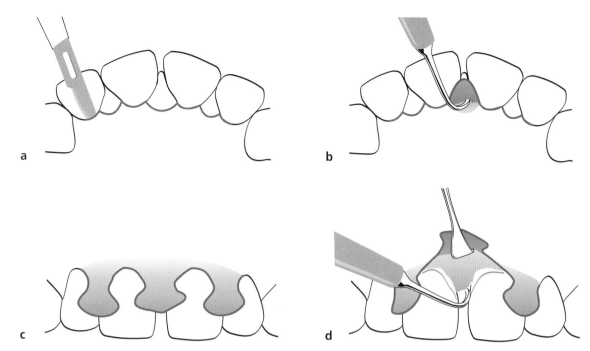

Fig. 38-31 Papilla preservation flap. (a) An intracrevicular incision is made along the lingual/palatal aspect of the teeth with a semilunar incision made across each interdental area. (b) A curette or a papilla elevator is used to carefully free the interdental papilla from the underlying hard tissue. (c,d) The detached interdental tissue is pushed through the embrasure with a blunt instrument to be included in the facial flap.

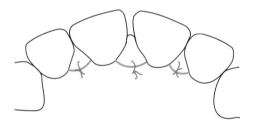

Fig. 38-32 Papilla preservation flap. The flap is replaced and sutures are placed on the palatal aspect of the interdental areas.

area. The dressing and sutures are removed after 1 week.

Regenerative procedures

In the 1980s treatment of periodontal pockets was given a new dimension when it was shown that, with specific surgical handling of the periodontal wound, a significant amount of new connective tissue attachment is achievable following surgical treatment (Nyman *et al*. 1982; Bowers *et al*. 1989).

Obtaining periodontal regeneration has always been a major challenge to the periodontist and several approaches to periodontal regeneration have been used throughout the years. The earliest attempts involved various bone-grafting procedures, such as the use of autogenous grafts from both extraoral and intraoral donor sites, allogenic marrow grafts, and non-decalcified/decalcified lyophilized bone grafts, or "implant" procedures utilizing slowly resorbable tricalcium phosphate and non-resorbable, non-

porous hydroxyapatite. Other approaches to periodontal regeneration involved the use of citric acid for root surface demineralization or the use of methods for improved root surface biocompatibility or to enhance cellular responses.

The use of physical barriers, such as membranes (non-biodegradable or biodegradable), to retard or prevent apical migration of epithelium as well as exclude gingival connective tissue from the healing wound, formed the basis for the concept known as "guided tissue regeneration" (Gottlow *et al*. 1986). The procedure can be described as a coronally repositioned flap procedure without bone recontouring, with the adjunctive use of a membrane tightened to the tooth to cover the exposed root surface and adjacent intrabony defect before repositioning the soft tissue flaps.

In the late 1990s a new approach to periodontal regeneration was presented, which involves the use of a derivative of enamel matrix proteins (Hammarström 1997; Heijl *et al*. 1997). These proteins are involved in the embryogenesis of cementum, periodontal ligament, and supporting bone, and when applied to the exposed root surface facing an intrabony periodontal defect they mediate regeneration of a new attachment apparatus. The surgical procedure is performed as a coronally repositioned flap procedure without bone recontouring. Before repositioning of the soft tissue flaps, the exposed roots are treated with EDTA for removal of the "smear layer", followed by the application of the derivative of enamel matrix proteins.

Various regenerative procedures for surgical treatment of periodontal lesions, as well as the biologic basis for periodontal regeneration, are discussed in detail in Chapters 25 and 43.

Distal wedge procedures

In many cases the treatment of periodontal pockets on the distal surface of distal molars is complicated by the presence of bulbous tissues over the tuberosity or by a prominent retromolar pad. The most direct approach to pocket elimination in such cases in the maxillary jaw is the gingivectomy procedure. The incision is started on the distal surface of the tuberosity and carried forward to the base of the pocket of the distal surface of the molar (Fig. 38-33).

However, when only limited amounts of keratinized gingiva are present, or none at all, or if a distal angular bony defect has been diagnosed, the bulbous tissue should be reduced in size rather than being

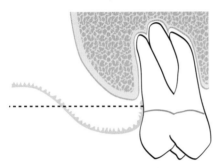

Fig. 38-33 Distal wedge procedure. Simple gingivectomy incision (broken line) can be used to eliminate a soft tissue pocket and adjacent fibrous tissue pad behind a maxillary molar.

removed *in toto*. This may be accomplished by the *distal wedge procedure* (Robinson 1966). This technique facilitates access to the osseous defect and makes it possible to preserve sufficient amounts of gingiva and mucosa to achieve soft tissue coverage.

Technique
- Buccal and lingual incisions are made in a vertical direction through the tuberosity or retromolar pad to form a triangular wedge (Fig. 38-34a). The facial and lingual incisions should be extended in a mesial direction along the buccal and lingual surfaces of the distal molar to facilitate flap elevation.
- The facial and lingual walls of the tuberosity or retromolar pad are deflected and the incised wedge of tissue is dissected and separated from the bone (Fig. 38-34b).
- The walls of the facial and lingual flaps are then reduced in thickness by undermining incisions (Fig. 38-34c). Loose tags of tissue are removed and the root surfaces are scaled and planed. If necessary, the bone is recontoured.
- The buccal and lingual flaps are replaced over the exposed alveolar bone, and the edges trimmed to avoid overlapping wound margins. The flaps are secured in this position with interrupted sutures (Fig. 38-34d). The sutures are removed after approximately 1 week.

The original distal wedge procedure may be modified according to individual requirements. Some commonly used modifications of the incision

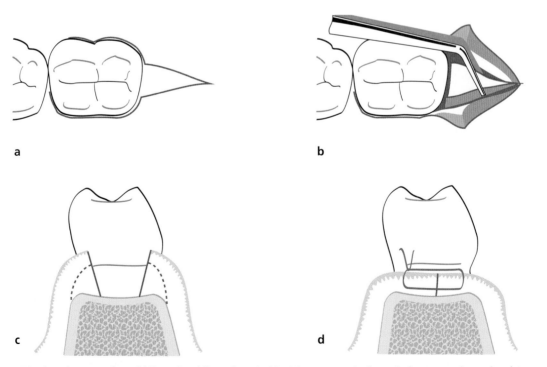

Fig. 38-34 Distal wedge procedure. (a) Buccal and lingual vertical incisions are made through the retromolar pad to form a triangle behind a manibular molar. (b) The triangular-shaped wedge of tissue is dissected from the underlying bone and removed. (c) The walls of the buccal and lingual flaps are reduced in thickness by undermining incisions (broken lines). (d) The flaps, which have been trimmed and shortened to avoid overlapping wound margins, are sutured.

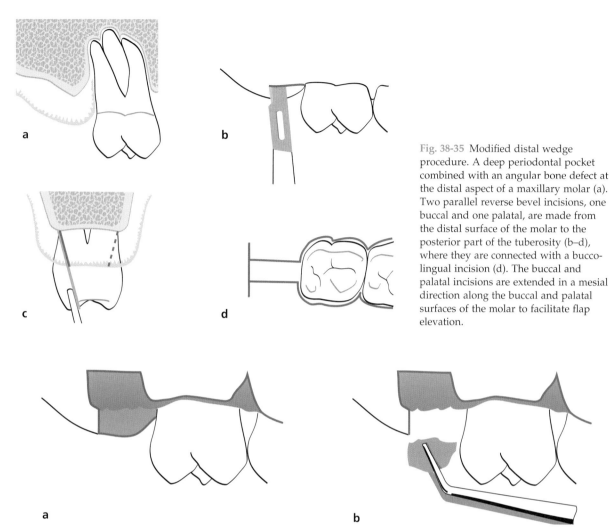

Fig. 38-35 Modified distal wedge procedure. A deep periodontal pocket combined with an angular bone defect at the distal aspect of a maxillary molar (a). Two parallel reverse bevel incisions, one buccal and one palatal, are made from the distal surface of the molar to the posterior part of the tuberosity (b–d), where they are connected with a bucco-lingual incision (d). The buccal and palatal incisions are extended in a mesial direction along the buccal and palatal surfaces of the molar to facilitate flap elevation.

Fig. 38-36 Modified distal wedge procedure. Buccal and palatal flaps are elevated (a) and the rectangular wedge is released from the tooth and underlying bone by sharp dissection and then removed (b).

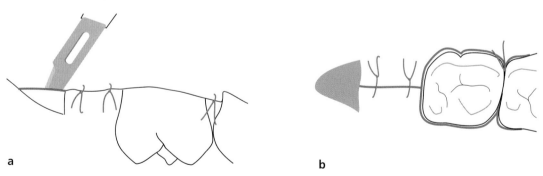

Fig. 38-37 Modified distal wedge procedure. Following bone recontouring and root debridement, the flaps are trimmed and shortened to avoid overlapping wound margins and sutured (a,b). A close soft tissue adaptation should be accomplished to the distal surface of the molar. The remaining fibrous tissue pad distal to the bucco-lingual incision line is "levelled" by the use of a gingivectomy incision.

technique are illustrated in Figs. 38-35 to 38-38, all having the goals of eliminating the deep pocket and achieving mucosal coverage of the remaining periodontium.

Osseous surgery

The principles of osseous surgery in periodontal therapy were outlined by Schluger (1949) and Goldman (1950). They pointed out that alveolar bone loss caused by inflammatory periodontal disease often results in an uneven outline of the bone crest. Since, according to these authors, the gingival contour is closely dependent on the contour of the underlying bone as well as the proximity and anatomy of adjacent tooth surfaces, the elimination of soft tissue pockets often has to be combined with osseous reshaping and the elimination of osseous craters and

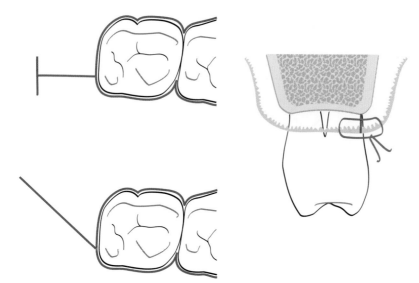

Fig. 38-38 Modified incision techniques in distal wedge procedures. To ensure optimal flap adaptation at the furcation site the incision technique may be modified. The amount of attached keratinized tissue present as well as the accessibility to the retromolar area has to be considered when placing the incision.

angular bony defects to establish and maintain shallow pockets and optimal gingival contour after surgery.

Osteoplasty

The term *osteoplasty* was introduced by Friedman in 1955. The purpose of osteoplasty is to create a physiologic form of the alveolar bone *without* removing any "supporting" bone. Osteoplasty therefore is a technique analogous to gingivoplasty. Examples of osteoplasty are the thinning of thick osseous ledges and the establishment of a scalloped contour of the buccal (lingual and palatal) bone crest (Fig. 38-39). In flap surgery without bone recontouring, interdental morphology may sometimes preclude optimal mucosal coverage of the bone post-surgically, even if pronounced scalloping of soft tissue flaps is performed. In such a situation removal of non-supporting bone by vertical grooving to reduce the facio-lingual dimension of the bone in the interdental areas may facilitate flap adaptation, thereby reducing the risk of bone denudation as well as reducing the risk of ischemic necrosis of unsupported mucosal flaps due to flap margin deficiencies.

Removal of non-supporting bone may sometimes also be required to gain access for intrabony root surface debridement. The leveling of interproximal craters and the elimination (or reduction) of bony walls of circumferential osseous defects are often referred to as "osteoplasty" since usually no resection of supporting bone is required (Fig. 38-40).

Ostectomy

In *ostectomy* supporting bone, i.e. bone directly involved in the attachment of the tooth, is removed to reshape deformities caused by periodontitis in the marginal and interdental bone. Ostectomy is considered to be an important part of surgical techniques aimed at pocket elimination. As a general rule, however, care must be exercised when supporting bone is to be removed.

After exposing the alveolar bone by elevation of a flap, buccal and/or lingual crater walls are reduced to the base of the osseous defect using bone chisels and bone rongeurs (Fig. 38-41). A round bur or a diamond stone under continuous saline irrigation

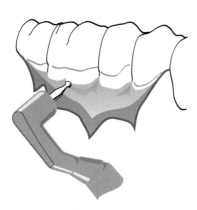

Fig. 38-39 Osteoplasty. Thick osseous ledges in a mandibular molar region area are eliminated with the use of a round bur to facilitate optimal flap adaptation.

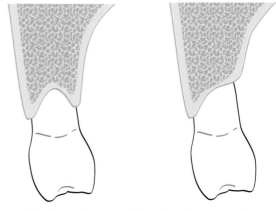

Fig. 38-40 Osteoplasty. Levelling of an interproximal bone crater through the removal of the palatal bone wall. For esthetic reasons the buccal bone wall is maintained to support the height of the soft tissue.

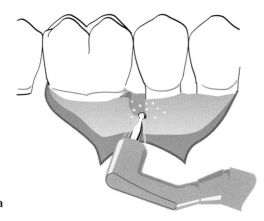
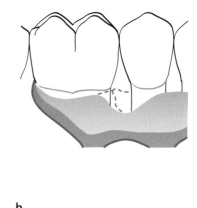

a   b

Fig. 38-41 Ostectomy. (a) A combined one- and two-wall osseous defect on the distal aspect of a mandibular bicuspid has been exposed following reflection of mucoperiosteal flaps. Since esthetics is not a critical factor to consider in the posterior tooth region of the mandible, the bone walls are reduced to a level close to the base of the defect using rotating round burs under continuous saline irrigation. (b) The osseous recontouring completed. Note that some supporting bone has to be removed from the buccal and lingual aspect of both the second bicuspid and the first molar in order to provide a hard tissue topography which allows a close adaptation of the covering soft tissue flap.

can also be used. If bone resection has been carried out in the interdental area, the buccal and lingual/palatal bone margins may subsequently have to be recontoured to compensate for discrepancies in bone height resulting from the interdental bone resection (Fig. 38-41b). It is considered important to remove the small peaks of bone, which often remain in the area of the line angles. The objective of bone surgery is thus to establish a "physiologic" anatomy of the alveolar bone, but at a more apical level.

General guidelines for periodontal surgery

Objectives of surgical treatment

Traditionally, *pocket elimination* has been the main objective of periodontal therapy. The removal of the pocket by surgical means served two purposes: (1) the pocket, which established an environment conducive to progression of periodontal disease, was eliminated and (2) the root surface was made accessible for scaling and for self-performed tooth cleaning after healing.

While these objectives cannot be entirely discarded today, the necessity for pocket elimination in periodontal therapy has been challenged. During recent years our understanding of the biology of the periodontium, the pathogenesis of periodontal disease and the healing capacity of the periodontium has markedly increased. This new information has thus formed the basis for a more differentiated understanding of the role played by periodontal surgery in the preservation of teeth.

In the past, *increased pocket depth* was the main indication for periodontal surgery. However, pocket depth is no longer as unequivocal a concept as it used to be. The *probeable depth*, i.e. the distance from the gingival margin to the point where tissue resistance

stops further periodontal probe penetration, may only rarely correspond to the "true" depth of the pocket (see Chapter 26). Furthermore, regardless of the accuracy with which pockets can be measured, there is no established correlation between probeable pocket depths and the presence or absence of active disease. This means that symptoms other than increased probing depth should be present to justify surgical therapy. These include clinical signs of inflammation, especially exudation and bleeding on probing (to the bottom of the pockets), as well as aberrations of gingival morphology. Finally, the fact that proper infection control, maintained by the patient, is a decisive factor for a good prognosis (Rosling *et al.* 1976a; Nyman *et al.* 1977; Axelsson & Lindhe 1981) must be considered prior to the initiation of surgery.

In conclusion, the main objective of periodontal surgery is to contribute to the long-term preservation of the periodontium by facilitating plaque removal and infection control, and periodontal surgery can serve this purpose by:

- Creating accessibility for proper professional scaling and root planing
- Establishing a gingival morphology which facilitates the patient's self-performed infection control.

In addition to this, periodontal surgery may aim at regeneration of periodontal attachment lost due to destructive disease. (New attachment procedures in periodontal therapy are discussed in Chapter 43.)

Indications for surgical treatment

Impaired access for scaling and root planing

Scaling and root planing are methods of therapy that are difficult to master. The difficulties in accomplishing proper debridement increase with (1) increasing depth of the periodontal pockets, (2) increasing width of the tooth surfaces, and (3) the presence of root fissures, root concavities, furcations, and defective margins of dental restorations in the subgingival area.

Provided a correct technique and suitable instruments are used, it is usually possible properly to debride pockets up to 5 mm deep (Waerhaug 1978; Caffesse *et al.* 1986). However, this 5 mm limit cannot be used as a universal rule of thumb. Reduced accessibility and the presence of one or several of the above-mentioned impeding conditions may prevent proper debridement of shallow pockets, whereas at sites with good accessibility and favorable root morphology, proper debridement can be accomplished even in deeper pockets (Badersten *et al.* 1981; Lindhe *et al.* 1982a).

It is often difficult to ascertain by clinical means whether subgingival instrumentation has been properly performed. Following scaling, the root surface should be smooth – roughness will often indicate the presence of remaining subgingival calculus. It is also important to monitor carefully the gingival reaction to subgingival debridement. If inflammation persists and if bleeding is elicited by gentle probing in the subgingival area, the presence of subgingival deposits should be suspected (Fig. 38-42). If such symptoms are not resolved by repeated subgingival instrumentation, surgical treatment should be performed to expose the root surfaces for proper cleaning.

Impaired access for self-performed plaque control

The level of infection control that can be maintained by the patient is determined not only by his/her interest and dexterity but also, to some extent, by the morphology of the dentogingival area. The patient's responsibility in an infection-control program must obviously include the cleansing of the supragingival tooth surfaces and the marginal part of the gingival sulcus. This means that the tooth area coronal to the gingival margin and at the entrance to the gingival sulcus should be the target for the patient's home care efforts.

Pronounced gingival hyperplasia and gingival craters (Fig. 38-43) are examples of morphologic aberrations, which may impede proper home care. Likewise, the presence of restorations with defective marginal fit or adverse contour and surface characteristics at the gingival margin may seriously compromise plaque removal.

By the professional treatment of periodontal disease, the dentist prepares the dentition in such a way that home care can be effectively managed. At the completion of treatment, the following objectives should have been met:

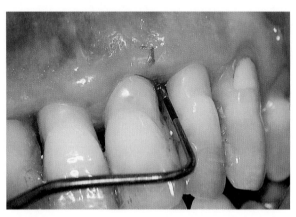

Fig. 38-42 Evaluation following non-surgical instrumentation reveals persistent signs of inflammation, bleeding following pocket probing and probing depth ≥6 mm. Flap elevation to expose the root surface for proper cleaning should be considered.

- No sub- or supragingival dental deposits
- No pathologic pockets (no bleeding on probing to the bottom of the pockets)
- No plaque-retaining aberrations of gingival morphology

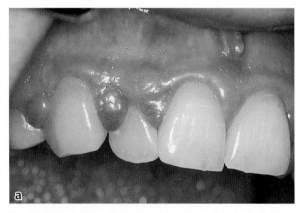

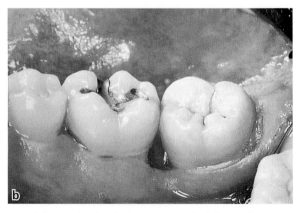

Fig. 38-43 Examples of gingival aberrations, (a) gingival enlargement and (b) proximal soft tissue crater, which favor plaque retention and thereby impede the patient's plaque control.

- No plaque-retaining parts of restorations in relation to the gingival margin.

These requirements lead to the following indications for periodontal surgery:

- Accessibility for proper scaling and root planing
- Establishment of a morphology of the dentogingival area conducive to infection control
- Pocket depth reduction
- Correction of gross gingival aberrations
- Shift of the gingival margin to a position apical to plaque-retaining restorations
- Facilitate proper restorative therapy.

Contraindications for periodontal surgery

Patient cooperation

Since optimal post-operative infection control is decisive for the success of periodontal treatment (Axelsson & Lindhe 1981), a patient who fails to cooperate during the cause-related phase of therapy should not be exposed to surgical treatment. Even though short-term post-operative infection control entails frequent professional treatments, the long-term responsibility for maintaining good oral hygiene must rest with the patient. Theoretically, even the poorest oral hygiene performance by a patient may be compensated for by frequent recall visits for supportive therapy (e.g. once a week), but it is unrealistic to consider larger groups of patients being maintained in this manner. A typical recall schedule for periodontal patients involves professional consultations for supportive periodontal therapy once every 3–6 months. Patients who cannot maintain satisfactory oral hygiene over such a period should normally be considered unsuited for periodontal surgery.

Cardiovascular disease

Arterial hypertension does not normally preclude periodontal surgery. The patient's medical history should be checked for previous untoward reactions to local anesthesia. Local anesthetics free from or low in adrenaline may be used and an aspirating syringe should be adopted to safeguard against intravascular injection.

Angina pectoris does not normally preclude periodontal surgery. The drugs used and the number of episodes of angina may indicate the severity of the disease. Premedication with sedatives and the use of local anesthesia low in adrenaline are often recommended. Safeguards should be adopted against intravascular injection.

Myocardial infarction patients should not be subjected to periodontal surgery within 6 months following hospitalization, and thereafter only in cooperation with the physician responsible for the patient.

Anticoagulant treatment implies increased propensity for bleeding. Periodontal surgery should be scheduled first after consultation with the patient's physician to determine whether modification of the anticoagulant therapy is indicated. In patients on moderate levels of anticoagulation and only requiring minor surgical treatment, no alteration of their anticoagulant therapy may be required. To keep the prothrombin time within a safety level for hemorrhage control during surgery in patients with higher levels of anticoagulation, adjustments of the anticoagulant drug therapy usually needs to be initiated 2–3 days prior to the dental appointment. Anticoagulation may be safely resumed immediately after the periodontal surgical procedure since several days are needed for full anticoagulation to return. Aspirin and other non-steroidal anti-inflammatory drugs should not be used for post-operative pain control since they increase bleeding tendency. Furthermore, tetracyclines are contraindicated in patients on anticoagulant drugs due to interference with prothrombin formation (Fay & O'Neil 1984).

Rheumatic endocarditis, congenital heart lesions, and *heart/vascular implants* involve risk for transmission of bacteria to heart tissues and heart implants during the transient bacteremia that follows manipulation of infected periodontal pockets. In patients with these conditions, as well as in patients at risk of hematogenous total prosthetic joint infection (for the first 2 years following joint placement), probing, scaling and root planing (including placement of antimocribial devices and prophylactic cleaning of implants and teeth where bleeding is anticipated), surgery and tooth extraction should be preceded by prescription and administration of an appropriate antibiotic at a high dose (American Dental Association – Position Statement on Antibiotic Prophylaxis 2003) and antiseptic mouth rinsing (0.2% chlorhexidine). According to the recommendations by the American Heart Association (Advisory Statement 1997), 2 grams of amoxicillin administrated orally 1 hour before the treatment is an adequate regimen. If the patient is allergic to penicillin, clindamycin (600 mg) orally 1 hour before the treatment is recommended as alternative. No second doses are recommended for any of the above dosing regimens. Tetracyclines and erythromycin are not recommended for prophylactic cardiovascular antibiotic coverage.

Organ transplantation

In organ transplantation medications are used to prevent transplant rejection. The drug of choice today is cyclosporine A, a potent immunosuppressant drug. The adverse effects seen following cyclosporine A treatment include an increased risk for gingival enlargement as well as hypertension. In addition, hypertension seen in renal transplant recipients is often treated with calcium channel blockers. These antihypertensive agents have also been associated with gingival enlargement. As in patients on phenytoin therapy, gingival enlargement in patients on cyclosporine A therapy or on antihypertensive therapy with calcium blockers may be corrected by means of periodontal surgery. However, due to the strong propensity for recurrence, the use of intensified conservative periodontal therapy to prevent gingival enlargement in susceptible patients should be encouraged.

Prophylactic antibiotics are recommended in transplant patients taking immunosuppressive drugs, and the patient's physician should be consulted before any periodontal therapy is performed. In addition, antiseptic mouth rinsing (0.2% chlorhexidine) should precede the surgical treatment.

Blood disorders

If the medical history includes blood disorders, the exact nature of these should be ascertained. Patients suffering from *acute leukemias*, *agranulocytosis*, and *lymphogranulomatosis* must *not* be subjected to periodontal surgery. *Anemias* in mild and compensated forms do not preclude surgical treatment. More severe and less compensated forms may entail lowered resistance to infection and increased propensity for bleeding. In such cases, periodontal surgery should only be performed after consultation with the patient's physician.

Hormonal disorders

Diabetes mellitus entails lowered resistance to infection, propensity for delayed wound healing, and predisposition for arteriosclerosis. Well compensated patients may be subjected to periodontal surgery provided precautions are taken not to disturb dietary and insulin routines.

Adrenal function may be impeded in patients receiving large doses of corticosteroids over an extended period. These conditions involve reduced resistance to physical and mental stress, and the doses of corticosteroid may have to be altered during the period of periodontal surgery. The patient's physician should be consulted.

Neurologic disorders

Multiple sclerosis and *Parkinson's disease* may, in severe cases, make ambulatory periodontal surgery impossible. Paresis, impaired muscular function, tremor, and uncontrollable reflexes may necessitate treatment under general anesthesia.

Epilepsy is often treated with *phenytoin* that, in approximately 50% of cases, may mediate the formation of gingival enlargement. These patients may, without special restrictions, be subjected to periodontal surgery for correction of the enlargement. There is, however, a strong propensity for recurrence of the

enlargement, which in many cases can be countered by intensifying plaque control.

Smoking

Although smoking negatively affects wound healing (Siana *et al.* 1989), it may not be considered as a contraindication for surgical periodontal treatment. The clinician should be aware, however, that less resolution of probing pocket depth and smaller improvement in clinical attachment may be observed in smokers than in non-smokers (Preber & Bergström 1990; Ah *et al.* 1994; Scabbia *et al.* 2001; Labriola *et al.* 2005).

Local anesthesia in periodontal surgery

Traditional views of pain and discomfort as an inevitable consequence of dental procedures, in particular surgical procedures (including scaling and root planing) and extractions, are no longer accepted by patients. Pain management is an ethical obligation and will improve patient satisfaction in general (e.g. increased confidence and improved cooperation) as well as patient recovery and short-term functioning after oral/periodontal surgical procedures. In order to prevent pain during the performance of a periodontal surgical procedure, the entire area of the dentition scheduled for surgery, the teeth as well as the periodontal tissues, require proper local anesthesia.

Mechanism of action

Local anesthesia is defined as a loss of feeling or sensation that is confined to a certain area of the body. All local anesthetics have a common mechanism of action. To produce their effect they block the generation and propagation of impulses along nerve fibers. Such impulses are transmitted by rapid depolarization and repolarization within the nerve axons. These changes in polarity are due to the passage of sodium and potassium ions across the nerve membrane through ionic channels within the membrane. Local anesthetics prevent the inward movement of sodium ions, which initiate depolarization, and as a consequence the nerve fiber cannot propagate any impulse. The potassium efflux, on the other hand, is influenced very little and there is no change in the resting potential. The mechanisms behind the activity of the local anesthetics are not fully understood, but the most plausible theory is that the lipid-soluble free base form of the local anesthetic, which is the form that penetrates biologic membranes most easily, penetrates the connective tissue to reach the axons and diffuses across the lipid membrane into the axon. Inside the axon the drug interacts with specific receptor sites on or within the sodium channels to exert an inhibitory effect on sodium influx and, consequently, on impulse conduction.

Dental local anesthetics

Anesthetics from the chemical group amino-amides, for example lidocaine, mepivacaine, prilocaine, and articaine, are more potent and significantly less allergenic than amino-esters (e.g. procaine and tetracaine) and have therefore replaced esters as the "gold standard" for dental local anesthetics.

Due to the specific need for bone penetration, dental local anesthetics contain high concentrations of the active agent. Although most amide local anesthetics may cause local vasoconstriction in low concentrations, the clinically used concentrations in dental solutions will cause an increase in the local blood flow. Significant clinical effects of this induced vasodilatation are an increased rate of absorption, thus decreasing the duration of anesthesia. Major benefits can therefore be obtained by adding relatively high concentrations of vasoconstrictors (e.g. epinephrine >1 : 200 000 or >5 mg/ml) to dental local anesthetic solutions; the duration is considerably prolonged, the depth of anesthesia may be enhanced, and the peak concentrations of the local anesthetic in blood can be reduced. Furthermore, in periodontal surgery incorporation of adrenergic vasoconstrictors into the local anesthetic is of considerable value to allow for only minimal bleeding during surgery (to avoid considerable blood loss, to visualize the surgical site, and shorten the time spent on the procedure maintaining surgical quality). As a matter of fact, the use of a dental local anesthetic without a vasoconstrictor during a periodontal surgical procedure is counterproductive because the vasodilating properties of such a local anesthetic will increase bleeding in the area of surgery.

Vasoconstrictors and local hemostasis

Epinephrine is the vasoconstrictor of choice for local hemostasis and is most commonly used in a concentration of 1 : 80 000 (12.5 mg/ml). However, 1 : 100 000 epinephrine also provides excellent hemostasis and most periodontists are unable to detect a clinical difference between the two concentrations. It therefore seems prudent to use the least concentrated form of epinephrine that provides clinically effective hemostasis (i.e. the 1 : 100 000 concentration).

Although the cardiovascular effects of the usually small amounts of epinehrine used during a periodontal surgical procedure are of little practical concern in most individuals, accidental intravascular injections, unusual patient sensitivity and unanticipated drug interactions (or excessive doses), can result in potentially serious outcomes. It must also be understood that the use of epinephrine for hemostasis during periodontal surgery has some potential drawbacks. Epinephrine will produce a rebound vasodilatation after the vasoconstriction has worn off leading to increased risk for bleeding in the immediate postoperative period. There is a greater potential for such undesirable delayed hemorrhage following the use of 1 : 80 000 epinephrine than after the use of 1 : 100 000.

Post-operative pain may increase and wound healing may be delayed when adrenergic vasoconstrictors are used because of local ischemia with subsequent tissue acidosis and accumulation of inflammatory mediators. Furthermore, the possibility of an ischemic necrosis of surgical flaps infiltrated with an adrenergic vasoconstrictor (especially if norepinephrine is used instead of epinephrine) cannot be discounted. For these reasons as well as for the possibility of systemic reactions eluded to above, dental local anesthetics containing adrenergic vasoconstrictors for hemostasis should be infiltrated *only* as needed and *not* merely by habit.

Felypressin, another commonly used vasoconstrictor, appears to act preferentially on the venous side of the microcirculation and is not very active in constricting the arteriolar circulation. Felypressin is therefore not nearly as effective as adrenergic vasoconstrictors in limiting hemorrhage during a surgical procedure.

Individual variability in response to dental local anesthetics

Although it is possible for the periodontist to choose from a broad spectrum of dental local anesthetics to achieve the expected clinical action, there is a number of other factors (i.e. not related to the drug) that can affect the drug action in a single patient. During clinical conditions the variability in response to dental local anesthetics administered can be expected to be great, for example with regard to depth and duration of anesthesia. The reasons for the great variation have not been adequately explained but have to be accepted as the variation may have significant implications in periodontal surgical procedures. A list of possible factors that may cause anesthetic failures include:

- Accuracy in administration of the drug
- Anatomic variation between patients (e.g. in elderly patients with bone resorption)
- Status of the tissues at the site of injection (vascularity, inflammation)
- General condition of patient
- Psychologic factors.

Inaccuracy in administration is a major factor causing anesthetic failures. Although not particularly significant in infiltration anesthesia, the mandibular block is a prime example of a technique in which duration of anesthesia is greatly influenced by accuracy of injection.

The general condition of the patient as well as psychologic factors may also affect the anticipated duration of action. Infection, stress or pain will usually lead to decreased duration of anesthesia, while an increase in the patient's own defense mechanisms against pain perception by, for example, release of endogenous endorphins, may provide for improved depth and/or duration of anesthesia.

Techniques for anesthesia in periodontal surgery

Injections of dental local anesthetics prior to a periodontal surgical procedure may be routine for the dentist, but is often a most unpleasant experience for the patient. Reassurance and psychologic support are essential and will increase the patient's confidence in his dentist. To create a relaxed atmosphere and to decrease the patient's fear in an unusual situation is of course also a useful way of increasing the patient's own defense mechanisms against pain perception (e.g. release of endogenous endorphins).

Anesthesia for periodontal surgery is obtained by nerve block and/or by local infiltration. In cases of flap surgery, complete anesthesia must be attained before commencing the operation, as it may be difficult to supplement the anesthesia after the bone surface has been exposed. In addition, the pain elicited by needle insertion can be significantly reduced if the mucosa at the puncture site is anesthetized in advance by the use of a suitable topical ointment or spray.

Local infiltration may have a greatly decreased rate of success in areas where inflammation remains in the periodontal tissues, in spite of optimal conservative periodontal therapy and good oral hygiene. The suggested reason being that tissue pH tends to be low in inflamed areas and anesthetic solutions are less potent at low pH because there is a greater proportion of charged cation molecules than of the uncharged base molecules. Because of this, diffusion of the local anesthetic into the axoplasm is slower with subsequent delayed onset and decreased efficacy. Another more recent hypothesis suggests that NGF (nerve growth factor) released during tissue inflammation will induce sprouting or proliferation of sensory nerve endings expressing a different (sub-) type of sodium channel than is expressed in normal tissues. Our presently used dental local anesthetics may not be selective enough for proper interaction with these sodium channel subtypes to induce anticipated anesthesia.

Local anesthesia in the mandible

As a rule, analgesia of the teeth and the soft and hard tissues of the mandible should be obtained by a mandibular block and/or a mental block. In the anterior region of the mandible, canines and incisors can often be anesthetized by infiltration, but there are often anastomoses over the midline. These anastomoses must be anaesthetized by bilateral infiltration, or by bilateral mental blocks. The buccal soft tissues of the mandible are anesthetized by local infiltration or by

blocking the buccal nerve. Local infiltration, performed as a series of injections in the buccal fold of the treatment area, has of course the added advantage of providing a local ischemic effect if a suitable anesthetic is used.

The lingual periodontal tissues must also be anesthetized. This is accomplished by blocking the lingual nerve and/or by infiltration in the floor of the mouth close to the site of operation. If necessary to obtain proper ischemia, and only then, supplementary injections may be made in the interdental papillae (intraseptal injections).

Local anesthesia in the maxilla

Local anesthesia of the teeth and buccal periodontal tissues of the maxilla can easily be obtained by injections in the muco-gingival fold of the treatment area. If larger areas of the maxillary dentition are scheduled for surgery, repeated injections (in the muco-gingival fold) have to be performed, e.g. at the central incisor, canine, second premolar, and second molar. In the posterior maxillary region a tuberosity injection can be used to block the superior alveolar branches of the maxillary nerve. However, because of the vicinity to the pterygoid venous plexus, this type of block anesthesia is not recommended due to the risk of intravenous injection and/or hematoma formation.

The palatal nerves are most easily anesthetized by injections made at right angles to the mucosa and placed around 10 mm apical to the gingival margin adjacent to teeth included in the operation. In cases of advanced bone loss, the pain produced by injecting into the non-resilient palatal mucosa can be minimized if the injections are performed from the buccal aspect, i.e. through the interdental gingiva. Sometimes blocks of the nasopalatine nerves and/or the greater palatine nerves can be applied. Supplementary blocking of the greater palatine nerve should be considered, especially for periodontal surgery involving molars.

Instruments used in periodontal surgery

General considerations

Surgical procedures used in periodontal therapy often involve the following measures (instruments):

- Incision and excision (periodontal knives)
- Deflection and re-adaptation of mucosal flaps (periosteal elevators)
- Removal of adherent fibrous and granulomatous tissue (soft tissue rongeurs and tissue scissors)
- Scaling and root planing (scalers and curettes)
- Removal of bone tissue (bone rongeurs, chisels, and files)
- Root sectioning (burs)

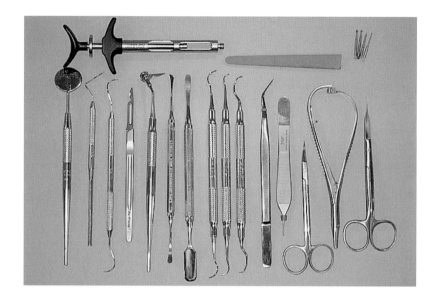

Fig. 38-44 Set of instruments used for periodontal surgery and included in a standard tray.

- Suturing (sutures and needle holders, suture scissors)
- Application of wound dressing (plastic instruments).

The set of instruments used for the various periodontal surgical procedures should have a comparatively simple design. As a general rule, the number and varieties of instruments should be kept to a minimum. In addition to particular instruments used for periodontal treatment modalities, equipment and instruments generally used in oral surgery are often needed. Within each category of surgical instruments used for periodontal therapy there are usually several brands available, varying in form and quality, leaving ample room for individual preferences.

The instruments should be stored in sterile "ready-to-use" packs or trays. Handling, storing, and labeling of surgical instruments and equipment must be managed in such a way that interchanging of sterile and non-sterile items is prevented.

It is also important that the instruments are kept in good working condition. The maintenance routine should ensure that scalers, curettes, knives with fixed blades, etc., are sharp and the hinges of scissors, rongeurs, and needle holders are properly lubricated. Spare instruments (sterile) should always be available to replace instruments found to be defective or accidentally contaminated.

The instrument tray

Instrument trays for periodontal surgery may be arranged in several ways. Different trays can be used for different procedures or a standard tray can be used for all procedures supplemented with the particular instruments that are needed for a specific procedure.

A commonly used standard tray combines the basic set of instruments used in oral surgery and a few periodontal instruments. The instruments listed below are often found on such a standard tray (Fig. 38-44):

- Mouth mirrors
- Graduated periodontal probe/explorer
- Handles for disposable surgical blades (e.g. Bard-Parker handle)
- Mucoperiosteal elevator and tissue retractor
- Scalers and curettes
- Cotton pliers
- Tissue pliers (*ad modum* Ewald)
- Tissue scissors
- Needle holder
- Suture scissors
- Plastic instrument
- Hemostat
- Burs.

Additional equipment may include:

- Syringe for local anesthesia
- Syringe for irrigation
- Aspirator tip
- Physiologic saline
- Drapings for the patient
- Surgical gloves, surgical mask, surgeon's hood.

Surgical instruments

Knives
Knives are available with fixed or replaceable blades. The advantage of the fixed blade versions is that the blade can be given any desired shape and orientation in relation to the handle. A disadvantage is that such instruments need frequent resharpening. Figure 38-45 shows examples of knives with fixed blades.

New disposable blades are always sharp. They can be rapidly replaced if found defective. The cutting edge of the blades normally follows the long axis of

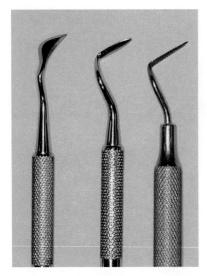

Fig. 38-45 Examples of gingivectomy knives with fixed blades. From left to right: Kirkland 15/16, Orban 1/2, and Waerhaug 1/2.

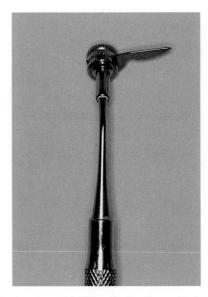

Fig. 38-47 A universal 360° handle for disposable blades, which allows the mounting of the blade in any angulated position of choice.

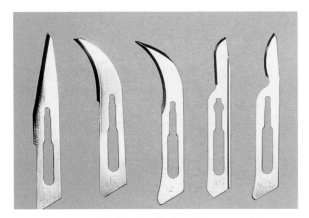

Fig. 38-46 Disposable blades which can be mounted in various types of handles. The shape of the blades are from left to right: No. 11, No. 12, No. 12D, No. 15, and No. 15C.

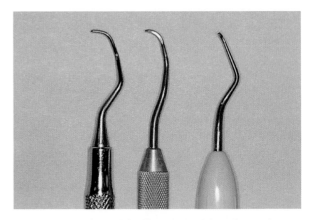

Fig. 38-48 Examples of double-ended sickle scalers and curettes useful for root debridement in conjunction with periodontal surgery. From left to right: Curette SG 215/16C Syntette, Sickle 215-216 Syntette, and mini-curette SG 215/16MC.

the handle, which limits their use. However, knives with disposable blades fitted at an angle to the handle are also available. Disposable blades are manufactured in different shapes (Fig. 38-46). When mounted in ordinary handles (Bard-Parker®), they are used for releasing incisions in flap operations and mucogingival surgery and for reverse bevel incisions where access is obtainable. Special handles (Fig. 38-47) make it possible to mount blades in angulated positions, which facilitate the use of such knives for both gingivectomy excisions and reverse bevel incisions.

Scalers and curettes

Scaling and root planing in conjunction with periodontal surgery take place on exposed root surfaces. Access to the root surfaces for debridement may therefore be obtained with the use of comparatively sturdy instruments (Fig. 38-48). Tungsten carbide curettes and scalers with durable cutting edges are often used when "access" is not a problem. Rotating fine-grained diamond stones (Fig. 38-49) may be used

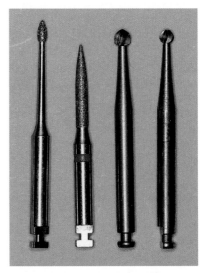

Fig. 38-49 A set of burs useful in periodontal surgery. The rotating fine-grained diamond stones may be used for debridement of infrabony defects. The round burs are used for bone recontouring.

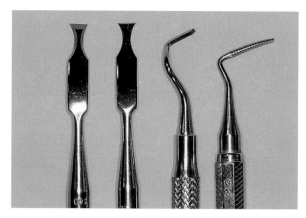

Fig. 38-50 Examples of instruments used for bone recontouring. From left to right: Bone chisels Ochsenbein no. 1 and 2 (Kirkland 13K/13KL), Bone chisel Ochsenbein no. 3, and Schluger curved file no. 9/10.

within infrabony pockets, root concavities, and entrances to furcations.

Instruments for bone removal

Sharp bone chisels or bone rongeurs (Fig. 38-50) cause the least tissue damage and should be employed whenever access permits. With reduced access, surgical burs or files may be used. The burs should operate at low speed and ample rinsing with sterile physiologic saline should ensure cooling and removal of tissue remnants.

Instruments for handling flaps

The proper healing of the periodontal wound is critical for the success of the operation. It is therefore important that the manipulations of soft tissue flaps are performed with the minimum of tissue damage. Care should be exercised in the use of periosteal elevators when flaps are deflected and retracted for optimal visibility. Surgical pliers and tissue retractors that pierce the tissues should not be used in the marginal area of the flaps. Needle holders with small beaks and atraumatic sutures should be used.

Additional equipment

Hemorrhage is rarely a problem in periodontal surgery. The characteristic oozing type of bleeding can normally be controlled by a pressure pack (sterile gauze moistened with saline). Bleeding from small vessels can be stopped by clamping and tying using a hemostat and resorbable sutures. If the vessel is surrounded by bone, bleeding may be stopped by crushing the nutrient canal in which the vessel runs with a blunt instrument.

Sterile physiologic saline is used for rinsing and moistening the field of operation and for cooling when burs are employed. The saline solution may be kept in a sterile metal cup on the instrument tray and may be applied to the wound by means of a sterile disposable plastic syringe and a needle with a blunt tip.

Visibility in the field of operation is secured by using effective suction. The lumen of the aspirator tip should have a smaller diameter than the rest of the tube, in order to prevent clogging.

The patient's head may be covered by autoclaved cotton drapings or sterile disposable plastic/paper drapings. The surgeon and all assistants should wear sterile surgical gloves, surgical mask, and surgeon's hood.

Selection of surgical technique

Many of the technical problems experienced in periodontal surgery stem from the difficulties in accurately assessing the degree and type of breakdown that has occurred prior to surgery. Furthermore, at the time of surgery, previously undiagnosed defects may be recognized or some defects may have a more complex outline than initially anticipated. Since each of the surgical procedures described above is designed to deal with a specific situation or to meet a certain objective, it must be understood that in most patients no single standardized technique alone can be applied when periodontal surgery is undertaken. Therefore, in each surgical field, different techniques are often used and combined in such a way that the overall objectives of the surgical part of the periodontal therapy are met. As a general rule, surgical modalities of therapy that preserve or induce the formation of periodontal tissue should be preferred over those that resect or eliminate tissue.

General indications for various surgical techniques

Gingivectomy

The obvious indication for gingivectomy is the presence of deep supra-alveolar pockets. In addition, the gingivectomy technique can be used to reshape abnormal gingival contours such as gingival craters and gingival hyperplasias (Fig. 38-43). In such cases the technique is often termed *gingivoplasty*.

Gingivectomy is usually not considered suitable in situations where the incision will lead to the removal of the entire zone of gingiva. This is the case when the bottom of the probeable pocket to be excised is located at or below the mucogingival junction. As an alternative in such a situation, an *internal beveled gingivectomy* may be performed (Fig. 38-51). Furthermore, since the gingivectomy procedure is aimed at the complete elimination of the periodontal pocket, the procedure cannot be used in periodontal sites where infrabony lesions or bony craters are present.

These limitations, combined with the development in recent years of surgical methods which have a broader field of application, have led to less frequent use of gingivectomy in the treatment of periodontal disease.

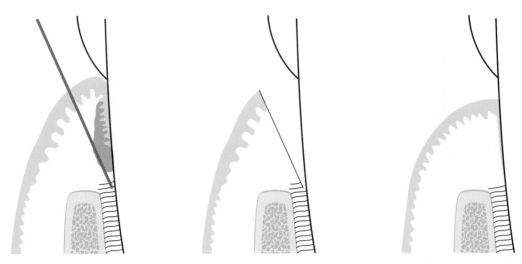

Fig. 38-51 Internal beveled gingivectomy. Schematic illustration of the incision technique in case of the presence of only a minimal zone of gingiva.

Flap operation with or without osseous surgery

Flap operations can be used in all cases where surgical treatment of periodontal disease is indicated. Flap procedures are particularly useful at sites where pockets extend beyond the muco-gingival border and/or where treatment of bony lesions and furcation involvements is required.

The advantages of flap operations include:

- Existing gingiva is preserved
- The marginal alveolar bone is exposed whereby the morphology of bony defects can be identified and the proper treatment rendered
- Furcation areas are exposed, the degree of involvement and the "tooth–bone" relationship can be identified
- The flap can be repositioned at its original level or shifted apically, thereby making it possible to adjust the gingival margin to the local conditions
- The flap procedure preserves the oral epithelium and often makes the use of surgical dressing superfluous
- The post-operative period is usually less unpleasant to the patient when compared to gingivectomy.

Treatment decisions for soft and hard tissue pockets in flap surgery

Classifications of different flap modalities used in the treatment of periodontal disease often make distinctions between methods involving the marginal tissues and those involving the muco-gingival area and, further, between tissue-eliminating/resective varieties and tissue-preserving/reconstructive types (access flaps for debridement). Such classifications appear less than precise since several techniques are often combined in the treatment of individual cases, and since there is no clear-cut relationship between disease characteristics and selection of surgical

methods. From a didactic point of view it seems more appropriate to discuss surgical therapy with regard to how to deal with (1) the soft tissue component and (2) the hard tissue component of the periodontal pocket at a specific tooth site (Fig. 38-52).

Soft tissue pockets

The description of the various flap procedures reveals that, depending on the surgical technique used, the soft tissue flap should either be apically positioned at the level of the bone crest (original Widman flap, Neumann flap, and apically repositioned flap) or maintained in a coronal position (Kirkland flap, modified Widman flap, and papilla preservation flap) at the completion of the surgical intervention. The maintenance of the pre-surgical soft tissue height is of importance from an esthetic point of view, particularly in the anterior tooth region. However, long-term results from clinical trials have shown that major differences in the final position of the soft tissue margin are not evident between surgical procedures involving coronal and apical positioning of the flap margin. The reported difference in final positioning of the gingival margin between surgical techniques is attributed to osseous recontouring (Townsend-Olsen et al. 1985; Lindhe et al. 1987; Kaldahl et al. 1996; Becker et al. 2001). In many patients it may be of significance to position the flap coronally in the anterior tooth region in order to give the patient a prolonged time of adaptation to the inevitable soft tissue recession. In the posterior tooth region, however, an apical position should be the standard.

Independent of flap position, the goal should be to achieve complete soft tissue coverage of the alveolar bone, not only at buccal/lingual sites but also in proximal sites. It is therefore of utmost importance to carefully plan the incisions in such a way that this goal can be achieved at the termination of the surgical intervention.

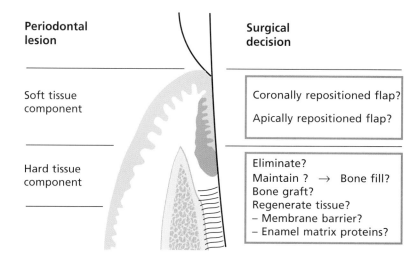

Periodontal lesion

Soft tissue component

Hard tissue component

Surgical decision

Coronally repositioned flap?

Apically repositioned flap?

Eliminate?
Maintain ? → Bone fill?
Bone graft?
Regenerate tissue?
– Membrane barrier?
– Enamel matrix proteins?

Fig. 38-52 Surgical decisions. Treatment decisions with respect to the soft and the hard tissue component of a periodontal pocket.

Hard tissue pockets

During conventional periodontal surgery one would usually opt for the conversion of an intrabony defect into a suprabony defect, which then is eliminated by apical repositioning of the soft tissues. Osseous recontouring of angular bony defects and craters are excisional techniques, which should be used with caution and discrimination. However, the therapist is often faced with the dilemma of deciding whether or not to eliminate an angular bony defect. There are a number of factors that should be considered in the treatment decision, such as:

- Esthetics
- Tooth/tooth site involved
- Defect morphology
- Amount of remaining periodontium.

Since alveolar bone supports the soft tissue, an altered bone level through recontouring will result in recession of the soft tissue margin. For esthetic reasons one may therefore be restrictive in eliminating proximal bony defects in the anterior tooth region. For example, in the case of an approximal crater it may often be sufficient to reduce/eliminate the bone wall on the lingual side of the crater, thereby maintaining the bone support for the soft tissue on the facial aspect (Fig. 38-40). In favor of esthetics one may even have to compromise the amount of bone removal and accept that some pocket depth will remain in certain situations. In addition to esthetics, the presence of furcations may limit the extent to which bone recontouring can be performed.

Defect morphology is a variable of significance for repair/regeneration during healing (Rosling *et al.* 1976a; Cortellini *et al.* 1993, 1995a). While two- and, especially, three-wall defects may show great potential for repair/regeneration, one-wall defects and approximal craters will rarely result in such good healing. Further, the removal of intrabony connective tissue/granulation tissue during a surgical procedure will always lead to crestal resorption of bone,

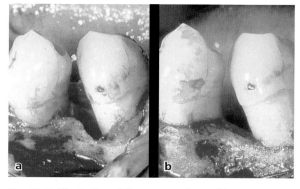

Fig. 38-53 Illustration of the amount of crestal bone resorption that may take place following a modified Widman flap procedure without bone recontouring. (a) View of the area at time of initial surgical treatment. (b) At the re-entry operation performed after 6 months of healing.

especially in sites with thin bony walls. This results in reduction of the vertical dimensions of the bone tissue at the site (Fig. 38-53). Thus, the potential for bone fill following a compromise in regard to osseous surgery is greater in areas with thick, non-supporting bone.

The various treatment options available for the hard tissue defect may include:

- Elimination of the osseous defect by resection of bone (osteoplasty and/or ostectomy)
- Maintenance of the area without osseous resection (hoping for some type of periodontal repair, e.g. bone fill leading to gain of clinical attachment)
- Compromising the amount of bone removal and accepting that a certain pocket depth will remain
- An attempt to improve healing through the use of a regenerative procedure
- Extract the involved tooth if the bony defect is considered too advanced.

After careful consideration, indications for osseous surgery in conjunction with apical repositioning of flaps may also include subgingival caries, perforations or root fractures in the coronal third of the root as well as inadequate retention for fixed prosthetic restorations due to a short clinical crown (crown-lengthening procedures). The "crown lengthening" needed in such cases is performed by removing often significant amounts of supporting bone and by recontouring. A "biologic width" of approximately 3 mm between the alveolar bone crest to be established and the anticipated restoration margin must be ensured for successful results (Brägger *et al.* 1992; Herrero *et al.* 1995; Pontoriero & Carnevale 2001).

Root surface instrumentation

Before incisions are made to excise or elevate the soft tissue, a careful examination should be carried out to identify at which tooth sites periodontal lesions remain. Only tooth sites with signs of pathology (bleeding following pocket probing) should be subjected to root instrumentation following surgical exposure. Further, at these sites root surface instrumentation should be limited to that part of the root that will be covered by the soft tissue following flap replacement and suturing. This is an important consideration since instrumentation of the supragingival portion of the root may lead to post-surgical root hypersensitivity, which in turn may impede proper oral hygiene measures. Before root instrumentation is executed, therefore, remaining granulation tissue must be removed, bone recontouring is carried out, if indicated, and the post-surgical soft tissue level is determined. If the intention is to reposition the flap apically at the level of the bone crest, only approximately 3 mm of the root surface coronal to the bone crest has to be carefully scaled and root planed, whereas if the flap is to be positioned coronally the entire exposed root has to be instrumented.

The root instrumentation can be performed with hand or ultrasonic instruments according to the operator's preferences. Ultrasonic (sonic) instrumentation offers the additional benefits of improved visibility due to the irrigating effect of the cooling water. For root instrumentation within intrabony defects, root concavities, and entrances to furcations, the use of rotating fine-grained diamond stones may be used.

Root surface conditioning/biomodification

An important consideration in periodontal surgery is to make the exposed root surface biologically compatible with a healthy periodontium. This so-called conditioning includes removing bacteria, endotoxins, and other antigens found within the cementum–dentin of a pathologically exposed root. In addition to scaling and root planing, agents such as citric acid/orthophosphoric acid, tetracycline, and EDTA are used for root surface conditioning. Root surface conditioning/biomodification by means of an etching procedure may serve several purposes:

- Removal of the smear layer following mechanical debridement
- Demineralization of the root surface (citric acid)
- Selective removal of hydroxyapatite and exposure of the collagenous matrix of the root surface (EDTA)
- Local delivery of antimicrobial compound (tetracycline HCL)
- Inhibition of collagenolytic activity (tetracycline HCL)
- Enhancing cellular responses
- Preventing of epithelial down-growth
- Improving retention of different biomolecules to exposed collagen
- To express a cementoblast phenotype for colonizing cells.

It should be noted that etching of a root surface with an agent operating at a low pH, e.g. citric acid or orthophosphoric acid, might exert immediate necrotizing effects on the surrounding periodontal ligament and other periodontal tissues, whereas agents operating at a neutral pH (e.g. EDTA) do not seem to have this negative effect (Blomlöf & Lindskog 1995a,b).

Although *in vitro* results have indicated possible benefits of the use of root surface conditioning/biomodification agents through enhanced cellular responses during wound healing, the usefulness of acids as well as other chemical agents for conditioning of root surfaces in conjunction with conventional periodontal surgery has been questioned (Blomlöf *et al.* 2000). Histologic evidence indicates that healing following root surface conditioning with acids or other chemical agents is generally dominated by a long junctional epithelium or connective tissue attachment without evidence of new cementum formation. However, root surface biomodification must still be regarded as an important method to facilitate regeneration. Thus, in this treatment the root represents one of the wound margins and must provide an appropriate surface for cell attachment, colonization, and proliferation.

Suturing

When a flap procedure has been employed it is important to ensure that, at the end of surgery, the flaps are placed in the intended position and that the flaps are properly adapted to each other and to the tooth surfaces. Preferably, full coverage of the buccal/lingual (palatal) and interdental alveolar bone should be obtained by full (primary) closure of the soft tissue flaps. If this can be achieved, healing by first intention results and post-operative bone resorption is minimal. Therefore, prior to suturing, the flap margins should be trimmed to properly fit the buccal and lingual (palatal) bone margin as well as the interproximal areas; excessive soft tissue must be removed. If the amount of flap tissue present is insufficient to cover the interproximal bone, the flaps at the buccal or lingual aspects of the teeth must be recontoured and, in some cases, even displaced coronally.

Following proper trimming, the flaps are secured in the correct position by sutures. Sutures should not interfere with incision lines and must not pass through the tissues near the flap margins or too close to a papilla, because this may result in tearing of the tissues. The use of non-irritating, mono-filamentous materials is recommended. These materials are non-resorbable and extremely inert, do not adhere to tissues, and are therefore easy to pull out. "Wicking", the phenomenon of bacteria moving along or within multi-stranded suture materials, particularly silk, is also avoided. The dimensions usually preferred are 4/0 to 5/0, but even finer suture material (6/0 or 7/0) may be used, particularly in conjunction with periodontal micro- and plastic surgical procedures. Sutures are removed after 7–14 days.

Since the flap tissue following the final preparation is thin, either curved or straight non-traumatic needles (eyeless), with a small diameter, should be used. Such needles are available as rounded (non-cutting) or with different cutting edges. In the latter case, a reverse-cutting needle should be selected.

Suturing technique

The three most frequently used sutures in periodontal flap surgery are:

- Interrupted interdental sutures
- Suspensory sutures
- Continuous sutures.

The *interrupted interdental suture* (Fig. 38-54) provides a close interdental adaptation between the buccal and lingual flaps with equal tension on both units. This type of suture is therefore not recommended when the buccal and lingual flaps are repositioned at different levels. When this technique of suturing is employed, the needle is passed through the buccal flap from the external surface, across the interdental area and through the lingual flap from the internal surface, or vice versa. When closing the suture, care must be taken to avoid tearing the flap tissues.

In order to avoid having the suture material between the mucosa and the alveolar bone in the interdental area, an alternative technique in the use of the interrupted interdental suture can be used if the flaps have not been elevated beyond the mucogingival line (Fig. 38-55). With the use of a curved needle the suture is anchored in the attached tissue on the buccal aspect of the proximal site, the suture brought to the lingual side through the proximal sites, and anchored in the attached tissue on the lingual side. The suture is then brought back to the starting point and tied (Fig. 38-55b). Hence, the suture will be lying on the surface of the interdental tissue,

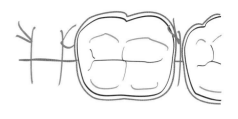

a

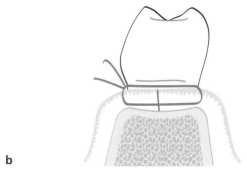

b

Fig. 38-54 Suturing. Interrupted interdental suture.

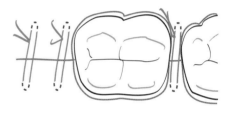

a

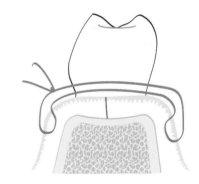

b

Fig. 38-55 Suturing. Modified interrupted interdental suture. Note that with this suturing technique the suture is laying on the surface of the interdental tissue keeping the soft tissue flaps in close contact with the underlying bone.

keeping the soft tissue flaps in close contact with the underlying bone.

In regenerative procedures, which usually require a coronal advancement of the flap, a *modified mattress suture* may be used to secure close flap adaptation (Fig. 38-56). The needle is passed through the buccal flap from the external surface, across the interdental area and through the lingual flap from the internal surface. The suture is run back to the buccal side by passing the needle through the lingual and buccal flaps. Thereafter, the suture is brought through the approximal site coronally to the tissue, passed

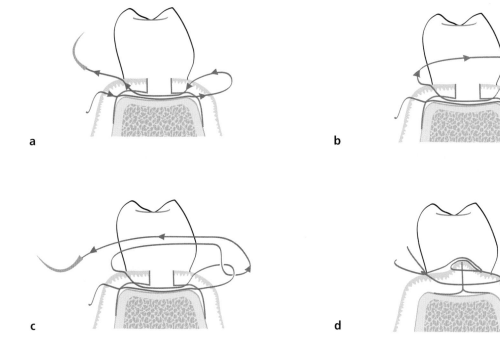

a

b

c

d

Fig. 38-56 Suturing. Modified mattress suture.

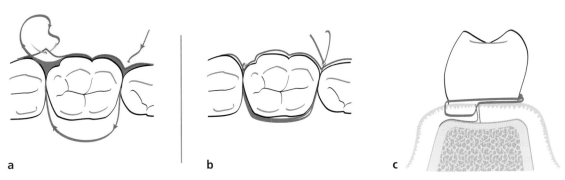

a

b

c

Fig. 38-57 Suturing. Suspensory suture.

through the loop of the suture on the lingual aspect, and then brought back to the starting point on the buccal side and tied.

The *suspensory suture* (Fig. 38-57) is used primarily when the surgical procedure is of limited extent and involves only the tissue of the buccal or lingual aspect of the teeth. It is also the suture of choice when the buccal and lingual flaps are repositioned at different levels. The needle is passed through the buccal flap from its external surface at the mesial side of the tooth, the suture is placed around the lingual surface of the tooth and the needle is passed through the buccal flap on the distal side of the tooth (Fig. 38-57a). The suture is brought back to the starting point via the lingual surface of the tooth and tied (Figs. 38-57b,c). If a lingual flap has been elevated as well, this is secured in the intended position using the same technique.

The *continuous suture* (Fig. 38-58) is commonly used when flaps involving several teeth are to be repositioned apically. When flaps have been elevated on both sides of the teeth, one flap at a time is secured

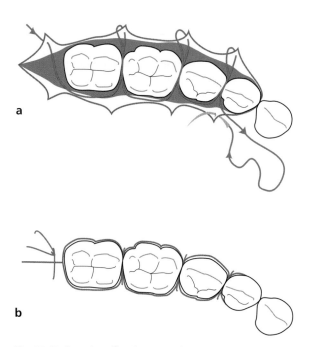

a

b

Fig. 38-58 Suturing. Continuous suture.

in its correct position. The suturing procedure is started at the mesial/distal aspect of the buccal flap by passing the needle through the flap and across the interdental area. The suture is laid around the lingual surface of the tooth and returned to the buccal side through the next interdental space. The procedure is repeated tooth by tooth until the distal/mesial end of the flap is reached. Thereafter, the needle is passed through the lingual flap (Fig. 38-58a), with the suture laid around the buccal aspect of each tooth and through each interproximal space. When the suturing of the lingual flap is completed and the needle has been brought back to the first interdental area, the positions of the flaps are adjusted and secured in their proper positions by closing the suture (Fig. 38-58b). Thus, only one knot is needed.

Periodontal dressings

Periodontal dressings are mainly used:

- To protect the wound post-surgically
- To obtain and maintain a close adaptation of the mucosal flaps to the underlying bone (especially when a flap has been repositioned apically)
- For the comfort of the patient.

In addition, periodontal dressings can prevent post-operative bleeding during the initial phase of healing and, if properly placed in the operated segment (especially interproximally), prevent the formation of excessive granulation tissue.

Periodontal dressings should have the following properties:

- The dressing should be soft, but still have enough plasticity and flexibility to facilitate its placement in the operated area and to allow proper adaptation.
- The dressing should harden within a reasonable time.
- After setting, the dressing should be sufficiently rigid to prevent fracture and dislocation.
- The dressing should have a smooth surface after setting to prevent irritation to the cheeks and lips.
- The dressing should preferably have bacteriocidal properties to prevent excessive plaque formation.
- The dressing must not detrimentally interfere with healing.

It has been suggested that antibacterial agents should be incorporated in periodontal dressings to prevent bacterial growth in the wound area during healing. Results from clinical studies and *in vitro* evaluation of the antibacterial properties of various periodontal dressings, however, suggest that the antibacterial activity of most commercial dressings probably is exhausted long before the end of the 7–14-day period during which the dressing is frequently

maintained in the operated segment (O'Neil 1975; Haugen *et al.* 1977).

Mouth rinsing with antibacterial agents such as chlorhexidine does not prevent the formation of plaque *under* the dressing (Plüss *et al.* 1975) and should therefore not be regarded as a means to improve or shorten the period of wound healing. On the other hand, results from clinical studies as well as clinical experience suggest that a periodontal dressing may often be unnecessary or even undesirable after periodontal flap procedures and may be usefully replaced by rinsing with chlorhexidine only (Sanz *et al.* 1989; Vaughan & Garnick 1989).

A commonly used periodontal dressing is Coe-Pak™ (Coe Laboratories Inc., Chicago, IL, USA), which is supplied in two tubes. One tube contains oxides of various metals (mainly zinc oxide) and lorothidol (a fungicide). The second tube contains non-ionizing carboxylic acids and chlorothymol (a bacteriostatic agent). Equal parts from both tubes are mixed together immediately prior to insertion. Adding a retarder can prolong the setting time of the dressing.

A light-cured dressing, e.g. Barricaid™ (Dentsply International Inc., Milford, DE, USA), is useful in the anterior tooth region and particularly following muco-gingival surgery, because it has a favorable esthetic appearance and it can be applied without dislocating the soft tissue. However, the light-cured dressing is not the choice of dressing for situations where the flap has to be retained apically, due to its soft state before curing.

Cyanoacrylates have also been used as periodontal dressings with varying success. Dressings of the cyanoacrylate type are applied in a liquid directly on to the wound, or sprayed over the wound surface. Although the application of this kind of dressing is simple, its properties often do not meet clinical demands, which is why its use is rather limited at present.

Application technique

- Ensure that bleeding from the operated tissues has ceased before the dressing material is inserted.
- Carefully dry teeth and soft tissue before the application for optimal adherence of the dressing.
- Moisten the surgical gloves to avoid the material sticking to the fingertips.
- When using the Coe-Pak™ dressing material, the interproximal areas are filled first. Thin rolls of the dressing, adjusted in length to cover the entire field of operation, are then placed against the buccal and lingual surfaces of the teeth. The rolls are pressed against the tooth surfaces and the dressing material is forced into the interproximal areas. Coe-Pak™ may also be applied to the wound surfaces by means of a plastic syringe. It is important to ensure that dressing material is never introduced between the flap and the underlying bone or root surface.

- The surface of the dressing is subsequently smoothened and excess material is removed with a suitable instrument. The dressing should not cover more than the apical third of the tooth surfaces. Furthermore, interference of the dressing with muco-gingival structures (e.g. vestibular fold, frenula) should be carefully checked to avoid displacement of the dressing during normal function.

The light-cured dressing (Barricaid™) is preferably applied with the supplied syringe, adjusted and then cured by light. It is important to dry teeth and soft tissue carefully before application for optimal adherence. Excess of dressing material can easily be removed following curing with a knife or finishing burs in a low-speed handpiece.

Post-operative pain control

In order to minimize post-operative pain and discomfort for the patient, surgical handling of the tissues should be as atraumatic as possible. Care should be taken during surgery to avoid unnecessary tearing of the flaps, to keep the bone moistened, and to secure complete soft tissue coverage of the alveolar bone at suturing. With a carefully performed surgical procedure most patients will normally experience only minimal post-operative problems. The pain experience is usually limited to the first days following surgery and of a level that in most patients can be adequately controlled with normally used drugs for pain control. However, it is important to recognize that pain threshold level is subjective and may vary between individuals. It is also important to give the patient information about the post-surgical sequence and that uncomplicated healing is the common event. Further, during the early phase of healing, the patient should be instructed to avoid chewing in the area subjected to surgical treatment.

Post-surgical care

Post-operative plaque control is the most important variable in determining the long-term result of periodontal surgery. Provided proper post-operative infection control levels are established, most surgical treatment techniques will result in conditions that favor the maintenance of a healthy periodontium. Although there are other factors of a more general nature affecting surgical outcome (e.g. the systemic status of the patient at time of surgery and during healing), disease recurrence is an inevitable complication, regardless of surgical technique used, in patients not given proper post-surgical and maintenance care.

Since self-performed oral hygiene is often associated with pain and discomfort during the immediate post-surgical phase, regularly performed professional tooth cleaning is a more effective means of mechanical infection control following periodontal surgery. In the immediate post-surgical period self-performed rinsing with a suitable antiplaque agent, e.g. twice daily rinsing with 0.1–0.2% chlorhexidine solution, is recommended. Although an obvious disadvantage with the use of chlorhexidine is the staining of teeth and tongue, this is usually not a deterrent for compliance. Nevertheless, it is important to return to and maintain good mechanical oral hygiene measures as soon as possible. This is especially important since rinsing with chlorhexidine, in contrast to properly performed mechanical oral hygiene, is not likely to have any influence on subgingival recolonization of plaque.

Maintaining good post-surgical wound stability is another important factor affecting the outcome of some types of periodontal flap surgery. If wound stability is judged an important part of a specific procedure, the procedure itself as well as the post-surgical care must include measures to stabilize the healing wound (e.g. adequate suturing technique, protection from mechanical trauma to the marginal tissues during the initial healing phase). If a muco-periosteal flap is replaced rather than repositioned apically, early apical migration of gingival epithelial cells will occur as a consequence of a break between root surface and healing connective tissue. Hence, maintenance of a tight adaptation of the flap to the root surface is essential and one may therefore consider keeping the sutures in place for longer than the 7–10 days usually prescribed following standard flap surgery.

Following suture removal, the surgically treated area is thoroughly irrigated with a dental spray and the teeth are carefully cleaned with a rubber cup and polishing paste. If the healing is satisfactory for starting mechanical tooth cleaning, the patient is instructed in gentle brushing of the operated area using a toothbrush that has been softened in hot water. Toothpicks are prescribed for cleaning the interdental area. In this early phase following surgical treatment the use of interdental brushes is abandoned due to the risk of traumatizing the interdental tissues. Visits are scheduled for supportive care at 2-week intervals to monitor the patient's plaque control closely. During this post-operative maintenance phase, adjustments of the methods for optimal self-performed mechanical cleaning are made depending on the healing status of the tissues. The time interval between visits for supportive care may gradually be increased, depending on the patient's plaque control standard.

Outcome of surgical periodontal therapy

Healing following surgical pocket therapy

Gingivectomy

Within a few days following excision of the inflamed gingival soft tissues coronal to the base of the periodontal pocket, epithelial cells start to migrate over the wound surface. The epithelialization of the gingivectomy wound is usually complete within 7–14 days following surgery (Engler *et al.* 1966; Stahl *et al.* 1968). During the following weeks a new dentogingival unit is formed (Fig. 38-59). The fibroblasts in the supra-alveolar tissue adjacent the tooth surface proliferate (Waerhaug 1955) and new connective tissue is laid down. If the wound healing occurs in the vicinity of a plaque-free tooth surface, a free gingival unit will form which has all the characteristics of a normal free gingiva (Hamp *et al.* 1975). The height of the newly formed free gingival unit may vary not only between different parts of the dentition but also from one tooth surface to another due to primarily anatomic factors.

The re-establishment of a new, free gingival unit by coronal regrowth of tissue from the line of the "gingivectomy" incision implies that sites with so-called "zero pockets" only occasionally occur following gingivectomy. Complete healing of the gingivectomy wound takes 4–5 weeks, although by clinical inspection the surface of the gingiva may appear to be healed already after approximately 14 days (Ramfjord *et al.* 1966). Minor remodeling of the alveolar bone crest may also occur post-operatively.

The apically repositioned flap

Following osseous surgery for elimination of bony defects and the establishment of "physiologic contours" and repositioning of the soft tissue flaps to the level of the alveolar bone, healing will occur primarily by first intention, especially in areas where proper soft tissue coverage of the alveolar bone has been obtained. During the initial phase of healing, bone resorption of varying degrees almost always occurs in the crestal area of the alveolar bone (Fig. 38-60)

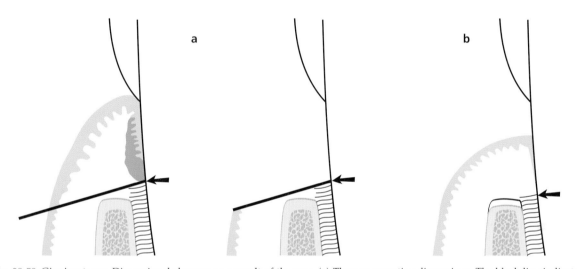

Fig. 38-59 Gingivectomy. Dimensional changes as a result of therapy. (a) The pre-operative dimensions. The black line indicates the location of the primary incision, i.e. the suprabony pocket is eliminated with the gingivectomy technique. (b) Dimensions following proper healing. Minor resorption of the alveolar bone crest as well as some loss of connective tissue attachment may occur during the healing.

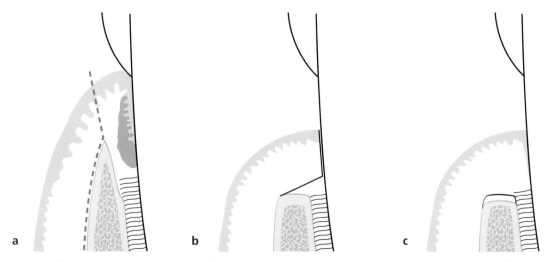

Fig. 38-60 Apically repositioned flap. Dimensional changes. (a) The pre-operative dimensions. The broken line indicates the border of the elevated mucoperiosteal flap. (b) Bone recontouring has been completed and the flap repositioned to cover the alveolar bone. (c) Dimensions following healing. Minor resorption of the marginal alveolar bone has occurred as well as some loss of connective tissue attachment.

(Ramfjord & Costich 1968). The extent of the reduction of the alveolar bone height resulting from this resorption is related to the thickness of the bone in each specific site (Wood *et al.* 1972; Karring *et al.* 1975).

During the phase of tissue regeneration and maturation a new dentogingival unit will form by coronal growth of the connective tissue. This regrowth occurs in a manner similar to that which characterized healing following gingivectomy.

The modified Widman flap

If a "modified Widman flap" procedure is carried out in an area with a deep infrabony lesion, bone repair may occur within the boundaries of the lesion (Rosling *et al.* 1976a; Polson & Heijl 1978). However, crestal bone resorption is also seen. The amount of bone fill obtained is dependent upon (1) the anatomy of the osseous defect (e.g. a three-walled infrabony defect often provides a better mould for bone repair than two- or one-walled defects), (2) the amount of crestal bone resorption, and (3) the extent of chronic inflammation, which may occupy the area of healing. Interposed between the regenerated bone tissue and the root surface, a long junctional epithelium is always found (Fig. 38-61) (Caton & Zander 1976; Caton *et al.* 1980). The apical cells of the newly formed junctional epithelium are found at a level on the root that closely coincides with the presurgical attachment level.

Soft tissue recession will take place during the healing phase following a modified Widman flap procedure. Although the major apical shift in the position of the soft tissue margin will occur during the first 6 months following the surgical treatment (Lindhe *et al.* 1987), the soft tissue recession may often continue for a time period of more than 1 year. Among factors influencing the degree of soft tissue recession as well as the time period for soft tissue remodeling are the initial height and thickness of the supracrestal flap tissue and the amount of crestal bone resorption.

Clinical outcome of surgical access therapy in comparison to non-surgical therapy

Surgical treatment of periodontal lesions mainly serves the purpose of (1) creating accessibility for proper professional debridement of the infected root surfaces and (2) establishing a gingival morphology that facilitates the patient's self-performed plaque control, in order to enhance the long-term preservation of the dentition. Hence, the amount of tooth loss would be the most relevant criterion in an evaluation of the relative importance of surgical access therapy in the overall treatment of periodontal disease. However, this would require studies with extremely long follow-up periods and, therefore, other criteria are commonly used to evaluate the efficacy of periodontal therapy, even if these may only be considered as surrogate end-points. The most commonly used outcome criteria in clinical research have been resolution of gingivitis (bleeding on probing), probing pocket depth reduction, and clinical attachment level change. An additional variable often of concern is gingival recession, since this outcome variable may affect the patient's overall appreciation of the treatment result. With regard to changes in probing attachment levels, it should be recalled that healing following conventional surgical access therapy consistently results in the formation of a junctional epithelium to a level on the root that closely coincides with the presurgical attachment level. Hence, when

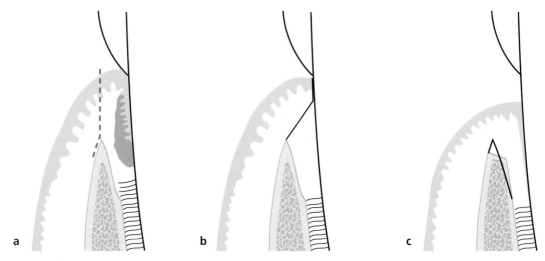

Fig. 38-61 Modified Widman flap. Dimensional changes. (a) The pre-operative dimensions. The broken line indicates the border of the elevated mucoperiosteal flap. (b) Surgery (including currettage of the angular bone defect) is completed with the mucoperiosteal flap repositioned as close as possible to its presurgical position. (c) Dimensions following healing. Osseous repair as well as some crestal bone resorption can be expected during healing with the establishment of a "long" junctional epithetium interposed between the regenerated bone tissue and the root surface. An apical displacement of the soft tissue margin has occurred.

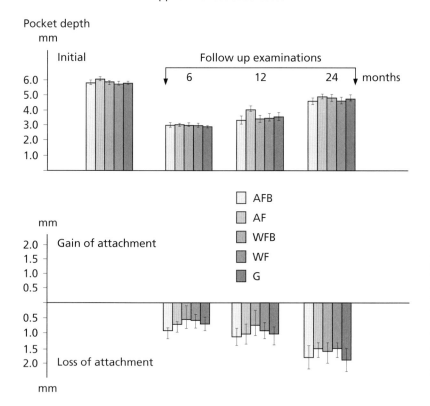

Fig. 38-62 Average approximal pocket depth at the initial examination and 6, 12, and 24 months after surgery (top) and alterations in approximal attachment levels from the initial examination immediately prior to surgery to the re-examinations 6, 12, and 24 months post-operatively (bottom). Note that only areas with pockets that at the initial examination had a depth of 3 mm or more are included in the analysis. I = standard error; AFB = apically repositioned flap with bone recontouring; AF = apically repositioned flap; WFB = modified Widman flap with bone recontouring; WF = modified Widman flap; G = gingivectomy including curettage of bone defects. (Data from Nyman *et al.* 1977.)

evaluating the outcome of various therapeutic approaches the magnitude of *gain* of clinical attachment may be of less importance since it mainly is a measure of "pocket closure". Instead maintained probing attachment levels or further loss should be focused on as the pertinent outcome variable.

Pioneering contributions to the understanding of the relative importance of the surgical component of periodontal therapy were generated by the classical longitudinal studies by the Michigan group (Ramfjord and co-workers) and the Gothenburg group (Lindhe and co-workers). Subsequently, several other clinical research centers contributed with important data regarding the efficacy of surgical access therapy in comparison to non-surgical periodontal therapy. The topic has been extensively reviewed in several recent publications (e.g. Kaldahl *et al.* 1993; Palcanis 1996) and some of the general conclusions from these reviews will be highlighted below.

Plaque accumulation

An important factor to consider in the evaluation of the relative effect of the surgical component of periodontal therapy is the standard of post-operative infection control. Nyman *et al.* (1977) reported on a clinical study in which the patients received only a single episode of oral hygiene instruction before the surgical treatment and no specific post-operative supportive care. As a consequence both plaque and gingival indices remained relatively high during the 2 years of post-operative follow-up. Independent of

surgical technique used, the patients showed a rebound of pocket depths to more or less pre-treatment levels and further deterioration of clinical attachment levels at both proximal and lingual tooth sites (Fig. 38-62). In contrast, in a parallel study in which the patients received repeated oral hygiene instructions and professional tooth-cleaning once every 2 weeks during the post-operative period (Rosling *et al.* 1976b), the patients maintained the surgically reduced pocket depth throughout the 2-year follow-up period and clinical attachment level gains were observed for most of the surgical procedures evaluated (Fig. 38-63). The fact that the standard of post-operative oral hygiene is decisive for the outcome of surgical pocket therapy is further underlined by data from a 5-year longitudinal study by Lindhe *et al.* (1984), which showed that patients with a high standard of infection control maintained clinical attachment levels and probing depth reductions following treatment more consistently than patients with poor plaque control. On the other hand, professional tooth cleaning, including subgingival scaling every 3 months, may partly compensate for the negative effects of variations in self-performed plaque control (Ramfjord *et al.* 1982; Isidor & Karring 1986).

With regard to post-treatment plaque accumulation, there is no evidence to suggest that differences exist between non-surgical or surgical treatment or between various surgical procedures. In addition, most studies have shown that the magnitude of gingivitis resolution is not influenced by the treatment modality.

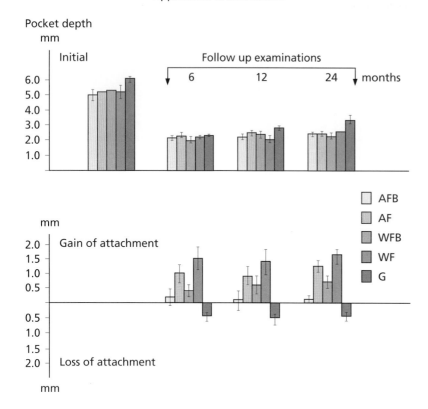

Fig. 38-63 Average approximal pocket depth at the initial examination and 6, 12, and 24 months after surgery (top) and alterations in approximal attachment levels from the initial examination immediately prior to surgery to the re-examinations 6, 12, and 24 months post-operatively (bottom). Note that only areas with pockets that at the initial examination had a depth of 3 mm or more are included in the analysis. I = standard error; AFB = apically repositioned flap with bone recontouring; AF = apically repositioned flap; WFB = modified Widman flap with bone recontouring; WF = modified Widman flap; G = gingivectomy including curettage of bone defects. (Data from Rosling *et al.* 1976b.)

Probing pocket depth reduction

All surgical procedures result in a decrease in probing pocket depths with greater reduction occurring at initially deeper sites (Knowles *et al.* 1979; Lindhe *et al.* 1984; Ramfjord *et al.* 1987; Kaldahl *et al.* 1996; Becker *et al.* 2001). Furthermore, surgical therapy generally creates greater short-term reduction of probing depth than non-surgically performed scaling and root planing. Flap surgery with bone recontouring (pocket elimination surgery) usually results in the most pronounced short-term pocket reduction. Long-term (5–8 years) results show various outcomes. Some studies reported greater probing depth reduction following surgery while others reported no differences in relation to non-surgical therapy. Also, the magnitude of the initial probing depth reduction shows a tendency to decrease with time, independent of treatment modality.

Clinical attachment level change

In sites with shallow initial probing depth, both short- and long-term data demonstrate that surgery creates a greater loss of clinical attachment than non-surgical treatment, whereas in sites with initially deep pockets (≥7 mm), a greater gain of clinical attachment is generally obtained (Knowles *et al.* 1979; Lindhe *et al.* 1984; Ramfjord *et al.* 1987; Kaldahl *et al.* 1996; Becker *et al.* 2001) (Fig. 38-64). When clinical attachment levels following surgery with and without osseous resection were compared, either no differ-

ence was found between therapies, or flap surgery without osseous resection produced a greater gain. In addition, there was no difference in the longitudinal maintenance of clinical attachment levels between sites treated non-surgically and those treated surgically, with or without osseous resection.

Based on data generated from a clinical trial comparing non-surgical and surgical (modified Widman flap) approaches to root debridement, Lindhe *et al.* (1982b) developed the concept of *critical probing depth* in relation to clinical attachment level change. For each treatment approach, the clinical attachment change was plotted against the initial pocket depth and regression lines were calculated (Fig. 38-65). The point where the regression line crossed the horizontal axis (initial probing depth) was defined as the *critical probing depth* (CPD), i.e. the level of pocket depth below which clinical attachment loss would occur as the result of the treatment procedure performed. The CPD was consistently found to be greater for the surgical approach than for the non-surgical treatment. Furthermore, at incisors and premolars the surgical therapy showed superior outcome only when the initial probing depth was greater than 6–7 mm, while at molars the corresponding cut-off point was 4.5 mm. The interpretation of the latter finding would be that, in the molar tooth regions, the surgical approach to root debridement offers advantages over the non-surgical approach. This interpretation is supported by the observation that inferior results are obtained by non-surgical therapy in molars compared to single-rooted teeth (Nordland *et al.*

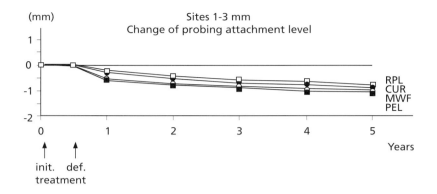

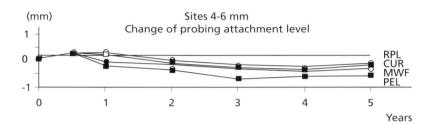

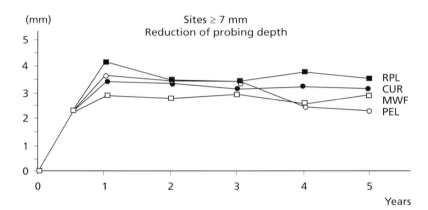

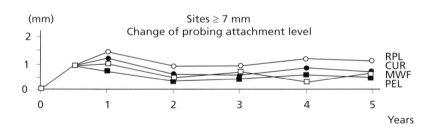

Fig. 38-64 Longitudinal evaluation of four treatment modalities in the three categories of initial probing depth; 1–3 mm, 4–6 mm and ≥7 mm. RPL = scaling and root planning; CUR = subgingival curettage; MWF = modified Widman flap; PEL = pocket elimination surgery. (Data from Ramfjord *et al.* 1987, presented by Egelberg 1995.)

1987; Loos *et al.* 1988). Also data generated from studies comparing closed and open root debridement in furcation sites favor surgical access therapy in the treatment of molar tooth regions (Matia *et al.* 1986).

The removal of the pocket epithelium and the soft tissue lesion by curettage (Echeverria & Caffesse 1983; Ramfjord *et al.* 1987) or surgical excision (Lindhe & Nyman 1985) is not a prerequisite for proper healing of the treated periodontal site. In the study by Lindhe and Nyman (1985) three treatment modalities were used, i.e. excision of the soft tissue lesion during flap surgery (modified Widman flap procedure), surgery without removal of the soft tissue lesion (Kirkland flap), and non-surgical scaling and

root planing. The 1-year follow-up examination revealed about 1 mm of gain in clinical attachment level for all three procedures. Thus, deliberate excision of the soft tissue lesion did not improve the healing result.

Gingival recession

Gingival recession is an inevitable consequence of periodontal therapy. Since it occurs primarily as a result of resolution of the inflammation in the periodontal tissues, it is seen both following non-surgical and surgical therapy. Irrespective of treatment modality used, initially deeper pocket sites will experience

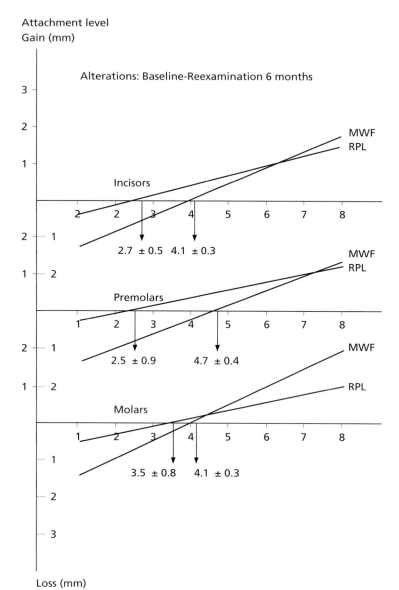

Fig. 38-65 Diagram illustrating the gain and loss of clinical attachment (Y-axis) at incisors, premolars, and molars, calculated from measurements taken prior to and 6 months after treatment. RPL = scaling and root planing; MWF = modified Widman flap surgery. The non-surgical approach (RPL) consistently yielded lower critical probing depth (CPD) values than the surgical approach. (Data from Lindhe *et al.* 1982b.)

more pronounced signs of recession of the gingival margin than sites with shallow initial probing depths (Badersten *et al.* 1984; Lindhe *et al.* 1987; Becker *et al.* 2001).

A general finding in short-term follow-up studies of periodontal therapy is that non-surgically performed scaling and root planing causes less gingival recession than surgical therapy, and that surgical treatment involving osseous resection results in the most pronounced recession. However, data obtained from long-term studies reveal that the initial differences seen in amount of recession between various treatment modalities diminish over time due to a coronal rebound of the soft tissue margin following surgical treatment (Kaldahl *et al.* 1996; Becker *et al.* 2001) (Fig. 38-66). Lindhe and Nyman (1980) found that after an apically repositioned flap procedure the buccal gingival margin shifted to a more coronal position (about 1 mm) during 10–11 years of maintenance. In interdental areas denuded following surgery, van der Velden (1982) found an upgrowth of around 4 mm of gingival tissue 3 years after

surgery, while no significant change in attachment levels was observed. A similar finding was reported by Pontoriero and Carnevale (2001) 1 year after an apically positioned flap procedure for crown lengthening.

Bone fill in angular bone defects

The potential for bone formation in angular defects following surgical access therapy has been demonstrated in a number of studies. Rosling *et al.* (1976a) studied the healing of two- and three-wall angular bone defects following a modified Widman flap procedure, including careful curettage of the bone defect and proper root debridement, in 24 patients with multiple osseous defects. Following active treatment, patients assigned to the test group received supportive periodontal care once every 2 weeks for a 2-year period, while the patients in the control group were only recalled once a year for prophylaxis. Re-examination carried out 2 years after therapy demonstrated that the patients who had been subjected to the inten-

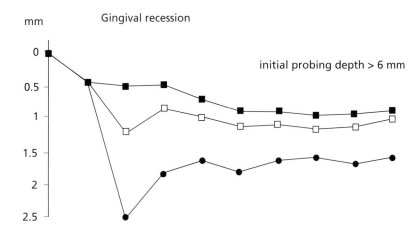

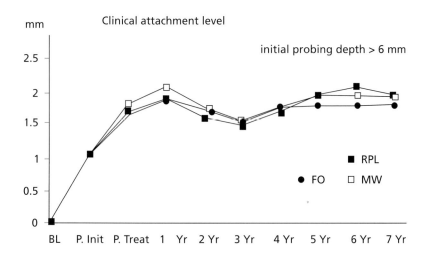

Fig. 38-66 Longitudinal changes over 7 years in recession (top diagram) and clinical attachment levels (bottom diagram) at sites with initial probing pocket depth of >6 mm following three different periodontal treatment modalities. RPL = scaling and root planing; MWF = modified Widman flap procedure; FO = flap and osseous surgery. (Data from Kaldahl *et al.* 1996.)

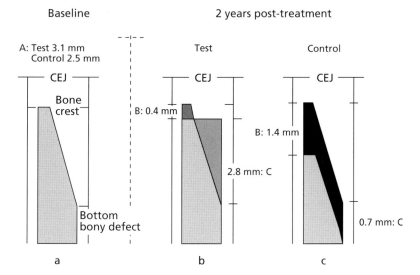

Fig. 38-67 Schematic drawing illustrating alterations in the level of the marginal bone crest and the level of the bottom of the bone defects in the test and control groups of the study by Rosling *et al.* (1976a). Distance A denotes the depth of the bone defects at the initial examination; test group 3.1 mm, control 2.5 mm. Distance B denotes resorption of the alveolar crest (b,c), which amounted to 0.4 mm in the test patients (b) and 1.4 mm in the controls (c). Distance C denotes gain or loss of bone in the apical portion of the defect. There was a refill of bone in the test patients (b) amounting to 2.8 mm, whereas a further 0.7 mm loss of bone occurred in the control patients (c).

sive professional tooth-cleaning regimen had experienced a mean gain of clinical attachment in the angular bone defects amounting to 3.5 mm. Measurements performed on radiographs revealed a marginal bone loss of 0.4 mm, but the remaining portion of the original bone defect (2.8 mm) was refilled with bone (Fig. 38-67). All the 124 bone defects treated were completely resolved. In the control group most of the sites treated showed signs of recurrent periodontitis,

including further loss of clinical attachment and alveolar bone. Similar healing results were reported by Polson and Heijl (1978). They treated 15 defects (two- and three-wall) in nine patients using a modified Widman flap procedure. Following curettage of the bone defect and root planing, the flaps were closed to achieve complete soft tissue coverage of the defect area. All patients were enrolled in a professional tooth-cleaning program. The healing was evaluated at a re-entry operation 6–8 months after the initial surgery. Eleven of the 15 defects had resolved completely. The healing was characterized by a combination of coronal bone regeneration (77% of the initial depth of the defects) and marginal bone resorption (18%). The authors concluded that intrabony defects might predictably remodel after surgical debridement and establishment of optimal plaque control.

The results from the studies referred to demonstrate that a significant bone fill may be obtained in two- and three-wall intrabony defects at single-rooted teeth, provided the post-operative supportive care is of very high quality. Two recent reviews (Laurell *et al.* 1998; Lang 2000), focusing on the outcome of surgical access therapy in angular bone defects, give additional information regarding expected bone regeneration in angular defects following open-flap debridement (modified Widman flap). In the review by Laurell *et al.* (1998) 13 studies were included representing a total of 278 treated defects with a mean depth of 4.1 mm. The weighted mean bone

fill in the angular defects amounted to 1.1 mm. Lang (2000) reported an analysis of 15 studies providing data generated from radiographic assessments of the healing of 523 angular bone defects. The analysis yielded a weighted mean of 1.5 mm of bone gain. Since the included studies in these reviews showed great variability in bone fill, one may assume that the standard of post-surgical plaque control varied between the studies. As shown in the study by Rosling *et al.* (1976a), meticulous post-surgical plaque control and close professional supervision of the patients are critical for optimal healing conditions. One also has to consider that the potential for bone fill may differ depending on the morphology of the angular bone defect. Most angular defects appear as combinations of one-, two- and three-wall defects and whereas the two- and three-wall component of an angular bone defect may show great potential for bone fill during healing, the one-wall component will rarely demonstrate this type of healing.

References

Ah, M.K.B., Johnson, G.K., Kaldahl, W.B., Patil, K.D. & Kalkwarf, K.L. (1994). The effect of smoking on the response to periodontal therapy. *Journal of Clinical Periodontology* **21**, 91–97.

American Dental Association; American Academy of Orthopaedic Surgeons (2003). Advisory statement – Antibiotic prophylaxis for dental patients with total joint replacements. *Journal of the American Dental Association* **134**, 895–899.

Ariaudo, A.A. & Tyrell, H.A. (1957). Repositioning and increasing the zone of attached gingiva. *Journal of Periodontology* **28**, 106–110.

Axelsson, P. & Lindhe, J. (1981). The significance of maintenance care in the treatment of periodontal disease. *Journal of Clinical Periodontology* **8**, 281–294.

Badersten, A., Nilveus, R. & Egelberg, J. (1981). Effect of nonsurgical periodontal therapy. I. Moderately advanced periodontitis. *Journal of Clinical Periodontology* **8**, 57–72.

Badersten, A., Nilveus, R. & Egelberg, J. (1984). Effect of nonsurgical periodontal therapy. II. Severely advanced periodontitis. *Journal of Clinical Periodontology* **11**, 63–76.

Becker, W., Becker, B.E., Caffesse, R., Kerry, G., Ochsenbein, C., Morrison, E. & Prichard, J. (2001). A longitudinal study comparing scaling, osseous surgery and modified Widman procedures: Results after 5 years. *Journal of Peridontology* **72**, 1675–1684.

Blomlöf, J. & Lindskog, S. (1995a). Root surface texture and early cell and tissue colonization after different etching modalities. *European Journal of Oral Sciences* **103**, 17–24.

Blomlöf, J. & Lindskog, S. (1995b). Periodontal tissue-vitality after different etching modalities. *Journal of Clinical Peridontology* **22**, 464–468.

Blomlöf, L., Jonsson, B., Blomlöf, J. & Lindskog, S. (2000). A clinical study of root surface conditioning with an EDTA gel. II. Surgical periodontal treatment. *International Journal of Periodontics and Restorative Dentistry* **20**, 566–573.

Bowers, G.M., Chadroff, B., Carnevale, R., Mellonig, J.T., Corio, R., Emerson, J., Stevens, M. & Romberg, E. (1989). Histologic evaluation of new human attachment apparatus formation in humans, Part III. *Journal of Periodontology* **60**, 683–693

Brägger, U., Lauchenauer, D. & Lang, N.P. (1992). Surgical lengthening of the clinical crown. *Journal of Clinical Periodontology* **19**, 58–63.

Caffesse, R.G., Sweeney, P.L. & Smith, B.A. (1986). Scaling and root planing with and without periodontal flap surgery. *Journal of Clinical Periodontology* **13**, 205–210.

Caton, J., Nyman, S. & Zander, H. (1980). Histometric evaluation of periodontal surgery. II. Connective tissue attachment levels after four regenerative procedures. *Journal of Clinical Periodontology* **7**, 224–231.

Caton, J.G. & Zander, H.A. (1976). Osseous repair of an infrabony pocket without new attachment of connective tissue. *Journal of Clinical Periodontology* **3**, 54–58.

Cortellini, P., Pini Prato, G. & Tonetti, M.S. (1993). Periodontal regeneration of human infrabony defects. I. Clinical measures. *Journal of Periodontology* **64**, 254–260.

Cortellini, P., Pini Prato, G. & Tonetti, M.S. (1995a). Periodontal regeneration of human intrabony defects with titanium reinforced membranes. A controlled clinical trial. *Journal of Periodontology* **66**, 797–803.

Cortellini, P., Pini Prato, G. & Tonetti, M. (1995b). The modified papilla preservation technique. A new surgical approach for interproximal regenerative procedures. *Journal of Periodontology* **66**, 261–266.

Cortellini, P., Pini Prato, G. & Tonetti, M. (1999). The simplified papilla preservation flap. A novel surgical approach for the management of soft tissues in regenerative procedures. *International Journal of Periodontics and Restorative Dentistry* 1999; **19**, 589–599.

Dajani, A.S., Taubert, K.A., Wilson, W., Bolger, A.F., Bayer, A., Ferrieri, P., Gewitz, M.H., Shulman, S.T., Nouri, S., Newburger, J.W., Hutto, C., Pallasch, T.J., Gage, T.W., Levison, M.E., Peter, G. & Zuccaro, G. Jr. (1997). Prevention of bacterial endocarditis: recommendations by the American Heart Association. *Journal of the American Dental Association* **128**, 1142–1151.

Echeverria, J.J. & Caffesse, R.G. (1983). Effects of gingival curettage when performed 1 month after root instrumentation. A biometric evaluation. *Journal of Clinical Periodontology* **10**, 277–286.

Egelberg, J. (1995). *Periodontics: the Scientific Way. Synopsis of Human Clinical Studies*, 2nd edn. Malmö: Odonto Science, p. 113.

Engler, W.O., Ramfjord, S.P. & Hiniker, J.J. (1966). Healing following simple gingivectomy. A tritiated thymidine radioautographic study. I. Epithelialization. *Journal of Periodontology* **37**, 298–308.

Fay, J.T. & O'Neal, R.B. (1984). Dental responsibility for the medically compromised patient. *Journal of Oral Medicine* **39**, 218–255.

Friedman, N. (1955). Periodontal osseous surgery: osteoplasty and ostectomy. *Journal of Periodontology* **26**, 257–269.

Friedman, N. (1962). Mucogingival surgery. The apically repositioned flap. *Journal of Periodontology* **33**, 328–340.

Goldman, H.M. (1950). Development of physiologic gingival contours by gingivoplasty. *Oral Surgery, Oral Medicine and Oral Pathology* **3**, 879–888.

Goldman, H.M. (1951). Gingivectomy. *Oral Surgery, Oral Medicine and Oral Pathology* **4**, 1136–1157.

Gottlow, J., Nyman, S., Lindhe, J., Karring, T. & Wennström, J. (1986). New attachment formation in the human periodontium by guided tissue regeneration. *Journal of Clinical Periodontology* **13**, 604–616.

Grant, D.A., Stern, I.B. & Everett, F.G. (1979). *Periodontics in the Tradition of Orban and Gottlieb*, 5th edn. St. Louis: C.V. Mosby Co.

Hammarström, L. (1997). Enamel matrix, cementum development and regeneration. *Journal of Clinical Periodontology* **24**, 658–668.

Hamp, S.E., Rosling, B. & Lindhe, J. (1975). Effect of chlorhexidine on gingival wound healing in the dog. A histometric study. *Journal of Clinical Periodontology* **2**, 143–152.

Haugen, E., Gjermo, P. & Ørstavik, D. (1977). Some antibacterial properties of periodontal dressings. *Journal of Clinical Periodontology* **4**, 62–68.

Heijl, L., Heden, G., Svärdström, G. & Östgren, A. (1997). Enamel matrix derivative (Emdogain®) in the treatment of intrabony periodontal defects. *Journal of Clinical Periodontology* **24**, 705–714.

Herrero, F., Scott, J.B., Maropis, P.S. & Yukna, R.A. (1995). Clinical comparison of desired versus actual amount of surgical crown lengthening. *Journal of Periodontology* **66**, 568–571.

Isidor, F. & Karring, T. (1986). Long-term effect of surgical and non-surgical periodontal treatment. A 5-year clinical study. *Journal of Periodontal Research* **21**, 462–472.

Kaldahl, W.B., Kalkwarf, K.L. & Patil, K.D. (1993). A review of longitudinal studies that compared periodontal therapies. *Journal of Periodontology* **64**, 243–253.

Kaldahl, W.B., Kalkwarf, K.L., Patil, K.D., Molvar, M.P. & Dyer, J.K. (1996). Long-term evaluation of periodontal therapy: I. Response to 4 therapeutic modalities. *Journal of Periodontology* **67**, 93–102.

Karring, T., Cumming, B.R., Oliver, R.C. & Löe, H. (1975). The origin of granulation tissue and its impact on postoperative results of mucogingival surgery. *Journal of Periodontology* **46**, 577–585.

Kirkland, O. (1931). The suppurative periodontal pus pocket; its treatment by the modified flap operation. *Journal of the American Dental Association* **18**, 1462–1470.

Knowles, J.W., Burgett, F.G., Nissle, R.R., Schick, R.A., Morrison, E.C. & Ramfjord, S.P. (1979). Results of periodontal treatment related to pocket depth and attachment level. Eight years. *Journal of Periodontology* **50**, 225–233.

Labriola, A., Needleman, I. & Moles, D.R. (2005). Systematic review of the effect of smoking on nonsurgical periodontal therapy. *Periodontology 2000* **37**, 124–137.

Lang, N.P. (2000). Focus on intrabony defects – conservative therapy. *Periodontology 2000* **22**, 51–58.

Laurell, L., Gottlow, J., Zybutz, M. & Persson, R. (1998). Treatment of intrabony defects by different surgical procedures. A literature review. *Journal of Periodontology* **69**, 303–313.

Lindhe, J. & Nyman, S. (1980). Alterations of the position of the marginal soft tissue following periodontal surgery. *Journal of Clinical Periodontology* **7**, 538–530.

Lindhe, J. & Nyman, S. (1985). Scaling and granulation tissue removal in periodontal therapy. *Journal of Clinical Periodontology* **12**, 374–388.

Lindhe, J., Westfelt, E., Nyman, S., Socransky, S.S., Heijl, L. & Bratthall, G. (1982a). Healing following surgical/non-surgical treatment of periodontal disease. *Journal of Clinical Periodontology* **9**, 115–128.

Lindhe, J., Nyman, S., Socransky, S.S., Haffajee, A.D. & Westfelt, E. (1982b). "Critical probing depth" in periodontal therapy. *Journal of Clinical Periodontology* **9**, 323–336.

Lindhe, J., Westfelt, E., Nyman, S., Socransky, S.S. & Haffajee, A.D. (1984). Long-term effect of surgical/non-surgical treatment of periodontal disease. *Journal of Clinical Periodontology* **11**, 448–458.

Lindhe, J., Socransky, S.S., Nyman, S. & Westfelt, E. (1987). Dimensional alteration of the periodontal tissues following therapy. *International Journal of Periodontics and Restorative Dentistry* **7**(2), 9–22.

Loos, B., Claffey, N. & Egelberg, J. (1988). Clinical and microbiological effects of root debridement in periodontal furcation pockets. *Journal of Clinical Periodontology* **15**, 453–463.

Matia, J.I., Bissada, N.F., Maybury, J.E. & Ricchetti, P. (1986). Efficiency of scaling of the molar furcation area with and without surgical access. *International Journal of Periodontics and Restorative Dentistry* **6**, 24–35.

Nabers, C.L. (1954). Repositioning the attached gingiva. *Journal of Periodontology* **25**, 38–39.

Neuman, R. (1920). *Die Alveolar-Pyorrhöe und ihre Behandlung*, 3rd edn. Berlin: Herman Meusser.

Nordland, P., Garrett, S., Kiger, R., Vanooteghem, R., Hutchens, L.H. & Egelberg, J. (1987). The effect of plaque control and root debridement in molar teeth. *Journal of Clinical Periodontology* **14**, 231–236.

Nyman, S., Lindhe, J. & Rosling, B. (1977). Periodontal surgery in plaque-infected dentitions. *Journal of Clinical Periodontology* **4**, 240–249.

Nyman, S., Lindhe, J., Karring, T. & Rylander, H. (1982). New attachment following surgical treatment of human periodontal disease. *Journal of Clinical Periodontology* **9**, 290–296.

O'Neil, T.C.A. (1975). Antibacterial properties of periodontal dressings. *Journal of Periodontology* **46**, 469–474.

Palcanis, K.G. (1996). Surgical pocket therapy. *Annals of Periodontology* **1**, 589–617.

Plüss, E.M., Engelberger, P.R. & Rateitschak, K.H. (1975). Effect of chlorhexidine on dental plaque formation under periodontal pack. *Journal of Clinical Periodontology* **2**, 136–142.

Polson, A.M. & Heijl, L. (1978). Osseous repair in infrabony periodontal defects. *Journal of Clinical Periodontology* **5**, 13–23.

Pontoriero, R. & Carnevale, G. (2001). Surgical crown lengthening: a 12-month clinical wound healing study. *Journal of Periodontology* **72**, 841–848.

Preber, H. & Bergström, J. (1990). Effect of cigarette smoking on periodontal healing following surgical therapy. *Journal of Clinical Periodontology* **17**, 324–328.

Ramfjord, S.P., Caffesse, R.G., Morrison, E.C., Hill, R.W., Kerry, G.J., Appleberry, E.A., Nissle, R.R. & Stults, D.L. (1987). Four modalities of periodontal treatment compared over 5 years. *Journal of Periodontology* **14**, 445–452.

Ramfjord, S.P. & Costich, E.R. (1968). Healing after exposure of periosteum on the alveolar process. *Journal of Periodontology* **38**, 199–207.

Ramfjord, S.P., Morrison, E.C., Burgett, F.G., Nissle, R.R., Schick, R.A., Zann, G.J. & Knowles, J.W. (1982). Oral hygiene and maintenance of periodontal support. *Journal of Periodontology* **53**, 26–30.

Ramfjord, S.P. & Nissle, R.R. (1974). The modified Widman flap. *Journal of Periodontology* **45**, 601–607.

Ramfjord, S.P., Engler, W.O. & Hiniker, J.J. (1966). A radioautographic study of healing following simple gingivectomy.

II. The connective tissue. *Journal of Periodontology* **37**, 179–189.

Robicsek, S. (1884). Ueber das Wesen und Entstehen der Alveolar-Pyorrhöe und deren Behandlung. The 3rd Annual Report of the Austrian Dental Association (Reviewed in *Journal of Periodontology* **36**, 265, 1965).

Robinson, R.E. (1966). The distal wedge operation. *Periodontics* **4**, 256–264.

Rosling, B., Nyman, S. & Lindhe, J. (1976a). The effect of systemic plaque control on bone regeneration in infrabony pockets. *Journal of Clinical Periodontology* **3**, 38–53.

Rosling, B., Nyman, S., Lindhe, J. & Jern, B. (1976b). The healing potential of the periodontal tissue following different techniques of periodontal surgery in plaque-free dentitions. A 2-year clinical study. *Journal of Clinical Peridontology* **3**, 233–255.

Sanz, M., Newman, M.G., Anderson, L., Matoska, W., Otomo-Corgel, J. & Saltini, C. (1989). Clinical enhancement of post-periodontal surgical therapy by a 0.12% chlorhexidine gluconate mouthrinse. *Journal of Periodontology* **60**, 570–576.

Scabbia, A., Cho, K.S., Sigurdsson, T.J., Kim, C.K. & Trombelli, L. (2001). Cigarette smoking negatively affects healing response following flap debridement surgery. *Journal of Periodontology* **72**, 43–49.

Schluger, S. (1949). Osseous resection – a basic principle in periodontal surgery? *Oral Surgery, Oral Medicine and Oral Pathology* **2**, 316–325.

Siana, J.E., Rex, S. & Gottrup, F. (1989). The effect of cigarette smoking on wound healing. *Scandinavian Journal of Plastic and Reconstructive Surgery and Hand Surgery* **23**, 207–209.

Stahl, S.S., Witkin, G.J., Cantor, M. & Brown, R. (1968). Gingival healing. II. Clinical and histologic repair sequences following gingivectomy. *Journal of Periodontology* **39**, 109–118.

Takei, H.H., Han, T.J., Carranza, F.A., Kennedy, E.B. & Lekovic, V. (1985). Flap technique for periodontal bone implants. Papilla preservation technique. *Journal of Periodontology* **56**, 204–210.

Townsend-Olsen, C., Ammons, W.F. & Van Belle, C.A. (1985). A longitudinal study comparing apically repositioned flaps with and without osseous surgery. *International Journal of Periodontics and Restorative Dentistry* **5**(4), 11–33.

van der Velden, U. (1982). Regeneration of the interdental soft tissues following denudation procedures. *Journal of Clinical Periodontology* **9**, 455–459.

Vaughan, M.E. & Garnick, J.J. (1989). The effect of a 0.125% chlorhexidine rinse on inflammation after periodontal surgery. *Journal of Periodontology* **60**, 704–708.

Wachtel, H.C. (1994). Surgical periodontal therapy. In: Lang, N.P. & Karring, T., eds. *Proceedings of the 1st European Workshop on Periodontology*. London: Quintessence Publishing Co. Ltd., pp. 159–171.

Waerhaug, J. (1955). Microscopic demonstration of tissue reaction incident to removal of subgingival calculus. *Journal of Periodontology* **26**, 26–29.

Waerhaug, J. (1978). Healing of the dentoepithelial junction following subgingival plaque control. II. As observed on extracted teeth. *Journal of Periodontology* **49**, 119–134.

Widman, L. (1918). The operative treatment of pyorrhea alveolaris. A new surgical method. *Svensk Tandläkaretidskrift* (reviewed in *British Dental Journal* **1**, 293, 1920).

Wood, D.L., Hoag, P.M., Donnenfeld, O.W. & Rosenfeld, L.D. (1972). Alveolar crest reduction following full and partial thickness flaps. *Journal of Periodontology* **42**, 141–144.

Zentler, A. (1918). Suppurative gingivitis with alveolar involvement. A new surgical procedure. *Journal of the American Medical Association* **71**, 1530–1534.

Chapter 39

Treatment of Furcation-Involved Teeth

Gianfranco Carnevale, Roberto Pontoriero, and Jan Lindhe

Terminology, 823
Anatomy, 824
    Maxillary molars, 824
    Maxillary premolars, 825
    Mandibular molars, 825
    Other teeth, 826
Diagnosis, 826
    Probing, 828
    Radiographs, 828

Differential diagnosis, 829
    Trauma from occlusion, 829
Therapy, 830
    Scaling and root planing, 830
    Furcation plasty, 830
    Tunnel preparation, 832
    Root separation and resection (RSR), 832
    Regeneration of furcation defects, 840
    Extraction, 843
Prognosis, 843

Detailed knowledge of the morphology of the multi-rooted teeth and their position in the dental arch is a fundamental prerequisite for a proper understanding of problems which may occur when such teeth become involved in destructive periodontal disease. The first part of this chapter therefore includes a brief description of some important anatomic features of the root complexes and related structures of premolars and molars.

Terminology

Root complex is the portion of a tooth that is located apical to the cemento-enamel junction (CEJ), i.e. the portion that normally is covered with a root cementum. The root complex may be divided into two parts: the *root trunk* and the *root cone(s)* (Fig. 39-1).

The *root trunk* represents the *undivided region* of the root. The height of the root trunk is defined as the distance between the CEJ and the separation line (furcation) between two root cones (roots). Depending on the position of the separation line the height of the root trunk may vary from one surface to the next in one given molar or premolar.

The *root cone* is included in the *divided region* of the root complex. The root cone (root) may vary in size and position and may at certain levels be connected to or separated from other root cones. Two or more root cones make up the *furcated region* of the root complex (Fig. 39-2a). The *furcation* is the area located between individual root cones.

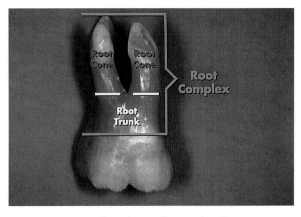

Fig. 39-1 Root complex of a maxillary molar. The root complex is separated into one undivided region: the root trunk, and one divided region: the (three) root cones.

The *furcation entrance* is the transitional area between the undivided and the divided part of the root (Fig. 39-2a,b). The *furcation fornix* is the roof of the furcation (Fig. 39-2b).

The d*egree of separation* is the angle of separation between two roots (cones) (Fig. 39-3a). *Divergence* is the distance between two roots; this distance normally increases in apical direction (Fig. 39-3a). The *coefficient of separation* is the length of the root cones in relation to the length of the root complex (Fig. 39-3b).

Fusion between divergent root cones may occur. The fusion may be complete or incomplete. In the

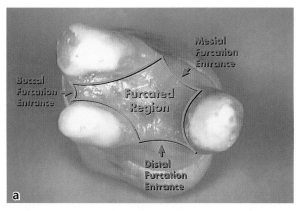 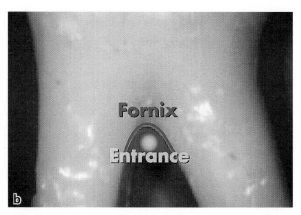

Fig. 39-2 (a) Apical-occlusal view of a maxillary molar where the three root cones make up the furcated region and the three furcation entrances. (b) A buccal view of the furcation entrance and of its roof.

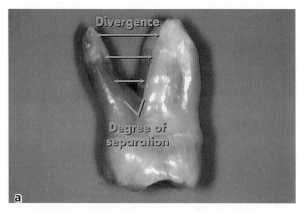 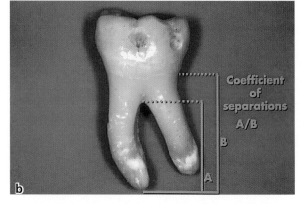

Fig. 39-3 (a) Photograph illustrating the angle (degree) of separation and the divergence between the mesio-buccal and the palatal roots of a maxillary molar. (b) The coefficient of separation (A/B) of the illustrated mandibular molar is 0.8 (A = 8 mm; B = 10 mm).

case of an incomplete fusion, the root cones may be fused in the area close to the CEJ but separated in a more apical region of the root complex.

Anatomy

Maxillary molars

As a general rule the maxillary first molar, in all respects – crown and individual roots – is larger than the second molar, which in turn is larger than the third molar.

The first and second molars most often have three roots; one mesio-buccal, one disto-buccal, and one palatal. The mesio-buccal root is normally vertically positioned while the disto-buccal and the palatal roots are inclined. The disto-buccal root projects distally and the palatal root projects in palatal direction (Fig. 39-4). The cross sections of the distobuccal and the palatal roots are generally circular. The palatal root is generally wider in the mesio-distal than in the bucco-palatal direction. The distal surface of the mesio-buccal root has a concavity which is about 0.3 mm deep (Bower 1979a,b). This concavity gives

the cross section of the mesio-buccal root an "hour-glass" configuration (Fig. 39-5).

The three furcation entrances of the maxillary first and second molars vary in width and are positioned at varying distances apical to the CEJ. As a rule, the first molar has a shorter root trunk than the second molar. In the first molar the mesial furcation entrance is located about 3 mm from the CEJ, while the buccal is 3.5 mm and the distal entrance about 5 mm apical to the CEJ (Abrams & Trachtenberg 1974; Rosenberg 1988). This implies that the furcation fornix is inclined; in the mesiodistal plane the fornix is comparatively close to the CEJ at the mesial but closer to the apex at the distal surface. The buccal furcation entrance is narrower than its distal and mesial counterparts.

The degree of separation between the roots and their divergence decreases from the first to the second, and from the second to the third maxillary molar.

The mesio-buccal root of the first molar is frequently located more buccally in the arch than the disto-buccal root. If the buccal bone plate is thin, the mesio-buccal root frequently projects through the outer surface of the alveolar bone and bone fenestrations and/or dehiscences may occur.

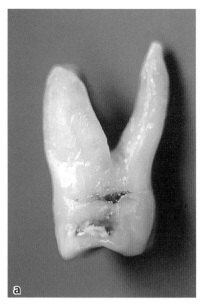
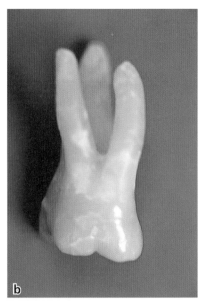
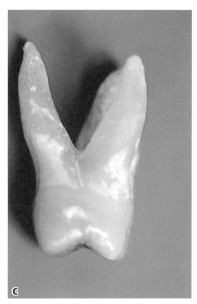

Fig. 39-4 Furcation entrances (a, mesial; b, buccal; c, distal) and the position of the roots of a maxillary first molar.

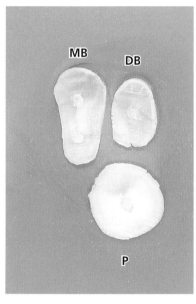

Fig. 39-5 Root-shape of a maxillary first molar in a horizontal cut at the level of the coronal third of the cones. Note the circular shape of the palatal root in comparison with the mesio-distally compressed shape of the mesio-buccal root, which also exhibits a concavity in the distal aspect.

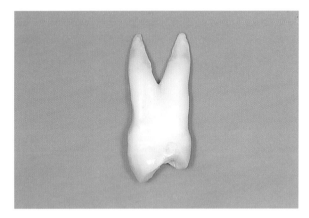

Fig. 39-6 A maxillary first premolar with the furcation located in the apical third of the root complex.

Maxillary premolars

In about 40% of cases the maxillary first premolars have two root cones, one buccal and one palatal, and hence have a mesiodistal furcation. A concavity (about 0.5 mm deep) is often present in the furcation aspect of the buccal root. In many cases the furcation is located in the middle or in the apical third of the root complex (Fig. 39-6). The mean distance between CEJ and the furcation entrance is about 8 mm. The width of the furcation entrance is about 0.7 mm.

Mandibular molars

The mandibular first molar is larger than the second molar, which in turn is larger than the third molar. In the first and second molars the root complex almost always includes two root cones, one mesial and one distal. The mesial root is larger than the distal. The mesial root has a position which is mainly vertical while the distal root projects distally. The mesial root is wider in the bucco-lingual direction and has a larger cross-sectional area than the distal root. The cross section of the distal root is circular while the mesial root has an "hour-glass" shape. In addition, furrows and concavities often occur on the distal surface of the mesial root (Fig. 39-7). The distal concavity of the mesial root is more pronounced than that of the distal root (Bower 1979a,b; Svärdström & Wennström 1988).

The root trunk of the first molar is often shorter than the trunk of the second molar. The furcation entrances of the mandibular first molar, similar to

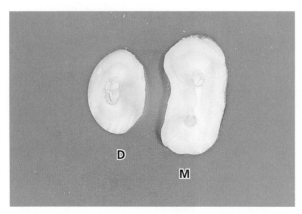

Fig. 39-7 "Hour-glass" shape of the mesial root – with a concavity in the distal aspect – and the circular shape of the distal root (horizontal section at the level of the coronal third of the cones).

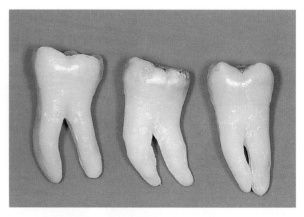

Fig. 39-8 From left to right, differences in degree of separation and in divergence between the root cones from the first to the mandibular third molar.

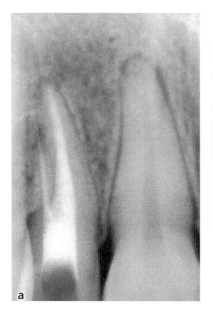

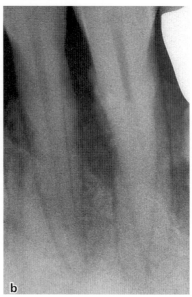

Fig. 39-9 Radiographs illustrating morphologic variations represented by two-rooted (a) maxillary lateral incisor and (b) mandibular canine.

those of the maxillary first molar, are located at different distances from the CEJ. Thus, the lingual entrance is frequently found more apical to the CEJ (>4 mm) than the buccal entrance (>3 mm). Thus, the furcation fornix is inclined in the bucco-lingual direction. The buccal furcation entrance is often <0.75 mm wide while the lingual entrance is >0.75 mm in most cases (Bower 1979a,b). The degree of separation and divergence between the roots decreases from the first to the third molar (Fig. 39-8).

It should also be observed that the buccal bone plate is thinner outside the roots of the first than of the second molar. Bone fenestrations and dehiscences are, as a consequence, more frequent in the first than in the second molar region.

Other teeth

Furcations may be present also in teeth which normally have only one root. In fact, two-rooted incisors (Fig. 39-9a), canines (Fig. 39-9b), and mandibular premolars may exist. Occasionally three-rooted maxillary premolars (Fig. 39-10a) and three-rooted mandibular molars can be found (Fig. 39-10b).

Diagnosis

The presence of furcation-involved teeth in a periodontal patient will influence the treatment plan (see Chapter 31). The selection of procedures to be used in the treatment of periodontal disease at multi-rooted teeth can first be made when the presence and depth of furcation lesions have been assessed. In this examination traditional measures of periodontal disease are used (see Chapter 26) but special attention is paid to findings from clinical *probing* and analysis of *radiographs* from the premolar–molar regions.

The classification description of the involved furcation is based on the amount of periodontal tissue destruction that has occurred in the inter-radicular area, i.e. degree of "horizontal root exposure" or

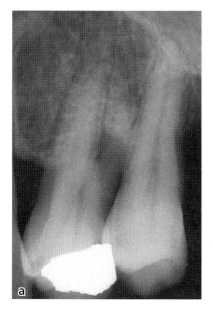
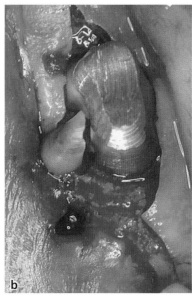

Fig. 39-10 (a) Anatomic variation represented in a radiograph of a three-rooted mandibular first premolar. (b) Clinical photograph illustrating, during surgery, the separation – before extraction – of an "abnormal" second mesial root of a mandibular molar.

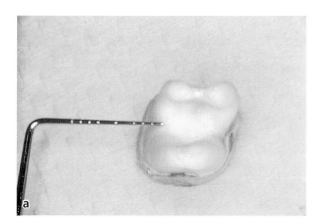
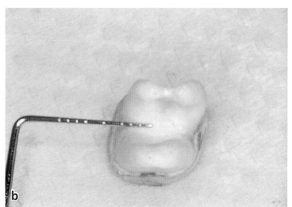
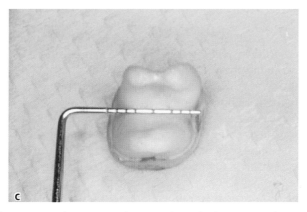

Fig. 39-11 Different degrees of furcation involvement in relation to the probe (penetration/superimposition) in the interradicular space of a mandibular molar. (a) Degree I. (b) Degree II. (c) Degree III.

attachment loss that exists within the root complex. Hamp *et al.* (1975) has suggested the following classification of the involved furcation:

- Degree I: horizontal loss of periodontal support not exceeding one third of the width of the tooth (Fig. 39-11a).
- Degree II: horizontal loss of periodontal support exceeding one third of the width of the tooth, but not encompassing the total width of the furcation area (Fig. 39-11b).
- Degree III: horizontal "through-and-through" destruction of the periodontal tissues in the furcation area (Fig. 39-11c).

It is important to understand that each furcation entrance must be examined and each entrance must be classified according to the above criteria.

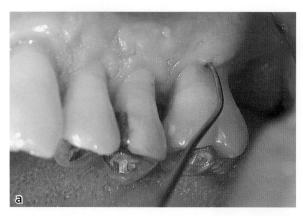
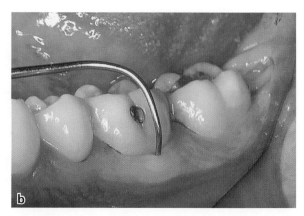

Fig. 39-12 Easily accessible vestibular furcation entrances for probing of a (a) maxillary molar and (b) mandibular molar.

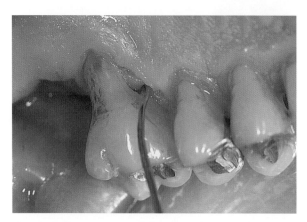

Fig. 39-13 Common access for probing of a mesial furcation entrance of a maxillary molar. The mesial furcation entrance is generally located at the palatal aspect of the tooth, while the distal entrance is located midway between the buccal and the palatal surface.

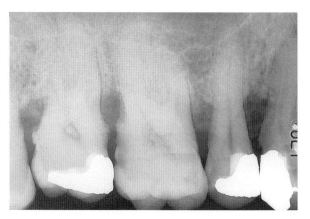

Fig. 39-14 Radiograph showing the location of the interdental bone level in relation to the furcation entrances of the maxillary first and second molar.

Probing

The buccal furcation entrance of the *maxillary molars* and the buccal and lingual furcation entrances of the *mandibular molars* are normally accessible for examination using a curved graduated periodontal probe (Fig. 39-12), an explorer or a small curette. The examination of approximal furcations is more difficult, in particular when neighboring teeth are present. Large contact areas between the teeth further impair access to approximal furcation entrances.

In maxillary molars the mesial furcation entrance is located much closer to the palatal than to the buccal tooth surface. Thus, the mesial furcation should be probed from the palatal aspect of the tooth (Fig. 39-13). The distal furcation entrance of a *maxillary molar* is generally located midway between the buccal and palatal surfaces and, as a consequence, this furcation could be probed from either the buccal or the palatal aspect of the tooth.

In *maxillary premolars* the root anatomy often varies considerably. The roots may also harbor irregularities such as longitudinal furrows, invaginations or true furcations, which may open at varying distances from the CEJ. Due to the above variations and limited access, the clinical assessment of a furcation involvement in maxillary premolars is often difficult. In some patients, a furcation involvement may, in such teeth, first be identified after the elevation of a soft tissue flap.

Radiographs

Radiographs must always be obtained to confirm findings made during probing of a furcation-involved tooth. The radiographic examination should include both paralleling "periapical" and vertical "bite-wing" radiographs. In the radiographs the location of the interdental bone as well as the bone level within the root complex should be examined (Fig. 39-14). Situations may occur when findings from clinical probing and from the radiographs are inconsistent. Thus, the localized but extensive attachment loss which may be detected within the root complex of a maxillary molar with the use of a probe, will not always appear in the radiograph. This may be due to the superimposition in the radiograph of the palatal root and of remaining bone structures (Fig. 39-15a). In such a case, additional radiographs with different angles of orientation of the central beam should be used to identify bone loss within the root complex (Fig. 39-15b).

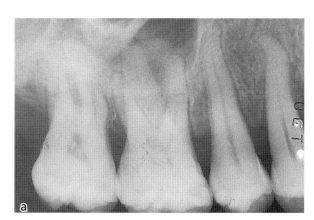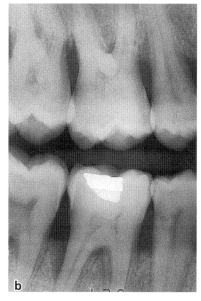

Fig. 39-15 (a) Radiographs of the right maxillary molar region where, with a normal bisecting projection, the furcation defect of the first molar is not evident. (b) It is, however, easily identified in a bitewing radiograph.

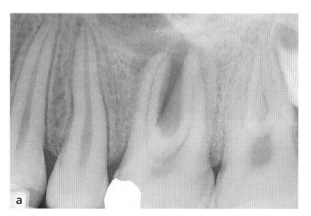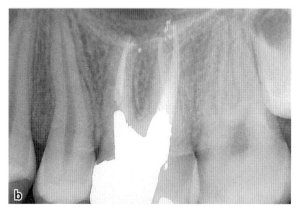

Fig. 39-16 (a) Radiograph demonstrating a destruction of inter-radicular bone and the presence of periapical defects at the mesial and distal roots of a maxillary first molar. (b) Radiographic appearance of complete healing of the inter-radicular and periapical lesions after endodontic treatment.

Differential diagnosis

A lesion in the inter-radicular space of a multi-rooted tooth may be associated with problems originating from the root canal or be the result of occlusal overload. The treatment of a furcation-involved tooth, therefore, should not be initiated until a proper differential diagnosis of the lesion has been made.

Pulpal pathosis may sometimes cause a lesion in the periodontal tissues of the furcation (see Chapter 23). The radiographic appearance of such a defect may have some features in common with a plaque-associated furcation lesion. In order to differentiate between the two lesions the vitality of the affected tooth must *always* be tested. If the tooth is vital, a plaque-associated lesion should be suspected. If the tooth is non-vital, the furcation involvement may have an endodontic origin. In such a case, proper endodontic treatment must *always* precede periodontal therapy. In fact, endodontic therapy may resolve

the inflammatory lesion, soft and hard tissue healing may occur and the furcation defect will disappear (Fig. 39-16). If signs of healing of a furcation defect fail to appear within 2 months of endodontic treatment, the furcation involvement is probably associated with marginal periodontitis.

Trauma from occlusion

Forces elicited by occlusal interferences, e.g. bruxers and clenchers (see Chapters 14 and 51), may cause inflammation and tissue destruction or adaptation within the inter-radicular area of a multi-rooted tooth. In such a tooth a radiolucency may be seen in the radiograph of the root complex. The tooth may exhibit increased mobility. Probing, however, fails to detect an involvement of the furcation. In this particular situation, occlusal adjustment must always precede periodontal therapy. If the defects seen

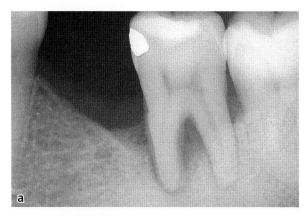 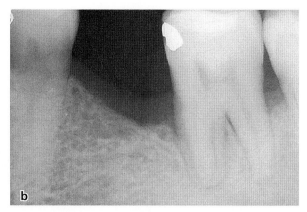

Fig. 39-17 (a) Radiographic appearance of a defect in the furcation area caused by occlusal overload. After occlusal adjustment the interradicular defect spontaneously healed, as documented 6 months after therapy in a radiograph (b). (Courtesy of M. Cattabriga.)

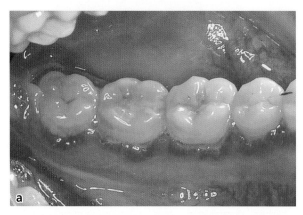 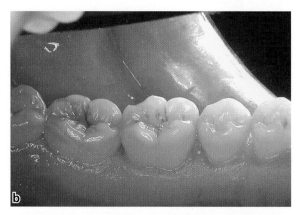

Fig. 39-18 Resolution of inflammatory lesions in the gingiva achieved by scaling, root planing and the re-establishment of a correct tissue morphology in the inter-radicular area of degree I furcation-involved mandibular molars. (a) Before therapy. (b) 6 months after therapy.

within the root complex are of "occlusal" origin, the tooth will become stabilized and the defects disappear within weeks following correction of the occlusal overload (Fig. 39-17).

Therapy

Treatment of a defect in the furcation region of a multi-rooted tooth is intended to meet two objectives:

1. The elimination of the microbial plaque from the exposed surfaces of the root complex.
2. The establishment of an anatomy of the affected surfaces that facilitates proper self-performed plaque control.

Different methods of therapy are recommended:

- Degree I furcation involvement. Recommended therapy: scaling and root planing; furcation plasty.
- Degree II furcation involvement. Recommended therapy: furcation plasty; tunnel preparation; root resection; tooth extraction; guided tissue regeneration at mandibular molars.

- Degree III furcation involvement. Recommended therapy: tunnel preparation; root resection; tooth extraction.

Scaling and root planing

Scaling and planing of the root surfaces in the furcation entrance of a degree I involvement in most situations result in the resolution of the inflammatory lesion in the gingiva. Healing will re-establish a normal gingival anatomy with the soft tissue properly adapted to the hard tissue walls of the furcation entrance (Fig. 39-18).

Furcation plasty

Furcation plasty (Fig 39-19) is a resective treatment modality which should lead to the elimination of the inter-radicular defect. Tooth substance is removed (odontoplasty) and the alveolar bone crest is remodeled (osteoplasty) at the level of the furcation entrance.

Furcation plasty is used mainly at buccal and lingual furcations. At approximal surfaces access is

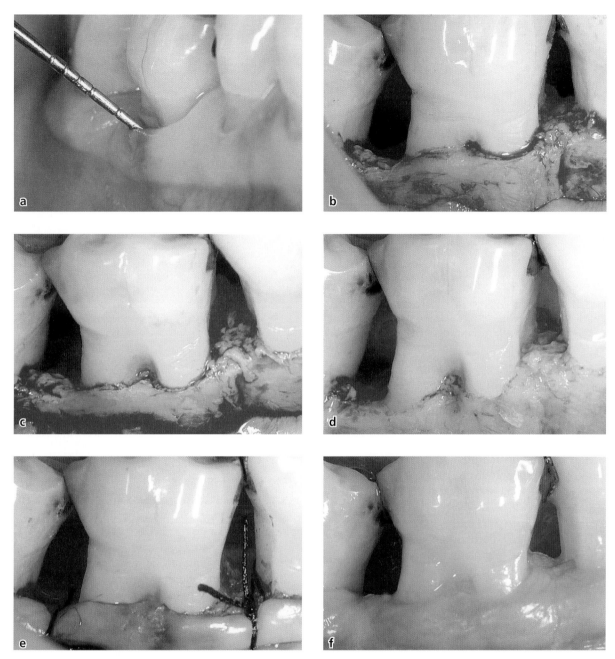

Fig. 39-19 Furcation plasty performed at the buccal aspect of a mandibular molar. (a) Initial degree II furcation involvement. (b) After flap elevation, removal of the granulation tissue and scaling of the exposed root surfaces. (c) After odontoplasty. (d) After osteoplasty. (e) Apical position of the flap managed by periosteal sutures. (f) Healing resulting in the elimination of the furcation defect and in the establishment of a proper soft tissue morphology.

often too limited for this treatment. Furcation plasty involves the following procedures:

- The dissection and reflection of a soft tissue flap to obtain access to the inter-radicular area and the surrounding bone structures.
- The removal of the inflammatory soft tissue from the furcation area followed by careful scaling and root planing of the exposed root surfaces.
- The removal of crown and root substance in the furcation area (odontoplasty) to eliminate or reduce the horizontal component of the defect and to widen the furcation entrance.

- The recontouring of the alveolar bone crest in order to reduce the buccal–lingual dimension of a bone defect in the furcation area.
- The positioning and the suturing of the mucosal flaps at the level of the alveolar crest in order to cover the furcation entrance with soft tissue. Following healing a "papilla-like" tissue should close the entrance of the furcation.

Care must be exercised when odontoplasty is performed on vital teeth. Excessive removal of tooth structure will enhance the risk for increased root sensitivity.

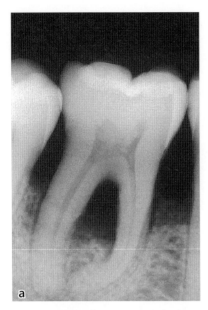

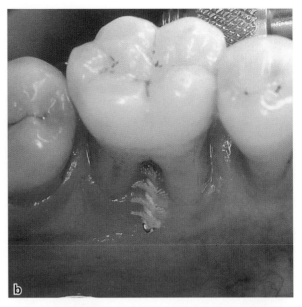

Fig. 39-20 Tunnel preparation of a degree III-involved mandibular molar. Radiograph (a) and photograph (b) showing a wide inter-radicular space where self-performed plaque control can be obtained by the use of an interproximal brush.

Tunnel preparation

Tunnel preparation is a technique used to treat deep degree II and degree III furcation defects in mandibular molars. This type of resective therapy can be offered at mandibular molars which have a short root trunk, a wide separation angle, and long divergence between the mesial and distal root. The procedure includes the surgical exposure and management of the entire furcation area of the affected molar.

Following the reflection of buccal and lingual mucosal flaps, the granulation tissue in the defect is removed and the root surfaces are scaled and planed. The furcation area is widened by the removal of some of the inter-radicular bone. The alveolar bone crest is recontoured; some of the interdental bone, mesial and distal to the tooth in the region, is also removed to obtain a flat outline of the bone. Following hard tissue resection enough space has been established in the furcation region to allow access for cleaning devices to be used during self-performed plaque-control measures (Fig. 39-20). The flaps are apically positioned to the surgically established inter-radicular and interproximal bone level.

During maintenance the exposed root surfaces should be treated by topical application of chlorhexidine digluconate and fluoride varnish. This surgical procedure should be used with caution, because there is a pronounced risk for root sensitivity and for carious lesions developing on the denuded root surfaces within artificially prepared tunnels (Hamp *et al.* 1975).

Root separation and resection (RSR)

Root separation involves the sectioning of the root complex and the maintenance of all roots. *Root resection* involves the sectioning and the removal of one or two roots of a multi-rooted tooth. RSR is frequently used in cases of deep degree II and degree III furcation-involved molars.

Before RSR is performed the following factors must be considered:

- *The length of the root trunk*. In a patient with progressive periodontal disease a tooth with a *short* root trunk may have an early involvement of the furcation (Larato 1975; Gher & Vernino 1980). A tooth with a short root trunk is a good candidate for RSR; the amount of remaining periodontal tissue support following separation and resection is often sufficient to ensure the stability of the remaining root cone. If the root trunk is *long*, the furcation involvement occurs later in the disease process, but, once established, the amount of periodontal tissue support left apical to the furcation may be insufficient to allow RSR.
- *The divergence between the root cones*. The distance between the root cones must be considered. Roots with a short divergence are technically more difficult to separate than roots which are wide apart. In addition, the smaller the divergence is, the smaller also is the inter-radicular (furcation) space. In cases where the divergence between two roots is small, the possibility of increasing the inter-radicular distance with an orthodontic root movement may be considered (Fig. 39-21). The furcation space may also be increased by odontoplasty performed during surgery. Figure 39-22 illustrates that *odontoplasty* was performed on (1) the distal part of the mesial root and (2) the mesial part of the distal root and deep finishing lines prepared for the subsequent restoration (Di Febo *et al.* 1985).
- *The length and the shape of the root cones*. Following separation, short and small root cones (Fig. 39-23)

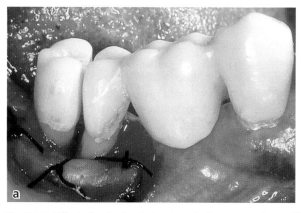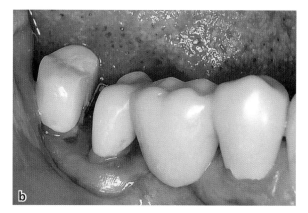

Fig. 39-21 Effect of orthodontic treatment of a separated mandibular molar with a small root divergence. (a) After root separation. (b) 3 months after completion of orthodontic therapy.

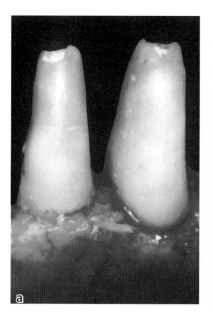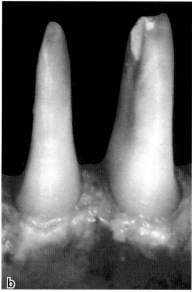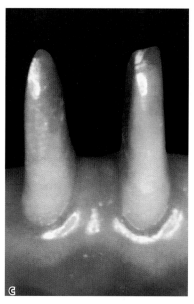

Fig. 39-22 Odontoplasty of a separated mandibular molar performed during surgery to increase the furcation space. After flap elevation and exposure of the alveolar bone, it is evident that the distance between the two roots is small (a). By preparing the inter-radicular surfaces during surgery (b) the furcation space is increased and is sufficient for self-performed plaque control measures (c).

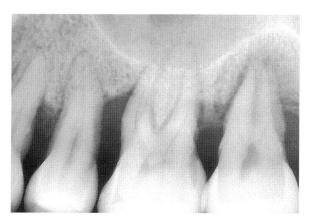

Fig. 39-23 Radiograph showing maxillary molars with thin, short, and conical roots.

tend to exhibit an increased mobility. Such roots, in addition, have narrow root canals which are difficult to ream. Short and small roots consequently should be regarded as poor abutments for prosthetic restorations.

• *Fusion between root cones*. When a decision has been made to perform RSR, it is important that the clinician first determines that the cones within the root complex are not fused. This is generally an uncomplicated diagnostic problem for mandibular molars or for the buccal furcation of maxillary molars (Fig. 39-24). At such teeth the separation area between the roots can easily be identified both with the probe and in a radiograph. It is more difficult to identify a separation line between mesio-buccal (or disto-buccal) and palatal roots of a maxillary molar or maxillary first premolar with a narrow root complex. In such situations, a soft tissue flap must often be raised to allow the operator to get proper access to the approximal tooth surfaces. The mesial (or distal) entrance of the furcation must be probed to a depth of 3–5 mm to ascertain that a fusion does *not* exist between the roots scheduled for RSR.

- *Amount of remaining support around individual roots.* This should be determined by probing the entire circumference of the separated roots. It should be observed that a localized deep attachment loss at one surface of one particular root (e.g. on the buccal surface of the palatal root, or the distal surface of the mesio-buccal root of a maxillary molar) may compromise the long-term prognosis for an otherwise ideal root.
- *Stability of individual roots.* This must be examined following root separation. Rule of thumb: the more mobile the root cone is, the less periodontal tissue support remains.
- *Access for oral hygiene devices.* After completion of therapy the site must have an anatomy which facilitates proper self-performed tooth cleaning.

Maxillary molars

General example

Several decisions must be made when RSR is planned for a furcation-involved maxillary molar. Since such teeth have three root cones, one or two cones may be retained after separation. Different treatment alternatives exist. They are listed in Table 39-1.

Prior to RSR, the morphology of the individual roots as well as the surface area of each root must be carefully analyzed.

The *disto-buccal root* of a maxillary molar (1) is the shortest of the three roots; (2) the root trunk is comparatively long. Thus, the distal root has a small quantity of bone support and once separated, the cone may exhibit increased mobility. The disto-buccal root is, therefore, often removed as part of RSR (Rosenberg 1978; Ross & Thompson 1980).

The *mesio-buccal root* has (1) a wide buccopalatal dimension, (2) an hour-glass cross section, and therefore a large root surface area. In fact, the mesio-buccal cone often has a total root surface area that is equal to or greater than that of the palatal root cone. The mesio-buccal root (1) is located centrally in the alveolar process, (2) is properly aligned with the maxillary premolars and is in an ideal position to function as a separate unit (Fig. 39-25). For these reasons, the mesio-buccal root may be preferred for retention when the clinician is selecting between the mesio-buccal or palatal root. It should be remembered, however, that the root canals of the mesio-buccal root are narrow and more difficult to treat than the single and wide canal of the palatal root.

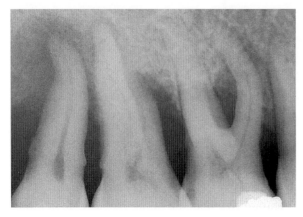

Fig. 39-24 Radiograph indicating the presence of a degree III involvement of the buccal furcation of the maxillary first molar. This tooth is a candidate for root resection.

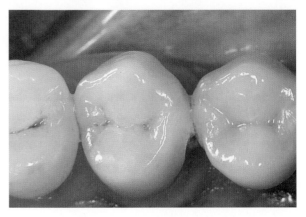

Fig. 39-25 Occlusal view of a restoration using the mesial root of a maxillary first molar as abutment. Note the alignment of the mesial root and the adjacent premolars.

Table 39-1 Root resective treatment possibilities in molars with furcation involvement

Furcation involvement	Root resection	Root resection plus separation of the remaining roots
1 Buccal	Mesio-buccal, disto-buccal	
Mesial	Mesio-buccal, palatal	
Distal	Disto-buccal, palatal	
2 Buccal & distal	Disto-buccal, mesio-buccal & palatal	Palatal
Buccal & mesial	Mesio-buccal, disto-buccal & palatal	Palatal, disto-buccal
Mesial & distal	Palatal, mesial & disto-buccal	Distobuccal
3 Buccal, distal & mesial	Disto-buccal & palatal, mesio-buccal & palatal, mesio- & disto-buccal	Palatal, disto-buccal

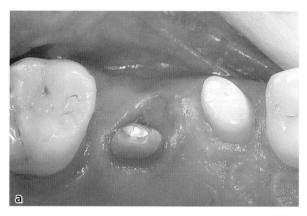 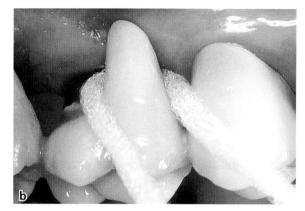

Fig. 39-26 (a) Palatal root of a root-resected maxillary molar serving as a single abutment for a crown restoration. (b) A mesio-buccal root was included in the restoration for esthetic reasons.

The tissue destruction in the furcation area often causes deep attachment and bone loss at the distal palatal surface of the mesio-buccal root. In such situations the palatal root remains as the only candidate for retention (Fig. 39-26).

The series of illustrations presented in Fig. 39-27 demonstrates two left maxillary molars (teeth 26 and 27) with degree III involvement of all six furcation entrances. Both teeth were, following a detailed examination and diagnosis, scheduled for treatment with RSR. Note that in this case the second premolar was missing. In cases of advanced periodontal disease at maxillary molars, it is often necessary to separate all three roots of the individual tooth to obtain access to the inter-radicular area for assessment of the height of the remaining bone at (1) the buccal surface of the palatal root and (2) the palatal surfaces of the buccal roots. Figure 39-27b illustrates the two maxillary molars with all six roots separated. Because of anatomic considerations and increased mobility, the distobuccal roots of 26 and 27 were extracted (Fig. 39-27c). The palatal root of the first molar had a deep area of localized attachment loss on its buccal surface, was considered to be a poor candidate for a bridge abutment, and was extracted. The mesio-buccal root of the first molar as well as the mesio-buccal and palatal roots of the second molar (27) were stable and exhibited moderate probing depth. It was anticipated that at all three roots the anatomy would allow proper plaque control following healing after treatment. The three roots were maintained (Fig. 39-27d). Figure 39-27e shows the area after 3 months' healing and Fig. 39-27f illustrates the segment properly restored. Since in this segment one premolar was missing, the mesio-buccal root of the first molar was used as second premolar in the prosthetic reconstruction and the two roots of the second molar served as abutments for a crown restoration in the position of a molar.

Maxillary premolars

Root resection of maxillary first premolars is possible only in rare instances due to the anatomy of the root

complex (Joseph *et al*. 1996) (Fig. 39-28). The furcation of this premolar is often located at such an apical level that the maintenance of one root serves no meaningful purpose. In most cases, therefore, the presence of a deep furcation involvement of degree II or degree III in a maxillary first premolar calls for tooth extraction.

Mandibular molars

If RSR must be applied in a furcation-involved mandibular molar, three treatment alternatives exist:

1. Separate the two roots, but maintain both roots (premolarization)
2. Separate and extract the mesial root
3. Separate and extract the distal root.

In some situations, both roots may be maintained following separation. If one root is to be removed, the following facts must be considered:

• The *mesial* root has a significantly greater root surface area than the distal root. The mesial root, however, has an hour-glass-shaped cross section which may be difficult to manage (1) in the self-performed plaque control and (2) in the restorative procedure. In addition, the mesial root frequently has two narrow root canals. The root canals are often close to the external root surface. This may complicate root preparation during the subsequent restorative treatment.
• The *distal* root has an oval cross section and, as a rule, only one, wide root canal. The distal root is: (1) comparatively large, providing a greater mass of dentin to resist root fracture (Langer *et al*. 1981); and (2) a good candidate for pin or post placement. Further, when the resected mandibular molar is a terminal abutment for a bridge, the retention of the distal root will result in a longer dental arch than would be the case had the mesial root been retained (Fig. 39-29).

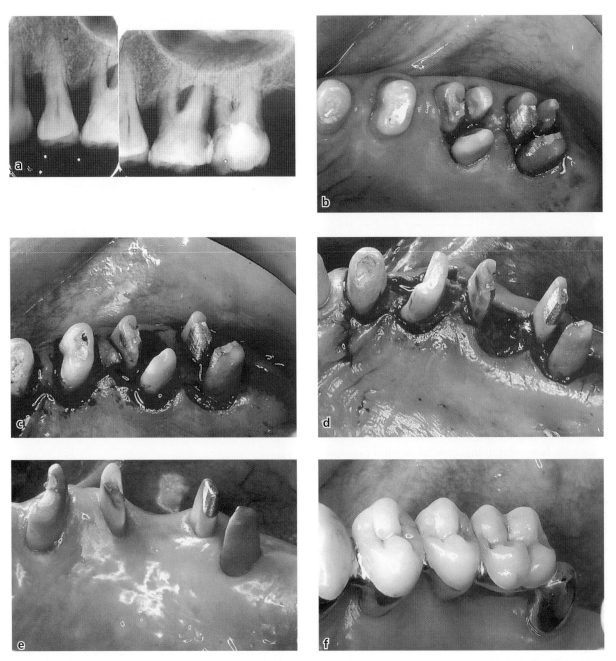

Fig. 39-27 The sequential stages of root resection of two maxillary molars with degree III involvement. (a) Radiograph showing the pre-RSR situation. (b)The roots were separated before flap elevation. (c,d) The distal roots of both molars and the palatal root of the first molar were extracted and the teeth prepared. (e) After 3 months of healing. (f) The final prosthetic restoration of the site.

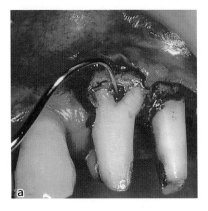

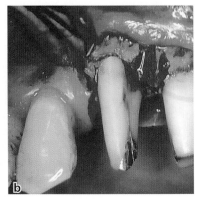

Fig. 39-28 Resection of the disto-buccal root of a three-rooted maxillary first premolar.

Sequence of treatment at RSR

Once anatomic and pathologic characteristics of the root complex(es) of multi-rooted teeth have been documented, treatment should follow a logical plan (see also Chapter 31).

Endodontic treatment

If the tooth to be resected is vital or if an improper root canal filling was placed in a non-vital tooth, RSR starts with endodontic therapy. Rubber dam can be placed, and optimal conditions thus be established for the important management (cleaning and shaping) of the root canal. The structural integrity of the root must be maintained and minimal amounts of root dentin should be removed (Fig. 39-30a,b). Direct filling with amalgam or chemically cured composite of the endodontically treated tooth should be performed before RSR (Fig. 39-30c). Each root should have individual retention for a restoration which should not break or detach during RSR, removal and relining of the provisional restorations, impressions, and prosthetic try-in. Endocanal posts or endodontic screws are used only if natural retention needs improvement.

Occasionally, a furcation involvement may first be identified during periodontal surgery. In this emergency situation RSR may be completed but the root canal entrance(s) of the remaining root(s) must be properly sealed. Definitive root canal therapy must be completed within 2 weeks (Smukler & Tagger 1976).

Provisional restoration

Alginate impressions of the area to be treated are taken and sent to the laboratory together with a wax record of the intercuspal position. A provisional restoration is prepared.

Root separation and resection

Root separation and root resection may be performed as part of the preparation of the segment for prosthetic rehabilitation ("prosthetic preparation"), i.e. prior to periodontal surgery (Carnevale *et al.* 1981). During the prosthetic preparation it is important to *avoid*

- Exposing the interradicular bone to undue mechanical trauma (Fig. 39-31)
- Leaving behind parts of the furcation fornix (Fig. 39-32)
- Perforating the root canals
- Preparing the vertical surfaces of the remaining roots with sharp angles (Fig. 39-33).

Situation 1: mandibular molar. Following separation, both roots are maintained. The distal surface of the distal root and the mesial surface of the mesial root must be prepared parallel to each other to increase the retention for a subsequent restoration. The mesial surface of the distal root and the distal surface of the mesial root should be prepared with diverging angles to increase the space available between the separated roots (Fig. 39-34).

Situation 2: maxillary molar. Following separation, the disto-buccal root was extracted. The distal surface of the crown is prepared with a bevel cut and in such

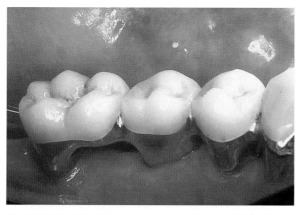

Fig. 39-29 Results of the root resection of a mandibular first molar of which the distal root was retained.

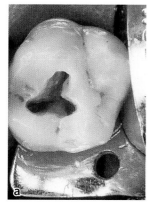
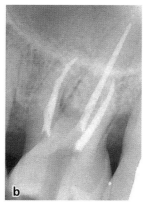
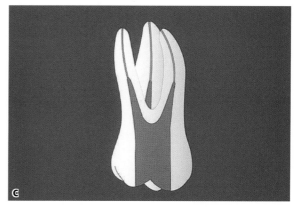

Fig. 39-30 Combined photograph and radiograph showing the "conservative" approach both regarding the access to the pulp chamber (a) and the shaping and filling of the root canal system (b). (c) Schematic illustration showing the temporary restoration of the endodontically treated tooth.

a way that the concave curvature (in apicocoronal direction) is eliminated (Fig. 39-35). If the mesio-buccal and the palatal roots of this molar must be separated but maintained, it is important that the buccal surface of the mesio-buccal root and the palatal surface of the palatal root are prepared parallel to each other. This will enhance the retention of the subsequent restoration. The palatal surface of the mesio-buccal root and the buccal surface of the palatal root must be prepared at diverging angles to increase

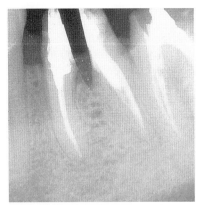

Fig. 39-31 Radiograph illustrating the damage which occurred to the inter-radicular septum during root separation.

the space available between the separated roots (Fig. 39-36). At this stage the provisional restoration is relined with cold cured acrylic and cemented after RSR.

Periodontal surgery

Following flap elevation, osseous resective techniques are used to eliminate angular bone defects that may exist around the maintained roots. Bone resection may also be performed to reduce the bucco-lingual dimension of the alveolar process of the extraction site. The remaining root(s) may be prepared with a bevel cut to the level of the supporting bone (Levine 1972; Ramfjord & Nissle 1974; Carnevale *et al*. 1983). This additional preparation may serve the purpose of (1) eliminating residual soft and hard deposits and (2) eliminating existing undercuts to facilitate the final impression (Fig. 39-37). The provisional restoration is relined. The margins of the provisional restoration must end ≥3 mm coronal of the bone crest. The soft tissue flaps are secured with sutures at the level of the bone crest. The relined provisional restoration is cemented and a periodontal dressing is applied to cover the surgical area. The dressing and the sutures are removed 1 week later. The roots are debrided and a new dressing applied. After another week, the dressing is finally removed

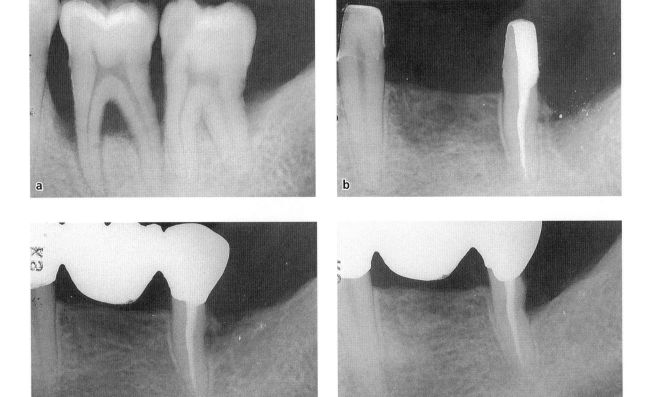

Fig. 39-32 (a) Radiographs of a mandibular first molar to be extracted and of a second molar to be root resected. (b) During hemisection an overhang is left behind as a result of an oblique sectioning of the tooth distal to the furcation. (c) In a radiograph obtained 2 years later, the presence of an angular bony defect can be seen adjacent to the "overhang". The lesion was resolved and the angular defect disappeared following removal of the "overhang". (d) Radiograph after 2 years.

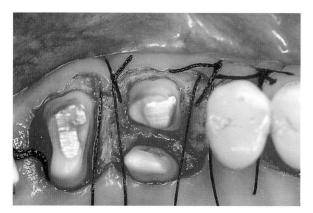

Fig. 39-33 Maintenance of the two fused buccal roots of a maxillary first molar. The buccal roots were separated from the palatal root. Note the rounded line angles and the wide space created between the separated roots.

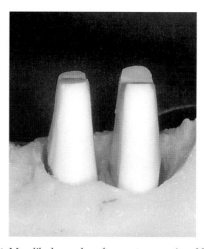

Fig. 39-34 Mandibular molar after root separation. Note the diverging angle of preparation performed to increase the inter-radicular space between the mesial and distal roots and the parallel approximal surfaces.

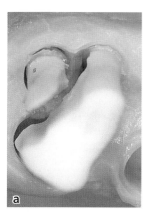
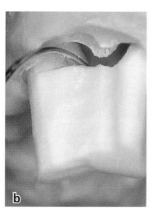
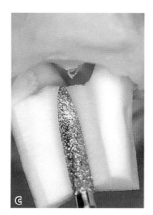
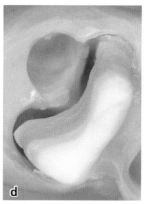

Fig. 39-35 (a,b) The sequential stages of root resection and extraction of the distal root of a maxillary molar. In order to minimize the concave outline of the cut surfaces, the sectioning should be performed with a straight line cut. (c, d) After extraction of the distal root, the furcation area of the remaining roots must be re-prepared to eliminate undercuts.

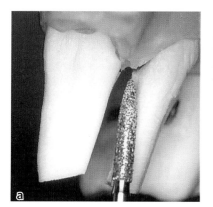
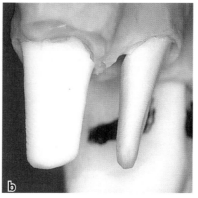
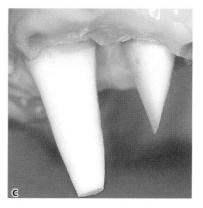

Fig. 39-36 (a,b) Preparation, during separation, of the mesio-buccal and palatal roots after the disto-buccal root of a maxillary molar had been extracted. The internal (furcation) surfaces of the two roots should be prepared with diverging angles to increase the inter-radicular space, while the external surfaces of the two roots should be prepared parallel to each other to increase the subsequent retention of the restoration. (c) When the palatal surface of the palatal root is not prepared parallel to the buccal surface, the palatal abutment will become shortened and not self-retentive.

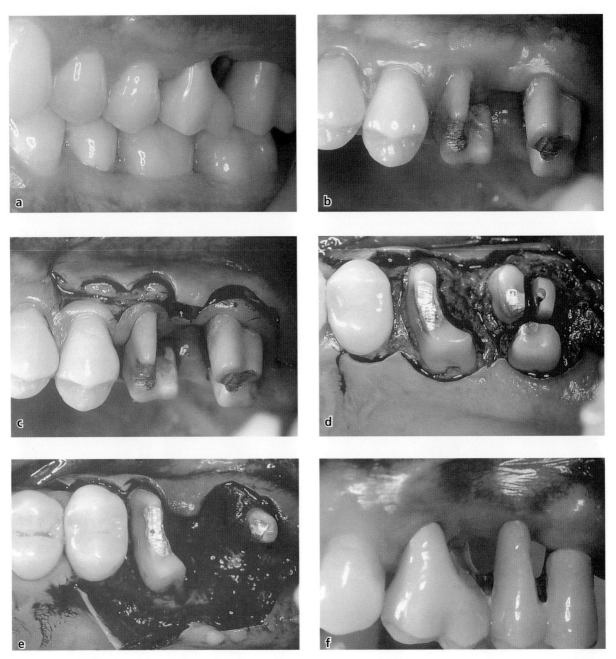

Fig. 39-37 (a,b) Sequential stages of root resection at maxillary first and second molars. The extraction of the distal root of the first molar was performed during tooth preparation and prior to the insertion of the provisional restoration. (c,d,e) During the surgical procedure, after flap elevation, the furcation-involved second molar was separated, the mesial and palatal roots were extracted and the osseous defects were eliminated. (f) Healing with the definitive prosthetic restoration in place.

and the patient instructed in proper plaque-control techniques.

Final prosthetic restoration
Since the prosthetic preparation of the roots was completed during surgery, the clinician concerns him-/herself only with minor adjustments. The preparation margins are located supragingivally, which improves the precision of the definitive crown restoration. The framework of the restoration must be rigid to compensate for the compromised abutments (roots) with a compromised periodontal tissue support. The occlusion should be designed to mini-mize the infliction of lateral deflective forces (see Chapter 51) (Fig. 39-38).

Regeneration of furcation defects

The possibility of regenerating and closing a furcation defect has been investigated (see Chapter 43). Following an early case report publication (Gottlow *et al.* 1986), where histologic documentation of new attachment formation in human furcation defects (Fig. 39-39) treated by "guided tissue regeneration" (GTR) therapy was provided, the results of several investigations on this form of treatment in furcation-

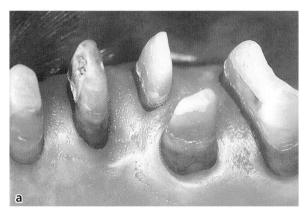 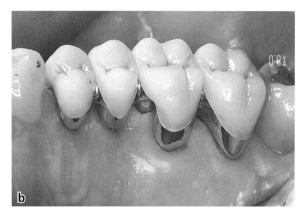

Fig. 39-38 (a) Soft tissue healing at a separated maxillary first molar and at a root-resected second molar. (b) The final prosthetic restoration in place with the occlusion designed to minimize the lateral stresses on the roots left as abutments.

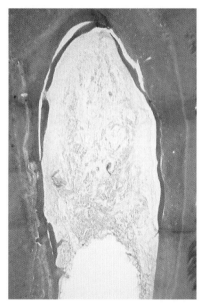 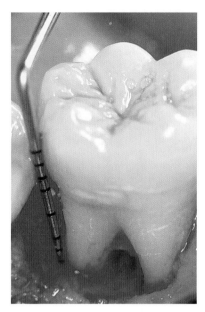

Fig. 39-39 Histologic mesiodistal section of a previous degree II furcation involvement of a human mandibular molar, treated with GTR. The section demonstrates that the newly formed cementum covers the entire circumference of the furcation defect.

Fig. 39-40 Position of the furcation fornix in relation to the level of the supporting bone and attachment apparatus in a lingual degree II furcation-involved mandibular molar.

involved teeth have been presented. In these reports, a reasonably predictable outcome of GTR therapy was demonstrated only in degree II furcation-involved mandibular molars, where a clinical soft tissue closure or a decreased probing depth of the furcation defect was recorded (Pontoriero *et al.* 1988; Lekovic *et al.* 1989; Caffesse *et al.* 1990).

Less favorable results have been reported when GTR therapy was used in other types of furcation defects such as degree III furcation-involved mandibular and maxillary molars (Pontoriero *et al.* 1989; Pontoriero & Lindhe 1995a) and degree II furcations in maxillary molars (Metzeler *et al.* 1991; Pontoriero & Lindhe 1995b).

The reason for the limited predictability of GTR therapy in furcation-involved teeth may be related to several factors:

- The morphology of the periodontal defect, which in the root complex often has the character of a "horizontal lesion". New attachment formation is hence dependent on coronal upgrowth of periodontal ligament tissue (Fig. 39-40).
- The anatomy of the furcation, with its complex internal morphology, may prevent proper instrumentation and debridement of the exposed root surface (Fig. 39-41).
- The varying and changing location of the soft tissue margins during the early phase of healing with a possible recession of the flap margin and early exposure of both the membrane material and the fornix of the furcation (Fig. 39-42).

GTR treatment could be considered in dentitions with isolated degree II furcation defects in mandibular molars. The predictability of this treatment outcome improves following GTR therapy if:

- The *interproximal* bone is located at a level which is close to the CEJ of the approximal surface. This "key-hole" type of degree II involvement allows for an effective retention of the membrane material and retention also of the position of the coronally placed flap margins (Fig. 39-43).
- The debridement of the exposed root surfaces in the furcation area is comprehensive. Since the width of the furcation entrance and the internal morphology of the inter-radicular area may limit

the access of curettes for proper debridement, the removal of hard and soft bacterial deposits from the root surfaces must frequently be made with ultrasonic instruments, rotating, flame-shaped fine diamond burs, and endodontic files (Fig. 39-44).

- The membrane material is properly placed and a "space" between the tooth and the material

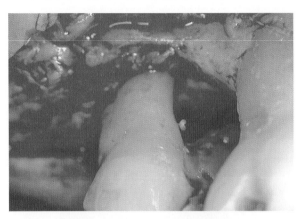

Fig. 39-41 Internal morphology of the furcation of a maxillary molar. Note the invagination of the palatal root.

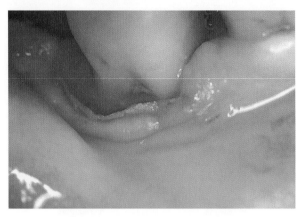

Fig. 39-42 Exposure of the membrane and of the furcation entrance as a consequence of recession of the flap margin. The photograph is taken at 3 weeks of healing after GTR treatment of a degree II buccal furcation of a mandibular molar.

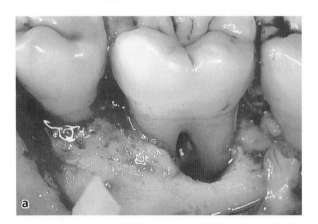
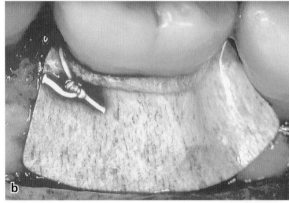
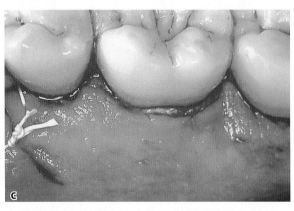
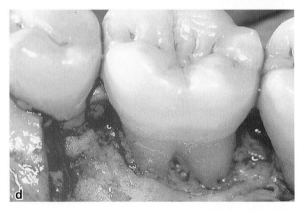

Fig. 39-43 Aspect of a lingual degree II furcation involvement in a mandibular first molar. (a) Note the infrabony component of the defect and the level of the approximal supporting bone in relation to the furcation fornix. (b) The Teflon membrane sutured in position and supported by the interproximal alveolar bone. (c) The flap positioned and sutured over the membrane. (d) At re-entry, after 6 months of healing, the previously exposed furcation defect was closed and filled with bone tissue.

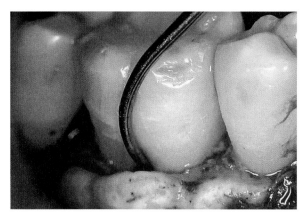

Fig. 39-44 Phase of debridment of a buccal degree II furcation defect by the use of an "extra-fine" ultrasonic tip.

established. A "primary" wound closure is thereby obtained, blood clot protection will occur, and recession of the soft tissue margin during the early phase of healing will be minimized (Fig. 39-45).
• A plaque-control program is put in place. This should include daily rinsing with a chlorhexidine solution and professional tooth cleaning once a week for the first month, and once every 2–3 weeks for at least another 6 months of healing following the surgical procedure.

Enamel matrix proteins included in a commercially available product (Emdogain®; Straumann, Basel, Switzerland) were used in the treatment of furcation defects in experimental studies in animals (Araùjo & Lindhe 1998) and in clinical trials in humans (Jepsen *et al.* 2004; Meyle *et al.* 2004). The ability of Emdogain® (EMD), applied to the root surfaces in the furcation area, to stimulate periodontal regeneration in surgically created degree III furcation defects in dogs was documented histologically by Araùjo and Lindhe (1998). In a multicenter randomized controlled clinical trial, including 45 subjects with 45 paired mandibular molars with buccal degree II furcation involvements, Jepsen *et al.* (2004) compared the EMD with GTR therapy. After 14 months of healing, the subjects were re-examined. The authors reported a mean reduction in the open horizontal furcation depth of 2.8 mm for EMD-treated sites and of 1.8 mm for GTR-treated defects. In addition the frequency of complete closed furcation defects was higher for EMD sites (8/45) than for GTR sites (3/45). It was concluded that both treatment modalities resulted in significant clinical improvements although the EMD method provided (1) greater reduction of the furcation depths, (2) a smaller incidence of post-operative pain/swelling, and (3) less gingival recession (Meyle *et al.* 2004) as compared to GTR therapy.
The outcome of the regenerative procedures at furcation-involved molars should result in the com-

plete elimination of the defect within the interradicular space in order to establish anatomic conditions which facilitate optimal self-performed plaque-control measures. In fact, partial gain of clinical attachment levels within the furcation defect, although statistically significant, will not necessarily improve the site's accessibility for plaque-control measures.

Extraction

The extraction of a furcation-involved tooth must be considered when the attachment loss is so extensive that no root can be maintained or when the treatment will not result in a tooth/gingival anatomy which allows proper self-performed plaque-control measures. Moreover, extraction can be considered as an alternative form of therapy when the maintenance of the affected tooth will not improve the overall treatment plan or when, due to endodontic or caries-related lesions, the preservation of the tooth will represent a risk factor for the long-term prognosis of the overall treatment.
The possibility of substituting a furcation-involved tooth with an osseointegrated implant should be considered with extreme caution and only if implant therapy will improve the prognosis of the overall treatment (see Chapter 32). In fact, the implant alternative has obvious anatomic limitations in the maxillary and mandibular molar regions.

Prognosis

Several studies have evaluated the long-term prognosis of multi-rooted teeth with furcation involvement that were treated in accordance with the principles described in this chapter (Table 39-2). In a 5-year study, Hamp *et al.* (1975) observed the outcome of treatment of 175 teeth with various degrees of furcation involvement in 100 patients. Of the 175 teeth, 32 (18%) were treated by scaling and root planing alone, 49 (28%) were subjected, in addition to scaling and root planing, to furcation plasty which included odonto- and/or osteoplasty. In 87 teeth (50%) root resection had been carried out and in seven teeth (4%) a tunnel had been prepared. At the completion of the active phase of therapy the patients were enrolled in a maintenance program which included a recall visit every 3–6 months. The plaque and gingivitis scores assessed immediately after treatment and once a year during maintenance indicated that the patients' oral hygiene was of high quality. None of the teeth treated was lost during the 5 years of study. Only 16 furcation sites exhibited probing depths exceeding 3 mm. During the observation period carious lesions were detected in 12 surfaces of the 32 teeth which had been treated by scaling and root planing, in three surfaces of the 49 teeth subjected to furcation plasty, in five surfaces of the

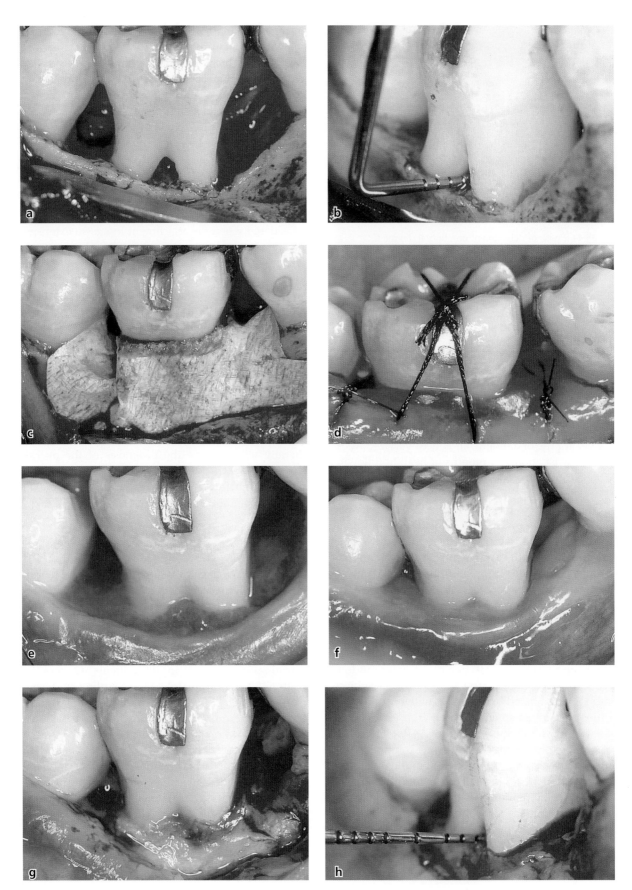

Fig. 39-45 The sequential stages of GTR treatment of a buccal degree II furcation-involved mandibular first molar. (a,b) The clinical appearance and the horizontal probing of the defect. (c,d) Membrane placement and retention. (e) The clinical aspect of the soft tissue at 4 weeks after membrane removal. (f) The clinical aspect after 6 months of healing. During the re-entry procedure the furcation defect appeared completely closed (g) and was not probeable (h).

Table 39-2 Long-term clinical studies on root resection therapy in molars with furcation involvement

Author	Observation period	No. of teeth examined	Causes of tooth loss					
			% teeth lost	% root/ tooth fracture	% periodontal	% endodontic	% caries or decementation	% strategic
Bergenholtz (1972)	21 teeth/2–5 yrs 17 teeth/5–10 yrs	45	6		4	2		
Klavan (1975)	3 yrs	34	3		3			
Hamp et al. (1975)	5 yrs	87	0					
Langer et al. (1981)	10 yrs	100	38	18	10	7	3	
Erpenstein (1983)	4–7 yrs	34	9		3	6		
Bühler (1988)	10 yrs	28	32	3.6	7.1	17.7	3.6	
Carnevale et al. (1991)	303 teeth/3–6 yrs 185 teeth/7–11 yrs	488	4	1.8	0.4	0.9	0.9	
Basten et al. (1996)	2–23 yrs	49	8			2	4	2
Carnevale et al. (1998)	10 yrs	175	7	1.1	1.8	2.3	1.8	

78 root-resected teeth, and in four surfaces of the seven teeth where a tunnel was prepared.

The results of this study were basically confirmed in a more recent investigation (Hamp et al. 1992). In this 7-year study, the authors followed 100 patients with 182 furcation-involved teeth. Out of the 182 furcation-involved teeth, 57 had been treated by scaling and root planing only, 101 were treated by furcation plasty, and 24 were subjected to root resection or hemisection. No tunnel preparation was performed. After the active phase of therapy, the patients were enrolled in a meticulous maintenance care program including recall appointments once every 3–6 months. During the course of the study, more than 85% of the furcations treated with scaling root planing alone, or in conjunction with furcation plasty, maintained stable conditions or showed signs of improvement. Only one tooth and one mesial root of a mandibular molar were extracted among the root-resected or hemisected teeth.

Carnevale et al. (1998), in a 10-year prospective controlled clinical trial, demonstrated a 93% survival rate of root resected furcation-involved teeth and a 99% survival rate of non-furcation-involved teeth.

More recently, Svärdström (2001) presented the results of a retrospective analysis on factors influencing the decision-making process regarding the treatment for 1313 molars with furcation involvement in 222 patients and the outcome of the treatment deci-sions after 8–12 years (mean 9.5 years) of regular maintenance care. The treatment options included were: tooth extraction, root separation/resection, and maintenance of the tooth with non-surgically/surgically performed scaling and root planing with or without furcation plasty. Of the 1313 furcation-involved molars, 366 (28%) were extracted during the active phase of therapy. The decision for tooth extraction was primarily influenced by factors such as tooth mobility, tooth position, absence of occlusal antagonism, the degree of furcation involvement, probing depth, and the amount of remaining periodontal support. Out of the 685 molars with furcation involvement and the 160 patients that were available for the follow-up examination 8–12 years after treatment, 47 teeth were root separated/resected and 638 teeth were considered to be maintainable after a non-surgical or conservative surgical therapy.

The factor found to have the strongest influence for the decision to perform root separation/resection was the degree of furcation involvement (degree II and III). Tooth position, probing depth, and tooth mobility were also factors of statistical significance. The author explained that other factors such as endodontic conditions, root anatomy, and overall treatment strategy may also have influenced the choice of treatment. The long-term outcome of the treatment decisions made for furcation-involved molars showed a favorable survival rate for both root resective (89%)

Table 39-3 Factors to consider in treatment of furcation-involved molars

Tooth-related factors

Degree of furcation involvement
Amount of remaining periodontal support
Probing depth
Tooth mobility
Endodontic conditions and root/root-canal anatomy
Available sound tooth substance
Tooth position and occlusal antagonisms

Patient-related factors

Strategic value of the tooth in relation to the overall plan
Patient's functional and esthetic demands
Patient's age and health conditions
Oral hygiene capacity

and non-resective (96%) therapy options in patients included in a proper maintenance care program. Of the 47 root separated/resected teeth, only five (11%) were lost during the 9.5 years of follow-up. Of the 638 molars initially considered to be maintainable by a non-resective treatment, 21 teeth (3.5%) were extracted and three teeth were root resected.

Conclusion

In treatment decisions for furcation-involved molars, it must be realized that there is no scientific evidence that a given treatment modality is superior to the others (Table 39-3).

References

Abrams, L. & Trachtenberg, D.I. (1974). Hemisection – technique and restoration. *Dental Clinics of North America* **18**, 415–444.

Araùjo, M. & Lindhe, J. (1998). GTR treatment of degree III furcation defects following application of enamel matrix proteins. An experimental study in dogs. *Journal of Clinical Periodontology* **25**, 524–530.

Basten, C.H.J., Ammons, W.F.J. & Persson, R. (1996). Long-term evaluation of root-resected molars: a retrospective study. *International Journal of Periodontics and Restorative Dentistry* **16**, 207–219.

Bergenholtz, G. (1972). Radectomy of multi-rooted teeth. *Journal of the American Dental Association* **85**, 870–875.

Bower, R.C. (1979a). Furcation morphology relative to periodontal treatment. Furcation entrance architecture. *Journal of Periodontology* **50**, 23–27.

Bower, R.C. (1979b). Furcation morphology relative to periodontal treatment. Furcation root surface anatomy. *Journal of Periodontology* **50**, 366–374.

Bühler, H. (1988). Evaluation of root resected teeth. Results after ten years. *Journal of Periodontology* **59**, 805–810.

Caffesse, R., Smith, B., Duff, B., Morrison, E., Merril, D. & Becker, W. (1990). Class II furcations treated by guided tissue regeneration in humans: case reports. *Journal of Periodontology* **61**, 510–514.

Carnevale, G., Di Febo, G. & Trebbi, L. (1981). A patient presentation: planning a difficult case. *International Journal of Periodontics and Restorative Dentistry* **6**, 51–63.

Carnevale, G., Di Febo, G., Tonelli, M.P., Marin, C. & Fuzzi, M. (1991). A retrospective analysis of the periodontal-prosthetic treatment of molars with interradicular lesions. *International Journal of Periodontics and Restorative Dentistry* **11**, 189–205.

Carnevale, G., Freni Sterrantino, S. & Di Febo, G. (1983). Soft and hard tissue wound healing following tooth preparation to the alveolar crest. *International Journal of Periodontics and Restorative Dentistry* **3**, 36–53.

Carnevale, G., Pontoriero, R. & Di Febo, G. (1998). Long-term effects of root-resective therapy in furcation-involved molars. A 10-year longitudinal study. *Journal of Clinical Periodontology* **25**, 209–214.

Di Febo, G., Carnevale, G. & Sterrantino, S.F. (1985). Treatment of a case of advanced periodontitis: clinical procedures utilizing the "combined preparation" technique. *International Journal of Periodontics and Restorative Dentistry* **1**, 52–63.

Erpenstein, H. (1983). A 3 year longitudinal study of hemisectioned molars. *Journal of Clinical Peridontology* **10**, 1–10.

Gher, M.E. & Vernino, A.R. (1980). Root morphology – clinical significance in pathogenesis and treatment of periodontal disease. *Journal of the American Dental Association* **101**, 627–633.

Gottlow, J., Nyman, S., Lindhe, J., Karring, T. & Wennström, J. (1986). New attachment formation in the human periodontium by guided tissue regeneration. Case reports. *Journal of Clinical Periodontology* **13**, 604–616.

Hamp, S.E., Nyman, S. & Lindhe, J. (1975). Periodontal treatment of multirooted teeth. Results after 5 years. *Journal of Clinical Periodontology* **2**, 126–135.

Hamp, S.E., Ravald, N., Tewik, A. & Lundström, A. (1992). Perspective a long terme des modalités de traitement des lesions inter-radiculaires. *Journal de Parodontologie* **11**, 11–23.

Jepsen, S., Heinz, B., Jepsen, K., Arjomand, M., Hoffmann, T., Richter, S., Reich, E., Sculean, A., Gonzales, J., Bodeker, R. & Meyle, J. (2004). A randomized clinical trial comparing enamel matrix derivative and membrane treatment of buccal Class II furcation involvement in mandibular molars. Part I: Study design and results for primary outcomes. *Journal of Periodontology* **75**, 1150–1160.

Joseph, I., Varma, B.R.R. & Bhat, K.M. (1996). Clinical significance of furcation anatomy of the maxillary first premolar: a biometric study on extracted teeth. *Journal of Periodontology* **67**, 386–389.

Klavan, B. (1975). Clinical observation following root amputation in maxillary molar teeth. *Journal of Periodontology* **46**, 1–5.

Langer, B., Stein, S.D. & Wagenberg, B. (1981). An evaluation of root resection. A ten year study. *Journal of Periodontology* **52**, 719–722.

Larato, D.C. (1975). Some anatomical factors related to furcation involvements. *Journal of Periodontology* **46**, 608–609.

Lekovic, V., Kenney, E.B., Kovacevic, K. & Carranza, F.A. Jr. (1989). Evaluation of guided tissue regeneration in class II furcation defects. A clinical re-entry study. *Journal of Periodontology* **60**, 694–698.

Levine, H.L. (1972). Periodontal flap surgery with gingival fiber retention. *Journal of Periodontology* **43**, 91–98.

Metzeler, D., Seamons, B.C., Mellonig, J.T., Marlin, G.E. & Gray, J.L. (1991). Clinical evaluation of guided tissue regeneration in the treatment of maxillary class II molar furcation invasion. *Journal of Periodontology* **62**, 353–360.

Meyle, J., Gonzales, J., Bodeker, R., Hoffmann, T., Richter, S., Heinz, B., Arjomand, M., Reich, E., Sculean, A., Jepsen, K. & Jepsen, S. (2004). A randomized clinical trial comparing enamel matrix derivative and membrane treatment of buccal Class II furcation involvement in mandibular molars. Part II: Secondary outcomes. *Journal of Periodontology* **75**, 1188–1195.

Pontoriero, R. & Lindhe, J. (1995a). Guided tissue regeneration in the treatment of degree III furcations defects in maxillary molars. *Journal of Clinical Periodontology* **22**, 810–812.

Pontoriero, R. & Lindhe, J. (1995b). Guided tissue regeneration in the treatment of degree II furcations in maxillary molars. *Journal of Clinical Periodontology* **22**, 756–763.

Pontoriero, R., Lindhe, J., Nyman, S., Karring, T., Rosenberg, E. & Sanavi, F. (1988). Guided tissue regeneration in degree II furcation involved mandibular molars. A clinical study. *Journal of Clinical Periodontology* **15**, 247–254.

Pontoriero, R., Lindhe, J., Nyman, S., Karring, T., Rosenberg, E. & Sanavi, F. (1989). Guided tissue regeneration in the treatment of furcation defects in mandibular molars. A clinical study of degree III involvements. *Journal of Clinical Periodontology* **16**, 170–174.

Ramfjord, S.P. & Nissle, L.L. (1974). The modified Widman flap. *Journal of Periodontology* **45**, 601–607.

Rosenberg, M.M. (1978). Management of osseous defects. *Clinical Dentistry* **3**, 103.

Rosenberg, M.M. (1988). Furcation involvement: periodontic, endodontic and restorative interrelationships. In: Rosenberg, M.M., Kay, H.B., Keough, B.E. & Holt, R.L., eds. *Periodontal and Prosthetic Management for Advanced Cases.* Chicago: Quintessence, pp. 249–251.

Ross, I.F. & Thompson, R.H. (1980). Furcation involvement in maxillary and mandibular molars. *Journal of Periodontology* **51**, 450–454.

Smukler, H. & Tagger, M. (1976). Vital root amputation. A clinical and histologic study. *Journal of Periodontology* **47**, 324–330.

Svärdström, G. (2001). *Furcation involvements in periodontitis patients. Prevalence and treatment decisions.* Thesis. Department of Periodontology, Institute of Odontology, Göteborg University, pp. 31.

Svärdström, G. & Wennström, J. (1988). Furcation topography of the maxillary and mandibular first molars. *Journal of Clinical Periodontology* **15**, 271–275.

Chapter 40

Endodontics and Periodontics

Gunnar Bergenholtz and Gunnar Hasselgren

Introduction, 848
Infectious processes in the periodontium of endodontic
  origin, 849
  General features, 849
  Clinical presentations, 850
  Distinguishing lesions of endodontic origin from
    periodontitis, 851
  Endo–perio lesions – diagnosis and treatment aspects, 856
  Endodontic treatments and periodontal lesions, 858
Iatrogenic root perforations, 858

Vertical root fractures, 859
  Mechanisms, 860
  Incidence, 861
  Clinical expressions, 861
  Diagnosis, 862
  Treatment considerations, 863
External root resorptions, 865
  Mechanisms of hard tissue resorption in general, 865
  Clinical presentations and identification, 866
  Different forms, 866

Introduction

Inflammatory lesions of the attachment apparatus of teeth involve a variety of etiologies other than plaque accumulations in the dentogingival region; these require attention in diagnosis and treatment planning processes. In fact, signs and symptoms, seen as typical of periodontitis, such as pocket probing depths, loss of attachment, increased tooth mobility, pain, swellings and suppurations, may reflect several tooth-associated infections including infections of endodontic origin (here termed endodontic lesion), infections initiated and maintained by iatrogenic root perforations, vertical root fractures, and external root resorption.

Differentiating between inflammatory disease conditions of the periodontium is not normally a thorny exercise. This is because symptoms of periodontitis usually affect several teeth in the dentition and are confined to the marginal periodontium. Other tooth-associated infections, by contrast, are usually isolated to a single tooth and display rather typical clinical and radiographic signs. These conditions can nevertheless produce confusing clinical expressions and lead to misinterpretation of their cause, especially when affecting teeth in dentitions diseased by periodontitis. Diagnostic difficulties particularly arise when lesions appear deep down the lateral aspects of roots in what can be designated a marginal–apical communication. These so-called

"endo–perio lesions" present the clinician with exceptional challenges in that the origin and thus the proper course of treatment are not readily revealed. An "endo–perio lesion", as the term implies, involves a condition where both the pulp and the periodontium are diseased simultaneously in what appears to be a single periodontal lesion. However, a complicating factor is that the process may be of periodontal origin in its entirety and may have caused the death of the pulp in the process or the lesion may just be a representation of a root canal infection alone. Hence, determination of causality is crucial in these cases not only to avoid unnecessary and possibly detrimental treatment, but also to assess whether the disease condition stands a reasonable chance of being successfully treated.

To guide clinical decision making on diagnosis and treatment of inflammatory lesions in the periodontium, the focus of this chapter is on various tooth-associated disorders that display similar signs and symptoms to periodontitis. Specifically addressed are the clinical presentations and the means by which endodontic infections and infections associated with root perforations, root fractures, and root resorptions can be identified and distinguished from manifestations of periodontitis. Management principles will be given where appropriate. Non-infectious processes *viz.* developmental cysts and tumors, which also can interfere with the supporting tissues, will not be discussed in this chapter.

Infectious processes in the periodontium of endodontic origin

General features

Disease conditions of the dental pulp are for the most part infectious in nature and involve inflammatory processes. Caries, restorative procedures, and traumatic injuries are common etiologies (see Chapter 23). In fact, any loss of hard tissue integrity of teeth, exposing dentin or the pulp directly to the oral environment, may allow bacteria and bacterial elements to adversely affect the normally healthy condition of the pulp. The resulting inflammatory lesion will then be directed towards the source of irritation and be confined for as long as the inflammatory defense does not collapse and convert into a major destructive breakdown of the pulpal tissue. Consequently, inflammatory alterations in the vital pulp will not normally produce lesions in the adjoining periodontium that can be detected by clinical means. Yet, disruption of the apical lamina dura or widening of the periodontal ligament space can occasionally be observed radiographically (Fig. 40-1a). Teeth, particularly in young individuals with large pulp chambers, may also display minor radiolucent areas either apically or laterally along the root surface at exits of accessory canals and apical foramina or both, in spite of the fact that vital pulp functions prevail (Langeland 1987; Gesi et al. 2006). In such cases, typical clinical signs of pulpitis, including spontaneous pain, thermal sensitivity or tenderness to percussion, may or may not be present.

Overt lesions in the periodontium, on the other hand, are common in teeth where the pulp has lost its vitality. In these cases the process is associated either with a non-treated necrotic pulp or a tooth that has been the subject of endodontic treatment. In the latter case, the cause of the lesion is usually to be found in an existing, although not successfully managed, root canal infection (Fig. 40-1b). Extrusion of toxic medicaments and root-filling materials into the periodontium in conjunction with endodontic treatments may also cause periodontal lesions. While severe damage of the periodontal tissue support formerly was a rather common complication following the use of arsenic- or formaldehyde-based preparations to devitalize pulps, medicate, and fill root canals (Fig. 40-2), modern day medicaments for canal irrigation and disinfection as well as materials for root canal filling are comparatively well tolerated (Geurtsen & Leyhausen 1997). However, acute toxic and allergic reactions may be encountered from the use of highly concentrated sodium hypochlorite (Pashley et al. 1985) and adverse components of root-filling material (Hensten-Pettersen et al. 1985).

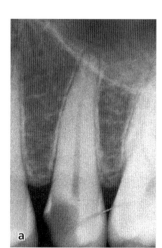
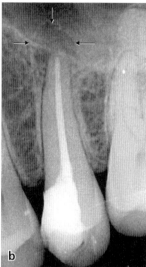

Fig. 40-1 (a) Radiograph of an upper second premolar with caries extending to the vicinity of the pulp. There is loss of lamina dura at the root tip. (b) The 3-year recall radiograph after pulpectomy of the vital pulp and root filling shows a periapical radiolucency suggesting existence of a persistent root canal infection in this case.

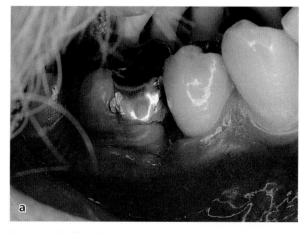
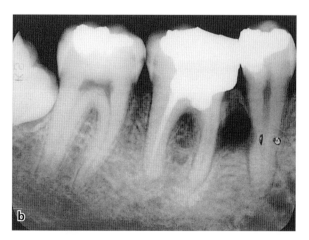

Fig. 40-2 (a) Clinical photograph showing a periodontal defect at the mesial aspect of tooth #46. The pulp had been subjected to devitalization by the use of a paraformaldehyde-containing paste. (b) Leakage of the agent along the temporary filling margins obviously occurred as suggested by the subsequent loss of proximal bone and the emergence of a bone sequestrum.

Conclusion

It is important to realize that as long as the pulp maintains vital functions, although inflamed or scarred, it is unlikely to produce irritants that cause overt periodontal tissue lesions. For clinically significant lesions to occur the pulp must have lost its vitality. Consequently no benefit will normally be gained from extirpation of vital pulps (pulpectomy) as an adjunct or alternative to the treatment of teeth for periodontal disease.

Clinical presentations

Inflammatory lesions in the periodontal tissues, induced and maintained by root canal infection, typically expand around the apex of teeth, where the root canal space interconnects with the periodontium along apical foramina. Lesions develop more seldom in a juxtaposition that is at the lateral aspects of roots (Fig. 40-3) and in furcations of multi-rooted teeth (Fig. 40-4). An important reason is that accessory canals that can mediate the release of bacterial elements from the pulpal chamber are relatively uncommon in cervical and mid-root portions (see Chapter 23). Another important factor is that an intact layer

of root cementum blocks potential dissemination of bacteria and their products along the dentinal tubules.

The clinical presentation varies. Lesions can either be in a silent, non-symptomatic state or appear with more or less salient signs of acute infection. In the former case a balanced host–parasite interrelationship has usually been established. The only means to diagnose the condition is then by radiography (Fig. 40-1b). Unless transformed to a cyst, the extension of such non-symptomatic lesions may remain limited and stable over many years. This applies in particular to lesions associated with root-filled teeth, where the persisting root canal infection has assumed a relatively low grade of metabolic activity (see Chapter 23).

Lesions associated with untreated infections of a necrotic pulp or with inadequately treated root canals may any time, either soon after pulp tissue breakdown or after a period of silence, turn into an exacerbating, acute inflammatory process. Exacerbating lesions may also be induced in conjunction with endodontic treatment from over-instrumentation along with extrusion of bacterial organisms and tissue-irritating medicaments. Exudation and pus production dictate the clinical course. Typical symptoms

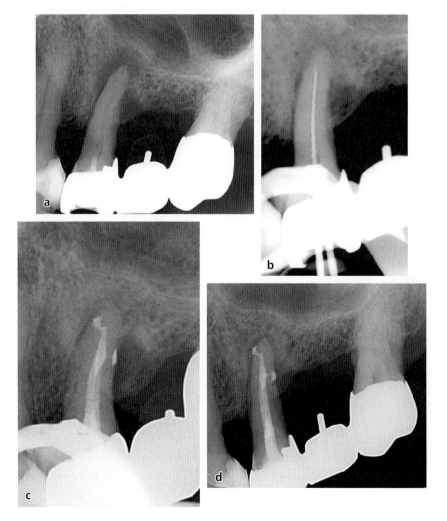

Fig. 40-3 Series of radiographs showing endodontic treatment of an upper premolar included as an abutment in a three-unit bridge. The patient, a 78-year-old male, had been treated and maintained for periodontal disease. (a) There are bone lesions both at the apical and at the distal aspect of the tooth. Following endodontic treatment of the necrotic pulp (b) and root filling (c), an accessory canal communicating with the lateral lesion became evident. (d) The 6-month recall radiograph shows substantial reduction of both bone lesions. Case kindly provided by Dr. Peter Jonasson.

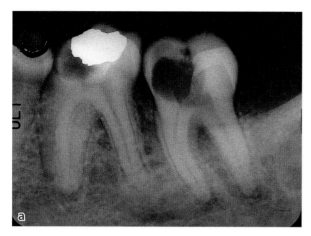 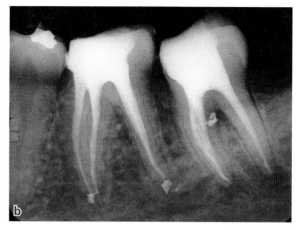

Fig. 40-4 (a) Bone loss of the furcal region in a second left molar in addition to apical bone lesions at both the mesial and the distal roots. (b) Upon endodontic treatment an accessory canal became filled, suggesting that the furcal lesion was of endodontic origin. Case kindly provided by Dr. Pierre Machtou.

include throbbing pain, pain on percussion, tenderness to palpation, increased tooth mobility, and apical as well as marginal swellings. The severity of these symptoms may have escalated successively over a period of time, although a single sign may be the only presenting symptom. It should be noted that the very same symptoms occur with some forms of aggressive periodontitis, iatrogenic root perforation, root fracture, and external root resorption (see below).

The pressure the exudative process exerts results in tissue destruction as a path for drainage is sought. This expansion of the lesion may take a variety of directions. Significant in the context of differential diagnosis to periodontitis are those lesions that drain at or near the gingival margin. The character of the accompanying bone lesion may add to the risk of misdiagnosis, as it may look similar to that of aggressive periodontitis (Fig. 40-5).

Several routes of drainage from an acute endodontic lesion should be recognized (Fig. 40-6):

1. The suppurative process may drain off along the periodontal ligament space and exit at the bottom of the sulcus (Fig. 40-6a). This usually results in only a narrow opening of the fistula into the gingival sulcus/pocket and may not be detected unless careful probing of the sulcus is carried out at multiple sites. Such a sinus tract may readily be probed down to the apex of the tooth, where no increased probing depth otherwise may exist around the tooth. In multi-rooted teeth a sinus tract along the periodontal ligament can drain into the furcation area as it exits along the root surface. The resulting bone lesion may then resemble a "through-and-through" furcation defect from periodontal disease (Figs. 40-7 and 40-8).
2. A periapical abscess can also perforate the cortical bone close to the apex. In this acute stage the soft tissue including the periosteum may be elevated from the bone surface to the extent that a wide

opening for drainage of pus is created in the gingival sulcus/pocket area (extraosseous drainage; Fig. 40-6b). Later this route of drainage may develop into in a chronic sinus tract that may remain in or near the sulcus, often at the buccal aspect of the involved tooth. Such a fistula may also emerge following a less aggressive process. It is important to note that this type of drainage is not associated with loss of bone tissue at the inner walls of the alveolus, and that a periodontal probe cannot penetrate into the periodontal ligament space.

Conclusion

Endodontic lesions either do not have overt clinical signs or may present with various acute manifestations of root canal infection. The asymptomatic lesions usually assume a limited extension around the apex, while rapid and extensive destruction that may extend marginally along the attachment apparatus may follow acute exacerbations. Exudation and pus formed in the process may drain off in different directions; pathways along the periodontal ligament space or following penetration of the alveolar bone at the apical region with drainage in or near the gingival sulcus/pocket warrant particular attention from a differential diagnostic point of view. In addition to deep pocket probing depths, the accompanying bone lesion may mimic that of periodontitis.

Distinguishing lesions of endodontic origin from periodontitis

Pulp vitality testing

Differential diagnosis is important because at times endodontic lesions may produce clinical signs and symptoms similar to those of periodontitis. Tools to distinguish the two disease conditions from each

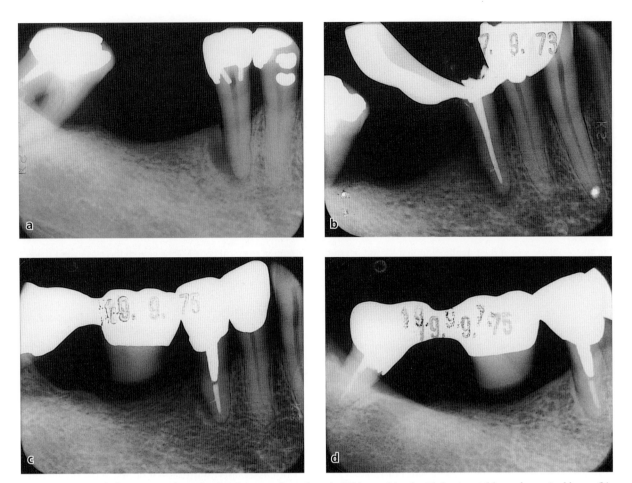

Fig. 40-5 (a) A radiolucent area along the distal root surface of tooth #45 is combined with horizontal loss of marginal bone. (b) As the pulp was non-vital it was subjected to endodontic treatment. After prosthodontic treatment (c) the 2-year recall radiograph (d) shows bone fill in the previous angular defect. Careful examination of the radiographs in (b) and (c) reveals a filled accessory canal communicating with the lateral bone defect.

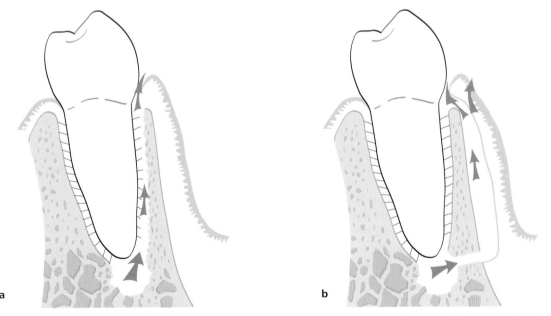

Fig. 40-6 Schematic illustrations demonstrating possible pathways for drainage of a periapical abscess. (a) Drainage along the periodontal ligament with an exit in the sulcus. (b) Extraosseous drainage with exits either in or near the sulcus.

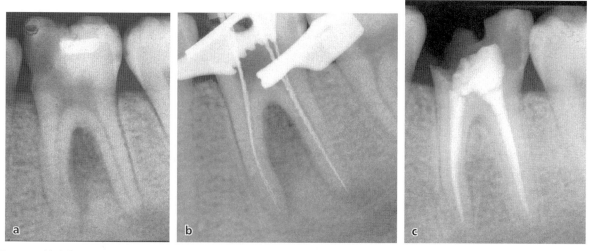

Fig. 40-7 (a) A large radiolucent area is present in the furcal region of a lower left first molar mimicking a furcation involvement caused by periodontal disease. In this case the lesion was of endodontic origin as indicated by the large caries lesion and necrosis of the pulp. (b) Endodontic treatment resulted in complete resolution of the bone lesion as demonstrated by the 18-month follow-up radiograph (c). Case kindly provided by Dr. Kevin Martin.

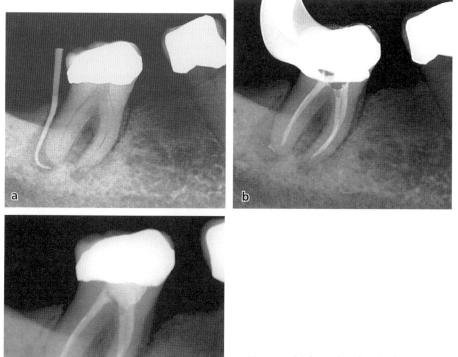

Fig. 40-8 (a) Second molar displaying an apical–marginal communication along the distal root surface. The communication was made visible by a gutta-percha point brought into the sulcus. Endodontic treatment (b) resulted in complete resolution of the bone lesions associated with the distal root (c). At an emergency visit 2 years later the patient complained of pain and tenderness that turned out to be caused by a longitudinal root fracture involving the mesial root. Case kindly provided by Dr. Peter Jonasson.

other, however, are limited as neither the patient's disease history, the clinical presentation nor the character of the radiographic signs invariably are clear-cut. As an endodontic lesion of clinical significance in this context cannot emerge unless the tissue has turned necrotic and become infected, determination of pulp vitality is a most important measure in cases where an endodontic etiology is suspected. Endo-

dontic lesions associated with root-filled teeth are discussed separately, below.

Pulp vitality implies that the tissue has an intact neurovascular supply to support cell and tissue functions. Although a vital pulp may be inflamed or display a variety of degenerative changes, the vasculature is still functioning in a vital pulp. Most methods of determining pulp vitality act by stimulating the pulp's sensory nerve function and presume that the provocation of a sharp pain sensation indicates a vital pulp. This means that in reality the *sensibility* of the pulp is tested rather than the *vitality* of it. However, there is ample documentation to support the concept that a tooth which responds to sensory stimuli has vital pulp functions. Conversely, if a tooth does not respond, the pulp may be non-vital (Petersson *et al.* 1999; Peters *et al.* 1994; Pitt Ford & Patel 2004). Means to detect blood flow within the pulp by non-invasive methods, for example by laser light scattering, have been developed and tested, but have so far gained limited clinical application (see review by Pitt Ford & Patel 2004).

Caution should be exercised in interpreting sensibility tests as findings can reflect both false-positive and false-negative readings (Mumford 1964; Petersson *et al.* 1989; Peters *et al.* 1994; Pitt Ford & Patel 2004). A combination of different test methods should be employed to ensure correct diagnosis, especially in doubtful cases. Also the equipment and the results should be tested for reliability by comparing results from tests of neighboring and contralateral teeth. No test has so far been advanced, which can identify the disease status of the pulp in other terms than vital or non-vital.

Testing non-restored or minimally restored teeth in dentitions affected by periodontitis can usually be successfully conducted by mechanical, thermal, and electric stimulation. Common methods utilize hydrodynamic forces to stimulate nociceptive mechanoreceptors at the pulp–dentin border, primarily the fast conducting A-delta fibers. Useful techniques include direction of a jet of compressed air against an exposed root surface, scratching such surfaces, use of a rubber wheel to generate frictional heat, and various cold tests; all intended to elicit movement of dentinal fluid. Highly effective and reliable are carbon dioxide snow (Fulling & Andreasen 1976) and dichlorodifluoro-methane sprayed on a cotton pledge. Boiling points of these two agents are at –72°C and –50°C, respectively. For this reason patients should be cautioned prior to application that an intense pain response might be elicited. Clues can also be obtained with less potent means such as ice sticks and ethyl chloride as well as heated gutta-percha sticks (for review see Pitt Ford & Patel 2004).

In dubious cases, mechanical and thermal provocation should be supplemented with electric pulp testing. Units are available which provide a read-out value of the voltage or micro-current being applied to generate the pain response. This function is important so that the test result can be repeated and compared for assessment of patient reliability. Electric pulp testing is technique sensitive and therefore warrants extra precaution to avoid leakage of current to the gingiva and neighboring teeth. To avoid this problem, the test should only be carried out on cleaned and dry teeth isolated from saliva and adjacent teeth with pieces of rubber dam placed in the

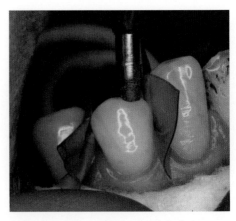

Fig. 40-9 Demonstration of proper tooth isolation to avoid leakage of current during pulp sensibility testing with an electric pulp tester.

tooth contacts (Fig. 40-9). The test further requires that the tooth electrode be provided with proper conducting medium and applied directly on to enamel or dentin.

Cases with extensive restorations and crowned teeth present special challenges as none of the normal test procedures are useful. Unless tooth substance can be reached underneath the restoration with a good margin to the gingiva, the restoration must be pierced to the extent that the test procedure can be conducted in a so-called test cavity. Even then a false-negative response can be obtained as extensive hard tissue repair may have developed in the pulp from previous disease and cutting traumas thus attenuating the stimulus.

Three cases are described below to illustrate the significance of pulp vitality testing in the process of distinguishing endodontic lesion from periodontitis. The cases demonstrate, in addition, that diagnostic entities such as location, form, and extension of radiolucencies, clinical symptoms of pain or swelling, and increased probing depths may not serve as precise diagnostic signs.

The clinical photograph in Fig. 40-10a shows swelling of the marginal gingiva on the buccal aspect of tooth #11. The swelling had been preceded by severe throbbing pain for a few days. Radiographic examination (Fig. 40-10b) disclosed the presence of an angular bone defect that involved the apical portions of the tooth. In this case the pulp clearly responded sensible on testing, indicating that the pathologic condition was not of endodontic origin. Pocket debridement was combined with irrigation with 0.2% chlorhexidine digluconate solution and systemic administration of an antibiotic. The lesion healed rapidly. Seven months following treatment new bone had formed around the apex and in the defect along the mesial root surface (Fig. 40-10c). In this case, therefore, the periodontal lesion was a manifestation of periodontal disease.

In Fig. 40-11a the radiograph taken of the lower front teeth demonstrates bone loss associated with

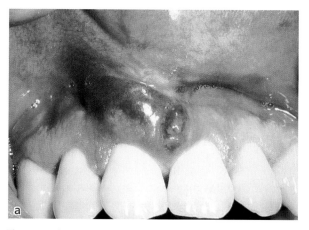
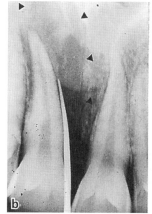
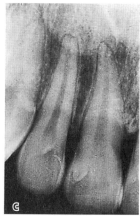

Fig. 40-10 (a) Gingival swelling at the buccal aspect of tooth #11. (b) There is advanced destruction of alveolar bone along the mesial aspect of the root (arrowheads). Following periodontal treatment bone lesion resolved. Case kindly provided by Dr. Harald Rylander.

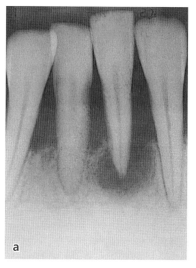
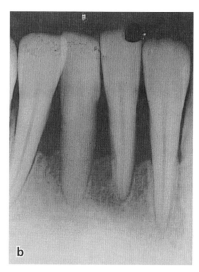
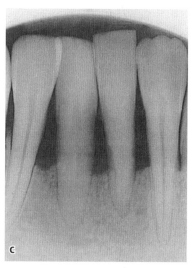

Fig. 40-11 Advanced bone destruction of alveolar bone including an angular bone defect simulating an endodontic periapical lesion around the root tip of tooth #31. The pulp responded vital on testing and the tooth was therefore not subjected to endodontic therapy but to periodontal treatment only. For further case history see the text. Case kindly provided by Dr. Ingvar Magnusson.

the apex of tooth #31 in addition to a generalized horizontal loss of alveolar bone in this young individual. The form and extension of the apical radiolucency around tooth #31 suggests an endodontic lesion. Clinically, a deep periodontal pocket could be probed along the disto-buccal aspect of the root. The patient had been on a recall program after treatment for periodontal disease and had previously shown excellent gingival conditions. Sensibility tests by cold and electricity indicated vital pulp. Therefore, endodontic treatment was not performed. On elevating a mucoperiosteal flap an angular bone defect was found at the buccal aspect of the root without involvement of the root tip. The wound area was debrided along with scaling of the root surface. Rapid bone fill followed surgery without undertaking any adjunctive measures to support tissue regeneration (Fig. 40-11b). The pulp maintained its vitality, although later the root canal became obliterated by hard tissue,

most likely as a consequence of the surgical trauma (Fig. 40-11c). The apically positioned radiolucency in Fig. 40-11a is explained by superimposition of the buccal loss of alveolar bone on the root tip of tooth #31, which went beyond its most apical level (Fig. 40-12) without interfering with the neurovascular supply of the pulp.

Figure 40-13 demonstrates a clinical case where pulp vitality testing was difficult to carry out and which gave inconclusive findings even upon the preparation of a test cavity. A swelling had appeared at the buccal aspect of tooth #46 (Fig. 40-13a) after the patient had experienced pain and tenderness in the area for approximately 1 week. Periodontal probing disclosed a deep facial pocket along the mesial root (Fig. 40-13b). Radiographic examination indicated a lesion that seemed to circumscribe the mesial root with a marginal extension into the furcation (Fig. 40-13c). Frictional heat by drilling, as well as cold and

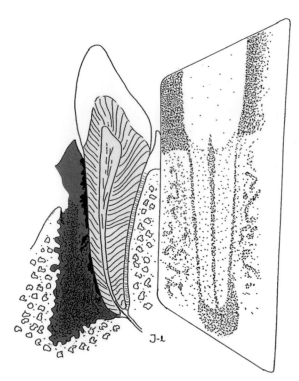

Fig. 40-12 Drawing depicting a potential mechanism for the radiographic lesion in tooth #31, Fig. 40-11. While there was substantial breakdown of alveolar bone there was no interference of the inflammatory lesion with the neurovascular supply of the pulp. The fact that the bone lesion appeared as an apical radiolucency is explained by the superimposition of the bone loss on the root tip. Courtesy of Dr. Mats Joatell.

electric tests, failed to give a positive response even in a test cavity preparation. After finding a sensitive and bleeding pulp in the distal root, a necrotic pulp with pus drainage was detected in the mesial root canals confirming an endodontic cause of the lesion. Endodontic treatment with a temporary intracanal dressing with calcium hydroxide over 3 months resulted in an obvious reduction of the bone lesion (Fig. 40-13d). The gingival lesion resolved with no abnormal pocket-probing depth (Fig. 40-13e), although a small bone defect remained in the furcation area (Fig. 40-13d). Treatment was then completed with root canal fillings. The 12-month recall radiograph demonstrates complete resolution of the bone defect (Fig. 40-13f).

Other indications of endodontic lesion

Except for a negative pulp test response, single-tooth lesions in a dentition otherwise free from periodontal disease strongly suggest an endodontic cause, provided other tooth-associated disorders such as external root resorption and root fracture can be excluded. An endodontic etiology should be explored particularly in cases with extensive restoration or a crowned tooth (Figs. 40-8 and 40-13), bridge abutment (Fig. 40-3), caries (Fig. 40-7), a root-filled tooth, and in patients with a history of a previous dental trauma. The character of the pocket probing depth should

also be taken into consideration. Endodontic lesions, when extending marginally, usually do not follow more than one root surface and then exit in a rather narrow area of the sulcus. Pocket probing depth may also be in an area uncharacteristic of periodontitis, for example at the buccal aspect, when all other sites display normal probing depths.

Conclusion

The clinical presentation and the character of radiographic findings may lead to erroneous diagnosis in cases, where an endodontic lesion emerges in a patient with periodontal disease. The recognition of pulp vitality is crucial because clinically significant lesions of endodontic origin rarely develop in teeth with vital but inflamed pulps. The clinician should always be watchful for false leads and consider features which normally are associated with diseased pulps, such as extensive restoration, previous pulp capping, history of dental trauma, and endodontic treatment.

Endo–perio lesions – diagnosis and treatment aspects

The potential for an infected, necrotic pulp to cause breakdown of the attachment apparatus with extension into the marginal periodontium has been addressed above, along with the measures to establish the diagnosis. Once confirmed, the mode of treatment in this type of case is simple and should involve only conservative root canal therapy. Following adequate treatment, directed to elimination of the root canal infection, the lesion should be expected to heal without a persistent periodontal defect (Figs. 40-3, 40-5, 40-8, and 40-13). Adjunctive periodontal therapy would have no treatment effect and would be inappropriate.

A more complex situation arises when a periodontal lesion is sustained by both plaque infection and a root canal infection concurrently. This kind of lesion is associated with a deep pocket probing depth and a lateral bone defect that extends to the apex (Fig. 40-8). The problem here is that it is not normally possible to determine how much of the lesion is sustained by one or the other infection. In fact there are three scenarios. Firstly, the entire lesion may be a manifestation of a root canal infection alone. Secondly, the entire lesion may be the result of plaque infection. Thirdly, there are, in fact, two disease processes, one marginal associated with a plaque infection and one apical associated with a root canal infection. It is just that the two soft tissue lesions have merged and there is no longer a clear demarcation zone between the two as a probe can penetrate both soft tissue lesions. This latter condition has been termed a "true endo–perio lesion".

Pulp vitality testing only partly settles the diagnostic quandary in this kind of case. Yet, if distinctly

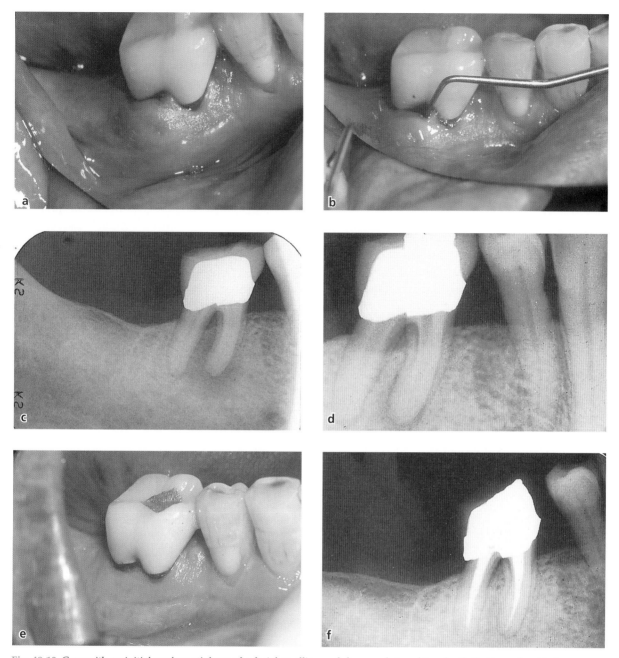

Fig. 40-13 Case with an initial unclear etiology of a facial swelling and deep pocket probing depth that turned out to have an endodontic etiology. The case history is given in the text. Diagnosis and treatment of this case was carried out by one of the authors (G.B.) in collaboration with Dr. David Simpson.

positive, one can exclude contribution of an endodontic infection and the process should be subject to periodontal therapy. Taking the pulp out and replacing it with a root filling is then a meaningless and unnecessary treatment effort. In the case of a negative pulp test, death of the pulp may have occurred as a direct result of the periodontal disease process or it may have developed independently as a separate condition. In the former case, prognosis for any other treatment than extraction must be regarded as bleak. A major reason is that not only may a substantial portion of the attachment apparatus be lost, but the root surface may be bacterially infected close to the root tip as well. In addition, the infection may have entered the root canal after necrosis of the pulp (see

Chapter 23). Accessing this kind of infection for treatment is therefore a very challenging task with a questionable outcome.

If a portion of the lesion is sustained by a root canal infection independent of periodontal disease, the potential for periodontal tissue regeneration is much increased. Because it is not possible to know beforehand how far the endodontic lesion has extended along the root, root canal treatment should be attempted first and periodontal treatment postponed until the result of the endodontic treatment can be evaluated. The part of the lesion sustained by root canal infection can usually be expected to heal rapidly (Fig. 40-3). Periodontal attachment along with bone healing can then be expected within a few

Table 40-1 Outline of treatment strategies

Cause	Condition of the pulp	Treatment
Endodontic	Non-vital	Endodontic
Periodontal	Vital	Periodontal
Endodontic/periodontal	Non-vital	Endodontic – first observe the result of this therapy and institute periodontal therapy later if necessary

months. The part of the lesion caused by plaque infection may also heal following adequate periodontal therapy. Yet little or no regeneration of the attachment apparatus should be anticipated. Table 40-1 outlines the strategy to be taken for treatment of "endo–perio lesions".

Conclusion

Deep pocket probing depths associated with angular bone defects may reflect a combined endodontic and periodontal lesion. Yet, the extent to which an endodontic infection has contributed to the attachment loss cannot normally be determined upon a negative sensibility test, as the entire loss might be caused by plaque infection. Therefore, a treatment strategy should be applied which includes endodontics in the first place, but only in cases where an endodontic etiology is reasonably plausible, that is in teeth with large restorations, full-coverage crowns or history of dental trauma. If the tooth is completely intact without major restoration, caries or history of trauma, the potential of an endodontic etiology of the process is remote.

Endodontic treatments and periodontal lesions

Periodontal lesions, as already stated, may be maintained by infectious elements released from endodontically treated teeth. The lesion may have never resolved or may have developed after the completion of treatment. Several routes for dissemination of bacterial products are possible. Except for apical foramina and accessory canals, another possible pathway is inadvertently produced communication by root perforation (see below). The clinical presentation is no different to the one described above and consequently may involve acute exacerbations with quite extensive breakdowns of the attachment apparatus as well as localized, non-symptomatic lesions, only apparent in radiographs.

A persistent infection in root-filled teeth may also impact on the periodontium along dentinal tubules in areas where cementum has been damaged or lost

(Hammarström *et al.* 1986; Blomlöf *et al.* 1988). The potential significance of such an avenue has been highlighted in clinical studies. Comparing teeth with healthy pulps, endodontically treated teeth with periapical pathology, indicating presence of persistent root canal infection, showed increased pocket probing depths (Jansson *et al.* 1993a), more marginal bone loss (Jansson *et al.* 1993b), and retarded or impaired periodontal tissue healing subsequent to periodontal therapy (Ehnevid *et al.* 1993a, b). Although the differences in probing depths and attachment losses in these studies were rather small, the observations suggest that endodontic re-treatment should be considered as an adjunct to periodontal therapy when a root canal filling is defective and/or displays signs of periapical inflammation. In individuals with no or minor evidence of periodontal disease, the root canal condition, whether root filled or not or infected or not, did not seem to affect the periodontal status in a controlled study (Miyashita *et al.* 1998).

Conclusion

Unfilled spaces in endodontically treated root canals can sustain bacterial growth, and infectious products from these may reach the periodontium along the very same pathways as in an untreated tooth with infected pulp. Endodontic re-treatment may be considered as an adjunct to periodontal therapy when a root canal filling is of poor quality and/or displays signs of periapical inflammation because of the potential that bacterial elements may become disseminated to the periodontium along dentinal tubules exposed by periodontal instrumentation.

Iatrogenic root perforations

During endodontic treatment, and in conjunction with preparation of root canals for insertion of posts, instrumentation can accidentally result in perforation of the root and wounding of the periodontal ligament (Sinai 1977; Kvinnsland *et al.* 1989; Eleftheriadis & Lambrianidis 2005). Perforations can be made through the lateral walls of the root or through the pulpal floor in multi-rooted teeth. The clinical course from then on depends largely on the extent the wound site becomes infected (Beavers *et al.* 1986). If made in the crestal bone area, a typical feature is epithelial proliferation and periodontal pocket formation (Lantz & Persson 1967; Petersson *et al.* 1985). If the perforation is more apical along the root, a wound site infection process may first lead to an acute pain condition, including abscess formation and drainage of pus, followed by further loss of fibrous attachment and periodontal pocketing (Fig. 40-14).

Early detection is critical for a successful outcome of treatment as long-standing perforations with a manifest infection have poor potential for repair.

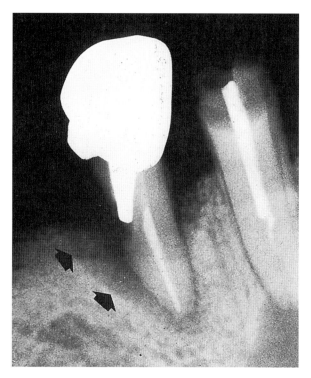

Fig. 40-14 Angular bone defect at the distal root surface of a mandibular molar (arrows). The root is perforated as indicated by the misaligned post. Clinical symptoms included drainage of pus from the pocket and increased tooth mobility. The tooth was extracted.

Successful treatments have, however, been attained in such cases (Tsesis & Fuss 2006).

Diagnosis is based on the occurrence of sudden pain and bleeding during preparation of root canals coronal to the working length. Such signs are likely to be less distinct, however, if the perforation occurs during a procedure conducted under local anesthesia. A perforation may also go undetected as bleeding may not invariably be provoked. For example, when post preparations are carried out by means of a machine-driven instrument, a smear layer is formed that may clog up the blood vessels. Thus, in many instances no bleeding will be noticed until the following visit, when granulation tissue has proliferated into the root canal space along the perforation defect. Granulation tissue usually bleeds profusely on attempts to remove it. Electronic apex locators are helpful in the confirmation of a root perforation, when readings obtained are substantially shorter than the root canal length (Fuss et al. 1996).

Over the years many therapeutic agents and methods have been proposed for the management of root perforations (reviewed by Tsesis & Fuss 2006). Materials proposed for sealing from the inside of the root canal space include amalgam, zinc oxide and eugenol cements, both chemically cured and light-cured calcium hydroxide-containing pastes, and plaster of Paris. More recently, mineral trioxide aggregate (MTA) based on Portland cement has shown great promise by its ability to permit cemen-

tum repair (Arens & Torabinejad 1996; Schwartz et al. 1999).

Regardless of the material used, healing of the lesion in the periodontium depends on whether bacterial infection can be excluded from the wound site by a tight seal of the perforation (Beavers et al. 1986) (Fig. 40-15). This may be difficult to achieve, particularly if the perforation is made deep into the root canal at an oblique angle giving it an oval-shaped orifice into the periodontium. Nevertheless, for mid-root and cervical perforations, non-surgical approaches, including placement of an internal seal, are preferable to a surgical approach, as the latter often results in persistent pocket formation and furcation involvement. Furthermore, surgical treatment is not always feasible because of the inherent difficulty of accessing many perforation sites. As a last resort, extraction followed by repair and re-implantation of the tooth may be attempted (Tsesis & Fuss 2006). In multi-rooted teeth, hemisection and extraction of one or two roots may be a treatment of choice.

Conclusion

Inflammatory lesions in the marginal periodontium, as manifested by increased probing depth, suppuration, increased tooth mobility, and loss of fibrous attachment, may result from an undetected or unsuccessfully treated root perforation. If an iatrogenic root perforation occurs during instrumentation of root canals, filling of the artificial canal to the periodontium should be carried out without delay to prevent granulation tissue formation and wound site infection. Outcome of treatment depends on how well the wound site can be sealed. The closer the perforation is to the bone margin, the greater the likelihood is for proliferation of epithelium at the perforation site with a deep, potentially suppurating pocket as a result.

Vertical root fractures

Clinical symptoms that are typical of tooth-associated infections such as endodontic lesions and plaque-induced periodontitis may also appear at teeth with vertical root fractures. A vertical root fracture is defined as a fracture of a root that is longitudinally oriented at a more or less oblique angle relative to the long axis of the tooth (Fig. 40-16). It can traverse the root in different directions mesially/distally or facially/lingually; it may, but does not always, engage the root canal space. A vertical root fracture can extend the entire length of a root and then involve the gingival sulcus/pocket area. It may also be incomplete and confined to either coronal or apical ends. It should be noted that vertical root fractures although expanding in opposite directions may extend to one root surface only.

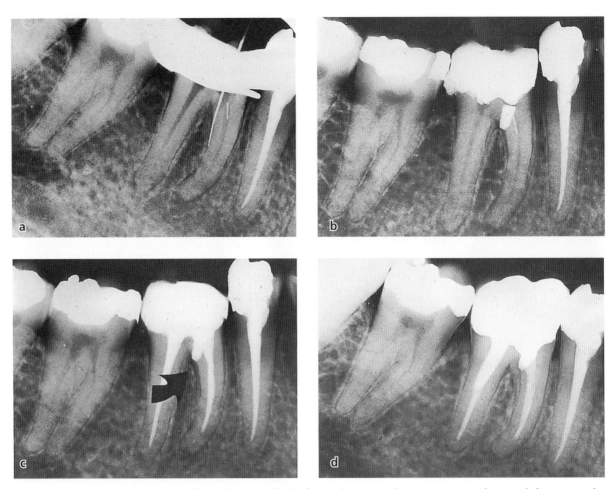

Fig. 40-15 (a) Perforation of the pulpal floor of the mandibular first molar occurred in conjunction with a search for root canal openings. There is also a file fragment in one of the mesial canals. (b) The perforation was immediately sealed with gutta-percha. (c) In a radiograph taken 1 month after treatment a slight radiolucency is seen at the site of the perforation (arrow). (d) Follow-up after 2 years showed normal periodontal conditions both clinically and radiographically. Case kindly provided by Dr. Gunnar Heden.

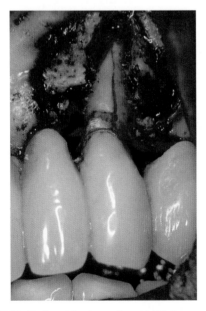

Fig. 40-16 Vertical root fracture of a root-filled upper canine included as an abutment in a prosthetic reconstruction. Due to inflammatory breakdown of the buccal plate a typical bone dehiscence is seen.

Mechanisms

Endodontically treated teeth appear over-represented among teeth with vertical root fracture in comparison to teeth with vital pulps (Meister *et al.* 1980; Gher *et al.* 1987; Patel *et al.* 1995). Generally the increased fracture propensity of root-filled teeth has been attributed to loss of tooth structure as a result of endodontic instrumentation and subsequent restorative procedures (Reeh *et al.* 1989; Sedgley & Messer 1992). Loss of fracture resistance increases especially after overzealous root canal preparation leaving thin dentin walls to the periodontium (Tjan & Whang 1985). Notches, ledges, and cracks induced by root canal preparation, root canal filling procedures, and seating of threaded pins and posts also contribute to sites of stress concentration during mastication that eventually may lead to fracture (Kishen 2006). Decrease of moisture content following root canal treatment is another claimed cause of increased fracture susceptibility of root-filled teeth; insignificant moisture differences were found, however, when dentin of teeth with vital pulps and dentin of root-filled teeth were compared (Papa *et al.* 1994). More recent observations have nevertheless demonstrated

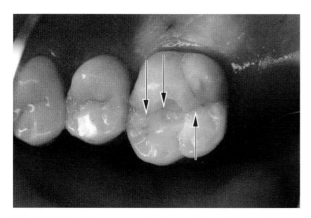

Fig. 40-17 Crack in an unrestored maxillay molar causing symptoms of pulpitis. The patient, a 47-year-old male, had thought the pain problem originated from the temporomandibular joint. Following the preparation of a test cavity, a clear split line was observed at the bottom of the cavity (arrows), confirming the cause of the pain condition. Case kindly provided by Dr. Hideaki Suda.

that biomechanical effects occur in dehydrated dentin that may render endodontically treated teeth prone to fracture (Kishen 2006). Dehydrated dentin *in vitro* was observed to assume increased stiffness as well as a decrease in toughness (e.g. the total energy a material can absorb before fracturing) in comparison to hydrated dentin (Jameson *et al.* 1994; Kahler *et al.* 2003; Kishen & Asundi 2005). Hence, fluid-filled dentinal tubules as well as a water-rich pulp tissue may give normal teeth better resistance to occlusal loading forces than root-filled teeth. It has also been speculated that, along with loss of vital pulp tissue, mechanoreceptive functions are lost concomitantly, allowing larger loads to be placed during mastication than the patient normally would feel tolerable (Löwenstein & Rathkamp 1955; Randow & Glantz 1986).

Vertical root fracture may also occur in clinically intact teeth with no or minor restoration (Fig. 40-17). As posterior teeth are exposed to more heavy occlusal forces, mandibular molars appear to be especially at risk for fracture (Yang *et al.* 1995; Chan *et al.* 1999). Subsequent to fracture of teeth with vital pulps, typical pulpitis symptoms may be initiated, together with pain on percussion and mastication.

Incidence

Data on the incidence of vertical root fractures are scarce in the literature. While it appears to be low, vertical root fractures probably occur more often than clinicians are able to diagnose (Tamse *et al.* 1999b). Molars and premolars appear more often affected than incisors and canines (Meister *et al.* 1980; Testori *et al.* 1993). In longitudinal clinical follow-up studies of patients treated with fixed prostheses, vertical root fractures were frequent in root-filled teeth with posts and especially so in teeth serving as terminal abutments in cantilever bridges (Randow *et al.* 1986).

It is important to recognize that root fracture of endodontically treated teeth may occur several years after the completion of endodontic therapy and final restoration of the tooth (Fig. 40-18). In a study comprising 32 vertical root fractures, the average time between the completion of endodontic treatment and diagnosis of fracture was 3.25 years, with a range varying between 3 days and 14 years (Meister *et al.* 1980). In another study comprising 36 teeth, symptoms of root fracture developed on average more than 10 years after completion of treatment (Testori *et al.* 1993).

Clinical expressions

Clinical signs and symptoms associated with vertical root fractures vary hugely. Occasionally, there may be pronounced pain symptoms and abscess formation because of active bacterial growth in the fracture space (Fig. 40-18). In other instances clinical symptoms may be limited to tenderness on mastication, mild pain, and dull discomfort. Sinus tracts may emerge near the gingival margin (Fig. 40-19). A strong indication of a vertical root fracture is sinus tracts occurring at both buccal and lingual/palatal sites (Tamse 2006). In other instances, a narrow, local deepening of a periodontal pocket in an area not typical for periodontal disease may be the only clinical finding (Fig. 40-20).

The osseous defect emanating from the periodontal tissue lesion may take different shapes depending on how the fracture extends. If there is a buccal extension, the thin alveolar bone plate readily resorbs and a typical bone cleft can be seen upon raising a mucoperiosteal flap (Fig. 40-16). At palatal or lingual extensions, the lesion may not resorb the entire bone wall. Therefore, the osseous defect may take a U-form shape with the height of the bone margin preserved. On fractures that are limited to the apical portion of the root, the bone defect may center on the root apex, similar to that of a periapical lesion associated with an infected root canal.

In conventional intraoral periapical radiographs these bone lesions may not be readily visible, depending on the location, character, and shape of the bone destruction (Fig. 40-20). Absence of lesion, even when taken at different angles, can also be explained by superimposition of roots and bone structures over the bone dehiscence. In yet other cases radiographic signs may be limited to widening of the periodontal ligament space. Lateral radiolucency along one or both of the lateral root surfaces may be discerned with more pronounced bone lesions. A thin halo-like apical radiolucency is another example of a radiographic lesion suggestive of a vertical root fracture (Pitts & Natkin 1983; Testori *et al.* 1993; Tamse *et al.* 1999a). Recent developments of tomographic techniques have brought valuable new diagnostic tools as they can remove interfering anatomic structures and thereby help to visualize presence, location, and

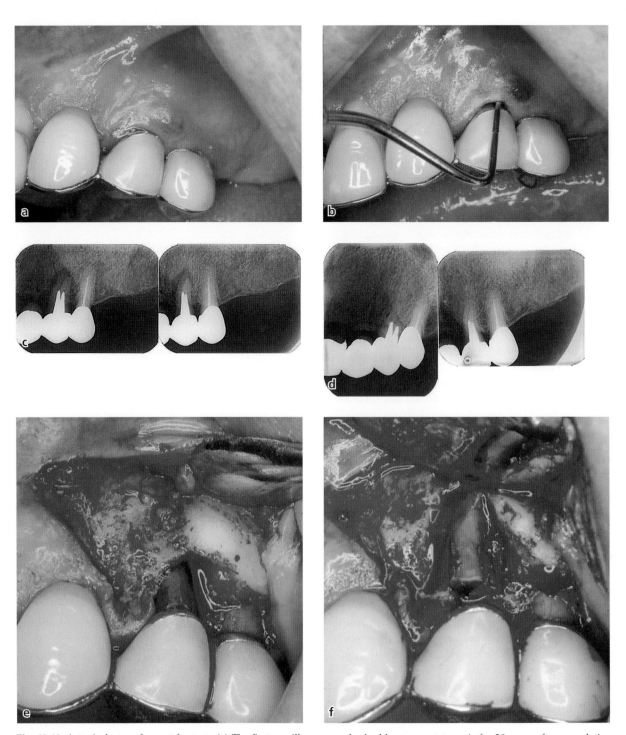

Fig. 40-18 A typical case of a root fracture. (a) The first maxillary premolar had been asymptomatic for 20 years after completion of endodontic treatment and bridge-work. Patient sought treatment because of suddenly appearing pain, tenderness and facial swelling. (b) A deep periodontal pocket could be probed at the buccal aspect of the tooth, while all other sites displayed normal pocket probing depths. (c) Radiographs revealed a radiolucent area along the mesial aspect of the root system. (d) A set of radiographs taken 6 months earlier showed no such lesion. (e) Elevation of a mucoperiosteal flap revealed substantial loss of marginal bone at the buccal aspect of the root. A fracture going in a mesio-distal direction was subsequently confirmed. (f) Following removal of bone tissue, the roots were separated from the crown and extracted.

extension of bone lesions (Gröndahl & Hummonen 2004) (Fig. 40-20e,f).

Diagnosis

The diagnosis of a vertical root fracture is often difficult to ascertain because the fracture is usually not readily detectable by clinical inspection unless there is a clear separation of the root fragments. To give a radiographic appearance of the fracture in the absence of separation, the central X-ray beam has to be parallel to the fracture plane (Fig. 40-21). This is rarely achieved. The suspicion of a vertical root fracture is often inferred from a pocket probing depth in an

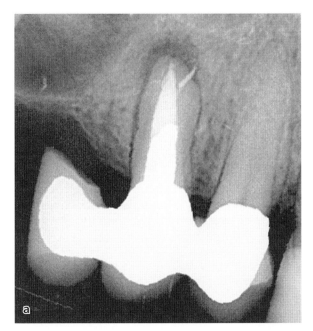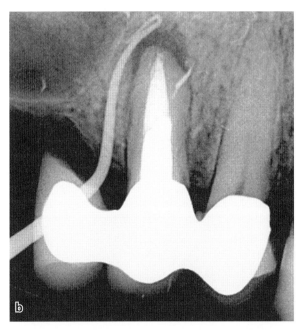

Fig. 40-19 (a) Periapical radiolucency associated with an upper second premolar that turned out to be caused by a vertical root fracture. There was a buccal, deep pocket-probing depth and a sinus tract near the gingival margin. (b) A gutta-percha point inserted in the fistulous tract points to the root apex but provided no additional clue in this case. The widely prepared root canal and the use of the tooth as an abutment in a cantilever bridge provided likely contributors to the fracture in this case kindly provided by Dr. Thomas Kvist.

aberrant position, for example at a buccal or lingual aspect of a tooth, in a dentition which otherwise is free from symptoms of periodontal disease. Another strong indication is the sudden appearance of clinical symptoms and/or radiographic lesion on a root-filled tooth that has remained asymptomatic and without lesion for years (Fig. 40-18).

A number of diagnostic procedures can be undertaken to confirm the diagnosis. Application of various dye solutions, e.g. methylene blue or iodine tincture, on to the crown and the root surface can sometimes be indicative. As the dye enters the fracture space, it will show up as a distinct line against the surrounding tooth substance. Indirect illumination of the root, using fiber-optic light, can also be of value. The fiber-optic probe should then be placed at various positions on the crown or the root, whereby the fracture line may clearly present itself. A surgical microscope or an endoscope, providing both enlargement and directed light, are other valuable tools to disclose vertical root fractures.

In premolars and molars the diagnosis may be supported from observation of varying pain sensations elicited by loading facial and lingual cusps. The procedure includes asking the patient to bite down on a rubber wheel or a specially designed plastic stick (FracFinder). Separate loading of either buccal or lingual cusps eliciting pain sensation from one, but not the other loaded cusp indicates the potential of a fracture. Often the diagnosis of a vertical root fracture has to be confirmed by surgical exposure of the root for direct visual examination (Walton *et al.* 1984) at which one may also discover a typical bone dehiscence (Fig. 40-16).

Treatment considerations

Vertical root fractures that involve the gingival sulcus/pocket area usually have a hopeless prognosis due to continuous bacterial invasion of the fracture space from the oral environment. While there are reports of successful management of fractured teeth by re-attaching the fragments with bonding resin or laser fusing after extraction followed by re-implantation, fractured teeth are normally candidates for extraction. In multi-rooted teeth a treatment alternative is hemisection and extraction of the fractured root.

Conclusion

Symptoms and signs associated with vertical root fractures vary and may be difficult to distinguish from those prevalent with other tooth-associated infections. A variety of diagnostic procedures should therefore be considered. Except for the leads obtained from anamnestic findings and pocket probing depths in buccal or lingual positions or both, clinical examination should include measures to make fracture lines visible *viz.* application of disclosing solutions, the use of fiber-optic light, inspection by a surgical microscope or endoscope, or by raising a surgical flap. Pain on selective loading of cusps may indicate root fracture. A vertical root fracture should be anticipated in root-filled teeth, which, after a long history of being asymptomatic and without signs of infection, suddenly present with tenderness, pain, and radiographic bone lesion (Fig. 40-18). Roots with vertical root fracture usually have a hopeless prognosis and are clear candidates for extraction.

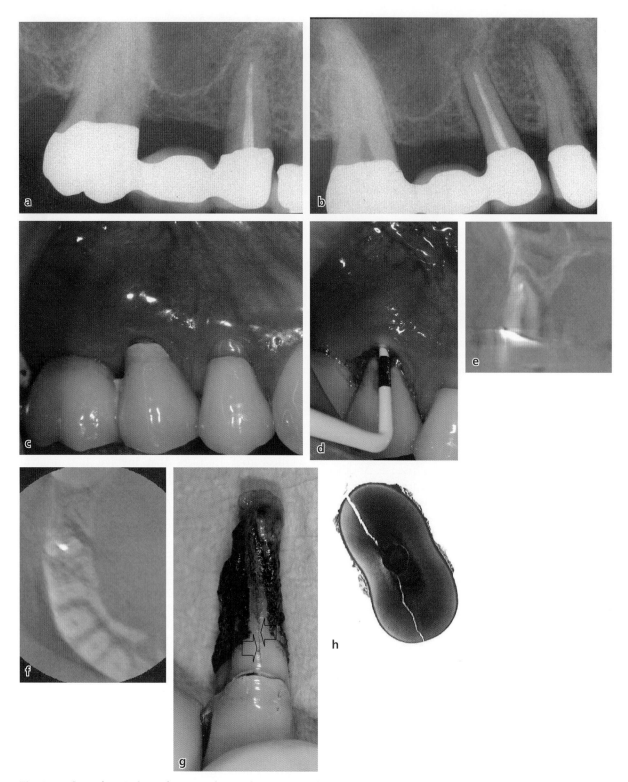

Fig. 40-20 Case of vertical root fracture, where ordinary intraoral radiographs failed to provide evidence of the associated bone lesion. (a) Radiograph shows normal periodontal contours. (b) A second radiograph indicates a widened periodontal ligament space. (c) The patient had complained of recurrent pain on occlusal load for several weeks and presented at the clinic with a light swelling on the buccal aspect that had appeared several weeks before. (d) Clinically there was an isolated 9 mm pocket probing depth mid-buccally, suggesting root fracture. (e,f) Limited cone beam computed tomography was helpful to reveal a bone lesion in this case along the palatal aspect of the tooth. (g) After extraction methylene blue staining visualized the fracture line (arrows) that turned out to extend to both the lingual and the buccal root surface (h). Case kindly provided by Dr. Thomas von Arx.

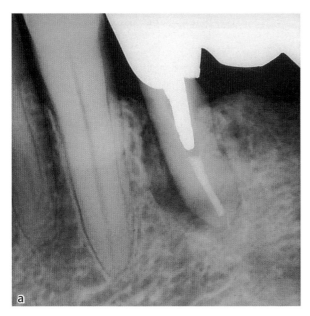
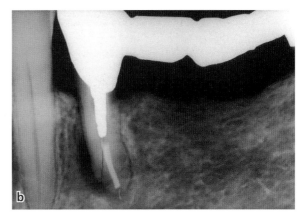

Fig. 40-21 (a) Mandibular premolar included in a four-unit bridge showing a bone lesion at the mesial aspect of the root. In this projection there is no sign of fracture, while in a radiograph (b) taken with a slight shift of angle, a fracture line is clearly visible. Case kindly provided by Dr. K-G. Olsson.

External root resorptions

Root surface resorptions, here termed external root resorptions, usually progress without producing clinical symptoms and may therefore go undetected unless observed radiographically. However, in advanced stages, the surface defect may interfere with the gingival sulcus and thereby initiate an infectious process. As such lesions can be associated with increased pocket probing depths as well as drainage of pus upon probing, this section of the chapter addresses various forms of external root resorptions, their mechanism, clinical features, and management.

Mechanisms of hard tissue resorption in general

The hard tissues of the body consist of two major components, mineral and matrix. While the ratio of these two components varies between bone, cementum, and dentin, the same tools – acids and enzymes – are used by nature to perform the degradation of these tissues. Bone is normally remodeled to adapt to functional changes. Resorption of dental hard tissues of permanent teeth, on the other hand, should be seen as an expression of a pathological process. Clast cells carry out resorption of bone as well as cementum, dentin, and enamel (Hammarström & Lindskog 1992; Suda *et al.* 1996). These cells are large, multinucleated, motile cells emanating from hematopoietic precursor cells in the bone marrow (Marks 1983; Vaes 1988; Pierce *et al.* 1991; Suda *et al.* 1996) and termed osteoclasts when involved in bone remodeling processes. Phenotypically the very same kind of clast cells conduct resorption of the hard tissues of the tooth. Mononucleated cells are also involved in the later phase of the resorption process by eliminating the organic matrix that became released follow-

ing dissolution of the mineral components (Wedenberg & Lindskog 1985; Lindskog *et al.* 1987; Brudvik & Rygh 1993; Lerner 2006).

Under normal, physiologic conditions, hard tissues are protected from resorption by their respective surface layers of blast cells; in the case of cementum by cementoblasts. As long as these blast cell layers remain intact with the unmineralized layer of osteoid or cementoid at the surface of the mineralized tissue, resorption will not occur. It is known that bone resorption is under hormonal regulation and is mediated by osteoblasts (Lerner 2006). Stimulation by parathyroid hormone makes the osteoblasts first degrade the osteoid and then contract to expose the bone surface for osteoclastic demineralization (Jones & Boyde 1976; Rodan & Martin 1981; Lerner 2006). However, parathyroid hormone exerts no influence on cementoblasts (Lindskog *et al.* 1987), which may explain why bone, but not teeth, is remodeled to adapt to functional changes. However, dental trauma, excessive orthodontic forces and aggressive scaling and root planing during periodontal therapy are examples of injuries that can initiate root resorption (Andreasen 1981; Rygh 1977). Subsequent to the injury, the denuded hard tissue surface, without its blast cell layer and cementoid, attracts motile clast cells (Chambers 1981), which seal themselves to the hard tissue surface and excrete acids for demineralization. Concomitantly an acid environment is created that is essential for the degradation of tissue matrix by lysosomal enzymes at low pH optima (Vaes 1988; Kremer *et al.* 1995; Pascoe & Oursler 2001; Czupalla *et al.* 2006; Henriksen *et al.* 2006).

Consequently, a trigger mechanism is required to set off root resorption. For the resorption process to continue, a lasting osteoclast stimulus is required, for example an infection or a continuous mechanical force such as the one elicited by orthodontic

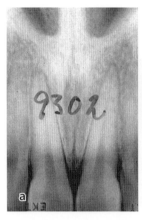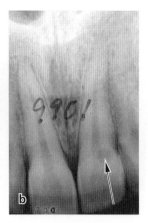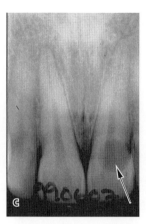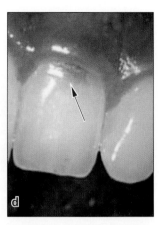

Fig. 40-22 Series of radiographs taken at different time intervals showing the appearance of an external root resorption in a young adult patient. (a) At the age of 15 years there is no sign of resorption. (b) Six years later a small radiolucency is seen (arrow). (c) In just 6 months the lesion expanded considerably (arrow). (d) The lesion appeared clinically as a pink spot in the cervical area of the tooth (arrow). Case kindly provided by Dr. Anders Molander.

treatment. In both instances the resorptive process may be halted if the cause for prolongation can be curbed; in the case of orthodontic tooth movement, by releasing the forces, and in the case of a root canal infection, by root canal therapy.

Conclusion

Two mechanisms are involved in resorption of a hard tissue: (1) a trigger mechanism and (2) a reason for the resorption to continue. Thus, treatment of active root resorption should be directed to eliminate the cause for its continuance.

Clinical presentations and identification

Root resorptions *per se* do not cause painful symptoms. Unless a resorptive process is located coronally and is undermining the enamel, giving it a pinkish appearance (Fig. 40-22), the only way to detect and diagnose dental resorption is by means of radiography (Fig. 40-22b,c). Only in very late stages, as the resorptive process engages the gingival sulcus, may an infectious process emerge with typical features of a periodontal abscess (Fig. 40-23).

A single radiograph is usually not sufficient to define a radiolucent area within the confines of a root as an external resorption. A radiolucency may portray a variety of conditions including a resorptive process inside the root canal (internal root resorption), or a resorptive defect located buccally or lingually as the image of the root is superimposed. It may also be an artifact and reflect a radiolucent bone area superimposed on the root. Therefore, one should always take more than one radiograph and use different angulations to observe whether the radiolucent area belongs to the root or not (Fig. 40-23). New tomographic techniques can be of great benefit to distinguish external from internal root resorptions.

The initial stage of a resorptive process usually passes undetected as radiographs can only present a resorptive cavity after a certain size has been reached (Andreasen *et al*. 1987) (Fig. 40-23). The location of the lesion is also important for detection. A facial or lingual root resorption defect is more difficult to visualize radiographically than a proximal cavity, unless tomography is used. Be aware that in the cervical region it may be difficult to differentiate radiographically between cavities caused by caries and those caused by resorption. To distinguish caries from resorption it is useful to recognize that bacterial acids that demineralize dentin leave a soft cavity surface. By contrast, clastic resorption removes both the mineral and the organic phases of the hard tissues resulting in a cavity floor that is hard to probing.

Different forms

There are different forms of external root resorption. The underlying mechanism is understood only for some of them. A genetic link can be seen in certain cases as external root resorptions run in families. There are also instances when only the enamel of an unerupted tooth is resorbed. Furthermore, external resorptions can be caused by precipitation of oxalate crystals in the hard tissues of patients as a result of increased concentration of oxalates in the blood due to kidney failure (Moskow 1989). Malignant tumors close to a tooth can also cause root resorption (Fig. 40-24).

Andreasen (1981) has published a classification of those external root resorptions that have a known etiology:

- Surface resorption
- Replacement resorption associated with ankylosis
- Inflammatory resorption associated with persistent inflammation in the periodontium adjacent to the resorption site.

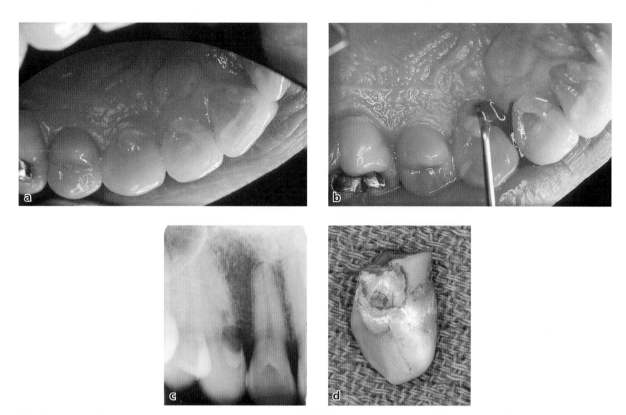

Fig. 40-23 Case of peripheral inflammatory root resorption (PIRR). Pain and tenderness of the right maxilla for several weeks prompted the 30-year-old male patient to seek treatment. (a) Clinical inspection revealed no obvious pathology. (b) Periodontal probing, however, released pus drainage from the lingual aspect of tooth #13. Pulp-vitality test of the tooth as well as neighboring teeth gave clear positive responses. (c) An angulated radiograph disclosed the presence of a resorptive defect. (d) The tooth was extracted as successful treatment was deemed unlikely. An extensive resorptive defect had undermined the clinical crown.

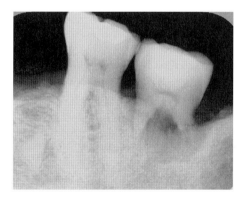

Fig. 40-24 External root resorption of a lower second molar caused by breast cancer metastasis. Case kindly provided by Dr. John Kuo-Hung Yu.

Subforms are:

- Peripheral inflammatory root resorption (PIRR)
- External inflammatory root resorption (EIRR).

Surface resorption

This type of resorption is common, self-limiting, and reversible (Harding 1878; Andreasen 1981). In a histologic study of human teeth from individuals varying in age from 16–58 years, only 10% of the teeth showed absence of active resorption or signs of healed resorptions (Henry & Weinman 1951). Resorptions were noted twice as often in older than in young subjects. Another study demonstrated up to 88% of teeth with active or, in most instances, healed resorptions (Hötz 1967).

The mechanisms behind surface resorptions are only partly understood. These resorptions are normally initiated in conjunction with a localized injury to the cementoblast cell layer, for example by external trauma (Andreasen 1981) or by trauma from occlusion. As clast cells are attracted to the denuded root surface, hard tissue is resorbed for as long as the activating factors are released at the site of injury (Hammarström & Lindskog 1992). The resorptive process then stops within a few days following the disappearance of clast cells along with the defect becoming populated with hard tissue repairing cells leading to cementum repair (Lindskog *et al.* 1983, 1987). The regulating factors governing this process are virtually unknown.

Surface resorption may also result from orthodontic forces. Light forces produce insignificant cemental cratering (root resorption) with rapid tooth movement. On the other hand, intermediate and heavy forces produce substantial cemental cratering and slower tooth movement (Rygh 1977). Following application of an orthodontic force three main stages for the tooth movement can be identified:

1. *Initial minor movement due to the compression of pliable tissues.* During the initial stage of tooth movement, osteoclasts, macrophages, fibroblasts, and resorption lacunae in bone increase on the pressure side (Kurihara 1977; Brudvik & Rygh 1993, 1995).
2. *Delay period with no movement.* The induced tissue damage to the periodontal ligament is resolved by macrophages and osteoclasts during a delay period (Rygh 1977; Brudvik & Rygh 1993, 1995). If excessive forces are placed on teeth, there is increased damage to the surrounding tissues, which prolongs the delay period (Storey 1973). In this phase, the tissues show signs of hyalinization, i.e. development of a cell-free, structureless zone (Sandstedt 1904; Reitan 1951; Kvam 1967; Brudvik & Rygh 1993) as compressed collagen fibers gradually unite to a more or less cell-free mass (Rygh 1972, 1977).
3. *Rapid tooth movement and extensive bone remodeling.* Elimination of the hyalinized tissue leads to removal of the mature collagen and cementoid layer leaving a raw root surface lacking a protective blast cell barrier. The denuded root surface subsequently attracts clast cells and root resorption continues for as long as the force is present (Storey 1973; Rygh 1977; Brudvik & Rygh 1993, 1995). Major loss of dental hard tissue may follow this kind of iatrogenic injury.

Conclusion

Signs of active or healed surface resorptions or both are common in the large majority of teeth of the adult dentition. It is conceivable that minor traumata caused by unintentional biting on hard objects, bruxism, high fillings, etc., cause localized damage to the periodontal ligament and trigger the initiation of this type of resorption. The process is self-limiting and self-healing and no active treatment is required. During orthodontic treatment caution should be exercised and the forces moderated so that the risk of root foreshortening is minimized. When heavy forces are used the involved teeth should be monitored radiographically.

Replacement resorption

This type of resorptive process involves replacement of the dental hard tissues by bone, hence the name (Andreasen 1981). When a surface resorption stops, cells from the periodontal ligament will proliferate and populate the resorbed area (Lindskog *et al.* 1983, 1987). If the surface resorption defect is large, it will take some time before periodontal ligament cells have covered the entire surface. In the interim period osteoblasts from the nearby bone tissue may then

arrive first and establish themselves at the resorbed surface (Andreasen & Kristerson 1981; Gottlow *et al.* 1986). Bone is thus being formed directly upon the dental hard tissue. This results in a fusion between the bone and the tooth substance, which is known as ankylosis. Note that replacement resorption and ankylosis are often erroneously used as synonyms. While replacement resorption describes the active process during which the tooth is resorbed and replaced by bone tissue, ankylosis is the Greek word for immobile. Thus, it describes the situation of a tooth lacking normal mobility due to the fusion between tooth and bone.

The fusion can be permanent or transient and appears to depend on the size of the resorbed area. If the ankylotic area is small, the bone on the tooth surface can resorb and be replaced with reparative cementum (Andreasen & Skougaard 1972; Andreasen & Kristerson 1981; Andersson *et al.* 1985; Hammarström *et al.* 1986). If the ankylotic area is large, a sufficient amount of bone will be formed on the root surface to make the fusion between bone and tooth permanent (Andreasen 1981; Andreasen & Kristersson 1981; Hammarström *et al.* 1986). It has been shown that long-term rigid splinting following external trauma results in a higher incidence of dentoalveolar ankylosis than with a short-term, less rigid fixation (Andreasen 1975).

Clinically, ankylosis is diagnosed by absence of tooth mobility and by a percussion tone that is higher than in a normal tooth (Andreasen 1975; Andersson *et al.* 1985). Radiographically, a local disappearance of the periodontal ligament contour may show an initial stage of fusion. However, even in non-ankylosed teeth it is not always possible to observe the entire contour of the periodontal ligament. Percussion and tooth mobility testing are therefore more sensitive diagnostic tools than radiography in the early stages of replacement resorption (Andersson *et al.* 1985). When dento-alveolar ankylosis occurs at a young age, the tooth will not erupt resulting in infra-occlusion (Andreasen & Hjörting-Hansen 1966; Malmgren *et al.* 1984; Kürol 1984).

The formation of bone on a dentin surface is not a pathologic process, but one to be regarded as a form of repair. The bone has accepted the dental hard tissue as a part of itself and the tooth becomes involved in the normal skeletal turnover (Löe & Waerhaug 1961; Hammarström *et al.* 1986). The turnover phase is fast in a growing child, but slower in an adult. Hence, the rate of bone replacement follows the pattern of bone remodeling. The detailed mechanism directing the resorptive process is not understood.

Conclusion

Ankylosis caused by apposition of bone to a root surface is a prerequisite for replacement resorption. The condition may be seen as a form of repair of root surface resorptions, albeit not desirable from a clinical standpoint as the root structure will become successively destroyed. No treatment is available for this condition.

External inflammatory resorption

The term external inflammatory resorption describes the presence of an inflammatory lesion in the periodontal tissues adjacent to a resorptive process (Andreasen 1985). There are two main forms – peripheral inflammatory root resorption (PIRR) and external inflammatory root resorption (EIRR). Both forms are triggered by destruction of cementoblasts and the cementoid. In PIRR the factor maintaining osteoclast activation is thought to be provided by an inflammatory lesion in the adjacent periodontal tissue (Andreasen 1985; Gold & Hasselgren 1992). EIRR, on the other hand, receives its stimulus from an infected necrotic pulp (Andreasen 1985; Andreasen & Andreasen 1992).

Peripheral inflammatory root resorption
The major feature of this type of resorption is its location close to the gingival margin and its invasive nature. In teeth with a normal height of bone crest it usually becomes localized cervically, whereas in cases where the periodontal tissue has receded it can

develop more apically. Different names have been proposed, including subosseous resorption (Antrim *et al*. 1982) and (the complete opposite) supraosseous extra-canal invasive resorption (Frank & Bakland 1987) reflecting the confusion that has surrounded the cause of this type of resorptive lesion. As it extends into the peripheral dentin towards the pulp, and as clast-activating factors seem to emanate from an inflammatory lesion in the periodontium, the term peripheral inflammatory root resorption (PIRR) was proposed to reflect the potential etiology of this phenomenon (Gold & Hasselgren 1992).

The clinical features of PIRR include a granulation tissue that bleeds freely on probing. Occasionally, a periodontal abscess may develop due to marginal infection, which may mimic a periodontal or endodontic condition (Fig. 40-23). When the lesion is located more apically or proximally, probing is usually difficult. Radiographically, the lesion may only be seen after a certain size has been reached (Fig. 40-22c). Sometimes the appearance is mottled due to the proliferation of bone tissue into the resorptive defect (Seward 1963) (Fig. 40-25). The outline of the root canal can often be seen within the radiolucent area (Figs. 40-22, 40-25 and 40-26) and this is a diagnostic feature for external root resorption in general. The presence of profuse bleeding upon probing and

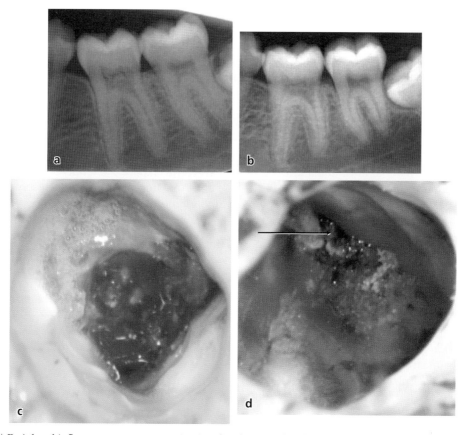

Fig. 40-25 (a,b) Peripheral inflammatory root resorption in a first lower molar showing a mottled appearance. There are pulp stones within the pulp tissue and bone tissue formation within the resorptive defect superimposed on the pulpal space. Following accessing both the pulp and the resorptive process (c) and removing the bleeding tissue, bone tissue appeared at the lingual wall of the cavity, where the resorptive process had entered the tooth (d). Arrow in (d) indicates the orifice of the root canal in the distal root. Case kindly provided by Dr. Magnus Fridjon Ragnarsson.

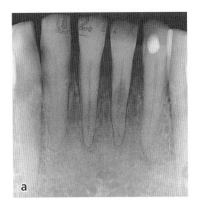
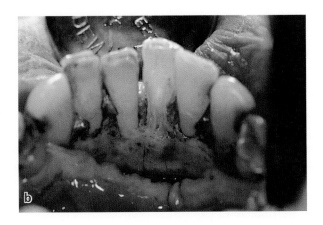
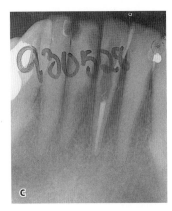
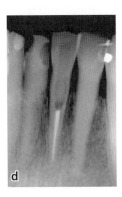

Fig. 40-26 Case with external root resorption on the lingual aspect of both central incisors. (a) The patient, a 78-year-old lady, had presented herself to the clinic after an episode of severe pain and development of a lingual periodontal abscess. The medical history was unremarkable. The patient was initially managed by antibiotic treatment. (b) Later, upon flap elevation and accessing the resorbing area and removal of the granulation tissue, exposure to a necrotic pulp of tooth #31 was noted. (c) Endodontic treatment was carried out during the surgery procedure. Tooth #41 was left without any further treatment and the case was followed clinically and radiographically. No recurrence of resorption occurred on either tooth and the patient remained comfortable. (d) Radiograph of the last follow-up is 8 years after treatment. Note that there is no progression of the resorptive process associated with tooth #41.

granulation tissue formation, in combination with a hard cavity bottom confirm the diagnosis of PIRR. Electric pulp test and cold tests are usually positive, but will not distinguish this condition from caries or internal resorption, the two major differential diagnostic options (Frank & Bakland 1987).

The mechanism for this form of resorption is far from completely understood. Predisposing factors seem to be orthodontic treatment, trauma, and intracoronal bleaching, while periodontal therapy had a low incidence among 222 analyzed cases (Heithersay 1999). The reason for the low incidence following periodontal treatment could be that, even upon excessive scaling and root planing, the damaged area of the root surface usually becomes covered by junctional epithelium. If a resorptive process is triggered it seems that its continuance has an infectious cause (Brosjö et al. 1990; Gold & Hasselgren 1992).

Unmineralized, newly formed tissue in cementum (Gottlieb 1942) and in predentin (Stenvik & Mjör 1970) appears resistant to resorption and explains why PIRR expands laterally without invading the pulp. Yet, this peripheral extension can markedly undermine the tooth structure (Fig. 40-23). If there is a non-vital pulp and thus no resorption inhibition in the form of odontoblast-supported predentin, PIRR may extend to the pulpal space. In root-filled teeth, which have been subjected to intracoronal bleaching, tissue toxic bleaching agents such as hydrogen peroxide have been found to be capable of penetrating through dentin and cementum (Fuss et al. 1989). If this occurs during the bleaching process, periodontal tissue injury will be inflicted and a resorptive processs may be initiated (Harrington & Natkin 1979; Montgomery 1984). The ensuing progression is thought to be a function of persisting inflammation as bacteria have colonized the chemically emptied dentinal tubules (Cvek & Lindvall 1985).

Obviously there are also different forms of this kind of resorption, some of which may be associated with a broad opening to the periodontium, as in the cases initiated by bleaching agents. Others may have smaller openings through the cementum layer along which the resorptive process continues inside the tooth structure without causing major peripheral breakdown. The two patterns dictate the choice of treatment attempt. Surgical exposure of the area including removal of the granulation tissue is the only reasonable option in the former case; a dental filling, e.g. a resin composite, is placed in the defect followed by resuturing the flap. Other treatment options include repositioning of the flap apical to the restoration or orthodontic extrusion of the tooth (Gold & Hasselgren 1992). Guided tissue regeneration has also been advocated after surgical removal of the granulation tissue, to promote ingrowth of periodontal ligament cells into the resorbed area (Rankow & Krasner 1996)

External inflammatory root resorption

This type of resorption usually occurs as a complication to luxation injuries in conjunction with dental traumata. It begins as a surface resorption due to damage of the periodontal ligament and the cementum layer. There is good support for the view that the stimulus for continuance is infectious in nature and that the source is an infected pulp that succumbed as a result of the traumatic injury (Bergenholtz 1974; Andreasen 1985; Andreasen & Andreasen 1992). Following the initial surface resorption the often rapid progression is then due to the release of bacterial elements into the periodontal tissue by way of the exposed dentinal tubules. While the inflammatory process is maintained, the resorptive process, aimed at eliminating the irritants in the dentin tubules, moves in the direction of the infected pulp. As dentin is further resorbed, more infectious products are released thus perpetuating the inflammatory reaction with acceleration of the resorptive process as a result (Andreasen 1985).

The earliest stages are not radiographically visible due to the small size of the resorptive cavity and the first radiographic signs following trauma cannot usually be seen for several weeks (Andreasen *et al.* 1987). Treatment is directed towards the cause of the resorption, that is, the root canal infection (Cvek 1993), and the procedure to be carried out is no different to the one applied in normal cases. While a successful halt of the resorption can be anticipated (Cvek 1973) there is always risk of ankylosis after the initial healing phase. The greater the resorbed area, the greater is the risk for this complication (Andreasen & Kristerson 1981; Andersson *et al.* 1985; Gottlow *et al.* 1986).

Conclusion

Peripheral inflammatory root resorption (PIRR) and external inflammatory root resorption (EIRR) are two forms of progressive external root resorption associated with persistent inflammation in the periodontal tissues. While the direct cause for progression is not well understood, infectious elements maintaining periodontal inflammation close to a root surface that is not covered by periodontal ligament or epithelium appear to drive PIRR. To remedy the condition it is necessary to remove all resorbing granulation tissue surgically and fill the resorption cavity. In certain cases it may be possible to carry out the treatment from the pulpal side (Fig. 40-25). Regardless of approach, periodontal tissue complications may ensue, including deep pockets and suppuration from such pockets. Treated cases should therefore be monitored by regular clinical/radiographic follow-ups to

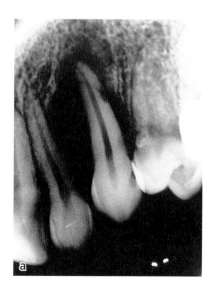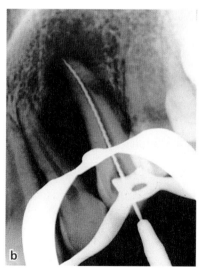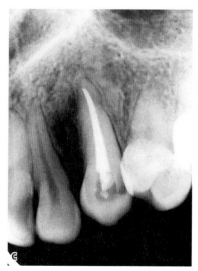

Fig. 40-27 Radiographs from a 27-year-old woman showing the emergence of external inflammatory root resorptions on the left maxillary canine, which had been autotransplanted into a surgically prepared socket 2 months earlier (a). Endodontic treatment of the necrotic pulp (b) halted the resorptive process. (c) Radiograph following root filling shows that the external resorption cavity is rounded. A normal contour of the periodontal ligament space can be seen between the root and bone, which has filled the prepared socket.

observe any signs of recurrence and how the periodontal tissue copes. In advanced cases extraction is the only reasonable treatment option. EIRR is usually seen as a complication to luxation injuries in conjunction with dental traumata. The primary impetus for its progression is an infected pulp that releases bacterial elements to the resorbing area along

exposed dentinal tubules by which an inflammatory lesion is also maintained in the periodontium. EIRR can usually be stopped by focusing the treatment on the endodontic infection (Fig. 40-27) although ankylosis and replacement resorption may appear as complications that may not be detected until years later.

References

Andersson, L., Lindskog, S., Blomlöf, L., Hedström, K-G. & Hammarström, L. (1985). Effect of masticatory stimulation on dentoalveolar ankylosis after experimental tooth replantation. *Endodontics and Dental Traumatology* **1**, 13–16.

Andreasen, J.O. (1975). Periodontal healing after replantation of traumatically avulsed human teeth. Assessment by mobility testing and radiography. *Acta Odontologica Scandinavica* **33**, 325–335.

Andreasen, J.O. (1981). Relationship between surface and inflammatory resorption and changes in the pulp after replantation of permanent incisors in monkeys. *Journal of Endodontics* **7**, 294–301.

Andreasen, J.O. (1985). External root resorptions: its implication in dental traumatology, paedodontics, periodontics, orthodontics and endodontics. *International Journal of Endodontics* **8**, 109–118.

Andreasen, J.O. & Andreasen, F.M. (1992). Root resorption following traumatic dental injuries. *Proceedings of the Finnish Dental Society* **88** (Suppl 1), 95–114.

Andreasen, J.O. & Hjörting-Hansen, E. (1966). Replantation of teeth. I. Radiographic and clinical study of human teeth replanted after accidental loss. *Acta Odontologica Scandinavica* **24**, 263–286.

Andreasen, J.O. & Kristerson, L. (1981). Evaluation of different types of autotransplanted connective tissues as potential periodontal ligament substitutes. *International Journal of Oral Surgery* **10**, 189–201.

Andreasen, F.M., Sewerin, I., Mandel, U. & Andreasen, J.O. (1987). Radiographic assessment of simulated root resorption cavities. *Endodontics and Dental Traumatology* **3**, 21–27.

Andreasen, J.O. & Skougaard, M. (1972). Reversibility of surgically induced dental ankylosis in rats. *International Journal of Oral Surgery* **1**, 98–102.

Antrim, D.D., Hicks, M.L. & Altaras, D.E. (1982). Treatment of subosseous resorption: a case report. *Journal of Endodontics* **8**, 567–569.

Arens, D.E. & Torabinejad, M. (1996). Repair of furcal perforations with mineral trioxide aggregate: two case reports. *Oral Surgery Oral Medicine Oral Pathology* **82**, 84–88.

Beavers, R.A., Bergenholtz, G. & Cox, C.F. (1986). Periodontal wound healing following intentional root perforations in permanent teeth of *Macaca mulatta*. *International Journal of Endodontics* **19**, 36–44.

Bergenholtz, G. (1974). Micro-organisms from necrotic pulp of traumatized teeth. *Odontologisk Revy* **25**, 347–358.

Blomlöf, L., Lindskog, S. & Hammarström, L. (1988). Influence of pulpal treatments on cell and tissue reactions in the marginal periodontium. *Journal of Periodontology* **59**, 577–583.

Brosjö, M., Andersson, K., Berg, J.O. & Lindskog, S. (1990). An experimental model for cervical resorption in monkeys. *Endodontics and Dental Traumatology* **6**, 118–120.

Brudvik, P. & Rygh, P. (1993). Non-clast cells start orthodontic root resorption in the periphery of hyalinazed zone. *European Journal of Orthodontics* **15**, 467–480.

Brudvik, P. & Rygh, P. (1995). Transition and determinants of orthodontic root resorption-repair sequence. *European Journal of Orthodontics* **17**, 177–188.

Chambers, T.J. (1981). Phagocytic recognition of bone by macrophages. *Journal of Pathology* **135**, 1–7.

Chan, C.P., Lin, C.P., Tseng, S.C. & Jeng, J.H. (1999). Vertical root fracture in endodontically versus nonendodontically treated teeth: a survey of 315 cases in Chinese patients. *Oral Surgery Oral Medicine Oral Pathology Oral Radiology and Endodontics* **87**, 504–507.

Cvek, M. (1973). Treatment of non-vital permanent incisors with calcium hydroxide. II. Effect on external root resorption in luxated teeth compared with effect of root filling with gutta-percha. *Odontologisk Revy* **25**, 343–354.

Cvek, M. (1993). Endodontic management of traumatized teeth. In: Andreasen, J.O. & Andreasen, F.M., eds. *Textbook and Color Atlas of Traumatic Injuries to the Teeth.* Copenhagen: Munksgaard, pp. 517–585.

Cvek, M. & Lindvall, A.M. (1985). External root resorption following bleaching of pulpless teeth with hydrogen peroxide. *Endodontics and Dental Traumatology* **1**, 56–60.

Czupalla, C., Mansukoski, H., Riedl, T., Krause, E. & Hoflack, B. (2006). Proteomic analysis of lysosomal acid hydrolases secreted by osteoclasts: implications for lytic enzyme transport and bone metabolism. *Molecular & Cellular Proteomics* **5**, 134–143.

Ehnevid, H., Jansson, L.E., Lindskog, S.F. & Blomlöf, L.B. (1993a). Periodontal healing in relation to radiographic attachment and endodontic infection. *Journal of Periodontology* **64**, 1199–1204.

Ehnevid, H., Jansson, L., Lindskog, S. & Blomlöf, L. (1993b). Periodontal healing in teeth with periapical lesions. A clinical retrospective study. *Journal of Clinical Periodontology* **20**, 254–258.

Eleftheriadis, G.I. & Lambrianidis, T.P. (2005). Technical quality of root canal treatment and detection of iatrogenic errors in an undergraduate dental clinic. *International Endodontic Journal* **38**, 725–734.

Frank, A.L. & Bakland, L.K. (1987). Nonendodontic therapy for supraosseous extracanal invasive resorption. *Journal of Endodontics* **13**, 348–355.

Fulling, H.J. & Andreasen, J.O. (1976). Influence of maturation status and tooth type of permanent teeth upon electrometric and thermal pulp testing. *Scandinavian Journal of Dental Research* **84**, 286–290.

Fuss, Z., Assooline, L.S. & Kaufman, A.Y. (1996). Determination of location of root perforations by electronic apex locators. *Oral Surgery Oral Medicine Oral Pathology Oral Radiology and Endodontics* **96**, 324–329.

Fuss, Z., Szjakis, S. & Tagger, M. (1989). Tubular permeability to calcium hydroxide and to bleaching agents. *Journal of Endodontics* **15**, 3362–3364.

Gesi, A., Hakeberg, M., Warfvinge, J. & Bergenholtz, G. (2006). Incidence of periapical lesions and clinical symptoms after pulpectomy – a clinical and radiographic evaluation of 1- versus 2-session treatment. *Oral Surgery Oral Medicine Oral Pathology Oral Radiology and Endodontics* **101**, 379–388.

Geurtsen, W. & Leyhausen, G. (1997). Biological aspects of root canal filling materials – histocompatibility, cytotoxicity, and mutagenicity. *Clinical Oral Investigations* **1**, 5–11.

Gher, M.E. Jr., Dunlap, M.R., Anderson, M.H. & Kuhl, L.V. (1987). Clinical survey of fractured teeth. *Journal of the American Dental Association* **14**, 174–177.

Gold, S. & Hasselgren, G. (1992). Peripheral inflammatory root resorption; a review of the literature with some case reports. *Journal of Clinical Periodontology* **19**, 523–534.

Gottlieb, B. (1942). Biology of the cementum. *Journal of Periodontology* **13**, 13–17.

Gottlow, J., Nyman, S., Lindhe, J., Karring T. & Wennström, J. (1986). New attachment formation in the human periodontium by guided tissue regeneration: Case reports. *Journal of Clinical Periodontology* **13**, 604–616.

Gröndahl, H.-G. & Hummonen, S. (2004). Radiographic manifestations of periapical inflammatory lesions. How new radiological techniques may improve endodontic diagnosis and treatment planning. *Endodontic Topics* **8**, 55–67.

Hammarström, L.E. & Lindskog, S. (1992). Factors regulating and modifying dental root resorption. *Proceedings of the Finnish Dental Society* **88** (Suppl 1), 115–123.

Hammarström, L.E., Pierce, A., Blomlöf, L., Feiglin, B. & Lindskog, S. (1986). Tooth avulsion and replantation – a review. *Endodontics and Dental Traumatology* **2**, 1–8.

Harding, G.H. (1878). The process of absorption in bone and tooth structure. *British Journal of Dental Science* **21**, 308–315.

Harrington, G.W. & Natkin, E. (1979). External resorption associated with bleaching of the pulpless teeth. *Journal of Endodontics* **5**, 344–348.

Hensten-Pettersen, A., Örstavik, D. & Wennberg, A. (1985). Allergic potential of root canal sealers. *Endodontics and Dental Traumatology* **1**, 61–65.

Heithersay, G.S. (1999). Invasive cervical resorption: An analysis of potential predisposing factors. *Quintessence International* **30**, 83–95.

Henriksen, K., Sörensen, M.G., Nielsen, R.H., Gram, J., Schaller, S., Dziegel, M.H., Everts, V., Bollerslev, J. & Karsdal, M.A. (2006). Degradation of the organic phase of bone by osteoclasts: a secondary role for lysosomal acidification. *Journal of Bone and Mineral Research* **21**, 58–66.

Henry, J.L. & Weinmann, J.P. (1951). The pattern of resorption and repair of human cementum. *Journal of the American Dental Association* **42**, 270–290.

Hötz, R. (1967). Wurzel Resorptionen an bleibenden Zähnen. *Fortschritte der Kieferorthopädie* **28**, 217–224.

Jameson, M.W., Tidmarsh, B.G. & Hood, J.A. (1994). Effect of storage media on subsequent water loss and regain by human and bovine dentine and on mechanical properties of human dentine in vitro. *Archives of Oral Biology* **39**, 759–767.

Jansson, L., Ehnevid, H., Lindskog, S. & Blomlöf, L. (1993a). Relationship between periapical and periodontal status. A clinical retrospective study. *Journal of Clinical Periodontology* **20**, 117–123.

Jansson, L., Ehnevid, H., Lindskog, S. & Blomlöf, L. (1993b). Radiographic attachment in periodontitis-prone teeth with endodontic infection. *Journal of Clinical Periodontology* **64**, 947–953.

Jones, S.J. & Boyde, A. (1976). Experimental study of changes in osteoblastic shape induced by calcitonin and parathyroid extract in an organ culture system. *Cellular Tissue Research* **169**, 449–465.

Kahler, B., Swain, M.V. & Moule, A. (2003). Fracture-toughening mechanisms responsible for differences in work to fracture of hydrated and dehydrated dentine. *Journal of Biomechanics* **36**, 229–237.

Kishen, A. (2006). Mechanisms and risk factors for fracture predilection in endodontically treated teeth. *Endodontic Topics* **13**, 57–83.

Kishen, A. & Asundi, A. (2005). Experimental investigation on the role of water in the mechanical behavior of structural dentine. *Journal of Biomedical Material Research A* **73**, 192–200.

Kremer, M., Judd, J., Rifkin, B., Auszman, J. & Oursler, M.J. (1995). Estrogen stimulation of osteoclast lysosomal enzyme secretion. *Journal of Cellular Biochemistry* **57**, 271–279.

Kurihara, S. (1977). An electron microscope observation on cells found in bone resorption area incident to experimental tooth movement. *Bulletin of Tokyo Medical and Dental University* **24**, 103–123.

Kürol, J. (1984). Infraocclusion of primary molars. An epidemiological, familial, longitudinal, clinical and histological study. Thesis. *Swedish Dental Journal*, Supplement.

Kvam, E. (1967). Tissue changes incident to movement of rat molars. Thesis. Oslo.

Kvinnsland, I., Oswald, R.J., Halse, A. & Grönningsaeter, A.G. (1989). A clinical and roentgenological study of 55 cases of root perforation. *International Endodontic Journal* **22**, 75–84.

Langeland, K. (1987). Tissue response to dental caries. *Endodontics and Dental Traumatology* **3**, 149–171.

Lantz, B. & Persson, P. (1967). Periodontal tissue reactions after root perforations in dogs teeth: a histologic study. *Odontologisk Tidskrift* **75**, 209–236.

Lerner, U.H. (2006). Bone remodeling in post-menopausal osteoporosis. *Journal of Dental Research* **85**, 584–595.

Lindskog, S., Blomlöf, L. & Hammarström, L. (1983). Repair of periodontal tissues *in vivo* and *in vitro*. *Journal of Periodontology* **10**, 188–205.

Lindskog, S., Blomlöf, L. & Hammarström, L. (1987). Comparative effects of parathyroid hormone on osteoblasts and cementoblasts. *Journal of Clinical Periodontology* **14**, 386–389.

Löe, H. & Waerhaug, J. (1961). Experimental replantation of teeth in dogs and monkeys. *Archives of Oral Biology* **3**, 176–184.

Löwenstein, N.R. & Rathkamp, R. (1955). A study on the pressoreceptive sensibility of the tooth. *Journal of Dental Research* **34**, 287–294.

Malmgren, B., Cvek, M., Lundberg, M. & Frykholm, A. (1984). Surgical treatment of ankylosed and infrapositioned reimplanted incisors in adolescents. *Scandinavian Journal of Dental Research* **92**, 391–399.

Marks, S.C. Jr. (1983). The origin of the osteoclast: Evidence, clinical implications and investigative challenges of an extraskeletal source. *Journal of Oral Pathology* **12**, 226–256.

Meister, F., Lommel, T.J. & Gerstein, H. (1980). Diagnosis and possible causes of vertical root fractures. *Oral Surgery Oral Medicine Oral Pathology* **49**, 243–253.

Miyashita, H., Bergenholtz, G. & Wennström, J. (1998). Impact of endodontic conditions on marginal bone loss. *Journal of Periodontology* **69**, 158–164.

Montgomery, S. (1984). External cervical resorption after bleaching a pulpless tooth. *Oral Surgery Oral Medicine Oral Pathology* **57**, 203–206.

Moskow, B.M. (1989). Periodontal manifestations of hyperoxaluria and oxalosis. *Journal of Periodontology* **60**, 271–278.

Mumford, J.M. (1964). Evaluation of gutta percha and ethyl chloride in pulp testing. *British Dental Journal* **116**, 338–342.

Papa, J., Cain, C. & Messer, H.H. (1994). Moisture content of vital vs endodontically treated teeth. *Endodontics and Dental Traumatology* **10**, 91–93.

Pascoe, D. & Oursler, M.J. (2001). The Scr signaling pathway regulates osteoclast lysosomal enzyme secretion and is rapidly modulated by estrogen. *Journal of Bone and Mineral Research* **16**, 1028–1036.

Pashley, E.L., Birdsong, N.L., Bowman, K. & Pashley, D.H. (1985) Cytotoxic effects of NaOCl on vital tissue. *Journal of Endodontics* **11**, 525–528.

Patel, D.K. & Burke, F.J. (1995). Fractures of posterior teeth: a review and analysis of associated factors. *Primary Dental Care* **2**, 6–10.

Peters, D.D., Baumgartner, J.C. & Lorton L. (1994). Adult pulpal diagnosis. I. Evaluation of the positive and negative responses to cold and electrical pulp tests. *Journal of Endodontics* **20**, 506–511.

Petersson, K., Hasselgren, G. & Tronstad, L. (1985). Endodontic treatment of experimental root perforations in dog teeth. *Endodontics and Dental Traumatology* **1**, 22–28.

Petersson, K., Söderström, C., Kiani-Anaraki, M. & Levy G. (1999). Evaluation of the ability of thermal and electrical tests to register pulp vitality. *Endodontics and Dental Traumatology* **15**, 127–131.

Pierce, A.M., Lindskog, S. & Hammarström, L.E. (1991). Osteoclasts: structure and function. *Electron Microscopical Reviews* **4**, 1–5.

Pitt Ford, T.R. & Patel, S. (2004). Technical equipment for assessment of pulp status. *Endodontic Topics* **7**, 2–13.

Pitts, D.L. & Natkin, E. (1983). Diagnosis and treatment of vertical root fractures. *Journal of Endodontics* **9**, 338–346.

Randow, K. & Glantz, P.-O. (1986). On cantilever loading of vital and non-vital teeth. An experimental clinical study. *Acta Odontologica Scandinavica* **44**, 271–277.

Randow, K., Glantz, P.O. & Zöger, B. (1986). Technical failures and some related clinical complications in extensive fixed prosthodontics. An epidemiological study of long-term clinical quality. *Acta Odontologica Scandinavica* **44**, 241–255.

Rankow, H.J. & Krasner, P.R. (1996). Endodontic applications of guided tissue regeneration in endodontic surgery. *Journal of Endodontics* **22**, 34–43.

Reeh, E.S., Messer, H.H. & Douglas, W.H. (1989). Reduction in tooth stiffness as a result of endodontic and restorative procedures. *Journal of Endodontics* **15**, 512–516.

Reitan, K. (1951). The initial tissue reaction incident to orthodontic tooth movement as related to the influence of function. *Acta Odontologica Scandinavica* Supplement 6.

Rodan, G.A. & Martin, T.J. (1981). Role of osteoblasts in hormonal control of bone resorption. A hypothesis. *Calcified Tissue Research* **33**, 349–355.

Rygh, P. (1972). Ultrastructural cellular reactions in pressure zones of rat molar perodontium incident to orthodontic tooth movement. *Acta Odontologica Scandinavica* **30**, 575–593.

Rygh, P. (1977). Orthodontic root resorption studied by electron microscopy. *Angle Orthodontist* **47**, 1–16.

Sandstedt, C. (1904). Einige Beitrage zur Theorie der Zahnregulierung. *Nordisk Tandläkare Tidskrift* **6**, 1–25.

Schwartz, R.S., Mauger, M., Clement, D.J. & Walker W.A. 3rd. (1999). Mineral trioxide aggregate: a new material for endodontics. *Journal of the American Dental Association* **130**, 967–975.

Sedgley, C.M. & Messer, H.H. (1992). Are endodontically treated teeth more brittle? *Journal of Endodontics* **18**, 332–335.

Seward, G.R. (1963). Periodontal disease and resorption of teeth. *British Dental Journal* **34**, 443–449.

Sinai, I. (1977). Endodontic perforations: their prognosis and treatment. *Journal of the American Dental Association* **95**, 90–95.

Stenvik, A. & Mjör, I.A. (1970). Pulp and dentin reactions to experimental tooth intrusion. *American Journal of Orthodontics* **57**, 370–385.

Storey, E. (1973). The nature of tooth movement. *American Journal of Orthodontics* **63**, 292–314.

Suda, T., Udagawa, N. & Takahashi, N. (1996). Osteoclast generation. In: Bilzekian, J.P., Raisz, L.G. & Rodan, G., eds. *Principles of Bone Biology*. San Diego: Academic, pp. 87–102.

Tamse, A. (2006). Vertical root fractures in endodontically treated teeth: diagnostic signs and clinical management. *Endodontic Topics* **13**, 84–94.

Tamse, A., Fuss, Z., Lustig, J., Ganor, Y. & Kaffe, I. (1999a). Radiographic features of vertically fractured, endodontically treated maxillary premolars. *Oral Surgery Oral Medicine Oral Pathology Oral Radiology and Endodontics* **88**, 348–352.

Tamse, A., Fuss, Z., Lustig, J. & Kaplavi, J. (1999b). An evaluation of endodontically treated vertically fractured teeth. *Journal of Endodontics* **25**, 506–508.

Testori, T., Badino, M. & Castagnola, M. (1993). Vertical root fractures in endodontically treated teeth. *Journal of Endodontics* **19**, 87–90.

Tjan, A.H. & Whang, S.B. (1985). Resistance to root fracture of dowel channels with various thicknesses of buccal dentin walls. *Journal of Prosthetic Dentistry* **53**, 496–500.

Tsesis, I. & Fuss, Z. (2006). Diagnosis and treatment of accidental root perforations. *Endodontic Topics* **13**, 95–107.

Vaes, G. (1988). Cellular biology and biochemical mechanism of bone resorption. A review of recent developments on the formation, activation, and mode of action of osteoclasts. *Clinical Orthopedics and Related Research* **231**, 239–271.

Walton, R.E., Michelich, R.J. & Smith, G.N. (1984). The histopathogenesis of vertical root fractures. *Journal of Endodontics* **10**, 48–56.

Wedenberg, C. & Lindskog, S. (1985). Experimental internal resorption in monkey teeth. *Endodontics and Dental Traumatology* **1**, 221–227.

Yang, S.F., Rivera, E.M. & Walton, R.E. (1995). Vertical root fracture in nonendodontically treated teeth. *Journal of Endodontics* **21**, 337–339.

Chapter 41

Treatment of Peri-implant Lesions

Tord Berglundh, Niklaus P. Lang, and Jan Lindhe

Introduction, 875
The diagnostic process, 875
Treatment strategies, 875
  Resolution of peri-implantitis lesions, 877
Cumulative Interceptive Supportive Therapy (CIST), 878

Preventive and therapeutic strategies, 878
Mechanical debridement; CIST protocol A, 878
Antiseptic therapy; CIST protocol A+B, 878
Antibiotic therapy; CIST protocol A+B+C, 879
Regenerative or resective therapy; CIST protocol A+B+C+D, 880

Introduction

Inflammatory lesions occurring in the peri-implant tissues were described in Chapter 24. Such processes are the result of opportunistic infections (see Chapter 10) and may, if left untreated, progress deep into the supporting bone and lead to implant loss. It is, therefore, imperative that the tissues around implants be monitored at regular intervals to discover arising biologic complications and to interfere with the disease process at an early stage. The appropriate therapy instituted following diagnosis must be aimed towards the reduction of the submucosal biofilm and the alteration of the ecologic conditions for the bacterial habitat.

The diagnostic process

The examination of the tissues around implants has many features in common with the periodontal examination and must include parameters relevant to the pathogenic process of the peri-implant lesion. It should be understood that, while advanced peri-implant lesions are easily recognized on radiographs, early alterations in the mucosa are often discrete (see also Chapter 24). Hence, a systematic examination for their detection is required that should include assessments of:

- Bleeding on probing (BoP)
- Suppuration
- Probing depth (PPD)
- Radiographic bone loss
- Implant mobility.

Assessments of BoP, suppuration, and PPD must be made at four surfaces (mesial, buccal, distal, and lingual) of each implant, while radiographic evaluation is limited to mesial and distal aspects.

Treatment strategies

The decision on treatment strategies is based on the diagnosis and the severity of the peri-implant lesion. Peri-implant mucositis and incipient forms of peri-implantitis require less extensive measures than advanced peri-implantitis lesions with severe bone loss. In all situations of peri-implant disease, however, the treatment strategies must include mechanical cleaning (infection control) procedures. Thus, information and instruction on the use of oral hygiene measures must be provided to the patient in combination with professional mechanical cleaning, including removal of plaque and calculus on implant surfaces. In this context it is important that the design of the implant-supported prosthesis allows access for oral hygiene. Thus, in cases where access for implant cleaning is obstructed, the prosthesis has to be modified to promote self-performed and professional mechanical infection control.

Two cases that illustrate the outcome of self-performed and professional mechanical cleaning are presented in Figs. 41-1 and 41-2. While plaque, calculus, and signs of inflammation are evident at implants in the initial examination, the follow-up visit at 3 months of infection control demonstrates improved oral hygiene and soft tissue conditions.

There are obvious similarities between teeth and implants regarding the strategies in treatment of

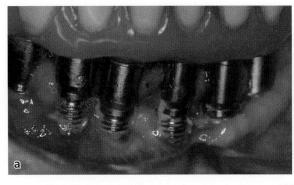
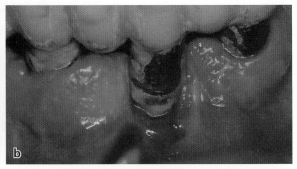

Fig. 41-1 Clinical photograph from implant sites in the mandible of a 75-year-old male (a) and a 62-year-old woman (b). Note the large amounts of plaque and calculus and the overt signs of inflammation in the peri-implant mucosa (a).

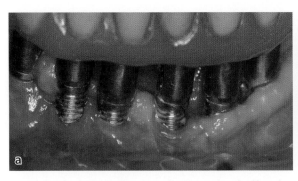
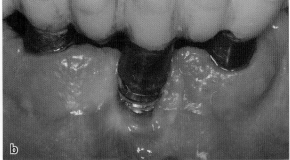

Fig. 41-2 Implant sites in Fig. 41-1 after 3 months of self-performed mechanical infection control combined with professional cleaning. Improved oral hygiene and soft tissue conditions.

periodontal and peri-implant infections. One important difference, however, relates to difficulties with instrumentation of the implant surface below the margin of the mucosa. Thus, subgingival scaling and root planing are well known procedures in the treatment of periodontitis, while in peri-implantitis the geometry of the implant with threads of different designs may impede the ability of the clinician to detect and remove calculus located below the mucosal margin. During such "blind" instrumentation at implants there is also a risk that deposits may be dislodged and become displaced into the mucosa. It is thus recommended that non-surgical debridement of implant surfaces, i.e. procedures that aim to remove calculus and plaque, should be restricted the portion of the implant located coronal to or at the level of the mucosal margin. While calculus may be chipped off using carbon fiber (Fig. 41-3) or plastic curettes, plaque is removed by polishing the implant surface with rubber cups and a polishing paste. Carbon fiber curettes do not damage the implant surface. They may be sharpened and are strong enough to remove most accumulations of calculus. Conventional steel curettes or ultrasonic instruments with metal tips should not be used because they may cause severe damage to the implant surface (Matarasso *et al.* 1996).

Peri-implant mucositis and incipient peri-implantitis lesions may be resolved using the cause-related measures described above. A re-examination

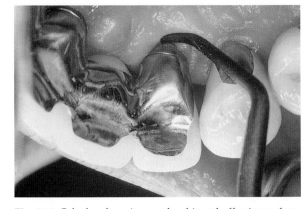

Fig. 41-3 Calculus deposits may be chipped off using carbon fiber curettes with the aim of not scratching the implant surface.

of peri-implant tissues following initial therapy that reveals absence of BoP and pocket closure indicates resolution of peri-implant lesions. On the other hand, if signs of pathology, i.e. BoP/suppuration in combination with deep pockets remain at the re-examination, additional therapy is required. Surgical procedures are one treatment option which provides access to the implant surfaces harboring biofilms. A prerequisite for surgical therapy in treatment of peri-implantitis is appropriate standards of self-performed infection control.

Surgical therapy of peri-implantitis lesions is illustrated in Figs. 41-4, 41-5, and 41-6. Clinical signs

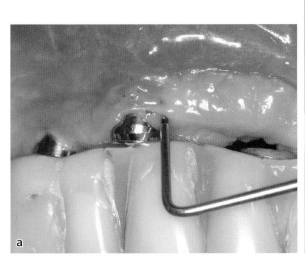
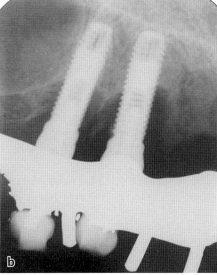

Fig. 41-4 Clinical photograph from implant sites with peri-implantitis. Note the PPD of 10 mm and suppuration (a) and the crater-formed defects in the radiograph (b).

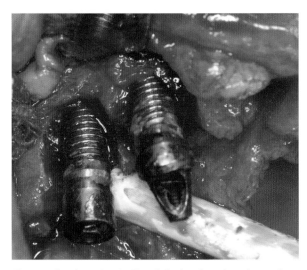

Fig. 41-5 Implant sites in Fig. 41-3 after flap elevation and removal of granulation tissue. Note the absence of buccal bone walls of the osseous defects. The implant surfaces are accessible for mechanical debridement.

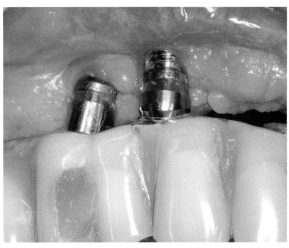

Fig. 41-6 Implant sites in Fig. 41-3 at 6 months after surgical therapy. Maintenance therapy with supervised infection control is provided. Note the soft tissue recession following the pocket elimination procedure.

of inflammation, PPD of about 10 mm in combination with BoP and suppuration were detected at the initial examination (Fig. 41-4). The radiograph revealed crater-formed defects around the two implants. Flap elevation allowed access to the area and granulation tissue in the defects was removed using steel curettes (Fig. 41-5). Mechanical debridement of the implant surface was performed using carbon fiber curettes and small pieces of gauze or pellets soaked in saline. The peri-implantitis associated bone defect may be treated using either resective or regenerative procedures (see also Chapter 46). In this case the morphology of the osseous defect was not suitable for regenerative techniques and, hence, resective procedures were performed to adjust the morphology of the interproximal bone walls. At the 6-month follow-up after surgery, PPD was reduced

and clinical signs of inflammation were absent (Fig. 41-6).

Recent reviews on treatment of peri-implant mucositis and peri-implantitis indicated that most articles in the literature consist mainly of case reports (Klinge et al. 2002; Roos-Jansåker et al. 2003). In addition to mechanical debridement a vast number of different treatment procedures have been suggested including antiseptic agents and local and/or systemic antibiotics. Klinge et al. (2002) concluded that there is insufficient evidence to support a specific treatment protocol.

Resolution of peri-implantitis lesions

In dog experiments by Ericsson et al. (1996) and Persson et al. (1996, 1999), peri-implantitis lesions were first produced according to the technique previously described (Lindhe *et al.* 1992). The peri-implantitis lesions were subsequently exposed to therapy. Antibiotics (amoxicillin and metronidazole) were administered to the animals via the systemic route but local treatment was provided to only some of the diseased implant sites. Following several months of healing, it was observed that in implant sites also given local therapy, i.e. submarginal debridement, the inflammatory lesions were resolved. In implant sites not exposed to local debridement, however, the inflammatory infiltrate persisted in the mucosa as well as in locations immediately adjacent to the bone tissue.

These observations clearly demonstrate that a treatment regimen that is restricted to systemic administration of antibiotics is not effective in the management of peri-implantitis, but must always be combined with meticulous removal of the biofilm from the contaminated implant surface. In this context it must be remembered that in the treatment of chronic periodontitis administration of systemic antibiotics without local therapy (i.e. scaling and root planing) will not resolve the inflammatory lesion in the gingiva and will also fail to arrest further progression of tissue breakdown (Lindhe *et al.* 1983a,b; Berglundh *et al.* 1998).

Cumulative Interceptive Supportive Therapy (CIST)

Preventive and therapeutic strategies

Depending on the clinical, and eventually the radiographic, diagnosis, protocols for preventive and therapeutic measures were designed to intercept the development of peri-implant lesions. This system of supportive therapy is cumulative in nature and includes four steps, which should not be used as single procedures, but rather as a sequence of therapeutic procedures with increasing anti-infective potential depending on the severity and extent of the lesion. Diagnosis, therefore, represents a key feature of this supportive therapy program (Lang *et al.* 2004).

The major clinical parameters to be used have been discussed above and include:

- Presence of a biofilm
- Presence or absence of BoP
- Presence or absence of suppuration
- Increased peri-implant probing depth
- Evidence and extent of radiographic alveolar bone loss.

Oral implants without plaque and calculus and surrounded by healthy peri-implant tissues, as evidenced by (1) absence of BoP, (2) absence of suppuration, and (3) probing depth usually not exceeding

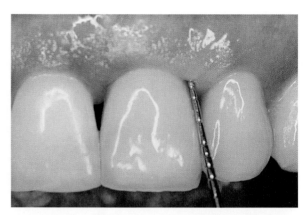

Fig. 41-7 Clinically stable implant with VMK crown (region 21) characterized by absence of bleeding on probing, suppuration, and a peri-implant probing depth not exceeding 3 mm.

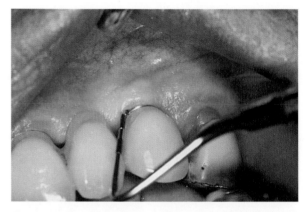

Fig. 41-8 Peri-implant mucositis characterized by presence of bleeding on probing, absence of suppuration, and a peri-implant probing depth of 4 mm.

3 mm, should be considered clinically stable. Such sites should not be exposed to therapeutic measures (Fig. 41-7).

Mechanical debridement; CIST protocol A

Implants with plaque and calculus deposits and surrounded by a mucosa that is BoP positive but suppuration negative and with a PPD ≤4 mm are to be subjected to mechanical debridement as described above (Fig. 41-8).

Antiseptic therapy; CIST protocol A+B

At implant sites which are BoP positive, exhibit an increased probing depth (4–5 mm) and may or may not demonstrate suppuration, antiseptic therapy is delivered in addition to mechanical debridement. A 0.2% solution of chlorhexidine digluconate is prescribed for daily rinsing, or a 0.2% gel of the same antiseptic is recommended for application to the affected site (Fig. 41-9). Generally, 3–4 weeks of antiseptic therapy are necessary to achieve positive treatment results.

Antibiotic therapy; CIST protocol A+B+C

At BoP-positive implant sites with deep pockets (PPD ≥6 mm) (suppuration may or may not be present), there are frequently also radiographic signs of bone loss. Such pockets represent an ecologic habitat which is conducive for the colonization of Gram-negative and anaerobic putative periodontal pathogens (Mombelli *et al*. 1987). Anti-infective treatment must include

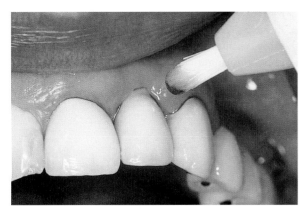

Fig. 41-9 Mechanical and antiseptic cleansing. Application of chlorhexidine gel (Plakout®, 0.2%) to a site with peri-implant mucositis.

the use of antibiotics to eliminate or reduce the pathogens in this habitat. This, in turn, will allow soft tissue healing as demonstrated in a clinical study by Mombelli and Lang (1992). Prior to administering antibiotics the mechanical (CIST A) and the antiseptic (CIST B) protocols have to be applied. During the last 10 days of the antiseptic treatment regimen, an antibiotic directed against anaerobic bacteria (e.g. metronidazole or ornidazole) is used. Thus for instance, 350 mg tid of Flagyl® (Rhone-Poulenc) or 500 mg bid of Tiberal® (Roche) is administered via the systemic route. A site treated according to the above protocol is depicted in Fig. 41-10. A fistula can be seen in the buccal aspect of implant site 45 (Fig. 41-10a). The site exhibited BoP and had a probing depth of 7 mm. After therapy the inflammation is resolved (Fig. 41-10b) and some recession of the mucosal margin has occurred. In Fig. 41-10c the bone fill that took place in the angular defect is illustrated in a subtraction radiography image using contrast enhancing. Figure 41-10d presents the site 8 years after active therapy.

An alternative to systemic administration is the controlled, local delivery of antibiotics. It must be realized, however, that only devices with proper release kinetics must be used to assure successful

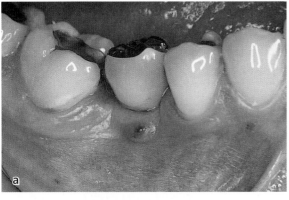

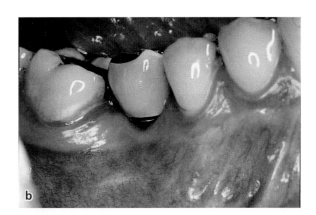

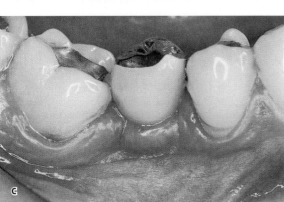

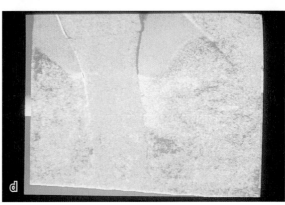

Fig. 41-10 Treatment of peri-implantitis according to the protocol of CIST (cumulative interceptive supportive therapy). (a) Clinical diagnosis of peri-implantitis: presence of bleeding on probing, suppuration, development of a fistula, loss of alveolar bone. Peri-implant probing depth 7 mm. (b) Clinical resolution of the peri-implant infection 1 year after mechanical and antiseptic cleansing, followed by the systemic application of antibiotics (500 mg Tiberal® bid for 10 days). Some recession is visible. (c) Absence of mucositis, reduced peri-implant probing depth to 3 mm, and bone fill of the lesion. (d) Documentation of the healed peri-implant infection by contrast-enhanced subtraction radiography. The intrabony crater has been completely filled 1 year after therapy.

clinical results. The antibiotic must thus remain at the site of action for at least 7–10 days and in a concentration high enough to penetrate the submucosal biofilm (Mombelli *et al.* 2001). An example of such a controlled-release device is the tetracycline-containing periodontal fiber (Actisite®; Alza). The therapeutic effect of this controlled-release device appears to be identical to the effect obtained by the systemic use of antibiotics (Mombelli *et al.* 2001).

In a more recent development, minocycline microspheres (1 mg Arestin®; Orapharma, Johnson & Johnson) have been used as a controlled-release device in a similar manner to the application of tetracycline fibers (Mombelli *et al.* 2001). These microspheres are easily applied into the peri-implant pocket by means of a syringe. The antibiotic is contained in very small beads that stick to the lateral walls of the pocket and to the implant surface providing enough substantivity (high enough concentration for up to 14 days) to penetrate the biofilm. The principle has been tested in a randomized controlled clinical trial with a 1% chlorhexidine gel as a control (Renvert *et al.* 2006) and a prospective cohort study in patients with peri-implantitis (Persson *et al.* 2006; Salvi *et al.* 2007). Both studies demonstrated reduction in bleeding on probing, pocket depth reduction, and slight recession. Significantly lower bacterial loads were seen after 10 days and up to 180 days for some presumptive pathogens (Persson *et al.* 2006). This indicates that the application of minocycline microspheres adjunctive to the CIST protocols A+B represents a valuable alternative to the administration of systemic antibiotics for the treatment of incipient peri-implant infections.

Regenerative or resective therapy; CIST protocol A+B+C+D

It is imperative to understand that regenerative or resective therapy is not instituted until the peri-implant infection is under control. Thus, before surgical intervention is planned, the previously diseased site should have become BoP negative, exhibit no suppuration, and have a reduced probing depth. Depending on the extent and severity of the local bone loss, a decision is made whether regenerative or resective measures are to be applied. In this context it must be realized that the goal of regenerative therapy, including the use of barrier membranes, is new bone formation in the crater-like defect around the implant, although *de novo* osseointegration may occur to a limited extent (Persson *et al.* 1999; Wetzel *et al.* 1999).

Conclusions

An implant patient must always be enrolled in a supportive therapy program that involves recall visits at regular intervals. Each recall visit must start with an examination to assess whether the implant sites are healthy or exhibit signs of inflammation. Cumulative Interceptive Supportive Therapy (CIST) includes a series of four protocols to be used when the examination and the diagnostic process are completed.

Figure 41-11 outlines (1) the decision process to be used for the peri-implant tissue diagnosis (Lang *et al.* 2004) and (2) the different therapeutic measures that are available to treat and/or prevent peri-implant infections.

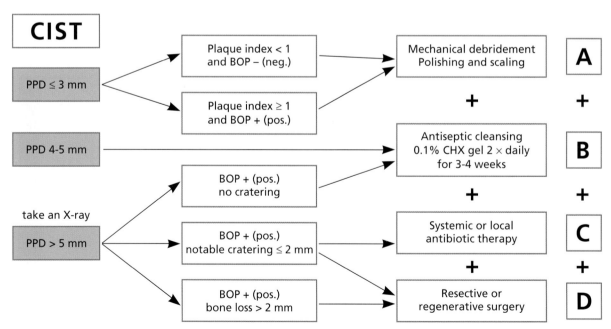

Fig. 41-11 Decision tree for cumulative interceptive supportive therapy (CIST). Depending on the mucosal condition and probing depth, either regime A or regime A+B, regime A+B+C or regime A+B+C+D are performed. A = Mechanical debridement; B = Antiseptic cleansing; C = Antibiotic therapy; D = Resective or regenerative surgery.

References

Berglundh, T., Krok, L., Liljenberg, B., Westfelt, E., Serino, G. & Lindhe, J. (1998). The use of metronidazole and amoxicillin in the treatment of advanced periodontal disease. A prospective, controlled clinical trial. *Journal of Clinical Periodontology* **25**, 354–362.

Ericsson, I., Persson, L.G., Berglundh, T., Edlund, T. & Lindhe, J. (1996). The effect of antimicrobial therapy on peri-implantitis lesions. An experimental study in the dog. *Clinical Oral Implants Research* **7**, 320–328.

Klinge, B., Gustavsson, A. & Berglundh, T. (2002). A systematic review on the effect of anti-infective therapy in the treatment of peri-implantitis. *Proceedings from the 4th European Workshop on Periodontology. Journal of Clinical Periodontology* **29** (Suppl), 213–225.

Lang, N.P., Berglundh, T., Heitz-Mayfield, L.J., Pjetursson, B.E., Salvi, G.E. & Sanz, M. (2004). Consensus statements and recommended clinical procedures regarding implant survival and complications. *International Journal of Oral and Maxillofacial Implants* **19**, 150–154.

Lindhe, J., Berglundh, T., Ericsson, I., Liljenberg, B. & Marinello, C.P. (1992). Experimental breakdown of periimplant and periodontal tissues. A study in the beagle dog. *Clinical Oral Implants Research* **3**, 9–16.

Lindhe, J., Liljenberg, B. & Adielsson, B. (1983b). Effect of long-term tetracycline therapy of human periodontal disease. *Journal of Clinical Periodontology* **10**, 590–601.

Lindhe, J., Liljenberg, B., Adielsson, B. & Börjesson, I. (1983a). Use of metronidazole as a probe in the study of human periodontal disease. *Journal of Clinical Periodontology* **10**, 100–112.

Matarasso, S., Quaremba, G., Coraggio, F., Vaia, E., Cafiero, C. & Lang, N.P. (1996). Maintenance of implants: an in vitro study of titanium implant surface modifications, subsequent to the application of different prophylaxis procedures. *Clinical Oral Implants Research* **7**, 64–72.

Mombelli, A., Feloutzis, A., Brägger, U. & Lang, N.P. (2001). Treatment of peri-implantitis by local delivery of tetracycline. Clinical, microbiological and radiological results. *Clinical Oral Implants Research* **12**, 287–294.

Mombelli, A. & Lang, N.P. (1992). Anti-microbial treatment of peri-implant infections. *Clinical Oral Implants Research* **3**, 162–168.

Mombelli, A., van Oosten, M.A.C., Schürch, E. & Lang, N.P. (1987). The microbiota associated with successful or failing osseointegrated titanium implants. *Oral Microbiology and Immunology* **2**, 145–151.

Persson, L.G., Araújo, M., Berglundh, T., Gröhndal, K. & Lindhe, J. (1999). Resolution of periimplantitis following treatment. An experimental study in the dog. *Clinical Oral Implants Research* **10**, 195–203.

Persson, L.G., Ericsson, I., Berglundh, T. & Lindhe, J. (1996). Guided bone generation in the treatment of periimplantitis, *Clinical Oral Implants Research* **7**, 366–372.

Persson, G.R., Salvi, G.E., Heitz-Mayfield, L.J.A. & Lang, N.P. (2006). Antimicrobial therapy using a local drug delivery system (Arestin®) in the treatment of peri-implantitis. I: Microbiological outcomes. *Clinical Oral Implants Research* **17**, 386–393.

Renvert, S., Lessem, J., Dahlén, G., Lindahl, C. & Svensson, M. (2006). Topical minocycline microspheres versus topical chlorhexidine gel as an adjunct to mechanical debridement of incipient peri-implant infections: a randomized clinical trial. *Journal of Clinical Periodontology* **33**, 362–369.

Roos-Jansåker, A-M., Renvert, S. & Egelberg, J. (2003). Treatment of peri-implant infections: a literature review. *Journal of Clinical Periodontology* **30**, 467–485.

Salvi, G.E., Persson, G.R., Heitz-Mayfield, L.J.A. & Lang, N.P. (2007). Antimicrobial therapy using a local drug delivery system (Arestin®) in the treatment of peri-implantitis. I: Clinical outcomes. *Clinical Oral Implants Research* **18** (in press).

Wetzel, A.C., Vlassis, J., Caffesse, R.J., Hämmerle, C.H.F. & Lang, N.P. (1999). Attempts to obtain re-osseointegration following experimental peri-implantitis in dogs. *Clinical Oral Implants Research* **10**, 111–119.

Chapter 42

Antibiotics in Periodontal Therapy

Andrea Mombelli

Principles of antibiotic therapy, 882
  The limitations of mechanical therapy: can antimicrobial agents
    help?, 882
  Specific characteristics of the periodontal
    infection, 883
  Drug delivery routes, 884

Evaluation of antibiotics for periodontal therapy, 886
  Systemic antimicrobial therapy in clinical trials, 888
  Systemic antibiotics in clinical practice, 889
  Local antimicrobial therapy in clinical trials, 890
  Local antibiotics in clinical practice, 893
  Overall conclusion, 893

Principles of antibiotic therapy

Antibiotics are drugs that can kill or stop the multiplication of bacterial cells, at concentrations that are relatively harmless to host tissues, and therefore can be used to treat infections caused by bacteria. The capacity of the drug to reach the infected site, and the ability of targeted bacteria to resist or inactivate the agent determine the effectiveness of therapy. Based on their effect at concentrations tolerated by the host, antibiotics can be categorized as "bactericidal" or "bacteriostatic", and, depending on the range of susceptible bacteria, "narrow-spectrum" or "wide-spectrum". Antibiotics are just one group of antimicrobial agents, which also comprise antiviral, antifungal, and antiparasitic chemicals. The term was originally applied to substances extracted from fungus or other living organisms, but today also includes synthetic products.

As antibiotics can kill or suppress bacteria, the recognition of periodontitis as an infection – caused or sustained by certain bacteria living and multiplying in diseased sites – is a fundamental issue for any antimicrobial treatment concept. Antibiotics do not remove calculus and bacterial residues, and this is traditionally perceived to be an essential part of periodontal therapy.

The limitations of mechanical therapy: can antimicrobial agents help?

The continued presence of large masses of bacteria on hard oral surfaces induces inflammation in adjacent soft tissues such as gingiva or mucosa, and the importance of removing bacterial plaque for resolution of gingivitis or mucositis is undisputed. The propensity of sites to undergo further periodontal destruction is felt to be more specific in nature, since not all sites with gingivitis invariably progress to periodontitis, and since increased proportions and detection frequencies of suspected oral pathogens are found in periodontitis lesions. Nevertheless, thorough mechanical cleaning of the root surfaces has also proven to be beneficial in the case of periodontitis, of whatever class, and under whatever clinical circumstances. Furthermore, it has been shown that the ability of the patient to prevent the re-formation of structured bacterial deposits by toothbrushing is crucial for long-term stability (for review see Chapter 59). However, this way of dealing with periodontal disease is time consuming, requires high levels of motivation and manual skills – of both the clinician and the patient – and has unwanted effects. It would be irrational to believe that mechanical instruments are able to completely remove periodontal pathogens from all infected sites (Mombelli *et al.* 2000). Bacteria may be inaccessible to mechanical instruments in concavities, lacunae, and dentin tubules, not to mention invaded soft tissues. Substantial hard tissue trauma may arise from repeated attempts at instrumentation in locally unresponsive sites, or sites with recurrent disease (Fig. 42-1). In addition, successfully treated sites may be recolonized by pathogens persisting in non-dental areas. Although we know that mechanical therapy can be clinically successful in many patients even if all putative pathogens are not completely eradicated, persistence or regrowth of certain microorganisms in treated sites should be

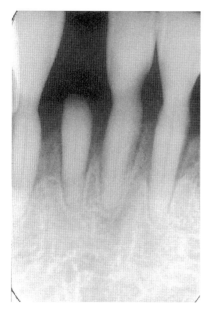

Fig. 42-1 Conventional periodontal therapy and maintenance imply repeated treatment of sites with localized unresponsive or recurrent disease, resulting in sometimes substantial hard tissue trauma.

considered as a cause of unsatisfactory treatment outcomes.

A closer look at the composition of the subgingival microbiota reveals that mechanical treatment is targeted at a variable mixture of different bacteria. The number of different species and subspecies occasionally identified in samples from human plaque by far exceeds 100, but only relatively few show a distinctive pattern of association with disease. While most frequently identified organisms are thought to harm tissues significantly only if present in high numbers over prolonged periods of time, in susceptible individuals certain species may have a negative effect even at relatively low numbers. On the basis of their pathogenicity, demonstrated in animal experiments, and the identification of virulence factors, a few organisms have been suggested to be specific periodontal pathogens (for review see Chapter 9). *Aggregatibacter actinomycetemcomitans* (formerly known as *Actinobacillus actinomycetemcomitans*) (Norskov-Lauritsen & Kilian 2006) and *Porphyromonas gingivalis* have attracted particular attention because longitudinal and retrospective studies have indicated an increased risk for periodontal breakdown in positive sites and because results of treatment have been better if the organisms could no longer be detected at follow-up (Bragd *et al.* 1987; Wennström *et al.* 1987; Carlos *et al.* 1988; Haffajee *et al.* 1991; Grossi *et al.* 1994; Haffajee & Socransky 1994; Dahlén *et al.* 1996; Rams *et al.* 1996; Chaves *et al.* 2000). If periodontal disease is in fact caused by a limited number of bacterial species, then non-specific continuous plaque removal is not the only possibility for prevention and therapy. Specific suppression of pathogenic bacteria becomes a valid alternative, and

antibiotic approaches to regain and maintain periodontal health may have a better efficiency ratio.

In the late 1930s and early 1940s, the appearance of powerful agents selectively active against bacteria – sulfonamides, penicillin, and streptomycin – revolutionized the treatment of bacterial infections. The phenomenal success of these agents in the treatment of formerly life-threatening diseases led many to believe that bacterial infections would never again be a major medical concern. More than six decades of experience with these, and hundreds of additionally developed antimicrobial drugs have shown that, despite all the success, this view was too optimistic. Emerging problems, resulting from the widespread use of antibiotics have modified the general perception of the capabilities of antimicrobial agents. Over the years, many bacteria have developed a remarkable ability to withstand or repel antibiotic agents and are increasingly resistant to formerly potent agents. It has been noted that the use of antibiotics may disturb the delicate ecologic equilibrium of the body, allowing the proliferation of resistant bacteria or non-bacterial organisms. Sometimes this may initiate new infections that are worse than the ones originally treated. In addition, no antibacterial drug is absolutely non-toxic and the use of any antimicrobial agent carries with it accompanying risks. Thus, before we can start to administer antibiotics routinely to our periodontal patients we need to be sure about the specific benefit in comparison to standard treatment approaches. To limit the development of microbial antibiotic resistance in general, and to avoid the risk of unwanted systemic effects of antibiotics for the treated individual, a precautionary, restrictive attitude towards using antibiotics is recommended.

Specific characteristics of the periodontal infection

The term infection refers to the presence and multiplication of microorganisms in or on body tissues. The uniqueness of plaque-associated dental diseases as infections relates to the lack of massive bacterial invasion of tissues. Although there is evidence for bacterial penetration in severely diseased periodontal tissues, notably in periodontal abscesses and in acute necrotizing ulcerative lesions (Listgarten 1965; Saglie *et al.* 1982a,b; Allenspach-Petrzilka & Guggenheim 1983; Carranza *et al.* 1983), it has not been generally accepted that true bacterial invasion (including multiplication of bacteria within tissues) is crucial for periodontal disease progression. Bacteria in the subgingival plaque obviously interact with host tissues even without direct tissue penetration. Thus, to have an effect, any antimicrobial agent used in periodontal therapy needs to be available at a sufficiently high concentration not only within the periodontal tissues, but also in the environment of the periodontal pocket (Fig. 42-2). Antibiotic resistance always occurs first in sites where penetration of the agent is restricted, and

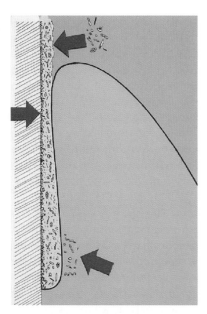

Fig. 42-2 Specific conditions for the use of antimicrobial agents in periodontal therapy. The periodontal pocket as an open site is subject to recolonization after therapy (top arrow). The subgingival bacteria are protected from antimicrobial agents in a biofilm (middle arrow). The agent must be available at a sufficiently high concentration not only within, but also in the subgingival environment, outside the periodontal tissues (bottom arrow).

therapeutic concentrations are difficult to achieve. A periodontal pocket may contain very large amounts of bacteria, and the antimicrobial agent may be inhibited, inactivated or degraded by non-target microorganisms.

The subgingival microbiota accumulate on the root surface to form an adherent layer of plaque. Accumulation of bacteria on solid surfaces can be observed on virtually all surfaces immersed in natural aqueous environments and is called "biofilm" formation. Extensive bacterial growth, accompanied by excretion of copious amounts of extracellular polymers, is a typical phenomenon in biofilms. Biofilms effectively protect bacteria from antimicrobial agents (Anwar et al. 1990, 1992). Bacteria involved in adhesion-mediated infections that develop on permanently or temporarily implanted materials, such as intravascular catheters, vascular prostheses or heart valves, are notoriously resistant to systemic antimicrobial therapy and tend to persist until the device is removed (Gristina 1987; Marshall 1992). Several mechanisms leading to this increased resistance of bacteria in biofilms have been proposed. Due to limited diffusion, antimicrobial agents may simply not reach deeper parts of a biofilm at sufficiently high levels during a given time of exposure. Within biofilms an unequal distribution of electrical charge may develop. Intrusion may thus be further complicated in certain areas of the biofilm depending on the charge of the penetrating molecule. Because of a limited availability of nutrients within the biofilm, bacteria may also reduce their metabolism, rendering

them less susceptible to killing by agents interfering with protein, DNA or cell wall synthesis. *In vitro* experiments indicate that the attachment of bacteria to surfaces can trigger genes, which activate specific resistance mechanisms. Since these mechanisms are switched on upon contact, they may occur already in newly forming, very thin biofilms (Costerton et al. 1995).

Recognizing the above described problems there is currently a general consensus that mechanical instrumentation must always precede antimicrobial therapy. First, we should quantitatively reduce the large mass of bacteria, which otherwise may inhibit or degrade the antimicrobial agent. Second, we should mechanically disrupt the structured bacterial aggregates that can protect the bacteria from the agent.

Since the periodontal flora never consists of one single species, synergistic, but also antagonistic, relationships between microorganisms could occur. Based on the concept that the presence of beneficial bacterial species may suppress the activity of pathogens, one can speculate that it may be advantageous specifically to eliminate target bacteria only and to allow the growth of potentially beneficial microorganisms. Such contemplations have been used as an argument to propagate narrow-spectrum antibiotics for periodontal therapy.

Drug delivery routes

Oral antibiotics (*per os*, by mouth, abbreviated "p.o.") are the most common approach for treating bacterial infections. Administration by means other than through the alimentary tract (as by intramuscular or intravenous injection) is usually reserved for serious medical conditions if the oral route is proven ineffective. Some local infections can be treated with topically administered antibiotics, as with eyedrops or ointments. In the therapy of periodontal diseases antibiotics may be delivered via the systemic route or by direct placement into the periodontal pocket. Each method of delivery has specific advantages and disadvantages (Table 42-1). Local therapy may allow the application of antimicrobial agents at levels that cannot be reached by the systemic route and may be suitable for agents, i.e. antiseptics, that are too toxic to be delivered by the systemic route. This form of application seems to be particularly promising if the presence of target organisms is confined to the clinically visible lesions. Systemic administration of antibiotics may be better if the targeted bacteria are distributed wider. Studies have shown that periodontal bacteria may in fact be distributed throughout the whole mouth in some patients (Mombelli et al. 1991a, 1994), including non-dental sites, such as the dorsum of the tongue or tonsillary crypts (Zambon et al. 1981; van Winkelhoff et al. 1988; Müller et al. 1993, 1995; Pavicic et al. 1994). Disadvantages of systemic antibiotic therapy relate to the fact that the

Table 42-1 Comparison of local and systemic antimicrobial therapy

Issue	Systemic administration	Local administration
Drug distribution	Wide distribution	Narrow effective range
Drug concentration	Variable levels in different body compartments	High dose at treated site, low levels elsewhere
Therapeutic potential	May reach widely distributed microorganisms better	May act locally on biofilm associated bacteria better
Problems	Systemic side effects	Re-infection from non-treated sites
Clinical limitations	Requires good patient compliance	Infection limited to the treated site
Diagnostic problems	Identification of pathogens, choice of drug	Distribution pattern of lesions and pathogens, identification of sites to be treated

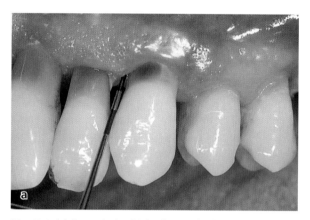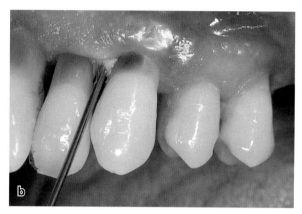

Fig. 42-3 (a) An antimicrobial gel is applied with a syringe inserted into a residual pocket. (b) For retention of the agent in the site, the viscosity of the carrier should change immediately. A large portion of the product may otherwise be expelled from the pocket quickly.

drug is dissolved by dispersal over the whole body, and only a small portion of the total dose actually reaches the subgingival microflora in the periodontal pocket. Adverse drug reactions are a greater concern and more likely to occur if drugs are distributed via the systemic route. Even mild forms of unwanted effects may severely decrease patient compliance (Loesche et al. 1993). Local delivery is independent of patient compliance.

Local drug delivery systems are means of drug application to confined areas. For the treatment of periodontal disease, local delivery of antimicrobial drugs ranges from simple pocket irrigation, over the placement of drug-containing ointments and gels, to sophisticated devices for sustained release of antibacterial agents. In order to be effective, the drug should not only reach the entire area affected by the disease, including especially the base of the pocket, but should also be maintained there at a sufficiently high local concentration for some time. With a mouth rinse or supragingival irrigation it is not possible to deliver an agent predictably to the deeper parts of a periodontal defect (Eakle et al. 1986; Pitcher et al. 1980). The crevicular fluid rapidly washes out agents brought into periodontal pockets by subgingival irrigation. Based on an assumed pocket volume of 0.5 ml and a crevicular fluid flow rate of 20 µl/hr, Goodson (1989) estimated that the half-time of a non-binding

drug placed into a pocket is about 1 minute. Even a highly concentrated, highly potent agent would thus be diluted below a minimal inhibitory concentration (MIC) for oral microorganisms within minutes. If an agent can bind to surfaces and be released in active form, a prolonged time of antibacterial activity could be expected. Such an effect has in fact been noted for salivary concentrations of chlorhexidine after use of chlorhexidine mouth rinse (Bonesvoll & Gjermo 1978). Although there are indications that this may also occur to a certain extent within the periodontal pocket, for instance after prolonged subgingival irrigation with tetracycline (Tonetti et al. 1990), the potential to create a drug reservoir of significant size on the small surface area available in a periodontal pocket is limited. To maintain a high concentration over a prolonged period, the flushing action of the crevicular fluid flow has to be counteracted by a steady release of the drug from a larger reservoir. Considering the small volume of a periodontal pocket and the pressure exerted by the tonus of the periodontal tissues on anything inserted, it appears unlikely that this task can be completed by a carrier that does not maintain its physical stability for some time and that cannot be secured against premature loss. Gels, for instance, rapidly disappear after instillation into periodontal pockets (Fig. 42-3), unless they change their viscosity immediately after

Concentration (µg/ml GCF)

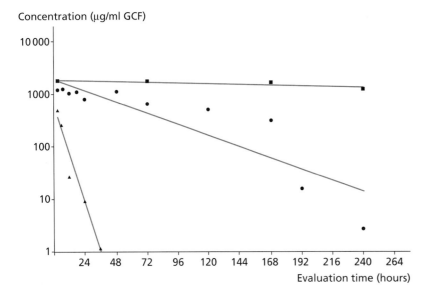

Fig. 42-4 Mean concentration of tetracycline (■) in gingival crevicular fluid (GCF) during tetracycline fiber treatment (Tonetti *et al.* 1990), of doxycycline hyclate (•) after application in a biodegradable polymer (Stoller *et al.* 1998), and of metronidazole (▲) after application of 25% metronidazole dental gel (Stoltze 1992).

placement (Oostervaal *et al.* 1990; Stoltze 1995). Viscous and/or biodegradable devices show an exponential decrease of their concentration in gingival fluid. In order to have sustained control over drug release it is necessary to have a matrix that lasts longer than the drug load. Controlled delivery of an antimicrobial agent over several days has been shown for tetracycline released from non-degradable monolithic ethylene vinyl acetate fibers (Fig. 42-4).

Evaluation of antibiotics for periodontal therapy

In the large range of antimicrobial agents, a limited number have been tested thoroughly for use in periodontal therapy. The drugs more extensively investigated for systemic use include tetracycline, minocycline and doxycycline, erythromycin, clindamycin, ampicillin, amoxicillin, and the nitro-imidazole compounds metronidazole and ornidazole. The drugs investigated for local application include tetracycline, minocycline, doxycycline, metronidazole, and chlorhexidine.

The first antibiotics used in periodontal therapy were mainly systemically administered penicillins. The choice was initially based exclusively on empiric evidence. Penicillins and cephalosporins act by inhibition of cell wall synthesis. They are narrow-spectrum and bactericidal. Among the penicillins, amoxicillin has been favored for treatment of periodontal disease because of its considerable activity against several periodontal pathogens at levels available in gingival fluid. The molecular structure of penicillins includes a β-lactam ring that may be cleaved by bacterial enzymes. Some bacterial β-lactamases have a high affinity for clavulanic acid, a β-lactam molecule without antimicrobial activity. To inhibit bacterial β-lactamase activity, clavulanic acid has been added successfully to amoxicillin. This combination (Augmentin®) has been tested for periodontal therapy in clinical studies.

Tetracycline-HCl became popular in the 1970s due to its broad-spectrum antimicrobial activity and low toxicity. The tetracyclines, clindamycin, and erythromycin are inhibitors of protein synthesis. They have a broad spectrum of activity and are bacteriostatic. In addition to their antimicrobial effect, tetracyclines are capable of inhibiting collagenase (Golub *et al.* 1985). This inhibition may interfere with tissue breakdown in periodontal disease. Furthermore they bind to tooth surfaces, from where they may be released slowly over time (Stabholz *et al.* 1993).

The nitro-imidazoles were introduced into the periodontal field in 1962 when *The Lancet* published the report of a female patient, who after a week of treatment for trichomonal vaginitis with metronidazole (200 mg tid) declared she had undergone "a double cure". The vaginitis was cured and the "acute marginal gingivitis" she was also suffering from was relieved (Shinn 1962). The nitro-imidazoles (metronidazole and ornidazole) and the quinolone antibiotics (e.g. ciprofloxacin) act by inhibiting DNA synthesis. Metronidazole is known to convert into several short-lived intermediates after diffusion into an anaerobic organism. These products react with the DNA and other bacterial macromolecules, resulting in cell death. The process involves reductive pathways characteristic of strictly anaerobic bacteria and protozoa, but not aerobic or microaerophilic organisms. Thus, metronidazole affects specifically the obligately anaerobic part of the oral flora, including *P. gingivalis* and other black-pigmenting Gram-negative organisms, but not *A. actinomycetemcomitans*, a facultative anaerobe.

The concentrations following systemic administration of the most common antimicrobial agents used in the treatment of periodontal disease are listed in Table 42-2. The *in vitro* susceptibility of *A. actinomycetemcomitans* to selected antimicrobial agents is given in Table 42-3 and the susceptibility of *P. gingivalis* is listed in Table 42-4. The data given in these tables may serve as a base for the choice of an

Table 42-2 Characteristics of antimicrobial agents used in the treatment of periodontal disease (adapted from Lorian 1986; Slots & Rams 1990)

Antibiotic	Dose (mg)	c serum (µg/ml)	c crevicular fluid (µg/ml)	t_{max} serum (h)	Half-life (h)
Penicillin	500	3	ND	1	0.5
Amoxicillin	500	8	3–4	1.5–2	0.8–2
Doxycycline	200	2–3	2–8	2	12–22
Tetracycline	500	3–4	5–12	2–3	2–3
Clindamycin	150	2–3	1–2	1	2–4
Metronidazole	500	6–12	8–10	1–2	6–12
Ciprofloxacin	500	1.9–2.9	ND	1–2	3–6

c = concentration; t_{max} = hours to reach peak serum concentration; ND = not determined.

Table 42-3 Susceptibility of *A. actinomycetemcomitans* to selected antimicrobial agents. MIC90: minimal inhibitory concentration for 90% of the strains (adapted from Mombelli & van Winkelhoff 1997)

Antibiotic	MIC90 (µg/ml)	Reference
Penicillin	4.0	Pajukanta et al. (1993b)
	1.0	Walker et al. (1985)
	6.25	Höffler et al. (1980)
Amoxicillin	1.0	Pajukanta et al. (1993b)
	2.0	Walker et al. (1985)
	1.6	Höffler et al. (1980)
Tetracycline	0.5	Pajukanta et al. (1993b)
	8.0	Walker (1992), Walker et al. (1985)
Doxycycline	1.0	Pajukanta et al. (1993b)
	3.1	Höffler et al. (1980)
Metronidazole	32	Pajukanta et al. (1993b)
	32	Jousimies-Somer et al. (1988)
	12.5	Höffler (1980)

Table 42-4 Susceptibility of *P. gingivalis* to selected antimicrobial agents (adapted from Mombelli & van Winkelhoff 1997)

Antibiotic	MIC90 (µg/ml)	Reference
Penicillin	0.016	Pajukanta et al. (1993a)
	0.29	Baker et al. (1983)
Amoxicillin	0.023	Pajukanta et al. (1993a)
	<1.0	Walker (1992)
Doxycycline	0.047	Pajukanta et al. (1993a)
Metronidazole	0.023	Pajukanta et al. (1993a)
	2.1	Baker et al. (1983)
	2.0	Walker (1992)
Clindamycin	0.016	Pajukanta et al. (1993a)
	<1.0	Walker (1992)

appropriate agent. However, it is important to remember that *in vitro* tests do not reflect the true conditions found in periodontal pockets. In particular, they do not account for the biofilm effect. One should add that MIC values depend on technical details that may vary between laboratories. As a consequence, demonstration of *in vitro* susceptibility is no proof that an agent will work in treatment of periodontal disease.

Since the subgingival microbiota in periodontitis often harbors several putative periodontopathic species with different antimicrobial susceptibility, combination drug therapy may be useful. A combination of antimicrobial drugs may have a wider spectrum of activity than a single agent. Overlaps of the antimicrobial spectrum may reduce the possible development of bacterial resistance. For some combinations of drugs there may be synergy in action against target organisms, allowing a lower dose of the single agents. A synergistic effect against *A. acti-*

nomycetemcomitans has been noted *in vitro* between metronidazole and its hydroxy metabolite (Jousimies-Somer et al. 1988; Pavicic et al. 1991) and between these two compounds and amoxicillin (Pavicic et al. 1992). With some drug combinations there may, however, also be antagonistic drug interaction. For instance, bacteriostatic agents such as tetracyclines, which suppress cell division, may decrease the antimicrobial effect of bactericidal antibiotics such as β-lactam drugs or metronidazole, which act during bacterial cell division. Combination drug therapy may also lead to increased adverse reactions.

Table 42-5 lists common adverse reactions to systemic antibiotic therapy (for a detailed overview the reader is referred to Walker 1996). The penicillins are among the least toxic antibiotics. Hypersensitivity reactions are by far the most important and most common adverse effects of these drugs. Most reactions are mild and limited to a rash or skin lesion in the head or neck region. More severe reactions may induce swelling and tenderness of joints. In highly sensitized patients a life-threatening anaphylactic reaction may develop. The systemic use of tetracyclines may lead to epigastric pain, vomiting or

Table 42-5 Adverse effects of antibiotics used in the treatment of periodontal diseases

Antibiotic	Frequent effects	Infrequent effects
Penicillins	Hypersensitivity (mainly rashes), nausea, diarrhea	Hematologic toxicity, encephalopathy, pseudomembranous colitis (ampicillin)
Tetracyclines	Gastrointestinal intolerance, candidiasis, dental staining and hypoplasia in childhood, nausea, diarrhea, interaction with oral contraceptives	Photosensitivity, nephrotoxicity, intracranial hypertension
Metronidazole	Gastrointestinal intolerance, nausea, antabus effect, diarrhea, unpleasant metallic taste	Peripheral neuropathy, furred tongue
Clindamycin	Rashes, nausea, diarrhea	Pseudomembranous colitis, hepatitis

diarrhea. Tetracyclines can induce changes in the intestinal flora, and superinfections with non-bacterial microorganisms (i.e. *Candida albicans*) may emerge. Tetracyclines are deposited in calcifying areas of teeth and bones where they cause yellow discoloration. Systemic administration of clindamycin may be accompanied by gastrointestinal disturbances, leading to diarrhea or cramps, and may cause mild skin rashes. The suppression of the normal intestinal flora increases the risk for colonization of *Clostridium difficile*, which may cause a severe colon infection (antibiotic-associated colitis). Although not related to *C. difficile*, gastrointestinal problems are also the most frequent adverse event of systemic metronidazole therapy. Nausea, headache, anorexia, and vomiting may be experienced. Symptoms may be more pronounced with alcohol consumption, because imidazoles affect the activity of liver enzymes. Because some cases have developed permanent peripheral neuropathies (numbness or paresthesia), patients should be advised to stop therapy immediately if such symptoms occur.

Systemic antimicrobial therapy in clinical trials

Although clinical efficacy is not an absolute proof for bacteriologic efficacy (Marchant *et al.* 1992), the ultimate evidence to advocate the use of systemic antibiotics must come from clinical trials in humans with periodontitis. A large number of reports suggesting beneficial effects in various clinical situations have been published. However, many of them score low when evaluated by established study quality criteria, e.g. those proposed by the Oxford Centre for Evidence-based Medicine (http://www.cebm.net/levels_of_evidence.asp). Studies may be difficult to interpret due to an unclear status of patients at baseline (treatment history, disease activity, composition of subgingival microbiota), insufficient or non-standardized maintenance after therapy, short observation periods, or lack of randomization and controls. Comparisons may be possible because studies not only vary with regard to the treatment provided, but also in the selection of subjects, sample size, range of study parameters, outcome variables, the duration of

the study, and the control to which the test procedure is compared. In most trials, systemic antibiotics have been used as an adjunct to scaling and root planing. Typically, the effect of mechanical therapy plus the antimicrobial agent has been compared to mechanical treatment alone. In studies evaluating the effect of antimicrobial therapy in patients with refractory periodontitis or with recurrent abscess formation, placebo control is often lacking for ethical reasons.

In recent years systematic reviews have become the preferred method of analyzing the medical literature. They use explicit procedures to perform a thorough literature search, critically appraise individual reports, and try to combine valid studies by applying appropriate statistical techniques. Two systematic reviews have been conducted to determine whether systemically administered antibiotics improve the clinical outcome of periodontal therapy (Herrera *et al.* 2002; Haffajee *et al.* 2003). Both have been prepared in the context of structured consensus conferences, where the findings have been translated into consensus statements on periodontal therapy.

Herrera *et al.* (2002) sought studies of at least 6 months' duration, designed as controlled clinical trials, in which systemically healthy subjects with either chronic or aggressive periodontitis had been treated with scaling and root planing, with or without systemic antibiotics. Main outcome variables were changes in clinical attachment level and pocket probing depth. Twenty-five papers were eligible for inclusion, but due to difficulties encountered when pooling the data, only limited meta-analyses could be performed. Overall, antibiotic groups showed better results than control groups. A specific benefit in change of attachment level was found in deep pockets for the combination of metronidazole plus amoxicillin.

Haffajee *et al.* (2003) sought clinical trials in periodontitis patients of more than 1 month duration, comparing systemic antibiotic therapy with non-antibiotic therapy, and using mean attachment level change as primary outcome. A meta-analysis included the data from 27 eligible studies. The authors noted that by and large therapeutic procedures were diverse, although metronidazole, alone or in combination with amoxicillin, was the most frequently used drug. In all studies the antibiotic groups showed significantly better mean attachment level changes than the control groups, and this benefit averaged 0.45 mm. Although tests of heterogeneity were not significant, indicating that the outcomes were consistent, differences in the magnitude of the effect were noted in some patient populations: aggressive periodontitis groups had a larger adjunctive benefit than patients with chronic periodontitis. Results varied more between trials in which antibiotics had been used adjunctively to surgery than in trials where antibiotics had been tested adjunctively to scaling and root planing. Where it was possible to discriminate, sites with deep pockets seemed to show the greatest improvements. The reviews were unable to clarify which agents should be used for which infection, and what the optimal dosage and duration of antibiotic therapy should be. Furthermore it remained open how long the benefit would persist, and to what extent the antibiotics induced resistance or other changes in the oral microbiota. The low level of evidence with regards to the dosing regimen is very regrettable since the amount of drug administered is known to be a critical determinant of antimicrobial efficacy (Craig 1998).

In many trials the antibiotic has not been chosen based on a microbiologic analysis. This approach does not consider the possibility that some pathogens may be resistant to the tested drugs. We have mentioned *A. actinomycetemcomitans*, which is not susceptible to metronidazole when used as a monotherapy. Therefore, clinical studies including patients for an antibiotic therapy irrespective of their microbiologic status may underestimate the potential of the tested drug. Some studies have in fact indicated that systemic antibiotics were only effective in patients with a specific microbial profile (Flemmig *et al.* 1998; Winkel *et al.* 2001). Others, however, have demonstrated considerable adjunctive benefits to mechanical treatment even in the absence of specific target organisms (e.g. Rooney *et al.* 2002), and one could argue that nobody has ever shown certain patients to be better off, if treated *without* antibiotics.

In recent years the combination of metronidazole and amoxicillin has become the favorite treatment modality for many practitioners and clinical researchers. Studies corroborating the benefit of this regime, for example in non-surgical treatment of generalized aggressive periodontitis (Guerrero *et al.* 2005), continue to be published. Its remarkable ability to suppress or even eliminate *A. actinomycetemcomitans* and other subgingival organisms from periodontitis lesions and other oral sites (Christersson *et al.* 1989; Kornman *et al.* 1989; van Winkelhoff *et al.* 1989, 1992; Goené *et al.* 1990; Pavicic *et al.* 1992, 1994) has made it the first choice especially for the treatment of advanced periodontitis associated with *A. actinomycetemcomitans*. Gastrointestinal disturbances (diarrhea, nausea, and vomiting) have been noted as the most frequent side effects.

Systemic antibiotics in clinical practice

Overall, it can be stated that systemic antibiotic therapy can improve the clinical conditions and microbiologic status of periodontal patients. There is evidence to support the use of systemic antibiotics in cases of aggressive forms of periodontitis associated with *P. gingivalis* and/or *A. actinomycetemcomitans*. Systemic antibiotics are also indicated in generalized refractory periodontitis patients with evidence of ongoing disease despite previous mechanical therapy. Although some studies have shown a certain benefit of antibiotics even when administered without thorough subgingival debridement (Berglundh *et al.* 1998; Lopez & Gamonal 1998; Lopez *et al.* 2000, 2006) there is a general consensus that whenever possible antibiotics should not be administered before completion of root surface debridement (Mombelli 2006). Patients with acute signs of disease such as periodontal abscesses, or acute necrotizing gingivitis, with fever and malaise, may be the exception. Systemic antibiotics, given after scaling and root planing, provide an additional treatment benefit especially in deep pockets, and can reduce the need for further, surgical therapy (Loesche *et al.* 1992). In most cases however, mechanical therapy is initially carried out without antibiotics and evaluated after an appropriate period of time. The original treatment plan is then adapted, to account for the degree of clinical improvement already obtained. Immediately before starting the antibiotic regime the subgingival area should be reinstrumented once more to reduce the bacterial mass as much as possible and to disrupt the subgingival biofilm. This may be accomplished during a surgical intervention but is indicated also if no further mechanical therapy seems necessary from a clinical point of view.

Table 42-6 lists adjunctive systemic antibiotic regimens currently recommended for the therapy of periodontal diseases. Metronidazole alone has proven to be effective against *P. gingivalis*, *Tannerella forsythia*, spirochetes, and other strictly anaerobic Gramnegative bacteria. Clindamycin and tetracyclines have also been shown to act on a broad range of periodontal bacteria. Monotherapy with one antibiotic as an adjunct to mechanical instrumentation can change the composition of the subgingival microbiota significantly, but certain periodontal organisms cannot be eliminated predictably. For maximal suppression of subgingival *A. actinomycetemcomitans* the combination of metronidazole and amoxicillin is recommended. For patients who cannot tolerate amoxicillin it has been suggested to combine metronidazole with cefuroximaxetil or ciprofloxacin (Rams *et al.* 1992; van Winkelhoff & Winkel 2005).

Microbiologic tests can help to choose the appropriate antibiotic regimen. A microbial analysis should be comprehensive and sensitive enough to quantitatively identify the most important periodontal organisms. From the discussion above it follows that data

Table 42-6 Adjunctive systemic antibiotic regimens currently recommended for the therapy of periodontal diseases (adapted from van Winkelhoff & Winkel 2005)

Antibiotic	Usual dosage	Microbiology
Metronidazole	250–500 mg, tid 7–10 days	*P. gingivalis* *T. forsythia* *Treponema* spp.
Clindamycin	300 mg, qid 7–8 days	Gram-negative anaerobes Absence of *A. actinomycetemcomitans*
Doxycycline	100–200 mg, sid 7–14 days	Non-specific infection
Metronidazole + Amoxicillin	250–500 mg, tid 375–500 mg, tid 7 days	*A. actinomycetemcomitans* or *P. gingivalis* with high numbers of Gram-positive pathogens
Metronidazole + Cefuroximaxetil	250–500 mg, tid 250–500 mg, bid 7 days	*A. actinomycetemcomitans* Hypersensitivity towards amoxicillin
Metronidazole + Ciprofloxacin	250–500 mg, tid 500 mg, bid 7 days	*A. actinomycetemcomitans* Hypersensitivity towards β-lactams or presence of susceptible enteric microorganisms

indicating the involvement of *A. actinomycetemcomitans* and *P. gingivalis* have the highest practical utility. Microbial samples from the deepest pocket in each quadrant can give a good picture of the presence and relative proportion of these pathogens in the oral flora (Mombelli *et al.* 1991b, 1994). Since the antimicrobial profiles of most putative periodontal pathogens are quite predictable, susceptibility testing is not routinely performed. One should keep in mind, however, that some important microorganisms might demonstrate resistance to tetracyclines, β-lactam drugs or metronidazole.

As mentioned already, suboptimal dosage of antibiotics, caused by either inadequate prescribing or poor patient compliance, favors the spread of antibiotic-resistant bacterial clones. The classical oral dosage for metronidazole, used in most studies, has been 250 mg, three times a day, for 7–10 days. This dosage might not be sufficient in subjects with a high body mass. In addition, it has been proposed to prolong medication in smokers (van Winkelhoff & Winkel 2005), because smoking decreases the gingival blood flow and the amount of crevicular fluid, and hereby the availability of the drug in the subgingival environment (Morozumi *et al.* 2004). The specific conditions of smokers have become the subject of clinical research in recent time. The utilization of azithromycin, a macrolide antibiotic derived from erythromycin, has been advocated specifically for smokers (Mascarenhas *et al.* 2005). More research is however needed to substantiate the specific benefit of particular regimes for distinct groups of patients.

After resolution of the periodontal infection, the patient should be placed on an individually tailored maintenance care program. Optimal plaque control by the patient is of paramount importance for a favorable clinical response (Kornman *et al.* 1994) and long-term stability. Systemic antibiotics should never be applied as a means to compensate for inadequate oral hygiene.

Local antimicrobial therapy in clinical trials

Various methods to deliver antimicrobial agents into periodontal pockets have been devised and subjected to numerous kinds of experiments. The shortcomings of rinsing, irrigating, and similar forms of drug placement – rapid clearance resulting in inadequate exposure of subgingival bacteria to the drug and lack of significant clinical effects – have already been discussed. This section will deal with clinically tested drug delivery systems that fulfill at least the basic pharmacokinetic requirements of sustained drug release. Much of what has been stated about difficulties in the interpretation of studies dealing with the systemic use of antibiotics applies to the studies conducted with local delivery devices. Again, comparisons are complicated because studies vary with regard to sample size, selection of subjects, range of parameters, controls, duration of the study, and the inclusion of only one form of local drug delivery. Most of the evidence for a therapeutic effect of local delivery devices comes from trials involving patients with previously untreated adult periodontitis. Only few studies have addressed the use of local drug delivery in recurrent or persistent periodontal lesions – the potentially most valuable area for their application. Some protocols compare local drug delivery to a negative control, such as the application of only the carrier without the drug. These studies may be able to show a net effect of the drug, but they are not able to demonstrate a benefit over the most obvious alternative – scaling and root planing – and the question remains as to how much value the procedure has in addition to mechanical treatment. If a study is unable to demonstrate a significant difference between local drug delivery and scaling and root planing, this is not automatically a proof of equivalence of the two treatments (equivalence testing requires statistical testing of the power of the data, taking into account the size of the study sample).

The following paragraphs focus on minocycline ointment and microspheres, doxycycline hyclate in a biodegradable polymer, metronidazole gel, tetracycline in a non-resorbable plastic co-polymer, and chlorhexidine gluconate in a gelatin chip. These are the predominant commercial formulations adequately tested for local antimicrobial periodontal therapy. Unfortunately some of them are currently unavailable in certain regions of the world, or have disappeared completely, while other products without properly evaluated clinical efficacy continue to be introduced and utilized on an empiric basis.

Minocycline ointment and microspheres

The subgingival delivery of minocycline has been investigated in different forms. The efficacy of a 2% minocycline ointment (Dentomycin; Cyanamid, Lederle Division, Wayne, NJ, US) has been evaluated in a randomized, controlled trial of 103 adults with moderate to severe periodontitis (van Steenberghe *et al.* 1993). All patients were treated by conventional scaling and root planing. In addition, the patients received either the test or a control ointment in four consecutive sessions at baseline and weeks 2, 4, and 6. A significantly greater reduction of probing depths was noted in the test group at week 12. An additional study evaluating the repeated application of minocycline ointment as an adjunct to subgingival debridement in chronic periodontitis, demonstrated better clinical and microbiologic conditions over a 15-month period (van Steenberghe *et al.* 1999). One study assessed the effect of a weekly repeated local application of minocycline ointment for 8 weeks after placement of teflon membranes to guide regeneration of periodontal tissue. Although bacterial colonization of treated sites could not be prevented, the mean clinical attachment gain of the test group was significantly greater than that of the control group (Yoshinari *et al.* 2001).

Currently the major device for local minocycline application is a product with the physical properties of a powder, consisting of resorbable polymer microspheres (Arestin; OraPharma, Warminster, PA, US). The efficacy and safety of locally administered microencapsulated minocycline was shown in a multicenter trial including 748 patients with moderate to advanced periodontitis. Minocycline microspheres plus scaling and root planing provided substantially more probing depth reduction than either scaling and root planing alone or scaling and root planing plus vehicle. The difference reached statistical significance after the first month and was maintained throughout the 9 months of the trial (Williams *et al.* 2001; Paquette *et al.* 2004).

Doxycycline hyclate in a biodegradable polymer

A two-syringe mixing system for the controlled release of doxycycline (Atridox; Block Drug, Jersey City, NJ, US) has been evaluated in a number of investigations, and has been commercially available for a few years. One syringe contained the delivery vehicle, flowable bioabsorbable poly (DL-lactide) dissolved in N-methyl-2-pyrrolidone, and the other syringe contained doxycycline hyclate powder. The clinical efficacy and safety of Atridox was assessed in two multicenter studies. Each study entered 411 patients who demonstrated moderate to severe adult periodontitis. The treatment was statistically superior to placebo control and oral hygiene, and equally effective as scaling and root planing in reducing the clinical signs of adult periodontitis over a 9-month period (Garrett *et al.* 1999). In a group of patients undergoing supportive periodontal therapy, attachment level gains and probing depth reductions were similar at 9 months after local treatment with doxycycline or traditional scaling and root planing (Garrett *et al.* 2000).

The effect of Atridox, applied after no more than 45 minutes of debridement without analgesia in subjects with moderately advanced chronic periodontitis, was compared to 4 hours of thorough deep scaling and root planing in a study involving 105 patients at three centers. Interestingly, clinical parameters indicated a better result for the pharmacomechanical treatment approach after 3 months, although considerably less time had been invested than for conventional mechanical therapy (Wennström *et al.* 2001).

Metronidazole gel

Dialysis tubing, acrylic strips, and poly-OH-butyric acid strips have been tested as solid devices for delivery of metronidazole. The most extensively used device for metronidazole application is a gel consisting of a semi-solid suspension of 25% metronidazole benzoate in a mixture of glyceryl mono-oleate and sesame oil (Elyzol Dental Gel; Dumex, Copenhagen, Denmark). The gel is applied with a syringe into the pocket, and should increase its viscosity after placement. The clinical response to subgingival application of the metronidazole gel twice within 1 week was compared to the effect of subgingival scaling in several studies including subjects with untreated adult periodontitis (Ainamo *et al.* 1992; Pedrazzoli *et al.* 1992; Grossi *et al.* 1995). The results indicated no significant difference between metronidazole gel application and scaling and root planing. The fact that no significant difference between the two

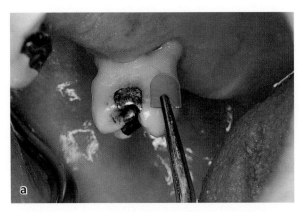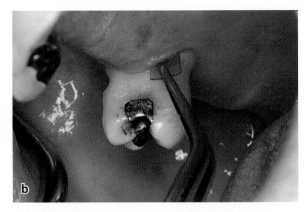

Fig. 42-5 Insertion of a chlorhexidine chip into a residual pocket mesial to an upper molar with a furcation involvement.

treatments was observed opened the question of equivalence between the two treatment modalities. Equivalence between scaling and root planing and metronidazole gel therapy has been evaluated using the lower bounds of confidence intervals in a parallel arm, multicenter, controlled clinical trial including 84 subjects (Pihlstrom *et al.* 1995). The estimates provided by this study indicated that metronidazole gel therapy is 82% as good as mechanical debridement at the 95% confidence level.

Tetracycline in a non-resorbable plastic co-polymer

Hollow devices, such as dialysis tubing, and solid devices, such as acrylic strips, collagen, or poly-OH-butyric acid strips, have been tested for tetracycline delivery in several experiments. Semi-solid viscous media include white petrolatum and poloxamer or carbopol gels. The most extensively tested tetracycline-releasing device is the Actisite periodontal fiber (ALZA, Palo Alto, CA, US). This currently unavailable product consists of a monolithic thread of a biologically inert, non-resorbable plastic co-polymer (ethylene and vinyl-acetate) containing 25% tetracycline hydrochloride powder. The fiber is packed into the periodontal pocket, secured with a thin layer of cyanoacrylate adhesive, and left in place for 7–12 days (Goodson *et al.* 1991a, 1983). By continuous delivery of tetracycline, a local concentration of the active drug in excess of 1000 mg/l can be maintained throughout that period (Fig. 42-4). Many clinical studies have been performed with Actisite, among them the following three large multicenter trials. The first showed better clinical results in deep pockets of 107 periodontitis patients 60 days after fiber therapy than control procedures (Goodson *et al.* 1991b). The second, conducted in periodontal maintenance patients needing treatment of localized recurrent periodontitis, demonstrated superiority after 6 months for scaling and root planing plus tetracycline fiber over scaling and root planing alone (Newman *et al.* 1994). The third indicated that the results obtained within 3 months after therapy were main-

tained over 1 year and that the combined treatment with fiber and scaling had a significantly lower incidence of disease recurrence than any of the other tested treatment modalities (Michalowicz *et al.* 1995).

Chlorhexidine gluconate in a gelatin chip

Several attempts have been made to develop local delivery devices for the subgingival application of antiseptic, rather than antibiotic agents. Acrylic strips and ethyl-cellulose compounds have been tested for this purpose. PerioChip (Perio Products, Jerusalem, Israel), a degradable gelatin chip containing 2.5 mg chlorhexidine, is the most extensively tested delivery device of this category (Fig. 42-5). Safety and efficacy of PerioChip were evaluated in a multicenter study of 118 patients with moderate periodontitis (Soskolne *et al.* 1997). The average pocket depth reduction in the treated sites with the chip was significantly greater than in the sites receiving mechanical treatment only. The efficacy of the chlorhexidine chip when used as an adjunct to scaling and root planing on reducing probing depth and improving clinical attachment level in adult periodontitis was evaluated in two double-blind, randomized, placebo-controlled multicenter clinical trials. At 9 months significant reductions from baseline were shown with the chlorhexidine chip compared with mechanical control treatments (Jeffcoat *et al.* 1998).

Comparison of treatment methods

Most studies have tested a single form of local drug delivery or systemic administration, instead of comparing various forms of therapy. Understandably, developers and distributors have the primary interest to register and promote their own product for the broadest possible usage, and not to differentiate specific benefits or shortcomings of various applications. The efficacy of three commercially available local delivery systems as adjuncts to scaling and root planing was tested in two trials including patients with persistent periodontal lesions: Actisite,

Dentomycin, Elyzol Dental Gel (Radvar et al. 1996; Kinane & Radvar 1999); Atridox, Elyzol Dental Gel, PerioChip (Salvi et al. 2002). One systematic review has tried to evaluate the combined literature-based evidence to determine the relative effect of local controlled release anti-infective drug therapy in patients with chronic periodontitis (Hanes & Purvis 2003). A meta-analysis including 19 studies, comparing scaling and root planing plus local sustained-release agents with scaling and root planing alone, confirmed the clinical advantages of minocycline gel, microencapsulated minocycline, doxycycline gel, and chlorhexidine chips over scaling and root planing alone. Due to the heterogeneity of the material the authors could not make any firm statements regarding the superiority of one system. A further systematic review looked at the relative adjunctive benefits of various locally applied agents (Bonito et al. 2005). Unfortunately data were combined from studies exploring various modes of local treatment, including irrigation, impregnated strips or pastes. Nonetheless, a statistically significant mean advantage resulted for four agents in terms of additional attachment gain, best for minocycline, followed by tetracycline, chlorhexidine, and metronidazole. One cannot exclude, however, that the differences noted between the drugs primarily reflect differences in modes of application and study populations, not the potency of the agent.

Few studies have addressed the problem of incorporating local or systemic antimicrobial therapy into an overall treatment strategy. As little direct evidence for a comparison of various methods of treatment is available so far, well founded decision algorithms to choose specific methods of intervention for distinct clinical situations are not yet available. A key issue requiring clarification refers to the selection of a local or a systemic delivery approach whenever the use of an antibiotic is indicated. One investigation addressed this question in patients with rapidly progressing periodontitis (Bernimoulin et al. 1995). Overall, no significant differences were noted between systemic administration of amoxicillin–clavulanic acid and tetracycline fibers as an adjunct to mechanical therapy. For patients with adult periodontitis, two studies reported better results of scaling and root planing supplemented with locally applied metronidazole than adjunctive systemic metronidazole (Paquette et al. 1994; Noyan et al. 1997).

As different oral distribution patterns can be recognized in periodontitis patients for microorganisms such as P. gingivalis (Mombelli et al. 1991a,b), local therapy may be less successful in patients where these organisms are widespread than in patients where the presence of pathogens is confined to isolated areas. This hypothesis was tested in a study comparing two extremes of local therapy. In one group of patients, a combination of measures including full mouth scaling and root planing, application of tetracycline fibers, and chlorhexidine rinse, was applied. In the other group, only two teeth were treated locally and no attempt was made to interfere with the overall conditions of the oral environment. Major clinical differences were found in the local healing response, depending on whether the rest of the dentition was left untreated or was also subjected to therapy (Mombelli et al. 1997). How can a clinician be sure that the areas he treats coincide with the sites harboring the pathogens? No diagnostic tool is available presently at a reasonable cost that could give the dentist a detailed distribution map of periodontal pathogens. Provided that such a tool would exist, could P. gingivalis and A. actinomycetemcomitans be eradicated from an infected dentition by microbiologically guided local antimicrobial therapy? A study evaluating the effect of local antibiotic therapy, given to every tooth with cultural evidence of P. gingivalis or A. actinomycetemcomitans after completion of conventional mechanical periodontal therapy demonstrated the limits of this approach (Mombelli et al. 2002). Even if a detailed microbiologic assessment provided information about the distribution pattern within the dentition, and all positive teeth were treated, the target organisms could be detected again after therapy in some sites in a considerable number of subjects.

Local antibiotics in clinical practice

To treat periodontal disease successfully, local delivery devices must provide therapeutic levels of antimicrobial agents in the subgingival area over several days. Clinical trials show the efficacy of local antibiotic therapy under these conditions. The current evidence suggests that local delivery may be most beneficial in the control of localized ongoing disease in otherwise stable patients. Maintenance patients with a few non-responding sites may therefore benefit most from local antimicrobial therapy. Local antibiotic therapy adds flexibility and improves efficacy of periodontal care by providing a non-surgical local treatment alternative with more powerful antibacterial effects than scaling and root planing. Potential uses for locally delivered antibiotics also include the treatment of peri-implant infections (Mombelli et al. 2001; Renvert et al. 2006). A comment made in the context of systemic antibiotics needs to be reiterated here with regards to local therapy: antibiotics are not a means to compensate for inadequate oral hygiene. For a maximal benefit, and a sustained local effect, patients should receive specific instructions on how to keep the treated sites plaque free with appropriate home care procedures.

Overall conclusion

Although mechanical periodontal treatment alone improves clinical conditions sufficiently in most cases, adjunctive antibiotics, delivered either systemically or locally, can enhance the effect of therapy. Systemic antibiotics may be a useful adjunct to the mechanical treatment of aggressive forms of periodontitis and for cases with evidence of ongoing disease despite previous mechanical therapy. By providing an additional treatment benefit especially in deep pockets, systemic antibiotics can reduce the need for further, surgical therapy. Localized nonresponding sites and localized recurrent disease may be treated with locally delivered antibiotics. Mechanical debridement before the application of antimicrobial agents, and mechanical plaque control after therapy, are essential for treatment success. To limit the development of microbial antibiotic resistance in general, and to avoid the risk of unwanted systemic effects of antibiotics for the treated individual, a precautionary, restrictive attitude towards using antibiotics is recommended.

References

Ainamo, J., Lie, T., Ellingsen, B.H., Hansen, B.F., Johansson, L.-Å., Karring, T., Kirsch, J., Paunio, K. & Stoltze, K. (1992). Clinical responses to subgingival placement of a metronidazole 25% gel compared to the effect of subgingival scaling in adult periodontitis. *Journal of Clinical Periodontology* **19**, 723–729.

Allenspach-Petrzilka, G.E. & Guggenheim, B. (1983). Bacterial invasion of the periodontium; an important factor in the pathogenesis of periodontitis? *Journal of Clinical Periodontology* **10**, 609–617.

Anwar, H., Dasgupta, M.K. & Costerton, J.W. (1990). Testing the susceptibility of bacteria in biofilms to antibacterial agents. *Antimicrobial Agents and Chemotherapy* **34**, 2043–2046.

Anwar, H., Strap, J.L. & Costerton, J.W. (1992). Establishment of aging biofilms: possible mechanism of bacterial resistance to antibiotic therapy. *Antimicrobial Agents and Chemotherapy* **36**, 1347–1351.

Baker, P.J., Slots, J., Genco, R.J. & Evans, R.T. (1983). Minimal inhibitory concentrations of various antimicrobial agents for human oral anaerobic bacteria. *Antimicrobial Agents and Chemotherapy* **24**, 420–424.

Berglundh, T., Krok, L., Liljenberg, B., Westfelt, E., Serino, G. & Lindhe, J. (1998). The use of metronidazole and amoxicillin in the treatment of advanced periodontal disease. A prospective, controlled clinical trial. *Journal of Clinical Periodontology* **25**, 354–362.

Bernimoulin, P., Purucker, H., Mertes, B. & Krüger, B. (1995). Local versus systemic adjunctive antibiotic therapy in RPP patients. *Journal of Dental Research* **74**, 481.

Bonesvoll, P. & Gjermo, P. (1978). A comparison between chlorhexidine and some quaternary ammonium compounds with regard to retention, salivary concentration and plaque-inhibiting effect in the human mouth after mouth rinses. *Archives of Oral Biology* **23**, 289–294.

Bonito, A.J., Lux, L. & Lohr, K.N. (2005). Impact of local adjuncts to scaling and root planing in periodontal disease therapy: a systematic review. *Journal of Periodontology* **76**, 1227–1236.

Bragd, L., Dahlén, G., Wikström, M. & Slots, J. (1987). The capability of *Actinobacillus actinomycetemcomitans, Bacteroides gingivalis* and *Bacteroides intermedius* to indicate progressive periodontitis; a retrospective study. *Journal of Clinical Periodontology* **14**, 95–99.

Carlos, J.P., Wolfe, M.D., Zambon, J.J. & Kingman, A. (1988). Periodontal disease in adolescents: Some clinical and microbiologic correlates of attachment loss. *Journal of Dental Research* **67**, 1510–1514.

Carranza, F.A. Jr., Saglie, R., Newman, M.G. & Valentin, P.L. (1983). Scanning and transmission electron microscopic study of tissue-invading microorganisms in localized juvenile periodontitis. *Journal of Periodontology* **54**, 598–617.

Chaves, E.S., Jeffcoat, M.K., Ryerson, C.C. & Snyder, B. (2000). Persistent bacterial colonization of *Porphyromonas gingivalis, Prevotella intermedia,* and *Actinobacillus actinomycetemcomitans* in periodontitis and its association with alveolar bone loss after 6 months of therapy. *Journal of Clinical Periodontology* **27**, 897–903.

Christersson, L., van Winkelhoff, A.J., Zambon, J.J., de Graaff, J. & Genco, R.J. (1989). Systemic antibiotic combination therapy in recalcitrant and recurrent localized juvenile periodontitis. *Journal of Dental Research* **68**, 197.

Costerton, J.W., Lewandowski, Z., Caldwell, D.E., Korber, D.R. & Lappin-Scott, H.M. (1995). Microbial biofilms. *Annual Reviews in Microbiology* **49**, 711–745.

Craig, W. (1998). Pharmacokinetic/pharmacodynamic parameters: rationale for antibacterial dosing of mice and men. *Clinical Infectious Diseases* **26**, 1–10.

Dahlén, G., Wikström, M. & Renvert, S. (1996). Treatment of periodontal disease based on microbiological diagnosis. A 5-year follow-up on individual patterns. *Journal of Periodontology* **67**, 879–887.

Eakle, W., Ford, C. & Boyd, R. (1986). Depth of penetration in periodontal pockets with oral irrigation. *Journal of Clinical Periodontology* **13**, 39–44.

Flemmig, T.F., Milian, E., Kopp, C., Karch, H. & Klaiber, B. (1998). Differential effects of systemic metronidazole and amoxicillin on *Actinobacillus actinomycetemcomitans* and *Porphyromonas gingivalis* in intraoral habitats. *Journal of Clinical Periodontology* **25**, 1–10.

Garrett, S., Adams, D.F., Bogle, G., Donly, K., Drisko, C.H., Hallmon, W.W., Hancock, E.B., Hanes, P., Hawley, C.E., Johnson, L., Kiger, R., Killoy, W., Mellonig, J.T., Raab, F.J., Ryder, M., Stoller, N., Polson, A., Wang, H.-L., Wolinsky, L.E., Yukna, R.A., Harrold, C.Q., Hill, M., Johnson, V.B. & Southard, G.L. (2000). The effect of locally delivered controlled-release doxycycline or scaling and root planing on periodontal maintenance patients over 9 months. *Journal of Periodontology* **71**, 22–30.

Garrett, S., Johnson, L., Drisko, C.H., Adams, D.F., Bandt, C., Beiswanger, B., Bogle, G., Donly, K., Hallmon, W.W., Hancock, E.B., Hanes, P., Hawley, C.E., Kiger, R., Killoy, W., Mellonig, J.T., Polson, A., Raab, F.J., Ryder, M., Stoller, N.H., Wang, H.L., Wolinsky, L.E., Evans, G.H., Harrold, C.Q., Arnold, R.M., Atack, D.F., Fitzgerald, B., Hill, M., Isaacs, R.L., Nasi, H.F., Newell, D.H., MacNeil, R.L., MacNeill, S., Spolsky, V.W., Duke, S.P., Polson, A. & Southard, G.L. (1999). Two multi-center studies evaluating locally delivered doxycycline hyclate, placebo control, oral hygiene, and scaling and root planing in the treatment of periodontitis. *Journal of Periodontology* **70**, 490–503.

Goené, R.J., Winkel, E.G., Abbas, F., Rodenburg, J.P., Van Winkelhoff, A.J. & De Graaff, J. (1990). Microbiology in diagnosis and treatment of severe periodontitis. A report of four cases. *Journal of Periodontology* **61**, 61–64.

Golub, L.M., Wolff, M., Lee, H.M., McNamara, T.F., Ramamurthy, N.S., Zambon, J. & Ciancio, S. (1985). Further evidence that tetracyclines inhibit collagenase activity in human crevicular fluid and other mammalian sources. *Journal of Periodontal Research* **20**, 12–23.

Goodson, J., Cugini, M., Kent, R., Armitage, G., Cobb, C., Fine, D., Fritz, M., Green, E., Imoberdorf, M., Killoy, W.,

Mendieta, C., Niederman, R., Offenbacher, S., Taggart, E. & Tonetti, M. (1991a). Multicenter evaluation of tetracycline fiber therapy: I. Experimental design, methods and baseline data. *Journal of Periodontal Research* **26**, 361–370.

Goodson, J., Cugini, M., Kent, R., Armitage, G., Cobb, C., Fine, D., Fritz, M., Green, E., Imoberdorf, M., Killoy, W., Mendieta, C., Niederman, R., Offenbacher, S., Taggart, E. & Tonetti, M. (1991b). Multicenter evaluation of tetracycline fiber therapy: II. Clinical response. *Journal of Periodontal Research* **26**, 371–379.

Goodson, J., Holborow, D., Dunn, R., Hogan, P. & Dunham, S. (1983). Monolithic tetracycline containing fibers for controlled delivery to periodontal pockets. *Journal of Periodontology* **54**, 575–579.

Goodson, J.M. (1989). Pharmacokinetic principles controlling efficacy of oral therapy. *Journal of Dental Research* **68**, 1625–1632.

Gristina, A.G. (1987). Biomaterial-centered infection: Microbial adhesion versus tissue integration. *Science* **237**, 1588–1595.

Grossi, S., Dunford, R., Genco, R.J., Pihlstrom, B., Walker, C., Howell, H. & Thorøe, U. (1995). Local application of metronidazole dental gel. *Journal of Dental Research* **74**, 468.

Grossi, S.G., Zambon, J.J., Ho, A.W., Koch, G., Dunford, R.G., Machtei, E.E., Norderyd, O.M. & Genco, R.J. (1994). Assessment of risk for periodontal disease. I. Risk indicators for attachment loss. *Journal of Periodontology* **65**, 260–267.

Guerrero, A., Griffiths, G.S., Nibali, L., Suvan, J., Moles, D.R., Laurell, L. & Tonetti, M.S. (2005). Adjunctive benefits of systemic amoxicillin and metronidazole in non-surgical treatment of generalized aggressive periodontitis: a randomized placebo-controlled clinical trial. *Journal of Clinical Periodontology* **32**, 1096–1107.

Haffajee, A.D. & Socransky, S.S. (1994). Microbial etiological agents of destructive periodontal diseases. *Periodontology 2000* **5**, 78–111.

Haffajee, A.D., Socransky, S.S. & Gunsolley, J.C. (2003). Systemic anti-infective periodontal therapy. A systematic review. *Annals of Periodontology* **8**, 115–181.

Haffajee, A.D., Socransky, S.S., Smith, C. & Dibart, S. (1991). Relation of baseline microbial parameters to future periodontal attachment loss. *Journal of Clinical Periodontology* **18**, 744–750.

Hanes, P.J. & Purvis, J.P. (2003). Local anti-infective therapy: pharmacological agents. A systematic review. *Annals of Periodontology* **8**, 79–98.

Herrera, D., Sanz, M., Jepsen, S., Needleman, I. & Roldán, S. (2002). A systematic review on the effect of systemic antimicrobials as an adjunct to scaling and root planing in periodontitis patients. *Journal of Clinical Periodontology* **29**, 136–159.

Höffler, U., Niederau, W. & Pulverer, G. (1980). Susceptibility of *Bacterium actinomycetemcomitans* to 45 antibiotics. *Antimicrobial Agents and Chemotherapy* **17**, 943–946.

Jeffcoat, M.K., Bray, K.S., Ciancio, S.G., Dentino, A.R., Fine, D.H., Gordon, J.M., Gunsolley, J.C., Killoy, W.J., Lowenguth, R.A., Magnusson, N.I., Offenbacher, S., Palcanis, K.G., Proskin, H.M., Finkelman, R.D. & Flashner, M. (1998). Adjunctive use of a subgingival controlled-release chlorhexidine chip reduces probing depth and improves attachment level compared with scaling and root planing alone. *Journal of Periodontology* **69**, 989–997.

Jousimies-Somer, H., Asikainen, S., Suomala, P. & Summanen, P. (1988). Activity of metronidazole and its hydroxymetabolite. *Oral Microbiology and Immunology* **3**, 32–34.

Kinane, D.F. & Radvar, M. (1999). A six-month comparison of three periodontal local antimicrobial therapies in persistent periodontal pockets. *Journal of Periodontology* **70**, 1–7.

Kornman, K.S., Newman, M.G., Flemmig, T., Alvarado, R. & Nachnani, S. (1989). Treatment of refractory periodontitis with metronidazole plus amoxicillin or Augmentin. *Journal of Dental Research* **68**, 917.

Kornman, K.S., Newman, M.G., Moore, D.J. & Singer, R.E. (1994). The influence of supragingival plaque control on clinical and microbial outcomes following the use of antibiotics for the treatment of periodontitis. *Journal of Periodontology* **65**, 848–854.

Listgarten, M.A. (1965). Electron microscopic observations on the bacterial flora of acute necrotizing ulcerative gingivitis. *Journal of Periodontology* **36**, 328–339.

Loesche, W.J., Giordano, J.R., Hujoel, P., Schwarcz, J. & Smith, B.A. (1992). Metronidazole in periodontitis: reduced need for surgery. *Journal of Clinical Periodontology* **19**, 103–112.

Loesche, W.J., Grossman, N. & Giordano, J. (1993). Metronidazole in periodontitis (IV). The effect of patient compliance on treatment parameters. *Journal of Clinical Periodontology* **20**, 96–104.

Lopez, N. & Gamonal, J. (1998). Effects of metronidazole plus amoxicillin in progressive untreated adult periodontitis: results of a single one-week course after 2 and 4 months. *Journal of Periodontology* **69**, 1291–1298.

Lopez, N., Socransky, S., Da Silva, I., Patel, M. & Haffajee, A. (2006). Effects of metronidazole plus amoxicillin as only therapy on the microbiological and clinical parameters of untreated chronic periodontitis. *Journal of Clinical Periodontology* **33**, 648–660.

Lopez, N.J., Gamonal, J.A. & Martinez, B. (2000). Repeated metronidazole and amoxicillin treatment of periodontitis. A follow-up study. *Journal of Periodontology* **71**, 79–89.

Lorian, V. (1986). *Antibiotics in Laboratory Medicine*, 2nd edn. Baltimore: Williams and Wilkins Co.

Marchant, C., Carlin, S., Johnson, C. & Shurin, P. (1992). Measuring the comparative efficacy of antibacterial agents for acute otitis media: the "Pollyanna phenomenon". *Journal of Pediatrics* **120**, 72–77.

Marshall, K.C. (1992). Biofilms: An overview of bacterial adhesion, activity, and control at surfaces. *ASM News* **58**, 202–207.

Mascarenhas, P., Gapski, R., Al-Shammari, K., Hill, R., Soehren, S., Fenno, J.C., Giannobile, W.V. & Wang, H.L. (2005). Clinical response of azithromycin as an adjunct to non-surgical periodontal therapy in smokers. *Journal of Periodontology* **76**, 426–436.

Michalowicz, B.S., Pihlstrom, B.L., Drisko, C.L. *et al.* (1995). Evaluation of periodontal treatments using controlled release tetracycline fibers: Maintenance response. *Journal of Periodontology* **66**, 708–715.

Mombelli, A. (2006). Heresy? Treatment of chronic periodontitis with systemic antibiotics only. *Journal of Clinical Periodontology* **33**, 661–662.

Mombelli, A., Feloutzis, A., Brägger, U. & Lang, N.P. (2001). Treatment of peri-implantitis by local delivery of tetracycline. Clinical, microbiological and radiological results. *Clinical Oral Implants Research* **12**, 287–294.

Mombelli, A., Gmür, R., Gobbi, C. & Lang, N.P. (1994). *Actinobacillus actinomycetemcomitans* in adult periodontitis. I. Topographic distribution before and after treatment. *Journal of Periodontology* **65**, 820–826.

Mombelli, A., Lehmann, B., Tonetti, M. & Lang, N.P. (1997). Clinical response to local delivery of tetracycline in relation to overall and local periodontal conditions. *Journal of Clinical Periodontology* **24**, 470–477.

Mombelli, A., McNabb, H. & Lang, N.P. (1991a). Black-pigmenting Gram-negative bacteria in periodontal disease. I. Topographic distribution in the human dentition. *Journal of Periodontal Research* **26**, 301–307.

Mombelli, A., McNabb, H. & Lang, N.P. (1991b). Black-pigmenting Gram-negative bacteria in periodontal disease. II. Screening strategies for *P. gingivalis*. *Journal of Periodontal Research* **26**, 308–313.

Mombelli, A., Schmid, B., Rutar, A. & Lang, N.P. (2000). Persistence patterns of *Porphyromonas gingivalis*, *Prevotella intermedia/nigrescens*, and *Actinobacillus actinomycetemcomitans* after mechanical therapy of periodontal disease. *Journal of Periodontology* **71**, 14–21.

Mombelli, A., Schmid, B., Rutar, A. & Lang, N.P. (2002). Local antibiotic therapy guided by microbiological diagnosis. Treatment of *Porphyromonas gingivalis* and *Actinobacillus actinomycetemcomitans* persisting after mechanical therapy. *Journal of Clinical Periodontology* **29**, 743–749.

Mombelli, A. & van Winkelhoff, A.J. (1997). The systemic use of antibiotics in periodontal therapy. In: Lang, N.P., Karring, T. & Lindhe, J., eds. *Proceedings of the Second European Workshop on Periodontology*. Berlin: Quintessenz Verlag, pp. 38–77.

Morozumi, T., Kubota, T., Sato, T., Okuda, K. & Yoshie, H. (2004). Smoking cessation increases gingival blood flow and gingival crevicular fluid. *Journal of Clinical Periodontology* **31**, 267–272.

Müller, H.P., Eickholz, P., Heinecke, A., Pohl, S., Müller, R.F. & Lange, D.E. (1995). Simultaneous isolation of *Actinobacillus actinomycetemcomitans* from subgingival and extracrevicular locations of the mouth. *Journal of Clinical Periodontology* **22**, 413–419.

Müller, H.P., Lange, D.E. & Müller, R.F. (1993). Failure of adjunctive minocycline-HCl to eliminate oral *Actinobacillus actinomycetemcomitans*. *Journal of Clinical Periodontology* **20**, 498–504.

Newman, M.G., Kornman, K.S. & Doherty, F.M. (1994). A 6-month multi-center evaluation of adjunctive tetracycline fiber therapy used in conjunction with scaling and root planing in maintenance patients: Clinical results. *Journal of Periodontology* **65**, 685–691.

Norskov-Lauritsen, N. & Kilian, M. (2006). Reclassification of *Actinobacillus actinomycetemcomitans, Haemophilus aphrophilus, Haemophilus paraphrophilus* and *Haemophilus segnis* as *Aggregatibacter actinomycetemcomitans gen. nov., comb. nov., Aggregatibacter aphrophilus comb. nov.* and *Aggregatibacter segnis comb. nov.*, and emended description of *Aggregatibacter aphrophilus* to include V factor-dependent and V factor-independent isolates. *International Journal of Systematic and Evolutionary Microbiology* **56**, 2135–2146.

Noyan, Ü., Yilmaz, S., Kuru, B., Kadir, T., Acar, O. & Büget, E. (1997). A clinical and microbiological evaluation of systemic and local metronidazole delivery in adult periodontitis patients. *Journal of Clinical Periodontology* **24**, 158–165.

Oostervaal, P.J., Mikx, F.H. & Renggli, H.H. (1990). Clearance of a topically applied fluorescein gel from periodontal pockets. *Journal of Clinical Periodontology* **17**, 613–615.

Pajukanta, R., Asikainen, S., Forsblom, B., Saarela, M. & Jousimies-Somer, H. (1993a). β-Lactamase production and *in vitro* antimicrobial susceptibility of *Porphyromonas gingivalis*. *FEMS Immunology and Medical Microbiology* **6**, 241–244.

Pajukanta, R., Asikainen, S., Saarela, M., Alaluusua, S. & Jousimies-Somer, H. (1993b). *In vitro* antimicrobial susceptibility of different serotypes of *Actinobacillus actinomycetemcomitans*. *Scandinavian Journal of Dental Research* **101**, 299–303.

Paquette, D., Ling, S., Fiorellini, J., Howell, H., Weber, H. & Williams, R. (1994). Radiographic and BANA test analysis of locally delivered metronidazole: a phase I/II clinical trial. *Journal of Dental Research* **73**, 305.

Paquette, D.W., Hanlon, A., Lessem, J. & Williams, R.C. (2004). Clinical relevance of adjunctive minocycline microspheres in patients with chronic periodontitis: secondary analysis of a phase 3 trial. *Journal of Periodontology* **75**, 531–536.

Pavicic, M.J.A.M.P., van Winkelhoff, A.J. & de Graaff, J. (1991). Synergistic effects between amoxicillin, metronidazole, and the hydroxymetabolite of metronidazole against *Actinobacillus actinomycetemcomitans*. *Antimicrobial Agents and Chemotherapy* **35**, 961–966.

Pavicic, M.J.A.M.P., van Winkelhoff, A.J. & de Graaff, J. (1992). *In vitro* susceptibilities of *Actinobacillus actinomycetemcomitans* to a number of antimicrobial combinations. *Antimicrobial Agents and Chemotherapy* **36**, 2634–2638.

Pavicic, M.J.A.M.P., van Winkelhoff, A.J., Douqué, N.H., Steures, R.W.R. & de Graaff, J. (1994). Microbiological and clinical effects of metronidazole and amoxicillin in *Actinobacillus actinomycetemcomitans*-associated periodontitis. *Journal of Clinical Periodontology* **21**, 107–112.

Pedrazzoli, V., Kilian, M. & Karring, T. (1992). Comparative clinical and microbiological effects of topical subgingival application of metronidazole 25% dental gel and scaling in the treatment of adult periodontitis. *Journal of Clinical Periodontology* **19**, 715–722.

Pihlstrom, B., Michalowicz, B., Aeppli, D., Genco, R., Walker, C., Howell, H. & Mørup-Jensen, A. (1995). Equivalence in clinical trials. *Journal of Dental Research* **74**, 530.

Pitcher, G., Newman, H. & Strahan, J. (1980). Access to subgingival plaque by disclosing agents using mouthrinsing and direct irrigation. *Journal of Clinical Periodontology* **7**, 300–308.

Radvar, M., Pourtaghi, N. & Kinane, D.F. (1996). Comparison of 3 periodontal local antibiotic therapies in persistent periodontal pockets. *Journal of Periodontology* **67**, 860–865.

Rams, T.E., Feik, D. & Slots, J. (1992). Ciprofloxacin/metronidazole treatment of recurrent adult periodontitis. *Journal of Dental Research* **71**, 319.

Rams, T.E., Listgarten, M.A. & Slots, J. (1996). The utility of 5 major putative periodontal pathogens and selected clinical parameters to predict periodontal breakdown in adults on maintenance care. *Journal of Clinical Periodontology* **23**, 346–354.

Renvert, S., Lessem, J., Dahlen, G., Lindahl, C. & Svensson, M. (2006). Topical minocycline microspheres versus topical chlorhexidine gel as an adjunct to mechanical debridement of incipient peri-implant infections: a randomized clinical trial. *Journal of Clinical Periodontology* **33**, 362–369.

Rooney, J., Wade, W.G., Sprague, S.V., Newcombe, R.G. & Addy, M. (2002). Adjunctive effects to non-surgical therapy of systemic metronidazole and amoxicillin alone and combined. A placebo controlled study. *Journal of Clinical Periodontology* **29**, 342–350.

Saglie, F.R., Carranza, F.A. Jr., Newman, M.G., Cheng, L. & Lewin, K.J. (1982a). Identification of tissue-invading bacteria in human periodontal disease. *Journal of Periodontal Research* **17**, 452–455.

Saglie, R., Newman, M.G., Carranza, F.A. & Pattison, G.L. (1982b). Bacterial invasion of gingiva in advanced periodontitis in humans. *Journal of Periodontology* **53**, 217–222.

Salvi, G.E., Mombelli, A., Mayfield, L., Rutar, A., Suvan, J., Garrett, S. & Lang, N.P. (2002). Local antimicrobial therapy after initial periodontal treatment. A randomized controlled clinical trial comparing three biodegradable sustained release polymers. *Journal of Clinical Periodontology* **29**, 540–550.

Shinn, D.L.S. (1962). Metronidazole in acute ulcerative gingivitis. *The Lancet*, 1191.

Slots, J. & Rams, T.E. (1990). Antibiotics in periodontal therapy: advantages and disadvantages. *Journal of Clinical Periodontology* **17**, 479–493.

Soskolne, W.A., Heasman, P.A., Stabholz, A., Smart, G.J., Palmer, M., Flashner, M. & Newman, H.N. (1997). Sustained local delivery of chlorhexidine in the treatment of periodontitis: a multi-center study. *Journal of Periodontology* **68**, 32–38.

Stabholz, A., Kettering, J., Aprecio, R., Zimmerman, G., Baker, P.J. & Wikesjö, U.M.E. (1993). Antimicrobial properties of human dentin impregnated with tetracycline HCl or chlorhexidine. An *in vitro* study. *Journal of Clinical Periodontology* **20**, 557–562.

Stoller, N.H., Johnson, L.R., Trapnell, S., Harrold, C.Q. & Garrett, S. (1998). The pharmacokinetic profile of a biodegradable controlled-release delivery system containing doxycycline compared to systemically delivered doxycycline in gingival crevicular fluid, saliva, and serum. *Journal of Periodontology* **69**, 1085–1091.

Stoltze, K. (1992). Concentration of metronidazole in periodontal pockets after application of a metronidazole 25% dental gel. *Journal of Clinical Periodontology* **19**, 698–701.

Stoltze, K. (1995). Elimination of Elyzol® 25% Dentalgel matrix from periodontal pockets. *Journal of Clinical Periodontology* **22**, 185–187.

Tonetti, M., Cugini, M.A. & Goodson, J.M. (1990). Zero-order delivery with periodontal placement of tetracycline loaded ethylene vinyl acetate fibers. *Journal of Periodontal Research* **25**, 243–249.

van Steenberghe, D., Bercy, P., Kohl, J., De Boever, J., Adriaens, P., Vanderfaeillie, A., Adriaenssen, C., Rompen, E., De Vree, H., McCarthy, E.F. & Vandenhoven, G. (1993). Subgingival minocycline hydrochloride ointment in moderate to severe chronic adult periodontitis: A randomized, double-blind, vehicle-controlled, multicenter study. *Journal of Periodontology* **64**, 637–644.

van Steenberghe, D., Rosling, B., Soder, P.O., Landry, R.G., van der Velden, U., Timmerman, M.F., McCarthy, E.F., Vandenhoven, G., Wouters, C., Wilson, M., Matthews, J. & Newman, H.N. (1999). A 15-month evaluation of the effects of repeated subgingival minocycline in chronic adult periodontitis. *Journal of Periodontology* **70**, 657–667.

van Winkelhoff, A.J., Rodenburg, J.P., Goené, R.J., Abbas, F., Winkel, E.G. & de Graaff, J. (1989). Metronidazole plus amoxicillin in the treatment of *Actinobacillus actinomycetemcomitans* associated periodontitis. *Journal of Clinical Periodontology* **16**, 128–131.

van Winkelhoff, A.J., Tijhof, C.J. & de Graaff, J. (1992). Microbiological and clinical results of metronidazole plus amoxicillin therapy in *Actinobacillus actinomycetemcomitans*-associated periodontitis. *Journal of Periodontology* **63**, 52–57.

van Winkelhoff, A.J., van der Velden, U., Clement, M. & de Graaff, J. (1988). Intra-oral distribution of black-pigmented *Bacteroides* species in periodontitis patients. *Oral Microbiology and Immunology* **3**, 83–85.

van Winkelhoff, A.J. & Winkel, E.G. (2005). Microbiological diagnostics in periodontics. Biological significance and clinical validity. *Periodontology 2000* **39**, 40–52.

Walker, C.B. (1992). Antimicrobial agents and chemotherapy In: Slots, J. & Taubmann, M., eds. *Contemporary Oral Microbiology and Immunology.* St Louis: Mosby Yearbook, pp. 242–264.

Walker, C.B. (1996). Selected antimicrobial agents: mechanisms of action, side effects and drug interactions. *Periodontology 2000* **10**, 12–28.

Walker, C.B., Pappas, J.D., Tyler, K.Z., Cohen, S. & Gordon, J.M. (1985). Antibiotic susceptibilities of periodontal bacteria. *In vitro* susceptibilities to eight antimicrobial agents. *Journal of Periodontology* **56**, 67–74.

Wennström, J., Newman, H.N., MacNeill, S.R., Killoy, W.J., Griffiths, G.S., Gillam, D.G., Krok, L., Needleman, I.G., Weiss, G. & Garrett, S. (2001). Utilization of locally delivered doxycycline in non-surgical treatment of chronic periodontitis. A comparative multi-center trial of 2 treatment approaches. *Journal of Clinical Periodontology* **28**, 753–761.

Wennström, J.L., Dahlén, G., Svensson, J. & Nyman, S. (1987). *Actinobacillus actinomycetemcomitans, Bacteroides gingivalis* and *Bacteroides intermedius*: Predictors of attachment loss? *Oral Microbiology and Immunology* **2**, 158–163.

Williams, R.C., Paquette, D.W., Offenbacher, S., Adams, D.F., Armitage, G.C., Bray, K., Caton, J., Cochran, D.L., Drisko, C.H., Fiorellini, J.P., Giannobile, W.V., Grossi, S., Guerrero, D.M., Johnson, G.K., Lamster, I.B., Magnusson, I., Oringer, R.J., Persson, G.R., Van Dyke, T.E., Wolff, L.F., Santucci, E.A., Rodda, B.E. & Lessem, J. (2001). Treatment of periodontitis by local administration of minocycline microspheres: a controlled trial. *Journal of Periodontology* **72**, 1535–1544.

Winkel, E.G., Van Winkelhoff, A.J., Timmerman, M.F., Van der Velden, U. & Van der Weijden, G.A. (2001). Amoxicillin plus metronidazole in the treatment of adult periodontitis patients. A double-blind placebo-controlled study. *Journal of Clinical Periodontology* **28**, 296–305.

Yoshinari, N., Tohya, T., Kawase, H., Matsuoka, M., Nakane, M., Kawachi, M., Mitani, A., Koide, M., Inagaki, K., Fukuda, M. & Noguchi, T. (2001). Effect of repeated local minocycline administration on periodontal healing following guided tissue regeneration. *Journal of Periodontology* **72**, 284–295.

Zambon, J.J., Reynolds, H.S. & Slots, J. (1981). Black-pigmented *Bacteroides* spp. in the human oral cavity. *Infection and Immunity* **32**, 198–203.

Part 13: Reconstructive Therapy

43 Regenerative Periodontal Therapy, 901
Pierpaolo Cortellini and Maurizio S. Tonetti

44 Mucogingival Therapy – Periodontal Plastic Surgery, 955
Jan L. Wennström, Giovanni Zucchelli, and Giovan P. Pini Prato

45 Periodontal Plastic Microsurgery, 1029
Rino Burkhardt and Niklaus P. Lang

46 Re-osseointegration, 1045
Tord Berglundh and Jan Lindhe

Chapter 43

Regenerative Periodontal Therapy

Pierpaolo Cortellini and Maurizio S. Tonetti

Introduction, 901
Classification and diagnosis of periodontal osseous defects, 901
Clinical indications, 903
Long-term effects and benefits of regeneration, 903
Evidence for clinical efficacy and effectiveness, 905
Patient and defect prognostic factors, 909
  Patient factors, 911
  Defect factors, 911
  Tooth factors, 912
  Factors affecting the clinical outcomes of GTR in furcations, 913
The relevance of the surgical approach, 913
  Papilla preservation flaps, 916
  Modified papilla preservation technique, 917
  Simplified papilla preservation flap, 920

Minimally invasive surgical technique, 922
Post-operative regime, 925
Post-operative morbidity, 926
Barrier materials for regenerative surgery, 928
  Non-absorbable materials, 928
  Bioabsorbable materials, 930
  Membranes in intrabony defects, 930
  Membranes for furcation involvement, 932
  Surgical issues with barrier membranes, 937
Bone replacement grafts, 938
Biologically active regenerative materials, 938
Membranes combined with other regenerative procedures, 940
Root surface biomodification, 943
Clinical strategies, 944

Introduction

The advances in the understanding of the biology of wound healing and periodontal regenerative technologies are applied to improve long-term clinical outcomes of teeth which are periodontally compromised by intrabony or inter-radicular defects. The treatment objective is to obtain shallow, maintainable pockets by reconstruction of the destroyed attachment apparatus and thereby also limiting recession of the gingival margin. In general periodontal regeneration is selected to obtain: (1) an increase in the periodontal attachment of a severely compromised tooth; (2) a decrease in deep pockets to a more maintainable range; (3) a reduction of the vertical and horizontal component of furcation defects. Current approaches, however, remain technique sensitive and clinical success requires application of meticulous diagnostic and treatment strategies.

Classification and diagnosis of periodontal osseous defects

Site-specific periodontal breakdown compromises the long-term prognosis of teeth by producing three types of defects: suprabony (or horizontal) defects, infrabony (or vertical) defects, and inter-radicular (or furcation) defects.

According to the classification by Goldman and Cohen (1958), suprabony defects are those where the base of the pocket is located coronal to the alveolar crest. Infrabony defects, on the other hand, are defined by the apical location of the base of the pocket with respect to the residual alveolar crest. This chapter does not deal with suprabony defects. With regard to infrabony defects, two types of defects can be recognized: intrabony defects and craters. Intrabony defects are bony defects whose infrabony component affects primarily one tooth, while in craters the defect affects two adjacent root surfaces to a similar extent. Intrabony defects (Fig. 43-1) have been classified according to their morphology in terms of residual bony walls, width of the defect (or radiographic angle), and in terms of their topographic extension around the tooth. Three-wall, two-wall, and one-wall defects have been defined on the basis of the number of residual alveolar bone walls. This represents the primary classification system. Frequently, intrabony defects present a complex anatomy consisting of a three-wall component in the most apical portion of the defect, and two- and/or one-wall components in the more superficial portions. Hemiseptal defects, that is, vertical defects in the presence of adjacent roots and where half of a septum remains on one tooth, represent a special case of one-wall defects. Several authors have also used

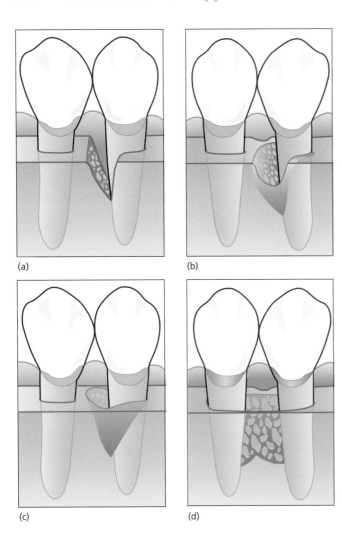

(a)

(b)

(c)

(d)

Fig. 43-1 Infrabony defects. (a) One-wall intrabony defect. (b) Two-wall intrabony defect. (c) Three-wall intrabony defect. (d) Interproximal crater. From Papapanou & Tonetti (2000).

descriptive terms to define special morphological characteristics: funnel-shaped defects, moat-like defects, trenches, etc. Of particular interest is a special morphology: the crater (Fig. 43-1). It is defined as a cup- or bowl-shaped defect in the interdental alveolar bone with bone loss nearly equal on the roots of two contiguous teeth and more coronal position of the buccal and lingual alveolar crest; the facial and lingual/palatal walls may be of unequal height. This defect can be considered as the result of the apical spread of periodontitis along two adjacent roots in a relatively narrow (mesiodistally) interproximal area. Notably, all the definitions above are not based on radiographic assessments but on the actual morphology of the defects after flap elevation. Conditions entailing pathologic resorption of bone within the furcation of a multi-rooted tooth, defined as furcation invasions, are also included in the group of periodontal bony defects; the reader however is referred to Chapter 39 for a discussion of the anatomy and classification of furcations.

The diagnosis of the presence and the morphology of periodontal osseous lesions represents a major clinical challenge. It is primarily performed combining clinical information derived from the evaluation of the attachment level with information derived from diagnostic-quality parallel-technique intraoral radiographs. A precise knowledge of root anatomy and its variations is also an important component for the diagnosis of periodontal osseous defects, and inter-radicular defects in particular. Diagnostic-quality radiographs provide additional information on the morphology of the alveolar bone resorption. In this context, interpretation of the radiographic image of the interdental septum is complicated, since the radiograph provides a two-dimensional illustration of a three-dimensional anatomy consisting of superimposed structures including alveolar bone, hard tooth substances, and soft tissue. This complexity of the visualized structures means that a certain amount of tissue destruction must occur before its radiographic detection becomes possible, often rendering incipient bone lesions obscure. Furthermore, even advanced lesions may be masked by the presence of superimposed structures. It is therefore generally stated that radiographic diagnosis has a high positive predictability (that is, the visualized lesions are indeed there) but a low negative predictability (that is, absence of radiographically detectable bone loss does not exclude the presence of an osseous lesion).

Clinical attachment level, on the other hand, is a highly sensitive diagnostic tool; its combination with radiographs, therefore, confers a higher degree of accuracy to the diagnostic approach (Tonetti *et al.* 1993b). In particular, the site-specific comparison of radiographic bone loss with clinical attachment loss allows the clinician to make a qualified guess of the true osseous architecture, whose exact morphology, however, can only be established after flap elevation. Detection of the defect, its location and extension, along with its major morphologic features, should be performed before flap elevation. A further aid to this end is the use of transgingival probing or bone sounding.

Clinical indications

Periodontal treatment, either surgical or non-surgical, results in recession of the gingival margin after healing (Isidor *et al.* 1984). In advanced cases of periodontitis, this may lead to poor esthetics in the front areas of the dentition, in particular when applying surgical procedures, including bone contouring, for the eradication of bone defects. Treatment of such cases without bone contouring, on the other hand, may result in residual pockets inaccessible to proper cleaning during post-treatment maintenance. These problems can be avoided or reduced by applying regenerative surgical procedures by which the lost periodontal attachment in the bone defects can be restored. Thus, the indication of applying regenerative periodontal therapy is often based on esthetic considerations, besides the fact that the function or long-term prognosis of the treated teeth may be improved.

Another indication for regenerative periodontal therapy are furcation-involved teeth. The furcation area is often inaccessible to adequate instrumentation and frequently the roots present concavities and furrows that make proper cleaning of the area after resective surgery impossible. Considering the long-term results and complications reported following treatment of furcation involvements by traditional resective therapy (Hamp *et al.* 1975; Bühler 1988), the long-term prognosis of furcation-involved teeth can be improved considerably by successful regenerative periodontal therapy.

Case reports also exist demonstrating that "hopeless" teeth with deep vertical defects, increased tooth mobility or through-and-through furcations can be successfully treated with regenerative periodontal therapy (Gottlow *et al.* 1986). However, controlled clinical trials or serial case reports presenting a reasonable predictability of treating such advanced cases are not available.

Long-term effects and benefits of regeneration

A pertinent question with respect to regenerative treatment is whether the achieved attachment level gains can be maintained over an extended period of time. In a long-term follow-up study, Gottlow *et al.* (1992) assessed the stability of new attachment gained

through guided tissue regeneration (GTR) procedures. Eighty sites in 39 patients, which 6 months after surgery exhibited a gain of clinical attachment of ≥2 mm (2–7 mm), were monitored during additional periods of 1–5 years. Of the 80 sites, 65 were monitored for 2 years, 40 for 3 years, 17 for 4 years, and 9 sites for 5 years. The results of this study and those of other trials indicate that attachment gain obtained following GTR treatment can be maintained on a long-term basis (Becker & Becker 1993; McClain & Schallhorn 1993).

An investigation on intrabony defects demonstrated that the stability of sites treated with GTR was dependent on participation of the patients in a recall program, and on the absence of bacterial plaque, bleeding on probing, and re-infection of the treated sites with periodontal pathogens (Cortellini *et al.* 1994). The susceptibility to disease recurrence at sites treated with non-bioabsorbable barrier membranes was assessed in a study comparing long-term changes in attachment levels at regenerated and non-regenerated sites in the same patient (Cortellini *et al.* 1996a). Results indicated that there was a high degree of concordance in the clinical outcomes (stability vs. recurrence of attachment loss) within the same patient suggesting that patient factors, rather than the site factors, including the specifics of the histologic type of expected wound healing, are associated with disease recurrence. Among patient factors, compliance with oral hygiene, smoking habits, and susceptibility to disease progression were the major determinants of stability of the treated sites, rather than the employed treatment modality.

Support for a limited impact of the histologic type of healing comes from an experimental study. In a study in monkeys (Kostopoulos & Karring 1994), periodontal breakdown was produced by the placement and retention of orthodontic elastics on experimental teeth until 50% bone loss was recorded. The experimental teeth were endodontically treated and subjected to a flap operation, and all granulation tissue was removed. The crowns of the teeth were resected at the level of the cemento-enamel junction and a barrier membrane was placed to cover the roots before they were submerged. Following 4 weeks of healing, the membranes were removed. At the same time the contralateral teeth that served as controls were endodontically treated and subjected to a sham operation during which the crowns were resected at the level of the cemento-enamel junction. Artificial composite crowns were then placed on both the experimental and the control roots. The sites were allowed to heal for 3 months during which period careful plaque control was performed. At the end of this period cotton-floss ligatures were placed on both experimental and control teeth to induce periodontal tissue breakdown. After another 6 months, the animals were sacrificed. With respect to attachment level, bone level, pocket depth, and gingival recession, similar results were recorded in histologic

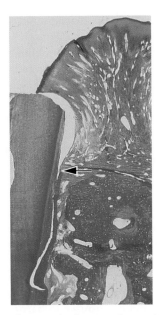

Fig. 43-2 Microphotograph of test specimen with a reformed connective tissue attachment. After 6 months of ligature-induced periodontitis, loss of attachment has occurred from the coronal cut root surface to the level indicated by the arrow.

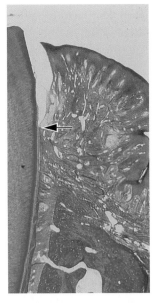

Fig. 43-3 Microphotograph of control specimen with a naturally existing periodontium. After 6 months of ligature-induced periodontitis, loss of attachment has occurred from the coronal cut tooth surface to the level indicated by the arrow.

specimens of experimental (Fig. 43-2) and control (Fig. 43-3) teeth. This indicates that the new connective tissue attachment formed with GTR is not more susceptible to periodontitis than the naturally existing periodontium.

A few studies have evaluated the long-term prognosis for furcation defects treated with regenerative therapy. Sixteen mandibular degree II furcation defects, following coronal flap positioning and citric acid root biomodification with and without implantation of demineralized freeze-dried bone allografts

(DFDBA), were determined as completely resolved with bone fill assessed by re-entry surgery. They were re-evaluated after 4–5 years (Haney *et al.* 1997), when 12 of the 16 sites exhibited recurrent degree II furcations and all 16 sites demonstrated probable buccal furcation defects. The investigators concluded that these findings question the long-term stability of bone regeneration in furcations following coronally advanced flap procedures.

The long-term stability of mandibular furcation defects regenerated following GTR alone or in combination with root surface biomodification with citric acid and bone grafting, was also evaluated by McClain and Schallhorn (1993). Out of the 57% of the furcation defects that were assessed as completely filled at 6 and 12 months, only 29% were completely filled after 4–6 years. However, 74% of the furcations treated with GTR in combination with the placement of DFDBA were completely filled at both the short and long-term evaluation, suggesting that the results obtained with the combined procedure were more stable over time. Long-term results of GTR treatment of mandibular degree II furcations with e-PTFE membranes were also reported by Machtei *et al.* (1996). The teeth were followed up to 4 years and compared with non-furcated molars. Improvements assessed in vertical (V-CAL) and horizontal (H-CAL) clinical attachment levels after treatment were also maintained after 4 years, suggesting that changes obtained in degree II furcation defects by GTR are stable. Only 9% of the treated defects were unstable, which was similar to that observed for non-furcated molars. Good oral hygiene, as reflected in low plaque scores and elimination of periodontal pathogens, was closely related to the long-term stability. On the basis of these results, it was concluded that furcation defects treated with membrane barriers can be maintained in health for at least 4 years, provided good oral hygiene and frequent recall visits are established.

In summary, several clinical studies addressing the long-term effects of periodontal regeneration show that, if the patient participates in a professionally delivered supportive periodontal care program and maintains good oral hygiene, the regenerated attachment can be maintained long term (Gottlow *et al.* 1992; MacClain & Schallhorn 1993; Cortellini *et al.* 1994, 1996a; Machtei *et al.* 1996; Christgau *et al.* 1997; Eickholz *et al.* 1997; Sculean *et al.* 2006). Risk factors for attachment loss are those associated with disease recurrence: poor compliance with supportive periodontal care, poor oral hygiene, and cigarette smoking (Cortellini *et al.* 1996a; Cortellini & Tonetti 2004).

Few investigations have looked at the long-term effects of periodontal regeneration on tooth survival. Cortellini and Tonetti (2004) performed a Kaplan Mayer analysis of tooth survival following periodontal regenerative treatment in a sample of 175 patients followed up for 2–16 years (average 8 ± 3.4 years) in a specialist environment. In this study, 96% of teeth

Table 43-1 Survival analysis of regenerated periodontal attachment over a 16-year follow-up period in 175 subjects treated with periodontal regeneration. In this survival analysis, the event is represented by clinical attachment level (CAL) loss of 2 mm or more from the level of attachment obtained at completion of healing 1 year after regeneration. No substantial recurrence of periodontitis (CAL loss) was observed in 92% of treated cases who participated in a secondary prevention program. (From Cortellini & Tonetti (2004) with permission)

Time at risk (years)	N CAL loss ≥2 mm	Censored	Effective sample size	Conditional probability CAL loss (%)	Survival (%)
0–2	2	0	175	1.1	100
2–4	3	0	166	1.7	98.9
4–6	2	0	155	1.2	97.1
6–8	1	55	119	0.7	96
8–10	0	47	70.5	0	95.3
10–12	2	16	41	3.5	95.3
12–14	0	25	24.5	0	92
14–16	0	21	8	0	92
16	0	1	0.5	0	92

treated by periodontal regeneration survived. Of interest was the observation that tooth loss was observed only among the 32% of the population that were smokers (tooth survival was 89% among smokers and 100% among non-smokers). Clinical attachment levels were located at the same level or coronal to the pre-treatment levels in 92% of cases up to 15 years after treatment (Table 43-1, Fig. 43-4).

The potential clinical benefits of periodontal regeneration can be best illustrated in a consecutive case series of strategic abutments severely compromised by the presence of deep intrabony defects with associated deep pockets with up to 8 years' follow-up following regenerative treatment (Tonetti *et al*. 1996a; Cortellini *et al*. 1998). At baseline, the periodontal defect rendered these teeth unsuitable as abutments to be included in a reconstruction. In all cases, periodontal regeneration with barrier membranes was able to change the clinical prognosis by providing both a 30% increase in radiographic bone support and shallow, maintainable probing depths. These outcomes remained stable during the follow-up period (Fig. 43-5). A similar benefit has been recently reported following use of combination therapy (barrier membranes and demineralized freeze-dried bone allograft) in teeth compromised by class II furcation defects (Bowers *et al*. 2003): 92% of class II defects were either closed or transformed into class I and thus at lower risk of tooth loss 1 year after therapy (McGuire & Nunn 1996a,b).

The limitation of recession of the gingival margin observed in controlled clinical trials when comparing a regenerative treatment with a non-regenerative surgical procedure is also an important benefit.

Evidence for clinical efficacy and effectiveness

Questions of efficacy relate to the added benefit of a treatment modality under ideal experimental conditions (such as those of a highly controlled research center environment). Effectiveness, on the other hand, relates to the benefit that can be achieved in a regular clinical setting where the procedure is likely to be performed in relation to morbidity and adverse events. Besides efficiency considerations, both evidence for efficacy and effectiveness need to be available in order to provide support for adoption of a novel approach in clinical practice.

The clinical efficacy of periodontal regenerative procedures has been extensively evaluated in randomized controlled clinical trials that have compared the regenerative procedure with a standard approach.

To limit sample size and study duration, these trials have utilized surrogate outcomes – clinical attachment level changes, decrease in pocket depths, furcation closure or radiographic measurements – rather than changes in tooth survival. These surrogate outcomes, however, are considered to be adequate proxies of the true outcome represented by tooth survival: persistence of deep pockets or furcation involvement are associated with higher risk of periodontal breakdown and tooth extraction.

The majority of clinical trials were small single-center studies. The evidence of these studies has been recently summarized in meta-analyses performed on data retrieved by systematic reviews of the published literature. In 2002 and 2003, the European Workshop on Periodontology and the Workshop on Emerging Technologies in Periodontics provided much of the systematic assessment of the evidence for currently available technologies. These include the use of barrier membranes (guided tissue regeneration, GTR), the use of bone replacement grafts, and the use of biologically active regenerative materials. The clinical evidence must be interpreted in the context of the biologic mechanisms and evidence for regeneration discussed in Chapter 25.

The evidence of clinical efficacy of barrier membranes has been assessed in the systematic reviews and meta-analyses performed by Needleman *et al*.

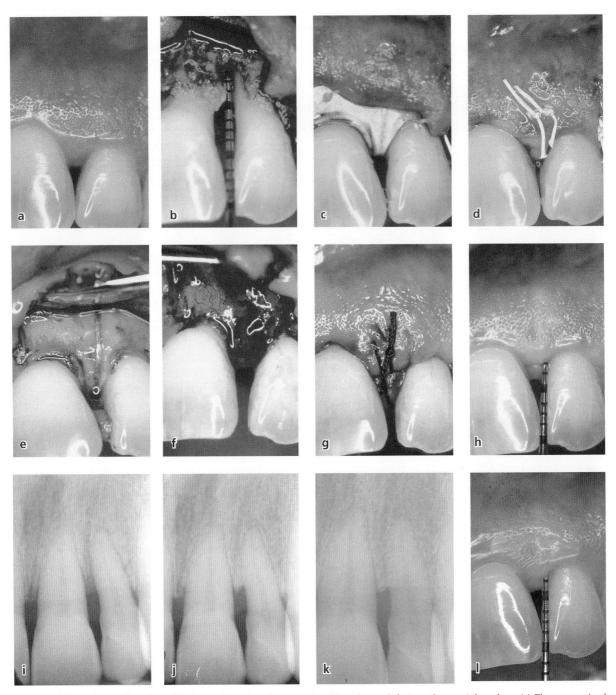

Fig. 43-4 (a,b) Left maxillary lateral incisor with a deep interproximal intrabony defect on the mesial surface. (c) Flaps are raised according to the modified papilla preservation technique, and a titanium-reinforced barrier membrane is placed over the defect. (d) By coronal displacement of the flap and preservation of the interdental papilla, the membrane is completely covered. (e,f) After 6 weeks of uneventful post-operative healing the membrane was removed, (g) and the newly formed tissue was completely covered. (h) At 1 year, residual probing pocket depth was 2 mm and no buccal or interdental recession had occurred. (i) The baseline radiograph shows radiolucency approaching the apex of the tooth, but after 1 year the intrabony defect is resolved and some supracrestal bone apposition seems to have occurred (j). The radiograph taken at 6 years confirms the supracrestal bone regeneration (k) and the clinical image shows the integrity of the interdental papilla with optimal preservation of the esthetic appearance (l).

(2002), Jepsen *et al.* (2002), and Murphy and Gunsolley (2003).

For intrabony defects, 26 controlled trials with 867 intrabony defects were included (Murphy & Gunsolley 2003). The application of barrier membranes resulted in an additional clinical attachment level gain of more than 1 mm compared to an access flap approach control (Fig. 43-6).

For class II furcation defects, 15 controlled trials with 376 involved teeth were included (Murphy & Gunsolley 2003). Membrane application resulted in additional vertical and horizontal (depth of the furcation involvement) clinical attachment level gains (Fig. 43-7).

These data alone, however, did not present conclusive evidence of efficacy as the possibility of bias

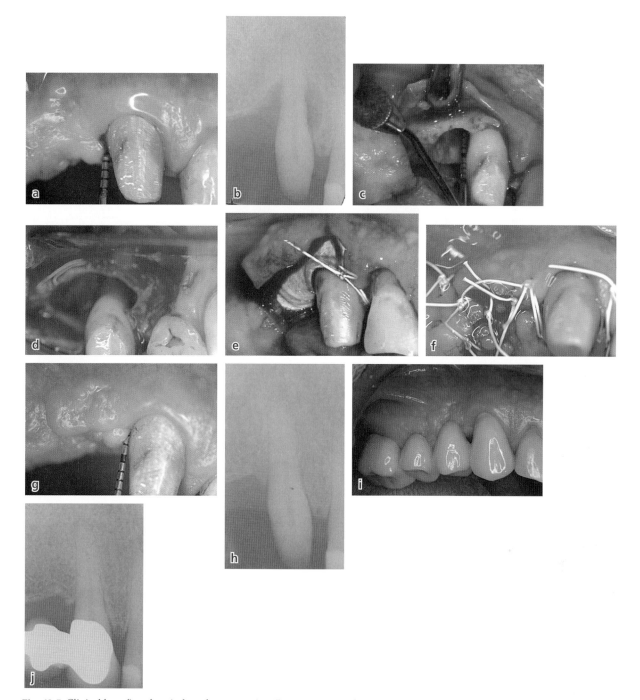

Fig. 43-5 Clinical benefits of periodontal regeneration. Patient presented with periodontally compromised mesial abutment of bridge: a 10-mm pocket was associated with a 10-mm intrabony defect extending on three of the four surfaces of the tooth (a–d). A barrier membrane was positioned and secured around the root of the tooth (e). Primary closure with internal mattress sutures was achieved (f) and maintained during the healing period. At 1 year, periodontal probing shows a shallow maintainable pocket (3 mm) (g) and the complete resolution of the defect (h). Clinical and radiographic stability of the outcome is illustrated 8 years following regenerative therapy (i,j): stability of the gingival margin, shallow pockets, good esthetics, and good periodontal support for the abutment are evident.

arising from a possible tendency to report studies with positive results could not be ruled out. Multi-center studies were designed to assess efficacy conclusively. These were performed in a private practice environment in order to assess also the generalizability of the benefit to this specific setting (effectiveness). The results of large prospective multi-center studies in private practice settings (Tonetti *et al.* 1998, 2004b; Cortellini *et al.* 2001) conclusively support the

additional benefit of membranes in improving clinical attachment levels in intrabony defects and thus their efficacy and effectiveness. More limited evidence is also available for combination therapy (bone replacement grafts and barrier membranes) in furcation defects (Bowers *et al.* 2003).

The efficacy of bone replacement graft materials has been assessed in two systematic reviews (Trombelli *et al.* 2002; Reynolds *et al.* 2003). As these two

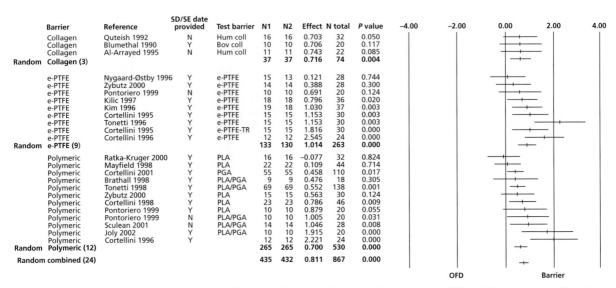

Barrier	Reference	SD/SE date provided	Test barrier	N1	N2	Effect	N total	P value
Collagen	Quteish 1992	N	Hum coll	16	16	0.703	32	0.050
Collagen	Blumethal 1990	Y	Bov coll	10	10	0.706	20	0.117
Collagen	Al-Arrayed 1995	N	Hum coll	11	11	0.743	22	0.085
Random Collagen (3)				37	37	0.716	74	0.004
e-PTFE	Nygaard-Østby 1996	Y	e-PTFE	15	13	0.121	28	0.744
e-PTFE	Zybutz 2000	Y	e-PTFE	14	14	0.388	28	0.300
e-PTFE	Pontoriero 1999	N	e-PTFE	10	10	0.691	20	0.124
e-PTFE	Kilic 1997	Y	e-PTFE	18	18	0.796	36	0.020
e-PTFE	Kim 1996	Y	e-PTFE	19	18	1.030	37	0.003
e-PTFE	Cortellini 1995	Y	e-PTFE	15	15	1.153	30	0.003
e-PTFE	Tonetti 1996	Y	e-PTFE	15	15	1.153	30	0.003
e-PTFE	Cortellini 1995	Y	e-PTFE-TR	15	15	1.816	30	0.000
e-PTFE	Cortellini 1996	Y	e-PTFE	12	12	2.545	24	0.000
Random e-PTFE (9)				133	130	1.014	263	0.000
Polymeric	Ratka-Kruger 2000	Y	PLA	16	16	-0.077	32	0.824
Polymeric	Mayfield 1998	Y	PLA	22	22	0.109	44	0.714
Polymeric	Cortellini 2001	Y	PGA	55	55	0.458	110	0.017
Polymeric	Brathall 1998	Y	PLA/PGA	9	9	0.476	18	0.305
Polymeric	Tonetti 1998	Y	PLA/PGA	69	69	0.552	138	0.001
Polymeric	Zybutz 2000	Y	PLA	15	15	0.563	30	0.124
Polymeric	Cortellini 1998	Y	PLA	23	23	0.786	46	0.009
Polymeric	Pontoriero 1999	Y	PLA	10	10	0.879	20	0.055
Polymeric	Pontoriero 1999	N	PLA/PGA	10	10	1.005	20	0.031
Polymeric	Sculean 2001	N	PLA/PGA	14	14	1.046	28	0.008
Polymeric	Joly 2002	Y	PLA/PGA	10	10	1.915	20	0.000
Polymeric	Cortellini 1996	Y		12	12	2.221	24	0.000
Random Polymeric (12)				265	265	0.700	530	0.000
Random combined (24)				435	432	0.811	867	0.000

Fig. 43-6 Meta-analysis of intrabony defect studies examining open flap debridement versus GTR with barrier, using clinical attachment level (CAL) gain as an outcome variable. Bov coll = bovine collagen; e-PTFE = expanded polytetrafluoroethylene; Hum coll = human collagen; PLA = polylactic acid; PLA/PGA = polylactic/polyglycolic acid; TR = titanium-reinforced. From Murphy & Gunsolley (2003) with permission from the American Academy of Periodontology.

Barrier	Reference	Location	SD/SE data provided	N1	N2	Effect	N total	P value
Collagen	Wang 1994	Mand	Y	12	12	0.516	24	0.204
Random Collagen (1)				12	12	0.516	24	0.228
e-PTFE	Pontoriero 1995	Max	N	8	8	0.000	16	1.000
e-PTFE	Lekovic 1989	Mand	Y	12	12	0.026	24	0.949
e-PTFE	Pontoriero 1995	Max	N	10	10	0.190	20	0.663
e-PTFE	Pontoriero 1995	Max	N	10	10	0.759	20	0.093
e-PTFE	Metzler 1991	Max	Y	17	17	1.172	34	0.001
e-PTFE	Pontoriero 1988	Mand	Y	21	21	1.450	42	0.000
e-PTFE	Avera 1998	Max	Y	8	8	9.115	16	0.000
Random e-PTFE (7)				86	86	0.930	172	0.025
Por coll	Flanary 1991	Mixed	Y	19	19	0.857	38	0.011
Peristeum	Lekovic 1991	Mand	Y	15	15	2.943	30	0.000
Random Other (2)				34	34	1.856	68	0.080
Random Combined (10)				132	132	1.063	264	0.001

Fig. 43-7 Forest plot of furcation defect studies examining open flap debridement (OFD) versus GTR with barrier, using HOPA gain as an outcome variable. e-PTFE = expanded polytetrafluoroethylene; Mand = mandibula; Max = maxilla. From Murphy & Gunsolley (2003) with permission from the American Academy of Periodontology.

systematic reviews used significantly different criteria for study inclusion, results did not fully overlap. Trombelli *et al.* (2002), who included only controlled studies that reported changes in clinical attachment level as the primary outcome, concluded that there was insufficient evidence to support clinical use of bone replacement graft materials in intrabony defects, since: (1) there was significant heterogeneity among included studies; (2) the size of the adjunctive effect was small; and (3) there were differences that did not allow pooling of results obtained with different materials. In the other meta-analysis for intrabony defects, 27 controlled trials with 797 intrabony defects were included (Reynolds *et al.* 2003). The application of bone replacement grafts resulted in an additional clinical attachment level gain of 0.5 mm compared to an access flap approach control (Fig. 43-8). Greater additional benefits from the application of bone replacement grafts were observed whenever hard

tissue measurements (bone fill or defect resolution) were utilized as outcome measures.

For furcation defects, the lack of consistent comparisons did not allow a meaningful assessment of the potential benefits of the use of bone replacement grafts alone (Reynolds *et al.* 2003). No large multi-center trials have provided definitive support for efficacy and/or effectiveness of the use of bone replacement grafts.

The evidence of clinical efficacy of biologically active regenerative materials has been summarized in meta-analyses only for enamel matrix derivative (Trombelli *et al.* 2002; Giannobile & Somerman 2003) and only for the application to intrabony defects. The outcomes of eight studies including 444 defects have indicated that enamel matrix derivative provides additional benefits of a magnitude of 0.75 mm in terms of clinical attachment level gains (Fig. 43-9). These data have been in accordance with those of a

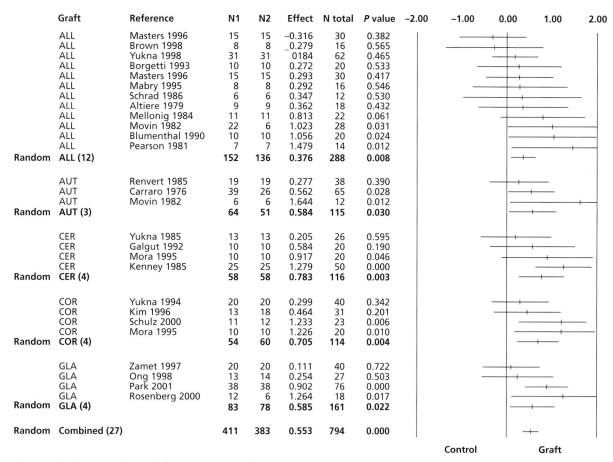

Fig. 43-8 Final meta-analysis of clinical attachment level in randomized controlled clinical studies comparing BRG to OFD in the treatment of intrabony defects. ALL = allograft; AUT = autograft; CER = calcium phosphate (hydroxyapatite) ceramic; COR = coralline calcium carbonate; GLA = bioactive glass. From Reynolds *et al.* (2003) with permission from the American Academy of Periodontology.

Fig. 43-9 Meta-analysis depicting the effectiveness of enamel matrix derivative (EMD) combined with surgery on clinical attachment level (CAL) gain as compared to control flap surgery alone. The use of EMD showed a significant improvement in CAL gain. Heterogeneity: Cohen's D, *P* = 0.04, Hedge's g, *P* = 0.16. From Giannobile & Somerman (2003) with permission from the American Academy of Periodontology.

large practice-based multi-center trial that demonstrated both efficacy and effectiveness of enamel matrix derivative in intrabony defects (Tonetti *et al.* 2002).

Patient and defect prognostic factors

The results reported in Table 43-2 indicate that clinical improvements beyond that of flap surgery can be obtained by treating intrabony defects with GTR, but

they also suggest a great variability in clinical outcomes among the different studies. In addition, it is apparent from the results that the complete resolution of the intrabony component of the defect is observed in only a minority of sites. A series of prognostic factors associated with the clinical outcomes were identified using multi-variate approaches (Tonetti *et al.* 1993a, 1995, 1996a; Cortellini *et al.* 1994; Machtei *et al.* 1994; Falk *et al.* 1997). Attention has focused on some important patient and defect factors.

Table 43-2 Clinical outcomes of GTR treatment of deep intrabony defects

Authors	Membranes	N	Gains in CAL ± SD (mm)	Residual PPD ± SD (mm)
Becker et al. 1988	e-PTFE	9	4.5 ± 1.7	3.2 ± 1.0
Chung et al. 1990	Collagen	10	0.6 ± 0.6	
Handelsman et al. 1991	e-PTFE	9	4.0 ± 1.4	3.9 ± 1.4
Kersten et al. 1992	e-PTFE	13	1.0 ± 1.1	5.1 ± 0.9
Proestakis et al. 1992	e-PTFE	9	1.2 ± 1.3	3.5 ± 0.9
Quteish & Dolby 1992	Collagen	26	3.0 ± 1.5	2.2 ± 0.4
Selvig et al. 1992	e-PTFE	26	0.8 ± 1.3	5.4
Becker & Becker 1993	e-PTFE	32	4.5	3.9 ± 0.3
Cortellini et al. 1993b	e-PTFE	40	4.1 ± 2.5	2.0 ± 0.6
Falk et al. 1993	Polylactic acid	25	4.5 ± 1.6	3.0 ± 1.1
Cortellini & Pini-Prato 1994	Rubber dam	5	4.0 ± 0.7	2.4 ± 0.5
Laurell et al. 1994	Polylactic acid	47	4.9 ± 2.4	3.0 ± 1.4
Al-Arrayed et al. 1995	Collagen	19	3.9	2.5
Chen et al. 1995	Collagen	10	2.0 ± 0.4	4.2 ± 0.4
Cortellini et al. 1995c	e-PTFE	15	4.1 ± 1.9	2.7 ± 1.0
Cortellini et al. 1995c	e-PTFE+titanium	15	5.3 ± 2.2	2.1 ± 0.5
Cortellini et al. 1995°	e-PTFE+FGG	14	5.0 ± 2.1	2.6 ± 0.9
Cortellini et al. 1995°	e-PTFE	14	3.7 ± 2.1	3.2 ± 1.8
Cortellini et al. 1995b	e-PTFE+fibrin	11	4.5 ± 3.3	1.7
Cortellini et al. 1995b	e-PTFE	11	3.3 ± 1.9	1.9
Mattson et al. 1995	Collagen	13	2.5 ± 1.5	3.6 ± 0.6
Mattson et al. 1995	Collagen	9	2.4 ± 2.1	4.0 ± 1.1
Mellado et al. 1995	e-PTFE	11	2.0 ± 0.9	
Becker et al. 1996	Polylactic acid	30	2.9 ± 2.0	3.6 ± 1.3
Cortellini et al. 1996c	Polylactic acid	10	4.5 ± 0.9	3.1 ± 0.7
Cortellini et al. 1996b	e-PTFE	12	5.2 ± 1.4	2.9 ± 0.9
Cortellini et al. 1996b	Polylactic acid	12	4.6 ± 1.2	3.3 ± 0.9
Gouldin et al. 1996	e-PTFE	25	2.2 ± 1.4	3.5 ± 1.3
Kim et al. 1996	e-PTFE	19	4.0 ± 2.1	3.2 ± 1.1
Murphy 1996	e-PTFE+ITM	12	4.7 ± 1.4	2.9 ± 0.8
Tonetti et al. 1996b	e-PTFE	23	5.3 ± 1.7	2.7
Benqué et al. 1997	Collagen	52	3.6 ± 2.2	3.9 ± 1.7
Caffesse et al. 1997	Polylactic acid	6	2.3 ± 2.0	3.8 ± 1.2
Caffesse et al. 1997	e-PTFE	6	3.0 ± 1.2	3.7 ± 1.2
Christgau et al. 1997	e-PTFE	10	4.3 ± 1.2	3.6 ± 1.1
Christgau et al. 1997	Polyglactin	10	4.9 ± 1.0	3.9 ± 1.1
Falk et al. 1997	Polylactic acid	203	4.8 ± 1.5	3.4 ± 1.6
Kilic et al. 1997	e-PTFE	10	3.7 ± 2.0	3.1 ± 1.4
Cortellini et al. 1998	Polylactic acid	23	3.0 ± 1.7	3.0 ± 0.9
Eickholz et al. 1998	Polylactic acid	14	3.4 ± 1.6	3.2 ± 0.7
Smith MacDonald et al. 1998	e-PTFE	10	4.3 ± 2.1	3.7 ± 0.9
Smith MacDonald et al. 1998	Polylactic acid	10	4.6 ± 1.7	3.4 ± 1.2
Parashis et al. 1998	Polylactic acid	12	3.8 ± 1.8	3.5 ± 1.4
Tonetti et al. 1998	Polylactic acid	69	3.0 ± 1.6	4.3 ± 1.3
Cortellini et al. 1999	Polylactic acid	18	4.9 ± 1.8	3.6 ± 1.2
Pontoriero et al. 1999	Diff. barriers	30	3.1 ± 1.8	3.3 ± 1.3
Sculean et al. 1999a	Polylactic acid	52	3.4 ± 1.4	3.6 ± 1.3
Dorfer et al. 2000	Polylactic acid	15	4.0 ± 1.2	2.7 ± 0.7
Dorfer et al. 2000	Polidiossanon	15	3.4 ± 1.9	3.1 ± 1.1
Eickholz et al. 2000	Polylactic acid	30	3.9 ± 1.2	2.6 ± 1.0
Karapataki et al. 2000	Polylactic acid	10	4.7 ± 0.7	4.2 ± 1.4
Karapataki et al. 2000	e-PTFE	9	3.6 ± 1.7	4.6 ± 1.3
Ratka-Kruger et al. 2000	Polylactic acid	23	3.1 ± 2.3	4.7 ± 1.4
Zybutz et al. 2000	Polylactic acid	15	2.4 ± 1.9	
Zubutz et al. 2000	e-PTFE	14	2.4 ± 0.8	
Cortellini & Tonetti 2001	Diff. barriers	26	5.4 ± 1.2	3.3 ± 0.6
Cortellini et al. 2001	Polylactic acid	55	3.5 ± 2.1	3.8 ± 1.5
Weighted mean		**1283**	**3.8 ± 1.7**	**3.4 ± 1.2**

FGG = free gingival graft; ITM = interproximal tissue maintenance.

Patient factors

Periodontal infection

Periodontal regeneration does not treat periodontitis, but rather is an approach for regenerating defects that have developed as a result of periodontitis. Therefore, appropriate periodontal treatment should always be completed before periodontal regeneration is initiated. In this context – i.e. in patients who underwent a cycle of cause-related periodontal therapy to the satisfaction of the treating clinician – evidence suggests that the level of control of periodontitis, achieved before a periodontal regenerative procedure is initiated, is associated with outcomes: the persistence of poor plaque control, high levels of bleeding upon probing in the dentition, as well as the persistence of high loads of total bacteria or of specific microbial pathogens (or complexes of pathogens) have all been associated in a dose-dependent manner with poor clinical outcomes (Tonetti *et al.* 1993a, 1995; Cortellini *et al.* 1994; Machtei *et al.* 1994; Heitz-Mayfield *et al.* 2006).

The level of self-performed plaque control has a great and dose-dependent effect on the outcome of periodontal regeneration. Better clinical attachment level gains were observed in patients with optimal levels of plaque control as compared with those in patients with less ideal oral hygiene (Cortellini *et al.* 1994; Tonetti *et al.* 1995, 1996a). Patients with plaque on <10% of the tooth surfaces (full mouth plaque score, FMPS) had a gain of clinical attachment which was 1.89 mm greater than that observed in patients with FMPS >20% (Tonetti *et al.* 1995).

Although not formally tested for efficacy in randomized trials, achieving high levels of plaque control and suppression of the pathogenic microflora through behavioral intervention and intensive anti-infective periodontal therapy are generally advocated before proceeding with periodontal regeneration. Furthermore, some proof of principle investigations have assessed the adjunctive effect of using an antibiotic locally delivered within the wound area or in the regenerative material (Yukna & Sepe 1982; Sanders *et al.* 1983; Stavropoulos *et al.* 2003). Results showed consistently better outcomes in the groups that received the antibiotic. At present, however, no regenerative device with enhanced antimicrobial activity is commercially available.

Smoking

A retrospective study found that cigarette smokers displayed significantly impaired regenerative outcomes compared to non-smokers (Tonetti *et al.* 1995). Data showed that cigarette smoking was associated with reduced attachment level gains. The attachment gain in subjects smoking more than ten cigarettes/day was 2.1 ± 1.2 mm versus 5.2 ± 1.9 mm observed in non-smokers (Tonetti *et al.* 1995). Thereafter a series of investigations has confirmed that cigarette smoking displays a dose-dependent detrimental effect on clinical attachment level gains.

Although no formal evidence is available, it is generally suggested that smoking cessation counseling should be initiated in the context of cause-related periodontal therapy and that patients who have been unable to quit the habit should be informed of the possibility of reduced outcomes and of the need to abstain from smoking during the peri-operative and early healing period.

Other patient factors

It has been suggested that other patient factors, such as age, genetics, systemic conditions or stress levels, may be associated with sub-optimal regenerative outcomes. In the light of the lack of evidence, however, no action is required with the exception of considering the patient characteristics that represent a contraindication to surgery (e.g. uncontrolled diabetes or unstable, severe diseases).

Clinical relevance of patient factors

The data discussed above indicates that patient factors play an important role in regenerative periodontal therapy (Fig. 43-10). Some of these factors can be modified by appropriate interventions in some patients. These interventions should be performed before periodontal regenerative therapy. Whenever modification is not possible, reduced outcomes in terms of extent and predictability should be considered.

Defect factors

Type of defect

With the currently available periodontal regenerative technologies, there is no evidence that suprabony (horizontal) defects, supracrestal components of intrabony defects or class III furcation involvements can be predictably treated with regenerative approaches. This limitation is also true for interdental craters, thus limiting the type of defects that can be treated to intrabony defects and class II furcation defects.

Morphology of the defect

Defect morphology plays a major role in healing following periodontal regenerative treatment of intrabony defects. This was demonstrated in studies showing that the depth and width of the intrabony component of the defect influence the amount of clinical attachment and bone gained at 1 year. The deeper the defect, the greater was the amount of clinical improvements, while the wider the defect, the

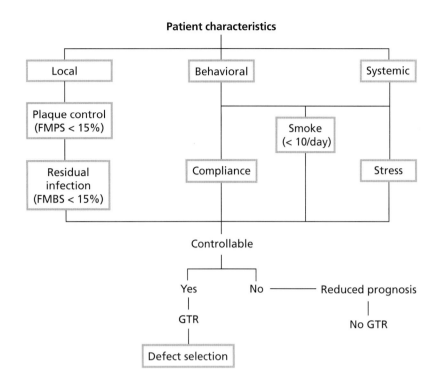

Patient characteristics

Fig. 43-10 Diagram illustrating patient selection criteria. It can be seen that control of local, behavioral, and systemic patient characteristics may improve the treatment outcomes. FMPS = full mouth plaque score; FMBS = full mouth bleeding score. Modified from Cortellini & Bowers (1995).

lower were the attachment and bone gains (Garrett *et al.* 1988; Tonetti *et al.* 1993a, 1996a).

In a controlled study, however, it was demonstrated that deep and shallow defects have the "same potential" for regeneration. In this study, deep defects (deeper than 3 mm) resulted in larger linear amounts of CAL gains than shallow defects (3.7 ± 1.7 mm versus 2.2 ± 1.3 mm), but the percentage of CAL gains as related to baseline defect depth was similar in deep (76.7 ± 27.7%) and in shallow (75.8 ± 45%) defects. The width of the intrabony component of the defects is measured as the angle that the bony wall of the defect forms with the long axis of the tooth. In a study on 242 intrabony defects treated with membranes, Cortellini and Tonetti (1999) demonstrated that defects with a radiographic angle of 25° or less gained consistently more attachment (1.6 mm on average) than defects of 37° or more.

Two recent follow-up studies have addressed the significance of the baseline radiographic angle of the intrabony defect following the use of either enamel matrix derivative (Tsitoura *et al.* 2004) or of a combination of bone replacement graft with a barrier membrane (Linares *et al.* 2006). The impact of the width of the baseline radiographic angle was confirmed for the non-space-making biological mediator but not for the more stable combination therapy. These data are consistent with the notion that choice of the regenerative technology may partially overcome negative morphologic characteristics of intrabony defects. An earlier secondary analysis of a controlled clinical trial using titanium-reinforced membranes (Tonetti *et al.* 1996a) indicated that the relevance of defect morphology parameters may be diminished with the use of supported membranes.

It was also shown that the number of residual bony walls was related to the outcomes of various regenerative approaches (Goldman & Cohen 1958; Schallhorn *et al.* 1970). This issue as related to GTR therapy was addressed in three investigations (Selvig *et al.* 1993; Tonetti *et al.* 1993a, 1996a). In one study, the reported 1-year mean clinical attachment level gain was 0.8 ± 1.3 mm. This gain corresponded to the depth of the three-wall intrabony component of the defect (Selvig *et al.* 1993). In the other two investigations, on the contrary, gains in attachment were not related to the defect configuration in terms of one-wall, two-wall, and three-wall subcomponents (Tonetti *et al.* 1993a, 1996a). A total of 70 defects were examined in these two latter studies, utilizing a multi-variate approach. The treatment resulted in mean attachment gains of 4.1 ± 2.5 mm and 5.3 ± 2.2 mm, and it was observed that the most coronal portion of the defects which is most susceptible to negative influences from the oral environment were often incompletely filled with bone, irrespective of whether these were one-wall, two-wall or three-wall defects. Thus, these studies questioned the impact of the number of residual bony walls of the defect on the clinical outcomes of periodontal regeneration with membranes and suggested that location of the one-wall subcomponent (the one most likely to be the most superficial one) may have acted as confounder in other studies and be an important predictor of the outcomes.

Tooth factors

The endodontic status of the tooth has been suggested as a potential relevant factor in periodontal therapy. Emerging evidence (see Chapter 40) indicates that root canal treated teeth may respond differently to periodontal therapy. A clinical study on 208 consecutive patients with one intrabony defect each demonstrated that properly performed root canal treatment does not negatively affect the healing response and the long-term stability of results of deep intrabony defects treated with membranes (Cortellini & Tonetti 2000b).

Tooth mobility has long been considered an important factor for periodontal regeneration (Sanders *et al.* 1983). Recently, a multi-variate analysis of a multi-center controlled clinical trial demonstrated that tooth hypermobility was negatively and dose-dependently associated with the clinical outcomes of regeneration (Cortellini *et al.* 2001). Though significant, the size of the effect was small within the range of physiologic mobility. Another recent secondary analysis of three previously reported trials assessed the regenerative outcomes of hypermobile teeth (Trejo & Weltman 2004). This report indicated that teeth with baseline mobility amounting to less than 1 mm horizontally could be successfully treated by periodontal regeneration. Although no intervention trial has been performed to date, these results are generally considered supportive of an approach that does not set the prognosis of the tooth or the regenerative procedure based on tooth mobility but rather considers splinting hypermobile teeth before periodontal regenerative surgery.

Based on these results, it can be concluded that deep and narrow intrabony defects at either vital or endodontically treated teeth are the ones in which the most significant and predictable outcomes can be achieved by GTR treatment. Severe, uncontrolled dental hypermobility (Miller class II or higher) may impair the regenerative outcomes.

Factors affecting the clinical outcomes of GTR in furcations

Significant evidence has demonstrated that treatment of maxillary degree II furcations and maxillary and mandibular degree III furcation involvements with GTR is unpredictable, while clinical improvements can be expected treating mandibular degree II furcations. The great variability in clinical outcomes, following treatment of mandibular degree II furcations with GTR, is probably related to the factors discussed relative to intrabony defects.

Regarding defect factors, it was shown that first and second mandibular molars and buccal and lingual furcations respond equally well to GTR treatment (Pontoriero *et al.* 1988; Machtei *et al.* 1994). It was also demonstrated that the pre-operative horizontal pocket depth is directly correlated with the magnitude of attachment gain and bone formation in the furcation area (Machtei *et al.* 1993, 1994). The deeper the baseline horizontal pocket, the greater was the H-CAL and bone gain. The anatomy of the

furcations in terms of height, width, depth, and volume, however, did not correlate with the clinical outcome (Machtei *et al.* 1994). Anderegg *et al.* (1995) demonstrated that sites with a gingival thickness of >1 mm exhibited less gingival recession post surgery than sites with a gingival thickness of <1 mm. The authors concluded that the thickness of the gingival tissue covering a barrier material must be considered if post-treatment recession is to be minimized or avoided.

The relevance of the surgical approach

At the beginning of the 1980s the need to modify standard periodontal surgical procedures to favor periodontal regeneration became apparent. In particular, the need to preserve soft tissues in order to attempt primary closure of the interdental space to contain grafts or coronally advanced flaps to cover furcation entrances led to the development of specific flap designs for periodontal regeneration (Takei *et al.* 1985; Gantes & Garret 1991).

In fact, graft exfoliation and membrane exposure with consequent bacterial contamination during healing represented the major complications of periodontal regenerative procedures at the time. Membrane exposure was reported to be a major complication with prevalence in the range of 50–100% (Becker *et al.* 1988; Cortellini *et al.* 1990, 1993b; Selvig *et al.* 1992, 1993; Murphy 1995a; DeSanctis *et al.* 1996a,b; Falk *et al.* 1997; Trombelli *et al.* 1997; Mayfield *et al.* 1998). Cortellini *et al.* (1995c,d) reported that the prevalence of membrane exposure could be greatly reduced with the use of access flaps, specifically designed to preserve the interdental tissues (modified papilla preservation technique) (Fig. 43-11).

Many studies have shown that the exposed membranes are contaminated with bacteria (Selvig *et al.* 1990, 1992; Grevstad & Leknes 1992; Machtei *et al.* 1993; Mombelli *et al.* 1993; Tempro & Nalbandian 1993; Nowzari & Slots 1994; Novaes *et al.* 1995; Nowzari *et al.* 1995; DeSanctis *et al.* 1996a,b). Contamination of exposed non-bioabsorbable as well as bioabsorbable membranes was associated with lower probing attachment level gains in intrabony defects (Selvig *et al.* 1992; Nowzari & Slots 1994; Nowzari *et al.* 1995; DeSanctis *et al.* 1996a,b). The impaired clinical results in some studies were associated with high counts of bacteria and with the presence of *P. gingivalis* and *A. actinomycetemcomitans* (Machtei *et al.* 1994; Nowzari & Slots 1994; Nowzari *et al.* 1995).

Bacterial contamination of the membrane may occur during surgery, but also during the post-operative healing phase. After placement, bacteria from the oral cavity may colonize the coronal part of the membrane. Frequently, this results in recession of the gingival tissues, which allows colonization of the membrane material further apically. In addition,

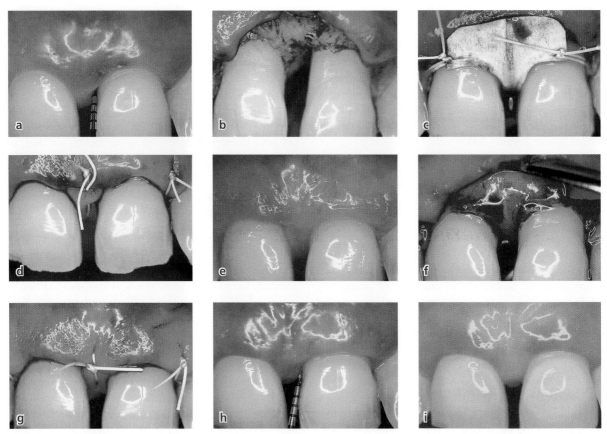

Fig. 43-11 (a) Left maxillary central incisor with a 10-mm pocket depth and 11 mm of clinical attachment loss on the mesial surface. A diastema is present between the two central incisors. (b) Full thickness buccal and palatal flaps have been raised and an intrabony defect can be seen. The interdental papilla has been incised on the buccal aspect and elevated with the palatal flap (modified papilla preservation technique). (c) A titanium-reinforced e-PTFE barrier membrane has been placed and fixed close to the level of the cemento-enamel junction. (d) The membrane is completely covered. This primary closure has been obtained by preserving the interdental papilla and by coronal displacement of the buccal tissue flap. (e) At 6 weeks, the membrane is completely covered with healthy tissue. (f) After membrane removal at 6 weeks, dense newly formed tissue is evident in the defect and in the supracrestal space maintained by the titanium-reinforced membrane. (g) The newly formed tissue is completely covered by the raised and well preserved tissue flaps. (h) The photograph after 1 year shows a 4 mm residual pocket depth. A gain of clinical attachment of 6 mm was recorded, and no recession has occurred compared to baseline. (i) Ten year photograph showing the optimal preservation of the interdental tissues.

"pocket" formation may occur on the outer surface of the membrane due to apical migration of the epithelium on the inner surface of the covering gingival tissue. This may allow bacteria from the oral cavity to colonize the subgingival area. The significance of bacterial contamination was addressed in an investigation in monkeys (Sander & Karring 1995). The findings of this study showed that new attachment and bone formation occurred consistently when bacteria were prevented from invading the membrane and the wound during healing.

In order to prevent wound infection, some investigators have administered systemic antibiotics to patients before and during the first weeks after membrane application (Demolon *et al.* 1993; Nowzari & Slots 1994). However, despite the application of systemic antibiotics, occurrence of post-operative wound infection related to implanted barrier membranes was noticed. This indicates that either the drug administered is not directed against the microorganisms responsible for the wound infection, or that the drug does not reach the infected site at a concentra-

tion sufficiently high to inhibit the target microorganisms. An improved effect on periodontal healing after GTR in association with local application of metronidazole was reported by Sander *et al.* (1994). Twelve patients with one pair of intrabony defects participated in the study. Metronidazole in a gel form was placed in the defects and on the membrane prior to wound closure, while the controls were treated with a membrane alone. Six months following membrane removal the medium gain in probing attachment level, presented as a percentage of the initial defect depth, was 92% for test defects versus 50% for the control defects. Other clinical parameters, like plaque index, bleeding on probing, pocket depth reduction or recession of the gingival margin, were similar in the test and control sites. Although the use of local or systemic antibiotics may reduce the bacterial load on exposed membranes, it seems ineffective in preventing the formation of a microbial biofilm (Frandsen *et al.* 1994; Nowzari *et al.* 1995). Apart from the erythema and swelling related to such infection of the wound, more severe post-operative complications such as suppuration, sloughing or perforation of the flap, membrane exfoliation, and post-operative pain have been reported (Murphy 1995a,b).

Another important issue associated with the clinical results is the coverage of the regenerated tissue after removal of a non-bioabsorbable membrane. Many authors have reported that the frequent occurrence of a gingival dehiscence over the membrane is likely to result in insufficient protection of the interdental regenerated tissue (Becker *et al.* 1988; Selvig *et al.* 1992; Cortellini *et al.* 1993b; Tonetti *et al.* 1993a). Exposure of the regenerated tissue to the oral environment entails the risks of mechanical and infectious insults that in turn may prevent complete maturation of the regenerated tissue into a new connective tissue attachment. In fact, incomplete coverage of the regenerated tissue was associated with

reduced attachment and bone gain at 1 year (Tonetti *et al.* 1993a). Recently, the positioning of a saddle-shaped free gingival graft over the regenerated interdental tissue (Fig. 43-12) was suggested to offer better coverage and protection than a dehiscent gingival flap (Cortellini *et al.* 1995a). In this randomized controlled study, more gain of attachment was observed in the 14 sites where a free gingival graft was positioned after membrane removal (5.0 ± 2.1 mm), than in the 14 sites where conventional protection of the regenerated tissue was accomplished (3.7 ± 2.1 mm).

The systematic assessment of the relevant factors associated with variability of periodontal regenerative outcomes performed at the beginning of the 1990s (Tonetti *et al.* 1993a, 1995, 1996a; Machtei *et al.* 1994; Falk *et al.* 1997) provided further evidence that

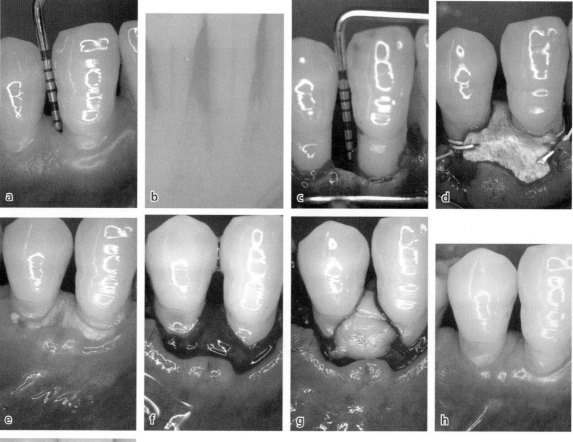

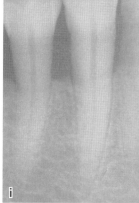

Fig. 43-12 Clinical case illustrating the management of the most common complication following application of non-resorbable barrier membrane: membrane exposure and consequent loss of interdental soft tissue. Upon completion of cause-related periodontal therapy, regenerative periodontal surgery was performed to resolve a deep pocket associated with a deep intrabony defect (a,b). The 7-mm intrabony defect was accessed with a modified papilla preservation flap (c) and a non-resorbable barrier membrane was placed (d). Primary closure with multilayered sutures was obtained, but 5 weeks after surgery, the membrane became exposed to the oral cavity (e). Upon membrane removal (f), a newly regenerated tissue completely filled the space below the membrane but inadequate amounts of soft tissue were available to completely cover the regenerated tissue in the interdental space. In order to protect the maturation of this tissue, a saddle-shaped interdental free gingival graft was harvested from the palate and shaped to precisely fit the interdental area (g). The graft healed well on the highly vascularized recipient bed and allowed good healing of the interdental tissues. Six years after completion of therapy, the clinical and radiographic outcomes show healing with shallow probing depths and elimination of the defect (h,i).

surgical factors had a great impact on regeneration and led the way to the development of procedures specifically designed for periodontal regeneration.

In general the development of new procedures was aimed at complete tissue preservation of the marginal tissue in order to achieve and maintain primary closure on top of the applied regenerative material during the critical stages of healing. Specifically, flap designs attempted to achieve passive primary closure of the flap combined with optimal wound stability.

Papilla preservation flaps

The modified papilla preservation technique (MPPT) was developed in order to increase the space for regeneration, and in order to achieve and maintain primary closure of the flap in the interdental area (Cortellini *et al.* 1995c,d). This approach combines special soft tissue management with use of a self-supporting titanium-reinforced membrane capable of maintaining a supra-alveolar space for regeneration. The MPPT allows primary closure of the interdental space, resulting in better protection of the membrane from the oral environment (Cortellini *et al.* 1995d). The technique involves the elevation of a full-thickness palatal flap which includes the entire interdental papilla. The buccal flap is mobilized with vertical and periosteal incisions, coronally positioned to cover the membrane, and sutured to the palatal flap through a horizontal internal crossed mattress suture over the membrane. A second internal mattress suture warrants primary closure between the flap and the interdental papilla. A representative case is shown in Figs. 43-4 and 43-11. In a randomized controlled clinical study on 45 patients (Cortellini *et al.* 1995c), significantly greater amounts of attachment gain were obtained with the MPPT (5.3 ± 2.2 mm), in comparison with either conventional GTR (4.1 ± 1.9 mm) or flap surgery (2.5 ± 0.8 mm), demonstrating that a modified surgical approach can result in improved clinical outcomes.

In this study 100% of the sites were closed on top of a titanium-reinforced membrane and 73% remained closed for up to 6 weeks, when the barrier membrane was removed. This study provided proof of principle of the benefit of specific flap designs for periodontal regeneration.

A recent meta-analysis (Murphy & Gunsolley 2003) showed the existence of a trend associating better clinical outcomes in studies using flap designs and closing techniques considered conducive to the achievement and maintenance of primary closure of the flap (Figs. 43-13, 43-14). The reported procedure can be successfully applied in sites where the interdental space width is at least 2 mm at the most coronal portion of the papilla.

When interdental sites are narrower, the reported technique is difficult to apply. In order to overcome this problem, a different papilla preservation proce-

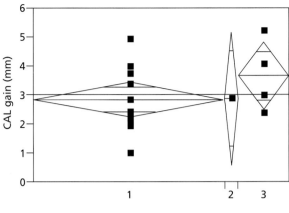

Ranks	Number of studies	Mean (mm)
1	15	2.84
2	1	2.90
3	4	3.68

Fig. 43-13 Means of intrabony defect studies examining the relationship between flap closure technique ranking and the gain in clinical attachment level (CAL) (in mm) considering only e-PTFE barrier types. Groupings were not statistically different from one another. From Murphy & Gunsolley (2003) with permission from the American Academy of Periodontology.

dure (the simplified papilla preservation flap) has been proposed for narrower interdental spaces (Cortellini *et al.* 1999). This approach includes an oblique incision across the defect-associated papilla, starting from the buccal angle of the defect-associated tooth to reach the mid-interdental part of the papilla at the adjacent tooth under the contact point. In this way, the papilla is cut into two equal parts of which the buccal is elevated with the buccal flap and the lingual with the lingual flap. In the cited study, 100% of the narrow interdental papillae could be closed on top of bioresorbable barriers, and 67% maintained primary closure over time, resulting in 4.9 ± 1.8 mm of clinical attachment level gains. This approach has been successfully applied in different multi-center randomized clinical trials designed to test the generalizability of the added benefits of using barrier membranes on deep intrabony defects (Tonetti *et al.* 1998; Cortellini *et al.* 2001).

In the cited studies, GTR therapy of deep intrabony defects performed by different clinicians on various patient populations resulted in both greater amounts and improved predictability of CAL gains than access flap alone. The issue of soft tissue manipulation to obtain stable protection of the regeneration site has been further explored, applying a microsurgical approach in the regenerative therapy of deep intrabony defects (Fig. 43-15). In a patient cohort study on 26 patients with 26 intrabony defects treated with papilla preservation techniques, primary closure on the barrier was obtained in 100% of the cases and maintained over time in 92.3% of the sites (Cortellini & Tonetti 2001). Treatment resulted in large amounts of CAL gains (5.4 ± 1.2 mm) and minimal gingival

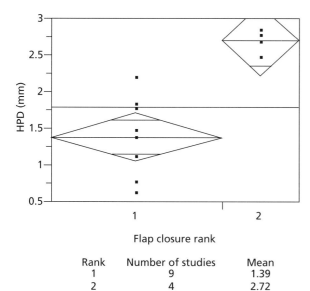

	Difference	*t* test	DF	Prob > |t|
Estimate	−1.3319	−7.014	10.538	< 0.0001
Std error	0.1899			
Lower 95%	−1.9277			
Upper 95%	−0.7361			

Rank	Number of studies	Mean
1	9	1.39
2	4	2.72

Fig. 43-14 Regression analysis of furcation defect studies examining the relationship between flap closure technique ranking and the reduction (in mm) in horizontal probing depth (HPD). Groups 1 and 2 are statistically different from one another. From Murphy & Gunsolley (2003) with permission from the American Academy of Periodontology.

recession (0.4 ± 0.7 mm). Thus, the improved vision and better soft tissue handling improved the predictability of periodontal regeneration.

Today, the use of papilla preservation flap designs and closure techniques has become the standard approach for regenerative periodontal surgery.

Modified papilla preservation technique

The rationale for developing this technique was to achieve and maintain primary closure of the flap in the interdental space over the membrane (Cortellini *et al.* 1995d) (Figs. 43-16 to 43-18). Access to the interdental defect consists of a horizontal incision traced in the buccal keratinized gingiva at the base of the papilla, connected with mesio-distal buccal intrasulcular incisions. After elevation of a full-thickness buccal flap, the residual interdental tissues are dissected from the neighboring teeth and the underlying bone and elevated towards the palatal aspect. A full-thickness palatal flap, including the interdental papilla, is elevated and the interdental defect exposed. Following debridement of the defect, the buccal flap is mobilized with vertical and periosteal incisions, when needed.

This technique was originally designed for use in combination with self-supporting barrier membranes. In fact, the suturing technique requires a supportive (or supported) membrane to be effective (Figs. 43-16, 43-17). To obtain primary closure of the interdental space over the membrane, a first suture (horizontal internal crossed mattress suture) is placed beneath the mucoperiosteal flaps between the base of the palatal papilla and the buccal flap. The interdental portion of this suture hangs on top of the membrane allowing the coronal displacement of the buccal flap. This suture relieves all the tension of the flaps. To

ensure primary passive closure of the interdental tissues over the membrane, a second suture (vertical internal mattress suture) is placed between the buccal aspect of the interdental papilla (i.e. the most coronal portion of the palatal flap which includes the interdental papilla) and the most coronal portion of the buccal flap. This suture is free of tension.

An alternative type of suture to close the interdental tissues has been proposed by Dr Lars Laurell. This modified internal mattress suture (see Fig. 38-56) starts from the external surface of the buccal flap, crosses the interdental area and gets through the lingual flap at the base of the papilla. The suture runs back through the external surface of the lingual flap and the internal surface of the buccal flap, about 3 mm apart from the first two bites. Finally, the suture is passed through the interdental area above the papillary tissues, passed through the loop of the suture on the lingual side, and brought back to the buccal side, where it is tied. This suture is very effective in ensuring stability and primary closure of the interdental tissues.

In a randomized controlled clinical study on 45 patients (Cortellini *et al.* 1995c), significantly greater amounts of PAL were gained with the MPPT (5.3 ± 2.2 mm), in comparison with either conventional GTR (4.1 ± 1.9 mm) or access flap surgery (2.5 ± 0.8 mm), demonstrating that a modified surgical approach can result in improved clinical outcomes. The sites accessed with the MPPT showed primary closure of the flap in all but one case, and no gingival dehiscence until membrane removal, in 73% of the cases.

This surgical approach has also been used in combination with non-supported bioresorbable barrier membranes (Cortellini *et al.* 1996c), with positive results. Clinical attachment level gains at 1 year were

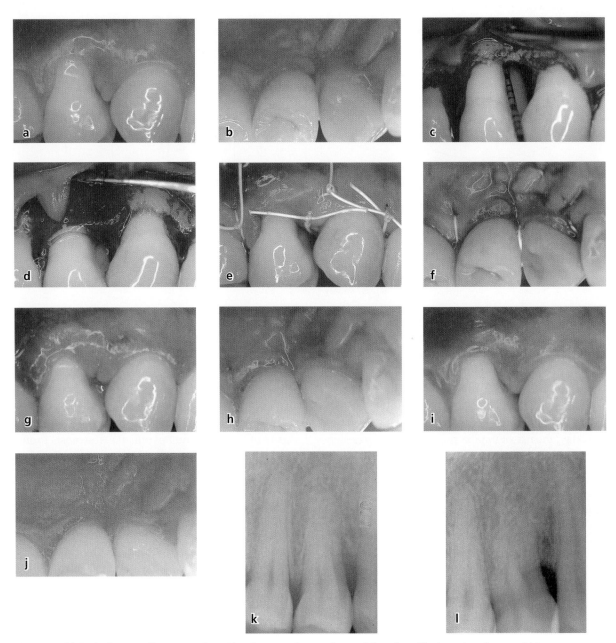

Fig. 43-15 (a) Right first maxillary premolar with a 7-mm pocket on the mesial surface. The interdental space (b) is very narrow (>2 mm), and is accessed with a simplified papilla preservation flap. The 5-mm deep intrabony defect (c) is covered with a bioresorbable barrier membrane (d). Primary closure of the flap over the membrane (e,f) is maintained over time (g,h). After 1 year, the interdental papilla is completely preserved and the residual pocket depth is 3 mm (i,j). The radiograph taken at baseline (k) compared with that taken 1 year after treatment (l) shows that the intrabony defect has healed completely.

4.5 ± 1.2 mm. In all the cases primary closure of the flap was achieved and about 80% of the sites maintained primary closure over time (Fig. 43-19). It should be underlined, however, that the horizontal internal crossed mattress suture most probably caused an apical displacement of the interdental portion of the membrane, thereby reducing the space for regeneration.

The MPPT can be successfully applied in conjunction with a variety of regenerative materials including biologically active materials such as enamel matrix derivative (EMD) (Tonetti *et al.* 2002) (Fig. 43-20) or growth factors and bone replacement grafts

(Fig. 43-21) (Tonetti *et al.* 2004b; Cortellini & Tonetti 2005).

The surgical access of the interdental space with the MPPT is technically very demanding, but it has been reported to be very effective and applicable in wide interdental spaces (wider than 2 mm at interdental tissue level), especially in the anterior dentition. In properly selected cases, large amounts of attachment gain, and consistent reduction of pocket depths associated with no or minimal recession of the interdental papilla are consistently expected. It is, therefore, indicated in cases in which esthetics are particularly important.

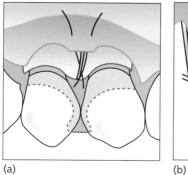 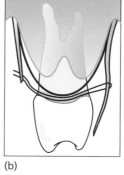 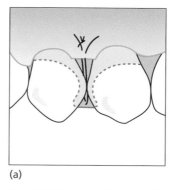 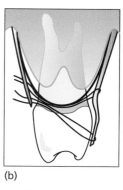

Fig. 43-16 Suture to obtain coronal positioning of the buccal flap: schematic illustration of the crossed horizontal internal mattress suture between the base of the palatal papilla and the buccal flap immediately coronal to the muco-gingival junction. Note that the suture crosses above the titanium reinforcement of the membrane. (a) Buccal view; (b) mesio-distal view. From Cortellini *et al.* (1995d) with permission from the American Academy of Periodontology.

Fig. 43-17 Suture to obtain tension-free primary closure of the interdental space: schematic illustration of the vertical internal mattress suture between the most coronal portion of the palatal flap (which includes the interdental papilla) and the most coronal portion of the buccal flap. (a) Buccal view; (b) mesio-distal view. From Cortellini *et al.* (1995d) with permission from the American Academy of Periodontology.

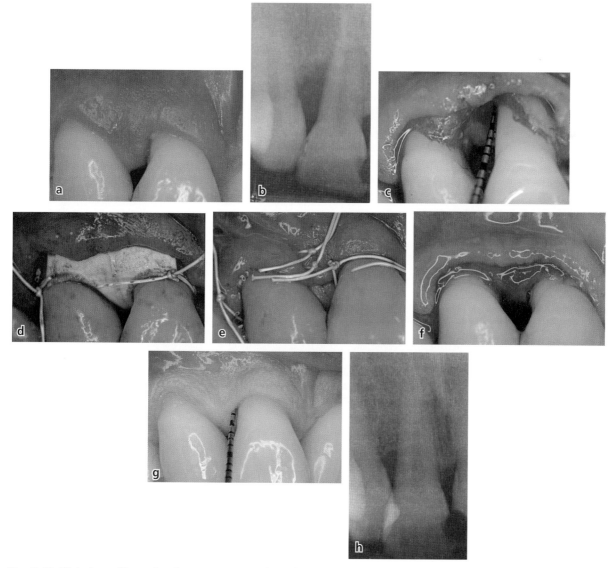

Fig. 43-18 Clinical case illustrating the operative procedure of the modified papilla preservation technique used to completely close the interdental space above a barrier membrane. Following completion of initial cause-related therapy, an 8-mm pocket associated with 2 mm of recession of the gingival margin was present on the distal of the central incisor (a). A wide intrabony defect was detectable on the radiograph (b). The defect was accessed with the modified papilla preservation technique keeping the whole interdental tissue connected with the palatal flap. A 7-mm intrabony defect was uncovered (c). Following root debridement, a titanium-reinforced barrier membrane was positioned (d). Primary closure of the interdental space was obtained by suturing back the papilla preservation flap using a multilayered suturing technique aimed at coronal advancement of the flap, complete relief of wound tension, and good flap stability (e). Six weeks thereafter, the same flap was elevated in order to remove the membrane that had remained completely submerged for the whole time. New tissue formed below the membrane was obtained with a shape that filled the space maintained under the membrane (f). Following completion of healing (1 year) a 3-mm probing depth and fill of the intrabony defect were observed. The results were maintained over time as indicated by the clinical and radiographic appearance 6 years after regeneration (g,h).

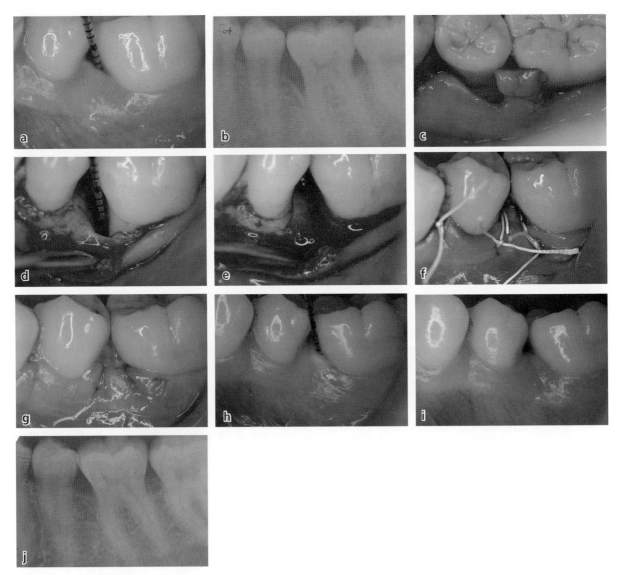

Fig. 43-19 Clinical case illustrating the application of the modified papilla preservation technique to a case treated with a resorbable barrier membrane. An 8-mm pocket associated with an intrabony defect persisted on the mesial aspect of the lower first molar following completion of initial cause-related therapy (a,b). The defect was accessed with the modified papilla preservation flap. Please note the papilla preserved attached to the lingual flap (c) as well as the presence of a 7-mm intrabony defect (d). Following root debridement, a bioresorbable barrier membrane was positioned and secured around the root of the tooth with bioresorbable sutures (e). Primary closure of the interdental space was obtained with multilayered sutures (f) and was fully maintained at the 1-week suture removal appointment (g). At 6 years, probing depths were 2–3 mm, the soft tissue profile was conducive to optimal self-performed oral hygiene measures and the radiograph showed elimination of the defect (h–j).

Simplified papilla preservation flap

To overcome some of the technical problems encountered with the MPPT (difficult application in narrow interdental spaces and in posterior areas, suturing technique not appropriate for use with non-supportive barriers) a different approach (simplified papilla preservation flap, SPPF) (Figs. 43-15, 43-22) was subsequently developed (Cortellini *et al*. 1999).

This different and simplified approach to the interdental papilla includes a first incision across the defect-associated papilla, starting from the gingival margin at the buccal-line angle of the involved tooth to reach the mid-interdental portion of the papilla under the contact point of the adjacent tooth. This

oblique incision is carried out keeping the blade parallel to the long axis of the teeth in order to avoid excessive thinning of the remaining interdental tissues. The first oblique interdental incision is continued intrasulcularly in the buccal aspect of the teeth neighboring the defect. After elevation of a full-thickness buccal flap, the remaining tissues of the papilla are carefully dissected from the neighboring teeth and the underlying bone crest. The interdental papillary tissues at the defect site are gently elevated along with the lingual/palatal flap to fully expose the interdental defect. Following defect debridement and root planing, vertical releasing incisions and/or periosteal incisions are performed, when needed, to improve the mobility of the buccal flap. After

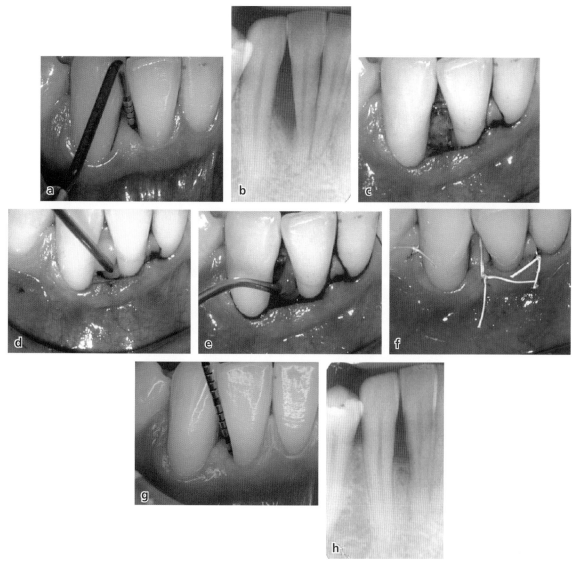

Fig. 43-20 Clinical case illustrating the application of the papilla preservation technique in conjunction with the application of enamel matrix derivative in gel form. A 10-mm pocket was detectable on the distal aspect of the lower lateral incisor following successful completion of initial cause-related therapy (a). The radiograph showed the presence of a deep intrabony defect extending to the apical third of the root (b). The defect was accessed with the modified papilla preservation technique (c) with limited mesial and distal extension of the flap. Following careful debridement, the root is conditioned with an EDTA gel according to the manufacturer's instructions for the application of enamel matrix derivative (d). After rinsing and drying of the defect and root surface, the enamel matrix derivative gel is applied on the root surface and to fill the defect (e), and flaps are sutured with a multilayer technique to achieve primary closure in the absence of tension (f). One year following regenerative surgery, shallow pockets and radiographic resolution of the defect are apparent (g,h).

application of a barrier membrane, primary closure of the interdental tissues above the membrane is attempted in the absence of tension, with the following sutures:

1. A first horizontal internal mattress suture (offset mattress suture) is positioned in the defect-associated interdental space running from the base (near to the mucogingival junction) of the keratinized tissue at the mid-buccal aspect of the tooth not involved with the defect to a symmetrical location at the base of the lingual/palatal flap. This suture frictions against the interdental root surface, hangs on the residual interdental bone crest and is anchored to the lingual/palatal flap. When tied, it

allows the coronal positioning of the buccal flap. A relevant notation is that this suture, lying on the interdental bone crest, does not cause any compression at the mid-portion of the membrane, therefore preventing its collapse into the defect.

2. The interdental tissues above the membrane are then sutured to obtain primary closure with one of the following approaches: (a) one interrupted suture whenever the interdental space is narrow and the interdental tissues thin; (b) two interrupted sutures, when the interdental space is wider and the interdental tissues thicker; (c) an internal vertical/oblique mattress suture, when the interdental space is wide and the interdental tissues are thick.

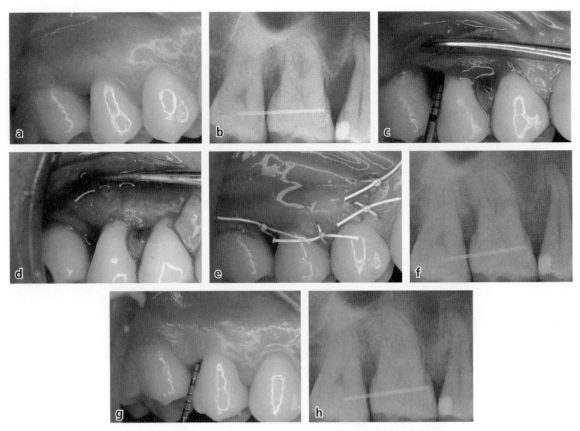

Fig. 43-21 Clinical case illustrating the application of the modified papilla preservation technique in conjunction with a bone replacement graft in combination with a bioresorbable membrane. After completion of initial cause-related therapy, a 9-mm pocket associated with an intrabony defect was present on the distal aspect of the upper second premolar (a,b). The defect reached the apical portion of the root and had a 9-mm intrabony component (c). Following careful root debridement, a bioresorbable membrane was adapted to the local anatomy and was positioned to contain the defect. A bone replacement graft was subsequently inserted under the membrane to provide additional support for the membrane and for the soft tissues (d). Primary closure was achieved with a single internal mattress suture (e). The control radiograph taken upon completion of the surgery shows the presence of the radio-opaque bone replacement graft in the defect (f). At 1-year follow-up, a 3-mm probing depth associated with resolution of the intrabony component of the defect is apparent (g,h). Please note that the radio-opaque bone replacement graft particles are still detectable but appear embedded in newly formed mineralized tissue.

Special care has to be paid to ensure that the first horizontal mattress suture would relieve all the tension of the flaps, and to obtain primary passive closure of the interdental tissues over the membrane with the last suture. When tension is observed, the sutures should be removed and the primary passive closure attempted a second time.

This approach has been preliminarily tested in a case series of 18 deep intrabony defects in combination with bioresorbable barrier membranes (Cortellini *et al*. 1999). The average clinical attachment level gain observed at 1 year was 4.9 ± 1.8 mm. In all the cases it was possible to obtain primary closure of the flap over the membrane, and 67% of the sites maintained primary closure over time. The same approach was then tested in a multi-center controlled randomized clinical trial involving 11 clinicians from seven different countries and a total of 136 defects (Tonetti *et al*. 1998). The average clinical attachment gain observed at 1 year in the 69 defects treated with the SPPF and a resorbable barrier membrane was 3 ± 1.6 mm. More than 60% of the treated sites maintained primary closure over time. It is important to

underline that these results were obtained by different clinicians treating different populations of patients and defects, also involving narrow spaces and posterior areas of the mouth. The SPPF was successfully applied in conjunction with a variety of regenerative materials including biologically active materials such as EMD (Tonetti *et al*. 2002) (Fig. 43-23) and bone replacement grafts (Fig. 43-24) (Tonetti *et al*. 2004b; Cortellini & Tonetti 2004).

Minimally invasive surgical technique

In order to provide even greater wound stability and to further limit patient morbidity, a papilla preservation flap can be used in the context of a minimally invasive, high-power magnification-assisted surgical technique (Cortellini & Tonetti 2007a). Such a minimally invasive approach is particularly suited for treatment in conjunction with biologically active agents such as EMD or growth factors.

The defect-associated interdental papilla is accessed either with the simplified papilla preservation flap (SPPF) (Cortellini *et al*. 1999) or the modified

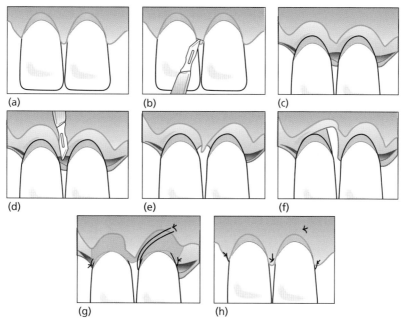

Fig. 43-22 (a) Pre-surgical appearance of the area that will be accessed with a simplified papilla preservation flap (SPPF). The defect is located on the mesial aspect of the maxillary right lateral incisor. (b) First oblique incision in the defect-associated papilla begins at the gingival margin of the mesio-buccal line angle of the lateral incisor. The blade is kept parallel to the long axis of the tooth and reaches the midpoint of the distal surface of the central incisor just below the contact point. (c) First oblique incision continues intrasulcularly in the buccal aspect of the lateral and central incisors, extending until the adjacent papillae, and a buccal full-thickness flap is elevated to expose 2–3 mm of bone. Note the defect-associated papilla still in place. (d) Bucco-lingual horizontal incision at the base of the papilla is as close as possible to the interproximal bone crest. Care is taken to avoid a lingual/palatal perforation. (e) Intrasulcular interdental incisions continue in the palatal aspect of the incisors until the adjacent partially dissected papillae. A full-thickness palatal flap including the interdental papilla is elevated. (f) Intrabony defect following debridement. Note the position of the bone crest on the distal aspect of the central incisor. (g) Membrane is positioned to cover the defect and 2–3 mm of remaining bone and secured to neighboring teeth. A horizontal internal mattress suture runs from the base of the keratinized tissue at the midbuccal side of the central incisor to a symmetric location at the base of the palatal flap. This suture causes no direct compression of the midportion of the membrane, preventing its collapse into the defect. (h) Primary closure and complete coverage of the membrane are obtained. From Cortellini *et al.* (1999) with permission from Quintessence Publishing Co. Inc.

papilla preservation technique (MPPT) (Cortellini *et al.* 1995d). The SPPF is performed whenever the width of the interdental space is 2 mm or narrower, while the MPPT is applied at interdental sites wider than 2 mm. The interdental incision (SPPF or MPPT) is extended to the buccal and lingual aspects of the two teeth adjacent to the defect. These incisions are strictly intrasulcular to preserve all the height and width of the gingiva, and their mesio-distal extension is kept at a minimum to allow the corono-apical elevation of a very small full-thickness flap with the objective of exposing just 1–2 mm of the defect-associated residual bone crest. When possible, only the defect-associated papilla is accessed and vertical releasing incisions are avoided. With these general rules in mind, different clinical pictures can be encountered in different defects.

The shortest mesio-distal extension of the incision and the minimal flap reflection occurs when the intrabony defect is a pure three-wall, or has shallow two- and/or one-wall subcomponents allocated entirely in the interdental area. In these instances the mesio-distal incision involves only the defect-associated papilla and part of the buccal and lingual aspects

of the two teeth neighboring the defect. The full-thickness flap is elevated minimally, just to expose the buccal and lingual bone crest delineating the defect in the interdental area (Fig. 43-25).

A larger corono-apical elevation of the full-thickness flap is necessary when the coronal portion of the intrabony defect has a deep two-wall component. The corono-apical extension of the flap is kept to a minimum at the aspect where the bony wall is preserved (either buccal or lingual), and extends more apically at the site where the bony wall is missing (lingual or buccal), the objective being to reach and expose 1–2 mm of the residual bone crest (Fig. 43-26).

When a deep one-wall defect is approached, the full-thickness flap is elevated to the same extent on both the buccal and the lingual aspects.

When the position of the residual buccal/lingual bony wall(s) is very deep and difficult or impossible to reach with the above described minimal incision of the defect-associated interdental space, the flap(s) is(are) further extended mesially or distally involving one extra interdental space to obtain a larger flap reflection. The same approach is used when the bony

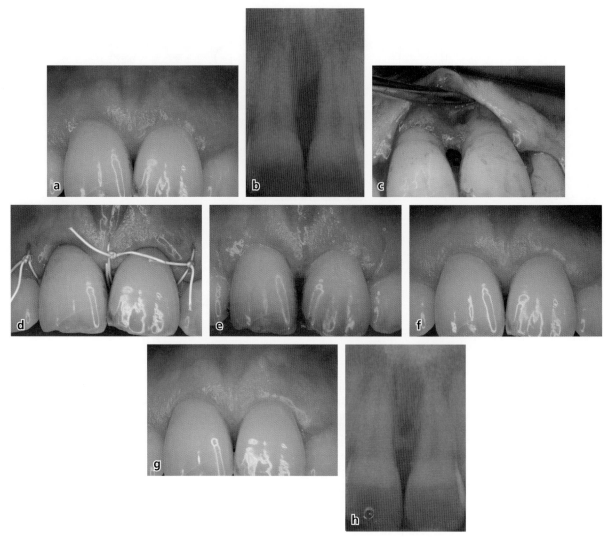

Fig. 43-23 Clinical case illustrating the clinical application of the simplified papilla preservation flap in conjunction with the application of a biologically active regenerative material (enamel matrix derivative in gel form). At re-evaluation following completion of successful initial cause-related therapy, an 8-mm pocket was detected on the mesial palatal aspect of the left central incisor (a). An angular defect was evidenced on a peri-apical radiograph (b). The complex anatomy of the defect is apparent following access to the defect with the modified papilla preservation technique: a buccal fenestration is apparent with the majority of the defect extending palatally to the apical third of the root (c). Following application of the enamel matrix derivative, primary closure of the flap was achieved with a multilayered suture (d). At the 1-week suture removal appointment, excellent maturation of the soft tissue healing is apparent (e). At 6 months, a well represented interdental papilla is present thanks to both the papilla preservation approach and the presence of a bony bridge that assisted in soft tissue support, in spite of the gel formulation of the enamel matrix derivative (f). Clinical and radiographic outcomes at 1 year show preservation of excellent esthetics and elimination of the defect (g,h). Probing depths were in the 2 to 3 mm range.

defect also extends to the buccal or the palatal side of the involved tooth, or when it involves the two interdental spaces of the same tooth (Fig. 43-27) or two approximal teeth (Fig. 43-28). In the latter instance a second interdental papilla is accessed, either with a SPPF or a MPPT, according to indications. Vertical releasing incisions are performed when flap reflection causes tension at the extremities of the flap(s). The vertical releasing incisions are always kept very short and within the attached gingiva (never involving the mucogingival junction). The overall aim of this approach is to avoid using vertical incisions whenever possible or to reduce their number and extent to a minimum when there is a clear

indication for them. Periosteal incisions are never performed.

The defects are debrided with a combined use of mini curettes and power-driven instruments and the roots carefully planed. During the instrumentation the flaps are slightly reflected, carefully protected with periosteal elevators and frequent saline irrigations. At the end of instrumentation the biologically active agent is applied. Then the flaps are repositioned.

The suturing approach in most of the instances consists of a single modified internal mattress suture at the defect-associated interdental area to achieve primary closure of the papilla in the absence of any

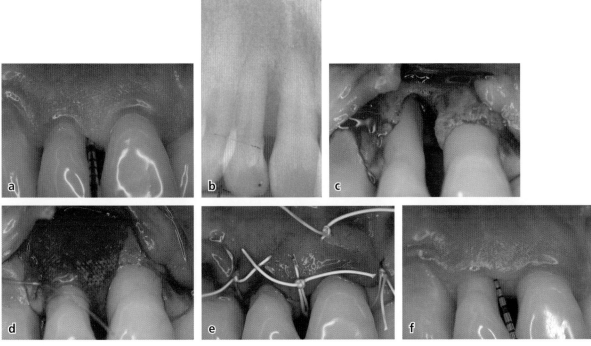

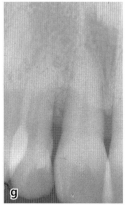

Fig. 43-24 Clinical case illustrating the application of the simplified papilla preservation flap in combination with a bioresorbable barrier membrane applied in combination with a bone replacement graft. At re-evaluation, a 9-mm pocket is detected on the mesial aspect of the lateral incisor (a). The radiograph shows the presence of a deep intrabony defect (b). Following access with a simplified papilla preservation flap, a predominantly two-wall intrabony defect was exposed (c). After careful root instrumentation, a bioresorbable membrane was placed on top of a bone replacement graft (d). Primary closure of the flap was obtained with a multilayered suture approach (e). At 6 years, shallow probing depths are present (f); note the moderate increase in recession of the gingival margin. The radiograph at 6 years shows elimination of the defect but persistence of mineralized granules of bone replacement graft embedded in the newly formed mineralized tissue (g).

tension (Cortellini & Tonetti 2001, 2005). When a second interdental space has been accessed, the same suturing technique is used to obtain primary closure in this area. Vertical releasing incisions are sutured with simple passing sutures. The buccal and lingual flaps are re-positioned at their original level, without any coronal displacement to avoid any additional tension in the healing area.

All the surgical procedures can be performed with the aid of an operating microscope or magnifying loops at a magnification of 4× to 16× (Cortellini & Tonetti 2001, 2005). Microsurgical instruments are utilized, whenever needed, as a complement to the normal set of periodontal instruments.

This approach has been preliminarily tested in two case series with a total of 53 deep intrabony defects (Cortellini & Tonetti 2007a,b). One-year results have shown clinically significant improvements (clinical attachment level gains of 4.8 ± 1.9 mm and 88.7 ± 20.7% clinical resolution of the defect) accompanied by greatly reduced morbidity.

Post-operative regime

The post-operative regime prescribed to the patients is aimed at controlling wound infection or contamination as well as mechanical trauma to the treated sites. A recent meta-analysis indicated that differences in regenerative outcomes are expected based on the post-operative care protocol: more frequent, intensive regimens were associated with better clinical attachment level gains in intrabony defects (Murphy *et al.* 2003) (Fig. 43-29). It generally includes the prescription of systemic antibiotics (doxycycline or amoxicillin) in the immediate post-operative period (1 week), 0.2 or 0.12% chlorhexidine mouthrinsing two or three times per day, and weekly professional tooth cleaning until the membrane is in place. Professional tooth cleaning consists of supragingival prophylaxis with a rubber cup and chlorhexidine gel. Patients are generally advised not to perform mechanical oral hygiene and not to chew in the treated area.

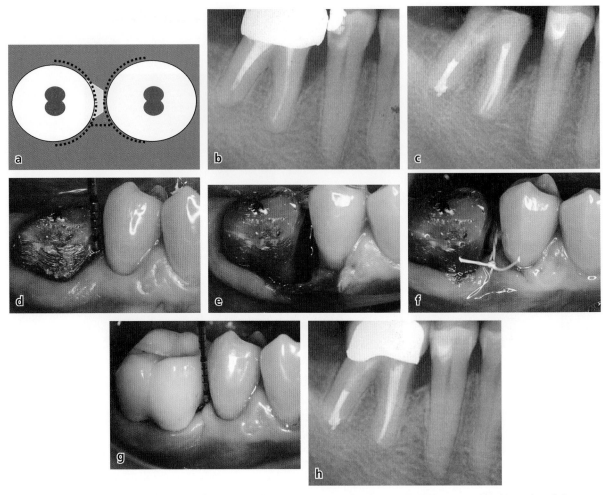

Fig. 43-25 Clinical illustration of the use of the minimally invasive surgical technique (MIST) in an isolated interdental three-wall defect. The diagram shows the extent of the incision performed according to the principles of the modified papilla preservation technique in the interdental space associated with the defect. Mesio-distal extension of the flap is limited to the buccal aspect of the teeth adjacent to the defect in order to optimize wound stability (a). The baseline radiograph shows the presence of dental diseases (peri-apical infection and caries) that need to be controlled during the initial cause-related phase of therapy (b). At re-evaluation, an 8-mm pocket associated with the presence of a deep intrabony defect was detected on the mesial aspect of the first molar (c,d). The defect was accessed in a minimally invasive fashion using a modified papilla preservation flap. The three-wall intrabony defect was exposed and carefully debrided (e). After application of enamel matrix derivative, primary closure was obtained with a single modified internal mattress suture (f). The 1-year outcomes show shallow probing depths and almost complete resolution of the defect (g,h).

Non-resorbable membranes are removed 4–6 weeks after placement, following elevation of partial-thickness flaps. Patients are re-instructed to rinse two or three times per day with chlorhexidine, not to perform mechanical oral hygiene and not to chew in the treated area for 3–4 weeks. In this period weekly professional control and prophylaxis are recommended. When bioresorbable membrane, bone replacement grafts or biologically active regenerative materials are used, the period of tight infection control regime is extended for 6–8 weeks. After this period, patients are re-instructed to resume mechanical oral hygiene gradually, including interdental cleaning, and to discontinue chlorhexidine. Patients are then enrolled in a periodontal care program on a monthly basis until 1 year. Probing or deep scaling in the treated area is generally avoided before the 1-year follow-up visit.

Post-operative morbidity

To date, little consideration has been given to critical elements that could contribute to the patient's assessment of the cost-benefit ratio of GTR procedures. These include post-operative pain, discomfort, complications, and the perceived benefits from the treatment. A parallel group, randomized, multicenter and controlled clinical trial designed to test the efficacy of GTR and flap surgery alone assessed these patient issues (Cortellini *et al.* 2001). During the procedure, 30.4% of the test and 28.6% of the controls reported moderate pain and subjects estimated the hardship of the procedure as 24 ± 25 units on a visual analog scale (VAS in a scale from 0 to 100) in the test group and 22 ± 23 VAS in the controls. Test surgery with membranes required longer chair time than flap surgery (on average 20 minutes longer). Among the

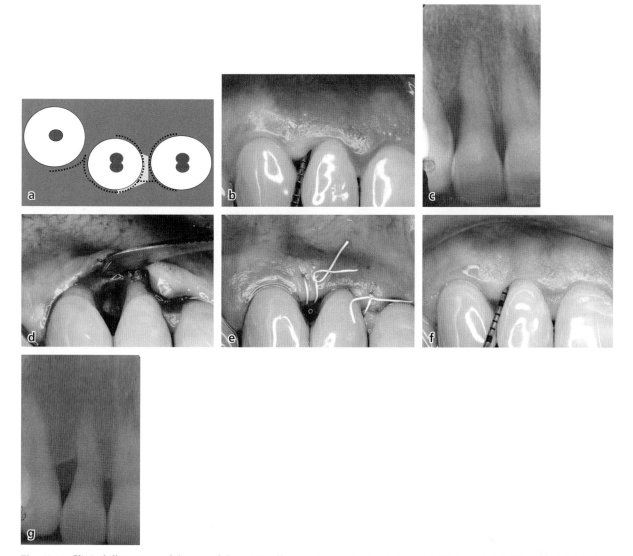

Fig. 43-26 Clinical illustration of the use of the minimally invasive surgical technique (MIST) in an isolated interdental defect extending towards the buccal aspect of the tooth. The diagram shows the extent of the incision performed according to the principles of the modified papilla preservation technique in the interdental space associated with the defect. Mesio-distal extension of the flap is limited to the buccal aspect of the teeth adjacent to the defect and to the interdental aspect adjacent to the buccal extension of the defect in order to optimize wound stability (a). Following completion of successful initial cause-related therapy, a 6-mm pocket associated with an intrabony defect was detected on the distal aspect of the lateral incisor (b,c). The attachment loss extended to the buccal aspect of the lateral incisor, suggesting the need to obtain access to the buccal aspect of this tooth. The defect was therefore accessed with a minimally invasive approach using the modified papilla preservation technique to access the interdental area and extending the incision to the papilla between the lateral and central incisors to ensure adequate access to the defect (d). Primary closure was obtained with a modified internal mattress suture and a simple passing suture (e). The 1-year outcomes show shallow probing depths, good preservation of the soft tissue heights, and resolution of the defect (f,g).

post-operative complications, edema was most prevalent at week 1 and most frequently associated with the GTR treatment, while post-operative pain was reported by fewer than 50% of both test and control patients. Pain intensity was described as mild and lasted on average 14.1 ± 15.6 hours in the test patients and 24.7 ± 39.1 hours in the controls. Post-operative morbidity was limited to a minority of subjects: 35.7% of the test and 32.1% of the controls reported that the procedures interfered with daily activities for an average of 2.7 ± 2.3 days in the test group and 2.4 ± 1.3 days in the control group. These data indicate that GTR adds almost 30 minutes to a flap procedure and

is followed by a greater prevalence of post-surgical edema, while no difference could be observed between GTR and flap surgery alone in terms of post-operative pain, discomfort, and interference with daily activities.

To date, no comparative study has reported the morbidity associated with various regenerative approaches. Reports of multi-center trials on application of enamel matrix derivative or barrier membranes using the same methodology, however, show similar results for the application of these two regenerative materials (Tonetti *et al.* 1998, 2004a; Cortellini *et al.* 2001).

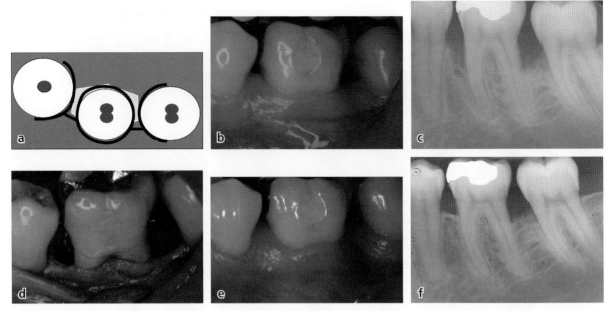

Fig. 43-27 Clinical illustration of the use of the minimally invasive surgical technique (MIST) in intrabony defects involving both interdental spaces of the same tooth. The diagram shows the extent of the incision performed according to the principles of the modified papilla preservation technique in the two interdental spaces associated with the defects. Mesio-distal extension of the flap is limited to the two interdental papillae associated with the defects (a) and reaches the line angle of the two adjacent teeth in order to limit the loss of wound stability while allowing adequate access to the defects. The clinical and radiographic appearance at baseline highlight the good control of inflammation obtained following completion of initial cause-related therapy and the presence of deep mesial and distal pockets with associated intrabony defects (b,c). Both the mesial and distal defects are accessed with papilla preservation flaps, the defects are debrided, and the root surfaces are carefully instrumented (d). Following application of enamel matrix derivative in the well contained defects, primary closure of the flap is achieved by modified internal mattress sutures. At 1-year follow-up, shallow pockets, preservation of soft tissues, and elimination of the defects are apparent (e,f).

Another important issue that has been addressed in a large multi-center trial has been the comparison of surgical complications (such as membrane exposure, flap dehiscence, or occurrence of suppuration) using resorbable barrier membranes or biologically active regenerative materials (EMD in gel form). Sanz *et al.* (2004) showed that all sites treated with membranes presented at least a surgical complication during healing, while this was observed in only 6% of sites treated with EMD. This study indicates that some regenerative materials/procedures may be less technique sensitive than others.

Barrier materials for regenerative surgery

In the first GTR attempts, a bacterial filter produced from cellulose acetate (Millipore®) was used as an occlusive membrane (Nyman *et al.* 1982; Gottlow *et al.* 1984; Magnusson *et al.* 1985b). Although this type of membrane served its purpose, it was not ideal for clinical application.

Non-absorbable materials

Later studies have utilized membranes of expanded polytetrafluoroethylene (e-PTFE) specially designed for periodontal regeneration (Gore Tex Periodontal Material®). The basic molecule of this material con-

sists of a carbon–carbon bond with four attached fluorine atoms to form a polymer. It is inert and does not result in any tissue reaction when implanted in the body. This type of membrane persists after healing and must be removed in a second operation. Membranes of e-PTFE have been used successfully in animal experiments and in several clinical studies. From such studies it was found that for a barrier material to function optimally, it has to meet certain essential design criteria:

1. To allow for good tissue acceptance it is important that the material is biocompatible. The material should not elicit an immune response, sensitization or chronic inflammation that may interfere with healing and present a hazard to the patient. Biocompatibility, however, is a relative term since practically no materials are completely inert.
2. The material should act as a barrier to exclude undesirable cell types from entering the secluded space adjacent to the root surface. It is also considered an advantage that the material would allow the passage of nutrients and gases.
3. Tissue integration is another important property of a barrier material. Thus, tissue may grow into the material without penetrating all the way through. The goal of tissue integration is to prevent rapid epithelial downgrowth on the outer surface of the material or encapsulation of the material,

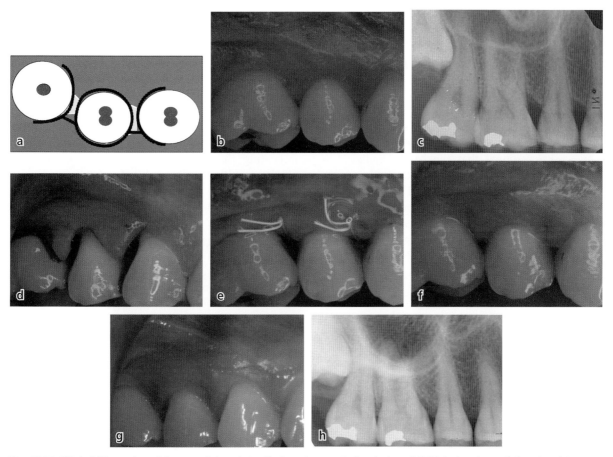

Fig. 43-28 Clinical illustration of the use of the minimally invasive surgical technique (MIST) in intrabony defects involving two adjacent teeth. The diagram shows the extent of the incision performed according to the principles of the papilla preservation flaps in the two interdental spaces associated with the defects. Mesio-distal extension of the flap is limited to the two interdental papillae associated with the defects (a) and reaches the line angle of the two adjacent teeth in order to limit the loss of wound stability and limit flap extension. After successful initial cause-related therapy, two defects are present on the mesial aspect of the first molar and second premolar (b,c). Simplified papilla preservation flaps are used to access the defects (d). Incisions are stopped at the distal line angle of the first premolar and on the buccal aspect of the first molar. Root debridement and application of enamel matrix proteins in gel form are performed before primary closure of the flap that was obtained by using two modified internal vertical mattress sutures (e). Excellent early healing in the absence of pain or discomfort is evident at the 1-week suture removal (f). At 1-year follow-up, absence of inflammation, shallow probing depths and resolution of the defects are evident (g,h).

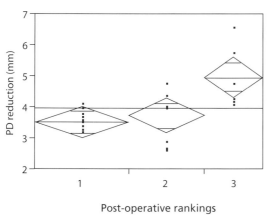

Source	DF	Sum of squares	Mean square	F ratio	Prob F
Post-op rank	2	8.45	4.22	7.21	0.004
Error	21	12.29	0.58		
C. Total	23	20.75			

Post-operative rankings

Rank	Number of studies	Mean
1	10	3.52
2	8	3.73
3	6	4.97

Fig. 43-29 Regression analysis of intrabony defect studies examining the relationship between post-operative care protocol ranking and the reduction (in mm) in probing depth (PD). Group 3 is statistically different from groups 1 and 2. From Murphy & Gunsolley (2003) with permission from the American Academy of Periodontology.

and to provide stability to the overlying flap. The importance of tissue integration was demonstrated in a study in monkeys (Warrer *et al.* 1992) in which bioabsorbable membranes of polylactic acid, a synthetic polymer, were used for treatment of circumferential periodontal defects. Due to the lack of tissue integration, the membranes in this study became surrounded by an epithelial layer and were often encapsulated and exfoliated.

4. It is also essential that the barrier material is capable of creating and maintaining a space adjacent to the root surface. This will allow the ingrowth of tissue from the periodontal ligament. Some materials may be so soft and flexible that they collapse into the defect. Other materials are too stiff and may perforate the overlying tissue.

5. Finally, there are clinical needs in the design of a barrier. It should be provided in configurations which are easy to trim and to place.

Bioabsorbable materials

In recent years, natural or synthetic bioabsorbable barrier materials for GTR have been introduced in order to avoid a second surgery for membrane removal. Barrier materials of collagen from different species and from different anatomic sites have been tested in animals and in humans (Blumenthal 1988, 1993; Pitaru *et al.* 1988; Tanner *et al.* 1988; Paul *et al.* 1992; Wang *et al.* 1994; Camelo *et al.* 1998; Mellonig 2000). Often the collagen used is a cross-linked variety of porcine or bovine origin. When a collagen membrane is implanted in the human body it is resorbed by the enzymatic activity of macrophages and polymorphnuclear leucocytes (Tatakis *et al.* 1999). Successful treatment following the use of such barrier materials has been demonstrated, but the results of the studies vary. Several complications, such as early degradation, epithelial downgrowth along the material, and premature loss of the material, were reported following the use of collagen materials. The varying results are probably due to differences in the properties of the material and the handling of the material at the time of implantation. Although probably very minimal, there is a risk that infectious agents from animal products can be transmitted to humans, and autoimmunization has also been mentioned as a risk.

Barrier materials of polylactic acid or copolymers of polylactic acid and polyglycolic acid were evaluated in animal and human studies and are commonly used (Magnusson *et al.* 1988; Caffesse *et al.* 1994; Caton *et al.* 1994; Gottlow *et al.* 1994; Laurell *et al.* 1994; Hugoson *et al.* 1995; Polson *et al.* 1995a; Hürzeler *et al.* 1997; Sculean *et al.* 1999a). These materials are biocompatible, but by definition they are not inert since some tissue reaction may be expected during degradation. The materials are degraded by hydrolysis and eliminated from the organism through the Krebs cycle as carbon dioxide and water (Tatakis *et al.* 1999).

The types of barrier materials tested in the studies differ regarding configuration and design. It appears that a number of bioabsorbable materials meet to a varying extent the requirements of a good barrier listed above. Indeed, there are several studies (Hugoson *et al.* 1995; Cortellini *et al.* 1996b; Smith *et al.* 1998; Tonetti *et al.* 1998; Cortellini & Tonetti 2000a) indicating that similar satisfactory results can be obtained with bioabsorbable barrier materials of polylactic and polyglycolic acid as with non-bioabsorbable materials.

Membranes in intrabony defects

Early evidence that GTR treatment of deep intrabony defects may produce clinical improvements in terms of clinical attachment gain was presented in several case reports (Nyman *et al.* 1982; Gottlow *et al.* 1986; Becker *et al.* 1988; Schallhorn & McClain 1988; Cortellini *et al.* 1990). In recent years, a number of clinical investigations have reported on a total of 1283 intrabony defects treated with GTR (Table 43-2). In these studies, the issue of evaluating the predictability of the clinical outcomes following application of GTR procedures was addressed. The weighted mean of the reported results indicates a mean gain in clinical attachment of 3.8 ± 1.7 mm, with a 95% confidence interval ranging from 3.7–4.0 mm (Cortellini & Tonetti 2000a). The reported clinical attachment gains following GTR treatment were significantly larger than the ones obtained from conventional flap surgery. A recent review (Lang 2000) on flap surgery reported a weighted mean of 1172 defects in 40 studies. CAL gains were 1.8 ± 1.4 mm, with a 95% confidence interval ranging from 1.6–1.9 mm.

Different types of non-bioabsorbable (Fig. 43-30) and bioabsorbable (Fig. 43-31) barrier materials were used in the studies summarized in Table 43-2. A subset analysis indicated that cases treated with non-bioabsorbable barrier materials (351 defects) showed a mean gain in clinical attachment of 3.7 ± 1.7 mm which did not differ from that obtained with bioabsorbable barrier materials of 3.6 ± 1.5 mm (592 defects).

Analysis of the results reported in some of the studies in Table 43-2 (i.e. 211 defects in 9 investigations: Proestakis *et al.* 1992; Cortellini *et al.* 1993b, 1995c, 1996b; Cortellini & Pini-Prato 1994; Laurell *et al.* 1994; Mattson *et al.* 1995; Mellado *et al.* 1995; Tonetti *et al.* 1996b) provides important information regarding the predictability of GTR in intrabony defects. Gains of 2–3 mm were observed in 29.2% of the defects, gains of 4–5 mm in 35.4% of the defects, and gains of 6 mm or more in 24.9% of the defects. Only in 10.5% of the treated defects was the gain less than 2 mm, while no change or attachment loss was observed in two cases.

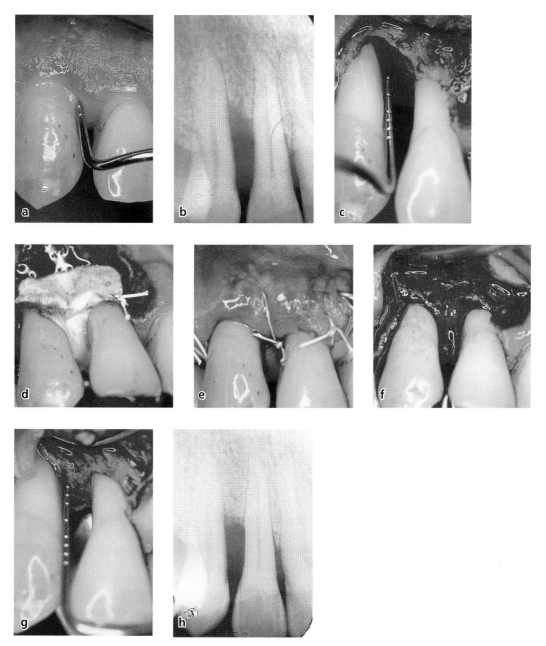

Fig. 43-30 Intrabony defect on the mesial aspect of a right maxillary canine treated with a non-bioabsorbable barrier membrane. (a) The pocket depth is 9 mm and the loss of clinical attachment is 10 mm. (b) Radiograph showing the presence of an interproximal intrabony defect. (c) After full-thickness flap elevation, defect debridement, and root planing, a 4-mm intrabony defect is evident. (d) An e-PTFE non-bioabsorbable barrier membrane has been tailored, positioned and tightly sutured around the teeth adjacent to the defect. (e) The flap has been repositioned and sutured to cover the membrane. Optimal preservation of the soft tissues has been accomplished with an intrasulcular incision. (f) After removal of the membrane at 5 weeks, the defect appears to be completely filled with newly formed tissue. (g) The treated site has been surgically re-entered after 1 year. The intrabony defect is completely filled with bone. (h) The 1-year radiograph confirms the complete resolution of the intrabony defect.

In some of the investigations, changes in bone levels were also reported (Becker *et al.* 1988; Handelsman *et al.* 1991; Kersten *et al.* 1992; Cortellini *et al.* 1993b,c; Selvig *et al.* 1993). Bone gains ranged between 1.1 and 4.3 mm and correlated with the reported gains in clinical attachment. In a study by Tonetti *et al.* (1993b), 1 year after GTR the bone was found to be located 1.5 mm apically to the position of the attained clinical attachment level.

Another important parameter related to the outcome of regenerative procedures is the residual

pocket depth. In the studies reported in Table 43-2, shallow pockets were consistently found at 1 year. The weighted mean of residual pocket depth was 3.4 ± 1.2 mm, with a 95% CI ranging from 2.3–3.5 mm.

The reported outcomes indicate that GTR procedures predictably result in clinical improvements in intrabony defects beyond that of flap surgery. This was further confirmed in 11 controlled randomized clinical trials in which guided tissue regeneration was compared with conventional flap surgery (Table 43-3). A total of 267 defects were treated with flap

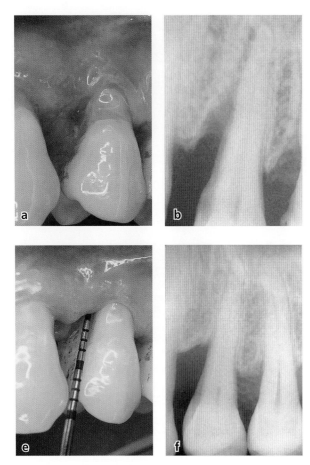
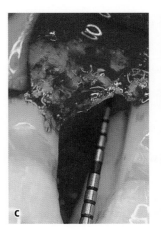
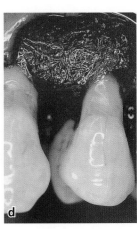

Fig. 43-31 Intrabony defect on the mesial aspect of a left maxillary premolar treated with a bioabsorbable barrier membrane. (a) Clinical attachment loss was 12 mm. (b) Radiograph showing the presence of a deep interproximal intrabony defect approaching the apex of the tooth. (c) A 7-mm interproximal intrabony defect was measured after flap elevation, defect debridement, and root planing. (d) A bioabsorbable barrier membrane has been placed and sutured to cover the defect. (e) At 1 year, a 4-mm pocket depth and 5-mm clinical gain of attachment were recorded. (f) The 1-year radiograph shows that the intrabony defect is almost resolved.

surgery and 317 with GTR. In 9 of the 11 investigations, GTR resulted in statistically significantly greater probing attachment level gains when compared to flap surgery. Similar results were also observed for residual pocket depth. It should be emphasized that one of the investigations reporting no significant differences between GTR and flap surgery was carried out in only nine pairs of defects (18 defects) located on maxillary premolars (Proestakis *et al.* 1992). In this study the intrabony component of the defects was shallow and 10 of the 18 defects had a furcation involvement. The weighted mean of the results reported in the 11 studies listed in Table 43-3 (Cortellini & Tonetti 2000a) indicated that the gain in clinical attachment in sites treated with GTR was 3.3 ± 1.8 mm (95% CI 2.8–3.6 mm), while the flap surgery resulted in a mean gain of 2.1 ± 1.5 mm (95% CI 1.8–2.4 mm). These clinical results strongly indicate that there is an added beneficial effect of placing a barrier material over an intrabony defect in conjunction with surgery.

Membranes for furcation involvement

The invasion of the furcation area of multi-rooted teeth by periodontitis represents a serious complication in periodontal therapy. The furcation area is often inaccessible to adequate instrumentation, and the roots frequently present concavities and furrows which make proper cleaning of the area impossible

(see Chapter 39). As long as the pathologic process only extends a small distance (<5 mm; degree I and II involvements) into the furcation area, further progress of the disease can usually be prevented by scaling and root planing, provided a proper oral hygiene program is established after treatment. In more advanced cases (5–6 mm; degree II involvements), the initial cause-related treatment is frequently supplemented with surgery involving contouring of the inter-radicular bone (osteoplasty) or reduction of the tooth prominence at the furcation entrance by grinding (odontoplasty), in order to reduce the horizontal extension of the furcation involvement. In cases where the involvement extends deeper into the furcation area (>5 mm; degree II involvements), or a through-and-through defect (degree III involvements) has developed, tunnel preparation or root resection have been advocated as the choice of treatment. However, both of these latter treatments involve a risk of complications on a long-term basis. Following tunnel preparation, caries frequently develops in the furcation area and root-resected teeth often present complications of non-periodontal nature, although controversial reports exist regarding the long-term results of these treatment modalities (Hamp *et al.* 1975; Langer *et al.* 1981; Erpenstein 1983; Bühler 1988; Little *et al.* 1995; Carnevale *et al.* 1998).

Considering the complexity of current techniques for the treatment of furcation problems, and in view

Table 43-3 Controlled clinical trials comparing clinical outcomes of GTR procedures with access flap procedures in deep intrabony defects

Authors	Membranes	N	Gains in CAL ± SD (mm)		Residual PPD ± SD (mm)	
			GTR	Access flap	GTR	Access flap
Chung et al. 1990	Collagen	10	0.6 ± 0.6			
	Collagen	9	2.4 ± 2.1		4.0 ± 1.1	
	Control	14		−0.7 ± 0.9		
Proestakis et al. 1992	e-PTFE	9	1.2 ± 1.3		3.5 ± 0.9	
	Control	9		0.6 ± 1.0		3.7 ± 3.0
Quteish & Dolby 1992	Collagen	26	3.0 ± 1.5		2.2 ± 0.4	
	Control	26		1.8 ± 0.9		3.4 ± 0.6
Al-Arrayed et al. 1995	Collagen	19	3.9		2.5	
	Control	14		2.7		3.5
Cortellini et al. 1995c	e-PTFE	15	4.1 ± 1.9		2.7 ± 1.0	
	e-PTFE+titanium	15	5.3 ± 2.2		2.1 ± 0.5	
	Control	15		2.5 ± 0.8		3.7 ± 1.3
Mattson et al. 1995	Collagen	13	2.5 ± 1.5		3.6 ± 0.6	
	Control	9		0.4 ± 2.1		4.5 ± 1.8
Cortellini et al. 1996b	e-PTFE	12	5.2 ± 1.4		2.9 ± 0.9	
	Polylactic acid	12		4.6 ± 1.2		3.3 ± 0.9
	Control	12		2.3 ± 0.8		4.2 ± 0.9
Tonetti et al. 1998	Polylactic acid	69	3.0 ± 1.6		4.3 ± 1.3	
	Control	67		2.2 ± 1.5		4.2 ± 1.4
Pontoriero et al. 1999	Diff. barriers	30	3.1 ± 1.8		3.3 ± 1.3	
	Control	30		1.8 ± 1.5		4.0 ± 0.8
Ratka-Kruger et al. 2000	Polylactic acid	23	3.1 ± 2.3		4.7 ± 1.4	
	Control	21		3.3 ± 2.7		4.9 ± 2.1
Cortellini et al. 2001	Polylactic acid	55	3.5 ± 2.1		3.8 ± 1.5	
	Control	54		2.6 ± 1.8		4.7 ± 1.4
Weighted mean		**584**	**3.3 ± 1.8**	**2.1 ± 1.5**	**3.5 ± 1.1**	**4.1 ± 1.3**

CAL = clinical attachment level; PPD = probing pocket depth; SD = standard deviation.

of the long-term results and complications reported following treatment of advanced furcation involvements by traditional resective therapy, predictable regeneration of the periodontium at furcation-involved sites would represent a considerable progress in periodontics.

Mandibular degree II furcations

Pontoriero et al. (1988) reported a controlled randomized clinical trial in which significantly greater amounts of horizontal clinical attachment (H-CAL) gain (3.8 ± 1.2 mm) were obtained in 21 mandibular degree II furcations treated with e-PTFE membranes compared to those in a control group treated with open flap debridement alone (H-CAL gains of 2.0 ± 1.2 mm). Complete closure of the furcation was observed in 67% of the test sites and in only 10% of the control sites. Other studies, however, have failed to confirm these promising results to the same extent (Becker et al. 1988; Lekovic et al. 1989; Caffesse et al.

1990). Analysis of a series of studies published between 1988 and 1996 demonstrates a great variability in the clinical outcomes (Figs. 43-32, 43-33). Table 43-4 summarizes the outcomes of 21 clinical trials in which a total of 423 mandibular degree II furcations were treated with different types of non-bioabsorbable and bioabsorbable barrier membranes. The weighted mean of the reported results shows a H-CAL gain of 2.3 ± 1.4 mm with a 95% confidence interval ranging from 2.0–2.5 mm in defects with a baseline horizontal probing depth of 5.4 ± 1.3 mm. The reported number of complete furcation closures after GTR range from 0–67%. In three studies none of the treated furcations were closed (Becker et al. 1988; Yukna 1992; Polson et al. 1995b), in seven studies fewer than 50% were closed (Schallhorn & McClain 1988; Blumenthal 1993; Bouchard et al. 1993; Parashis & Mitsis 1993; Laurell et al. 1994; Mellonig et al. 1994; Hugoson et al. 1995), and in only one study were more than 50% of the treated furcations completely resolved (Pontoriero et al. 1988).

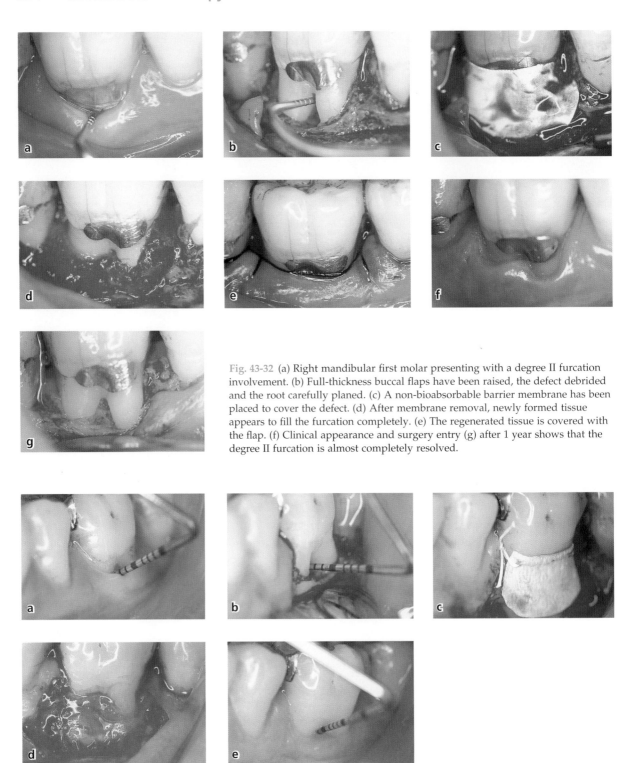

Fig. 43-32 (a) Right mandibular first molar presenting with a degree II furcation involvement. (b) Full-thickness buccal flaps have been raised, the defect debrided and the root carefully planed. (c) A non-bioabsorbable barrier membrane has been placed to cover the defect. (d) After membrane removal, newly formed tissue appears to fill the furcation completely. (e) The regenerated tissue is covered with the flap. (f) Clinical appearance and surgery entry (g) after 1 year shows that the degree II furcation is almost completely resolved.

Fig. 43-33 (a) Left mandibular first molar presenting with a deep degree II furcation involvement. (b) Horizontal loss of tooth support of 7 mm was probed. (c) An e-PTFE barrier membrane has been trimmed and sutured to cover the furcation. (d) At membrane removal after 5 weeks, newly formed tissue fills the furcation completely. (e) At 1 year, a 3-mm gain of tooth support was measured, but a residual 4-mm degree II furcation involvement was still present.

A subset analysis of the studies reported in Table 43-4 indicated that furcations treated with non-bioabsorbable barrier membranes (287) showed a gain in horizontal clinical attachment of 1.8 ± 1.4 mm (95% CI 1.5–2.1 mm) as compared with 2.3 ± 1.2 mm H-CAL gain (95% CI 2–2.6 mm) in 174 defects treated with bioabsorbable barrier membranes. Five controlled clinical trials compared treatment with

non-resorbable e-PTFE membranes and treatment with different types of bioabsorbable membranes (Table 43-5). In particular, one investigation reported significantly greater H-CAL gain in the non-bioabsorbable group (Bouchard *et al.* 1993), while another one (Hugoson *et al.* 1995) showed a significantly greater H-CAL gain in the bioabsorbable group. The remaining three investigations failed to

Table 43-4 Clinical outcomes and weighted mean of GTR treatment of mandibular degree II furcations

Authors	Type of study	Treatment	N	Defect depth (mm)	H-CAL gain (mm)	H-OPAL gain (mm)	No. of furca closed
Pontoriero et al. 1988	Controlled clinical trial	e-PTFE	21	4.4 ± 1.2	3.8 ± 1.2	NA	14 (67%)
Becker et al. 1988	Case cohort	e-PTFE	6	8.3 ± 2.3	NA	1.8 ± 1.5	0
Schallhorn & McClain 1988	Case cohort	e-PTFE	16	NA	NA	3.1 ± 1.7	5 (31%)
Lekovic et al. 1989	Controlled clinical trial	e-PTFE	6	NA	NA	0.2 ± 0.5	NA
Lekovic et al. 1990	Controlled clinical trial	e-PTFE	15	4.2 ± 0.2	NA	0.1 ± 0.1	NA
Caffesse et al. 1990	Controlled clinical trial	e-PTFE	9	4.8 ± ?	0.8 ± ?	NA	NA
Anderegg et al. 1991	Controlled clinical trial	e-PTFE	15	4.2 ± 2.2	NA	1.0 ± 0.8	NA
Yukna 1992	Controlled clinical trial	e-PTFE	11	3.0 ± ?	NA	1.0 ± ?	0
		FDDMA	11	4.0 ± ?	NA	2.0 ± ?	0
Blumenthal 1993	Controlled clinical trial	e-PTFE	12	4.4 ± 0.9	1.8 ± 1	1.7 ± 0.5	4 (33%)
		Collagen	12	4.5 ± 0.9	2.5 ± 0.8	2.5 ± 0.7	1 (8%)
Bouchard et al. 1993	Controlled clinical trial	e-PTFE	12	NA	2.8 ± 1.3	2.2 ± 1.4	4 (33%)
		Conn. graft	12	NA	1.5 ± 1.5	1.5 ± 1.1	2 (17%)
Machtei et al. 1993	Controlled clinical trial	e-PTFE	18	NA	2.3 ± 1.7	NA	NA
Parashis & Mitsis 1993	Controlled clinical trial	e-PTFE	9	5.7 ± 0.7	4.7 ± 1.5	NA	4 (44%)
Van Swol et al. 1993	Controlled clinical trial	Collagen	28	5.1 ± 1.4	2.3 ± 1	1.7 ± ?	NA
Wallace et al. 1994	Controlled clinical trial	e-PTFE	7	NA	NA	2.3 ± ?	NA
Black et al. 1994	Controlled clinical trial	e-PTFE	13	4.3 ± 2	0.8 ± 2.2	NA	NA
		Collagen	13	4.4 ± 1.5	1.5 ± 2	NA	NA
Laurell et al. 1994	Case cohort	Polylactic acid	19	NA	3.3 ± 1.4	NA	9 (47%)
Machtei et al. 1994	Controlled clinical trial	e-PTFE	30	7.7 ± 1.8	2.6 ± 1.7	NA	NA
Mellonig et al. 1994	Controlled clinical trial	e-PTFE	11	8.4 ± 1.2	NA	4.5 ± 1.6	1 (9%)
Wang et al. 1994	Controlled clinical trial	Collagen	12	6.0 ± 2.7	2.0 ± 0.4	2.5 ± ?	NA
Hugoson et al. 1995	Controlled clinical trial	e-PTFE	38	5.9 ± 1.3	1.4 ± 2.2	NA	4 (11%)
		Polylactic acid	38	5.6 ± 1.4	2.2 ± 2	NA	13 (34%)
Polson et al. 1995	Case cohort*	Polylactic Acid	29	5.4 ± 0.2	2.5 ± 0.1	NA	0
Weighted mean			**423**	**5.4 ± 1.3†**	**2.3 ± 1.4‡**	**1.9 ± 1§**	

H-CAL = horizontal clinical attachment; H-OPAL = horizontal open probing attachment; NA = data not available; e-PTFE = expanded polytetrafluoroethylene; FDDMA = freeze-dried dura mater allograft; Conn. graft = connective tissue graft.
* Mandibular and maxillary molars.
† N = Mean (340) ± S.D. (302); ‡ N = Mean (325) ± S.D. (316); § N = Mean (186) ± S.D. (177).

Table 43-5 Controlled clinical trials comparing clinical outcomes of GTR procedures with e-PTFE non-bioabsorbable barrier membranes with different types of bioabsorbable barrier membranes in mandibular degree II furcations

Authors	Design & treatment (GTR C/GTR T)	N C/T	Defect depth (mm)		H-CAL gain (mm)		H-OPAL gain (mm)	
			GTR C	GTR T	GTR C	GTR T	GTR C	GTR T
Yukna 1992	Intra-individual (e-PTFE/FDDMA)	11/11	3.0 ± ?	4.0 ± ?	NA	NA	1.0 ± ?	2.0 ± ?
Blumenthal 1993	Intra-individual (e-PTFE/collagen)	12/12	4.4 ± 0.9	4.5 ± 0.9	1.8 ± 1	2.5 ± 0.8	1.7 ± 0.5	2.5 ± 0.7
Bouchard et al. 1993	Intra-individual (e-PTFE/conn. graft)	12/12	NA	NA	2.8 ± 1.3*	1.5 ± 2	2.2 ± 1.4	1.5 ± 1.1
Black et al. 1994	Intra-individual (e-PTFE/collagen)	13/13	4.3 ± 2	4.4 ± 1.5	0.8 ± 2.2	1.5 ± 2	NA	NA
Hugoson et al. 1995	Intra-individual (e-PTFE/polytetrafluoroethylene)	38/38	5.9 ± 1.3	5.6 ± 1.4	1.4 ± 2.2*	2.2 ± 2.0*	NA	NA
Weighted mean		**86/86**	**4.9 ± 1.4†**	**5 ± 1.3†**	**1.6 ± 1.9‡**	**2 ± 1.7‡1**	**1.3 ± 1§**	**1.4 ± 0.9§**

GTR C = guided tissue regeneration control treatment; GTR T = guided tissue regeneration test treatment; N C/T = number of defects in the control (C) and in the test (T) treatment arm; H-CAL = horizontal clinical attachment; H-OPAL = horizontal open probing attachment; NA = data not available; e-PTFE = expanded polytetrafluoroethylene; FDDMA = freeze-dried dura mater allograft; Conn. graft = connective tissue graft.
* Difference between treatments statistically significant.
† N = Mean (74) ± S.D. (63); ‡ N = Mean (75) ± S.D. (75); § N = Mean (35) ± S.D. (24).

detect any significant differences between the outcomes of treatment with bioabsorbable or non-bioabsorbable membranes. Generally the results indicate that the predictability of GTR in the treatment of mandibular degree II furcations is questionable, if the treatment objective is the complete resolution of the furcation involvement.

Significant gain in vertical attachment level (VCAL) and reduction in pocket depth (PPD) was also reported by several investigators following treat-

Table 43-6 Controlled clinical trials comparing clinical outcomes of GTR procedures with access flap procedures in mandibular degree II furcations

Authors	Design (GTR treatment)	N C/T	Defect depth (mm)		H-CAL gain (mm)		H-OPAL gain (mm)	
			Access flap	GTR	Access flap	GTR	Access flap	GTR
Pontoriero et al. 1988	Intra-individual (e-PTFE)	21/21	4.0 ± 0.8	4.4 ± 1.2	2.0 ± 1.2*	3.8 ± 1.2*	NA	NA
Lekovic et al. 1989	Intra-individual (e-PTFE)	6/6	NA	NA	NA	NA	−0.1 ± 0.3	0.2 ± 0.5
Caffesse et al. 1990	Parallel (e-PTFE)	6/9	5.3 ± ?	4.8 ± ?	0.3 ± ?	0.8 ± ?	NA	NA
Van Swol et al. 1993	Parallel (collagen)	10/28	5.7 ± 2.5	5.1 ± 1.4	0.7 ± 1.2*	2.3 ± 1*	0.8 ± ?	1.7 ± ?
Mellonig et al. 1994	Intra-individual (e-PTFE)	6/6	7.5 ± 2.3	8.4 ± 1.2	NA	NA	1.1 ± 1.3*	4.5 ± 1.6*
Wang et al. 1994	Intra-individual (collagen)	12/12	5.6 ± 2.7	6.0 ± 2.7	1.1 ± 0.6*	2.0 ± 0.4*	1.5 ± ?	2.5 ± ?
Weighted mean		**66/87**	**5.4 ± 1.8†**	**5.5 ± 1.5‡**	**1.3 ± 1§**	**2.5 ± 1#**	**1 ± 1¶**	**2.3 ± 1.2****

N C/T = number of defects in the control (C) and in the test (T) treatment arm; H-CAL = horizontal clinical attachment; H-OPAL = horizontal open probing attachment; NA = data not available; e-PTFE = expanded polytetrafluoroethylene.
* Difference between treatments statistically significant.
† N = Mean (60) ± S.D. (54); ‡ N = Mean (81) ± S.D. (72); § N = Mean (49) ± S.D. (43); # N = Mean (70) ± S.D. (61); >3 N = Mean (39) ± S.D. (17);
** N = Mean (57) ± S.D. (17).

ment of mandibular degree II furcation defects (Pontoriero et al. 1988; Lekovic et al. 1989, 1990; Blumenthal 1993; Machtei et al. 1993, 1994; Black et al. 1994; Laurell et al. 1994; Mellonig et al. 1994; Wang et al. 1994; Hugoson et al. 1995; Polson et al. 1995b). The reported mean values ranged from 0.1 mm to 3.5 mm for V-CAL gain and from 1 mm to 4 mm for PPD reduction.

The effect of using barrier membranes for the treatment of mandibular degree II furcations was investigated in six controlled randomized clinical trials in which GTR procedures were directly compared to flap surgery (Table 43-6). Sixty-six furcations treated with flap surgery and 87 treated with GTR were included. Three of the four studies reporting H-CAL gains concluded that GTR resulted in statistically significantly greater horizontal attachment level gains than flap surgery (Pontoriero et al. 1988; Van Swol et al. 1993; Wang et al. 1994). The weighted mean of the results reported in Table 43-6 indicated that the H-CAL in furcations treated with GTR was 2.5 ± 1 mm (95% CI 2.1–2.9 mm) while the flap surgery resulted in a mean H-CAL gain of 1.3 ± 1 mm (95% CI 0.8–1.8 mm). These results indicate an added benefit from GTR in the treatment of mandibular degree II furcations.

Maxillary degree II furcations

Results reported in three controlled studies (Metzeler et al. 1991; Mellonig et al. 1994; Pontoriero & Lindhe 1995a) comparing GTR treatment of maxillary degree II furcations with non-bioabsorbable e-PTFE membranes and with open-flap debridement, indicate that GTR treatment of such defects is generally unpredictable. In a study including 17 pairs of degree II furcations Metzeler et al. (1991) measured CAL gains of 1.0 ± 0.9 mm in the GTR-treated sites versus 0.2 ± 0.6 mm in the control sites. Following re-entry, horizontal probing attachment gains (H-OPAL) of 0.9 ± 0.4 mm and 0.3 ± 0.6 mm were detected in the GTR- and flap-

treated furcations, respectively. No differences were found and none of the furcations of the two groups were completely resolved. Similarly, Mellonig et al. (1994) treated eight pairs of maxillary degree II furcations which resulted in H-OPAL gains of 1.0 mm (GTR sites) and 0.3 mm (flap-treated sites). No differences were found and none of the treated furcations were completely closed. On the other hand, in a study on 28 maxillary degree II furcations Pontoriero and Lindhe (1995a) found a significant gain in CAL (1.5 mm) and horizontal bone (1.1 mm) in buccal degree II furcations.

Although these three investigations show a slight clinical improvement following treatment of degree II maxillary furcations with GTR, the results are generally inconsistent.

Degree III furcations

Four investigations on the treatment of mandibular degree III furcations (Becker et al. 1988; Pontoriero et al. 1989; Cortellini et al. 1990; Pontoriero & Lindhe 1995b) indicate that the treatment of such defects with GTR is unpredictable. A controlled study of Pontoriero et al. (1989) showed that only eight out of 21 "through-and-through" mandibular furcations treated with non-bioabsorbable barrier membranes healed with complete closure of the defect. Another ten defects were partially filled, and three remained open. In the control group, treated with open flap debridement, 10 were partially filled and 11 remained open. Similar results were reported by Cortellini et al. (1990) who, in a case cohort of 15 degree III mandibular furcations, found that 33% of the defects had healed completely, 33% were partially closed, and 33% were still through-and-through following treatment. Becker et al. (1988) did not observe complete closure of any of 11 treated degree III mandibular furcations. Similarly, in a controlled clinical trial by Pontoriero and Lindhe (1995b) on 11 pairs of maxillary degree III furcations randomly assigned to GTR

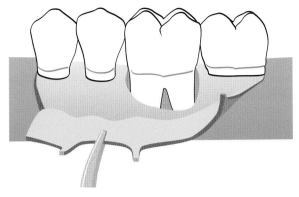

Fig. 43-34 Following marginal incisions and vertical releasing incisions on the buccal aspect of the jaw, buccal and lingual full-thickness flaps are elevated.

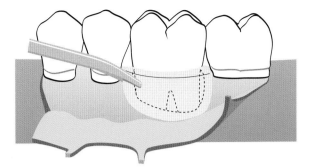

Fig. 43-35 The barrier material is placed in such a way that it completely covers the defect and extends at least 3 mm on the bone beyond the defect margin.

or flap surgery, none of the furcation defects were closed.

Based on present evidence, it seems that mandibular degree II furcations in the first or second molars, either buccal or lingual, with deep pockets at baseline and a gingival thickness of >1 mm, may benefit from GTR treatment.

Surgical issues with barrier membranes

Surgery is initiated by sulcular incisions at both the buccal and lingual aspect of the jaw, followed by buccal and vertical releasing incisions, if necessary. For intrabony defects, the releasing incisions must be placed a minimum of one tooth anterior and/or posterior to the tooth that is being treated (Fig. 43-34). Care should be taken during this procedure to preserve the interdental papillae. All pocket epithelium is excised so that fresh connective tissue is left on the full-thickness flaps following reflection. After elevation of the tissue flaps, all granulation tissue is removed and thorough debridement of the accessed root surfaces is carried out using curettes, burs, etc.

Various types of bioabsorbable and non-bioabsorbable barrier materials are available in a variety of configurations designed for specific applications. The configuration most suitable for covering the defect is selected and additional adaptation of the material to the shape and extent of the defect is performed. The shaping of the material is carried out in such a way that it adapts closely to the tooth and completely covers the defect, extending at least 3 mm on the bone beyond the defect margins after placement (Fig. 43-35). This assures good stability of the material and protects the underlying blood clot during healing. At placement it is essential to ensure good adaptation of the barrier material to the alveolar bone surrounding the defect and to avoid overlaps or folds of the material.

Although exceptions exist, the barrier materials available are fixed to the tooth with a suture using a sling technique. For optimal performance, the barrier should be placed with its margin 2–3 mm apical to

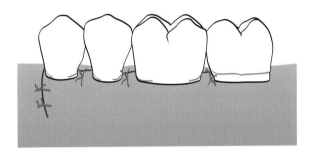

Fig. 43-36 The elevated tissue flaps are coronally displaced and sutured in such a way that the border of the barrier material is at least 2 mm below the flap margin.

the flap margin. To maximize coverage of the barrier, a horizontal releasing incision in the periosteum may assist in the coronal displacement of the flap at the suturing of the wound. However, care should be taken not to compromise the blood supply to the flap. The interdental space near the barrier should be closed first. In order to achieve good closure, an internal vertical mattress suturing technique is advocated (Fig. 43-36).

To reduce the risk of infection and to assure optimal healing, the patient should be instructed to brush the area gently post-operatively with a soft bristle toothbrush and to rinse with chlorhexidine (0.2%) for a period of 4–6 weeks. In addition, systemic antibiotics are frequently administered immediately prior to surgery and for 1–2 weeks after surgery. When a non-bioabsorbable barrier is used, it should be removed after 4–6 weeks. However, if complications develop it may be necessary to remove it earlier.

Removal of the material requires a minor surgical procedure (Fig. 43-37). To obtain access to the barrier material, a small incision is made extending one tooth mesial and distal to the border of the barrier. The soft tissue flap is gently reflected and the barrier material dissected free from the flap using a sharp blade. During this procedure it is essential not to compromise the newly regenerated tissue. At removal of the barrier material there will usually be some pocket formation on the outer surface of the material. It is important that this epithelium is removed so

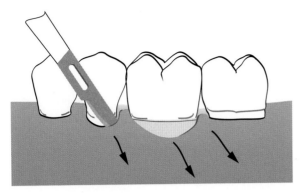

Fig. 43-37 In order to remove the barrier material an incision is made extending one tooth mesially and distally to the border of the barrier. After reflecting the covering tissue flaps, the barrier can be removed without compromising the newly regenerated tissue.

that fresh connective tissue is in contact with the newly regenerated tissue after wound closure. It is essential that the newly regenerated tissue is completely covered after suturing. The patient is instructed to rinse with chlorhexidine for 2–3 weeks during which period frequent visits for professional tooth cleaning are recommended. After this period, brushing and interdental cleaning can be resumed, chlorhexidine rinsing discontinued, and the patient enrolled in a regular periodontal maintenance program.

If the flap is excessively traumatized during surgery either part or all of it may slough during healing. Perforations may also occur, particularly in sites with sharp bony ledges. A minor osteoplasty during placement may help to allow the barrier to better follow the contours of the ridge. Abscess formation may also occur in the wound, probably due to severe bacterial contamination of the barrier. Dependent on the severity of such complications, early removal of the barrier may be indicated.

Bone replacement grafts

Bone replacement grafts (BRG) comprise a heterogeneous group of materials of human (autologous or allogeneic), animal or synthetic origin. Some consist of bone or exoskeletal mineral; others contain mainly bone matrix. Only few materials present evidence of periodontal regeneration. A randomized controlled clinical trial provided histologic support that the healing outcome following application of demineralized freeze-dried bone allograft (DFDBA) in intrabony defects has a regenerative component in the apical to middle portion of the depth of the defect (Bowers *et al.* 1989a,b,c). Isolated evidence also supports the fact that allograft and bovine bone mineral may yield a regenerative outcome when used alone (i.e. without other regenerative materials such as barrier membranes or biologically active regenerative materials (BARG) – see also Chapter 25) (Nevins *et al.* 2000).

Bone replacement grafts were the first periodontal regenerative materials to be applied clinically. Today they are widely used in North America as demineralized freeze-dried allografts and are frequently used in combination with other regenerative materials (GTR and/or BARG).

The clinical efficacy of allografts in terms of bone fill and clinical attachment level gains is supported by a meta-analysis indicating that an additional bone fill of 1 mm and additional clinical attachment level gains of 0.4 mm were observed (Reynolds *et al.* 2003). The total number of defects contributing to this meta-analysis however is relatively small (136 for clinical attachment level gain and 154 for bone fill). Furthermore no large-scale multi-center trial has ever been performed and hence the applicability of these results to clinical practice settings remains to be established.

As to their use, BRG can be applied alone following elevation of a papilla preservation flap for the treatment of intrabony defects. The graft is applied to overfill the defect to compensate for a degree of shedding of the graft expected in cases of imperfect containment of the graft by the closed flap. A study has suggested using BRG in combination with an antibiotic powder to enhance control of the bacterial contamination of the surgical wound (Yukna & Sepe 1982). This study reported improved outcomes from mixing the graft with tetracycline powder.

Biologically active regenerative materials

Preclinical and clinical evidence for the use of biologically active regenerative materials has been reviewed (see also Chapter 25). Currently, two preparations consisting of growth and/or differentiation factors are available for use in periodontal regeneration: enamel matrix derivative (EMD) in a gel form and platelet-derived growth factor (PDGF) mixed in a beta tricalcium phosphate bone replacement graft.

Significant preclinical evidence supports the positive effect of PDGF on periodontal wound healing and regeneration (Howell *et al.* 1997). Clinically, support for use of PDGF comes from a single multi-center trial performed in North America (Nevins *et al.* 2005). In that study 180 defects comprising both intrabony and furcation defects were treated with one of two concentrations of PDGF (0.3 mg/ml and 1.0 mg/ml) combined with the beta tricalcium phosphate delivery device or tricalcium phosphate alone. Results were assessed at 3 and 6 months and included both clinical and radiographic assessments. Clinical attachment level gains at 6 months failed to demonstrate a significant benefit of either concentration of PDGF compared to the bone replacement graft alone. With regards to radiographic assessments, however, the lower tested concentration of PDGF resulted in significantly higher percentages of radiographic bone

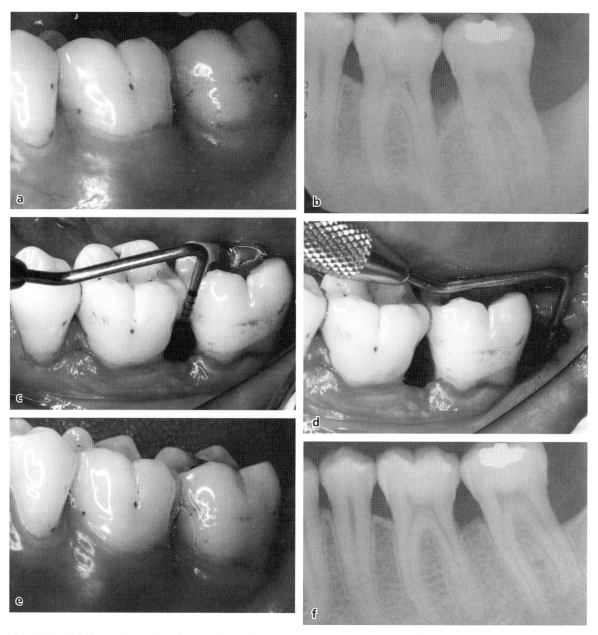

Fig. 43-38 Clinical case illustrating the use of enamel matrix derivative to regenerate defects located on two adjacent teeth. At re-evaluation, deep pockets associated with deep intrabony defects are evident on the distal aspect of the first and second molars (a,b). Defects were accessed with the modified papilla preservation technique on the distal aspect of the first molar and with the use of a crestal incision in the retromolar area (c,d). Deep defects were exposed following debridement and root instrumentation (c,d). Following application of enamel matrix derivative in gel form, primary closure was obtained with multilayered sutures. At 1-year follow-up, shallow probing depths associated with the elimination of the defects were observed (e,f).

fill of the defect (57% vs. 18%) and linear radiographic bone growth (2.6 mm vs. 0.9 mm). The results of this study led to the approval by the US Food and Drug Administration of this material. The authors interpreted the dichotomy represented by the significance of the added benefit in terms of radiographic parameters without the presence of significant changes in CAL as the result of biologic action of the growth factor formulation in shortening the healing time of the hard tissues. As of today, however, the results of this study have not been independently confirmed.

The benefit of use of EMD gel in the treatment of intrabony defects is supported by human histologic evidence, case report studies, meta-analysis of randomized controlled clinical trials, and a large multi-center trial (Heijl *et al.* 1997; Heden *et al.* 1999; Sculean *et al.* 1999b; Silvestri *et al.* 2000; Heden 2000; Tonetti *et al.* 2002; Giannobile & Somerman 2003; Heden & Wennstrom 2006) (Fig. 43-38).

Given their hydrophobic nature, enamel matrix proteins are mixed in a gel carrier at low pH for clinical use. Following an increase in pH in the periodontal wound and rapid elimination of the gel, EMD proteins (consisting mainly of amelogenins) are deposited in the wound environment and the root surface. While the mechanism(s) of action of EMD are not fully understood, significant evidence suggests that periodontal ligament cells exposed to EMD switch their phenotype by increasing expression of a host of growth and differentiation factor related genes (Brett *et al.* 2002; Parkar & Tonetti 2004), including transforming growth factor beta (Lyngstadaas *et al.* 2001).

A secondary analysis of a multi-center trial has shown that, in intrabony defects, the added benefit of EMD was greater in three-wall defects than in one-wall defects (Tonetti *et al.* 2002). Furthermore, another secondary analysis of the same material assessing the effect of the radiographic defect angle on the outcome (Tsitoura *et al.* 2004) has uncovered a negative association between the ragiographic angle of the defect and the clinical attachment level gains observed at 1 year. These data have questioned the suitability of the gel formulation of the EMD for the treatment of defects with a non-supporting anatomy (wide defects with missing bony walls).

These observations have spurred considerable research interest in the incorporation of EMD in a variety of bone replacement grafts in order to enhance wound stability and space maintenance. At this stage, however, no systematic evidence is available to support the use of such combinations.

Clinically, the rate of wound healing following application of EMD seems to be enhanced. A study looking at soft tissue density in the surgical site by using underexposed radiographs (Tonetti *et al.* 2004b) has found that the rate of increase in soft tissue density following application of EMD may be faster than in the access flap control. Such modulation has been interpreted as the outcome of the local release of growth and differentiation factors by the cells involved in local wound healing.

Membranes combined with other regenerative procedures

Compromised results after GTR may be obtained in cases where the membrane collapses/falls (partially or totally) into the defect and/or towards the root surface, thereby reducing the space available for invasion of new tissue capable of forming periodontal ligament and bone in particular. Reduced amounts of regenerated bone due to membrane collapse were noticed in early studies of GTR. In the study of Gottlow *et al.* (1984), it was observed that collapse of the membrane towards the root surface resulted in new cementum formation on the entire exposed root surfaces, whereas bone regeneration was minimal. Although the authors reported that the degree of coronal regrowth of bone was unrelated to the amount of new cementum formation, they did not comment on what effect membrane collapse might have had. Experimental studies, however, recognized the negative effect of membrane collapse on periodontal regeneration generally and on bone formation in particular (Caton *et al.* 1992; Haney *et al.* 1993;

Sigurdsson *et al.* 1994; Sallum *et al.* 1998). Haney *et al.* (1993) observed a highly significant correlation between the space provided by the membrane and the amount of regenerated alveolar bone using a supra-alveolar defect model in dogs. This finding corroborates that of Cortellini *et al.* (1995c) who reported that clinical application of self-supporting (reinforced with titanium) e-PTFE membranes, which could be positioned more coronally than ordinary e-PTFE membranes, yielded a statistically significant increase in PAL gain in intrabony defects. A particular risk for membrane collapse exists in cases where the configuration of the defect is incapable of supporting/preserving the membrane at the position where it was originally placed.

As already discussed, membrane materials must possess certain characteristics in order to be efficient. Among those it is important that the membrane is capable of keeping its shape and integral features, thereby maintaining the space created adjacent to the root surface. The e-PTFE membranes reinforced with titanium are the closest in meeting these requirements but they have the disadvantage that they are non-resorbable. At present there are no resorbable membranes available that fulfill this requirement sufficiently, which means that the placement of a resorbable membrane on, for instance, a wide one-wall defect involves the risk of membrane collapse. The collapse may be prevented by means of implantation of a biomaterial into the defect to support the membrane so that it maintains its original position (Fig. 43-39). However, the biomaterial to be used for this purpose must not interfere with the process of periodontal regeneration and ideally it may also promote bone regeneration.

As previously described, periodontal regeneration has been attempted with a variety of grafting materials, among which demineralized freeze-dried bone allografts (DFDBA) apparently facilitated regeneration in humans (Ouhayoun 1996). Schallhorn and McClain (1988) reported on improved clinical results in intrabony defects and degree II furcations, following a combination therapy including barrier membranes plus DFDBA and citric acid root conditioning.

In three controlled clinical trials, the treatment of a total of 45 pairs of intrabony defects with DFDBA grafting and GTR were compared to GTR alone (Table 43-7). The weighted mean of the results of the reported investigations showed similar gain in CAL in the GTR group (2.1 ± 1.1 mm, 95% CI 1.6–2.6 mm) and in the GTR plus DFDBA group (2.3 ± 1.4 mm, 95% CI 1.7–2.9 mm). The differences between the two treatments did not reach statistical significance, thus indicating no added effect of combining DFDBA with barrier materials in the treatment of intrabony defects. Guillemin *et al.* (1993) compared the effect of DFDBA alone with a combination of barrier materials and DFDBA in 15 pairs of intrabony defects. Both treatments resulted in significant amounts of CAL gains

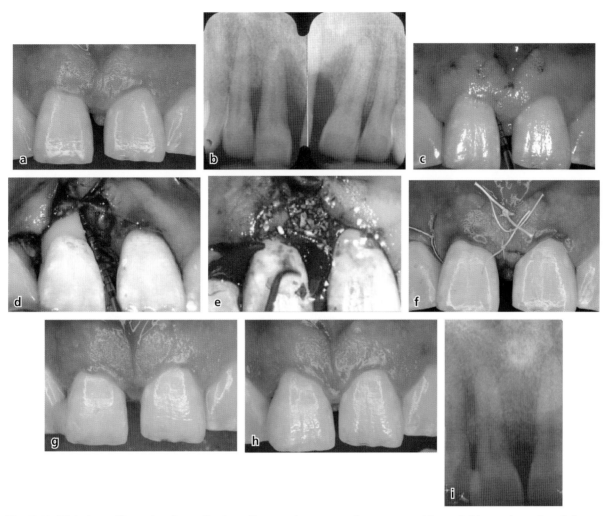

Fig. 43-39 Clinical case illustrating the application of bone replacement graft to support a bioresorbable membrane in a defect with poor space maintaining anatomy. Following control of periodontitis and risk factors, the upper right contral incisor presented with a 12-mm deep pocket associated with a defect extending close to the apex of the tooth (a–c). The defect was accessed with the modified papilla preservation flap to reveal an 8-mm intrabony component (d). A bone replacement graft was placed under a bioresorbable collagen membrane (e). Primary closure was achieved with a multilayered suture technique (f). Excellent early healing was observed already at the 2-week follow-up (g). At 1 year, periodontal regeneration resulted in shallow probing depths and good resolution of the intrabony defect (h,i). Radio-opaque bone replacement graft particles are visible within the newly formed mineralized tissue.

Table 43-7 Summary of controlled clinical trials evaluating the combined effects of decalcified freeze-dried bone allografts (DFDBA) and barrier membranes in deep intrabony defects

Authors	Design (GTR treatment)	N*	Gains in CAL (mm)		Significance	Residual PD (mm)		Significance
			GTR	GTR + DFDBA		GTR	GTR + DFDBA	
Chen et al. 1995	Intra-individual (Collagen)	8	2.0 ± 0.4	2.3 ± 0.5	P > 0.05, NS	4.2 ± 0.4	4.2 ± 0.5	P > 0.05, NS
Mellado et al. 1995	Intra-individual (e-PTFE)	11	2.0 ± 0.9	2.0 ± 1.4	P = 0.86, NS	NA	NA	NA
Gouldin et al. 1996	Intra-individual (e-PTFE)	26	2.2 ± 1.4	2.4 ± 1.6	NS	3.7 ± 1.6	3.7 ± 1.8	NS
Weighted mean		**45**	**2.1 ± 1.1**	**2.3 ± 1.4**		**3.8 ± 1.3**§	**3.8 ± 1.5**§	

* Defects per treatment arm.
CAL = clinical attachment level; PD = pocket depth; e-PTFE = expanded polytetrafluoroethylene; DFDBA = decalcified freeze-dried bone allograft; NS = not significant; NA = data not available.
§ N = mean (34) ± S.D. (34).

Table 43-8 Controlled clinical trials comparing clinical outcomes of GTR procedures with e-PTFE non-bioabsorbable barrier membranes with or without the adjunctive use of grafts in mandibular degree II furcations

Authors	Design & treatment (GTR C/GTR T)	N C/T	Defect depth (mm)		H-OPAL gain (mm)	
			GTR C	GTR T	GTR C	GTR T
Lekovic et al. 1990	Intra-individual (e-PTFE/e-PTFE + HA)	15/15	4.2 ± 0.2	4.3 ± 0.2	0.1 ± 0.1	1.6 ± 0.2
Anderegg et al. 1991	Intra-individual (e-PTFE/e-PTFE + DFDBA)	15/15	4.2 ± 2.2	5.3 ± 2.6	1.0 ± 0.8*	2.4 ± 1.5*
Wallace et al. 1994	Parallel (e-PTFE/e-PTFE + DFDBA)	7/10	6.0 ± ?	6.5 ± ?	2.3 ± ?	2.4 ± ?
Weighted Mean		**37/40**	**4.5 ± 1.2†**	**5.2 ± 1.4‡**	**0.9 ± 0.5†**	**2.1 ± 0.9§**

GTR C = guided tissue regeneration control treatment; GTR T = guided tissue regeneration test treatment; N C/T = number of defects in the control (C) and in the test (T) treatment arm; H-OPAL = horizontal open probing attachment; e-PTFE = expanded polytetrafluoroethylene; HA = hydroxyapatite; DFDBA = decalcified freeze-dried bone allograft.
* Difference between treatments statistically significant.
† N = Mean (37) ± S.D. (30); ‡ N = Mean (40) ± S.D. (30); § N = Mean (35) ± S.D. (24).

and bone fill at 6 months, but no difference was found between the treatments.

In three studies on mandibular degree II furcations, GTR treatment alone was compared with GTR treatment combined with hydroxyapatite or DFDBA (Table 43-8). In one of these investigations, a statistically significant improvement was found in terms of horizontal open probing attachment levels (H-OPAL) in the group of furcations treated with the combination therapy (Anderegg et al. 1991). In another of these three studies the difference between the two treatments was not statistically significant, but the combination therapy resulted in a greater extent of furcation fill (Lekovic et al. 1990). In the third investigation (Wallace et al. 1994), the two treatments were equivalent in terms of H-OPAL gains. The weighted mean of the cited studies showed greater H-OPAL gains in the cases treated with the combination therapy (2.1 ± 0.9 mm, 95% CI 1.6–2.6 mm) when compared to GTR treatment alone (0.9 ± 0.5 mm, 95% CI 0.6–1.1 mm), indicating a possible added benefit from the use of grafting materials in combination with non-bioabsorbable barrier membranes for the treatment of mandibular degree II furcations.

Promising clinical results with a PAL-gain of 1.0–5.5 mm were obtained in human case reports, in which the GTR technique was combined with grafting of Bio-Oss® for the treatment of intrabony periodontal defects (Lundgren & Slotte 1999; Mellonig 2000; Paolantonio et al. 2001). The combined Bio-Oss® and GTR treatment resulted in greater PPD reduction, PAL gain and defect fill than the mere implantation of Bio-Oss® in case series (Camelo et al. 1998) and than flap surgery alone in a split-mouth study (Camargo et al. 2000).

In a recent randomized controlled clinical study including 60 patients (Stavropoulos et al. 2003), Bio-Oss® alone or impregnated with gentamicin was used as an adjunct to GTR in the treatment of one-wall or two-wall intrabony defects, and the outcomes were compared to those obtained following GTR alone or flap surgery. Treatment with a membrane alone (Fig. 43-40) resulted in a mean PAL gain of 2.9 mm, while it was 3.8 and 2.5 mm, respectively, when Bio-Oss®

grafts with or without gentamicin were placed in the defects prior to membrane coverage (Fig. 43-41). The control defects treated with flap surgery demonstrated a gain of PAL of only 1.5 mm. The clinical improvements in defects treated with GTR alone or in combination with Bio-Oss® grafting were significantly better than those obtained with flap surgery, whereas the differences between the groups treated with membranes were not statistically significant.

In a controlled study (Pietruska 2001), similar clinical improvements were obtained when Bio-Oss® combined with GTR was compared with biomodification of the root surface with enamel matrix protein (Emdogain®).

Camelo et al. (1998) and Mellonig (2000) presented histologic data indicating that the use of Bio-Oss® under a membrane may result in partial regeneration of the periodontal apparatus, but in all the cases, most of the defect was still occupied by deproteinized bone particles. Bone was not observed near the root, and the connective tissue fibers of the "new" periodontal ligament were mostly oriented parallel to the root surface. These results corroborate findings reported by Paolantonio et al. (2001), who observed only limited bone formation in the vicinity of the pre-existing bone in a biopsy, taken from a site treated 8 months earlier with Bio-Oss® and a collagen membrane. Most of the space in the defect was occupied by Bio-Oss® particles embedded in connective tissue. However, in a case report where intrabony defects were treated with Bio-Oss® combined with intraoral autogenous bone and GTR, new attachment formation had occurred consistently, but a major portion of the regenerated osseous tissue consisted of deproteinized bone particles (Camelo et al. 2001). The effect of combining citric acid root biomodification with GTR treatment was evaluated in two randomized controlled clinical trials in intrabony defects. The first investigation (Handelsman et al. 1991) demonstrated significant amounts of CAL gains in both the test (e-PTFE membranes and citric acid; CAL gain 3.5 ± 1.6 mm) and control sites (e-PTFE membranes alone; CAL gain 4.0 ±

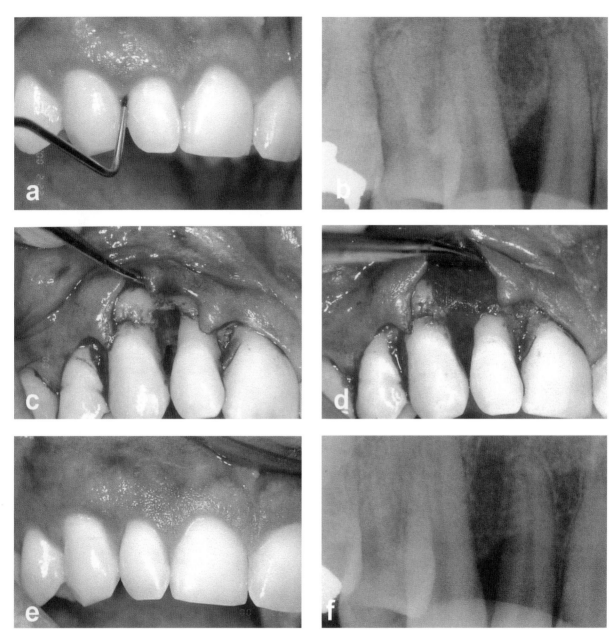

Fig. 43-40 Right lateral maxillary incisor with an 8-mm deep pocket associated with an intrabony defect on the distal aspect (a), as seen on the radiograph (b). Full-thickness buccal and palatal flaps have been raised and the defect has been debrided (c). A bioabsorbable membrane has been adopted over the defect (d). The level of the interdental gingiva is maintained after 1 year (e) and the intrabony defect (f) is resolved.

1.4 mm). Less favorable results following these two treatment modalities were reported by Kersten et al. (1992) who found CAL gains of 1.0 ± 1.1 mm in the test group, and CAL gains of 0.7 ± 1.5 mm in the control group. Both studies, however, failed to demonstrate any added effect of the use of citric acid in combination with non-bioabsorbable barrier membranes.

Root surface biomodification with tetracycline alone and in combination with GTR was evaluated in two controlled studies on degree II furcations (Machtei et al. 1993; Parashis & Mitsis 1993). Both investigations failed to show significant differences between sites treated with non-bioabsorbable barrier membranes alone or in combination with tetracycline

root surface biomodification. Similarly, the use of other surface active chemicals like EDTA also failed to provide a significant added effect to GTR treatment in humans (Lindhe & Cortellini 1996).

Root surface biomodification

The suggested role of root surface biomodification for improving periodontal regeneration has been recently assessed in a systematic review (Mariotti et al. 2003). The results of that exhaustive review of the evidence indicated that there was no evidence of a measurable improvement following root conditioning with agents like citric acid, tetracycline HCl, phosphoric acid, fibronectin or EDTA.

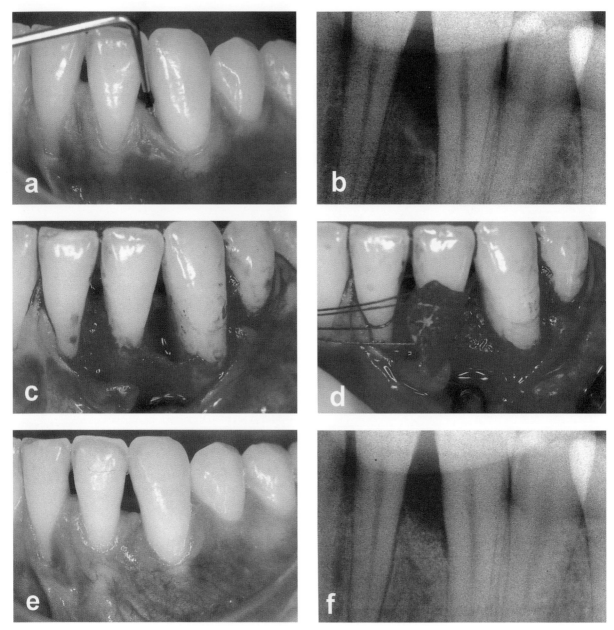

Fig. 43-41 Left mandibular canine with an 8-mm deep pocket (a) associated with an intrabony defect on its mesial aspect (b). The defect is debrided after flap elevation (c) and Bio-Oss® particles are placed in the defect (d) prior to placement of a bioabsorbable membrane. After 1 year (e), no gingival recession has occurred and the intrabony defect is almost resolved (f).

Clinical strategies

Periodontal regeneration in intrabony defects has been successfully attempted with a variety of different approaches. As discussed, meta-analyses of randomized controlled clinical trials as well as human and animal histologic findings support the potential of barrier membranes (Nyman *et al.* 1982; Gottlow *et al.* 1986), demineralized freeze dried bone allograft (DFDBA) (Bowers *et al.* 1989a,b,c), combination of barrier membranes and grafts (Camelo *et al.* 1998; Mellonig 2000), and the use of enamel matrix derivative (Mellonig 1999; Yukna & Mellonig 2000) to induce periodontal regeneration. Controlled clinical trials report that the above-mentioned approaches provide added benefits in terms of clinical attach-

ment level (CAL) gain as compared to open-flap debridement alone (Needleman *et al.* 2002; Murphy *et al.* 2003; Trombelli *et al.* 2002; Giannobile & Somerman 2003; Tonetti *et al.* 2004a). Comparisons among some of the cited regenerative approaches failed to demonstrate a clear superiority of one of the tested materials (Murphy *et al.* 2003; Giannobile & Somerman 2003; Reynolds *et al.* 2003).

The existing evidence, therefore, does not support the choice of a single approach among the different regenerative possibilities. In addition, all the cited studies have shown a substantial degree of variability, in terms of CAL gains, reporting failures or unsatisfactory outcomes in part of the treated population.

Research conducted mostly in the past decade has clearly established that the variability observed in outcomes of periodontal regenerative procedures is dependent on a variety of patient, defect, and surgical associated factors.

While relevant patient factors include cigarette smoking, residual periodontal infection, and oral hygiene, factors associated with the morphology of the defect are consistently found to be of relevance for the final outcome (Tonetti *et al.* 1998; Cortellini *et al.* 2001). Interestingly, however, the number of residual bony walls defining the defect seems to impact the outcomes of different periodontal regenerative materials in a divergent way. Non-resorbable (e-PTFE and titanium-reinforced e-PTFE) barrier membranes, and bioresorbable barriers supported by a graft do not seem to be affected by the number of residual bony walls of the defect (Tonetti *et al.* 1993a, 1996a, 2004b), while EMD results in better outcomes in three-wall defects (Tonetti *et al.* 2002). Furthermore, healing following application of bioresorbable barriers and non-resorbable e-PTFE barriers as well as EMD is associated with the radiographic width of the intrabony defect (Tonetti *et al.* 1993a; Falk *et al.* 1997; Tsitoura *et al.* 2004). No such association has been found for the use of a xenogenic bone replacement graft and resorbable barrier graft combination (Tonetti *et al.* 2004b).

Among the technical/surgical factors, membrane exposure and contamination have been associated with reduced outcomes (Selvig *et al.* 1992; Nowzari & Slots 1994; Nowzari *et al.* 1995; De Sanctis *et al.* 1996a,b). Similar problems were also encountered with bone grafting (Sanders *et al.* 1983). Reduced outcomes were also observed when the regenerated tissue was not properly protected with the flap at removal of non-resorbable barrier membranes (Tonetti *et al.* 1993a; Cortellini *et al.* 1995c).

A controlled clinical trial demonstrated that the combination of a papilla preservation flap and titanium-reinforced e-PTFE membrane resulted in greater amounts of clinical attachment level gains as compared to a conventional flap approach associated with an e-PTFE membrane (Cortellini *et al.* 1995c). This evidence, also partly supported by a systematic review (Murphy *et al.* 2003), strongly suggests that optimization of the surgical approach and control of surgical variables, particularly in relation to flap design and management and selection of the regenerative material, could improve outcomes. In the context of GTR, several specific flap designs aimed at the full preservation of the soft tissues during access to the defect have been described (Cortellini *et al.* 1995c,d, 1996c, 1999; Murphy 1996). Experimental testing of these regenerative flaps reported great improvements in achieving primary closure during the surgical session with optimal interdental closure being obtained in virtually all cases (Tonetti *et al.* 2004b; Cortellini *et al.* 1995c,d, 1999, 2001). During the subsequent healing, however, dehiscence of the interdental tissue and membrane exposure was observed in up to a third of the cases. The ability to accomplish

and maintain primary closure of the tissues over a GTR membrane was further improved by the use of a microsurgical approach that resulted in maintenance of primary wound closure in 92.3% of the treated sites for the whole healing period (Cortellini & Tonetti 2001, 2007a,b).

This body of evidence can be utilized together with a degree of clinical experience to develop an "evidence-based regenerative strategy" to guide clinicians through a decision-making process aimed at the optimization of the clinical outcomes of periodontal regeneration in intrabony defects (Cortellini & Tonetti 2000a, 2005). Key steps of this process are the careful evaluation of the patient and of the defect, the access of the defect with a papilla preservation flap, the possibility of choosing the most appropriate regenerative technology/material, and the ability to seal the regenerating wound from the contaminated oral environment with optimal suturing techniques.

Two to three months after completion of periodontal therapy, baseline clinical measurements are recorded. The regenerative strategy is selected according to a decision-making process. Surgical procedures, according to the principles of periodontal regeneration, are performed. Patients are then enrolled in a stringent periodontal supportive care program for 1 year followed by regular supportive periodontal care.

The appropriate regenerative strategy for the individual case is selected according to a recently modified, evidence-based operative decision tree (Cortellini & Tonetti 2000a, 2005) (Figs. 43-42, 43-43, 43-44).

The surgical access to the intrabony defects is selected from among three different surgical approaches: the simplified papilla preservation flap (SPPF) (Cortellini *et al.* 1999), the modified papilla preservation technique (MPPT) (Cortellini *et al.* 1995d), and the crestal incision (Cortellini & Tonetti 2000a). The SPPF is chosen whenever the width of the interdental space is 2 mm or less, as measured at the level of the papilla; the MPPT is used at sites with an interdental width greater than 2 mm (Fig. 43-42); the crestal incision is applied next to an edentulous area.

Selection of the regenerative material is based on the defect anatomy (Figs. 43-43, 43-44). A non-resorbable titanium-reinforced e-PTFE membrane is used when the defect anatomy is not "supportive", such as in wide and one- or two-wall defects. Alternatively, a bioresorbable membrane supported with a bone replacement graft material can be used in these instances. The latter is preferred to titanium-reinforced e-PTFE when the non-supportive defects are associated with narrow interdental spaces. A bioresorbable membrane is applied alone in "supportive" defects, like the narrow and the two-to-three-wall ones. EMD is preferred in defects with a prevalent three-wall morphology or in well supported two-wall defects.

The suturing approach is chosen according to the defect anatomy and to the type of

Surgical access

Interdental space width

Width >2mm — MPPT

Width ≥2mm — SPPF

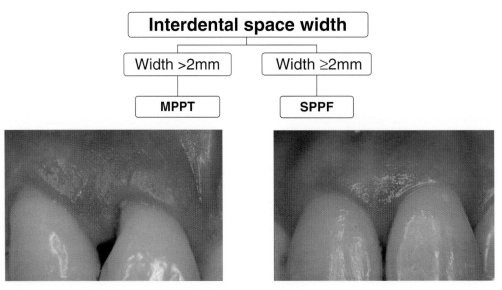

Fig. 43-42 Decision-making algorithm illustrating the parameters to take into account when deciding how to access an interdental intrabony defect: the simplified papilla preservation flap (SPPF) is used for narrow interdental spaces (2 mm or narrower), while the modified papilla preservation technique (MPPT) is used to access defect associated with wider interdental spaces (3 mm or wider).

Regenerative approach

Deep intrabony component

Wide and/or non-supportive anatomy   Narrow and/or supportive anatomy

Titanium e-PTFE   3 walls   Bioresorbable

EMD

BRG and bioresorbable

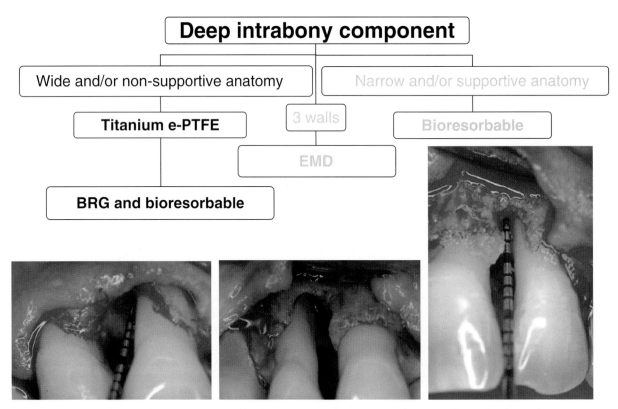

Fig. 43-43 Decision-making algorithm discussing the choice of currently available technologies for application in the treatment of intrabony defects with wide, non-space supporting anatomy. Either titanium-reinforced membranes or bioresorbable membranes are used to obtain a stable regenerative environment, provide space, and support the soft tissues.

Regenerative approach

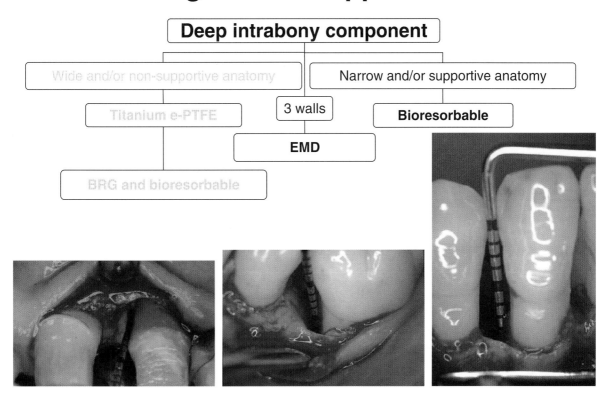

Fig. 43-44 Decision-making algorithm discussing the choice of currently available technologies for application in the treatment of intrabony defects with narrow, space-supporting anatomy. Enamel matrix derivative in gel form is preferred for three-wall defects, while bioresorbable membranes are used for the other narrow type of defects.

regenerative strategy used in each case. It consists of the combination of two sutures applied in the defect-associated interdental area to reach primary closure of the papilla in the absence of any tension. The first interdental suture is positioned between the apical part of the buccal gingiva, near the mucogingival junction, and an apical area of the lingual/palatal flap. In supportive defects (three-wall defects) or in the presence of a supportive membrane (titanium e-PTFE membrane), or a supported membrane (bioresorbable and bone replacement graft), an internal horizontal crossed mattress suture is used. In non-supportive defects and in the presence of bioresorbable membranes or EMD, an offset internal mattress suture is preferred. When a crestal incision is performed, internal horizontal mattress sutures can be conveniently applied. The aims of this first suture are to relieve the residual tension of the flaps in the defect-associated area and to displace the buccal flap coronally. A second, more coronal internal mattress suture is placed to close the interdental papilla passively over the regenerative material.

The surgical procedures can be performed with the aid of magnification such as loupes or an operating microscope. Microsurgical instruments can be utilized to complement the normal periodontal set of instruments.

An empirical protocol for the control of bacterial contamination consisting of doxycycline (100 mg bid for 1 week), 0.12% chlorhexidine mouth rinsing three times per day, and weekly prophylaxis is prescribed. Patients are requested to avoid brushing, flossing, and chewing in the treated area for 6–10 weeks. Non-resorbable membranes are removed after 6 weeks. Patients can resume full oral hygiene and chewing function in the treated area 2–4 weeks after membrane removal or when bioresorbable membranes are fully resorbed. Patients treated with EMD resume full oral hygiene after a period of 4–5 weeks. At the end of the "early healing phase", patients are placed on monthly recall for 1 year.

The performance of this clinical strategy has been recently assessed in a 40-patient consecutive case series (Cortellini & Tonetti 2005). Following completion of initial, cause-related periodontal therapy, subjects presented full-mouth plaque scores of $10.2 \pm 2.7\%$ and full-mouth bleeding scores at baseline of $7.9 \pm 2.8\%$. At the intrabony defects, clinical attachment levels (CAL) were 10.2 ± 2.4 mm and probing depths (PD) amounted to 8.9 ± 1.8 mm. The radiographic defect angle was $29° \pm 5.9°$. Distance from the cemento-enamel junction to the bottom of the defect (CEJ-BD) was 11.2 ± 2.7 mm and the intrabony component of the defects (INFRA) was 6.6 ± 1.7 mm.

In this population the simplified papilla preservation flap could be used in 37.5% of sites, while the modified papilla preservation technique was selected in 45% of cases. The remaining sites, presenting with defects adjacent to edentulous areas, were accessed with a crestal incision.

Based on defect anatomy, non-resorbable titanium-reinforced e-PTFE barrier membranes were used in 30% of cases. In these cases defect angles ranged from 27–42° (average 32.4° ± 4.3°), and two out of three of the selected defects had a one-wall intrabony sub-component of 1–3 mm (average one-wall component of the 12 sites was 1.4 ± 1.2 mm).

Ten of the 11 defects treated with bioresorbable membranes supported with a bone replacement graft, presented a one-wall sub-component of 1–5 mm (average one-wall component of the 11 sites 1.8 ± 1.3 mm); defect angles in this group ranged from 21–45° (average 31.4° ± 7°).

Bioresorbable barriers alone were used in seven sites presenting with a prevalent two- and three-wall morphology and narrow defect angles, ranging from 20–28° (average 24.1° ± 3.7°). EMD was applied to ten defects with a prevalent three-wall component. The defect angle in this group ranged from 19–31° (average 26.5° ± 4.3°).

In all treated sites primary closure was obtained at completion of the surgical procedure. At the 1-week follow-up, when sutures were removed, two sites, both accessed with a SPPF, presented with a small interdental wound dehiscence: one had been treated with a bioresorbable membrane and bone replacement graft, the other with EMD. At week 2, two additional small wound dehiscences were detected: one accessed with MPPT and treated with a bioresorbable membrane and bone replacement graft, the other accessed with SPPF and treated with a bioresorbable barrier alone. All the other sites (90%) remained closed during the whole early healing phase.

The 40 patients presented at the 1-year follow-up visit with excellent levels of plaque control and low levels of bleeding on probing. The 1-year CAL clinical attachment gain was 6 ± 1.8 mm (range 4–11 mm). No sites gained less then 4 mm of CAL; 77.5% gained 5 mm or more and 40% more then 6 mm. Residual probing depths were 2.7 ± 0.6 mm, with an average pocket depth reduction of 6.1 ± 1.9 mm. Only four sites showed a residual probing depth of 4 mm; all the other sites resulted with a 1-year PPD of 3 mm or less. A minimal increase of 0.1 ± 0.7 mm in gingival recession between baseline and 1 year was recorded.

The performance of each of the four treatments was described in the study and it indicated that, whenever the choices were made according to the protocol (i.e. based on: width of the interdental space to chose the papilla preservation surgery; morphology of the defect to choose the regenerative material; and choice of the material and local anatomy to select the suturing approach) all four approaches gave excellent results with clinical attachment level gains equal to 88–95% resolution of the original depth of the intrabony component of the defect (Cortellini & Tonetti 2005).

The use of this decision-making protocol in the reported case series resulted in 6 ± 1.8 mm of CAL gain at 1 year. These results were obtained in defects with an intrabony component of 6.6 ± 1.7 mm. The percentage clinical attachment gain therefore was 92.1 ± 12%. This indicates that a large part of the intrabony component of the defects was resolved. Using the Ellegaard criteria (Ellegaard *et al.* 1971), resolution of the intrabony component of the defect was either satisfactory or complete in all treated cases. In particular 40.5% of defects had attachment level gains equal to or greater then the baseline depth of the intrabony component, while the defect with the worst response showed a 71.4% CAL gain. Historical comparison with clinical experiments using bone grafting or GTR clearly indicates that the results of this trial approach were in the top percentiles in terms of clinical attachment level gains and defect resolution (Cortellini & Tonetti 2000a; Rosen *et al.* 2000).

Conclusions

GTR represents the best documented regenerative procedure for obtaining periodontal regeneration in intrabony defects and in degree II furcations. GTR has demonstrated significant clinical improvement beyond that achieved with only debridement in such defects. Regarding degree II maxillary furcations, the results following GTR treatment are inconsistent, and the treatment of degree III furcation defects is unpredictable. An added benefit may be obtained by the use of grafting materials in combination with GTR in some situations: in particular in furcation defects or to support bioresorbable membranes.

DFDBA alone gives documented improvements in some type of intrabony defects, in particular three-wall and two-wall defects.

EMD in gel formulation gives significant benefits in the treatment of intrabony defects, particularly those with a supportive anatomy (three-wall defects and narrow two-wall defects).

Differences between individuals and studies regarding the results of treating intrabony defects and class II furcations are related to patient compliance, maintenance procedures, selection of defects, surgical management, etc.

Periodontal regeneration obtained following GTR is stable on a long-term basis, provided good oral hygiene is maintained and a proper recall program is established. Current data indicate that, in patients participating in a supportive periodontal care program, 96% of teeth with severe intrabony defects and treated with a periodontal regenerative procedure could be retained for a period up to 15 years.

References

Al-Arrayed, F., Adam, S., Moran, J. & Dowell, P. (1995). Clinical trial of cross-linked human type I collagen as a barrier material in surgical periodontal treatment. *Journal of Clinical Periodontology* **22**, 371–379.

Anderegg, C., Martin, S., Gray, J., Mellonig, J., & Gher, M. (1991). Clinical evaluation of the use of decalcified freeze-dried bone allograft with guided tissue regeneration in the treatment of molar furcation invasions. *Journal of Periodontology* **62**, 264–268.

Anderegg, C., Metzeler, D. & Nicoll, B. (1995). Gingival thickness in guided tissue regeneration and associated recession at facial furcation defects. *Journal of Periodontology* **66**, 397–402.

Becker, W. & Becker, B. (1993). Treatment of mandibular three-wall intrabony defects by flap debridement and expanded polytetrafluoroethylene barrier membranes. Long term evaluation of 32 treated patients. *Journal of Periodontology* **64**, 1138–1144.

Becker, W., Becker, B.E., Berg, L., Pritchard, J., Caffesse, R. & Rosenberg, E. (1988). New attachment after treatment with root isolation procedures: Report for treated class III and class II furcations and vertical osseous defects. *International Journal of Periodontics and Restorative Dentistry* **8**, 2–16.

Becker, W., Becker, B.E., Mellonig, J. Caffesse, R.G., Warrer, K., Caton, J.G. & Reid, T. (1996). A prospective multicenter study evaluating periodontal regeneration for class II furcation invasions and intrabony defects after treatment with a biosorbable barrier membrane: 1 year results. *Journal of Periodontology* **67**, 641–649.

Benqué, E., Zahedi, S., Brocard, D., Oscaby, F., Justumus, P. & Brunel, G. (1997). Guided tissue regeneration using a collagen membrane in chronic adult and rapidly progressive periodontitis patients in the treatment of 3-wall intrabony defects. *Journal of Clinical Periodontology* **24**, 544–549.

Black, S., Gher, M., Sandifer, J., Fucini, S. & Richardson, C. (1994). Comparative study of collagen and expanded polytetrafluoroethylene membranes in the treatment of human class II furcation defects. *Journal of Periodontology* **65**, 598–604.

Blumenthal, N.M. (1988). The use of collagen membranes to guide regeneration of new connective tissue attachment in dogs. *Journal of Periodontology* **59**, 830–836.

Blumenthal, N.M. (1993). A clinical comparison of collagen membranes with e-PTFE membranes in the treatment of human mandibular Class II furcation defects. *Journal of Periodontology* **64**, 925–933.

Bouchard, P., Ouhayoun, J. & Nilveus, R. (1993). Expanded polytetrafluorethylene membranes and connective tissue grafts support bone regeneration for closing mandibular class II furcations. *Journal of Periodontology* **64**, 1193–1198.

Bowers, G.M., Chadroff, B., Carnevale, R., Mellonig, J., Corio, R., Emerson, J., Stevens, M. & Romberg, E. (1989a). Histologic evaluation of new attachment apparatus formation in humans. Part I. *Journal of Periodontology* **60**, 664–674.

Bowers, G.M., Chadroff, B., Carnevale, R., Mellonig, J., Corio, R., Emerson, J., Stevens, M. & Romberg, E. (1989b). Histologic evaluation of new human attachment apparatus formation in humans. Part II. *Journal of Periodontology* **60**, 675–682.

Bowers, G.M., Chadroff, B., Carnevale, R., Mellonig, J., Corio, R., Emerson, J., Stevens, M. & Romberg, E. (1989c). Histologic evaluation of a new attachment apparatus formation in humans. Part III. *Journal of Periodontology* **60**, 683–693.

Bowers, G.M., Schallhorn, R.G., McClain, P.K., Morrison, G.M., Morgan, R. & Reynolds, M.A. (2003). Factors influencing the outcome of regenerative therapy in mandibular Class II furcations: Part I. *Journal of Periodontology* **74**, 255–268.

Brett, P.M., Parkar, M., Olsen, I. & Tonetti, M. (2002). Expression profiling of periodontal ligament cells stimulated with enamel matrix proteins in vitro: a model for tissue regeneration. *Journal of Dental Research* **81**, 776–783.

Bühler, H. (1988). Evaluation of root-resected teeth. Results after 10 years. *Journal of Periodontology* **59**, 805–810.

Caffesse, R., Mota, L., Quinones, C. & Morrison, E.C. (1997). Clinical comparison of resorbable and non-resorbable barriers for guided tissue regeneration. *Journal of Clinical Periodontology* **24**, 747–752.

Caffesse, R.G., Nasjleti, C.E., Morrison, E.C. & Sanchez, R. (1994). Guided tissue regeneration: comparison of bioabsorbable and non-bioabsorbable membranes. Histologic and histometric study in dogs. *Journal of Periodontology* **65**, 583–591.

Caffesse, R.G., Smith, B.A., Castelli, W.A. & Nasjleti, C.E. (1988). New attachment achieved by guided tissue regeneration in beagle dogs. *Journal of Periodontology* **59**, 589–594.

Caffesse, R., Smith, B., Duff, B., Morrison, E., Merril, D. & Becker, W. (1990). Class II furcations treated by guided tissue regeneration in humans: case reports. *Journal of Periodontology* **61**, 510–514.

Camargo, P.M., Lekovic, V., Weinlander, M., Nedic, M., Vasilic, N., Wolinsky, L.E. & Kenney, E.B. (2000). A controlled re-entry study on the effectiveness of bovine porous bone mineral used in combination with a collagen membrane of porcine origin in the treatment of intrabony defects in humans. *Journal of Clinical Periodontology* **27**, 889–986.

Camelo, M., Nevins, M.L., Lynch, S.E., Schenck, R.K., Simion, M. & Nevins, M. (2001). Periodontal regeneration with an autogenous bone-Bio-Oss composite graft and a Bio-Gide membrane. *International Journal of Periodontics and Restorative Dentistry* **21**, 109–119.

Camelo, M., Nevins, M., Schenk, R., Simion, M., Rasperini, C., Lynch, S. & Nevins, M. (1998). Clinical radiographic, and histologic evaluation of human periodontal defects treated with Bio-Oss® and Bio-Gide. *International Journal of Periodontics and Restorative Dentistry* **18**, 321–331.

Carnevale, G., Pontoriero, R. & di Febo, G. (1998). Long-term effects of root-resective therapy in furcation-involved molars. A 10-year longitudinal study. *Journal of Clinical Periodontology* **25**, 209–214.

Caton, J., Greenstein, G. & Zappa, U. (1994). Synthetic bioabsorbable barrier for regeneration in human periodontal defects. *Journal of Periodontology* **65**, 1037–1045.

Caton, J., Wagener, C., Polson, A., Nyman, S., Frantz, B., Bouwsma, O. & Blieden, T. (1992). Guided tissue regeneration in interproximal defects in the monkey. *International Journal of Periodontics and Restorative Dentistry* **12**, 266–277.

Chen, C., Wang, H., Smith, F., Glickman, G., Shyr, Y. & O'Neal, R. (1995). Evaluation of a collagen membrane with and without bone grafts in treating periodontal intrabony defects. *Journal of Periodontology* **66**, 838–847.

Christgau, M., Schamlz, G., Wenzel, A. & Hiller, K.A. (1997). Periodontal regeneration of intrabony defects with resorbable and non-resorbable membranes: 30 month results. *Journal of Clinical Periodontology* **24**, 17–21.

Chung, K.M., Salkin, L.M., Stein, M.D. & Freedman, A.L. (1990). Clinical evaluation of a biodegradable collagen membrane in guided tissue regeneration. *Journal of Periodontology* **61**, 732–736.

Cortellini, P. & Bowers, G.M. (1995). Periodontal regeneration at intrabony defects: an evidence-based treatment approach. *International Journal of Periodontics and Restorative Dentistry* **15**, 128–145.

Cortellini, P., Carnevale, G., Sanz, M. & Tonetti, M.S. (1998). Treatment of deep and shallow intrabony defects. A multicenter randomized controlled clinical trial. *Journal of Clinical Periodontology* **25**, 981–987.

Cortellini, P. & Pini-Prato, G. (1994). Guided tissue regeneration with a rubber dam; A five case report. *International Journal of Periodontics and Restorative Dentistry* **14**, 9–15.

Cortellini, P., Pini-Prato, G., Baldi, C. & Clauser, C. (1990). Guided tissue regeneration with different materials. *International Journal of Periodontics and Restorative Dentistry* **10**, 137–151.

Cortellini, P., Pini-Prato, G. & Tonetti, M. (1993b). Periodontal regeneration of human infrabony defects. I. Clinical Measures. *Journal of Periodontology* **64**, 254–260.

Cortellini, P., Pini-Prato, G. & Tonetti, M. (1993c). Periodontal regeneration of human infrabony defects. II. Re-entry procedures and bone measures. *Journal of Periodontology* **64**, 261–268.

Cortellini, P., Pini-Prato, G. & Tonetti, M. (1994). Periodontal regeneration of human infrabony defects. V. Effect of oral hygiene on long term stability. *Journal of Clinical Periodontology* **21**, 606–610.

Cortellini, P., Pini-Prato, G. & Tonetti, M. (1995a). Interproximal free gingival grafts after membrane removal in GTR treatment of infrabony defects. A controlled clinical trial indicating improved outcomes. *Journal of Periodontology* **66**, 488–493.

Cortellini, P., Pini-Prato, G. & Tonetti, M. (1995b). No detrimental effect of fibrin glue on the regeneration of infrabony defects. A controlled clinical trial. *Journal of Clinical Periodontology* **22**, 697–702.

Cortellini, P., Pini-Prato, G. & Tonetti, M. (1995c). Periodontal regeneration of human infrabony defects with titanium reinforced membranes. A controlled clinical trial. *Journal of Periodontology* **66**, 797–803.

Cortellini, P., Pini-Prato, G. & Tonetti, M. (1995d). The modified papilla preservation technique. A new surgical approach for interproximal regenerative procedures. *Journal of Periodontology* **66**, 261–266.

Cortellini, P., Pini-Prato, G. & Tonetti, M. (1996a). Long term stability of clinical attachment following guided tissue regeneration and conventional therapy. *Journal of Clinical Periodontology* **23**, 106–111.

Cortellini, P., Pini-Prato, G. & Tonetti, M. (1996b). Periodontal regeneration of human intrabony defects with bioresorbable membranes. A controlled clinical trial. *Journal of Periodontology* **67**, 217–223.

Cortellini, P., Pini-Prato, G. & Tonetti, M. (1996c). The modified papilla preservation technique with bioresorbable barrier membranes in the treatment of intrabony defects. Case reports. *International Journal of Periodontics and Restorative Dentistry* **14**, 8–15.

Cortellini, P., Prato, G.P. & Tonetti, M.S. (1999). The simplified papilla preservation flap. A novel surgical approach for the management of soft tissues in regenerative procedures. *International Journal of Periodontics and Restorative Dentistry* **19**, 589–599.

Cortellini, P. & Tonetti, M. (1999). Radiographic defect angle influences the outcome of GTR therapy in intrabony defects. *Journal of Dental Research* **78**, 381 (abstract).

Cortellini, P. & Tonetti, M.S. (2000a). Focus on intrabony defects: guided tissue regeneration (GTR). *Periodontology 2000* **22**, 104–132.

Cortellini, P. & Tonetti, M. (2000b). Evaluation of the effect of tooth vitality on regenerative outcomes in intrabony defects. *Journal of Clinical Periodontology* **28**, 672–679.

Cortellini, P. & Tonetti, M.S. (2001). Microsurgical approach to periodontal regeneration. Initial evaluation in a case cohort. *Journal of Periodontology* **72**, 559–569.

Cortellini, P., Tonetti, M.S., Lang, N.P., Suvan, J.E., Zucchelli, G., Vangsted, T., Silvestri, M., Rossi, R., McClain, P., Fonzar, A., Dubravec, D. & Adriaens, P. (2001). The simplified papilla preservation flap in the regenerative treatment of deep intrabony defects: clinical outcomes and postoperative morbidity. *Journal of Periodontology* **72**, 1701–1712.

Cortellini, P. & Tonetti, M.S. (2004). Long-term tooth survival following regenerative treatment of intrabony defects. *Journal of Periodontology* **75**, 672–678.

Cortellini, P. & Tonetti, M.S. (2005). Clinical performance of a regenerative strategy for intrabony defects: scientific evidence and clinical experience. *Journal of Periodontology* **76**, 341–350.

Cortellini, P. & Tonetti, M.S. (2007a). A minimally invasive surgical technique (MIST) with enamel matrix derivate in the regenerative treatment of intrabony defects: a novel approach to limit morbidity. *Journal of Clinical Periodontology* **34**, 87–93.

Cortellini, P. & Tonetti, M.S. (2007b). Minimally invasive surgical technique (M.I.S.T.) and enamel matrix derivative (EMD) in intrabony defects. (I) Clinical outcomes and intra-operative and post-operative morbidity. *Journal of Clinical Periodontology* (in press).

Demolon, I.A., Persson, G.R., Johnson, R.H. & Ammons, W.F. (1993). Effect of antibiotic treatment of clinical conditions and bacterial growth with guided tissue regeneration. *Journal of Periodontology* **64**, 609–616.

DeSanctis, M., Clauser, C. & Zucchelli, G. (1996a). Bacterial colonization of barrier material and periodontal regeneration. *Journal of Clinical Periodontology* **23**, 1039–1046.

DeSanctis, M., Zucchelli, G. & Clauser, C. (1996b). Bacterial colonization of bioabsorbable barrier material and periodontal regeneration. *Journal of Periodontology* **67**, 1193–1200.

Dorfer, C.E., Kim, T.S., Steinbrenner, H., Holle, R. & Eickholz, P. (2000). Regenerative periodontal surgery in interproximal intrabony defects with biodegradable barriers. *Journal of Clinical Periodontology* **27**, 162–168.

Eickholz, P., Kim, T.S., Steinbrenner, H., Dorfer, C. & Holle, R. (2000). Guided tissue regeneration with bioabsorbable barriers: intrabony defects and class II furcations. *Journal of Periodontology* **71**, 999–1008.

Eickholz, P., Lenhard, M., Benn, D.K. & Staehle, H.J. (1998). Periodontal surgery of vertical bony defects with or without synthetic bioabsorbable barriers. 12-month results. *Journal of Periodontology* **69**, 1210–1217.

Ellegaard, B. & Löe, H. (1971). New attachment of periodontal tissues after treatment of intrabony lesions. *Journal of Periodontology* **42**, 648–652.

Erpenstein, H. (1983). A three year study of hemisectioned molars. *Journal of Clinical Periodontology* **10**, 1–10.

Falk, H., Fornell, J. & Teiwik, A. (1993). Periodontal regeneration using a bioresorbable GTR device. *Journal of the Swedish Dental Association* **85**, 673–681.

Falk, H., Laurell, L., Ravald, N., Teiwik, A. & Persson, R. (1997). Guided tissue regeneration therapy of 203 consecutively treated intrabony defects using a bioabsorbable matrix barrier. Clinical and radiographic findings. *Journal of Periodontology* **68**, 571–581.

Frandsen, E., Sander, L., Arnbjerg, D. & Theilade, E. (1994). Effect of local metronidazole application on periodontal healing following guided tissue regeneration. Microbiological findings. *Journal of Periodontology* **65**, 921–928.

Gantes, B.G. & Garrett, S. (1991). Coronally displaced flaps in reconstructive periodontal therapy. *Dental Clinics of North America* **35**, 495–504.

Garrett, S., Loos, B., Chamberlain, D. & Egelberg, J. (1988). Treatment of intraosseous periodontal defects with a combined therapy of citric acid conditioning, bone grafting and placement of collagenous membranes. *Journal of Clinical Periodontology* **15**, 383–389.

Giannobile, W.V. & Somerman, M.J. (2003). Growth and amelogenin-like factors in periodontal wound healing. A systematic review. *Annals of Periodontology* **8**, 193–204.

Goldman, H. & Cohen, W. (1958). The infrabony pocket: classification and treatment. *Journal of Periodontology* **29**, 272–291.

Gottlow, J., Laurell, L., Lundgren, D., Mathiesen, T., Nyman, S., Rylander, H. & Bogentoft, C. (1994). Periodontal tissue response to a new bioresorbable guided tissue regeneration device. A longitudinal study in monkeys. *Interna-*

tional Journal of Periodontics and Restorative Dentistry **14**, 437–449.

Gottlow, J., Nyman, S. & Karring, T. (1992). Maintenance of new attachment gained through guided tissue regeneration. *Journal of Clinical Periodontology* **19**, 315–317.

Gottlow, J., Nyman, S., Karring, T. & Lindhe, J. (1984). New attachment formation as the result of controlled tissue regeneration. *Journal of Clinical Periodontology* **11**, 494–503.

Gottlow, J., Nyman, S., Lindhe, J., Karring, T. & Wennström, J. (1986). New attachment formation in the human periodontium by guided tissue regeneration. *Journal of Clinical Periodontology* **13**, 604–616.

Gouldin, A., Fayad, S. & Mellonig, J. (1996). Evaluation of guided tissue regeneration in interproximal defects. II. Membrane and bone versus membrane alone. *Journal of Clinical Periodontology* **23**, 485–491.

Grevstad, H. & Leknes, K.N. (1992). Epithelial adherence to polytetrafluoroethylene (PTFE) material. *Scandinavian Journal of Dental Research* **100**, 236–239.

Guillemin, M., Mellonig, J. & Brunswold, M. (1993). Healing in periodontal defects treated by decalcified freeze-dried bone allografts in combination with e-PTFE membranes. (I) Clinical and scanning electron microscope analysis. *Journal of Clinical Periodontology* **20**, 528–536.

Hamp, S.E., Nyman, S. & Lindhe, J. (1975). Periodontal treatment of multirooted teeth after 5 years. *Journal of Clinical Periodontology* **2**, 126–135.

Handelsman, M., Davarpanah, M. & Celletti, R. (1991). Guided tissue regeneration with and without citric acid treatment in vertical osseous defects. *International Journal of Periodontics and Restorative Dentistry* **11**, 351–363.

Haney, J.M., Leknes, K.N. & Wikesjö, U.M.E. (1997). Recurrence of mandibular molar furcation defects following citric acid root treatment and coronally advanced flap procedures. *International Journal of Periodontics and Restorative Dentistry* **17**, 3–10.

Haney, J.M., Nilveus, R.E., McMillan, P.J. & Wikesjö, U.M.E. (1993). Periodontal repair in dogs: expanded polytetrafluoroethylene barrier membranes support wound stabilization and enhance bone regeneration. *Journal of Periodontology* **64**, 883–890.

Heden, G. (2000). A case report study of 72 consecutive Emdogain-treated intrabony periodontal defects: clinical and radiographic findings after 1 year. *International Journal of Periodontics and Restorative Dentistry* **20**, 127–139.

Heden, G., Wennström, J. & Lindhe, J. (1999). Periodontal tissue alterations following Emdogain treatment of periodontal sites with angular bone defects. A series of case reports. *Journal of Clinical Periodontology* **26**, 855–860.

Heden, G. & Wennstrom, J.L. (2006). Five-year follow-up of regenerative periodontal therapy with enamel matrix derivative at sites with angular bone defects. *Journal of Periodontology* **77**, 295–301.

Heijl, L., Heden, G., Svärdström, C. & Ostgren, A. (1997). Enamel matrix derivate (EMDOGAIN®) in the treatment of intrabony periodontal defects. *Journal of Clinical Periodontology* **24**, 705–714.

Heitz-Mayfield, L., Tonetti, M.S., Cortellini, P., Lang, N.P. and European Research Group on Periodontology (ERGOPERIO) (2006). Microbial colonization patterns predict the outcomes of surgical treatment of intrabony defects. *Journal of Clinical Periodontology* **33**(1), 62–68.

Howell, T.H., Fiorellini, J.P., Paquette, D.W., Offenbacher, S., Giannobile, W.V. & Lynch, S. (1997). A phase I/II clinical trial to evaluate a combination of recombinant human platelet-de-rived growth factor-BB and recombinant human insulin-like growth factor-I in patients with periodontal disease. *Journal of Periodontology* **68**, 1186–1193.

Hugoson, A., Ravald, N., Fornell, J., Johard, G., Teiwik, A. & Gottlow, J. (1995). Treatment of class II furcation involvements in humans with bioresorbable and nonresorbable guided tissue regeneration barriers. A randomized multicenter study. *Journal of Periodontology* **66**, 624–634.

Hürzeler, M.B., Quinones, C.R., Caffesse, R.G., Schupback, P. & Morrison, E.C. (1997). Guided periodontal tissue regeneration in interproximal intrabony defects following treatment with a synthetic bioabsorbable barrier. *Journal of Periodontology* **68**, 489–497.

Isidor, F., Karring, T. & Attström, R. (1984). The effect of root planing as compared to that of surgical treatment. *Journal of Clinical Periodontology* **11**, 669–681.

Jepsen, S., Eberhard, J., Herrera, D. & Needleman, I. (2002). A systematic review of guided tissue regeneration for periodontal furcation defects. What is the effect of guided tissue regeneration compared with surgical debridement in the treatment of furcation defects? *Journal of Clinical Periodontology* **29** (Suppl 3), 103–116; discussion 160–162.

Karapataki, S., Hugoson, A., Falk, H., Laurell, L. & Kugelberg, C.F. (2000). Healing following GTR treatment of intrabony defects distal to mandibular second molars using resorbable and non-resorbable barriers. *Journal of Clinical Periodontology* **27**, 333–340.

Kersten, B., Chamberlain, A., Khorsandl, S., Wikesjö, U.M.E., Selvig, K. & Nilveus, R. (1992). Healing of the intrabony periodontal lesion following root conditioning with citric acid and wound closure including an expanded PTFE membrane. *Journal of Periodontology* **63**, 876–882.

Kilic, A., Efeoglu, E. & Yilmaz, S. (1997). Guided tissue regeneration in conjunction with hydroxyapatite-collagen grafts for intrabony defects. A clinical and radiological evaluation. *Journal of Clinical Periodontology* **24**, 372–383.

Kim, C., Choi, E., Chai, J.K. & Wikesjö, U.M. (1996). Periodontal repair in intrabony defects treated with a calcium carbonate implant and guided tissue regeneration. *Journal of Periodontology* **67**, 1301–1306.

Kostopoulos, L. & Karring, T. (1994). Resistance of new attachment to ligature induced periodontal breakdown. An experiment in monkeys. *Journal of Dental Research* **73**, 963 (abstract).

Lang, N.P. (2000). Focus on intrabony defects – conservative therapy. *Periodontology 2000* **22**, 51–58.

Langer, B., Stein, S.D. & Wagenberg, B. (1981). An evaluation of root resection. A ten year study. *Journal of Periodontology* **52**, 719–722.

Laurell, L., Falk, H., Fornell, J., Johard, G. & Gottlow, J. (1994). Clinical use of a bioresorbable matrix barrier in guided tissue regeneration therapy. Case series. *Journal of Periodontology* **65**, 967–975.

Lekovic, V., Kenney, E.B., Carranza, F.A. & Danilovic, V. (1990). Treatment of class II furcation defects using porous hydroxylapatite in conjunction with a polytetrafluoroethylene membrane. *Journal of Periodontology* **61**, 575–578.

Lekovic, V., Kenney, E., Kovacevic, K. & Carranza, F. (1989). Evaluation of guided tissue regeneration in class II furcation defects. A clinical re-entry study. *Journal of Periodontology* **60**, 694–698.

Linares, A., Cortellini, P., Lang, N.P., Suvan, J., Tonetti, M.S. and European Research Group on Periodontology (ErgoPerio) (2006). Guided tissue regeneration/deproteinized bovine bone mineral or papilla preservation flaps alone for treatment of intrabony defects. II: radiographic predictors and outcomes. *Journal of Clinical Periodontology* **33**(5), 351–358.

Lindhe, J. & Cortellini, P. (1996). Consensus report of session 4. In: Lang, N.P., Karring, T. & Lindhe, J., eds. *Proceedings of the 2nd European Workshop on Periodontology*. London: Quintessence Publishing Co. Ltd, pp. 359–360.

Little, L.A., Beck, F.M., Bugci, B. & Horton, J.E. (1995). Lack of furcal bone loss following the tunneling procedure. *Journal of Clinical Periodontology* **22**, 637–641.

Lundgren, D. & Slotte, C. (1999). Reconstruction of anatomically complicated periodontal defects using a bioresorbable GTR barrier supported by bone mineral. A 6-months follow-

up study of 6 cases. *Journal of Clinical Periodontology* **26**, 56–62.

Lyngstadaas, S.P., Lundberg, E., Ekdahl, H., Andersson, C. & Gestrelius, S. (2001). Autocrine growth factors in human periodontal ligament cells cultured on enamel matrix derivative. *Journal of Clinical Periodontology* **28**(2), 181–188.

Machtei, E., Cho, M., Dunford, R., Norderyd, J., Zambon, J. & Genco, R. (1994). Clinical, microbiological, and histological factors which influence the success of regenerative periodontal therapy. *Journal of Periodontology* **65**, 154–161.

Machtei, E., Dunford, R., Norderyd, J., Zambon, J. & Genco, R. (1993). Guided tissue regeneration and anti-infective therapy in the treatment of class II furcation defects. *Journal of Periodontology* **64**, 968–973.

Machtei, E., Grossi, S., Dunford, R., Zambon, J. & Genco, R. (1996). Long-term stability of class II furcation defects treated with barrier membranes. *Journal of Periodontology* **67**, 523–527.

Machtei, E. & Schallhorn, R.G. (1995). Successful regeneration of mandibular class II furcation defects. An evidence-based treatment approach. *International Journal of Periodontics and Restorative Dentistry* **15**, 146–167.

Magnusson, I., Batich, C. & Collins, B.R. (1988). New attachment formation following controlled tissue regeneration using biodegradable membranes. *Journal of Periodontology* **59**, 1–6.

Magnusson, I., Nyman, S., Karring, T. & Egelberg, J. (1985). Connective tissue attachment formation following exclusion of gingival connective tissue and epithelium during healing. *Journal of Periodontal Research* **20**, 201–208.

Mattson, J., McLey, L. & Jabro, M. (1995). Treatment of intrabony defects with collagen membrane barriers. Case reports. *Journal of Periodontology* **66**, 635–645.

Mayfield, L., Söderholm, G., Hallström, H., Kullendorff, B., Edwardsson, S., Bratthall, G., Brägger, U. & Attström, R. (1998). Guided tissue regeneration for the treatment of intraosseous defects using a bioabsorbable membrane. A controlled clinical study. *Journal of Clinical Periodontology* **25**, 585–595.

McClain, P. & Schallhorn, R.G. (1993). Long term assessment of combined osseous composite grafting, root conditioning and guided tissue regeneration. *International Journal of Periodontics and Restorative Dentistry* **13**, 9–27.

McGuire, M.K. & Nunn, M.E. (1996). Prognosis versus actual outcome. III. The effectiveness of clinical parameters in accurately predicting tooth survival. *Journal of Periodontology* **67**(7), 666–674.

McGuire, M.K. & Nunn, M.E. (1996). Prognosis versus actual outcome. II. The effectiveness of clinical parameters in developing an accurate prognosis. *Journal of Periodontology* **67**(7), 658–665.

Mellado, J., Salkin, L., Freedman, A. & Stein, M. (1995). A comparative study of e-PTFE periodontal membranes with and without decalcified freeze-dried bone allografts for the regeneration of interproximal intraosseous defects. *Journal of Periodontology* **66**, 751–755.

Mellonig, J.T. (1999). Enamel matrix derivate for periodontal reconstructive surgery: Technique and clinical and histologic case report. *International Journal of Periodontics and Restorative Dentistry* **19**, 9–19.

Mellonig, J.T. (2000). Human histologic evaluation of a bovine-derived bone xenograft in the treatment of periodontal osseous defects. *International Journal of Periodontics and Restorative Dentistry* **20**, 18–29.

Mellonig, J.T., Semons, B., Gray, J. & Towle, H. (1994). Clinical evaluation of guided tissue regeneration in the treatment of grade II molar furcation invasion. *International Journal of Periodontics and Restorative Dentistry* **14**, 255–271.

Metzeler, D.G., Seamons, B.C., Mellonig, J.T., Gher, M.E. & Gray, J.L. (1991). Clinical evalution of guided tissue regen-

eration in the treatment of maxillary class II molar furcation invasions. *Journal of Periodontology* **62**, 353–360.

Mombelli, A., Lang, N. & Nyman, S. (1993). Isolation of periodontal species after guided tissue regeneration. *Journal of Periodontology* **64**, 1171–1175.

Murphy, K. (1995a). Post-operative healing complications associated with Gore-tex periodontal material. Part 1. Incidence and characterization. *International Journal of Periodontics and Restorative Dentistry* **15**, 363–375.

Murphy, K. (1995b). Post-operative healing complications associated with Gore-tex periodontal material. Part 2. Effect of complications on regeneration. *International Journal of Periodontics and Restorative Dentistry* **15**, 549–561.

Murphy, K. (1996). Interproximal tissue maintenance in GTR procedures: description of a surgical technique and 1 year reentry results. *International Journal of Periodontics and Restorative Dentistry* **16**, 463–477.

Murphy, K.G. & Gunsolley, J.C. (2003). Guided tissue regeneration for the treatment of periodontal intrabony and furcation defects. A systematic review. *Annals of Periodontology* **8**, 266–302.

Needleman, I., Tucker, R., Giedrys-Leeper, E. & Worthington, H. (2002). A systematic review of guided tissue regeneration for periodontal infrabony defects. *Journal of Periodontal Research* **37**, 380–388

Nevins, M., Giannobile, W.V., McGuire, M.K., Kao, R.T., Mellonig, J.T., Hinrichs, J.E., McAllister, B.S., Murphy, K.S., McClain, P.K., Nevins, M.L., Paquette, D.W., Han, T.J., Reddy, M.S., Lavin, P.T., Genco, R.J. & Lynch, S.E. (2005). Platelet-derived growth factor stimulates bone fill and rate of attachment level gain: results of a large multicenter randomized controlled trial. *Journal of Periodontology* **76**(12), 2205–2215.

Nevins, M.L., Camelo, M., Nevins, M., King, C.J., Oringer, R.J., Schenk, R.K. & Fiorellini, J.P. (2000). Human histologic evaluation of bioactive ceramic in the treatment of periodontal osseous defects. *International Journal of Periodontics and Restorative Dentistry* **20**, 458–467.

Novaes, A. Jr., Gutierrez, F., Francischetto, I. & Novaes, A. (1995). Bacterial colonization of the external and internal sulci and of cellulose membranes at times of retrieval. *Journal of Periodontology* **66**, 864–869.

Nowzari, H., Matian, F. & Slots, J. (1995). Periodontal pathogens on polytetrafluoroethylene membrane for guided tissue regeneration inhibit healing. *Journal of Clinical Periodontology* **22**, 469–474.

Nowzari, H. & Slots, J. (1994). Microorganisms in polytetrafluoroethylene barrier membranes for guided tissue regeneration. *Journal of Clinical Periodontology* **21**, 203–210.

Nyman, S., Lindhe, J., Karring, T. & Rylander, H. (1982). New attachment following surgical treatment of human periodontal disease. *Journal of Clinical Periodontology* **9**, 290–296.

Ouhayoun, J. (1996). Biomaterials used as bone graft substitutes. In: Lang, N.P., Karring, T. & Lindhe, J., eds. *Proceedings of the 2nd European Workshop on Periodontology*. London: Quintessence Publishing Co. Ltd, pp. 313–358.

Paolantonio, M., Scarano, A., DiPlacido, G., Tumini, V., D'Archivio, D. & Piattelli, A. (2001). Periodontal healing in humans using anorganic bovine bone and bovine peritoneum-derived collagen membrane: a clinical and histologic case report. *International Journal of Periodontics and Restorative Dentistry* **21**, 505–515.

Papananou, P.N. & Tonetti, M.S. (2000). Diagnosis and epidemiology of periodontal osseous lesions. *Periodontology 2000* **22**(1), 8–21.

Parashis, A., Andronikaki-Faldami, A. & Tsiklakis, K. (1998). Comparison of two regenerative procedures – guided tissue regeneration and demineralized freeze-dried bone allograft – in the treatment of intrabony defects: a clinical and radiographic study. *Journal of Periodontology* **69**, 751–758.

Parashis, A. & Mitsis, F. (1993). Clinical evaluation of the effect of tetracycline root preparation on guided tissue regeneration in the treatment of class II furcation defects. *Journal of Periodontology* **64**, 133–136.

Parkar, M.H. & Tonetti, M. (2004). Gene expression profiles of periodontal ligament cells treated with enamel matrix proteins in vitro: analysis using cDNA arrays. *Journal of Periodontology* **75**(11), 1539–1546.

Paul, B.F., Mellonig, J.T., Towle, H.J. & Gray, J.L. (1992). The use of a collagen barrier to enhance healing in human periodontal furcation defects. *International Journal of Periodontics and Restorative Dentistry* **12**, 123–131.

Pietruska, M.D. (2001). A comparative study on the use of Bio-Oss and enamel matrix derivative (Emdogain) in the treatment of periodontal bone defects. *European Journal of Oral Science* **109**, 178–181.

Pitaru, S., Tal, H., Soldinger, M., Grosskopf, A. & Noff, M. (1988). Partial regeneration of periodontal tissues using collagen barriers. Initial observations in the canine. *Journal of Periodontology* **59**, 380–386.

Polson, A.M, Garrett, S., Stoller, N.H., Greenstein, G., Polson, A., Harrold, C. & Laster, L. (1995b). Guided tissue regeneration in human furcation defects after using a biodegradable barrier: a multi-center feasibility study. *Journal of Periodontology* **66**, 377–385.

Polson, A.M., Southard, G.L., Dunn, R.L., Polson, A.P., Yewey, G.L., Swanbom, D.D., Fulfs, J.C. & Rodgers, P.W. (1995a). Periodontal healing after guided tissue regeneration with Atrisorb barriers in beagle dogs. *International Journal of Periodontics and Restorative Dentistry* **15**, 574–589.

Pontoriero, R. (1996). *Studies on regenerative therapy in furcation defects*. Thesis. Department of Periodontology, Faculty of Odontology, University of Gothenburg, p. 44.

Pontoriero, R. & Lindhe, J. (1995a). Guided tissue regeneration in the treatment of degree II furcations in maxillary molars. *Journal of Clinical Periodontology* **22**, 756–763.

Pontoriero, R. & Lindhe, J. (1995b). Guided tissue regeneration in the treatment of degree III furcations in maxillary molars. Short communication. *Journal of Clinical Periodontology* **22**, 810–812.

Pontoriero, R., Lindhe, J., Nyman, S., Karring, T., Rosenberg, E. & Sanavi, F. (1988). Guided tissue regeneration in degree II furcation-involved mandibular molars. A clinical study. *Journal of Clinical Periodontology* **15**, 247–254.

Pontoriero, R., Lindhe, J., Nyman, S., Karring, T., Rosenberg, E. & Sanavi, F. (1989). Guided tissue regeneration in the treatment of furcation defects in mandibular molars. A clinical study of degree III involvements. *Journal of Clinical Periodontology* **16**, 170–174.

Pontoriero, R., Nyman, S., Ericsson, I. & Lindhe, J. (1992). Guided tissue regeneration in surgically produced furcation defects. An experimental study in the beagle dog. *Journal of Clinical Periodontology* **19**, 159–163.

Pontoriero, R., Wennström, J. & Lindhe, J. (1999). The use of barrier membranes and enamel matrix proteins in the treatment of angular bone defects. A prospective controlled clinical study. *Journal of Clinical Periodontology* **26**, 833–840.

Proestakis, G., Bratthal, G., Söderholm, G., Kullendorff, B., Gröndahl, K., Rohlin, M. & Attström, R. (1992). Guided tissue regeneration in the treatment of infrabony defects on maxillary premolars. A pilot study. *Journal of Clinical Periodontology* **19**, 766–773.

Quteish, D. & Dolby, A. (1992). The use of irradiated-cross-linked human collagen membrane in guided tissue regeneration. *Journal of Clinical Periodontology* **19**, 476–484.

Ratka-Kruger, P., Neukranz, E. & Raetzke, P. (2000). Guided tissue regeneration procedure with bioresorbable membranes versus conventional flap surgery in the treatment of infrabony periodontal defects. *Journal of Clinical Periodontology* **27**, 120–127.

Reynolds, M.A., Aichelmann-Reidy, M.E., Branch-Mays, G.L. & Gunsolley, J.C. (2003). The efficacy of bone replacement grafts in the treatment of periodontal osseous defects. A systematic review. *Annals of Periodontology* **8**(1), 227–265.

Rosen, P.S., Reynolds, M.A. & Bowers, G.M. (2000). The treatment of intrabony defects with bone grafts. *Periodontology 2000* **22**, 88–103.

Sallum, E.A., Sallum, A.W., Nociti, F.H. Jr., Marcantonio, R.A. & de Toledo, S. (1998). New attachment achieved by guided tissue regeneration using a bioresorbable polylactic acid membrane in dogs. *International Journal of Periodontics and Restorative Dentistry* **18**, 502–510.

Sander, L., Frandsen, E.V.G., Arnbjerg, D., Warrer, K. & Karring, T. (1994). Effect of local metronidazol application on periodontal healing following guided tissue regeneration. Clinical findings. *Journal of Periodontology* **65**, 914–920.

Sander, L. & Karring, T. (1995). New attachment and bone formation in periodontal defects following treatment of submerged roots with guided tissue regeneration. *Journal of Clinical Periodontology* **22**, 295–299.

Sanders, J.J., Sepe, W.W., Bowers, G.M., Koch, R.W., Williams, J.E., Lekas, J.S., Mellonig, J.T., Pelleu, G.B. Jr. & Gambill, V. (1983). Clinical evaluation of freeze-dried bone allografts in periodontal osseous defects. Part III. Composite freeze-dried bone allografts with and without autogenous bone grafts. *Journal of Periodontology* **54**, 1–8.

Sanz, M., Tonetti, M.S., Zabalegui, I., Sicilia, A., Blanco, J., Rebelo, H. Rasperini, G., Merli, M., Cortellini, P. & Suvan, J.E. (2004). Treatment of intrabony defects with enamel matrix proteins or barrier membranes: results from a multicenter practice-based clinical trial. *Journal of Periodontology* **75**(5), 726–733.

Schallhorn, R.G., Hiatt, W.H, & Boyce, W. (1970). Iliac transplants in periodontal therapy. *Journal of Periodontology* **41**, 566–580.

Schallhorn, R.G. & McClain, P.K. (1988). Combined osseous composite grafting, root conditioning, and guided tissue regeneration. *International Journal of Periodontics and Restorative Dentistry* **4**, 9–31.

Sculean, A., Donos, N., Chiantella, G.C., Windisch, P., Reich, E. & Brecx, M. (1999a). GTR with bioresorbable membranes in the treatment of intrabony defects: a clinical and histologic study. *International Journal of Periodontics and Restorative Dentistry* **19**, 501–509.

Sculean, A., Donos, N., Windisch, P. Brecx, M., Gera, I., Reich, E. & Karring, T. (1999b). Healing of human intrabony defects following treatment with enamel matrix proteins or guided tissue regeneration. *Journal of Periodontal Research* **34**, 310–322.

Sculean, A., Schwarz, F., Miliauskaite, A., Kiss, A., Arweiler, N., Becker, J. & Brecx, M. (2006). Treatment of intrabony defects with an enamel matrix protein derivative or bioabsorbable membrane: an 8-year follow-up split-mouth study. *Journal of Periodontology* **77**, 1879–1886.

Selvig, K., Kersten, B., Chamberlain, A., Wikesjo, U.M.E. & Nilveus, R. (1992). Regenerative surgery of intrabony periodontal defects using e-PTFE barrier membranes. Scanning electron microscopic evaluation of retrieved membranes vs. clinical healing. *Journal of Periodontology* **63**, 974–978.

Selvig, K., Kersten, B. & Wikesjö, U.M.E. (1993). Surgical treatment of intrabony periodontal defects using expanded polytetrafluoroethylene barrier membranes: influence of defect configuration on healing response. *Journal of Periodontology* **64**, 730–733.

Selvig, K.A., Nilveus, R.E., Fitzmorris, L., Kersten, B. & Thorsandi, S.S. (1990). Scanning electron microscopic observations of cell population and bacterial contamination of membranes used for guided periodontal tissue regeneration in humans. *Journal of Periodontology* **61**, 515–520.

Sigurdsson, J.T., Hardwick, R., Bogle, G.C. & Wikesjö, U.M.E. (1994). Periodontal repair in dogs: space provision by reinforced e-PTFE membranes enhances bone and cementum regeneration in large supraalveolar defects. *Journal of Periodontology* **65**, 350–356.

Silvestri, M., Ricci, G., Rasperini, G., Sartori, S. & Cattaneo, V. (2000). Comparison of treatments of infrabony defects with enamel matrix derivate, guided tissue regeneration with a nonresorbable membrane and Widman modified flap. A pilot study. *Journal of Clinical Periodontology* **27**, 603–610.

Smith MacDonald, E., Nowzari, H., Contreras, A., Flynn, J., Morrison, J. & Slots, J. (1998). Clinical evaluation of a bioabsorbable and a nonresorbable membrane in the treatment of periodontal intraosseous lesions. *Journal of Periodontology* **69**, 445–453.

Stavropoulos, A., Karring, E.S., Kostopoulos, L. & Karring, T. (2003). Deproteinized bovine bone and gentamicin as an adjunct to GTR in the treatment of intrabony defects: a randomized controlled clinical study. *Journal of Clinical Periodontology* **30**(6), 486–495.

Takei, H.H., Han, T.J., Carranza, F.A. Jr., Kenney, E.B. & Lekovic, V. (1985). Flap technique for periodontal bone implants. Papilla preservation technique. *Journal of Periodontology* **56**(4), 204–210.

Tanner, M.G., Solt, C.W. & Vuddhakanok, S. (1988). An evaluation of new attachment formation using a microfibrillar collagen barrier. *Journal of Periodontology* **59**, 524–530.

Tatakis, D.N., Promsudthi, A. & Wikesjö, U.M.E. (1999). Devices for periodontal regeneration. *Periodontology 2000* **19**, 59–73.

Tempro, P. & Nalbandian, J. (1993). Colonization of retrieved polytetrafluoroethylene membranes: morphological and microbiological observations. *Journal of Periodontology* **64**, 162–168.

Tonetti, M., Cortellini, P., Suvan, J.E., Adriaens, P., Baldi, C., Dubravec, D., Fonzar, A., Fourmosis, I., Magnani, C., Muller-Campanile, V., Patroni, S., Sanz, M., Vangsted, T., Zabalegui, I., Pini Prato, G. & Lang, N.P. (1998). Generalizability of the added benefits of guided tissue regeneration in the treatment of deep intrabony defects. Evaluation in a multi-center randomized controlled clinical trial. *Journal of Periodontology* **69**, 1183–1192.

Tonetti, M., Lang, N.P., Cortellini, P. *et al.* (2002). Enamel matrix proteins in the regenerative therapy of deep intrabony defects. A multicenter randomized controlled clinical trial. *Journal of Clinical Periodontology* **29**, 317–325

Tonetti, M., Pini-Prato, G. & Cortellini, P. (1993a). Periodontal regeneration of human infrabony defects. IV. Determinants of the healing response. *Journal of Periodontology* **64**, 934–940.

Tonetti, M., Pini-Prato, G. & Cortellini, P. (1995). Effect of cigarette smoking on periodontal healing following GTR in infrabony defects. A preliminary retrospective study. *Journal of Clinical Periodontology* **22**, 229–234.

Tonetti, M., Pini-Prato, G. & Cortellini, P. (1996a). Factors affecting the healing response of intrabony defects following guided tissue regeneration and access flap surgery. *Journal of Clinical Periodontology* **23**, 548–556.

Tonetti, M., Pini-Prato, G. & Cortellini, P. (1996b). Guided tissue regeneration of deep intrabony defects in strategically important prosthetic abutments. *International Journal of Periodontics and Restorative Dentistry* **16**, 378–387.

Tonetti, M. S., Pini-Prato, G. P., Williams, R. C. & Cortellini, P. (1993b). Periodontal regeneration of human infrabony defects. III. Diagnostic strategies to detect bone gain. *Journal of Periodontology* **64**, 269–277.

Tonetti, M.S., Fourmousis, I., Suvan, J., Cortellini, P., Bragger, U., Lang, N.P.; European Research Group on Periodontology (ERGOPERIO) (2004a). Healing, post-operative morbidity and patient perception of outcomes following regenerative therapy of deep intrabony defects. *Journal of Clinical Periodontology* **31**(12), 1092–1098.

Tonetti, M.S., Cortellini, P., Lang, N.P., Suvan, J.E., Adriaens, P., Dubravec, D., Fonzar, A., Fourmousis, I., Rasperini, G., Rossi, R., Silvestri, M., Topoll, H., Wallkamm, B. & Zybutz, M. (2004b). Clinical outcomes following treatment of human intrabony defects with GTR/bone replacement material or access flap alone. A multicenter randomized controlled clinical trial. *Journal of Clinical Periodontology* **31**(9), 770–776.

Trejo, P.M. & Weltman, R.L. (2004). Favorable periodontal regenerative outcomes from teeth with presurgical mobility: a retrospective study. *Journal of Periodontology* **75**(11), 1532–1538.

Trombelli, L., Kim, C.K., Zimmerman, G.J. & Wikesjö, U.M.E. (1997). Retrospective analysis of factors related to clinical outcome of guided tissue regeneration procedures in intrabony defects. *Journal of Clinical Periodontology* **24**, 366–371.

Trombelli, L., Heitz-Mayfield, L.J., Needleman, I., Moles, D. & Scabbia, A. (2002). A systematic review of graft materials and biological agents for periodontal intraosseous defects. *Journal of Clinical Periodontology* **29** (Suppl 3), 117–135; discussion 160–162.

Tsitoura, E., Tucker, R., Suvan, J., Laurell, L., Cortellini, P. & Tonetti, M. (2004). Baseline radiographic defect angle of the intrabony defect as a prognostic indicator in regenerative periodontal surgery with enamel matrix derivative. *Journal of Clinical Periodontology* **31**(8), 643–647.

Van Swol, R., Ellinger, R., Pfeifer, J., Barton, N. & Blumenthal, N. (1993). Collagen membrane barrier therapy to guide regeneration in class II furcations in humans. *Journal of Periodontology* **64**, 622–629.

Wallace, S., Gellin, R., Miller, C. & Miskin, D. (1994). Guided tissue regeneration with and without decalcified freeze-dried bone in mandibular class II furcation invasions. *Journal of Periodontology* **65**, 244–254.

Wang, H., O'Neal, R., Thomas, C., Shyr, Y. & MacNeil, R. (1994). Evaluation of an absorbable collagen membrane in treating Class II furcation defects. *Journal of Periodontology* **65**, 1029–1036.

Warrer, K., Karring, T., Nyman, S. & Gogolewski, S. (1992). Guided tissue regeneration using biodegradable membranes of polylactic acid or polyurethane. *Journal of Clinical Periodontology* **19**, 633–640.

Yukna, R.A. & Sepe, W.W. (1982). Clinical evaluation of localized periodontosis defects treated with freeze-dried bone allografts combined with local and systemic tetracyclines. *International Journal of Periodontics and Restorative Dentistry* **2**(5), 8–21.

Yukna, R. (1992). Clinical human comparison of expanded polytetrafluoroethylene barrier membrane and freeze dried dura mater allografts for guided tissue regeneration of lost periodontal support. *Journal of Periodontology* **63**, 431–442.

Yukna, R. & Mellonig, J.T. (2000). Histologic evaluation of periodontal healing in humans following regenerative therapy with enamel matrix derivative. A 10-case series. *Journal of Periodontology* **71**, 752–759.

Zybutz, M.D., Laurell, L., Rapoport, D.A. & Persson, G.R. (2000). Treatment of intrabony defects with resorbable materials, non-resorbable materials and flap debridement. *Journal of Clinical Periodontology* **27**, 167–178.

Chapter 44

Mucogingival Therapy – Periodontal Plastic Surgery

Jan L. Wennström, Giovanni Zucchelli, and Giovan P. Pini Prato

Introduction, 955
Gingival augmentation, 955
  Gingival dimensions and periodontal health, 956
  Marginal tissue recession, 958
  Marginal tissue recession and orthodontic treatment, 961
  Gingival dimensions and restorative therapy, 964
  Indications for gingival augmentation, 965
  Gingival augmentation procedures, 965
  Healing following gingival augmentation procedures, 968
Root coverage, 970
  Root coverage procedures, 971
  Clinical outcome of root coverage procedures, 990

Soft tissue healing against the covered root surface, 992
Interdental papilla reconstruction, 996
  Surgical techniques, 997
Crown-lengthening procedures, 997
  Excessive gingival display, 997
  Exposure of sound tooth structure, 1002
  Ectopic tooth eruption, 1005
The deformed edentulous ridge, 1008
  Prevention of soft tissue collapse following
    tooth extraction, 1009
  Correction of ridge defects by the use of soft tissue grafts, 1010
  Surgical procedures for ridge augmentation, 1011

Introduction

Mucogingival therapy is a general term used to describe periodontal treatment involving procedures for correction of defects in morphology, position, and/or amount of soft tissue and underlying bone support at teeth and implants (*Glossary of Terms in Periodontology* 2001).

A more specific term, *mucogingival surgery*, was introduced in the 1950s by Friedman (1957) and was defined as "surgical procedures designed to preserve gingiva, remove aberrant frenulum or muscle attachments, and increase the depth of the vestibule". Frequently, however, the term "mucogingival surgery" was used to describe all surgical procedures that involved both the gingiva and the alveolar mucosa. Consequently, not only were techniques designed (1) to enhance the width of the gingiva and (2) to correct particular soft tissue defects regarded as mucogingival procedures but (3) certain pocket elimination approaches were also included in this group of periodontal treatment modalities. In 1993 Miller proposed the term *periodontal plastic surgery*, considering that mucogingival surgery had moved beyond the traditional treatment of problems associated with the amount of gingivae and recession type defects to also include correction of ridge form and soft tissue esthetics. Periodontal plastic surgery would accordingly be defined as "surgical procedures performed to prevent or correct anatomic, developmental, traumatic or disease-induced defects of the gingiva, alveolar mucosa or bone" (Proceedings of the World Workshop in Periodontics 1996). Among treatment procedures that may fall within this definition are various soft and hard tissue procedures aimed at:

- Gingival augmentation
- Root coverage
- Correction of mucosal defects at implants
- Crown lengthening
- Gingival preservation at ectopic tooth eruption
- Removal of aberrant frenulum
- Prevention of ridge collapse associated with tooth extraction
- Augmentation of the edentulous ridge.

The focus of this chapter is mainly on treatment procedures for corrections of soft tissue defects in relation to the tooth and the edentulous ridge, while bone augmentation procedures are covered in Chapter 49.

Gingival augmentation

A review of the literature on gingival augmentation reveals that the rationale for increasing the width of gingiva as a means of promoting gingival health and improving attachment levels is poorly supported by scientific evidence. Usually clinical impressions, case reports, and anecdotal information have been used as the main reference to justify surgical intervention. In this perspective a discussion of the scientific evidence forming the basis for our current understanding of the role played by the gingiva in the protection of the periodontium proper seems appropriate.

Gingival dimensions and periodontal health

For many years the presence of an "adequate" zone of gingiva was considered critical for the maintenance of marginal tissue health and for the prevention of continuous loss of connective tissue attachment (Nabers 1954; Ochsenbein 1960; Friedman & Levine 1964; Hall 1981; Matter 1982). Clinicians had the "impression" that sites with a narrow zone of gingiva (Fig. 44-1) were often inflamed while the wide zone of gingiva found at neighboring teeth remained healthy. The prevailing concept was thus that a narrow zone of gingiva was insufficient (1) to protect the periodontium from injury caused by friction forces encountered during mastication and (2) to dissipate the pull on the gingival margin created by the muscles of the adjacent alveolar mucosa (Friedman 1957; Ochsenbein 1960). Moreover it was believed that an "inadequate" zone of gingiva would (1) facilitate subgingival plaque formation because of improper pocket closure resulting from the movability of the marginal tissue (Friedman 1962) and (2) favor attachment loss and soft tissue recession because of less tissue resistance to apical spread of plaque-associated gingival lesions (Stern 1976; Ruben 1979). It was also considered that a narrow gingiva in combination with a shallow vestibular fornix might (1) favor the accumulation of food particles during mastication, and (2) impede proper oral hygiene measures (Gottsegen 1954; Rosenberg 1960; Corn 1962; Carranza & Carraro 1970).

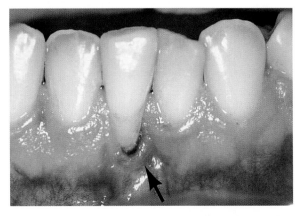

Fig. 44-1 A clinical photograph of a mandibular front tooth region. The gingiva on the buccal aspect of tooth 41 has a narrow width and shows more pronounced signs of inflammation than adjacent gingival units with a wider zone of gingiva.

The opinions expressed concerning what could be regarded as being an "adequate" or "sufficient" dimension of the gingiva varied. While some authors suggested that less than 1 mm of gingiva may be sufficient (Bowers 1963), others claimed that the apico-coronal height of keratinized tissue ought to exceed 3 mm (Corn 1962). A third category of authors had a more biologic approach to the question and stated that an adequate amount of gingiva is any dimension of gingiva which (1) is compatible with gingival health or (2) prevents retraction of the gingival margin during movements of the alveolar mucosa (Friedman 1962; De Trey & Bernimoulin 1980).

One of the first studies in which attempts were made to evaluate the significance of the gingival zone for the maintenance of periodontal health was carried out by Lang and Löe (1972) on dental students who had their teeth professionally cleaned once a day for 6 weeks. All buccal and lingual sites were examined for plaque, gingival conditions, and apico-coronal height of gingiva. The results showed that despite the fact that the tooth surfaces were free from plaque, all sites with less than 2 mm of gingiva exhibited persisting clinical signs of inflammation. Based on this observation the authors suggested that 2 mm of gingiva is an adequate width for maintaining gingival health. Subsequent clinical trials (Miyasato et al. 1977; Grevers 1977), however, failed to substantiate this concept of a required minimum dimension of gingiva. In fact, these clinical trials demonstrated that it is possible to maintain clinically healthy marginal tissues even in areas with less than 1 mm of gingiva.

The question whether a firmly attached portion of gingiva is critical for the protection of the periodontium proper was addressed by Wennström and Lindhe (1983a,b) utilizing the beagle dog model. In these studies dentogingival units with different clinical characteristics were experimentally established; (1) units with only a narrow and mobile zone of keratinized tissue and (2) units with a wide, firmly attached gingiva (Fig. 44-2). With daily performed mechanical plaque-control measures, the gingival units could be maintained free from clinical as well as histologic signs of inflammation irrespective of the presence or absence of an attached portion of gingiva. When bacterial plaque was allowed to accumulate (for 40 days), clinical signs of inflammation (redness and swelling) developed that were more pronounced in tooth regions with mobile gingiva (Fig. 44-3a) than in areas with presence of a wide and firmly attached gingival zone (Fig. 44-3b). However, histologic analysis revealed that the size of the inflammatory cell infiltrate and its extension in an apical direction (an assessment which indirectly may be used as an estimate of the apical migration of the bacterial plaque) were similar in the two categories of dentogingival units. The finding that the clinical signs of gingival inflammation did not correspond with the size of the inflammatory cell infiltrate illustrates the difficulties

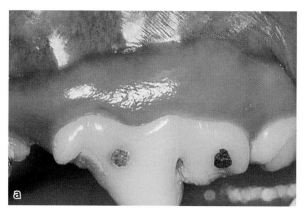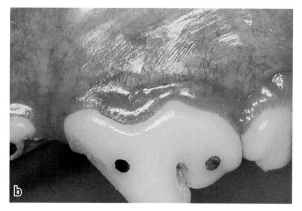

Fig. 44-2 Two teeth in a dog with varying dimensions of the marginal gingiva. (a) A buccal tooth site with a wide zone of attached gingiva. (b) A site with an unattached, narrow band of gingiva.

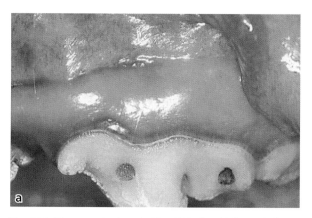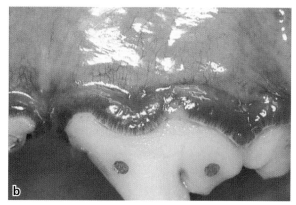

Fig. 44-3 The same teeth as in Fig. 44-2 after 40 days of plaque accumulation. The clinical signs of inflammation are more pronounced at the site with the narrow band of gingiva (b) than at the site with the wide zone of attached gingiva (a).

inherent in the interpretation of data from clinical examinations made in areas with varying width of gingiva. This should be kept in mind when interpreting the data by Lang and Löe (1972) showing that clinically visible signs of inflammation, such as redness and swelling, were more frequent in areas with less than 2 mm of gingiva than in areas with a wider zone of gingiva.

The necessity for and effectiveness of gingival augmentation in maintaining periodontal attachment was examined by Dorfman et al. (1980). Ninety-two patients with bilateral facial tooth surfaces exhibiting minimal keratinized tissue (i.e. less than 2 mm) had a free gingival graft placed on one side, while the contralateral side served as the untreated control. Prior to and after surgery the patients were subjected to scaling and root planing and instruction in oral hygiene measures. Not surprisingly, the investigators found a significant increase (approximately 4 mm) in the width of keratinized tissue at the grafted sites. This increased width of gingiva, as well as the clinical attachment level, was maintained throughout the 2 years of follow-up. In the control sites the width of gingiva was less than 2 mm and did not vary significantly during the observation period. However, the attachment level was also maintained unchanged

in the non-grafted areas. Thus, the resistance to continuous attachment loss was not linked to the height (width) of gingiva, a conclusion that was further substantiated by subsequent 4- and 6-year follow-up reports of this patient material (Dorfman et al. 1982; Kennedy et al. 1985).

Further support for the conclusion that a minimal zone of gingiva may not compromise periodontal health is available in a number of other longitudinal clinical studies (e.g. Hangorsky & Bissada 1980; De Trey & Bernimoulin 1980; Lindhe & Nyman 1980; Schoo & van der Velden 1985; Kisch et al. 1986; Wennström 1987; Freedman et al. 1999). Hence, Hangorsky and Bissada (1980), who evaluated the long-term clinical effect of free soft tissue grafts, concluded that while the free gingival graft is an effective means to widen the zone of the gingiva, there is no indication that this increase has direct influence upon periodontal health.

Conclusion

Gingival health can be maintained independent of its dimensions. Furthermore, there is evidence from both experimental and clinical studies that, in the presence of plaque, areas with a narrow zone of

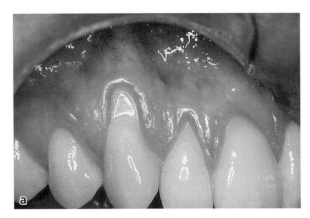 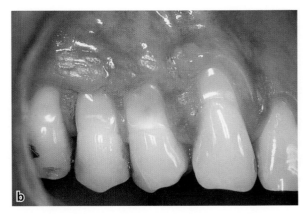

Fig. 44-4 Recessions associated with toothbrushing trauma. The marginal gingiva is clinically healthy and abrasion defects of various extension can be noted in the exposed roots.

gingiva possess the same "resistance" to continuous attachment loss as teeth with a wide zone of gingiva. Hence, the traditional dogma of the need of an "adequate" width (in millimeters) of gingiva, or attached portion of gingiva, for prevention of attachment loss is not scientifically supported.

Marginal tissue recession

Marginal tissue recession, i.e. displacement of the soft tissue margin apical to the cemento-enamel junction (CEJ) with exposure of the root surface, is a common feature in populations with high standards of oral hygiene (e.g. Sangnes & Gjermo 1976; Murtomaa *et al.* 1987; Löe *et al.* 1992; Serino *et al.* 1994), as well as in populations with poor oral hygiene (e.g. Baelum *et al.* 1986; Yoneyama *et al.* 1988; Löe *et al.* 1992; Susin *et al.* 2004). In populations maintaining high standards of oral hygiene, loss of attachment and marginal tissue recession are predominantly found at buccal surfaces (Löe *et al.* 1992; Serino *et al.* 1994), and are frequently associated with the presence of a "wedge-shaped defect in the crevicular area of one or several teeth" (Sangnes & Gjermo 1976). In contrast, all tooth surfaces are usually affected with soft tissue recession in periodontally untreated populations, although the prevalence and severity is more pronounced at single-rooted teeth than at molars (Löe *et al.* 1978; 1992; Miller *et al.* 1987; Yoneyama *et al.* 1988).

Tissue trauma caused by vigorous toothbrushing is considered to be a predominant causative factor for the development of recessions, particularly in young individuals. Traumatizing toothbrushing and tooth malposition are the factors most frequently found to be associated with marginal tissue recession (Sangnes 1976; Vekalahti 1989; Checchi *et al.* 1999). In addition, Khocht *et al.* (1993) showed that recessions are related to the use of hard toothbrushes. Other local factors that have been associated with marginal tissue recession are (1) alveolar bone dehiscences (Bernimoulin & Curilivic 1977; Löst 1984), (2) high muscle attachment and frenal pull (Trott & Love 1966), (3) plaque

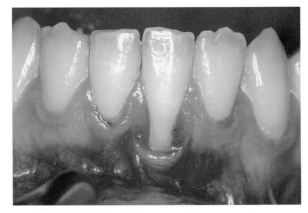

Fig. 44-5 A recession associated with localized plaque-induced inflammatory lesion.

and calculus (van Palenstein Helderman *et al.* 1998; Susin *et al.* 2004), and (4) iatrogenic factors related to restorative and periodontal treatment procedures (Lindhe & Nyman 1980; Valderhaug 1980).

At least three different types of marginal tissue recessions may exist:

- *Recessions associated with mechanical factors, predominately toothbrushing trauma* (Fig. 44-4). Recessions resulting from improper toothbrushing techniques are often found at sites with clinically healthy gingiva and where the exposed root has a wedge-shaped defect, the surface of which is clean, smooth and polished.
- *Recessions associated with localized plaque-induced inflammatory lesions* (Fig. 44-5). Such recessions may be found at teeth that are prominently positioned, i.e. the alveolar bone is thin or absent (bone dehiscence), and where in addition the gingival tissue is thin (delicate). An inflammatory lesion that develops in response to subgingival plaque occupies the connective tissue adjacent to the dentogingival epithelium. Measurements made by Waerhaug (1952) suggest that the distance between the periphery of microbial plaque on the tooth surface and the lateral and apical extension of the

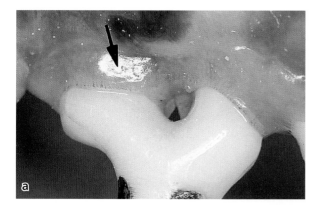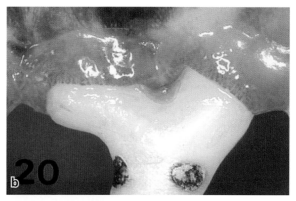
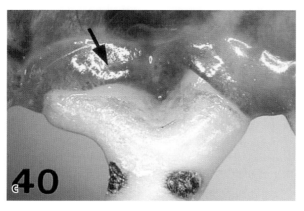

Fig. 44-6 Clinical photographs illustrating the development of a soft tissue recession as a result of plaque-induced inflammation in a beagle dog. (a) Note the thin but healthy gingiva (arrow) at the start of the plaque accumulation period. (b) Pronounced clinical signs of inflammation are seen after 20 days. (c) After 40 days of no tooth cleaning, the gingival margin has receded.

inflammatory cell infiltrate seldom exceeds 1–2 mm. Thus, if the free gingiva is voluminous the infiltrate will occupy only a small portion of the connective tissue. In a thin and delicate gingiva, on the other hand, the entire connective tissue portion may be engaged. Proliferation of epithelial cells from the oral as well as the dentogingival epithelium into the thin and degraded connective tissue may bring about a subsidence of the epithelial surface which clinically becomes manifest as recession of the tissue margin (Baker & Seymour 1976) (Fig. 44-6).

• *Recessions associated with generalized forms of destructive periodontal disease* (Fig. 44-7). The loss of periodontal support at proximal sites may result in compensatory remodeling of the support at the buccal/lingual aspect of the teeth leading to an apical shift of the soft tissue margin (Serino *et al.* 1994).

Cross-sectional studies showing that a correlation exists between the presence of recession defects and the height (width) of the gingiva (e.g. Stoner & Mazdyasna 1980; Tenenbaum 1982) have often been interpreted as an evidence that a narrow zone of gingiva is a contributing factor in the development of soft tissue recessions (Fig. 44-8). It should be realized, however, that data derived from cross-sectional studies can neither prove nor disprove a cause–effect

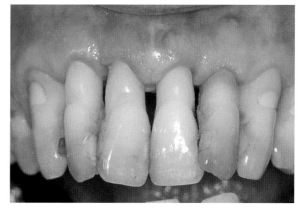

Fig. 44-7 Recessions associated with generalized forms of destructive periodontal disease. Recession of the soft tissue is found not only at the facial aspect of the teeth but also at proximal sites.

relationship. Consequently, the data reported from such studies may equally well be interpreted to demonstrate that the formation of a recession defect results in a reduced height of the gingiva. Fig. 44-1 illustrates a lower incisor tooth region with a localized gingival recession at the buccal aspect of tooth 41. The gingiva apical to the recession defect is narrow ("insufficient") while at neighboring teeth the gingival height may be considered "adequate". It is reasonable to assume that the gingiva at tooth 41, *before*

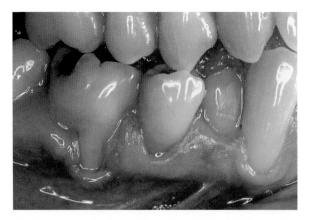

Fig. 44-8 A mandibular tooth segment with multiple buccal recessions illustrating the association proposed between recession depth and height of gingiva.

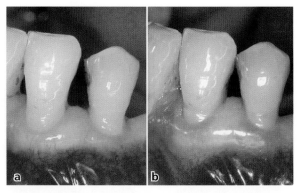

Fig. 44-9 (a) Clinical photographs of a canine and a first premolar in the mandibular jaw with <1 mm of attached portion of gingiva 6 months after surgical treatment. (b) Note the increase of the width of the gingiva at the facial aspect of the teeth and the more coronally positioned gingival margin 5 years later.

the recession defect developed, had a height that was similar to that found at tooth 31 and tooth 42. In other words, the narrow zone of gingiva found at tooth 41 may be the result of *loss of gingival tissue during the period of recession development*, rather than being the cause of the formation of the defect. If this interpretation is valid, the rationale for increasing the height of the gingiva in an area *apical to the existing defect* as a means of preventing further recession may appear somewhat obscure. In fact, data obtained from prospective, longitudinal studies of patients showing areas with only a minimal zone of gingiva favor the conclusion that a certain quantity of gingiva is not essential for the preclusion of soft tissue recessions.

Lindhe and Nyman (1980) examined the alterations of the position of the gingival margin following periodontal surgery in 43 patients with advanced periodontal breakdown. Following active treatment, all patients were recalled once every 3–6 months for maintenance care. The position of the soft tissue margin in relation to the CEJ was assessed on the facial aspect of all teeth after initial healing and after 10–11 years of maintenance. The presence or absence of keratinized tissue after surgical treatment was also determined. The results showed that both in areas with and without visible keratinized tissue after healing, a small coronal regrowth (≈1 mm) of the soft tissue margin had occurred during the period of maintenance. In other words, no recession was observed in this group of patients maintained on a careful prophylaxis program.

Dorfman *et al.* (1982) reported a 4-year follow-up study including 22 patients with bilateral tooth areas exhibiting gingival recession and lack of firmly attached marginal soft tissue. In conjunction with scaling and root planing a free gingival graft was placed on one side, while the contralateral control side was treated by scaling and root planing only. All patients were recalled for prophylaxis once every 3–6 months during a 4-year period. The data obtained from the examinations of the non-grafted control

areas revealed that no further recession of the soft tissue margin or loss of probing attachment had occurred despite the lack of attached marginal tissue. In fact, there was a slight gain of probing attachment. The authors concluded that recession sites without attached gingiva might not experience further attachment loss and recession if the inflammation is controlled. In a subsequent report (Kennedy *et al.* 1985), the authors reported data on 10 patients who had not participated in the maintenance program for a period of 5 years. In these patients plaque and clinical signs of inflammation as well as some further recession were noted at the 5-year examination as compared with the data obtained after termination of active treatment. However, except for the clinical signs of inflammation, which were more pronounced in non-grafted sites, no differences were observed between control sites with <1 mm or complete lack of attached gingiva and grafted sites.

The lack of relationship between the height of gingiva and the development of soft tissue recession is further validated by results from longitudinal clinical studies (Schoo & van der Velden 1985; Kisch *et al.* 1986; Wennström 1987; Freedman *et al.* 1999). The study by Wennström (1987) reports observations made at 26 buccal sites surgically deprived of all keratinized tissue. A baseline examination carried out 6 months after treatment revealed that these sites had regained a zone of gingiva which was, however, not attached or had only a minimal (<1 mm) portion attached to the underlying hard tissues (Figs. 44-9a and 44-10a). Adjacent teeth with a broad zone of attached gingiva were also included in the examinations. In most sites the position of the soft tissue margin had been maintained unchanged over 5 years (Figs. 44-9b and 44-10b). A further apical displacement of the soft tissue margin had occurred at two out of 26 sites with no/minimal attached portion of gingiva and at three out of 12 adjacent control sites with a wide attached zone of gingiva. Since four of these five sites were found in one patient (Fig. 44-11), and all sites were free from clinical signs of inflammation, excessive toothbrushing was considered to be the causative factor, and following correction of the brushing technique no further progression was observed. Furthermore, the development of soft tissue recession at the control sites resulted in a decreased width of the gingiva, an observation that supports the concept that a narrow zone of gingiva apical to a localized recession is a consequence rather than a cause of the recession.

Conclusion

Marginal soft tissue recession is a common feature in populations with good as well as poor standards of oral hygiene. There is evidence to suggest that the predominant cause for localized recessions in young individuals is toothbrushing trauma, while periodontal disease may be the primary cause in older adults. Evidence from prospective longitudinal studies shows that the gingival height is not a critical factor for the prevention of marginal tissue recession, but that the development of a recession will result in loss of gingival height.

Marginal tissue recession and orthodontic treatment

Results from clinical and experimental research have documented that most forms of orthodontic therapy are innocuous to the periodontium (see Chapter 57). The clinician may experience, however, that some patients respond to frontal movements of incisors and lateral movements of posterior teeth by gingival recession and loss of attachment (Maynard & Ochsenbein 1975; Coatoam *et al.* 1981; Foushee *et al.* 1985) (Fig. 44-12). Based on the clinical observation that recession may occur during orthodontic therapy involving sites that have an "insufficient" zone of gingiva, it was suggested that a grafting procedure to increase the gingival dimensions should precede the initiation of orthodontic therapy in such areas (Boyd 1978; Hall 1981; Maynard 1987).

As discussed previously, the presence of an alveolar bone dehiscence is considered to be a prerequisite for the development of a marginal tissue recession, i.e. a root dehiscence may establish an environment that is conducive for loss of gingival tissue. With respect to orthodontic therapy, this would imply that as long as a tooth is moved exclusively within the alveolar bone, soft tissue recession will not develop (Wennström *et al.* 1987). On the other hand, predisposing alveolar bone dehiscences may be induced by uncontrolled facial expansion of a tooth through the cortical plate, thereby rendering the tooth liable to development of soft tissue recession. In this context it is interesting to note that experimental studies have shown that labial bone will reform in the area of a dehiscence when the tooth is retracted towards a proper positioning of the root within the alveolar process (Engelking & Zachrisson 1982; Karring *et al.* 1982) (Fig. 44-13). It is therefore likely that the reduction in recession seen at a previously prominently positioned tooth that has been moved into a more proper position within the alveolar process (Fig. 44-14) is also accompanied by bone formation.

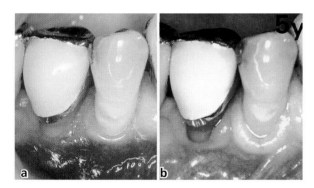

Fig. 44-10 (a) A mandibular canine and first premolar tooth region showing a very narrow zone of gingiva 6 months after surgical therapy. (b) No major change in the position of the soft tissue margin has occurred during a 5-year period despite the lack of attached gingiva.

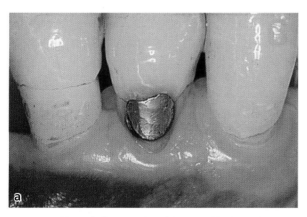
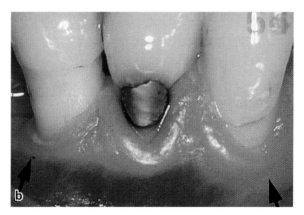

Fig. 44-11 Clinical photographs of the mandibular right canine–premolar tooth region in a patient showing several sites with apical displacement of the soft tissue margin during the 5 years of observation. (a) At the initial examination the two premolars had <1 mm and the canine >1 mm of attached portion of gingiva. (b) After 5 years, recession and loss of keratinized tissue can be seen on the buccal aspect of the canine, which initially had a broad zone of gingiva (black arrow). The second premolar also showed further apical displacement of the soft tissue margin (white arrow).

Alterations occurring in gingival dimensions and marginal tissue position in conjunction with orthodontic therapy are related to the *direction of tooth movement*. Facial movement results in reduced facial gingival dimensions, while an increase is observed following lingual movement (Coatoam *et al.* 1981;

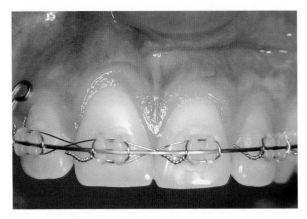

Fig. 44-12 Soft tissue recession at tooth 11 observed during the course of active orthodontic treatment.

Andlin-Sobocki & Bodin 1993). Recession of the labial gingival margin and loss of attachment was demonstrated in experimental studies in the monkey following either tipping and extrusion movements or bodily movements of incisors (Batenhorst *et al.* 1974; Steiner *et al.* 1981). However, similarly designed studies carried out in dogs (Karring *et al.* 1982; Nyman *et al.* 1982) and humans (Rateitschak *et al.* 1968) failed to demonstrate that labial tooth movement is accompanied by marginal tissue recession and attachment loss. The conflicting results may be related to differences with respect to e.g. (1) the amount of labial tooth displacement, (2) the presence/absence of plaque and gingival inflammation in the regions subjected to tooth movement, and/or (3) differences in gingival dimensions. Steiner *et al.* (1981) speculated on mechanisms by which gingival tissue could be lost as a result of labial tooth movement and suggested that tension in the marginal tissue created by the forces applied to the teeth could be an important factor. If this hypothesis were valid, obviously the volume (thickness) of the gingival tissue at the pres-

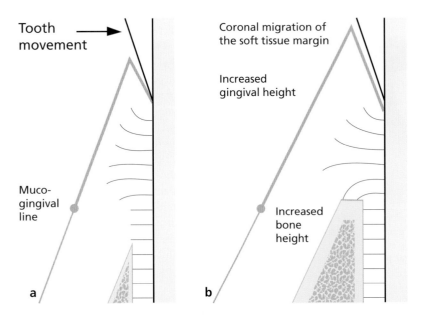

Fig. 44-13 (a) Schematic drawing illustrating alterations occurring in the marginal periodontal tissues following lingual movement of a tooth prominently positioned in the arch and having a bone dehiscence. (b) An increase in bone height and gingival height will be seen as well as a coronal migration of the soft tissue margin following lingual positioning of the tooth.

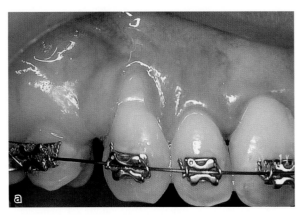

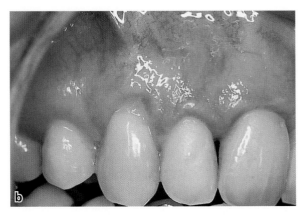

Fig. 44-14 (a) A prominently positioned 13 showing soft tissue recession. (b) The same tooth following the completion of the orthodontic tooth movement. Note the reduction of the recession that has taken place as a consequence of the changed position of the tooth.

sure side, rather than its apico-coronal height, would determine whether or not marginal tissue recession develops during orthodontic therapy.

Support for the hypothesis is obtained from an experimental study in monkeys (Wennström *et al.* 1987) in which teeth were orthodontically moved into areas with varying thickness and quality of the marginal soft tissue. Following extensive bodily movement of incisors in a labial direction through the alveolar bone (Fig. 44-15), most teeth showed a small apical displacement of the soft tissue margin but no loss of connective tissue attachment (Fig. 44-16). In other words, the apical displacement of the gingival margin was the result of a reduced height of the free gingiva (Fig. 44-17), which in turn may be related to tension ("stretching") in the soft tissues during the facial tooth movement and reduced bucco-lingual tissue thickness. Similar to results presented by

Foushee *et al.* (1985) from a study in humans, no relationship was found between the initial apico-coronal width (height) of the gingiva and the degree of apical displacement of the soft tissue margin during orthodontic therapy. Thus, the findings do not lend support to the concept of a certain zone of gingiva as essential for the prevention of recession during orthodontic therapy, but rather collaborate observations reported by Coatoam *et al.* (1981) that the integrity of the periodontium can also be maintained during orthodontic therapy in areas which have only a minimal zone of gingiva.

In the experimental studies by Steiner *et al.* (1981) and Wennström *et al.* (1987) it was observed that teeth, which experienced loss of connective tissue attachment when orthodontically moved facially, showed obvious clinical signs of inflammation throughout the experimental period. Since it has been demonstrated that, in presence of plaque-induced suprabony lesions, orthodontic forces generating bodily tooth movement are not capable of causing accelerated destruction of the connective tissue attachment (Ericsson *et al.* 1978), a decreased bucco-lingual dimension of the border tissue due to "stretching" of the facial gingiva may have favored the destructive effect of the plaque-associated inflammatory lesion. This assumption is validated by the observations that, in the presence of plaque-induced gingivitis, a thin marginal soft tissue is more susceptible to complete breakdown than a thick one (Baker & Seymour 1976). Furthermore, no difference in attachment loss was observed at plaque-infected teeth that were bodily moved *within the alveolar bone*, irrespective of the type of bordering soft tissue (gingiva or lining mucosa) (Wennström *et al.* 1987). Hence, the *thickness rather than the quality* of the marginal soft tissue on the pressure side of the tooth may be the determining factor for the development of the recession. The interpretation is supported by findings of recent clinical studies in humans analyzing factors of importance for the development of recessions during labial movement of mandibular incisors. Melsen and Allais (2005) found that gingival inflammation and a "thin gingival

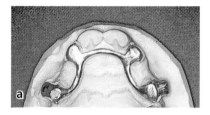
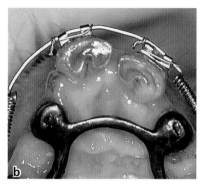

Fig. 44-15 Occlusal view of the maxillary jaw in a monkey showing the position of the central incisors before (a) and after (b) bodily movement in labial direction. The canines and lateral incisors were joined in an individual fabricated silver splint and used as anchorage teeth.

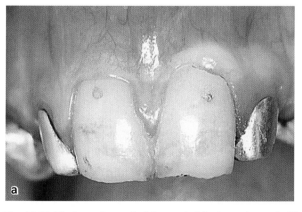
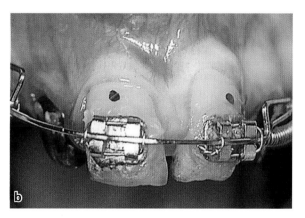

Fig. 44-16 The buccal aspect of the central incisors shown in Fig. 44-15, before (a) and after (b) the labial tooth movement. No obvious change in the location of the gingival margin has occurred despite the pronounced labial displacement of the incisors.

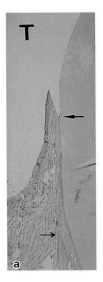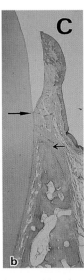

Fig. 44-17 Histologic specimens showing (a) reduced alveolar bone height at an incisor bodily moved in labial direction and (b) normal alveolar bone height at a non-moved control tooth. Note the maintained level of connective tissue attachment and the reduced height of the free gingiva at the labially displaced incisor (a). Large arrows indicate the position of the cemento-enamel junction and small arrows the position of the alveolar bone crest.

biotype" were significant predictors for gingival recession, and Yared *et al.* (2006) reported that 93% of the teeth that developed recession had a gingival thickness less than 0.5 mm. Hence, the observations made in the studies discussed strongly emphasize the importance of adequate infection control during orthodontic treatment.

Conclusion

The clinical implication of the results from the studies discussed is that labial tooth movement should be preceded by careful examination of the dimensions of the tissues covering the facial aspect of the teeth to be moved. As long as the tooth can be moved within the envelope of the alveolar process, the risk of harmful side effects in the marginal tissue is minimal, irrespective of the dimensions and quality of the soft tissue surrounding the tooth. If, however, the tooth movement is expected to result in the establishment of an alveolar bone dehiscence, the volume (thickness) of the covering soft tissue should be considered as a factor that may influence the development of soft tissue recession during, as well as after, the phase of active orthodontic therapy. A thin gingiva may serve as a *locus minorus resistentia* to developing soft tissue defects in the presence of plaque-induced inflammation or toothbrushing trauma.

Gingival dimensions and restorative therapy

The placement of restoration margins subgingivally may not only create a direct operative trauma to the tissues (Donaldson 1974), but may also facilitate subgingival plaque accumulation, with resultant inflammatory alterations in the adjacent gingiva and recession of the soft tissue margin (Parma-Benfenati *et al.* 1985; Lang 1995; Günay *et al.* 2000). Over a 10-year period, Valderhaug (1980) evaluated longitudinally the soft tissue alterations taking place at facial sites of 286 teeth with subgingivally or supragingivally placed crown margins in 82 patients. The re-examination performed 1 year after insertion of the restorations revealed that the gingivae at teeth with subgingival restoration margins were more inflamed than at those with supragingivally placed borders. Of the 150 teeth which had the facial crown margin located subgingivally at the time of cementation, 40% already showed supragingival exposure of the crown margin after 1 year, and at the 10-year examination as many as 71% had become supragingivally positioned due to recession of the soft tissue margin. Compared to teeth with supragingivally placed crown margins the amount of recession and clinical attachment loss was greater at sites with subgingivally placed restoration margins.

Stetler and Bissada (1987) evaluated the periodontal conditions at teeth with subgingivally placed restoration margins on teeth with varying apico-coronal height of gingiva and found that teeth having a narrow (<2 mm) band of gingiva showed more pronounced clinical signs of inflammation than restored teeth with a wide gingival zone, but that there was no difference in loss of probing attachment. However, if subgingivally placed restorations favor plaque accumulation and the adjacent gingiva is thin, there may be a potential risk for the development of soft tissue recession. In fact, an experimental study in the beagle dog (Ericsson & Lindhe 1984), in which metallic strips were inserted subgingivally in areas with varying width of gingiva, showed that in sites with a thin gingival margin, recession was a more likely consequence of the combined tissue trauma caused by the insertion of the strip and subsequent plaque accumulation during a 6-month period than in sites with a broad gingival zone. The authors suggested that the placement of restorations in a subgingival position might favor plaque retention and at sites with a thin gingiva this will lead to loss of tissue height, i.e. an apical displacement of the soft tissue margin. Accordingly, if such an apical displacement as a consequence of plaque-induced inflammation is to be prevented, either the plaque-control standard has to be improved or the *thickness* of the gingival margin has to be increased. However, an increased gingival dimension will not prevent the apical propagation of the plaque-associated lesion and the associated loss of periodontal attachment.

Conclusion

Subgingival placement of the margin of a restoration is likely to result in soft tissue recession over time.

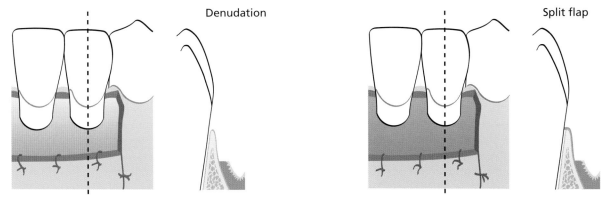

Fig. 44-18 The use of vestibular extension operations for increasing the width of the gingiva involves the production of a wound extending from the gingival margin to a level some millimeters apical to the mucogingival junction. With the "denudation" technique all soft tissue is removed leaving the alveolar bone exposed. With the "split flap" procedure only the superficial portion of the oral mucosa is removed leaving the bone covered with connective tissue.

Experimental and clinical data suggest that the thickness of the marginal gingiva, but not the apico-coronal width of the gingiva, may influence the magnitude of recession taking place as a result of direct mechanical trauma during tooth preparation and bacterial plaque retention.

Indications for gingival augmentation

Scientific data obtained from well controlled clinical and experimental studies have unequivocally demonstrated that the apico-coronal width of gingiva and the presence of an attached portion of gingiva are not of decisive importance for the maintenance of gingival health and the height of the periodontal tissues. Consequently, the presence of a narrow zone of gingiva *per se* cannot justify surgical intervention (Proceedings of the 1st European Workshop on Periodontology 1994; Proceedings of the World Workshop in Periodontics 1996). However, gingival augmentation should be considered in situations where, for example, the patient experiences discomfort during toothbrushing and/or chewing due to an interfering lining mucosa. Furthermore, when orthodontic tooth movement is planned and the final positioning of the tooth can be expected to result in an alveolar bone dehiscence, an increase of the *thickness* of the covering soft tissue may reduce the risk for development of soft tissue recession. An increase of the *thickness* of the gingival margin may also be considered in certain situations when subgingival restorations are placed in areas with a thin marginal tissue.

Gingival augmentation procedures

Gingival augmentation operations comprise a number of surgical techniques, the majority of which have been developed mainly on an empiric basis and without sufficient knowledge about the biology of the involved tissues. The earliest of these techniques are the "vestibular extension operations" which were designed mainly with the objective of extending the depth of the vestibular sulcus (Bohannan 1962a,b). In recent years, however, the use of pedicle or free soft tissue grafts have become the most commonly used techniques in the management of "insufficient" gingival dimensions, because of higher predictability of the healing result.

Vestibular/gingival extension procedures

The "denudation techniques" included the removal of all soft tissue within an area extending from the gingival margin to a level apical to the mucogingival junction leaving the alveolar bone completely exposed (Ochsenbein 1960; Corn 1962; Wilderman 1964) (Fig. 44-18). Healing following this type of treatment resulted often in an increased height of the gingival zone, although in some cases only a very limited effect was observed. However, the exposure of alveolar bone produced severe bone resorption with permanent loss of bone height (Wilderman *et al.* 1961; Costich & Ramfjord 1968). In addition, the recession of marginal gingiva in the surgical area often exceeded the gain of gingiva obtained in the apical portion of the wound (Carranza & Carraro 1963; Carraro *et al.* 1964). Due to these complications and severe postoperative pain for the patient, the use of the "denudation technique" can hardly be justified.

With the "periosteal retention" procedure or "split flap" procedure (Fig. 44-18) only the superficial portion of the oral mucosa within the wound area was removed leaving the bone covered by periosteum (Staffileno *et al.* 1962, 1966; Wilderman 1963; Pfeifer 1965). Although the preservation of the periosteum implies that less severe bone resorption will occur than following the "denudation technique", loss of crestal bone height was also observed following this type of operation unless a relatively thick layer of connective tissue was retained on the bone surface (Costich & Ramfjord 1968). If a thick layer was not secured, the periosteal connective tissue tended to undergo necrosis and the subsequent healing closely resembled that following the "denudation technique" described above.

Other described gingival extension procedures may be considered as modifications of the "denudation" and "split flap" techniques or combinations of these procedures. The apically repositioned flap procedure (Friedman 1962), for instance, involved the elevation of soft tissue flaps and their displacement during suturing in an apical position, often leaving 3–5 mm of alveolar bone denuded in the coronal part of the surgical area. This resulted in the same risk for extensive bone resorption as other "denudation techniques". It was proposed by Friedman (1962) that a post-surgical increase of the width of the gingiva can be predicted with the "apically repositioned flap", but several studies indicated that the presurgical width most often was retained or became only slightly increased (Donnenfeld *et al.* 1964; Carranza & Carraro 1970).

The vestibular/gingival extension procedures referred to were based on the assumption that it is the frictional forces encountered during mastication that determines the presence of a keratinized tissue adjacent to the teeth (Orban 1957; Pfeifer 1963). Therefore, it was believed that by the displacement of muscle attachments and the extension of vestibular depth, the regenerating tissue in the surgical area would be subjected to physical impacts and adapt to the same functional requirements as those met by "normal" gingiva (Ivancie 1957; Bradley *et al.* 1959; Pfeifer 1963). Later studies, however, showed that the characteristic features of the gingiva are determined by some inherent factors in the tissue rather than being the result of functional adaptation and that the differentiation (keratinization) of the gingival epithelium is controlled by morphogenetic stimuli from the underlying connective tissue (see Chapter 1).

Grafting procedures

The gingival and palatal soft tissues will maintain their original characteristics after transplantation to areas of the alveolar mucosa (see Chapter 1). Hence, the use of transplants offers the potential to predict the post-surgical result. The type of transplants used can be divided into (1) pedicle grafts, which maintain their connection with the donor site after placement at the recipient site (Fig. 44-19), and (2) free grafts that are completely deprived of their connection with the donor area (Fig. 44-20). For gingival augmentation free grafts have been used most commonly (Haggerty 1966; Nabers 1966; Sullivan & Atkins 1968a; Hawley & Staffileno 1970; Edel 1974). Acellular freeze-dried dermal matrix (ADM) allografts may be utilized

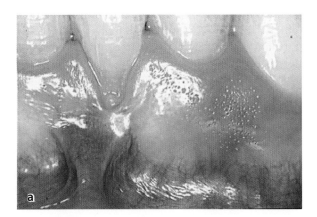
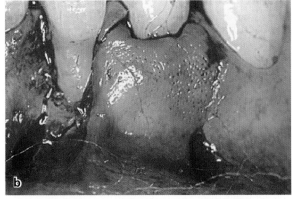
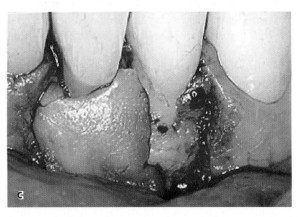
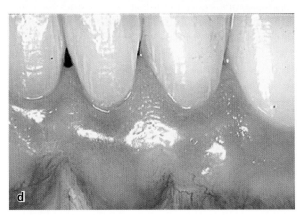

Fig. 44-19 Pedicle graft procedure for gingival augmentation. (a) A lower central incisor with facial soft tissue recession associated with high attachment of a frenulum. (b) The frenulum is released and a split flap of keratinized tissue is dissected from the area of the neighboring tooth. (c) The mobilized soft tissue flap is laterally moved and secured in position at the recipient site. (d) The healing result 1 year post-treatment shows the establishment of a broad zone of keratinized tissue without interfering frenulum.

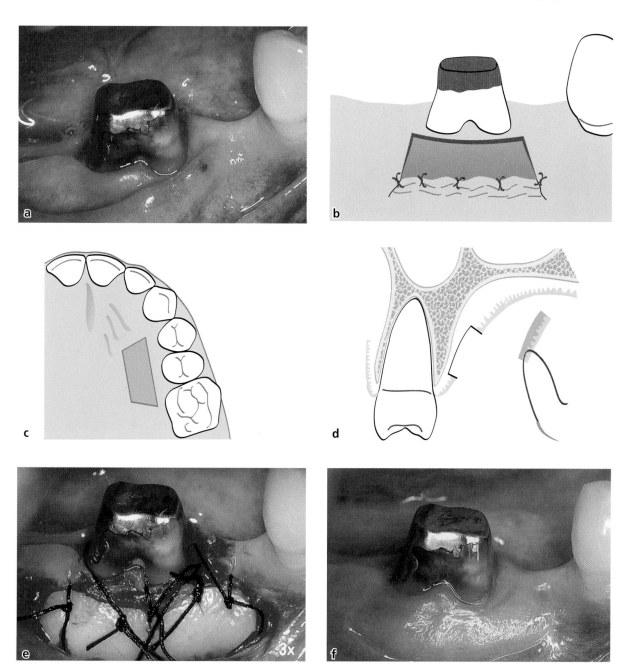

Fig. 44-20 Grafting procedure for gingival augmentation. (a) A lower molar at which the patient experiences discomfort during toothbrushing due to interfering lining mucosa and high attachment of a frenulum. Decision was made to displace the attachment of the frenulum apically and augment the gingival zone through the placement of a free graft. (b) A partial-thickness flap is dissected to prepare a recipient bed. The flap is displaced apically and sutured. (c,d) A graft with a thickness of 1.5–2 mm and of sufficient size and contour (a foil template of the recipient site may be used) is dissected from the palatal mucosa in the region of the premolars. (e) The graft is immediately transferred to the prepared recipient bed and anchored by sutures to secure a close adaptation of the graft to the recipient bed. (f) A periodontal dressing is applied to protect the graft. Following healing a broad zone of keratinized tissue has been established.

as an alternative to the use of an autogenous mucosal graft from the palate (Wei *et al.* 2000; Harris 2001), but the increase in the width of keratinized tissue following the use of these grafts may not be as predictable as with the use of autogenous grafts.

Technique

• The surgical procedure is initiated with the preparation of the recipient site (Fig. 44-20a-b). A periosteal bed free from muscle attachment and of sufficient size is prepared by sharp dissection. The partial-thickness flap is displaced apically and sutured.

• In order to ensure that a graft of sufficient size and proper contour is removed from the donor area, usually the palatal mucosa in the region of the premolars, it is recommended to produce a foil template over the recipient site. The template is transferred to the donor site where it is outlined by a shallow incision (Fig. 44-20c). A graft with a thickness of approximately 1.5–2 mm is then dissected from the donor area (Fig. 44-20d). It is

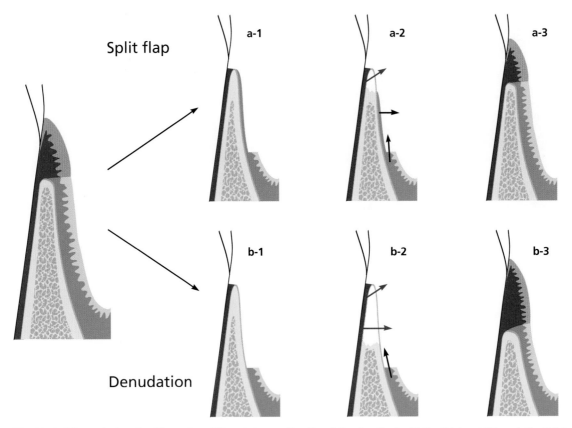

Split flap

a-1 a-2 a-3

b-1 b-2 b-3

Denudation

Fig. 44-21 Schematic drawing illustrating different stages of healing following the "split-flap" (a) and "denudation" (b) techniques. Cells from the oral mucosa, bone, and periodontal ligament (arrows) participate in granulation tissue formation. Due to the difference in the degree of bone resorption (a-2, b-2), a larger area of the coronal portion of the wound is filled with granulation tissue from the periodontal ligament following "denudation" than following the "split-flap" technique. Since granulation tissue from the periodontal ligament possesses the ability to induce a keratinized epithelium, "denudation" usually results in a wider zone of keratinized tissue than is the case following the "split-flap" technique (a-3, b-3).

advocated to place the sutures in the graft before it is cut completely free from the donor area since this may facilitate its transfer to the recipient site.

• The graft is immediately transferred to the prepared recipient bed and sutured (Fig. 44-20e). In order to immobilize the graft at the recipient site the sutures must be placed in the periosteum or the adjacent attached gingiva. After suturing, pressure is exerted against the graft for 5 minutes in order to eliminate blood and exudate from between the graft and the recipient bed. The graft and the palatal wound are protected with a periodontal dressing. To retain the dressing in the palatal site, a stent usually has to be used.

• The sutures and periodontal dressing are removed after 1–2 weeks.

For description of the pedicle graft procedure, see "Root coverage procedures".

Healing following gingival augmentation procedures

Vestibular/gingival extension procedures

Since the specificity of the gingiva is determined by some inherent factor in the tissues, the post-operative results of vestibular extension procedures depend on the degree to which the various tissues contribute to the formation of granulation tissue in the wound area (Karring *et al*. 1975). Following the "denudation" or "split flap technique", the wound area is filled with granulation tissue derived from the periodontal ligament, the tissue of the bone marrow spaces, the retained periosteal connective tissue, and the surrounding gingiva and lining mucosa (Fig. 44-21). The degree of bone resorption induced by the surgical trauma influences the relative amount of granulation tissue that grows into the wound from these various tissue sources. The resorption of crestal bone exposes varying amounts of the periodontal ligament tissue in the marginal area allowing granulation tissue from the periodontal ligament to fill out the coronal portion of the wound. The greater the bone loss, the greater is the portion of the wound that becomes filled with granulation tissue from the periodontal ligament. This particular tissue possesses the capability to induce keratinization of the covering epithelium. This means that the widening of the keratinized tissue following "denudation" and "split flap" operations is achieved at the expense of a reduced bone height. The "denudation technique" usually results in more bone loss than the "split flap technique". Therefore, a greater amount of granulation tissue

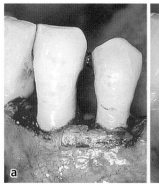
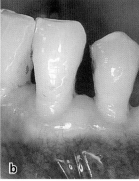

Fig. 44-22 (a) Clinical photograph of the buccal aspect of a canine and a premolar following the removal of the entire zone of gingiva by a gingivectomy procedure. (b) The healing result 9 months after surgery shows the regain of keratinized tissue.

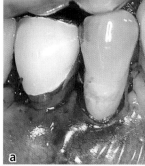
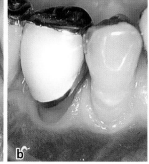

Fig. 44-23 Clinical photographs of a tooth region subjected to excision of the entire zone of gingiva by a flap procedure. (a) The alveolar mucosa has been displaced coronally to achieve complete coverage of the surgically exposed alveolar bone. (b) Healing has resulted in the reformation of a narrow zone of gingiva on the buccal aspect of the teeth, 9 months post surgery.

with the capability of inducing a keratinized epithelium develops in the marginal area following the "denudation technique" than following the "split flap technique". This is in accordance with the clinical observation that the "denudation technique" usually is superior to the "split flap technique" in increasing the width of keratinized tissue (Bohannan 1962a,b).

In a clinical study by Wennström (1983) periodontal pockets were eliminated by the use of a "gingivectomy" or a "flap" procedure which both involved the complete removal of the keratinized tissue. In the "gingivectomy" procedure the wounded area was left to heal by second intention, while in the "flap" procedure the alveolar mucosa was repositioned to achieve complete coverage of the surgically exposed alveolar bone (Figs. 44-22a and 44-23a). Irrespective of the surgical technique used, healing resulted in the reformation of keratinized tissue, the width of which, however, was greater following the "gingivectomy" procedure than following the "flap" procedure (Figs. 44-22b and 44-23b). The gingiva was formed because granulation tissue from the periodontal ligament,

with the capacity of inducing a keratinized epithelium, had proliferated coronally along the root surface. This granulation tissue formation was obviously favored by a more pronounced bone resorption during the healing following the "gingivectomy" procedure.

It can be concluded that the success or failure in extending the width of keratinized tissue by the "denudation" or "split flap" techniques rests with the origin of granulation tissue, which is related to the extent of bone loss induced by the surgical trauma. This in turn means that the result with respect to increasing the gingival width by methods involving periosteal exposure or denudation of the alveolar bone is unpredictable. The use of such methods is therefore not justified in periodontal therapy. The procedures discussed merely represent examples on how lack of knowledge about basic biologic principles may lead to the development of inappropriate therapeutic methods.

Grafting procedures

Healing of free soft tissue grafts placed entirely on a connective tissue recipient bed were studied in monkeys by Oliver *et al.* (1968) and Nobuto *et al.* (1988). According to these authors healing can be divided into three phases (Fig. 44-24):

1. *The initial phase (from 0–3 days)*. During these first days of healing a thin layer of exudate is present between the graft and the recipient bed. During this period the grafted tissue survives with an avascular "plasmatic circulation" from the recipient bed. Therefore, it is essential for the survival of the graft that a close contact is established to the underlying recipient bed at the time of operation. A thick layer of exudate or a blood clot may hamper the "plasmatic circulation" and result in rejection of the graft. The epithelium of the free graft degenerates early in the initial healing phase, and subsequently it becomes desquamated. In placing a graft over a recession, part of the recipient bed will be the avascular root surface. Since the graft is dependent on the nature of its bed for diffusion of plasma and subsequent revascularization, the utilization of free grafts in the treatment of gingival recessions involves a great risk of failure. The area of the graft over the avascular root surface must receive nutrients from the connective tissue bed that surrounds the recession. Thus, the amount of tissue that can be maintained over the root surface is limited by the size of the avascular area.

2. *Revascularization phase (from 2–11 days)*. After 4–5 days of healing, anastomoses are established between the blood vessels of the recipient bed and those in the grafted tissue. Thus, the circulation of blood is re-established in the pre-existing blood vessels of the graft. The subsequent time period is

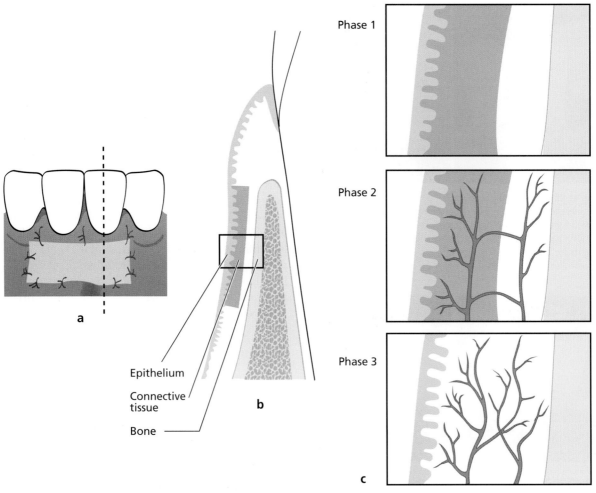

Fig. 44-24 Schematic drawings illustrating healing of a free gingival graft placed entirely on a connective tissue recipient bed (a). A cross-section through the area is shown in (b). The framed areas (c) illustrate the three phases into which the healing process can be divided.

characterized by capillary proliferation, which gradually results in a dense network of blood vessels in the graft. At the same time a fibrous union is established between the graft and the underlying connective tissue bed. The re-epithelialization of the graft occurs mainly by proliferation of epithelium from the adjacent tissues. If a free graft is placed over the denuded root surface, apical migration of epithelium along the tooth-facing surface of the graft may take place at this stage of healing.

3. *Tissue maturation phase (from 11–42 days)*. During this period the number of blood vessels in the transplant becomes gradually reduced, and after approximately 14 days the vascular system of the graft appears normal. Also, the epithelium gradually matures with the formation of a keratin layer during this stage of healing.

The establishment and maintenance of a "plasmatic circulation" between the recipient bed and the graft during the initial phase of healing is critical for the result of this kind of therapy. Therefore, in order to ensure ideal conditions for healing, blood between the graft and the recipient site must be removed by exerting pressure against the graft following suturing.

Root coverage

The main indications for root coverage procedures are esthetic/cosmetic demands (Fig. 44-25) and root sensitivity. Changing the topography of the marginal soft tissue in order to facilitate plaque control is also a common indication for root coverage procedures (Fig. 44-26).

It should be recalled that the two major causative factors in the development of marginal tissue recession are trauma caused by toothbrushing and plaque-induced periodontal inflammation. The control of these factors will prevent further progression of the recession in most cases. This means that in tooth regions with a thin covering soft tissue, with or without an incipient recession, the patient should be encouraged to carry out effective but at the same time non-traumatic plaque-control measures. With respect to toothbrushing, the Bass method (Chapter 35) should be avoided and the patient should be

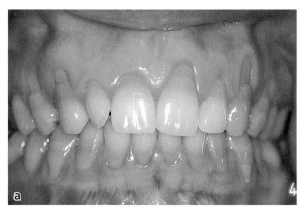
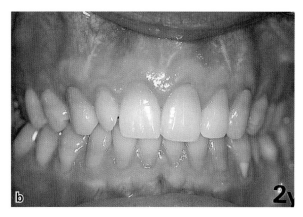

Fig. 44-25 (a) A 25-year-old woman with esthetic concerns due to multiple soft tissue recessions in the maxilla and a high lip line. The gingiva is healthy and several of the exposed root surfaces show abrasion defects, indicating toothbrushing trauma as the causative factor for the development of the recessions. The brushing technique was altered and root coverage was achieved surgically. (b) The 2-year post-treatment view.

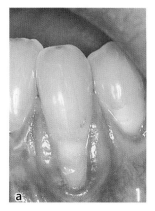
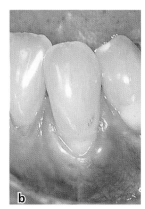

Fig. 44-26 (a) A mandibular canine with a deep recession, which offers problems with respect to self-performed plaque control. (b) To facilitate plaque control the position of the soft tissue margin was altered surgically.

instructed to use a technique creating as little apically directed pressure on the soft tissue margin as possible. A soft toothbrush should, of course, be used.

Miller (1985a) described a useful classification of recession defects taking into consideration the anticipated root coverage that is possible to obtain (Fig. 44-27):

- Class I: marginal tissue recession not extending to the mucogingival junction. No loss of interdental bone or soft tissue.
- Class II: marginal tissue recession extends to or beyond the mucogingival junction. No loss of interdental bone or soft tissue.
- Class III: marginal tissue recession extends to or beyond the mucogingival junction. Loss of interdental bone or soft tissue is apical to the CEJ, but coronal to the apical extent of the marginal tissue recession.
- Class IV: marginal tissue recession extends beyond the mucogingival junction. Loss of interdental bone extends to a level apical to the extent of the marginal tissue recession.

While complete root coverage can be achieved in class I and II defects, only partial coverage may be expected in class III. Class IV recession defects are not amenable to root coverage. Consequently, the critical clinical variable to assess in order to determine the possible outcome of a root coverage procedure is the level of periodontal tissue support at the proximal surfaces of the tooth.

Recession defects in the child need particular attention. In the growing child recession defects may be eliminated spontaneously, provided adequate plaque control is established and maintained (Fig. 44-28). Andlin-Sobocki *et al.* (1991) reported from a 3-year prospective study that 25 out of 35 recession defects with an initial depth of 0.5–3.0 mm healed spontaneously following improvement of the oral hygiene standard. Furthermore, all but three remaining recessions showed a decrease and no site demonstrated an increase in depth. Hence, reparative surgical treatment of soft tissue recessions in the developing dentition may not be necessary and should preferably be postponed until the growth is completed.

In an orthodontic case showing a recession defect and a thin (delicate) gingiva associated with a prominent, facially positioned tooth (Fig. 44-29a), surgical treatment for root coverage should be postponed until the orthodontic therapy is completed. The recession, as well as the dehiscence, will decrease as a consequence of the lingual movement of the tooth into a more proper position within the alveolar bone (Fig. 44-29b), and, if still indicated, the root coverage procedure will show higher predictability if performed after rather than before the tooth movement.

Root coverage procedures

Surgical procedures used in the treatment of recession defects may basically be classified as (1) *pedicle soft tissue graft procedures* and (2) *free soft tissue graft procedures*.

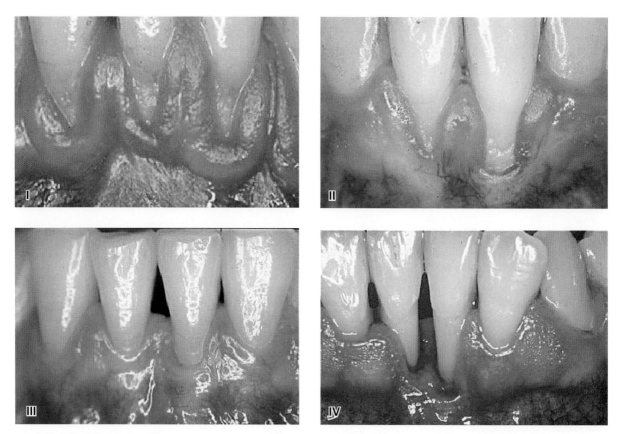

Fig. 44-27 The Miller classification of recession defects (see text).

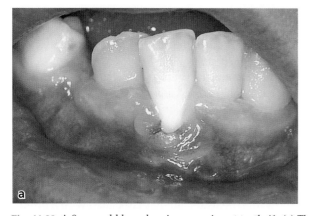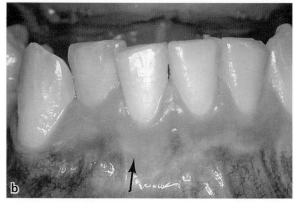

Fig. 44-28 A 9-year-old boy showing recession at tooth 41. (a) The tooth is rotated and buccally positioned. The minimal amount of gingiva found apical to the recession shows pronounced signs of inflammation. The plaque control in the region was improved but surgical intervention was postponed. (b) The same tooth area at the age of 14 years. Note the spontaneous soft tissue repair that has taken place at tooth 41 as a consequence of the improved plaque control and the growth in the alveolar process.

The pedicle graft procedures are, depending on the direction of transfer, grouped as (1) *rotational flap procedures* (e.g. laterally sliding flap, double papilla flap, oblique rotated flap) or (2) *advanced flap procedures* (e.g. coronally repositioned flap, semilunar coronally repositioned flap). The latter procedures do not include rotation or lateral movement of the pedicle graft. Regenerative procedures are also included within the group of pedicle graft procedures, i.e. rotational and advanced flap procedures

involving the placement of a barrier membrane between the graft and the root or the application of enamel matrix proteins.

The autogenous free soft tissue graft procedure may be performed as (1) an epithelialized graft or as (2) a subepithelial connective tissue graft (non-epithelialized graft), both usually taken from the area of the masticatory mucosa in the palate.

Factors, such as depth and width of recession, availability of donor tissue, presence of muscle

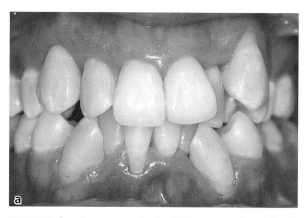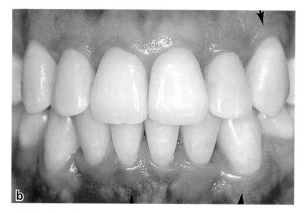

Fig. 44-29 Spontaneous repair of soft tissue recessions following orthodontic tooth movement. (a) A 22-year-old woman showing recessions and thin marginal tissues at prominently positioned teeth, particularly 23, 33, 41, and 43. (b) Following proper alignment of the teeth, the recessions have spontaneously been resolved and an increased gingival height can be noted.

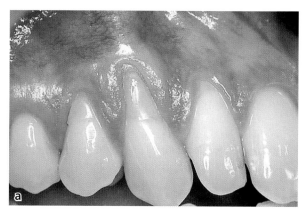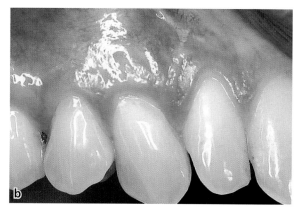

Fig. 44-30 (a) A canine showing pronounced recession and a composite resin restoration in the exposed root. Following removal of the restoration the exposed root was surgically covered with soft tissue (pedicle graft). (b) 2-year post-operative healing result.

attachments, and esthetics, have to be taken into consideration in the selection of treatment procedure.

Treatment of the exposed root surface

Before root coverage is attempted the exposed portion of the root should be rendered free from bacterial plaque. Preferably, this is achieved by the use of a rubber cup and a polishing paste. Controlled clinical trials have shown no differences in terms of root coverage or residual probing depth between teeth that had been instrumented (root planed) or polished only (Oles *et al*. 1988; Pini Prato *et al*. 1999). Extensive root planing may therefore only be performed in situations where a reduced root prominence would be considered beneficial for graft survival or tissue regeneration, or if a shallow root caries lesion is diagnosed. The presence of a filling in the root does not preclude the possibility for root coverage (Fig. 44-30), but the filling should be removed before the root is covered with soft tissue.

The use of root surface demineralization agents has been advocated as important not only for the removal of the smear layer, but also to facilitate the

formation of a new fibrous attachment through exposure of collagen fibrils of the dentine matrix and to allow subsequent interdigitation of these fibrils with those in the covering connective tissue. However, controlled clinical trials comparing the clinical outcome of root coverage procedures with and without root conditioning (Ibbott *et al*. 1985; Oles *et al*. 1985; Bertrand & Dunlap 1988; Laney *et al*. 1992; Bouchard *et al*. 1997; Caffesse *et al*. 2000) failed to demonstrate a beneficial effect from the use of acid root biomodification. Gottlow *et al*. (1986) evaluated the healing following treatment of localized gingival recessions with coronally positioned flaps and citric acid root biomodification in a controlled study in dogs. Histologic analysis after 3 months of healing disclosed no differences in the amount of root coverage or new connective tissue attachment between citric acid-treated sites and saline-treated control sites. Although root resorption was a common finding among the citric acid-treated teeth in this dog model, such a finding has not been reported to be common in humans. In conclusion, the literature clearly indicates that the inclusion of root conditioning does not improve the healing outcome of root coverage procedures.

Pedicle soft tissue graft procedures

Rotational flap procedures

The use of a laterally repositioned flap to cover areas with localized recession was introduced by Grupe and Warren (1956). This technique, which was called *the laterally sliding flap* operation, involved the reflection of a full-thickness flap in a donor area adjacent to the defect and the subsequent lateral displacement of this flap to cover the exposed root surface (Fig. 44-19). In order to reduce the risk for recession on the donor tooth, Grupe (1966) suggested that the marginal soft tissue should not be included in the flap. Staffileno (1964) and Pfeifer and Heller (1971) advocated the use of a split-thickness flap to minimize the potential risk for development of dehiscence at the donor tooth. Other modifications of the procedure presented are *the double papilla flap* (Fig. 44-31) (Cohen & Ross 1968), *the oblique rotational flap* (Pennel *et al.* 1965), *the rotation flap* (Patur 1977), and *the transpositioned flap* (Bahat *et al.* 1990).

The technique is as follows:

- The rotational flap procedure (Fig. 44-32) is initiated with the preparation of the recipient site. A reverse bevel incision is made all along the soft tissue margin of the defect (Fig. 44-32a). After removal of the dissected pocket epithelium, the exposed root surface is thoroughly curetted.

- At a distance of approximately 3 mm from the wound edge, which delineates the defect at the side opposite the donor area, a superficial incision is performed extending from the gingival margin to a level approximately 3 mm apical to the defect (Fig. 44-32b). Another superficial incision is placed horizontally from this incision to the opposite wound edge. The epithelium together with the outer portion of the connective tissue within the area delineated by these incisions and the wound edges is removed by sharp dissection (Fig. 44-32c). In this way a 3 mm wide recipient bed is created at the one side of the defect, as well as apical to the defect.

- A tissue flap to cover the recession is then dissected in the adjacent donor area. The preparation of this flap is initiated by a vertical superficial incision placed parallel to the wound edge of the recession and at a distance that exceeds the width of the recipient bed and the exposed root surface by approximately 3 mm (Fig. 44-32c). This incision is extended beyond the apical level of the recipient bed and is terminated within the lining mucosa with an oblique releasing incision directed towards the recession site. An incision connecting the vertical incision and the incision previously made around the recession is placed approximately 3 mm apical to the gingival margin of the donor site.

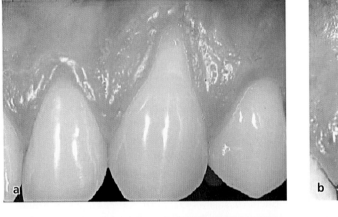

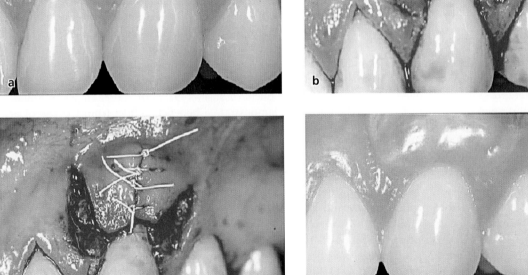

Fig. 44-31 Double papilla flap procedure. (a) Pre-treatment view of a maxillary canine with facial soft tissue recession. Using split incisions, soft tissue flaps are mobilized from both sides of the recession (b) and sutured together for coverage of the exposed root (c). The healing result 6-month post-operatively shows complete root coverage (d).

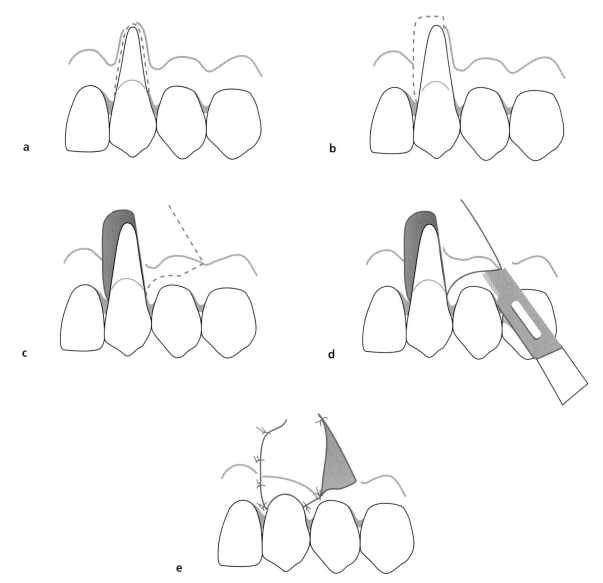

Fig. 44-32 Rotational flap procedure. Schematic drawings illustrating the surgical technique in utilizing rotational pedicle grafts to cover localized recession defects (see the text for explanation).

- A split-thickness flap is then prepared by sharp dissection within the area delineated by these incisions so that a layer of connective tissue is left covering the bone in the donor area when the flap is displaced laterally over the denuded root surface (Fig. 44-32d). It is important that the oblique releasing incision is made so far apically that the tissue flap can be placed on the recipient bed without being subjected to tearing forces when adjacent soft tissues are moved. The prepared tissue flap is rotated about 45° when sutured at the recipient bed (Fig. 44-32e).
- The suturing of the flap should secure a close adaptation of the pedicle graft to the underlying recipient bed. Pressure is applied against the flap for 2–3 minutes in order to further secure a good adaptation. To protect the surgical area during the initial phase of healing, a periodontal dressing may be applied. A light-cured dressing material, e.g. Barricaid™ (Dentsply International Inc.,

Milford, DE, USA), is preferably used since this can be applied without dislocating the flap and has, in addition, a favorable esthetic appearance.
- Following removal of the dressing and the sutures, usually after 10–14 days, the patient is instructed to avoid mechanical tooth cleaning for further 2 weeks, but to use twice daily rinsing with a chlorhexidine solution as a means of infection control.

Advanced flaps

Since the lining mucosa is elastic, a mucosal flap raised beyond the mucogingival junction can be stretched in coronal direction to cover exposed root surfaces (Harvey 1965; Sumner 1969; Brustein 1979; Allen & Miller 1989; Wennström & Zucchelli 1996; De Sanctis & Zucchelli 2007). The coronally advanced flap can be used for root coverage of a single tooth as well as multiple teeth, provided suitable donor tissue is available. In situations with only shallow

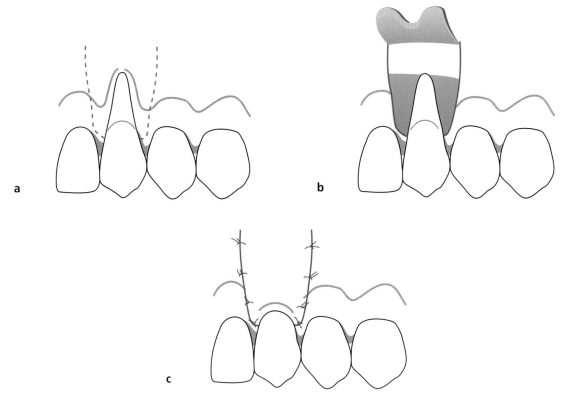

Fig. 44-33 Coronally advanced flap procedure. Schematic drawings illustrating the surgical technique in utilizing coronally advanced pedicle grafts to cover localized recession defects (see the text for explanation).

recession defects and minimal probing pocket depth labially, the *semilunar coronally repositioned flap* may offer an alternative approach (Harlan 1907; Tarnow 1986). For the treatment of an isolated deep gingival recession affecting a lower incisor, or the mesial root of the first maxillary molar, Zucchelli *et al.* (2004) suggested the use of a *laterally moved and coronally advanced flap*.

The technique for a *coronally advanced flap procedure* is as follows (Fig. 44-33):

- The coronally advanced flap procedure is initiated with the placement of two apically divergent vertical releasing incisions, extending from a point coronal to the CEJ at the mesial and distal line axis of the tooth and apically into the lining mucosa (Fig. 44-33a).
- A split-thickness flap is prepared by sharp dissection mesial and distal to the recession and connected with an intracrevicular incision. Apical to the receded soft tissue margin on the facial aspect of the tooth, a full-thickness flap is elevated to maintain maximal thickness of the tissue flap to be used for root coverage (Fig. 44-33b). Approximately 3 mm apical to the bone dehiscence, a horizontal incision is made through the periosteum, followed by blunt dissection into the vestibular lining mucosa to release muscle tension. The blunt dissection is extended buccally and laterally to such an extent that the mucosal graft is tension-free when positioned coronally at the level of the

CEJ. The facial portion of the interdental papillae may be de-epithelialized to allow for a final placement of the flap margin coronal to the CEJ.
- The tissue flap is coronally advanced, adjusted for optimal fit to the prepared recipient bed, and secured at the level of the CEJ by suturing the flap to the connective tissue bed in the papilla regions (Fig. 44-33c). Additional lateral sutures are placed to carefully close the wound of the releasing incisions. Mechanical tooth cleaning is avoided during the first 3–4 weeks of healing (rinsing with a chlorhexidine solution is prescribed), and when re-instituted, instructions in the use of a toothbrushing technique creating minimal apically directed trauma to the soft tissue margin is given.

Figure 44-34 illustrates the treatment of a recession defect with the use of the coronally advanced flap procedure. To allow the positioning of the flap margin coronal to the CEJ at the buccal surface the interdental papillae have to be de-epithelialized before suturing (Fig. 44-35).

The technique for a *laterally moved, coronally advanced flap* is as follows (Fig. 44-36):

- A vertical incision is made approximately 3 mm from the lateral edge of the recession defect at the side opposite the donor area, and parallel to the lateral border of the recession defect. The incision is extended from the level of the CEJ to a point

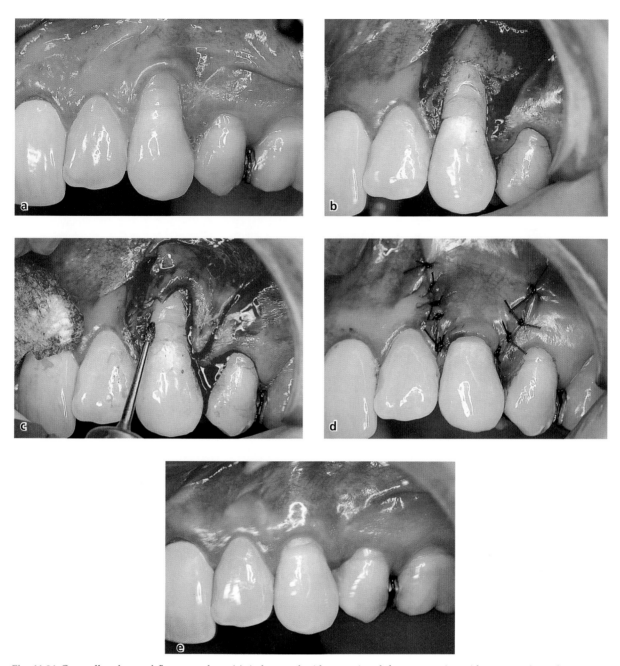

Fig. 44-34 Coronally advanced flap procedure. (a) A deep and wide recession defect on a canine with a composite resin restoration in the exposed root portion. Before preparation of the pedicle graft, the root is polished with pumice and a rubber cup. (b) A split flap has been dissected mesial and distal to the root, and a full-thickness flap apical to the recession. Approximately 4 mm apical to the bone dehiscence the periosteum has been cut and a blunt dissection performed to facilitate the coronal positioning of the pedicle graft. (c) The composite resin restoration is removed. (d) Close suturing of the pedicle graft to cover the exposed root surface. (e) Healing outcome 1 year post-operatively.

approximately 3 mm apical to the defect. At the marginal end of the vertical incision (at the level of the CEJ), a horizontal incision is made towards the recession defect. A third incision is made parallel to the lateral soft tissue margin of the recession defect on the donor side, from the bottom of the defect to the apical termination of the vertical incision on the recipient side. The area delineated by these incisions is de-epithelialized. In this way a 3 mm wide recipient bed is created lateral as well as apical to the defect.

- A pedicle graft is harvested from the adjacent tooth site by the use of three incisions: (1) a beveled intrasulcular incision along the lateral edge of the recession defect, (2) a horizontal submarginal incision with a 6 mm greater length than the width of the recession defect, and (3) a beveled oblique vertical incision extending into the alveolar mucosa and parallel to the first incision. The outline of the submarginal incision should preserve 3 mm of marginal soft tissue at the donor tooth, and preferably provide at least 2 mm of keratinized tissue

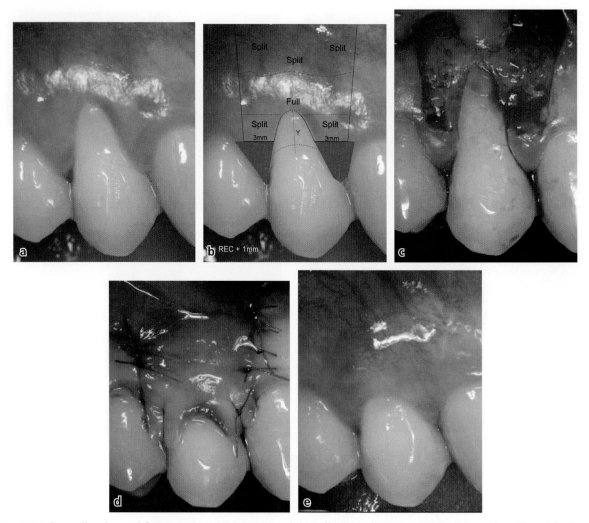

Fig. 44-35 Coronally advanced flap procedure. (a) A recession defect affecting a first premolar. (b) Schematic outline of the flap preparation. Blue line = amount (in mm) of intended coronal advancement of the flap; dotted red area = de-epithelialized papillae; Split = split-thickness elevation; Full = full-thickness elevation. (c) Flap elevated. The papilla areas are then de-epithelialized to allow anchorage of the flap coronal to the cemento-enamel junction (CEJ). (d) The flap is advanced and anchored at a level coronal to the CEJ with a sling suture. (e) Clinical healing at 1 year.

along the entire mesial–distal extension of the flap.

- The flap is mobilized as a split-thickness flap in its lateral parts, while the center part, which will be placed over the exposed root, is elevated as a full-thickness flap. Apical to the mucogingival line, the elevation is continued as split-thickness until it is possible to passively move the mucosal graft laterally to the recipient site.
- Blunt dissection is performed into the vestibular mucosa to release muscle tension to permit coronal advancement and passive adaptation of the flap to a level coronal to the CEJ.
- The facial surface of the interdental papillae is de-epithelized to create connective tissue beds to which the laterally moved, coronally advanced flap can be sutured.
- The suturing of the flap starts with the placement of two interrupted periosteal sutures in the most apical end of the vertical releasing incisions, and

continues with a series of interrupted sutures, directed in a apical–coronal direction from the flap to the adjacent wound edge. A horizontal double mattress periosteal suture is placed apical to the vertical incisions to reduce lip tension on the root coverage portion of the flap. The coronal suture is a sling suture, which permits a precise adaptation of the flap against the root surface and the interdental connective tissue beds.

Figure 44-37 illustrates the treatment of a recession defect at a maxillary molar with the use of the *laterally moved, coronally advanced flap* procedure.

Zucchelli and De Sanctis (2000) described a flap design for the treatment of multiple recessions, which allows for optimal adaptation of the flap following its coronal advancement without placement of vertical releasing incisions. The technique for this *coronally advanced flap procedure for multiple recessions* is as follows (Fig. 44-38):

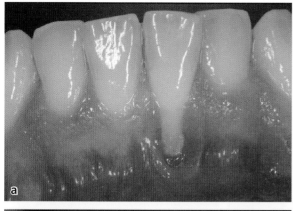

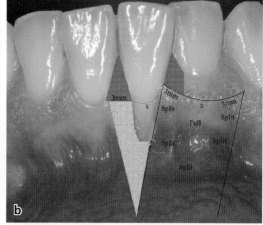

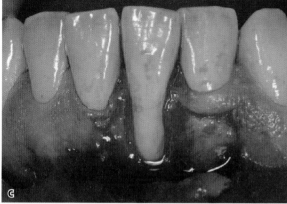

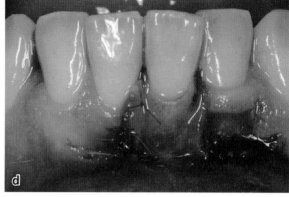

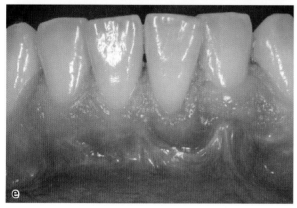

Fig. 44-36 The laterally moved, coronally advanced flap (see text for explanation). (a) A cenral insicor with recession defect. (b) Schematic outline of the preparation of the recipient site and the pedicle graft. Dotted pink area = receiving area for lateral flap; dotted red area = de-epithelialized papillae; x = recession width at the level of the cemento-enamel junction; Split = split-thickness elevation; Full = full-thickness elevation. (c,d) The flap is transpositioned laterally and coronally, and secured in position by sutures. A horizontal double mattress suture is performed to reduce lip tension on the marginal portion of the flap. (e) Clinical healing at 1 year.

- Oblique submarginal incisions are made in the interdental areas and connected with intracrevicular incisions at the recession defects. The incisions are extended to include one tooth on each side of the teeth to be treated to facilitate coronal repositioning of the flap. The oblique incisions over the interdental areas are placed in such a manner that the "surgically created papillae" mesial to the midline of the surgical field are dislocated apically and distally, while the papillae of the flap distal to the midline are shifted in a more apical and mesial position (Fig. 44-37a).
- Starting at the oblique interdental incisions, a split-thickness flap is dissected (Fig. 44-38c). Apical to the level of the root exposures, a full-thickness flap is raised to provide maximum soft tissue thickness of the flap to be positioned coronally over the roots (Fig. 44-38d).

- At the most apical portion of the flap, the periosteum is incised and followed by dissection into the vestibular lining mucosa to eliminate all muscle tension. The mobilized flap should be able to passively reach a level coronal to the CEJ at each single tooth in the surgical field.
- The remaining facial portion of the interdental papillae is de-epithelialized to create connective tissue beds to which the flap can be sutured.
- Sutures are placed to accomplish a precise adaptation of the coronally advanced flap against the teeth and to the interdental connective tissue beds (Fig. 44-38e). In addition, a horizontal double mattress suture is placed to reduce lip tension on the marginal portion of the flap.

The technique for a *semilunar coronally repositioned flap procedure* is as follows (Fig. 44-39):

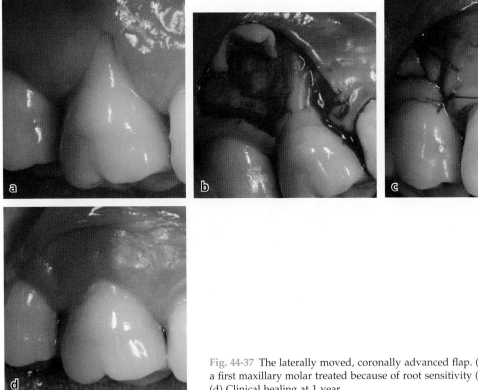

Fig. 44-37 The laterally moved, coronally advanced flap. (a–c) A recession defect at a first maxillary molar treated because of root sensitivity (see text for explanation). (d) Clinical healing at 1 year.

- A semilunar incision is placed apical to the recession and at a distance from the soft tissue margin, which should be approximately 3 mm greater than the depth of the recession. The outline of the incision should be parallel to the curvature of the gingival margin (Fig. 44-39a). The incision is extended into the papilla region on each side of the tooth, but care should be taken to maintain a broad base of anchorage to secure a collateral blood supply to the pedicle graft.
- A split-thickness dissection of the facially located tissue is then made by an intracrevicular incision extending apically to the level of the semilunar incision (Fig. 44-39b). The mid-facial soft tissue graft is coronally repositioned to the level of the CEJ (Fig. 44-39c) and stabilized by light pressure for 5 minutes.
- No suturing is needed but a light-cured dressing may be applied for wound protection.

Pedicle soft tissue graft procedures combined with a barrier membrane

The use of a barrier membrane, according to the principles of guided tissue regeneration (GTR, see Chapter 25), in conjunction with pedicle soft tissue graft procedures was introduced as a treatment modality for root coverage by Pini Prato *et al.* (1992). In order create space for tissue formation between the facial root surface and the membrane Pini Prato *et al.* (1992) suggested that extensive root planing should be carried out to produce concave root morphology. Specially designed membranes for the treatment of

recession type defects are available, such as non-absorbable titanium-reinforced expanded polytetrafluoroethylene (e-PTFE) membranes (Fig. 44-40c). In addition, a variety of bioabsorbable membranes are commercially available, but many of these may not be rigid enough for maintaining required space during healing.

The pedicle graft used in the GTR procedure is generated through the preparation of a coronally advanced flap (Fig. 44-40):

- Apically divergent vertical releasing incisions are made at the mesial and distal line axis of the tooth, extending from a point coronal to the CEJ and apically into the lining mucosa. A trapezium-shaped full-thickness flap is raised beyond the bone dehiscence (Fig. 44-40b). The periosteum at the base of the raised mucoperiosteal flap is incised, followed by a blunt supraperiosteal dissection to such a depth that the trapezoidal flap easily can be advanced coronally to the desired position. Depending on the degree of coronal repositioning, the facial portion of the interdental papillae may need to be de-epithelialized to prepare proper recipient beds for the pedicle graft.
- The root is extensively planed or ground to obtain a concave profile of the root surface, thereby providing space for tissue formation. If a titanium-reinforced membrane is used, the root profile may not need to be changed to establish the required space between the root and the membrane.

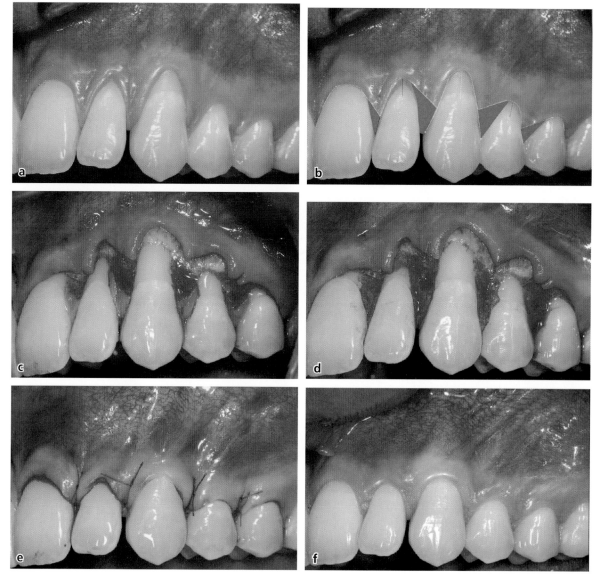

Fig. 44-38 Coronally advanced flap procedure for multiple recessions (see text for explanation). (a–e) The oblique incisions over the interdental areas are placed in such a manner that the "surgically created papillae" mesial to the midline of the surgical field are dislocated apically and distally, while the papillae of the flap distal to the midline are shifted in a more apical and mesial position. (f) The 1-year post-treatment view.

- The membrane barrier to be used is trimmed to cover the exposed root and approximately 3 mm of the bone lateral and apical to the dehiscence (Fig. 44-40c) and anchored to the tooth by a sling suture placed at the level of the CEJ.
- The mobilized flap is positioned coronally and secured by interdentally placed interrupted sutures (Fig. 44-40d). The membrane should be completely covered by the flap to reduce the risk for bacterial contamination during healing. Additional sutures are placed to close the lateral wound of the releasing incisions.
- The patient is advised to use a chlorhexidine mouth rinse for infection control and not to use any mechanical cleaning devices for at least 6 weeks in the tooth region subjected to surgery.
- The use of non-biodegradable membrane barriers requires a second surgery for membrane removal,

usually after 5–6 weeks (Fig. 44-40e,f). A partial-thickness trapezoidal flap is raised to expose the membrane. Following its removal, the flap is repositioned at the level of the CEJ to completely cover the newly formed tissue. Mechanical plaque control is reinstituted 4 weeks after membrane removal.

Pedicle soft tissue graft procedures combined with enamel matrix proteins

Abbas *et al.* (2003) described a surgical procedure for periodontal regenerative therapy of recession defects utilizing enamel matrix derivative bioactive material (Emdogain®):

- The surgical technique utilized is the coronally advanced flap as described above (Fig. 44-33). The interdental papillae should be de-epithelialized to

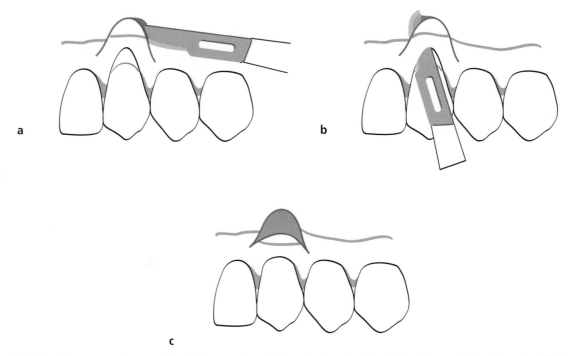

Fig. 44-39 Semilunar coronally repositioned flap procedure. Schematic drawings illustrating the surgical technique in utilizing coronally displaced pedicle grafts to cover shallow localized recession defects (see text for explanation).

allow for maximum coronal positioning of the tissue flap over the exposed root surface at suturing.

- Following preparation of the coronally advanced flap, the exposed root surface is conditioned with PrefGel™ (24% EDTA-gel, pH 6.7; Straumann Biologics, Switzerland) for 2 minutes to remove the smear layer.
- After thorough rinsing with sterile saline, the enamel matrix protein gel (Emdogain®, Straumann Biologics, Switzerland) is applied to the exposed root surface. The pedicle graft is advanced coronally and secured at a level slightly coronal to the CEJ by suturing the flap to the de-epithelialized papilla regions using non-irritating sutures. The vertical incisions are then closed with two to three sutures. Mechanical tooth cleaning is avoided during the first 3–4 weeks of healing (rinsing with a chlorhexidine solution is prescribed), and when re-instituted, a toothbrushing technique creating minimal apically directed trauma to the soft tissue margin is used.

Free soft tissue graft procedures

A free soft tissue graft of masticatory mucosa is usually selected when there is no acceptable donor tissue present in the area adjacent to the recession defect or when a thicker marginal tissue is desirable. The procedure can be used for the treatment of a single tooth as well as for groups of teeth. The graft used may either be (1) an *epithelialized graft* or (2) a *subepithelial connective tissue graft* of palatal masticatory mucosa.

Epithelialized soft tissue graft

The epithelialized free soft tissue graft procedure can be performed either as a two-step surgical technique, where an epithelialized free soft tissue graft is placed apical to the recession and following healing is positioned coronally over the denuded root (Fig. 44-41) (Bernimoulin *et al.* 1975; Guinard & Caffesse 1978), or as a one-step technique by which the graft is placed directly over the root surface (Sullivan & Atkins 1968a,b; Miller 1982) (Fig. 44-42). The latter of the two techniques has been most commonly used.

The principles of utilizing free mucosal grafts were outlined by Sullivan and Atkins (1968a,b) and later modified by Miller (1982):

- Before any incisions the exposed root surface is carefully scaled and root planed (Fig. 44-42a). The convexity of the root may be reduced to minimize the mesio-distal avascular recipient bed.
- As in the treatment with pedicle grafts, the preparation of *the recipient bed* is crucial for the success of free graft procedure. A 3–4 mm wide recipient connective tissue bed should be prepared apical and lateral to the recession defect (Fig. 44-42b). The area is demarcated by first placing a horizontal incision, at the level of the CEJ, in the interdental tissue on each side of the tooth to be treated. Subsequently, two vertical incisions, extending from the incision line placed in the interdental tissue to a level approximately 4–5 mm apical to the recession, are placed. A horizontal incision is then made connecting the two vertical incisions at their apical termination. Starting from an intracrevicular incision, a split incision is made to sharply dissect the

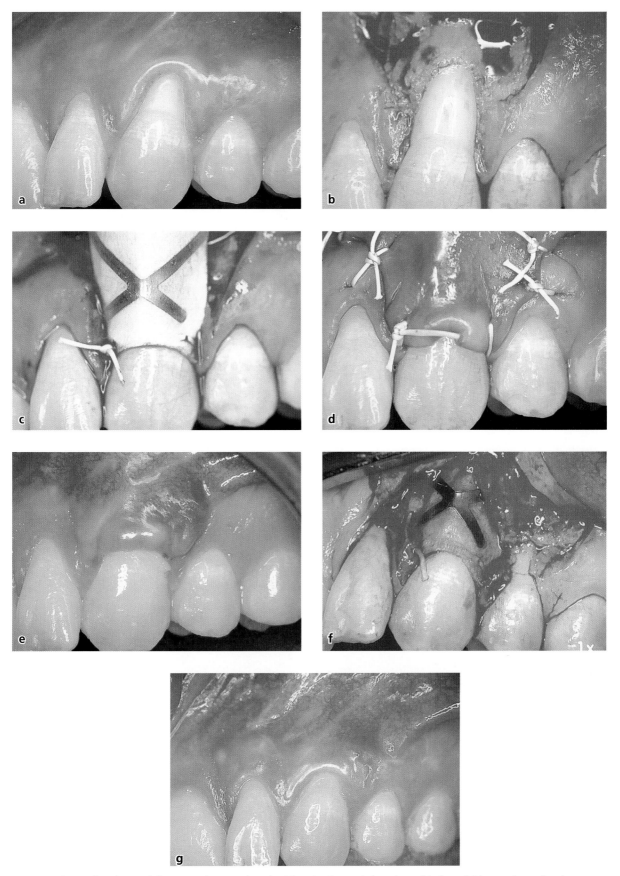

Fig. 44-40 Coronally advanced flap procedure combined with a titanium-reinforced non-biodegradable membrane barrier. (a–f) A recession defect at tooth 23 requiring treatment due to the patient's esthetic demands (see the text for explanation). (g) The 1-year post-operative result.

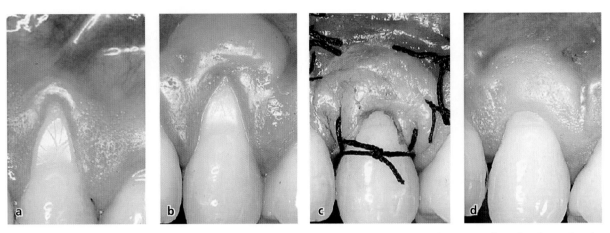

Fig. 44-41 Two-stage epithelialized free soft tissue graft procedure. (a–c) An epithelialized soft tissue graft is placed apical to the recession and allowed to heal. At a second stage surgery, a coronally advanced flap procedure is performed to achieve coverage of the denuded root. (d) The 1-year post-operative result.

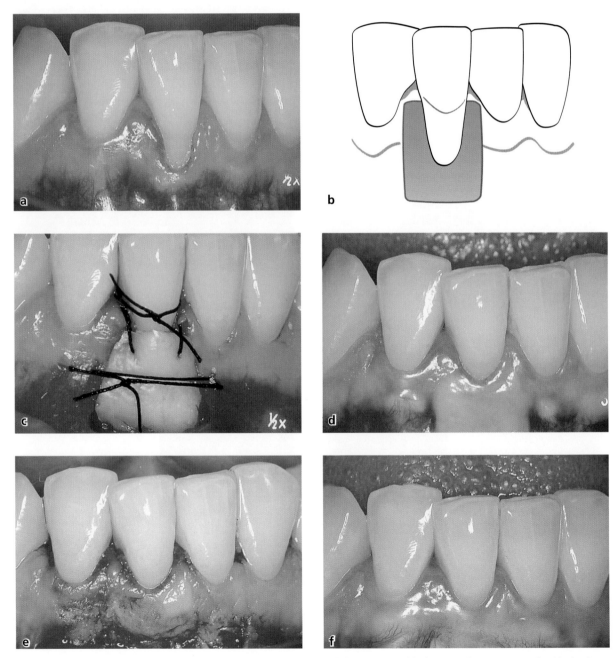

Fig. 44-42 Epithelialized free soft tissue graft procedure. A recession defect at a mandibular central incisor treated with the free graft procedure (see the text for explanation).

epithelium and the outer portion of the connective tissue within the demarcated area.

- To ensure that a graft of sufficient size and proper contour is removed from the donor area, a foil template of the recipient site is prepared. This template is transferred to the donor site, the palatal mucosa in the region of the premolars, and the required size of the graft is outlined by a shallow incision. A graft with a thickness of 2–3 mm is then dissected from the donor area (Fig. 44-20c–d). It is advocated to place sutures in the graft before it is cut completely free from the donor area since this may facilitate its transfer to the recipient site. Following the removal of the graft, pressure is applied to the wound area for control of bleeding.
- The graft is immediately placed on the prepared recipient bed. In order to immobilize the graft at the recipient site, sutures must be anchored in the periosteum or in the adjacent attached gingiva. Adequate numbers of sutures are placed to secure close adaptation of the graft to the underlying connective tissue bed and root surface (Fig. 44-42c). Before the placement of a periodontal dressing, pressure is exerted against the graft for some minutes in order to eliminate blood from between the graft and the recipient bed. Following the control of bleeding, the wound in the donor area

in the palate is covered by a periodontal dressing. An acrylic plate may be required to maintain the dressing in place during healing phase.
- The sutures and periodontal dressing are usually maintained for 2 weeks. The appearance of a grafted area after 3 months of healing is shown in Fig. 44-42d. A gingivoplasty may be indicated to achieve a satisfactory esthetic appearance of the grafted area (Fig. 44-42e,f).

Connective tissue graft

The techniques utilizing a subepithelial soft tissue graft, i.e. the connective tissue, involve the placement of the graft directly over the exposed root and the mobilization of a mucosal flap coronally (Fig. 44-43) or laterally (Fig. 44-44) for coverage of the graft (Langer & Langer 1985; Nelson 1987; Harris 1992; Bruno 1994; Zucchelli *et al.* 2003). An alternative technique is to place the base of the connective tissue graft within an "envelope" prepared by an undermining partial-thickness incision from the soft tissue margin, i.e. part of the graft will rest on the root surface coronal to the soft tissue margin (Fig. 44-45) (Raetzke 1985; Allen 1994). For the treatment of multiple adjacent recessions, a multi-envelope recipient bed ("tunnel") may be prepared (Zabalegui *et al.* 1999). The subepithelial connective tissue graft is harvested from the palate or the retromolar pad by the

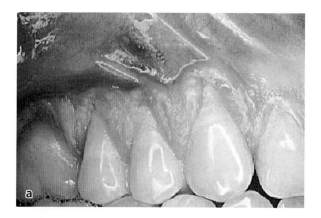
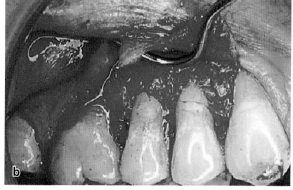
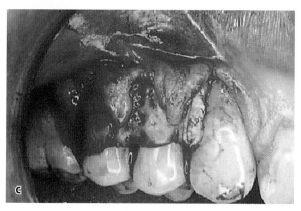
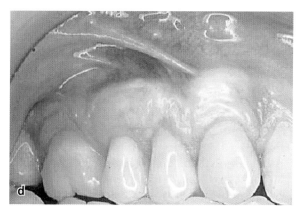

Fig. 44-43 Free connective tissue graft combined with a coronally advanced flap procedure – single recession (see the text for explanation). (a) Deep gingival recession at a cuspid with minimal height of keratinized tissue apical to the root exposure. (b) The graft has been sutured to leave an area between the cemento-enamel junction and the graft available for the marginal keratinized tissue of the flap. (c) The flap has been advanced coronally and sutured. (d) Clinical healing at 1 year.

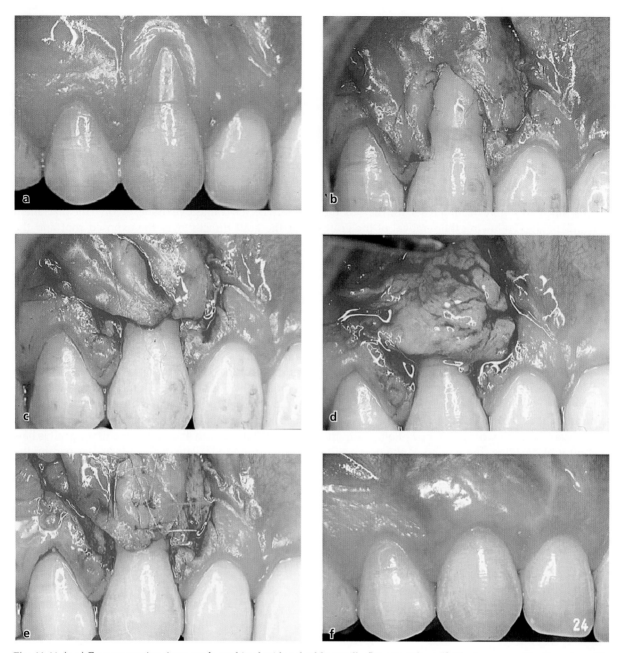

Fig. 44-44 (a–e) Free connective tissue graft combined with a double papilla flap procedure. (f) The 1-year post-treatment result.

use of a "trap door" approach (Fig. 44-46). Compared to the epithelialized graft, the connective tissue graft is preferable due to a less invasive palatal wound and an improved esthetic result.

The technique for the *connective tissue graft combined with a coronally advanced flap* is as follows (Fig. 44-43):

• The surgical technique utilized is the coronally advanced flap as described above, but with the difference that the flap is elevated entirely as a split-thickness flap. The interdental papillae should be de-epithelialized to allow for maximum coronal positioning of the tissue flap over the exposed root surface at suturing (Fig. 44-43b).
• A subepithelial connective tissue graft of masticatory mucosa is harvested on the palatal aspect of

the maxillary premolars/first molar (or from the retromolar pad) by the use of a "trap door" approach (Fig. 44-46). Before incisions are placed, the available thickness of the mucosa is estimated by the use of the tip of the syringe. A horizontal incision, perpendicular to the underlying bone surface, is made approximately 3 mm apical to the soft tissue margin (Fig. 44-46a). The mesio-distal extension of the incision is determined by the graft size required, which is 6 mm longer than the width of the dehiscence measured at the level of the CEJ. To facilitate the removal of the graft, a vertical releasing incision may be made at the mesial termination of the primary incision. An incision is then placed from the line of the first incision and directed apically to perform a split incision of the palatal mucosa (Fig. 44-46b–f). A small periosteal

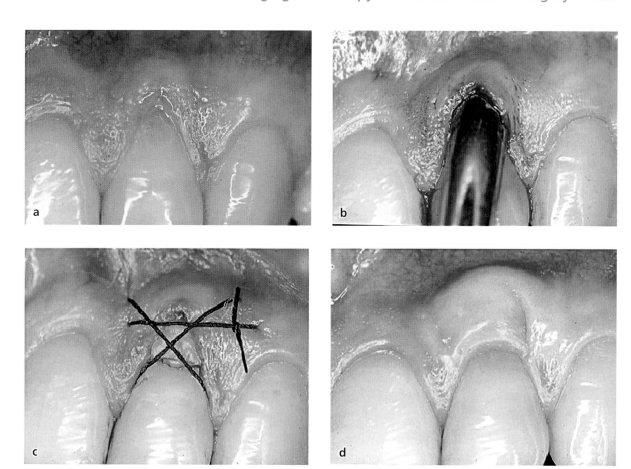

Fig. 44-45 (a–c) Free connective tissue graft procedure – the "envelope technique" (see text for explanation). (d) The 1-year post-treatment result. (Courtesy of Dr. P. Cortellini, Italy.)

elevator or scalpel is used to release the connective tissue graft from the bone.

- The graft is immediately transferred to the recipient site and positioned at a distance from the CEJ equal to the height of keratinized tissue originally present apical to the recession defect. The graft is secured in position with two double vertical mattress sutures to adjacent soft tissue lateral to the dehiscence (Fig. 44-43c). A sling suture is placed in the papilla regions to position the margin of the covering advanced flap about 1 mm coronal to the CEJ. Interrupted sutures are used to close the wound along the vertical incisions (Fig. 44-43d).

Figure 44-47 illustrates the procedure applied to a case with multiple recession sites.

The "envelope" technique (Fig. 44-48) is as follows:

- With the use of the "envelope" technique the recipient site is prepared by first eliminating the sulcular epithelium by an internal beveled incision (Fig. 44-48a). Secondly, an "envelope" is prepared apically and laterally to the recession by split incisions (Fig. 44-48b). The depth of the preparation should be 3–5 mm in all directions. In an apical direction, the preparation of the site should extend beyond the mucogingival junction to facilitate the placement of the connective tissue graft and to allow for coronal advancement of the mucosal flap at time of suturing.

- A foil template may be used for the harvest of an appropriately sized connective tissue graft. The graft, which is obtained by the "trap door" approach described above (Fig. 44-46), is inserted into the prepared "envelope" and positioned to cover the exposed root surface (Fig. 44-48c–d).

- Sutures are placed to secure graft in position (Fig. 44-48d). A crossed sling suture may be placed to advance the mucosal flap coronally. Pressure is applied for 5 minutes to adapt the graft closely to the root surface and covering soft tissue.

Figure 44-45 shows the treatment of a recession defect with the "envelope" technique.

The "tunnel" technique (Fig. 44-49) is as follows:

- In case multiple adjacent recessions are to be treated, "envelopes" are prepared for each tooth as described above. However, the lateral split incisions are extended so that the multi-envelopes are connected mesially and distally to form a mucosal tunnel. Care should be taken to avoid detachment of the papillae.

- The graft is gently positioned inside the tunnel and its mesial and distal extremities are fixed with two interrupted sutures. Sling sutures may be placed

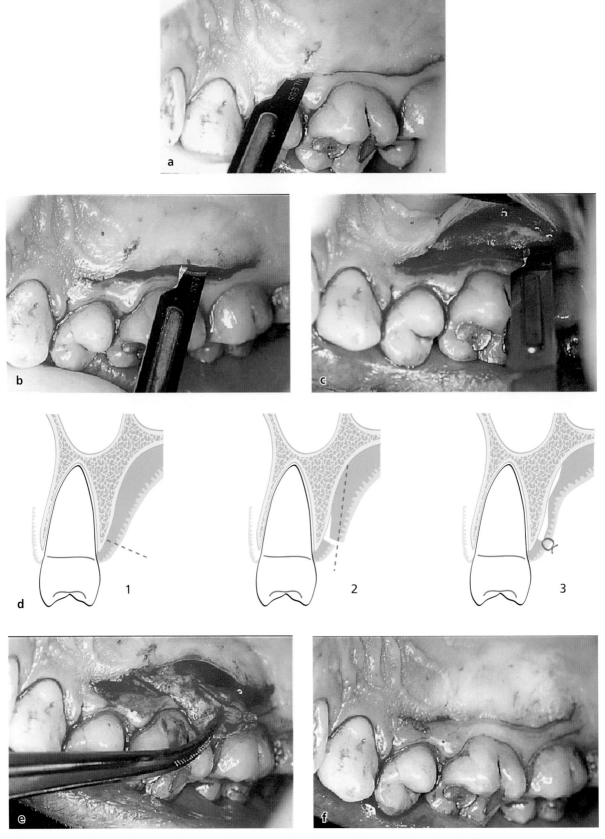

Fig. 44-46 "Trap-door" technique for harvest of a free connective tissue graft (see text for explanation).

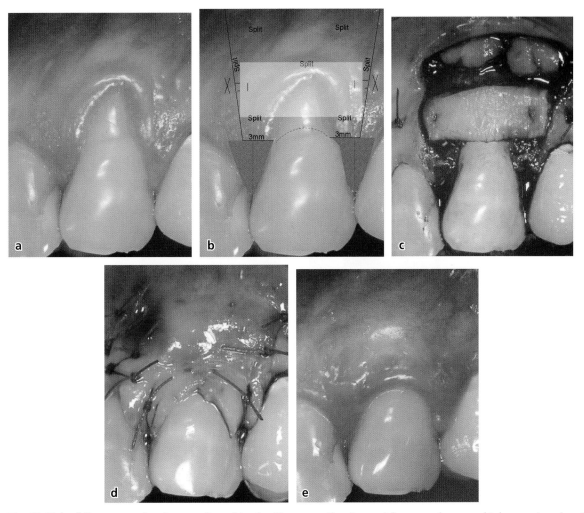

Fig. 44-47 (a–d) Free connective tissue graft combined with a coronally advanced flap procedure – multiple recessions (see the text for explanation). (e) The 1-year post-treatment result.

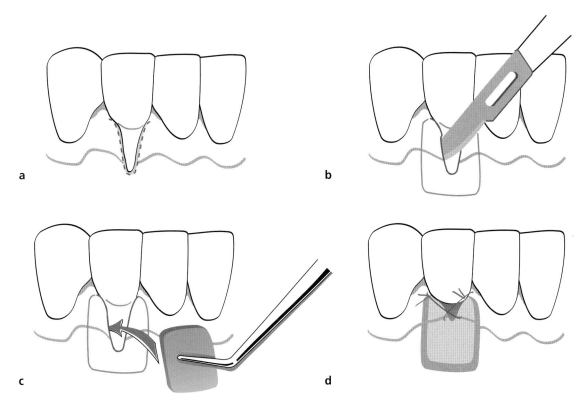

Fig. 44-48 Free connective tissue graft procedure – the "envelope technique". Schematic drawings illustrating the surgical technique (see the text for explanation).

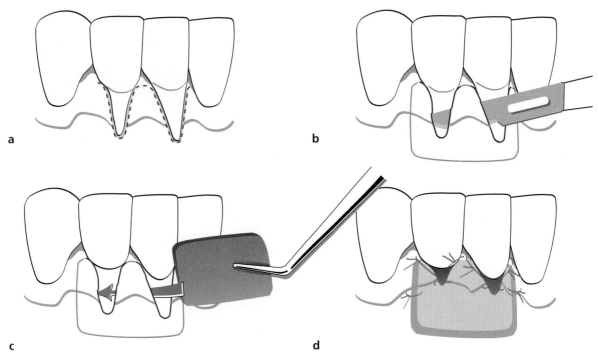

Fig. 44-49 Free connective tissue graft procedure – the "tunnel technique". Schematic drawings illustrating the surgical technique (see the text for explanation).

Table 44-1 Summary of the data available in the literature on the amount of root coverage obtainable with various procedures (Miller class I–II defects)

Root coverage procedure	No. of studies	No. of patients/teeth	Root coverage	
			Mean % of initial recession	Range
Rotational flaps	10	222/235	68	41–74
Coronally advanced flap	17	315/527	79	55–99
Guided tissue regeneration	35	589/695	75	48–94
Enamel matrix proteins	10	207/219	86	72–94
Free connective tissue graft	33	683/890	86	53–98
Epithelialized free soft tissue graft	16	335/491	63	11–87

to advance the mucosal flap coronally over the exposed portions of the connective tissue graft. Pressure is applied for 5 minutes to closely adapt the graft to the root surface and covering soft tissue. Application of a periodontal dressing is often not required.

Clinical outcome of root coverage procedures

Independent of the modality of surgical procedure used to obtain soft tissue root coverage, shallow residual probing depths, gain in clinical attachment, and an increase in gingival height are the common characteristics of treatment outcome. Although the major indication for performing root coverage procedures is esthetic/cosmetic demands by the patient, few studies have included assessments of esthetics as an end-point of success. Instead, the common outcome variables used are the amount of root coverage achieved, expressed in percentage of the initial depth of the recession defect, and the proportion of treated sites showing complete root coverage.

Root coverage

An overall comparison of the treatment outcome of various root coverage procedures is hampered by the fact that comparatively few studies have presented well documented clinical data and that there is substantial heterogeneity between studies (Roccuzzo *et al.* 2002; Oates *et al.* 2003). A summary with regard to the average amount of initial Miller class I–II recession defects that was successfully covered following treatment, based on the data published in a systematic review by Pagliaro *et al.* (2003) and relevant data from studies published between 2003 and 2006 (Table 44-1), shows that an average of 63–86% root coverage may be expected. However, the variability in the treatment outcome for the various procedures, both within and between studies, is large. This indicates that the procedures are operator sensitive and/or that various factors influencing the treatment outcome have not been adequately considered.

Complete coverage of the recession defect is the ultimate goal of the therapy. Table 44-2 summarizes

Table 44-2 Summary of the data available in the literature on the predictability of complete root coverage following the use of various procedures (Miller class I–II defects)

Root coverage procedure	No. of studies	No. of patients/teeth	Complete root coverage	
			Mean % of teeth	Range
Rotational flaps	1	30/30	43	–
Coronally advanced flap	15	287/499	48	9–95
Guided tissue regeneration	24	357/453	36	0–75
Enamel matrix proteins	7	138/150	72	53–90
Free connective tissue graft	26	549/732	61	0–93
Epithelialized free soft tissue graft	10	253/380	28	0–90

data on the predictability of this event with the use of the various surgical procedures. The average percentage of complete root coverage following pedicle or free graft procedures varies between 28 and 72%, with large variability between studies irrespective of surgical procedure used. According to the systematic reviews by Roccuzzo *et al.* (2002) and Oates *et al.* (2003), coronally advanced flaps with connective tissue grafts result in significantly greater root coverage compared to guided tissue regeneration. The lower mean predictability of complete root coverage achieved with the GTR procedure has been associated with the problem of membrane exposure during healing (Trombelli *et al.* 1995), but whether a bioabsorbable or a non-biodegradable barrier membrane is used does not seem to affect the treatment outcome (Roccuzzo *et al.* 1996).

Factors influencing the degree of root coverage

Patient-related factors. As with other surgical periodontal treatment procedures, poor oral hygiene is a factor that will negatively influence the success of root coverage procedures (Caffesse *et al.* 1987). Further, the predominant causative factor in the development of gingival recession is toothbrushing trauma, and hence this factor has to be corrected to secure an optimal outcome of any root coverage procedure. Treatment outcome in terms of root coverage is usually less favorable in smokers than in non-smokers (Trombelli & Scabbia 1997; Zucchelli *et al.* 1998; Martins *et al.* 2004; Erley *et al.* 2006; Silva *et al.* 2006), although some studies showed no differences (Tolmie *et al.* 1991; Harris 1994).

Site related factors. Among site-specific factors, the level of interdental periodontal support may be of greatest significance for the outcome of root coverage procedures. From a biological point of view complete root coverage is achievable in class I–II recession defects (Fig. 44-50), while when loss of connective tissue attachment also involves proximal tooth sites (class III–IV recession defects), only partial facial root coverage is obtainable (Miller 1985b) (Fig. 44-51).

An additional factor shown to influence the degree of attainable root coverage is the dimensions of the recession defect. Less favorable treatment outcome has been reported at sites with wide (>3 mm) and

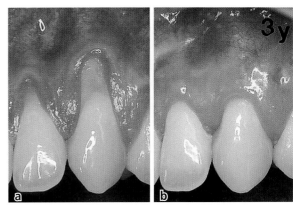

Fig. 44-50 (a) Buccal recession defects but no loss of periodontal support at proximal surfaces. Complete root coverage can be achieved. (b) 3-year follow-up.

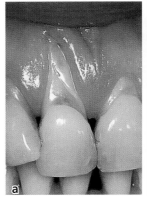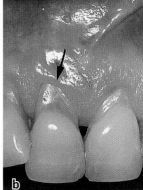

Fig. 44-51 (a) A deep buccal recession at tooth 11. The tooth has loss of support at proximal sites (Miller class III) and complete root coverage is not achievable. Also neighboring teeth show recessions at all tooth surfaces. (b) 2-year healing result following attempted root coverage at the facial aspect of tooth 11. The coronal position of the soft tissue margin is defined by the extension of proximal loss of periodontal support.

deep (≥5 mm) recessions (Holbrook & Ochsenbein 1983; Pini Prato *et al.* 1992; Trombelli *et al.* 1995). In a study comparing the treatment effect of coronally advanced flap and free connective tissue graft procedures, Wennström and Zucchelli (1996) reported that complete root coverage was observed in only 50% of the defects with an initial depth of ≥5 mm compared to 96% in shallower defects. Pini Prato *et al.* (1992) suggested, based on clinical observations in a controlled clinical trial, that a more favorable result with respect to root coverage might be obtained with the GTR procedure in sites with deep (≥5 mm) recession defects as compared to the coronally advanced flap. At the 18-month examination the average coverage was 77% with and 66% without the inclusion of a membrane barrier. However, data presented from recent systematic reviews and meta-analyses (Roccuzzo *et al.* 2002; Oates *et al.* 2003) showing that the predictability of root coverage is significantly reduced with the use of barrier membranes, limit the justification of using the GTR procedure in the treatment of recession defects. The pre-treatment gingival height apical to the recession defect is not correlated to the amount of root coverage obtained (Romanos *et al.* 1993; Harris 1994).

Technique-related factors. Several technique-related factors may influence the treatment outcome of a pedicle graft procedure. In a systematic review including data from 15 studies (Hwang & Wang 2006) a positive correlation was demonstrated between the thickness of the tissue flap and recession reduction. For complete root coverage the critical threshold thickness was found to be about 1 mm. However, whether a full- or split-thickness pedicle graft is used for root coverage may not influence the treatment outcome (Espinel & Caffesse 1981).

Elimination of flap tension is considered an important factor for the outcome of the coronally advanced flap procedure. Pini Prato *et al.* (2000a) measured the tension in coronally advanced flaps to compare the amount of root coverage in sites with and without residual flap tension. At sites that had residual tension (mean 6.5 g) the root coverage amounted to 78% 3 months post-surgically and 18% of the treated sites showed complete root coverage. Sites without tension demonstrated mean root coverage of 87% and complete root coverage in 45% of the cases. Furthermore, a statistically significant negative association was shown between the magnitude of residual tension in the flap and the amount of recession reduction.

Although the connective tissue areas lateral to the recession defect are considered important for the retention of the advanced flap when positioned over the root surface, the dimension of the interdental papilla is not a prognostic factor for the clinical outcome of the root coverage procedure (Saletta *et al.* 2001). As can be expected, the position of the gingival margin relative to the CEJ after suturing affects the probability of complete root coverage following healing. Pini Prato *et al.* (2005) demonstrated that for 100% predictability of complete root coverage in the treatment of Miller class I recessions with a coronally advanced flap procedure the flap margin has to be positioned at least 2 mm coronal to the CEJ.

With regard to free graft procedures, the thickness of the graft is a factor influencing the success of treatment procedure (Borghetti & Gardella 1990).

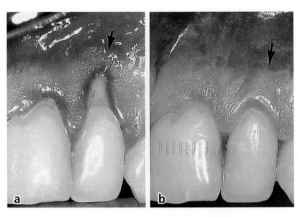

Fig. 44-52 Increased dimension of keratinized tissue 1 year following root coverage with a coronally advanced flap procedure. Before (a) and 1-year post-operatively (b). Arrows indicate the position of the mucogingival line.

A thickness of the free graft of about 2 mm is recommended.

Increased gingival height

An increased apico-coronal height of the gingiva is found following all procedures in which pedicle grafts of adjacent gingiva or free grafts from the palate have been placed over the recession defect. It is interesting to note, however, that an increased gingival height is also a common finding following a coronally advanced flap procedure only involving the existing gingiva apical to the recession (Fig. 44-52). This finding may be explained by several events taking place during the healing and maturation of the marginal tissue. Granulation tissue formation derived from the periodontal ligament tissue will form a connective tissue similar to the one of gingiva and with the potential to induce keratinization of the covering epithelium (Karring *et al.* 1971). A second factor to consider is the tendency of the mucogingival line to regain its "genetically" defined position following its coronal "dislocation" with the coronally advanced flap procedure used to achieve root coverage. Support for the concept that the mucogingival line will regain its original position over time is generated from a study by Ainamo *et al.* (1992). The authors performed an apically repositioned flap procedure in the lower anterior tooth region, which resulted in a 3 mm apical displacement of the mucogingival line. Re-examination after 18 years showed no differences in position of the mucogingival line between sites treated with the apically repositioned flap and contralateral control sites treated with a procedure not interfering with the mucogingival line, indicating that the mucogingival line had regained its original position.

Soft tissue healing against the covered root surface

Treatment of gingival recessions by pedicle grafts or free grafts may be clinically successful, but does the treatment result in a healing characterized by the formation of a connective tissue attachment or an epithelial attachment? Independent of the quality of attachment formed, however, root coverage procedures evidently rarely result in the formation of a deep periodontal pocket.

Healing of pedicle soft tissue grafts

In the areas surrounding the recession defect, i.e. where the recipient bed consists of bone covered by connective tissue, the pattern of healing is similar to that observed following a traditional flap operation. Cells and blood vessels from the recipient bed as well as from the tissue graft invade the fibrin layer, which gradually becomes replaced by connective tissue. After 1 week a fibrous reunion is already established between the graft and the underlying tissue.

Healing in the area where the pedicle graft is in contact with the denuded root surface was studied by Wilderman and Wentz (1965) in dogs. According to these authors the healing process can be divided into four different stages (Fig. 44-53):

1. *The adaptation stage (from 0–4 days).* The laterally repositioned flap is separated from the exposed root surface by a thin fibrin layer. The epithelium covering the transplanted tissue flap starts to proliferate and reaches contact with the tooth surface at the coronal edge of the flap after a few days.

2. *The proliferation stage (from 4–21 days).* In the early phase of this stage the fibrin layer between the root surface and the flap is invaded by connective tissue proliferating from the subsurface of the flap. In contrast to areas where healing occurs between two connective tissue surfaces, growth of connective tissue into the fibrin layer can only take place from one surface. After 6–10 days a layer of fibroblasts is seen in apposition to the root surface. These cells are believed to differentiate into cementoblasts at a later stage of healing. At the end of the proliferation stage, thin collagen fibers are formed adjacent to the root surface, but a fibrous union between the connective tissue and the root has not been observed. From the coronal edge of the wound, epithelium proliferates apically along the root surface. According to Wilderman and Wentz (1965), the apical proliferation of epithelium may stop within the coronal half of the defect although further downgrowth of epithelium was also frequently observed.

3. *The attachment stage (from 27–28 days).* During this stage of healing thin collagen fibers become inserted in a layer of new cementum formed at

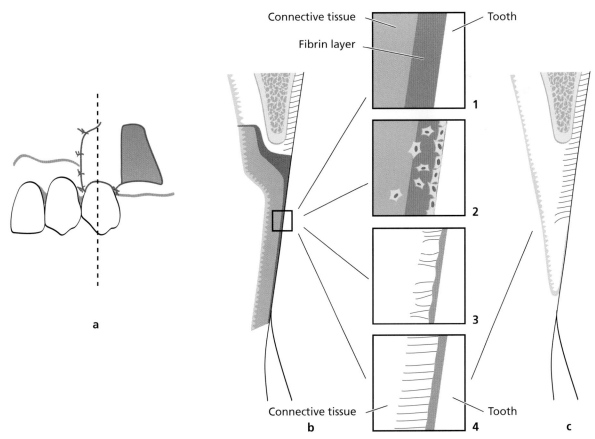

Fig. 44-53 (a) Schematic drawing illustrating healing following treatment of a localized soft tissue recession with a pedicle graft. (b) Cross section through the area immediately after operation. The framed areas (1–4) illustrate the four stages into which the healing process can be divided. (c) Area after healing. Approximately 50% of the successfully covered defect may show new connective tissue attachment.

the root surface in the apical portion of the recession.

4. *The maturation stage.* This last stage of healing is characterized by continuous formation of collagen fibers. After 2–3 months bundles of collagen fibers insert into the cementum layer on the curetted root surface in the apical portion of the recession.

Results of experimental studies in monkeys and dogs on the healing characteristics of the periodontal wound have been interpreted to indicate that gingival connective tissue lacks the ability to form a new connective tissue attachment to the root, but may induce root resorption (see Chapter 25). This finding is of particular interest when considering the rationale for the treatment of recession defects by free or pedicle soft tissue grafts. Since, in these surgical procedures, gingival connective tissue is placed in contact with a denuded root surface, root resorption should be expected to occur. The reason why it is not a common complication following this type of treatment can be explained by two possible events. Either cells from the periodontal ligament form a fibrous attachment to the root surface or epithelial cells proliferate apically, forming a root-protective barrier (long junctional epithelium) towards the gingival connective tissue.

Histologic studies on whether it is the one or the other type of attachment that results following treatment of recessions with pedicle grafts indicate that new connective tissue attachment may be formed in part of the defect. In the study by Wilderman and Wentz (1965) a connective tissue attachment of around 2 mm and an epithelial attachment of the same height had formed in the soft tissue covered portion of the defect, i.e. about 50% of the successfully covered defect showed new connective tissue attachment. Gottlow *et al.* (1986) examined the result of healing following treatment of experimentally produced recession type defects with a coronally advanced flap in dogs (Fig. 44-54). The histologic analysis after 3 months of healing disclosed that, on average, 20% of the apico-coronal length of the original defect had been exposed due to recession during healing (i.e. about 80% root coverage was achieved), 40% was covered by epithelium and 40% demonstrated connective tissue attachment with cementum formation (Fig. 44-55). Determining factors for the type of healing result were the size and the shape of the defect. The possibility of achieving a new connective tissue attachment in the apical portion of the defect seemed to be considerably better in narrow recession defects than in wider ones, most likely because the periodontal ligament at the lateral parts of the defect will serve as a source of granulation

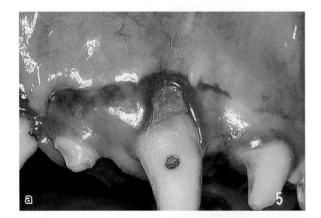
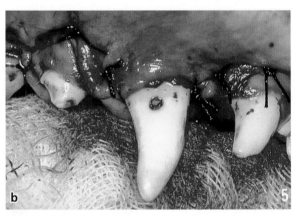
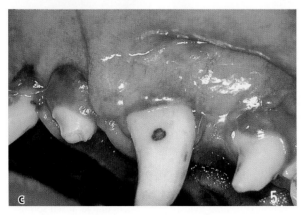

Fig. 44-54 Clinical photographs illustrating the treatment of an experimentally induced localized recession defect in a dog with a coronally displaced flap. (a) Presurgical appearance of the localized recession defect. (b) The site following flap closure of the defect and (c) following 3 months of healing.

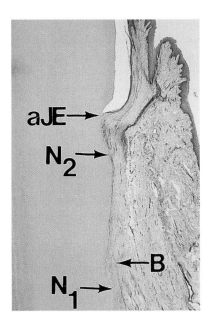

Fig. 44-55 Microphotograph of the healing following a coronally displaced flap in the dog as illustrated in Fig. 44-54. A new connective tissue attachment is formed and extends coronally from the apical border of the notch prepared at the bottom of the bone dehiscence (N_1) to the apical termination of the epithelium (aJE) located within the notch indicating the presurgical level of the soft tissue margin (N_2). B = alveolar bone crest.

tissue from which a new connective tissue attachment can develop.

Healing following pedicle graft procedures has also been histologically studied in monkeys (Caffesse *et al.* 1984; Gottlow *et al.* 1990), and in these studies 38–44% of the successfully covered recession defects demonstrated formation of new connective tissue attachment. The study by Gottlow *et al.* (1990) also showed that the use of a GTR membrane between the root surface and the pedicle graft generated significantly more new connective tissue attachment (79% of the covered part of the recession defect). A significantly increased amount of cementum formation with inserting collagen fibers was also demonstrated following the utilization of enamel matrix proteins in combination with a coronally advanced flap for treatment of experimentally produced recession defects in dogs (Sallum *et al.* 2004).

Some case reports with human block sections provide further evidence that new connective tissue attachment may be formed following pedicle graft procedures. Histologic evaluation of two teeth treated with a laterally positioned flap revealed that connective tissue attachment was re-established in the apical quarter of the successfully covered portion of the root (Sugarman 1969). Cortellini *et al.* (1993) examined histologically a tooth treated with the GTR procedure and showed that connective tissue faced 74% of the length of the recession defect. New cementum with inserting collagen fibers, i.e. new connective tissue attachment, covered 48% of the distance between the apical border of the root instrumentation and the soft

tissue margin. In addition, histomorphometric assessments of a tooth treated with enamel matrix proteins revealed that new cementum covered 73% of the original defect (Heijl 1997).

Healing of free soft tissue grafts

Survival of a free soft tissue graft placed over a denuded root surface depends on diffusion of plasma and subsequent revascularization from those parts of the graft that are resting on the connective tissue bed surrounding the dehiscence. The establishment of collateral circulation from adjacent vascular borders of the bed allows the healing phenomenon of "bridging" (Sullivan & Atkins 1968a). Hence, the amount of tissue that can be maintained over the root surface is limited by the size of the avascular area (Oliver *et al.* 1968; Sullivan & Atkins 1968). Other factors considered critical for the survival of the tissue graft placed over the root surface are that a sufficient vascular bed is prepared around the dehiscence and that a thick graft is used (Miller 1985b).

Another healing phenomenon frequently observed following free graft procedures is "creeping attachment", i.e. coronal migration of the soft tissue margin. This occurs as consequence of tissue maturation during a period of about 1 year post treatment.

There are few histologic evaluations of the nature of the attachment established to the root surface following the use of free grafts for root coverage. Sugarman (1969) reported from a histologic evaluation of a human tooth treated with a free soft tissue graft that new connective tissue attachment was found in the apical quarter of the successfully covered recession defect. Harris (1999) and Majzoub *et al.* (2001), each reporting the histologic outcome of free connective tissue grafts in two cases, found only minimal amounts of new cementum formation in the most apical part of the recession defect and that healing resulted in a long junctional epithelium occupying the interface between the covering soft tissue and the root. Carnio *et al.* (2002) performed histologic evaluation of four cases of root coverage with a connective tissue graft combined with application of enamel matrix proteins (Emdogain®). They reported that the healing resulted in connective tissue adhesion to the root surface and that the formation of new cementum was observed only in the most apical end of the grafted area.

Thus, the limited histologic information available from humans on the healing of free soft tissue grafts indicates that a healing pattern similar to the one discussed above following pedicle graft procedures may result, namely that connective tissue attachment may be established in the most apical and lateral parts of the recession defect, but that an epithelial attachment is formed along the major portion of the root. Further, the application of enamel matrix proteins may prevent the apical migration of the epithelium but may not favor the formation of a true connective tissue attachment between the free graft and the root surface.

Interdental papilla reconstruction

There may be several reasons for loss of papilla height and the establishment of "black triangles" between teeth. The most common reason in the adult individual is loss of periodontal support due to plaque-associated lesions. However, abnormal tooth shape, improper contours of prosthetic restorations, and traumatic oral hygiene procedures may also negatively influence the outline of the interdental soft tissues.

Nordland and Tarnow (1998) proposed a classification system regarding the papillary height adjacent to natural teeth, based on three anatomic landmarks: the interdental contact point, the apical extent of the facial CEJ, and the coronal extent of the proximal CEJ (Fig. 44-56):

- *Normal*: the interdental papilla occupies the entire embrasure space apical to the interdental contact point/area.
- *Class I*: the tip of the interdental papilla is located between the interdental contact point and the level of the CEJ on the proximal surface of the tooth.
- *Class II*: the tip of the interdental papilla is located at or apical to the level of the CEJ on the proximal surface of the tooth but coronal to the level of the CEJ mid-buccally.
- *Class III*: the tip of the interdental papilla is located at or apical to the level of the CEJ mid-buccally.

In an observational study in humans, Tarnow *et al.* (1992) analyzed the correlation between the presence of interproximal papillae and the vertical distance between the contact point and the interproximal bone crest. When the vertical distance from the contact point to the crest of bone was 5 mm or less, the papilla was present almost 100% of the time, whereas if the distance was 6 mm or more only partial papilla fill of the embrasure between the teeth was most commonly found. Considering that a supracrestal connective tissue attachment zone of approximately 1 mm is normally found (Gargiulo 1961), the observation indicates that the biologic height of the interdental papilla may be limited to about 4 mm. This interpretation is supported by the observation that in interdental areas denuded following an apically repositioned flap procedure, an up-growth of around 4 mm of soft tissue had taken place 3 years after surgery (Van der Velden 1982). Hence, before attempts are made to surgically reconstruct an interdental papilla, it is important to carefully assess both (1) the vertical distance between the bone crest and the apical point of the contact area between the crowns and (2) the soft tissue height in the interdental area. If the distance bone crest–contact point is ≤5 mm and the papilla height is less than 4 mm, surgical intervention for increasing the volume of the papilla could be justified in order to solve the problem of an interdental "black triangle". However, if the contact point is located >5 mm from the bone crest, because of loss of periodontal support and/or an inappropriate interdental contact relationship between the crowns, means to lengthen the contact

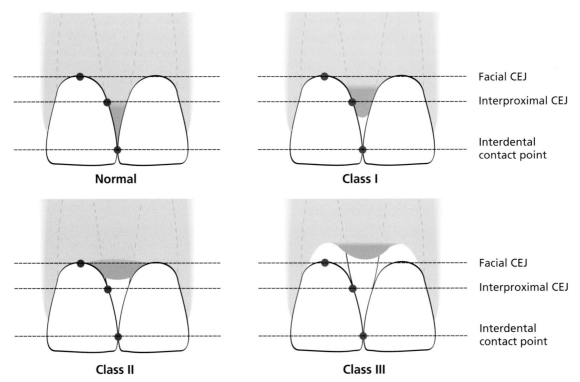

Normal

Class I

Facial CEJ

Interproximal CEJ

Interdental contact point

Class II

Class III

Facial CEJ

Interproximal CEJ

Interdental contact point

Fig. 44-56 Schematic drawing illustrating the classification system for papilla height (Nordland & Tarnow 1998).

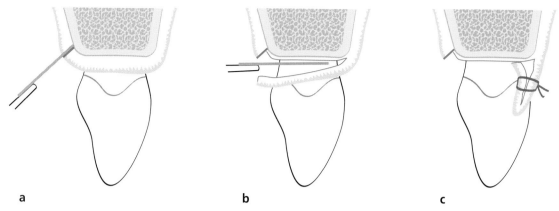

a   b   c

Fig. 44-57 Papilla reconstruction – pedicle graft technique. Schematic drawings illustrating the surgical technique (see the text for explanation).

area apically between the teeth should be selected rather than a surgical attempt to improve the topography of the papilla.

If loss of papilla height is only caused by soft tissue damage from oral hygiene devices, interproximal hygiene procedures must be initially discontinued to allow soft tissue recovery and then successively modified in order to eliminate/minimize traumatic injury to the papillae.

Surgical techniques

Several case reports have been published regarding surgical techniques for reconstruction of deficient papillae (e.g. Beagle 1992; Han & Takei 1996; Azzi et al. 1999). However, the predictability of the various procedures has not been documented and no data are available in the literature providing information on the long-term stability of surgically regained interdental papillae.

Beagle (1992) described a pedicle graft procedure utilizing the soft tissues palatal to the interdental area (Fig. 44-57). A split-thickness flap is dissected on the palatal aspect of the interdental area. The flap is elevated labially, folded, and sutured to create the new papilla at the facial part of the interdental area. A periodontal dressing is applied on the palatal aspect only, in order to support the papilla.

Han and Takei (1996) proposed an approach for papilla reconstruction ("semilunar coronally repositioned papilla") based on the use of a free connective tissue graft (Fig. 44-58). A semilunar incision is placed in the alveolar mucosa facial to the interdental area and a pouch-like preparation is performed into the interdental area. Intrasulcular incisions are made around the mesial and distal half of the two adjacent teeth to free the connective tissue from the root surfaces to allow coronal displacement of the gingival–papillary unit. A connective tissue graft, taken from the palate, is placed into the pouch to support the coronally positioned interdental tissue.

Azzi et al. (1999) described a technique in which an envelope-type flap is prepared for coverage of a connective tissue graft (Fig. 44-59). An intrasulcular

incision is made at the tooth surfaces facing the interdental area to be reconstructed. Subsequently, an incision is placed across the facial aspect of the interdental area and an envelope-type split-thickness flap is elevated into the proximal site as well as apically to a level beyond the mucogingival line. A connective tissue graft is harvested from the tuberosity area, trimmed to adequate size and shape, and placed under the flaps in the interdental papilla area. The flaps are brought together and sutured with the connective tissue graft underneath.

Crown-lengthening procedures

Excessive gingival display

In most patients, the lower edge of the upper lip assumes a "gum-wing" profile which limits the amount of gingiva that is exposed when a person smiles. Patients who have a high lip line expose a broad zone of gingival tissue and may often express concern about their "gummy smile" (Fig. 44-60a). The form of the lips and the position of the lips during speech and smiling cannot be easily changed, but the dentist may, if necessary, modify/control the form of the teeth and interdental papillae as well as the position of the gingival margins and the incisal edges of the teeth. In other words, it is possible by a combination of periodontal and prosthetic treatment measures to improve dentofacial esthetics in this category of patient.

As a base for treatment decisions, a careful analysis of the dentofacial structures and how they may affect esthetics should be performed. It should include the following features:

- Facial symmetry
- Interpupillary line; even or uneven
- Smile line: low, median or high
- Dental midline in relation to facial midline
- Gingival display during speech and during broad, relaxed smile
- Harmony of gingival margins

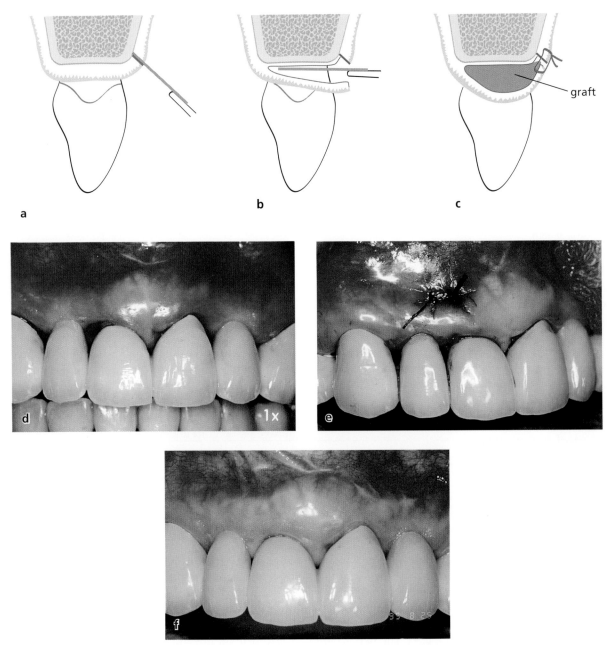

Fig. 44-58 Papilla reconstruction – the "semilunar coronally repositioned papilla" technique. (a–c) Schematic drawings illustrating the surgical technique (see the text for explanation). (d–f) Reconstruction of papillae distal to the central incisors with the use of the semilunar coronally repositioned papilla technique in a patient with a fixed bridge reconstruction.

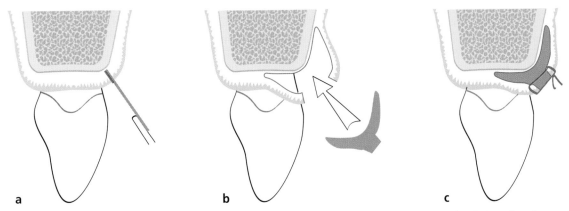

Fig. 44-59 Papilla reconstruction – "envelope" technique. Schematic drawings illustrating the surgical technique (see the text for explanation).

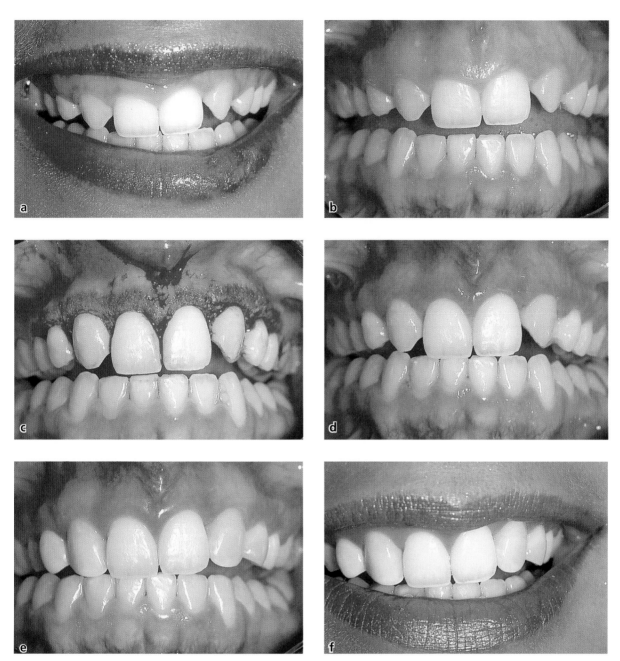

Fig. 44-60 Crown-lengthening procedure. (a,b) Pretreatment views. The clinical crowns are considerably shorter than the anatomic crowns. The lateral incisors were congenitally missing and orthodontic treatment had been carried out to move the posterior teeth anteriorly. The canine teeth in the position of the lateral incisors added to the esthetic disharmony. (c) A gingivectomy was performed to expose the anatomic crowns of the teeth. (d) One month post surgery. At this appointment, the canine and first premolar teeth were reshaped and bonded. (e) Tooth form and proportional balance were improved by bonding. (f) At 3 years post-treatment, the gingival tissues exhibited no rebound and retained the architectural form sculpted into the tissue at the time of the surgical procedure.

- Location of gingival margins in relation to the CEJs
- Tooth size and proportions/harmony
- Incisal plane/occlusal plane.

If excessive gingival exposure is due to insufficient length of the clinical crowns, a crown-lengthening procedure is indicated to reduce the amount of gingiva exposed, which in turn will favorably alter the shape and form of the anterior teeth. To select the proper treatment approach for crown lengthening,

an analysis of the individual case with regard to crown–root–alveolar bone relationships should also be included.

In the young adult with an intact periodontium the gingival margin normally resides about 1 mm coronal to the CEJ. However, some patients may have a height of free gingiva that is greater than 1 mm, resulting in an disproportional appearance of the clinical crown. If such a patient complains about their "small front teeth" and the periodontium is of a thin biotype, full exposure of the anatomic crown

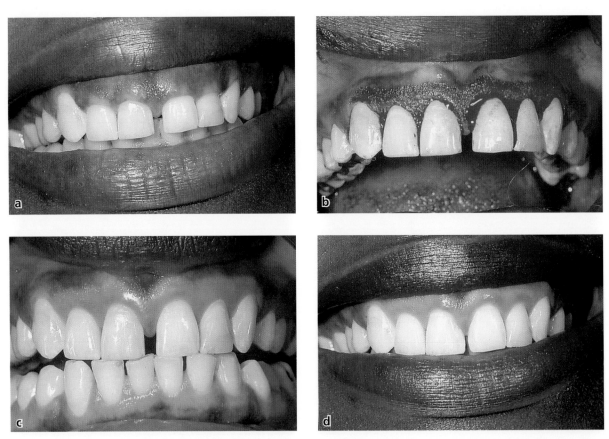

Fig. 44-61 (a) Pretreatment view. The patient disliked her "small front teeth" and diastema. Radiographs and probing indicated the gingival tissues were covering the cervical one third of the crowns. Crestal bone was thin and in normal relationship to the cemento-enamel junctions. The patient preferred "pink gums" if she could possibly have them. (b) A long externally beveled path of incision was used to accomplish the gingivectomy. (c) This view shows the color changes and pleasing architecture produced in the anterior gingiva at 2 months post surgery. The diastema was partially closed by direct bonding at this time. (d) Post-treatment view showing the enhancement of esthetic values for the patient.

can be accomplished by a gingivectomy/gingivoplasty procedure (Fig. 44-60).

An assessment should also be made regarding the amount and pattern of pigmentation existing within the gingival tissues, and the patient's desire to maintain or lessen the pigmentation contained within the tissues. The externally beveled path of incision that is usually employed in a gingivectomy procedure will remove the pigmentation and produce pink gingival tissue upon initial healing (Fig. 44-61). The surgically induced color change in the tissues comes about rapidly and markedly affects esthetic values. For this reason, an externally beveled gingivectomy procedure should not be terminated at the midline in patients that have pigmented gingival tissues. It should be extended across the midline to the premolar area to avoid a color mismatch in the esthetic zone of the anterior teeth. The color change may be permanent or the pigmentation may slowly return over a period of a year or more. Patients should be informed of the changes in tissue color that will occur and be allowed to make a choice as to the color of the tissue they will have post-surgically. If they wish to maintain their pigmentation, an internally beveled path of incision (internal gingivectomy) should be employed (Fig. 44-62).

If the periodontium is of the thick biotype and there is a bony ledge at the osseous crest, an apically positioned flap procedure (see Chapter 38) should be performed. This will allow for osseous recontouring (Fig. 44-63).

More extensive bone recontouring is required to solve esthetic problems found in patients who do indeed have short anatomic crowns in the anterior section of the dentition. In this category of patients, prosthetic measures must be used after resective periodontal therapy to increase the apico-coronal dimension of the crowns (Fig. 44-64). Patients who are candidates for this kind of resective therapy can be divided into two categories:

1. Subjects who have normal occlusal relationships and incisal guidance. In this category the incisal line of the front teeth must remain unaltered but the clinical crowns can be made longer by surgically exposing root structure and by locating the cervical margins of the restorations apical to the CEJ (Fig. 44-64).
2. Subjects who have abnormal occlusal relationships with excessive interocclusal space in the posterior dentition when the anterior teeth are in edge-to-edge contact. In this category of patients

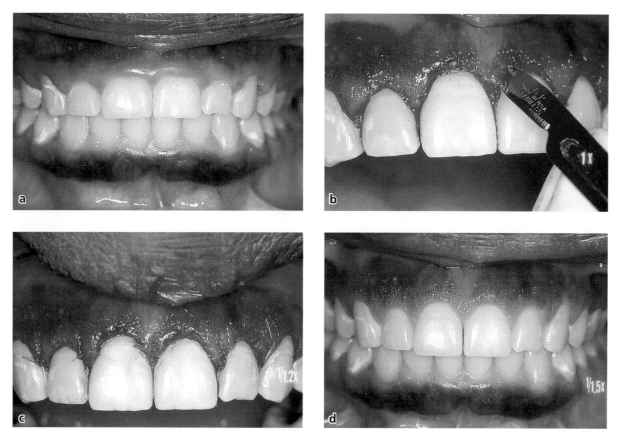

Fig. 44-62 (a) Pretreatment view. This patient disliked the looks of her "small front teeth"; she sought consultation to have her teeth made longer by crowning them. Probing and radiographs revealed normal osseous morphology and a wide zone of attached gingiva that covered the cervical one third of the incisors. It was explained to the patient that a surgical solution was preferred to restorative procedures to make her teeth longer. The patient made a request that the color of her gingival tissues remain unchanged. (b) An internally beveled path of incision was use to effect an "internal gingivectomy" to maintain the pigmentation in the tissues. This created mini flaps in the areas of the papillae. (c) 5-0 gut sutures were used to stabilize the papillae. (d). The crown lengthening that was achieved with maintenance of color harmony can be seen in this view at 3 months post surgery. (Courtesy of Dr. E. Saacks, Pennsylvania, USA.)

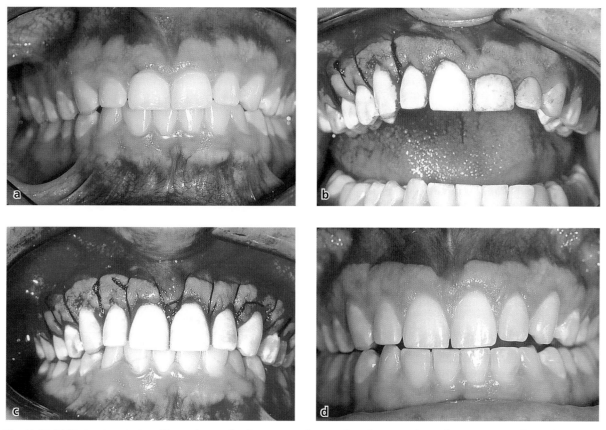

Fig. 44-63 (a) Pretreatment view. The patient, a dentist, requested crown lengthening to lessen his "gummy smile" and give him a more masculine appearance. The patient had a wide zone of attached gingiva and thick crestal bone. Palpation indicated bony exostoses. (b) An apically positioned flap and osseous resective surgery, from second premolar to second premolar, were used to lengthen the teeth. The surgery was confined to the labial surfaces. This view shows one half of the surgery completed. (c) Vertical mattress sutures were utilized to hold the flap apically. (d) Three years post-treatment. Note that the gingival tissues retain the morphology created at the time of surgery.

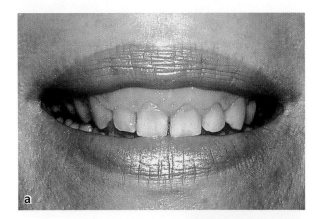
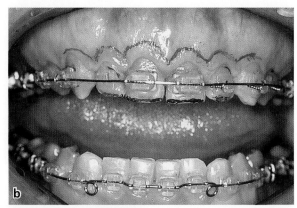
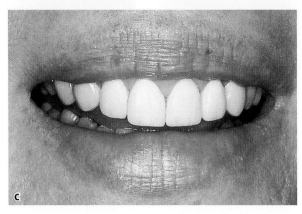

Fig. 44-64 Crown lengthening by surgical and prosthetic procedures. (a) Pretreatment view. The patient displayed "short front teeth" and a broad exposure of gum tissue. The full anatomic crown is exposed in this case and the surgically induced recession will expose root structure. (b) The patient had an unusually wide zone of attached gingiva. The gingival margins were positioned apically by making an internally beveled flap with a submarginal entrance incision as outlined in red ink. The crest of the bone was reduced in height. (c) After the tissues had matured following surgery, individual crowns were prepared for each of the anterior teeth. Crown lengthening was achieved and the patient no longer exposed a broad expanse of gum tissue. (Courtesy of Dr. D. Garber, Atlanta, GA, USA.)

the length of the maxillary front teeth can be reduced without inducing posterior occlusal interferences. In addition, the marginal gingiva can be resected or relocated to an apical position before crown restorations are made.

In some individuals with an excessive display of gingiva, the size and shape of the teeth and the location of the gingival margins may be perfectly normal. The excessive display of gingiva in these cases is often caused by vertical maxillary excess and a long mid-face (Fig. 44-65). Periodontal crown lengthening procedures will not suffice to solve their problems, but rather the maxilla must be altered by a major maxillofacial surgical procedure. The risk–benefit and cost–benefit ratios must be thoroughly evaluated before recommending this type of surgical therapy to correct esthetic problems.

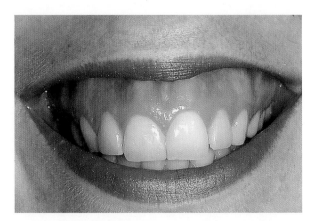

Fig. 44-65 This patient displays a large expanse of gingival tissue when smiling or speaking. The patient has a long mid-face and vertical maxillary excess. The gingival margins reside 1 mm coronal to the cemento-enamel junction and the anatomic and clinical crowns are approximately equal.

Exposure of sound tooth structure

Crown-lengthening procedures may be required to solve problems such as (1) inadequate amount of tooth structure for proper restorative therapy, (2) subgingival location of fracture lines, and (3) subgin-gival location of carious lesions. The techniques used to accomplish crown lengthening include (1) apically positioned flap procedure including bone resection and (2) forced tooth eruption with or without fiberotomy.

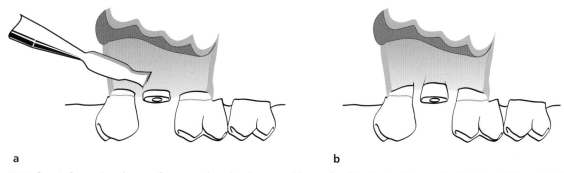

a   b

Fig. 44-66 Surgical resective therapy for crown lengthening cannot be confined to the tooth in need of treatment. The principles of osseous resection require that bone be removed from the adjacent teeth to create a gradual rise and fall in the profile of the osseous crest. This causes a loss of attachment apparatus and recession of the adjacent teeth as well.

Apically positioned flap with bone recontouring

The apically positioned flap technique with bone recontouring (resection) may be used to expose sound tooth structure. As a general rule, at least 4 mm of sound tooth structure must be exposed at the time of surgery. During healing the supracrestal soft tissues will proliferate coronally to cover 2–3 mm of the root (Herrero *et al.* 1995; Pontoriero & Carnevale 2001; Lanning *et al.* 2003), thereby leaving only 1–2 mm of supragingivally located sound tooth structure. When this technique is used for crown lengthening it must also be realized that gingival tissues have an inherent tendency to bridge abrupt changes in the contour of the bone crest. Thus, in order to retain the gingival margin at its new and more apical position, bone recontouring must be performed not only at the problem tooth but also at the adjacent teeth to gradually reduce the osseous profile (Fig. 44-66). Consequently, substantial amounts of attachment may have to be sacrificed when crown lengthening is accomplished with an apically positioned flap technique. It is also important to remember that, for esthetic reasons, symmetry of tooth length must be maintained between the right and left sides of the dental arch. This may, in some situations, call for the inclusion of even more teeth in the surgical procedure.

- *Indication:* crown lengthening of multiple teeth in a quadrant or sextant of the dentition.
- *Contraindication:* surgical crown lengthening of single teeth in the esthetic zone (Fig. 44-67).
- *Technique:* The apically positioned flap technique and methods used for bone recontouring are discussed in Chapter 38.

Forced tooth eruption

Orthodontic tooth movement can be used to erupt teeth in adults (Reitan 1967; Ingber 1974, 1976; Potashnick *et al.* 1982). If moderate eruptive forces are used, the entire attachment apparatus will move in

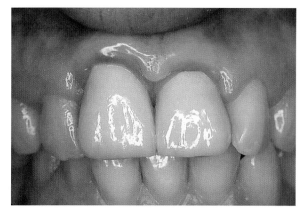

Fig. 44-67 A deformity which interfered with dentofacial esthetics was created at the right central incisor by using a surgical crown lengthening procedure at one single tooth to expose sound tooth structure. The soft tissues cannot follow the abrupt and steep changes in the osseous profile. The crown preparation invaded the zone of normal supracrestal connective tissue. This created a chronic periodontal pocket and adversely affected esthetics. (Courtesy of Dr. A. Winnick, Toronto, Canada.)

unison with the tooth. The tooth must be extruded a distance equal to or slightly longer than the portion of sound tooth structure that will be exposed in the subsequent surgical treatment. After the tooth has reached the intended position and has been stabilized, a full-thickness flap is elevated and bone recontouring is performed to expose sound root structure. For esthetic reasons it is important that the bone and soft tissue levels at adjacent teeth remain unchanged.

Forced tooth eruption can also be used to level and align gingival margins and the crowns of teeth to obtain esthetic harmony. Instead of using surgical procedures to position the gingival margins of unaffected normal teeth apically to the level of a tooth with recession or orthodontic malalignment, the tooth that is malpositioned or has sustained recession is erupted to the level of the normally positioned teeth. The entire attachment apparatus and dentogingival junction will follow the root of the tooth as it is moved coronally (Fig. 44-68).

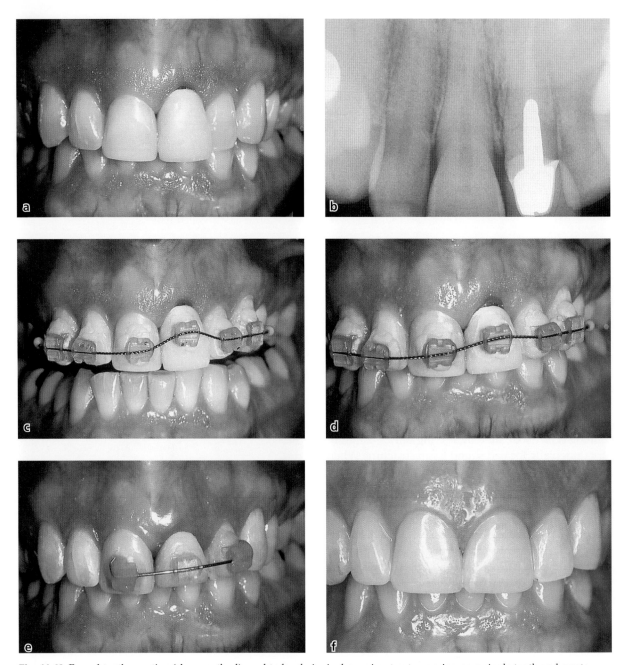

Fig. 44-68 Forced tooth eruption (show method) used to level gingival margins, treat recession on a single tooth and create esthetic harmony. (a,b) Recession on the left central incisor exposed the root surface darkened from root canal treatment. The uneven gingival margins and dark root surface detracted from an otherwise attractive smile. (c) A nitol wire with an offset bracket was used to slowly extrude the incisor. (d) Occlusal adjustment was done on the lingual side of the crown to create room for the tooth to erupt. This view, at 1 month in tooth movement, shows the gingival tissues moving with the root of the tooth. (e) Sufficient eruption had occurred by 3 months to level the gingival margins. The orthodontic brackets were used for temporary stabilization and a new crown was prepared. (f) The new crown masked the show-through of the dark root. The even gingival margins and beautiful crown created esthetic harmony. (Courtesy of Dr. J. Ingber, Philadelphia, PA, USA.)

- *Indication:* crown lengthening at sites where removal of attachment and bone from adjacent teeth must be avoided. The forced eruption technique can also be used as a means of reducing pocket depth at sites with angular bony defects (Brown 1973; Ingber 1974, 1976). The angular bony defect at the problem tooth can be reduced while the attachment level at the adjacent tooth surface remains unchanged (Fig. 44-69).
- *Contraindication:* the forced eruption technique requires the use of fixed orthodontic appliances.

Thus, in patients who only have a few teeth remaining, an alternative approach for crown lengthening has to be selected.
- *Technique:* orthodontic brackets are bonded to the problem tooth and to adjacent teeth and are combined with an arch wire. Another type of mechanical system can be utilized by placing a heavy gauge bar or wire in grooves prepared in the adjacent teeth and over the problem tooth. A power elastic is tied from the bracket to the arch wire (or the bar), which pulls the tooth coronally. If most of the

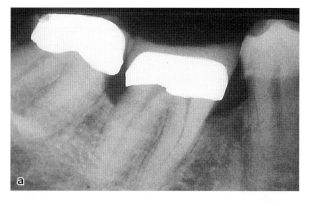
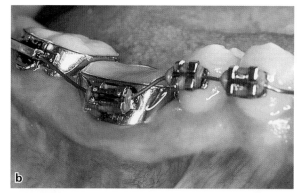
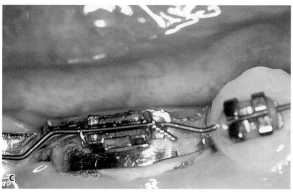
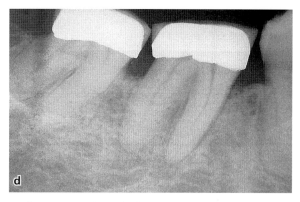

Fig. 44-69 Slow tooth eruption procedure used to level cemento-enamel junctions and angular bone crests. (a) Pretreatment radiograph. (b) A nitol wire was used to erupt the molar. (c) The crown was shortened over a period of 4 months by selective grinding. (d) Radiograph taken 8 months after the start of treatment. The angular bone defects were leveled.

crown structure is lost, root canal therapy is required. A post placed in the root canal is fitted with a power elastic, which is also joined with the arch wire. The direction of the tooth movement must be carefully checked to ensure that the problem tooth is not tilted or moved toward the adjacent tooth surfaces.

Forced tooth eruption with fiberotomy

If fiberotomy is performed during the forced tooth eruption procedure the crestal bone and the gingival margin are retained at their pre-treatment locations, and the tooth–gingiva interface at adjacent teeth is unaltered. Fiberotomy is performed by the use of a scalpel at 7–10-day intervals during the forced eruption to sever the supracrestal connective tissue fibers, thereby preventing the crestal bone from following the root in coronal direction. In the case presented in Fig. 44-70, fiberotomy was performed only at the mesial half of the root. Radiographs obtained after 9 weeks demonstrate that crestal bone migration has occurred at the distal but not at the mesial surface of the erupted tooth (Pontoriero *et al.* 1987).

- *Indication:* crown lengthening at sites where it is important to maintain the location of the gingival margin at adjacent teeth unchanged.
- *Contraindication:* fiberotomy should not be used at teeth associated with angular bone defects.

- *Technique:* similar to the technique described for the forced tooth eruption procedure. Fiberotomy is performed once every 7–10 days during the phase of forced tooth eruption.

Ectopic tooth eruption

Surgical intervention is often indicated for teeth erupting ectopically, i.e. with an eruption position facial to the alveolar ridge (Fig. 44-71). To create a satisfactory width of the gingiva for the permanent tooth, the tissue entrapped between the erupting tooth and the deciduous tooth is usually utilized as donor tissue (Agudio *et al.* 1985; Pini Prato *et al.* 2000b).

Three different techniques have been described for the interceptive mucogingival treatment of buccally erupting teeth, depending on the distance from the donor site (entrapped gingiva) to the recipient site (area located facially–apically to the erupting permanent tooth) (Agudio *et al.* 1985; Pini Prato *et al.* 2000b):

- *Double pedicle graft* (Fig. 44-72). This flap procedure is indicated when the permanent tooth erupts within the zone of keratinized tissue but close to the mucogingival junction. An intrasulcular incision is performed at the deciduous tooth and extended laterally to the gingival crevice of the adjacent teeth and apically to the erupting

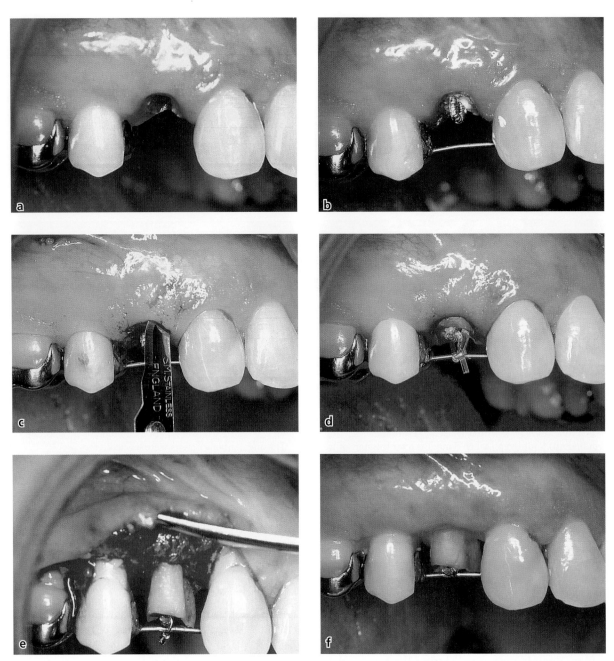

Fig. 44-70 Rapid tooth eruption procedure in conjunction with fiberotomy procedure. (a) Buccal view, the fracture on the first premolar extended subgingivally. (b) Soft tooth structure was excavated and a twisted wire with an occlusal hook was temporarily cemented in the root canal. A bar was placed into the amalgam restoration on the premolar and bonded to the lingual surface of the canine. (c,d) Sulcular fiber resection was performed at the mesial half of the tooth to the level of the bone crest. The distal half remained as a control surface. The fiber resection was repeated once a week during the 3-week eruption phase. (e) The tooth was stabilized for 6 weeks, and at that time a full-thickness flap was raised. The bone crest had a "positive" angulation at the distal surface and remained unchanged at the "test" mesial surface. Osseous resection was used to level the bony septum on the distal surface. (f) Ample crown lengthening was obtained and the gingival margins healed to their former shape and location. (g) Pretreatment radiograph enlarged to show the normal shape of the crests of the interdental septae. (h) Enlargement of the post-eruption radiograph (3 weeks of rapid eruption and 6 weeks of stabilization) to show the "positive" angular crest on the "control" distal side and the unchanged crest on the mesial "test" side. (Courtesy of Dr. R. Pontoriero, Milan, Italy.)

permanent tooth. By mobilization of the flap apical to the mucogingival line, the entrapped gingiva can be elevated and transposed for positioning apically to the erupting tooth. Sutures may be placed to secure the position of the gingival tissue facial to the erupting tooth.

• *Apically positioned flap* (Fig. 44-73). When the permanent tooth is erupting apical to the mucogingival junction, vertical releasing incisions have to be placed to allow for apical positioning of the keratinized tissue. Two lateral releasing incisions are made and extended apically beyond the mucogin-

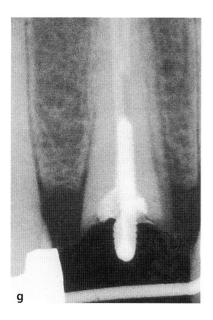

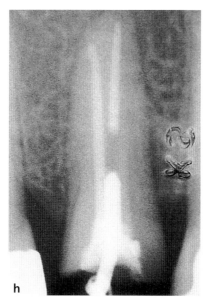

g

h

Fig. 44-70 *Continued*

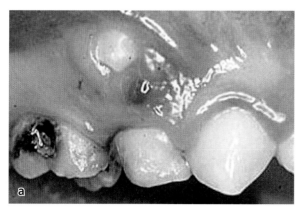

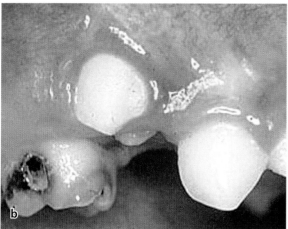

Fig. 44-71 Ectopic tooth eruption. The permanent tooth is erupting close to the mucogingival junction.

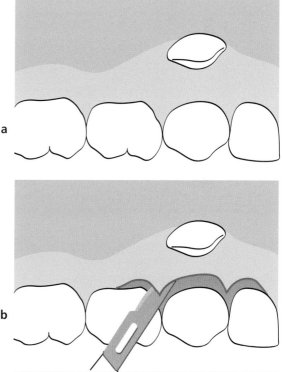

a

b

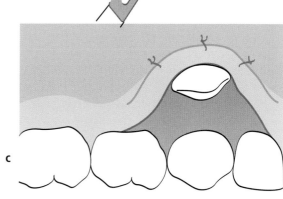

c

Fig. 44-72 Ectopically erupting tooth – double pedicle graft. Schematic drawings illustrating the surgical technique (see text for explanation).

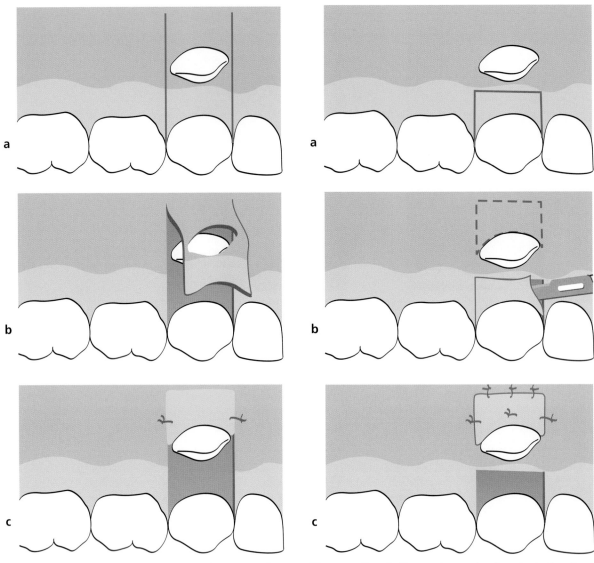

Fig. 44-73 Ectopically erupting tooth – apically positioned flap. Schematic drawings illustrating the surgical technique (see text for explanation).

Fig. 44-74 Ectopically erupting tooth – free gingival graft. Schematic drawings illustrating the surgical technique (see text for explanation).

gival junction. An intrasulcular incision is performed at the deciduous tooth and a partial-thickness flap is elevated beyond the ectopically erupting tooth. The mobilized gingival flap is moved apical to the erupting tooth and secured in position by sutures.

- *Free gingival graft* (Fig. 44-74). If the tooth is erupting within the alveolar mucosa distant to the mucogingival junction, a free gingival graft procedure may be selected. The entrapped gingiva is removed by a split incision and used as an epithelialized connective tissue graft. The free gingival graft is placed at a prepared recipient site facial/apical of the erupting tooth. Careful suturing is performed to secure close adaptation of the graft to the underlying connective tissue bed.

All the described procedures have been proven to be effective in establishing a facial zone of gingiva

following the alignment of teeth erupting in an ectopic position (Pino Prato *et al.* 2000b,c).

The deformed edentulous ridge

A partially edentulous ridge may retain the general shape of the alveolar process. Such a ridge is traditionally referred to as a normal ridge. Even though this normal ridge has retained the bucco-lingual and apico-coronal dimensions of the alveolar process, it is not normal in many other respects; the eminences that existed in the bone over the roots are no longer present, and the interdental papillae are missing.

The smooth contours of the normal ridge create problems for the restorative dentist. In a fixed bridge the pontics (1) frequently give the impression that they rest on the top of the ridge rather than emerge from within the alveolar process, (2) lack a root eminence, and (3) lack marginal gingivae and interdental papillae. Dark triangles, which almost always interfere with dentofacial esthetics, are present in the embrasure area between the pontics and between the abutments and the pontics. In other words, in the presence of a normal ridge it may be difficult or impossible to produce a fixed prosthesis which truly restores the esthetics and function of the natural dentition.

Prevention of soft tissue collapse following tooth extraction

Following extraction of a tooth, the topography of the surrounding soft and hard tissues will be altered. The soft tissue margin will collapse and the height of the adjacent papillae will be reduced. This soft tissue collapse may be prevented by immediate post-extraction placement of an ovate pontic to support the soft tissues. Figure 44-75 illustrates such a situation where

a central incisor had to be extracted due to root fracture. With the immediate placement of the pontic the facial soft tissue margin and the papillae were maintained almost unchanged following the healing of the extraction site. Also, in situations where several adjacent teeth have to be extracted, insertion of ovate pontics may facilitate the preservation of the outline of the soft tissue ridge (Fig. 44-76).

Prevention of ridge collapse due to alveolar bone resorption following tooth extractions must also be considered. Borghetti and Laborde (1996) recommended means for prevention of bone ridge collapse after tooth extraction in any case of:

1. Fracture of the vestibular osseous plate during tooth extraction or due to trauma
2. Resorption of the vestibular osseous plate
3. Presence of a thin vestibular bone plate.

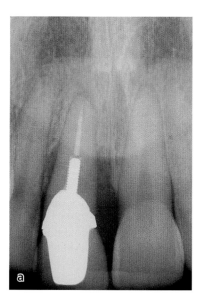

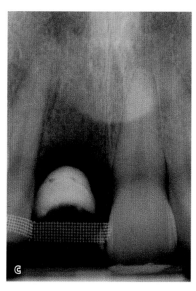

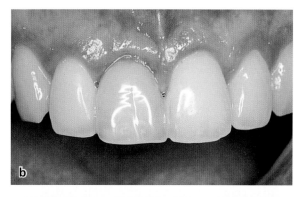

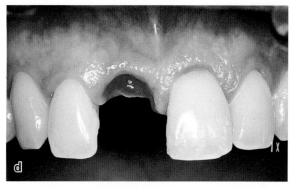

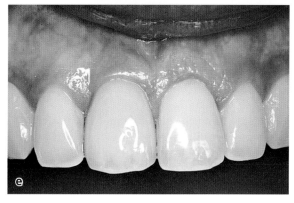

Fig. 44-75 (a) A central incisor that cannot be maintained because of root fracture which also caused pronounced periodontal destruction. (b) Immediately following tooth extraction, an ovate pontic was inserted to support the facial and proximal soft tissues. (c,d) Radiographic and clinical view of the area 6 weeks after tooth extraction. (e) Follow-up 1 year after the placement of permanent prosthetic reconstruction (single implant).

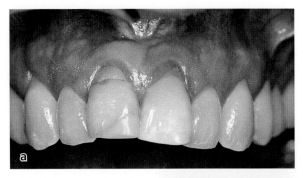
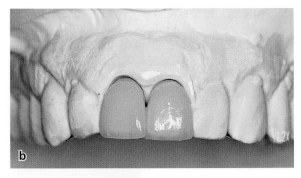
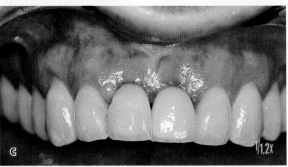

Fig. 44-76 (a) A 26-year-old female patient who had a trauma against the maxillary central incisors. Due to root fracture and endodontic complications both central incisors had to be extracted. (b) A Rochette bridge with ovate pontics was fabricated as a temporary replacement for the incisors. (c) Clinical view if the front tooth region 8 weeks after tooth extraction and placement of the resin bonded temporary bridge.

Among procedures proposed for prevention of ridge collapse in conjunction with tooth extractions are (1) flap elevation for complete soft tissue closure of the extraction sites (Borghetti & Glise 2000), (2) placement of connective tissue grafts over the extraction sites (Nevins & Mellonig 1998), (3) placement of bone grafts (Becker *et al.* 1994), and (4) utilization of barrier membranes (Lekovic *et al.* 1997). Procedures for preservation of the bone dimensions following tooth extraction are discussed in Chapter 49.

Correction of ridge defects by the use of soft tissue grafts

A deformed ridge may result from tooth extractions, advanced periodontal disease, abscess formations, etc. The deformity that exists in the ridge is directly related to the volume of root structure and associated bone that is missing or has been destroyed. According to Siebert (1983) ridge defects can be divided into three classes:

- Class I: loss of bucco-lingual width but normal apico-coronal height
- Class II: loss of apico-coronal height but normal bucco-lingual width
- Class III: a combination of loss of both height and width of the ridge.

Ridge augmentation procedures should be preceded by careful surgical–prosthetic treatment planning with joint consultations involving the surgeon and the restorative dentist in order to attain an optimal esthetic result. The following factors should be determined prior to the initiation of therapy:

- Volume of tissue required to eliminate the ridge deformity
- Type of graft procedure to be used
- Timing of various treatment procedures
- Design of the provisional restoration
- Potential problems with tissue discolorations and matching tissue color.

Ideally, a provisional restoration should be made prior to surgery. The shape of the teeth in the provisional restoration, the axial inclination and emergence profile of the teeth, and embrasure form should be an exact prototype of the final prosthesis that is to be constructed. It is the task of clinician performing the surgery to augment the tissues to meet the provisional prosthesis in the most exact manner possible. If a gingival flange of pink-colored acrylic is used around single or multiple pontics on a temporary removable partial denture, the flange must be cut away in order to avoid pressure on the graft and give the tissues room to swell during the immediate post-surgical phase of healing. The soft tissue at the surgically treated recipient site for a graft will undergo considerable swelling during the early phase of healing and the tissues will conform to the tissue-facing surfaces of the bridge or partial denture. The prosthesis is thus used to help in shaping the outline of the augmented ridge to the desired form. The location and shape of interproximal embrasure areas in the provisional bridge will determine where the "papillae" created in the ridge will be located.

Surgical procedures for ridge augmentation

Numerous surgical graft and implant procedures attempting to reconstruct a partially edentulous ridge or ridge defect have been described in the literature over the years. The procedures may be grouped according to the means used for ridge augmentation as (1) soft tissue augmentation procedures and (2) hard tissue augmentation procedures. In this chapter only soft tissue augmentation procedures will be addressed, while hard tissue augmentation procedures are covered in Chapter 49. To illustrate various approaches for utilization of soft tissues for ridge augmentation, the following procedures will be discussed:

- Pedicle graft procedure:
  - Roll flap procedure
- Free graft procedures:
  - Pouch graft procedure
  - Interpositional graft procedure
  - Onlay graft procedure.

Studer *et al.* (1997) proposed the use of the pedicle graft procedure for correction of a single-tooth ridge defect with minor horizontal and vertical loss, whereas submerged free connective tissue graft procedures should be selected for larger defects. The onlay full-thickness graft procedure is indicated pri-marily for ridge augmentation in the presence of additional mucogingival problems such as insuffi-cient gingival width, high frenum, gingival scarring, or tattoo. These recommendations were based on short-term evaluation of the obtained volumetric increase of the edentulous ridge following various augmentation procedures, which demonstrated superior results with the use of submerged connec-tive tissue grafts compared to the use of full-thickness grafts (Studer *et al.* 2000).

The "roll flap procedure"

Surgical concept
The "roll flap procedure" (Abrams 1980) involves the preparation of a de-epithelialized connective tissue pedicle graft, which is subsequently placed in a sub-epithelial pouch (Fig. 44-77). This procedure is used in the treatment of small to moderate class I ridge defects, primarily in cases with a single-tooth space. The technique enables the surgeon to augment tissue apically and labially to the cervical area of a pontic and to give the recipient site the appearance of a normal tooth–gingiva interface. Hence, a bucco-lingual ridge concavity can be converted into a ridge convexity resembling the eminence produced by the roots of the adjacent teeth (Fig. 44-78).

Technique
A rectangular pedicle of connective tissue is prepared on the palatal side of the defect (Fig. 44-77). The length of the pedicle must match the amount of

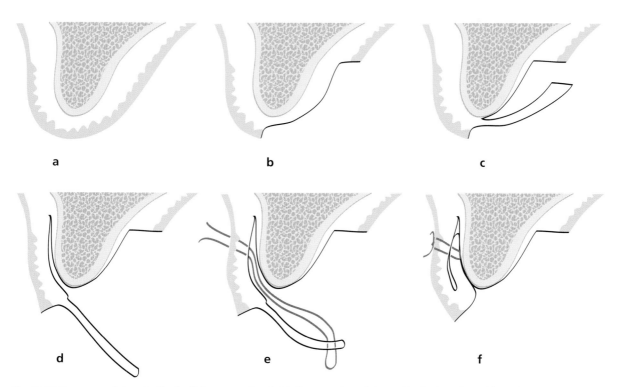

Fig. 44-77 Sequence of steps in the "roll flap procedure". (a) Cross section of the residual edentulous ridge prior to treatment. (b) The removal of the epithelium. (c) The elevation of the pedicle. (d) The pouch is created. (e) Sutures are placed at the mucogingival junction to catch the tip of the pedicle flap and pull it into place in the pouch. (f) The flap is secured. A convexity in the ridge was created.

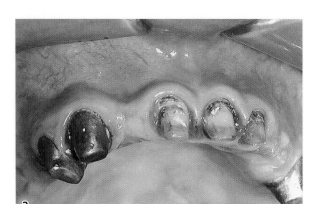
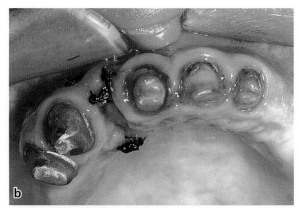
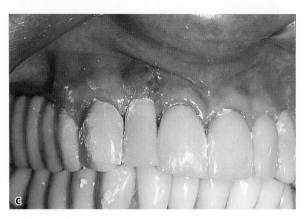
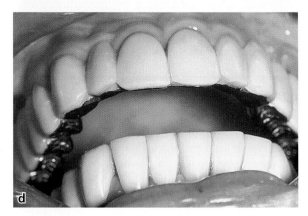

Fig. 44-78 "Roll flap procedure". (a) Pretreatment view of a class I ridge defect in the area of the right lateral incisor. Note the marked concavity in the ridge. (b) This view shows the surgical site 1 week after surgery and prior to the removal of the sutures. (c) The tissue surface of the pontic was relined with autopolymerizing resin. (d) Final prosthesis in place. Note the illusion of a root eminence and a free gingival margin apical to the lateral incisor pontic tooth. (Courtesy of Dr. L. Abrams, Philadelphia, PA, USA.)

apico-coronal augmentation that is planned. This, in turn, is related to the amount of root eminence that exists on either side of the defect. If a two- or three-tooth pontic space is treated with the roll technique, two or three separate pedicles are raised. Each of these pedicles will form a new "root–cervical margin".

The epithelium on the palatal surface of the donor site is first removed. A maximum amount of supraperiosteal connective tissue is raised from the palate using sharp dissection. The void that is produced at the donor site will gradually fill in with granulation tissue. Caution must be exercised in dissection of the pedicle flap so that tissue perforation is avoided when the plane of dissection approaches the facial (labial) surface. A pouch is made in the supraperiosteal connective tissue at the facial (labial) surface of the ridge. In order to preserve as much connective tissue and blood supply as possible at the recipient site, the dissection must be made as close as possible to the periosteum of the facial bone.

The pedicle is tucked into the pouch as a try-in procedure. Adjustment of pedicle size should now be made. Once the pedicle fits as desired, it is made ready for the stabilizing suture. The suturing scheme is illustrated in Fig. 44-77. The suture must be posi-tioned close to the mucobuccal fold. This enables the surgeon to pull the pedicle to the apical portion of the pouch. The suture should not be tied tightly, since it only serves as a positioning and stabilizing device. The use of a resorbable suture material is recommended.

Adjustment of pontic contours
Measures used to adapt the tissue surface of the pontic to the contour of the surgically treated ridge are common to all soft tissue ridge augmentation procedures in patients with fixed bridgework. A light contact is maintained between the pedicle graft and the tissue surface of the pontics. The post-operative swelling will cause the tissue to conform to the shape of the pontic. This enables the clinician to shape the soft tissue into a form that is intended for the aug-mented site. Autopolymerizing resin is added to the tissue surface of the pontics and is allowed to cure until the resin reaches a dough-like state. The bridge is then seated and pressed into the grafted site. When the resin has set to a firm consistency, the bridge is removed and placed in hot water to complete the process of polymerization (Fig. 44-78). The tissue surface of the pontics and the embrasure areas are then carved to the shape that is intended for the final bridge. The surface of the pontic is polished and the

bridge put in place using appropriate temporary cement.

Post-operative care

A periodontal dressing is placed over the donor site. No dressing should be placed over the facial (labial) surface of the grafted area where swelling will occur. The dressing at the donor site should be changed at weekly intervals and maintained until wound healing has progressed to a point where the tissue is no longer tender to touch.

Pouch graft procedures

Surgical concept

A subepithelial pouch is prepared in the area of the ridge deformity, into which a free graft of connective tissue is placed and molded to create the desired contour of the ridge. The entrance incision and the plane of dissection may be made in different ways (Kaldahl *et al.* 1982; Seibert 1983; Allen *et al.* 1985; Miller 1986; Cohen 1994):

- Coronal–apically: the horizontal incision is made on the palatal or lingual side of the defect and the plane of dissection carried in an apical direction (Fig. 44-79).

- Apical–coronally: the horizontal incision is made high in the vestibule near the mucobuccal fold and the plane of dissection is carried coronally to the crest of the ridge.
- Laterally: one or two vertical entrance incisions are started from either side of the defect (Fig. 44-80). The plane of dissection is made laterally across the span of the deformity.

Indication

The technique is used to correct class I defects. Patients with large-volume defects may have thin palatal tissues, which are insufficient to provide the volume of the donor tissue necessary to fill the deformity. In such cases, various procedures for hard tissue augmentation may be selected (see Chapter 49).

Technique

The pouch is prepared as described above. The mesio-distal entrance incision for the edge of the pouch should be made with a long bevel and must be started well to the palatal (lingual) side of the defect (Fig 44-79). After the pouch has been filled with graft, the facial tissue will be stretched. The long bevel of the entrance incision permits the palatal edge of the flap to slide toward the facial surface

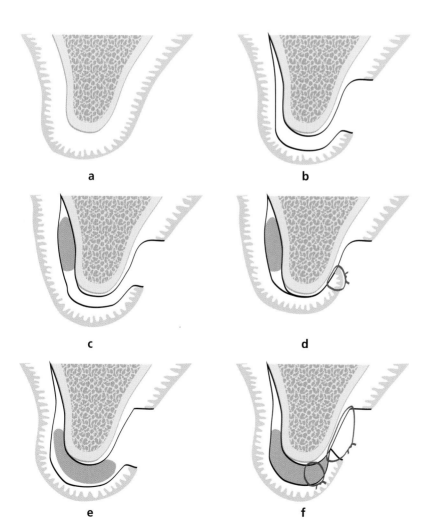

Fig. 44-79 Sequence of steps in the "pouch graft procedure" utilizing a free graft of connective tissue (CT) to expand the ridge. (a) Cross section of the residual edentulous ridge prior to treatment. (b) The horizontal incision to create the pouch is made well to the palatal side of the defect. The incision is started partial-thickness to leave CT to suture to when the flap is closed. The dissection is made supraperiosteal on the labial side of the ridge to (1) ensure an adequate blood supply within the pedicle and (2) permit the flap to expand labially or labially and coronally free of tension. (c,d) The CT graft can be placed as shown for maximal bucco-lingual augmentation. (e,f) If vertical augmentation is desired, the CT implant can be placed closer to the crest of the ridge. As is shown in (d) and (f), the more the flap is stretched or extended to gain augmentation, the more difficult it is to gain primary flap closure.

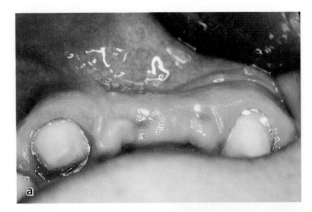
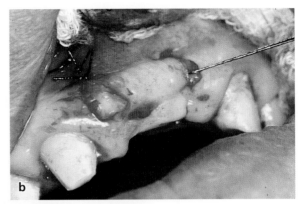
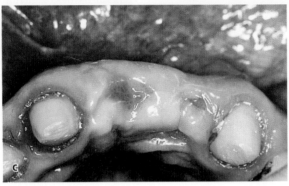

Fig. 44-80 Pouch graft procedure. (a) Pretreatment view of a class I ridge deformity. (b) Placement of the free connective tissue graft in a tunnel prepared by split incision between the two vertical incisions. The graft is brought into position by the use of a suture placed in one end of the free graft. (c) Four months post treatment showing restored facial dimension of the edentulous ridge.

without opening a gap at the incision line. Sometimes vertical releasing incisions have to be made lateral to the border of the defect.

A suitable donor site is selected in the palate, the tuberosity area, or in an edentulous area and a free graft of connective tissue is excised by the use of a "trap-door" approach. The graft is immediately transferred to the recipient site and properly positioned. The palatal entrance incision and the releasing incisions are closed with sutures.

Interpositional graft procedure

Surgical concept

Interpositional grafts are not completely submerged and covered in the manner that a subepithelial connective tissue graft is placed (Fig. 44-81) (Seibert 1991, 1993a,b). Therefore, there is no need to remove the epithelium from the surface of the donor tissue. If augmentation is required not only in the bucco-lingual but also in the apico-coronal direction, a portion of the graft must be positioned above the surface of the tissue surrounding the recipient site (Fig. 44-82). A certain amount of the grafted connective tissue will thus be exposed in the oral cavity.

Indications

Interpositional graft procedures are used to correct class I as well as small and moderate class II defects.

Technique

An envelope flap, or a split-thickness flap with releasing incisions, is prepared at the facial surface of the defect area. The provisional bridge is placed in position to serve as a reference when estimates are made regarding the amount of tissue that has to be grafted to fill the defect. A periodontal probe may be used to measure the length, width and depth of the void of the pouch. A suitable donor site is selected in the palate or the tuberosity area, and a free graft of epithelium–connective tissue is excised (Fig. 44-81).

The donor tissue is transferred to the recipient site and placed in position. If gain in ridge height is not intended, the epithelial surface for the graft is placed flush with the surrounding epithelium. The graft is sutured along its entire circumference to the tissues of the recipient site. The provisional bridge is placed in position and the pontics are trimmed and adjusted as discussed above. No dressing is used to cover the recipient site.

If gain also in ridge height is intended, a certain portion of the graft has to be kept above the surface of the surrounding tissue (Fig. 44-82d). Granulation tissue formed during healing will eventually make the border between the graft and the adjacent tissue smooth and properly epithelialized. The swelling, which occurs post-operatively, will assist in sculpting the contour of the ridge.

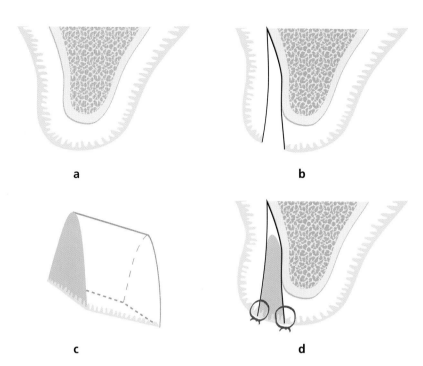

a

b

c

d

Fig. 44-81 Schematic illustrations of the interpositional graft procedure. (a) Cross section of class I ridge defect. (b) A labial flap (partial-thickness dissection preferred) is used to create the pouch. (c) A wedge-shaped graft is removed from the palate. (d) The epithelial surface of the graft is placed flush with the surface of the tissue surrounding the pouch and sutured around its circumference.

Onlay graft procedures

Surgical concept

The onlay procedure was designed to augment ridge defects in the apico-coronal plane, i.e. to gain ridge height (Meltzer 1979; Seibert 1983). Onlay grafts are epithelialized free grafts which, following placement, receive their nutrition from the de-epithelialized connective tissue of the recipient site. The amount of apico-coronal augmentation that can be obtained is related to the initial thickness of the graft, the events of the wound healing process, and the amount of graft tissue that survives (Figs. 44-82, 44-83, 44-84). If necessary, the grafting procedure can be repeated at 2-month intervals to gradually increase the ridge height.

Indications

Onlay graft procedures are used in the treatment of large class II and III defects. They are not suitable in areas where the blood supply at the recipient site has been compromised by scar tissue formation from previous wound healing.

Technique

An attempt must be made to retain as much of the lamina propria of the recipient site as possible. The anesthetic solution should be placed high in the vestibular fornix and in the palate, thus keeping vasoconstriction in the recipient site to a minimum. A scalpel blade is used to remove the epithelium. The scalpel is moved with short, saw-like strokes across the recipient site at a level approximately 1 mm below the outer surface of the epithelium. The least amount of connective tissue possible should be excised. The margins of the recipient site can be prepared with either a butt joint or a beveled margin.

The prepared recipient site should be covered with a surgical gauze moistened with isotonic saline while the donor tissue is dissected (Fig. 44-82g–i).

Selection of donor site

Onlay graft procedures, as well as interpositional graft procedures, require large amounts of donor tissue. As a general rule, the palatal vault region of premolars and first molars, midway between the gingival margin and the midline raphae, is the only area in the maxilla that contains the necessary volume of tissue required to augment large ridge defects. During the presurgical planning phase, the tissue of the palate should be probed with a 30-gauge syringe needle to ensure that an acceptable volume of tissue can be obtained at the time of surgery.

The major palatine artery emerges from the posterior palatine foramen located adjacent to the distal surface of the maxillary second molar, midway between the gingival margin and the midline raphae (Fig. 44-85). The artery passes in an anterior direction close to the surface of the palatal bone. It is important therefore that the second and third molar regions are not used as donor sites for large volume grafts.

Planning in graft preparation

As a rule the graft should be made a few millimeters wider and longer than the dimensions required at the recipient site. The dimensions of the graft are outlined on the palate with the use of a scalpel and light bleeding is provoked to define the surface borders. In order to avoid interference with the palatine artery, the borders of the graft must be planned in such a way that its thinner portions are located high in the palatal vault or in the first molar area. The thicker

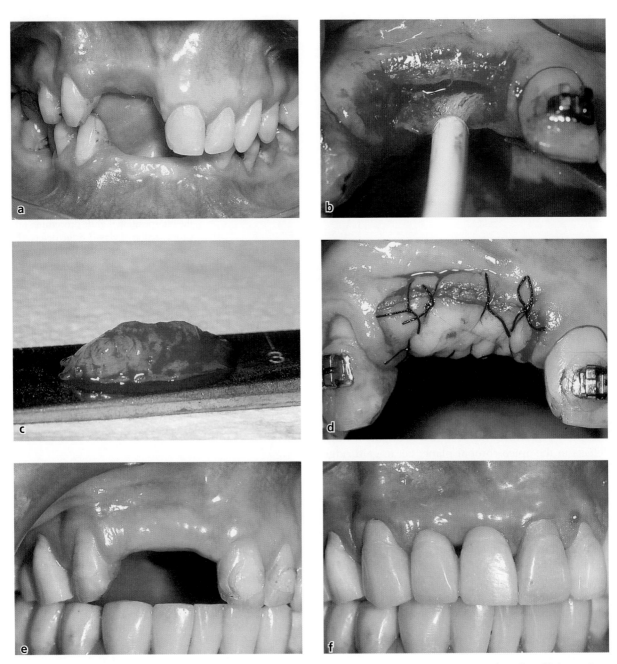

Fig. 44-82 (a) Pretreatment view, class III ridge defect. A two-stage procedure will be used to augment the ridge. (b) A pouch was prepared to receive an interpositional graft. Epithelium was removed from the borders of the recipient site to permit some of the graft to be placed above the level of the surrounding tissue in order to gain apico-coronal augmentation. (c) The wedge-shaped graft was 10 mm thick at its center. (d) The interpositional graft is both displacing the labial surface of the pouch in the labial direction as well as adding height to the ridge. (e) Two months post-treatment. Additional augmentation is needed apico-coronally. (f) A second-stage onlay graft will be used to create a papilla and fill the dark triangle between the pontics. (g) Two months after the first surgical procedure, the ridge was de-epithelialized and cuts were made into the connective tissue prior to placing the second-stage onlay graft into position. (h) The onlay graft was sutured into position. (i) The pontics were adjusted and brought into light contact with the graft. (j) Marked swelling occurred within the graft at 14 days post surgery. (k) Two months following the second surgical procedure, a gingivoplasty was performed to deepen the pontic receptacle sites for the ovate pontics. (l) Post-treatment view 1 year after the final surgical procedure. (Courtesy of Dr. J. Seibert & Dr. P. Malpeso, USA.)

portions should be harvested from the premolar areas.

Dissection of donor tissue

The base of the graft should be V- or U-shaped to match the shape of the defect in the ridge. The different planes of incision prepared in the palate must therefore converge towards an area under the center or toward one edge of the donor site. It is comparatively easy, with the use of a scalpel, to dissect in an antero-posterior or, from an area high in the palate, in a lateral direction towards the teeth. It is, however, difficult to dissect in an anterior direction from the distal edge of the donor site. There is a variety of

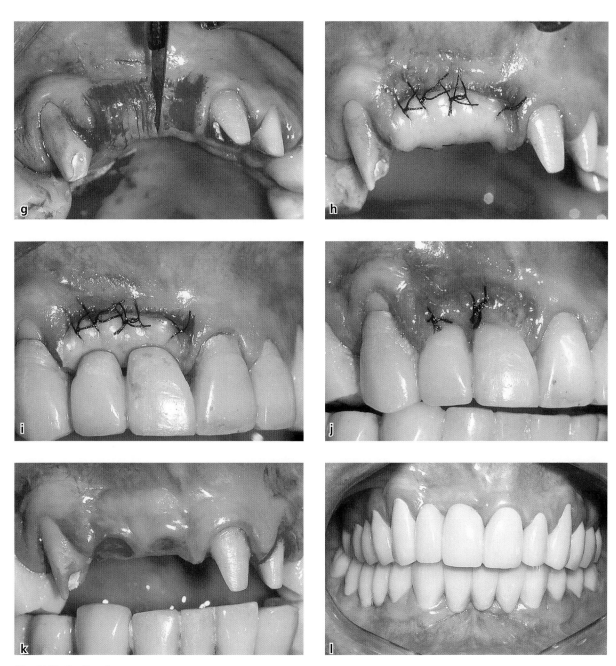

Fig. 44-82 *Continued*

blade holders available which permit the scalpel blade to be positioned at different angles to the holder and which enable the surgeon to cut with a back-action. When the donor tissue has been removed, it must be stored in pieces of surgical gauze moistened in isotonic saline at all times.

Treatment of the donor site
Since it is difficult to anchor and maintain a periodontal dressing at the donor site in the palatal vault, an acrylic stent should be fabricated prior to surgery. The stent should be made with wrought wire clasps on each side to add retention and to aid the patient in removing and inserting the device.

The donor site must be inspected carefully for signs of arterial bleeding. If any small vessel bleeding is observed, a circumferential suture must be placed around the vessel distal to the bleeding point. Immediately thereafter, the void at the donor site should be packed with a suitable hemostatic agent and the edges of the wound be brought closer together with sutures. The stent is then put into position.

Try-in and stabilization of graft
The graft is transferred with tissue forceps to the recipient site for a try-in. The graft is trimmed to the proper shape and adjusted to fit the connective tissue surface of the prepared ridge. A series of parallel cuts may be made deep into the exposed lamina propria of the recipient site to sever large blood vessels (Fig. 44-82g) immediately before suturing. A series of interrupted sutures is placed along the borders of the

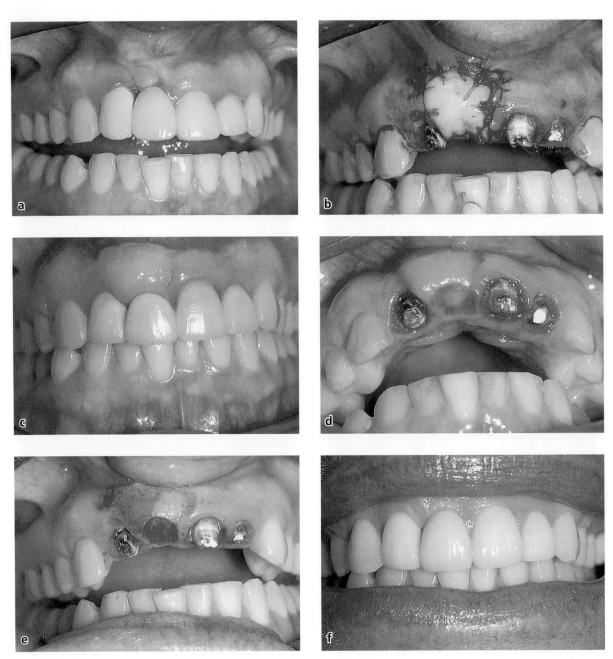

Fig. 44-83 Onlay graft procedure. (a) Pretreatment view. The gingival tissues were distorted from previous attempts at esthetic reconstruction. The patient wished to have a papilla between the right maxillary lateral and central incisor and a natural looking bridge. (b) The pontic area, including the papilla on the mesial of the right lateral incisor, was de-epithelialized and a thick (5 mm) onlay graft was sutured into position. (c) The pontic was shortened at the time of surgery to accommodate the thick graft. At 3 months post surgery the graft had undergone maximum shrinkage and gingivoplasty could now be done. (d) Incisal view at 3 months post surgery. Note the "papilla" that has been created. The indentation in the ridge was naturally created by the tissue swelling against the pontic tooth. (e) Rotary diamond point gingivoplasty was done to reshape the bulky graft to normal contours, deepen the receptacle site for the ovate pontic and level the gingival margins. (f) This view shows the esthetic harmony that was obtained in the soft tissues and tooth form at 2 years post treatment. (Courtesy of Dr. J. Seibert & Dr. C. Williams, USA.)

Fig. 44-84 Onlay graft procedures utilized to augment ridge and create papillae. (a) Pretreatment view. The left lateral incisor was extracted after a traumatic injury. The patient detested the dark triangle on the mesial of the pontic, the poor tooth form in the bridge and the irregular contours in her gingival tissue. (b,c) An onlay graft was used to gain apico-coronal and bucco-lingual ridge augmentation as well as to develop papillae. Note how the graft was extended to the palatal side of the ridge to gain greater blood supply from a larger connective tissue base. (d,e) At 2 months post surgery, a second-stage veneer graft was used to eliminate the surface irregularities on the surface of the gingiva and gain greater bucco-lingual augmentation. (f) At 4 months post second-stage surgery, gingivoplasty was done to prepare the area for an ovate form pontic. (g–h) 1 year post treatment, esthetics have been restored for this patient. (Courtesy of Dr. J. Seibert & Dr. D. Garber, USA.)

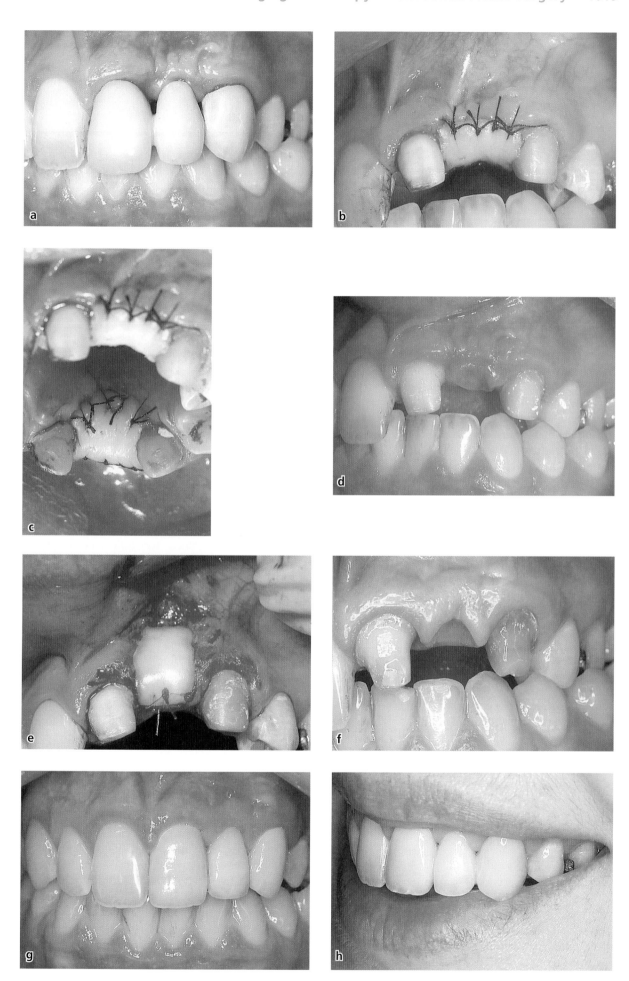

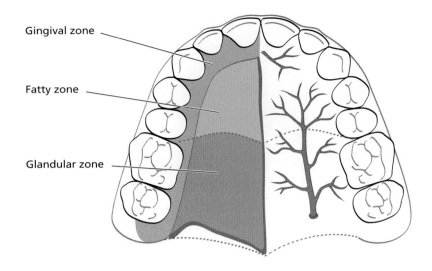

Gingival zone

Fatty zone

Glandular zone

Fig. 44-85 Basic anatomic–histologic zones of the palate. Note the normal location of the greater palatine foramen.

graft. The dental assistant should stabilize the onlay graft against the surface of the recipient site, while the surgeon completes the placement of sutures.

Wound healing in the recipient site

Considerable post-operative swelling often occurs during the first week after pouch and onlay augmentation procedures. The epithelium of the graft will slough to form a white film on the surface of the graft. Patients should rinse two to four times per day with an antimicrobial mouthwash during the first week after surgery and refrain from mechanical cleaning measures in the area until a new epithelial covering has formed over the graft, which will not occur until a functional capillary circulation has been re-established in the graft (4–7 days after the surgery). The grafted tissue will assume a normal color as the epithelium thickens via stratification. Tissue form is usually stable after 3 months, but further shrinkage may occur over a period of several months. Final restorative measures should therefore not be initiated until after 6 months.

Wound healing in the donor site

Granulation tissue will gradually fill the donor site. Initial healing is usually complete within 3–4 weeks after the removal of a 4–5 mm thick graft. Patients should wear the surgical stent for about 2 weeks to protect the healing wound. The palate returns to its presurgical contour after about 3 months.

Combined onlay–interpositional graft procedures

Class III ridge defects pose a major challenge to the clinician since the ridge has to be augmented in both vertical and horizontal dimensions. The combined onlay–interpositional graft procedure (Fig. 44-86 and 44-87) may successfully be used in such a situation (Seibert & Louis 1996). The combined graft procedure may offer the following advantages:

- The submerged connective tissue section of the interpositional graft aids in the revascularization of the onlay section of the graft, thereby gaining a greater percentage of take of the overall graft.
- A smaller post-operative open wound in the palate donor site.
- Faster healing in the palate donor site with less patient discomfort.
- Greater latitude or ability to control the degree of bucco-lingual and apico-coronal augmentation within a single procedure.
- Vestibular depth is not decreased and the muco-gingival junction is not moved coronally, thereby eliminating the need for follow-up corrective procedures.

Refinement of pontic contours and gingivoplasty soft tissue sculpting procedures

It is desirable, when reconstructing defects within a partially edentulous ridge, to moderately over-correct the ridge in the area of the deformity. This will compensate for wound contraction and provide the necessary bulk of tissue within the ridge to sculpt the ridge to its final form. Gingivoplasty techniques using rotary coarse diamond stones in an ultraspeed handpiece with copious water spray are used to smooth out incision lines and perfect the fit and shape of the pontic teeth to the crest of the ridge (Figs. 44-83, 44-87). Adjustments are made to shape the cervical contour and emergence profile of the pontic teeth to match that of the contralateral teeth. The tissue-contacting surfaces of the pontic teeth are immediately rebased with autopolymerizing resin and polished. This final tissue sculpting procedure and reshaping of the provisional prosthesis is minor in nature but aids greatly in defining the shape of the papillae and creating the illusion of the presence of a cuff of free gingiva at the pontic–ridge interface.

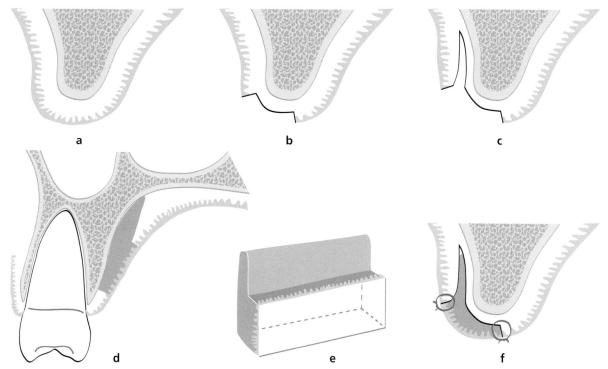

Fig. 44-86 Diagram of the combination onlay-interpositional graft procedure. (a) Cross section of a class III ridge defect. (b) Epithelium is removed on the labial–crestal side of the ridge to prepare the recipient bed for the onlay segment of the graft. (c) Partial-thickness dissection was then used to create a pouch for the interpositional section of the graft. (d) The dissection for the graft is started at right angles to the surface of the palate. The scalpel blade is then angled to remove a long connective tissue segment for the graft. (e) Three-dimensional view of the onlay section of the graft (including epithelium) and the connective tissue segment for buccolingual augmentation. (f) Graft sutured into position. (Reprinted with permission from *The International Journal of Periodontics and Restorative Dentistry*.)

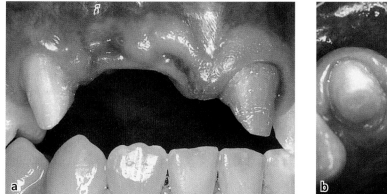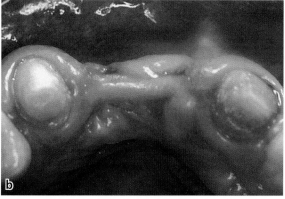

Fig. 44-87 (a,b) The right maxillary lateral and central incisors were lost due to trauma. These views show the horizontal and vertical loss of ridge tissue 10 months after the extractions. (c) A partial-thickness path of incision was extended labially and apically to create a pouch. The amount of space created within the pouch and the degree of relaxation of the flap was then tested with a periosteal elevator. (d) The epithelialized section of the graft can be seen in this view. (e) The premolar area, maxillary right side, was used as a donor area. The area of exposed connective tissue corresponds to the onlay section of the graft. The incisions were extended another 5–7 mm towards the midline on a long bevel to obtain the interpositional segment of the graft. (f) The graft was tucked into the labial pouch and sutured first along its palatal border. The labial flap was then sutured along the epithelial connective border of the graft. The residual labial socket defect in the flap created a soft tissue discontinuity defect along the labial margin of the flap. (g) At 6 weeks post surgery, it can be seen that further augmentation would be required to gain additional soft tissue in both the vertical and horizontal planes. A second-stage procedure was done at this time. (h) An incision 1.5 mm in depth was utilized to de-epithelialize the crestal surface of the ridge. Note that the papillae were not included within the surgical field. The mesial and distal borders of the onlay section of the recipient site were then extended apically to create vertical releasing incisions. The overall recipient site was to be trapezoidal in shape. A labial flap to create the pouch section of the recipient site was made using partial-thickness dissection. (i) The left maxillary premolar area was used as the donor site for the second-stage surgery. (j) This side view clearly shows the epithelialized onlay section of the graft and the de-epithelialized connective tissue section of the graft, as well as tissue thickness. (k) The graft was sutured first along the fixed palatal border to gain initial stabilization. Then the connective tissue interpositional section was sutured along the lateral borders. The flap was then sutured over the interpositional section of the graft at the epithelialized edge of the onlay section of the graft and along the vertical incisions. (l) At 6 weeks post surgery, the provisional prosthesis was modified to bring the tissue surface of the pontics into contact with the healing ridge. (m) At 2 months post surgery, tooth form was further modified on the provisional prosthesis and gingivoplasty was done to sculpt the tissues to final form and smooth out surface irregularities. (n) The final ceramo-metal prosthesis was inserted 4 months later. The life-like reconstruction of the soft tissues and dentition restored dentofacial esthetics for the patient. (Courtesy of Dr. J. Seibert, Dr. J. Louis & Dr. D. Hazzouri, USA. Reprinted with permission from *The International Journal of Periodontics and Restorative Dentistry*.)

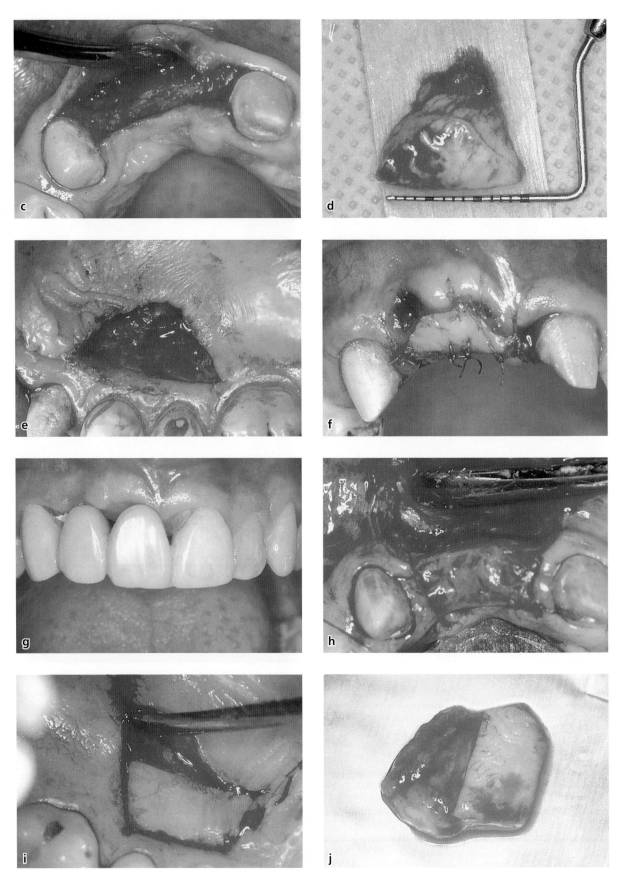

Fig. 44-87 *Continued*

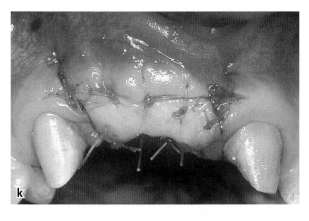
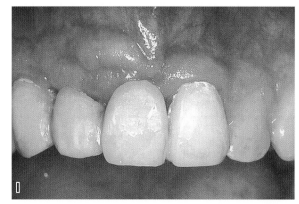
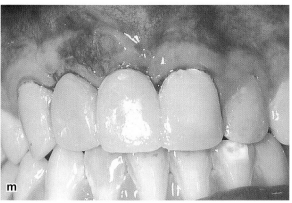
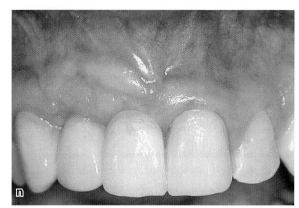

Fig. 44-87 *Continued*

References

Abbas, F., Wennström, J., Van der Weijden, F., Schneiders, T. & Van der Velden, U. (2003). Surgical treatment of gingival recessions using Emdogain gel: clinical procedure and case reports. *International Journal of Periodontics & Restorative Dentistry* **23**, 607–613.

Abrams, L. (1980). Augmentation of the residual edentulous ridge for fixed prosthesis. *Compendium of Continuing Education in General Dentistry* **1**, 205–214.

Agudio, G., Pini Prato, G., De Paoli, S. & Nevins, M. (1985). Mucogingival interceptive therapy. *International Journal of Periodontics & Restorative Dentistry* **5**, 49–59.

Ainamo, A., Bergenholtz, A., Hugoson, A. & Ainamo, J. (1992). Location of the mucogingival junction 18 years after apically repositioned flap surgery. *Journal of Clinical Periodontology* **19**, 49–52.

Allen, A.L. (1994). Use of the supraperiosteal envelope in soft tissue grafting for root coverage. I. Rationale and technique. *International Journal of Periodontics & Restorative Dentistry* **14**, 217–227.

Allen, E.P., Gainza, C.S., Farthing, G.G. *et al.* (1985). Improved technique for localized ridge augmentation. *Journal of Periodontology* **56**, 195–199.

Allen, E.P. & Miller, P.D. (1989). Coronal positioning of existing gingiva. Short term results in the treatment of shallow marginal tissue recession. *Journal of Periodontology* **60**, 316–319.

Andlin-Sobocki, A. & Bodin, L. (1993). Dimensional alterations of the gingiva related to changes of facial/lingual tooth position in permanent anterior teeth of children. A 2-year longitudinal study. *Journal of Clinical Periodontology* **20**, 219–224.

Andlin-Sobocki, A., Marcusson, A. & Persson, M. (1991). 3-year observation on gingival recession in mandibular incisors in children. *Journal of Clinical Periodontology* **18**, 155–159.

Azzi, R., Etienne, D. & Carranza, F. (1998). Surgical reconstruction of the interdental papilla. *International Journal of Periodontics & Restorative Dentistry* **18**, 467–473.

Baelum, V., Fejerskov, O. & Karring T. (1986). Oral hygiene, gingivitis and periodontal breakdown in adult Tanzanians. *Journal of Periodontal Research* **21**, 221–232.

Bahat, O., Handelsman, M. & Gordon, J. (1990). The transpositional flap in mucogingival surgery. *International Journal of Periodontics & Restorative Dentistry* **10**, 473–482.

Baker, D.L. & Seymour, G.J. (1976). The possible pathogenesis of gingival recession. A histological study of induced recession in the rat. *Journal of Clinical Periodontology* **3**, 208–219.

Batenhorst, K.F., Bowers, G.M. & Williams, J.E. (1974). Tissue changes resulting from facial tipping and extrusion of incisors in monkeys. *Journal of Periodontology* **45**, 660–668.

Beagle, J.R. (1992). Surgical reconstruction of the interdental papilla: case report. *International Journal of Periodontics & Restorative Dentistry* **12**, 144–151.

Becker, W., Becker, B.E. & Caffesse, R. (1994). A comparison of demineralized freeze-dried bone and autologous bone to induce bone formation in human extraction sockets. *Journal of Periodontology* **65**, 1128–1133.

Bernimoulin, J.P. & Curilivic, Z. (1977). Gingival recession and tooth mobility. *Journal of Clinical Periodontology* **4**, 208–219.

Bernimoulin, J.P., Lüscher, B. & Mühlemann, H.R. (1975). Coronally repositioned periodontal flap. Clinical evaluation after one year. *Journal of Clinical Periodontology* **2**, 1–13.

Bertrand, P.M. & Dunlap, R.M. (1988). Coverage of deep, wide gingival clefts with free gingival autografts: root planing with and without citric acid demineralization. *International Journal of Periodontics & Restorative Dentistry* **8** (1), 65–77.

Bohannan, H.M. (1962a). Studies in the alteration of vestibular depth. I. Complete denudation. *Journal of Periodontology* **33**, 120–128.

Bohannan, H.M. (1962b). Studies in the alteration of vestibular depth. II. Periosteum retention. *Journal of Periodontology* **33**, 354–359.

Borghetti, A. & Gardella, J-P. (1990). Thick gingival autograft for the coverage of gingival recession: A clinical evaluation. *International Journal of Periodontics & Restorative Dentistry* **10**, 217–229.

Borghetti, A. & Glise, J.M. (2000). Aménagement de la crête édentée pour la prothèse fixéesur pilers naturales. In: Borghetti, A. & Monnet-Corti, V., eds. *Chirurgie Plastique Parodontale*. Rueil-Malmaison Cedex: Editions CdP Groupe Liaisons SA, pp. 391–422.

Borghetti, A. & Laborde, G. (1996). La chirurgie parodontale pro-prothétique. *Actualités Odonto-Stomatologiques* **194**, 193–227.

Bouchard, P., Nilveus, R. & Etienne, D. (1997). Clinical evaluation of tetracycline HCL conditioning in the treatment of gingival recessions. A comparative study. *Journal of Periodontology* **68**, 262–269.

Bowers, G.M. (1963). A study of the width of attached gingiva. *Journal of Periodontology* **34**, 201–209.

Boyd, R.L. (1978). Mucogingival considerations and their relationship to orthodontics. *Journal of Periodontology* **49**, 67–76.

Bradley, R.E., Grant, J.C. & Ivancie, G.P. (1959). Histologic evaluation of mucogingival surgery. *Oral Surgery* **12**, 1184–1199.

Brown, S.I. (1973). The effect of orthodontic therapy on certain types of periodontal defects. I. Clinical findings. *Journal of Periodontology* **44**, 742–756.

Bruno, J.F. (1994). Connective tissue graft technique assuring wide root coverage. *International Journal of Periodontics & Restorative Dentistry* **14**, 127–137.

Brustein, D. (1979). Cosmetic periodontics. Coronally repositioned pedicle graft. *Dental Survey* **46**, 22.

Caffesse, R.G., Alspach, S.R., Morrison, E.C. & Burgett, F.G. (1987). Lateral sliding flaps with and without citric acid. *International Journal of Periodontics & Restorative Dentistry* **7**, 44–57.

Caffesse, R.G., De LaRosa, M., Garza, M., Munne-Travers, A., Mondragon, J.C. & Weltman, R. (2000). Citric acid demineralization and subepithelial connective tissue grafts. *Journal of Periodontology* **71**, 568–572.

Caffesse, R.G., Kon, S., Castelli, W.A. & Nasjleti, C.E. (1984). Revascularization following the lateral sliding flap procedure. *Journal of Periodontology* **55**, 352–359.

Carnio, J., Camargo, P.M., Kenney, E.B. & Schenk, R.K. (2002). Histological evaluation of 4 cases of root coverage following a connective tissue graft combined with an enamel matrix derivative preparation. *Journal of Periodontology* **73**, 1534–1543.

Carranza, F.A. & Carraro, J.J. (1963). Effect of removal of periosteum on post-operative results of mucogingival surgery. *Journal of Periodontology* **34**, 223–226.

Carranza, F.A. & Carraro, J.J. (1970). Mucogingival techniques in periodontal surgery. *Journal of Periodontology* **41**, 294–299.

Carraro, J.J., Carranza, F.A., Albano, E.A. & Joly, G.G. (1964). Effect of bone denudation in mucogingival surgery in humans. *Journal of Periodontology* **35**, 463–466.

Checchi, L., Daprile, G., Gatto, M.R. & Pelliccioni, G.A. (1999). Gingival recession and toothbrushing in an Italian School of Dentistry: a pilot study. *Journal of Clinical Periodontology* **26**, 276–280.

Coatoam, G.W., Behrents, R.G. & Bissada, N.F. (1981). The width of keratinized gingiva during orthodontic treatment: its significance and impact on periodontal status. *Journal of Periodontology* **52**, 307–313.

Cohen, D. & Ross, S. (1968). The double papillae flap in periodontal therapy. *Journal of Periodontology* **39**, 65–70.

Cohen, E.S. (1994). Ridge augmentation utilizing the subepithelial connective tissue graft: Case reports. *Practical Periodontics and Aesthetic Dentistry* **6**, 47–53.

Corn, H. (1962). Periosteal separation – its clinical significance. *Journal of Periodontology* **33**, 140–152.

Cortellini, P., Clauser, C. & Pini Prato, G.P. (1993). Histologic assessment of new attachment following the treatment of a human buccal recession by means of a guided tissue regeneration procedure. *Journal of Periodontology* **64**, 387–391.

Costich, E.R. & Ramfjord, S.F. (1968). Healing after partial denudation of the alveolar process. *Journal of Periodontology* **39**, 5–12.

De Sanctis, M. & Zucchelli, G. (2007). Coronally-advanced flap: a modified surgical approach for isolated recession type defects. 3-year results. *Journal of Clinical Periodontology* **34**, 262–268.

De Trey, E. & Bernimoulin, J. (1980). Influence of free gingival grafts on the health of the marginal gingiva. *Journal of Clinical Periodontology* **7**, 381–393.

Donaldson, D. (1974). The etiology of gingival recession associated with temporary crowns. *Journal of Periodontology* **45**, 468–471.

Donnenfeld, O.W., Marks, R.M. & Glickman, I. (1964). The apically repositioned flap – a clinical study. *Journal of Periodontology* **35**, 381–387.

Dorfman, H.S., Kennedy, J.E. & Bird, W.C. (1980). Longitudinal evaluation of free autogenous gingival grafts. *Journal of Clinical Periodontology* **7**, 316–324.

Dorfman, H.S., Kennedy, J.E. & Bird, W.C. (1982). Longitudinal evaluation of free gingival grafts. A four-year report. *Journal of Periodontology* **53**, 349–352.

Edel, A. (1974). Clinical evaluation of free connective tissue grafts used to increase the width of keratinized gingiva. *Journal of Clinical Periodontology* **1**, 185–196.

Engelking, G. & Zachrisson, B.U. (1982). Effects of incisor repositioning on monkey periodontium after expansion through the cortical plate. *American Journal of Orthodontics* **82**, 23–32.

Ericsson, I. & Lindhe, J. (1984). Recession in sites with inadequate width of the keratinized gingiva. An experimental study in the dog. *Journal of Clinical Periodontology* **11**, 95–103.

Ericsson, I., Thilander, B. & Lindhe, J. (1978). Periodontal condition after orthodontic tooth movement in the dog. *Angle Orthodontics* **48**, 210–218.

Erley, K.J., Swiec, G.D., Herold, R., Bisch, F.C. & Peacock, M.E. (2006). Gingival recession treatment with connective tissue grafts in smokers and non-smokers. *Journal of Periodontology* **77**, 1148–1155.

Espinel, M.C. & Caffesse, R.G. (1981). Lateral positioned pedicle sliding flap – revised technique in the treatment of localized gingival recession. *International Journal of Periodontics & Restorative Dentistry* **1**, 44–51.

Foushee, D.G., Moriarty, J.D. & Simpson, D.M. (1985). Effects of mandibular orthognatic treatment on mucogingival tissue. *Journal of Periodontology* **56**, 727–733.

Freedman, A.L., Green, K., Salkin, L.M., Stein, M.D. & Mellado, J.R. (1999). An 18-year longitudinal study of untreated mucogingival defects. *Journal of Periodontology* **70**, 1174–1176.

Friedman, N. & Levine, H.L. (1964). Mucogingival surgery: Current status. *Journal of Periodontology* **35**, 5–21.

Friedman, N. (1957). Mucogingival surgery. *Texas Dental Journal* **75**, 358–362.

Friedman, N. (1962). Mucogingival surgery: The apically repositioned flap. *Journal of Periodontology* **33**, 328–340.

Gargiulo, A.W. (1961). Dimensions and relations of the dentogingival junction in humans. *Journal of Periodontology* **32**, 261–267.

Glossary of Terms in Periodontology. (2001). The American Academy of Periodontology, Chicago, USA.

Gottlow, J., Karring, T. & Nyman, S. (1990). Guided tissue regeneration following treatment of recession-type defects in the monkey. *Journal of Periodontology* **61**, 680–685.

Gottlow, J., Nyman, S., Karring, T. & Lindhe, J. (1986). Treatment of localized gingival recessions with coronally displaced flaps and citric acid. An experimental study in the dog. *Journal of Clinical Periodontology* **13**, 57–63.

Gottsegen, R. (1954). Frenulum position and vestibular depth in relation to gingival health. *Oral Surgery* **7**, 1069–1078.

Grevers, A. (1977). Width of attached gingiva and vestibular depth in relation to gingival health. Thesis. University of Amsterdam.

Grupe, J. (1966). Modified technique for the sliding flap operation. *Journal of Periodontology* **37**, 491–495.

Grupe, J. & Warren, R. (1956). Repair of gingival defects by a sliding flap operation. *Journal of Periodontology* **27**, 290–295.

Guinard, E.A. & Caffesse, R.G. (1978). Treatment of localized gingival recessions. III. Comparison on results obtained with lateral sliding and coronally repositioned flaps. *Journal of Periodontology* **49**, 457–461.

Günay, H., Tschernitschek, H. & Geurtsen, W. (2000). Placement of the preparation line and periodontal health – a prospective 2-year clinical study. *International Journal of Periodontics & Restorative Dentistry* **20**, 173–181.

Haggerty, P.C. (1966). The use of a free gingival graft to create a healthy environment for full crown preparation. *Periodontics* **4**, 329–331.

Hall, W.B. (1981). The current status of mucogingival problems and their therapy. *Journal of Periodontology* **52**, 569–575.

Han, T.J. & Takei, H.H. (1996). Progress in gingival papilla ceconstruction. *Periodontology 2000* **11**, 65–68.

Hangorsky, U. & Bissada, N.B. (1980). Clinical assessment of free gingival graft effectiveness on maintenance of periodontal health. *Journal of Periodontology* **51**, 274–278.

Harlan, A.W. (1907). Discussion of paper: Restoration of gum tissue. *Dental Cosmos* **49**, 591–598.

Harris, R.J. (1992). The connective tissue and partial thickness double pedicle graft: a predictable method of obtaining root coverage. *Journal of Periodontology* **63**, 477–486.

Harris, R.J. (1994). The connective tissue with partial thickness double pedicle graft: the results of 100 consecutively-treated defects. *Journal of Periodontology* **65**, 448–461.

Harris, R.J. (1999). Human histologic evaluation of root coverage obtained with a connective tissue with prtial thickness double pedicle graft: a case report. *Journal of Periodontology* **70**, 813–821.

Harris, R.J. (2001). Clinical evaluation of 3 techniques to augment keratinized tissue without root coverage. *Journal of Periodontology* **72**, 932–938.

Harvey, P. (1965). Management of advanced periodontitis. Part I. Preliminary report of a method of surgical reconstruction. *New Zealand Dental Journal* **61**, 180–187.

Hawley, C.E. & Staffileno, H. (1970). Clinical evaluation of free gingival grafts in periodontal surgery. *Journal of Periodontology* **41**, 105–112.

Heijl, L. (1997). Periodontal regeneration with enanel matrix derivative in one human experimental defect. A case report. *Journal of Periodontology* **24**, 693–696.

Herrero, F., Scott, J.B., Maropis, P.S. & Yukna, R.A. (1995). Clinical comparison of desired versus actual amount of surgical crown lengthening. *Journal of Periodontology* **66**, 568–571.

Holbrook, T. & Ochsenbein, C. (1983). Complete coverage of the denuded root surface with a one-stage gingival graft. *International Journal of Periodontics & Restorative Dentistry* **3**, 9–27.

Hwang, D. & Wang, H.L. (2006). Flap thickness as a predictor of root coverage: a systematic review. *Journal of Periodontology* **77**, 1625–1634.

Ibbott, C.G., Oles, R.D. & Laverty, W.H. (1985). Effects of citric acid treatment on autogenous free graft coverage of localized recession. *Journal of Periodontology* **56**, 662–665.

Ingber, J.S. (1974). Forced eruption: Part I. A method of treating isolated one and two wall infrabony osseous defects – rationale and case report. *Journal of Periodontology* **45**, 199–206.

Ingber, J.S. (1976). Forced eruption: Part II. A method of treating non-restorable teeth – periodontal and restorative considerations. *Journal of Periodontology* **47**, 203–216.

Ivancie, G.P. (1957). Experimental and histological investigation of gingival regeneration in vestibular surgery. *Journal of Periodontology* **28**, 259–263.

Kaldahl, W.B., Tussing, G.J., Wentz, F.M. & Walker, J.A. (1982). Achieving an esthetic appearance with a fixed prosthesis by submucosal grafts. *Journal of the American Dental Association* **104**, 449–452.

Karring, T., Cumming, B.R., Oliver, R.C. & Löe, H. (1975). The origin of granulation tissue and its impact on postoperative results of mucogingival surgery. *Journal of Periodontology* **46**, 577–585.

Karring, T., Nyman, S., Thilander, B., Magnusson, I. & Lindhe, J. (1982). Bone regeneration in orthodontically produced alveolar bone dehiscences. *Journal of Periodontal Research* **17**, 309–315, 1982.

Karring, T., Ostergaard, E. & Löe, H. (1971). Conservation of tissue specificity after heterotopic transplantation of gingiva and alveolar mucosa. *Journal of Periodontal Research* **6**, 282–293.

Kennedy, J.E., Bird, W.C., Palcanis, K.G. & Dorfman, H.S. (1985). A longitudinal evaluation of varying widths of attached gingiva. *Journal of Clinical Periodontology* **12**, 667–675.

Khocht, A., Simon, G., Person, P. & Denepitiya, J.L. (1993). Gingival recession in relation to history of hard toothbrush use. *Journal of Periodontology* **64**, 900–905.

Kisch, J., Badersten, A. & Egelberg, J. (1986). Longitudinal observation of "unattached", mobile gingival areas. *Journal of Clinical Periodontology* **13**, 131–134.

Laney, J.B., Saunders, V.G. & Garnick, J.J. (1992). A comparison of two techniques for attaining root coverage. *Journal of Periodontology* **63**, 19–23.

Lang, N.P. (1995). Periodontal considerations in prosthetic dentistry. *Periodontology 2000* **9**, 118–131.

Lang, N.P. & Löe, H. (1972). The relationship between the width of keratinized gingiva and gingival health. *Journal of Periodontology* **43**, 623–627.

Langer, B. & Langer, L. (1985). Subepithelial connective tissue graft technique for root coverage. *Journal of Periodontology* **56**, 715–720.

Lanning, S.K., Waldrop, T.C., Gunsolley, J.C. & Maynard, G. (2003). Surgical crown lengthening: evalusion of the biological width. *Journal of Periodontology* **74**, 468–474.

Lekovic, V., Kenney, E.B., Weinlaender, M., Han, T., Klokkevold, P., Nedic, M. & Orsini, M. (1997). A bone regenerative approach to alveolar ridge maintenance following tooth extraction. Report of 10 cases. *Journal of Periodontology* **68**, 563–570.

Lindhe, J. & Nyman, S. (1980). Alterations of the position of the marginal soft tissue following periodontal surgery. *Journal of Clinical Periodontology* **7**, 525–530.

Löe, H., Ånerud, Å. & Boysen H. (1992). The natural history of periodontal disease in man: prevalence, severity, extent of gingival recession. *Journal of Periodontology* **63**, 489–495.

Löe, H., Ånerud, A., Boysen, H. & Smith, M. (1978). The natural history of periodontal disease in man. The rate of periodontal destruction before 40 years of age. *Journal of Periodontology* **49**, 607–620.

Löst, C. (1984). Depth of alveolar bone dehiscences in relation to gingival recessions. *Journal of Clinical Periodontology* **11**, 583–589.

Martins, A.G., Andia, D.C., Sallum, A.W., Sallum, E.A., Casati, M.Z. & Nociti, F.H. Jr. (2004). Smoking may affect root coverage outcome: a prospective clinical study in humans. *Journal of Periodontology* **75**, 586–591.

Matter, J. (1982). Free gingival grafts for the treatment of gingival recession. A review of some techniques. *Journal of Clinical Periodontology* **9**, 103–114.

Maynard, J.G. (1987). The rationale for mucogingival therapy in the child and adolescent. *International Journal of Periodontics & Restorative Dentistry* **7**, 37–51.

Maynard, J.G. & Ochsenbein, D. (1975). Mucogingival problems, prevalence and therapy in children. *Journal of Periodontology* **46**, 544–552.

Majzoub, Z., Landi, L., Grusovin, G. & Cordioli, G. (2001). Histology of connective tissue graft. A case report. *Journal of Periodontology* **72**, 1607–1615.

Melsen, B. & Allais, D. (2005). Factors of importance for the development of dehiscences during labial movement of mandibular insicors: a retrospective study of adult orthodontic patients. *American Journal of Orthodontics and Dentofacial Orthopedics* **127**, 552–561.

Meltzer, J.A. (1979). Edentulous area tissue graft correction of an esthetic defect. A case report. *Journal of Periodontology* **50**, 320–322.

Miller, A.J., Brunelle, J.A., Carlos, J.P., Brown, L.J. & Löe, H. (1987). Oral health of United States adults. Bethesda, Maryland: NIH Publication No. 87–2868, National Institute of Dental Research.

Miller, P.D. (1982). Root coverage using a free soft tissue autograft following citric acid application. I. Technique. *International Journal of Periodontics & Restorative Dentistry* **2**, 65–70.

Miller, P.D. (1985a). A classification of marginal tissue recession. *International Journal of Periodontics & Restorative Dentistry* **5**, 9–13.

Miller, P.D. (1985b). Root coverage using a free soft tissue autograft following citric acid application. III. A successful and predictable procedure in areas of deep-wide recession. *International Journal of Periodontics & Restorative Dentistry* **5**, 15–37.

Miller, P.D. Jr. (1986). Ridge augmentation under existing fixed prosthesis. Simplified technique. *Journal of Periodontology* **57**, 742–745.

Miller P.D. (1993). Root coverage grafting for regeneration and aesthetics. *Periodontology 2000* **1**, 118–127

Miyasato, M., Crigger, M. & Egelberg, J. (1977) Gingival condition in areas of minimal and appreciable width of keratinized gingiva. *Journal of Clinical Periodontology* **4**, 200–209.

Murtomaa, H., Meurman, J.H., Rytömaa, I. & Turtola, L. (1987). Periodontal status in university students. *Journal of Clinical Periodontology* **14**, 462–465.

Müller, H.P., Eger, T. & Schorb, A. (1998). Gingival dimensions after root coverage with free connective tissue grafts. *Journal of Clinical Periodontology* **25**, 424–430.

Nabers, C.L. (1954). Repositioning the attached gingiva. *Journal of Periodontology* **25**, 38–39.

Nabers, C.L. (1966). Free gingival grafts. *Periodontics* **4**, 244–245.

Nelson, S.W. (1987). The subpedicle connective tissue graft. A bilaminar reconstructive procedure for the coverage of denuded root surfaces. *Journal of Periodontology* **58**, 95–102.

Nevins, M. & Mellonig, J.T. (1998). *Periodontal Therapy: Clinical Approaches and Evidence of Success.* Quintessence Publishing Co, Inc.

Nobuto, T., Imai, H. & Yamaoka, A. (1988). Microvascularization of the free gingival autograft. *Journal of Periodontology* **59**, 639–646.

Nordland, W.P. & Tarnow, D.P. (1998). A classification system for loss of papillary height. *Journal of Periodontology* **69**, 1124–1126.

Nyman, S., Karring, T. & Bergenholtz, G. (1982). Bone regeneration in alveolar bone dehiscences produced by jiggling forces. *Journal of Periodontal Research* **17**, 316–322.

Oates, T.W., Robinson, M. & Gunsolley, J.C. (2003). Surgical therapies for the treatment of gingival recession. A systematic review. *Annals of Periodontology* **8**, 303–320.

Ochsenbein, C. (1960). Newer concept of mucogingival surgery. *Journal of Periodontology* **31**, 175–185.

Oles, R.D., Ibbott, C.G. & Laverty, W.H. (1985). Effects of citric acid treatment on pedicle flap coverage of localized recession. *Journal of Periodontology* **56**, 259–261.

Oles, R.D., Ibbott, C.G. & Laverty, W.H. (1988). Effects of roor curettage and sodium hypochlrite on pedicle flap coverage of localized recession. *Journal of the Canadian Dental Association* **54**, 515–517.

Oliver, R.G., Löe, H. & Karring, T. (1968). Microscopic evaluation of the healing and re-vascularization of free gingival grafts. *Journal of Periodontal Research* **3**, 84–95.

Orban, B.J. (1957). *Oral Histology and Embryology*, 4th edn. St. Louis: C.V. Mosby Company, pp. 221–264.

Pagliaro, U., Nieri, M., Franceschi, D., Clauser, C. & Pini Prato, G. (2003). Evidence-based mucogingival therapy. Part 1: A critical review of the literature on root coverage procedures. *Journal of Periodontology* **74**, 709–740.

Parma-Benfenati, S., Fugazzato, P.A. & Ruben, M.P. (1985). The effect of restorative margins on the postsurgical development and nature of the periodontium. *International Journal of Periodontics & Restorative Dentistry* **5**, 31–51.

Patur, B. (1977). The rotation flap for covering denuded root surfaces. A closed wound technique. *Journal of Periodontology* **48**, 41–44.

Pennel, B.M., Higgison, J.D., Towner, T.D., King, K.O., Fritz, B.D. & Salder, J.F. (1965). Oblique rotated flap. *Journal of Periodontology* **36**, 305–309.

Pfeifer, J.S. (1963). The growth of gingival tissue over denuded bone. *Journal of Periodontology* **34**, 10–16.

Pfeifer, J.S. (1965). The reaction of alveolar bone to flap procedures in man. *Periodontics* **3**, 135–140.

Pfeifer, J. & Heller, R. (1971). Histologic evaluation of full and partial thickness lateral repositioned flaps. A pilot study. *Journal of Periodontology* **42**, 331–333.

Pini Prato, G.P., Baccetti, T., Magnani, C., Agudio, G. & Cortellini, P. (2000b). Mucogingival interceptive surgery of buccally-erupted premolars in patients scheduled for orthodontic treatment. I. A seven-year longitudinal study. *Journal of Periodontology* **71**, 172–181.

Pini Prato, G.P., Baccetti, T., Giorgetti, R., Agudio, G. & Cortellini, P. (2000c). Mucogingival interceptive surgery of buccally-erupted premolars in patients scheduled for orthodontic treatment. II. Surgically treated versus nonsurgically treated cases. *Journal of Periodontology* **71**, 182–187.

Pini Prato, G.P., Baldi, C., Nieri, M. *et al.* (2005). Coronally advanced flap: The post-surgical position of the gingival margin is an important factor for achieving complete root coverage. *Journal of Periodontology* **76**, 713–722.

Pini Prato, G., Baldi, C., Pagliaro, U., Nieri, M., Saletta, D., Rotundo, R. & Cortellini, P. (1999). Coronally advanced flap procedure for root coverage. Treatment of root surface: Root planing versus polishing. *Journal of Periodontology* **70**, 1064–1076.

Pini Prato, G.P., Clauser, C., Cortellini, P., Tinti, C., Vincenzi, G. & Pagliaro, U. (1996). Guided tissue regeneration versus mucogingival surgery in the treatment of human buccal recessions. A 4-year follow-up. *Journal of Periodontology* **67**, 1216–1223.

Pini Prato, G., Pagliaro, U., Baldi, C., Nieri, M., Saletta, D., Cairo, F. & Cortellini, P. (2000a). Coronally advanced flap procedure for root coverage. Flap with tension versus flap without tension: A randomized controlled clinical study. *Journal of Periodontology* **71**, 188–201

Pini Prato, G.P., Tinti, C., Vincenzi, G., Magnani, C., Cortellini, P. & Clauser, C. (1992). Guided tissue regeneration versus mucogingival surgery in the treatment of human buccal gingival recession. *Journal of Periodontology* **63**, 919–928.

Pontoriero, R. & Carnevale, G. (2001). Surgical crown lengthening: A 12-month clinical wound healing study. *Journal of Periodontology* **72**, 841–848.

Pontoriero, R., Celenza, F. Jr., Ricci, G. & Carnevale, M. (1987). Rapid extrusion with fiber resection: A combined orthodontic-periodontic treatment modality. *International Journal of Periodontics and Restorative Dentistry* **5**, 30–43.

Potashnick, S.R. & Rosenberg, E.S. (1982). Forced eruption: Principles in periodontics and restorative dentistry. *Journal of Prosthetic Dentistry* **48**, 141–148.

Proceedings of 1st European Workshop on Clinical Periodontology (1994). Eds Lang, N.P. & Karring, T. Quintessence Publ. Co., Ltd., London, Consensus report of session II, pp. 210–214.

Proceedings of the World Workshop on Periodontics (1996). Consensus report on mucogingival therapy. *Annals of Periodontology* **1**, 702–706.

Raetzke, P.B. (1985). Covering localized areas of root exposure employing the "envelope" technique. *Journal of Periodontology* **56**, 397–402.

Rateitschak, K.H., Herzog-Specht, F. & Hotz, R. (1968). Reaktion und Regeneration des Parodonts auf Behandlung mit festsitzenden Apparaten und abnehmbaren Platten. *Fortschritte der Kieferorthopädie* **29**, 415–435.

Reitan, K. (1967). Clinical and histologic observations on tooth movement during and after orthodontic treatment. *American Journal of Orthodontics* **53**, 721–745.

Roccuzzo, M., Bunino, M., Needleman, I. & Sanz, M. (2002). Periodontal plastic surgery for treatment of localized gingival recessions: a systematic review. *Journal of Clinical Periodontology* **29** (Suppl 3), 178–194.

Roccuzzo, M., Lungo, M., Corrente, G. *et al.* (1996). Comparative study of a bioresorbable and a non-resorbable membrane in the treatment of human buccal gingival recessions. *Journal of Periodontology* **67**, 7–14.

Romanos, G.E., Bernimoulin, J.P. & Marggraf, E. (1993). The double lateral bridging flap for coverage of denuded root surface: Longitudinal study and clinical evaluation after 5 to 8 years. *Journal of Periodontology* **64**, 683–688.

Rosenberg, N.M. (1960). Vestibular alterations in periodontics. *Journal of Periodontology* **31**, 231–237.

Ruben, M.P. (1979). A biological rationale for gingival reconstruction by grafting procedures. *Quintessence International* **10**, 47–55.

Saletta, D., Pini Prato, G.P., Pagliaro, U., Baldi, C., Mauri, M. & Nieri M. (2001). Coronally advanced flap procedure: Is the interdental papilla a prognostic factor for root coverage? *Journal of Periodontology* **72**, 760–766.

Sallum, E.A., Pimentel, S.P., Saldanha, J.B., Nogueira-Filho, G.R., Casati, M.Z., Nociti, F.H. Jr. & Sallum, A.W. (2004). Enamel matrix derivative and guided tissue regeneration in the treatment of deshicence-type defects: A histomorphometric study in dogs. *Journal of Periodontology* **75**, 1357–1363.

Sangnes, G. & Gjermo, P. (1976). Prevalence of oral soft and hard tissue lesions related to mechanical tooth cleaning procedures. *Community Dentistry and Oral Epidemiology* **4**, 77–83.

Sangnes, G. (1976). Traumatization of teeth and gingiva related to habitual tooth cleaning procedures. *Journal of Clinical Periodontology* **3**, 94–103.

Schoo, W. H. & van der Velden, U. (1985). Marginal soft tissue recessions with and without attached gingiva. *Journal of Periodontal Research* **20**, 209–211.

Seibert, J.S. (1983). Reconstruction of deformed, partially edentulous ridges, using full thickness onlay grafts: I. Technique and wound healing. *Compendium of Continuing Education in General Dentistry* **4**, 437–453.

Seibert, J.S. (1991). Ridge augmentation to enhance esthetics in fixed prosthetic treatment. *Compendium of Continuing Education in General Dentistry* **12**, 548–561.

Seibert, J.S. (1993a). Treatment of moderate localized alveolar ridge defects: Preventive and reconstructive concepts in therapy. *Dental Clinics of North America* **37**, 265–280.

Seibert, J.S. (1993b). Reconstruction of the partially edentulous ridge: Gateway to improved prosthetics and superior esthetics. *Practical Periodontics and Aesthetic Dentistry* **5**, 47–55.

Seibert, J.S. & Louis, J. (1996). Soft tissue ridge augmentation utilizing a combination onlay-interpositional graft procedure: case report. *International Journal of Periodontics and Restorative Dentistry* **16**, 311–321.

Serino, G., Wennström, J.L., Lindhe, J. & Eneroth, L. (1994). The prevalence and distribution of gingival recession in subjects with high standard of oral hygiene. *Journal of Clinical Periodontology* **21**, 57–63.

Silva, C.O., Sallum, A.W., de Lima, A.F.M. & Tatakis, D.N. (2006). Coronally positioned flap for root coverage: Poorer outcomes in smokers. *Journal of Periodontology* **77**, 81–87.

Staffileno, H. (1964). Management of gingival recession and root exposure problems associated with periodontal disease. *Dental Clinics of North America* March, 111–120.

Staffileno, H., Levy, S. & Gargiulo, A. (1966). Histologic study of cellular mobilization and repair following a periosteal retention operation via split thickness mucogingival surgery. *Journal of Periodontology* **37**, 117–131.

Staffileno, H., Wentz, F. & Orban, B. (1962). Histologic study of healing of split thickness flap surgery in dogs. *Journal of Periodontology* **33**, 56–69.

Steiner, G.G., Pearson, J.K. & Ainamo, J. (1981). Changes of the marginal periodontium as a result of labial tooth movement in monkeys. *Journal of Periodontology* **52**, 314–320.

Stern, J.B. (1976). Oral mucous membrane. In: Bhaskar, S.N., ed. *Orban's Oral Histology and Embryology*. St. Louis: C.V. Mosby, Ch 8.

Stetler, K.J. & Bissada, N.B. (1987). Significance of the width of keratinized gingiva on the periodontal status of teeth with submarginal restorations. *Journal of Periodontology* **58**, 696–700.

Stoner, J. & Mazdyasna, S. (1980). Gingival recession in the lower incisor region of 15-year old subjects. *Journal of Periodontology* **51**, 74–76.

Studer, S.P., Lehner, C., Bucher, A. & Schärer, P. (2000). Soft tissue correction of a single-tooth pontic space: a comparative quantitative volume assment. *Journal of Prosthetic Dentistry* **83**, 402–411.

Studer, S., Naef, R. & Schärer, P. (1997). Adjustment of localized alveolar ridge defects by soft tissue transplantation to improve mucogingival esthetics: a proposal for clinical classification and an evaluation of procedures. *Quintessence International* **28**, 785–805.

Sugarman, E.F. (1969). A clinical and histological study of the attachment of grafted tissue to bone and teeth. *Journal of Periodontology* **40**, 381–387.

Sullivan, H.C. & Atkins, J.H. (1968a). Free autogenous gingival grafts. I. Principles of successful grafting. *Periodontics* **6**, 121–129.

Sullivan, H.C. & Atkins, J.H. (1968b). Free autogenous gingival grafts. III. Utilization of grafts in the treatment of gingival recession. *Periodontics* **6**, 152–160.

Sumner, C.F. (1969). Surgical repair of recession on the maxillary cuspid: incisionally repositioning the gingival tissues. *Journal of Periodontology* **40**, 119–121.

Susin, C., Haas, A.N., Oppermann, R.V., Haugejorden, O. & Albandar, J.M. (2004). Gingival recession: epidemiology and risk indicators in a representative urban Brazilian population. *Journal of Periodontology* **75**, 1377–1386.

Tarnow, D.P. (1986). Similunar coronally repositioned flap. *Journal of Clinical Periodontology* **13**, 182–185.

Tarnow, D.P., Magner, A.W. & Fletcher, P. (1992). The effect of the distance from the contact point to the crest of bone on the presence or absence of the interproximal dental papilla. *Journal of Periodontology* **63**, 995–996.

Tenenbaum, H. (1982) A clinical study comparing the width of attached gingiva and the prevalence of gingival recessions. *Journal of Clinical Periodontology* 9, 86–92.

Tolmie, P.N., Rubins, R.P., Buck, G.S., Vagianos, V. & Lanz, J.C. (1991). The predictability of root coverage by way of free gingival autografts and citric acid application: An evaluation by multiple clinicians. *International Journal of Periodontics & Restorative Dentistry* 11, 261–271

Trombelli, L. & Scabbia, A. (1997). Healing response of gingival recession defects following guided tissue regeneration procedures in smokers and non-smokers. *Journal of Clinical Periodontology* 24, 529–533.

Trombelli, L., Schincaglia, G.P., Scapoli, C. & Calura, G. (1995). Healing response of human buccal gingival recessions treated with expanded polytetrafluoroethylene membranes. A retrospective report. *Journal of Periodontology* 66, 14–22.

Trott, J.R. & Love, B. (1966). An analysis of localized recession in 766 Winnipeg high school students. *Dental Practice* 16, 209–213.

Valderhaug, J. (1980). Periodontal conditions and caries lesions following the insertion of fixed prostheses: a 10-year follow-up study. *International Dental Journal* 30, 296–304.

Van der Velden, U. (1982). Regeneration of the interdental soft tissues following denudation procedures. *Journal of Clinical Periodontology* 9, 455–459.

Van Palenstein Helderman, W.H., Lembariti, B.S., van der Weijden, G.A. & van't Hof, M.A. (1998). Gingival recession and its association with calculus in subjects deprived of prophylactic dental care. *Journal of Clinical Periodontology* 25, 106–111.

Vekalahti, M. (1989). Occurrence of gingival recession in adults. *Journal of Periodontology* 60, 599–603.

Waerhaug, J. (1952). The gingival pocket. Anatomy, pathology, deepening and elimination. *Odontologisk Tidskrift* 60, Suppl.

Wei, P-C., Laurell, L., Geivelis, M., Lingen, M.W. & Maddalozzo, D. (2000). Acellular dermal matrix allografts to achieve increased attached gingival. Part 1. A clinical study. *Journal of Periodontology* 71, 1297–1305.

Wennström, J.L. (1983). Regeneration of gingiva following surgical excision. A clinical study. *Journal of Clinical Periodontology* 10, 287–297.

Wennström, J.L. (1987). Lack of association between width of attached gingiva and development of gingival recessions. A 5-year longitudinal study. *Journal of Clinical Periodontology* 14, 181–184.

Wennström J.L. (1996). Mucogingival therapy. In: *Proceedings of the World Workshop on Periodontics. Annals of Periodontology* 1, 671–701.

Wennström, J.L. & Lindhe, J. (1983a). The role of attached gingiva for maintenance of periodontal health. Healing following excisional and grafting procedures in dogs. *Journal of Clinical Periodontology* 10, 206–221.

Wennström, J.L. & Lindhe, J. (1983b). Plaque-induced gingival inflammation in the absence of attached gingiva in dogs. *Journal of Clinical Periodontology* 10, 266–276.

Wennström, J.L., Lindhe, J., Sinclair, F. & Thilander, B. (1987). Some periodontal tissue reactions to orthodontic tooth movement in monkeys. *Journal of Clinical Periodontology* 14, 121–129.

Wennström, J.L. & Zucchelli, G. (1996). Increased gingival dimensions. A significant factor for successful outcome of root coverage procedures? A 2-year prospective clinical study. *Journal of Clinical Periodontology* 23, 770–777.

Wilderman, M.N. (1963). Repair after a periosteal retention procedure. *Journal of Periodontology* 34, 484–503.

Wilderman, M.N. (1964). Exposure of bone in periodontal surgery. *Dental Clinics of North America* March, 23–26.

Wilderman, M.N. & Wentz, F.M. (1965). Repair of a dentogingival defect with a pedicle flap. *Journal of Periodontology* 36, 218–231.

Wilderman, M.N., Wentz, F.M. & Orban, B.J. (1961). Histogenesis of repair after mucogingival surgery. *Journal of Periodontology* 31, 283–299.

Yared, K.F.G., Zenobio, E.G. & Pacheco, W. (2006). Periodontal staus of mandibular central incisors after orthodontic proclination in adults. *American Journal of Orthodontics and Dentofacial Orthopedics* 130, 6.e1–6.e8.

Yoneyama, T., Okamoto, H., Lindhe, J., Socransky, S.S. & Haffajee, A.D. (1988). Probing depth, attachment loss and gingival recession. Findings from a clinical examination in Ushiku, Japan. *Journal of Clinical Periodontology* 15, 581–591.

Zabalegui, I., Sicilia, A., Cambra, J., Gil, J. & Sanz, M. (1999). Treatment of multiple adjacent gingival recessions with the tunnel subepithelial connective tissue graft: a clinical report. *International Journal of Periodontics & Restorative Dentistry* 19, 199–206.

Zucchelli, G., Amore C., Montebugnoli, L. & De Sanctis, M. (2003). Bilaminar techniques for the treatment of recession type defects. A comparative clinical study. *Journal of Clinical Periodontology* 30, 862–870.

Zucchelli, G., Cesari, C., Amore C., Montebugnoli, L. & De Sanctis, M. (2004). Laterally moved, coronally advanced flap: a modified surgical approach for isolated recession-type defects. *Journal of Periodontology* 75, 1734–41.

Zucchelli, G., Clauser, C., De Sanctis, M. & Calandriello, M. (1998). Mucogingival versus guided tissue regeneration procedures in the treatment of deep recession type defects. *Journal of Periodontology* 69, 138–145.

Zucchelli, G. & De Sanctis, M. (2000). Treatment of multiple recession-type defects in patients with esthetic demands. *Journal of Periodontology* 71, 1506–1514.

Chapter 45

Periodontal Plastic Microsurgery

Rino Burkhardt and Niklaus P. Lang

Microsurgical techniques in dentistry (development of
  concepts), 1029
Concepts in microsurgery, 1030
  Magnification, 1030
  Instruments, 1035

Suture materials, 1035
Training concepts (surgeons and assistants), 1038
Clinical indications and limitations, 1039
Comparison to conventional mucogingival
  interventions, 1040

Microsurgical techniques in dentistry (development of concepts)

In general, the main aim of a surgical intervention is no longer only the survival of the patient or one of his organs, but the effort to preserve a maximum amount of function and to improve patient comfort. In many surgical specialties, these demands are met owing to a minimally invasive surgical approach.

Microsurgery in general is not an independent discipline, but is a technique that can be applied to different surgical disciplines. It is based on the fact that the human hand, by appropriate training, is capable of performing finer movements than the naked eye is able to control. First reports on microsurgery go back to the nineteenth century when a microscope was developed for use in ophthalmology (Tamai 1993). Later, the first surgical operation with a microscope was performed in Sweden to correct otosclerotic deafness (Nylén 1924). Microsurgical technique, however, did not attract the interest of surgeons until the 1950s, when the first surgical microscope, OPMI 1, with a coaxial lighting system and the option for stereoscopic view, was invented and commercialized by the Carl Zeiss company.

The micro vessel surgery that later revolutionized plastic and transplantation surgery was mainly developed by neurosurgeons (Jacobsen & Suarez 1960; Donaghy & Yasargil 1967). Applying microsurgically modified techniques, small vessels of a diameter of less than 1 mm could be successfully anastomosed on a routine basis (Smith 1964). As a consequence, a completely amputated thumb was successfully replanted for the first time in 1965 (Komatsu & Tamai 1968). Between 1966 and 1973, a total of 351 fingers were replanted at the Sixth People's Hospital in Shanghai without magnification, resulting in a healing rate of 51% (Zhong-Wei *et al.* 1981). From 1973, the interventions mentioned were solely performed with surgical microscopes and the corresponding success rates of replanted fingers increased to 91.5%. These results documented the importance of a fast and successful restoration of the blood circulation in replanted extremities and free tissue grafts. Further achievements of the microsurgical technique in plastic reconstructive surgery included transplantation of toes to replace missing thumbs (Cobbett 1969), interfascicular nerve transplantation (Millesi 1979), microvascular transplantation of toe joints (Buncke & Rose 1979), micro neurovascular transplantation of the pulp of a toe to restore the sensitivity of the finger tips (Morrison *et al.* 1980), and microvascular transplantation of the nail complex (Foucher 1991). Positive results of microsurgically modified interventions have led to today's clinical routine applications in orthopedics, gynecology, urology, plastic–reconstructive and pediatric surgery.

After a few early single reports (Baumann 1977; Apotheker & Jako 1981), the surgical microscope was introduced in dentistry in the 1990s. Case reports and the applications of the microscope were described in the prosthetic (Leknius & Geissberger 1995; Friedman & Landesman 1997, 1998; Mora 1998), endodontic (Carr 1992; Pecora & Andreana 1993; Ruddle 1994; Mounce 1995; Rubinstein 1997), and periodontal literature (Shanelec 1991; Shanelec & Tibbetts 1994, 1996; Tibbetts & Shanelec 1994; Burkhardt & Hürzeler 2000).

Treatment outcomes have been statistically analyzed in prospective studies in endodontics, since the introduction of microendodontic techniques (Rubinstein & Kim 1999, 2002). Within 1 year after apical microsurgery, 96.8% of the cases were considered to be healed. At re-evaluation, 5–7 years after the first post-operative year, a success rate of 91.5% measured by clinical and radiographic parameters was still evident (Rubinstein & Kim 2002). The corresponding percentage of healed cases, treated without a surgical microscope, yielded only 44.1%, 6 months to 8 years after conventional apical surgery (Friedman *et al.* 1991).

Despite the positive results in prospective studies (Rubinstein & Kim 2002; Cortellini & Tonetti 2001; Burkhardt & Lang 2005), the surgical microscope experiences a slow acceptance in prosthodontics, endodontics (Seldon 2002), and periodontal surgery. Possible reasons are the long learning curve, the impaired maneuverability of the devices and the high cost of purchasing the instrument.

Concepts in microsurgery

The continuous development of operating microscopes, refinement of surgical instruments, production of improved suture materials and suitable training laboratories have played a decisive role for the worldwide establishment of the microsurgical technique in many specialties. The three elements, i.e. *magnification*, *illumination*, and *instruments* are called the *microsurgical triad* (Kim *et al.* 2001), the improvement of which is a prerequisite for improved accuracy in surgical interventions. Without any one of these, microsurgery is not possible.

Magnification

An optimal vision is a stringent necessity in periodontal practice. More than 90% of the sensations of the human body are perceived by visual impressions. Vision is a complex process that involves the cooperation of multiple links between the eye, the retina, the optic nerve, and the brain. An important element to assess in human eyesight is visual acuity, measured in angular degrees. If necessary, it may be improved by corrective lenses. It is defined by the ability to perceive two objects separately. Visual acuity is influenced by anatomic and physiologic factors, such as the density of cells packed on the retina and the electrophysiologic process of the image on the retina.

Another important factor influencing visual acuity is the lighting. The relation between visual acuity and light density is well established: a low light density decreases visual acuity. The best eyesight can be achieved at a light density of 1000 cd/m^2. At higher densities, visual acuity decreases. This, in turn, means that claims for optimal lighting conditions have to be implemented.

Visualization of fine details is enhanced by increasing the image size of the object. Image size can be increased in two ways: (1) by getting closer to the objects and (2) by magnification. Using the former method, the ability of the lens of the eye to accommodate becomes important and has a relevant influence on the visual capacity. By changing the form of the lens, the refraction of the optical apparatus increases, allowing it to focus on nearer objects. During ageing, the ability to focus at closer distances is compromised because the lens of the eye loses its flexibility (Burton & Bridgeman 1990). This phenomenon is called presbyopia. Presbyopia affects all people in middle age, and becomes especially noticeable when the nearest point at which the eye can focus accurately exceeds ideal working distances (Burton & Bridgeman 1991). To see small objects accurately, the focal length must be increased. As an example, an older individual reading without glasses must hold the reading matter farther from the eyes to see the print. Increasing the distance enables the person to see the words, but the longer working distance results in a smaller size of the written text. This decrease in image size, resulting from the increased working distance, needs to accommodate the limitations of presbyopia and is especially hindering in clinical practice. In periodontal practice, the tissues to manipulate are usually very fine resulting in a situation in which the natural visual capacity reaches its limits. Therefore, the clinical procedure may only be performed successfully with the use of magnification improving precision and, hence, the quality of work.

Optical principles of loupes

In dentistry, two basic types of magnification systems are commonly used: the surgical microscope and loupes. The latter can further be classified as (1) single-lens magnifiers (clip-on, flip-up, jeweller's glasses) and (2) multi-lens telescopic loupes. Single-lens magnifiers produce the described diopter magnification that simply adjust the working distance to a set length. As diopters increase, the working distances decrease. With a set working distance, there is no range and no opportunity for movement; this can create difficulty in maintaining focus and, therefore, may cause neck and back strain from poor posture (Basset 1983; Diakkow 1984; Shugars *et al.* 1987). Additionally, diopter magnifiers also give poor image quality, which restricts the quality of the work (Kanca & Jordan 1995). These types of glasses cannot be considered to be a true means of magnification.

Telescopic loupes (compound or prism loupes), however, offer improved ergonomic posture as well as significant advancements in optical performance (Shanelec 1992). Instead of increasing the thickness of a single lens to increase magnification, compound loupes use multiple lenses with intervening air spaces (Fig. 45-1). These allow an adjustment of magnification, working distance, and depth of the field without excessive increase in size or weight. Prism loupes are

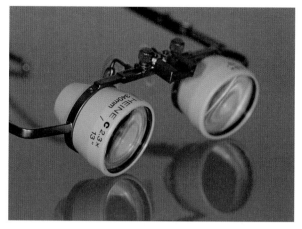

Fig. 45-1 Fixed compound loupe, adjustable only in the interpupilary distance (Galilean principle).

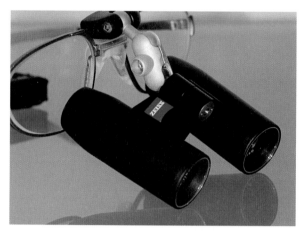

Fig. 45-2 Prism loupe, sealed to avoid leakage of moisture, front frame mounted and fully adjustable (Prism principle).

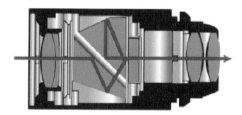

Fig. 45-3 Light path through prism loupe. Even though the distance the light travels has increased, there is no decrease in brightness or image contrast, even at 4× or 5×. This is because the light does not travel through air but instead through the glass of the prism.

the most optically advanced type of loupe magnification available (Fig. 45-2). While compound loupes use multiple refracting surfaces with intervening air spaces to adjust optical properties, prism loupes are actually low-power telescopes. They contain Pechan or Schmidt prisms that lengthen the light path through a series of mirror reflections within the loupes (Fig. 45-3). Prism loupes produce better magnification, larger fields of view, wider depths of field, and longer working distances than do other loupes. To guarantee proper adjustment of loupes, the knowl-

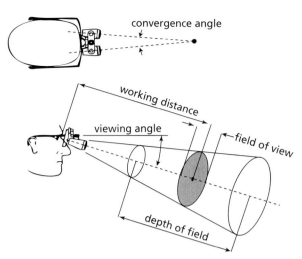

Fig. 45-4 Diagram indicating the principal optical features of loupes.

edge of some basic definitions and key optical features of loupes is necessary (Fig. 45-4).

Working distance

The working distance is the distance measured from the eye lens location to the object in vision. There is no set rule for how much the working distance may be increased. Depending on the height and the resulting length of the arms, the working distance with slightly bended arms usually ranges from 30 to 45 cm. At this distance, postural ergonomics are greatly improved and eye strain reduced due to lessened eye convergence. The multitude of back, neck, shoulder, and eye problems that dentists suffer, working without using loupes, frequently originate from the need to assume a short working distance to increase visual acuity (Coburn 1984; Strassler 1989). By wearing surgical loupes, the head is placed in the centre of its balance over the spine and stabilized against gravity.

Working range

The working range (depth of field) (Fig. 45-4) is the range within which the object remains in focus. The depth of field of normal vision ranges from working distance to infinity. Moving back from a close working distance, the eyes naturally accommodate and refocus to the new distance. Normally, eye position and body posture are not frozen in one place for an extended period, but vary constantly. Wearing loupes changes this geometry. Body posture and position of the extraocular muscles are confined to a range determined by the loupe's characteristics. It is important to understand that each individual's vision is limited to his/her own internal working range, which means that one may only be able to maintain focus on an object within a 15 cm range, even though the loupes have a 23 cm depth of field. With any brand of loupe, the depth of field decreases as the magnification increases.

Convergence angle

The convergence angle (Fig. 45-4) is the pivotal angle aligning the two oculars, such that they are pointing at the identical distance and angle. At a defined working distance, the convergence angle varies with interpupillary distance. Wider-set eyes will have more eye convergence at short working distances. Therefore, the convergence angle defines the position of the extraocular muscles that may result in tension of the internal and external rectus muscles; this may be an important source of eye fatigue.

Field of view

The field of view (Fig. 45-4) is the linear size or angular extent of an object when viewed through the telescopic system. It also varies depending on the design of the optic lens system, the working distance, and the magnification. As with depth of field, when magnification increases, the field of view decreases.

Interpupillary distance

The interpupillary distance (Fig. 45-4) depends on the position of the eyes of each individual and is a key adjustment that allows long-term, routine use of loupes. The ideal setting, as with binoculars, is to create a single image with a slightly oval-shaped viewing area. If the viewing area is adjusted to a full circle, excess eye muscle strain would limit the ability to use loupes for long periods.

Viewing angle

The viewing angle (Fig. 45-4) is the angular position of the optics allowing for comfortable working. The shallower the angle, the greater the need to tilt the neck to view the object being worked at. Therefore, loupes for dental clinicians should have a greater angulation than loupes designed for industrial workers. A slight or no angulation, which results when magnifiers are embedded in the lenses of the eyeglasses, may cause the operator to unduly tilt his or her head to view a particular object. This, again, may lead not only to neck discomfort, but also to pain in the shoulder muscles and possibly to a headache. As the working posture is likely to change over time, the loupes should be adjustable to any posture change.

Illumination

Most of the manufacturers offer collateral lighting systems or suitable fixing options. These systems may be helpful, particularly for higher magnification in the range of 4× and more. Loupes with a large field of view will have better illumination and brighter images than those with narrower fields of view. Important considerations in the selection of an accessory lighting source are total weight, quality, and the brightness of the light, ease of focusing and directing the light within the field of view of the magnifiers, and ease of transport between surgeries (Strassler *et al.* 1998).

It should be realized that each surface refraction in a lens will result in a 4% loss in transmitted light due to reflection. In telescopic loupes, this could amount to as much as 50% reduction in brightness. Anti-reflective coatings have been developed to counteract this effect by allowing lenses to transmit light more efficiently. The quality of lens coatings also varies and should be evaluated when selecting loupes (Shanelec 1992).

Choice of loupes

Before choosing a magnification system, different loupes and appropriate time for a proper adjustment have to be considered. Ill fitting or improperly adjusted loupes and the quality of the optics will influence the performance. For the use in periodontal surgery, an adjustable, sealed prism loupe with high-quality, coated lenses offering a magnification between 4× and 4.5×, either headband- or front frame-mounted, with a suitable working distance and a large field of view, seems to be the instrument of choice. The information in Table 45-1 serves as a basic guide to making an adequate selection.

Optical principles and components of a surgical microscope

The surgical microscope is a complicated system of lenses that allows stereoscopic vision at a magnification of approximately 4–40× with an excellent illumination of the working area. In contrast to loupes, the light beams fall parallel onto the retinas of the observer so that no eye convergence is necessary and the demand on the lateral rectus muscles is minimal (Fig. 45-5). The microscope

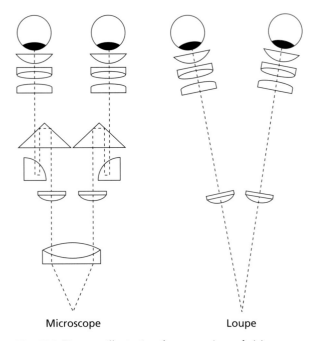

Microscope   Loupe

Fig. 45-5 Diagram illustrating the comparison of vision enhancement with loupes and a microscope. The loupes necessitate eye convergence while vision is paralleled through the microscope.

Table 45-1 Features to consider in the selection of a magnifying loupe system

Compound loupes (Galilean)	• Magnification range 2–3.5× • Lighter in weight • Shorter working distance • Shorter loupe barrel
Prism loupes (Keplerian)	• Magnification range 3–5× • Heavier in weight • Longer working distance • Longer loupe barrel
Front-frame mounted	• Allow up to 90% of peripheral vision • No prescription glasses • Require soft and cushioned nose piece • Better weight distribution
Head-band mounted	• Restricted peripheral vision • Allow to use prescription glasses • Better weight distribution • Require adjustment more often
Fixed-lens magnifiers	• No adjustment options when changing posture • Minimum weight
Flip-up capability	• Require removable, sterilizable handle • Allow switch from magnified to regular vision
Quality of the lenses	• Corrected for chromatic and spherical aberration • No drop-off in clarity when approaching the edges • Sealed system to avoid leakage of moisture • Option for disinfection
Adjustment options	• Interpupillary distance • Viewing angle • Vertical adjustment • Lock in adjusted position • Convergence angle (preset angle may be more user-friendly)
Lens coating	• Brighter image • More light
Accessories	• Transportation box • Side and front shields for protection • Mounted light source • Removable cushions

consists of the optical components, the lighting unit, and a mounting system. To avoid an unfavorable vibration of the microscope during use, the latter should be firmly attached to the wall, the ceiling or a floor stand. Mounted on the floor, the position of the microscope in the room must provide quick and easy access.

The optical unit includes the following components (Fig. 45-6): (1) magnification changer, (2) objective lenses, (3) binocular tubes, (4) eyepieces, and (5) lighting unit (Burkhardt & Hürzeler 2000).

Magnification changer

The magnification changer or "Galilean" changer consists of one cylinder, into which two Galilean telescope systems (consisting of a convex and concave lens) with various magnification factors are built. These systems can be used in either direction depending on the position of the magnification changer. A total of four different magnification levels are available. Straight transfer without any optics yields no magnification. The combination of the magnification changer with varying objective lenses and eyepieces yields an increasing magnification line when the control is adjusted.

The stepless motor-driven magnification changer must achieve a magnification of 0.5–2.5× with one optical system, which is operated by either a foot pedal or an electric rotating control, mounted on the microscope. The operator should decide whether to use the manual or motorized magnification changer. If the magnification must be changed frequently, it can be accomplished more quickly with the manual than with the motorized changer, the former not having in-between levels. While the motorized system improves the focus and comfort compared to the manual system, the former is more expensive.

Objective lenses

As processed by a magnification changer, the image is only projected by a single objective. This simultaneously projects light from its source twice for deflection by the prisms into the operation area (i.e. coaxial lighting). The most frequently used objective is 200 mm (f = 200 mm). The focal length of the objective generally corresponds to the working distance of the object.

Binocular tubes

Depending on the area of use, two different binocular tubes are attached (i.e. straight and inclined tubes). With straight tubes, the view direction is parallel to the microscope axis. Using inclined tubes, an angulation to the microscope axis of 45° is achieved. In dentistry, only inclined, swivelling tubes, that permit continuously adjustable viewing, are feasible for ergonomic reasons (Fig. 45-7). The precise adjustment of the interpupillary distance is the basic prerequisite for the stereoscopic view of the operation area.

Eyepieces

The eyepieces magnify the interim image generated in the binocular tubes. Varying magnifications can be achieved (10×, 12.5×, 16×, 20×) using different eyepieces. Eyepiece selection not only determines the magnification, but also the size of the field of view. Corresponding to the loupe spectacles, an indirect relationship exists between the magnification and the field of view. The 10× eyepiece generally provides a sufficient compromise between magnification and field of view. Modern eyepieces allow a correction

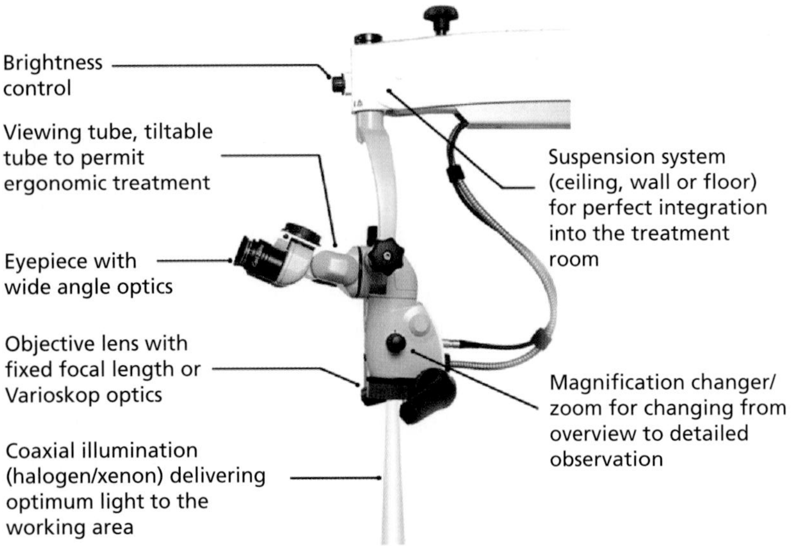

Brightness control

Viewing tube, tiltable tube to permit ergonomic treatment

Eyepiece with wide angle optics

Objective lens with fixed focal length or Varioskop optics

Coaxial illumination (halogen/xenon) delivering optimum light to the working area

Suspension system (ceiling, wall or floor) for perfect integration into the treatment room

Magnification changer/ zoom for changing from overview to detailed observation

Fig. 45-6 System components of a surgical microscope.

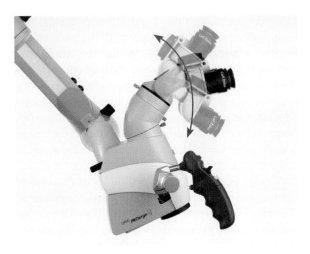

Fig. 45-7 Tiltable viewing tube which provides an ergonomic posture during clinical work, a prerequisite for optimal performance using microsurgical technique.

facility within –8 to +8 diopters that is a purely spherical correction.

The majority of surgical microscopes consist of modules and can be equipped with attachments that include integrated video systems, photographic adapters for cameras, units for image storage, colour printers, and powerful lighting sources. Prior to purchasing accessories, inexperienced clinicians should gather information about the needed equipment. The use of magnifying loupes is recommended prior to purchasing a microscope to accustom oneself to working under magnification.

Lighting unit
Optimal illumination is necessary with high magnifications. In recent years, the use of halogen lamps became popular. These lamps provide a whiter light than do lamps using conventional bulbs due to their higher colour temperature. As halogen lamps emit a considerable portion of their radiation within the

infrared part of the spectrum, microscopes are equipped with cold-light mirrors to keep this radiation from the operation area. An alternative to the halogen light is the xenon lamp that functions up to ten times longer than the halogen lamp. The light has daylight characteristics with even a whiter colour and delivers a brighter, more authentic image with more contrast.

Advantages and disadvantages of loupes and surgical microscopes

A substantial number of periodontists have already adopted the use of low magnification in their practices and recognize its great benefits. Most of the present results are based on subjective statements of patients or observations of the attending surgeons. At present, it can only be speculated how significantly the selection of magnification influences the result of the operation. The magnification recommended for surgical interventions ranges from 2.5–20× (Apotheker & Jako 1981; Shanelec 1992). In periodontal surgery, magnifications of 4–5× for loupe spectacles and 10–20× for surgical microscopes appear to be ideal depending on the kind of intervention. As the depth of field decreases with increasing magnification, the maximum magnification for a surgical intervention is limited to about 12–15×, when dealing with a localized problem such as the coverage of a single soft tissue recession or interdental wound closure after guided tissue regeneration of an infrabony defect. A magnification range of 6–8× seems appropriate for clinical inspections or surgical interventions when the entire quadrant is under operation. Higher magnifications such as 15–25× are more likely limited to the visual examination of clinical details only, such as in endodontic interventions.

Loupes have the advantage over the microscope in that they reduce technique sensitivity, expense, and learning phase. The lighting of the operation field is often insufficient, however, and that may limit magnifications more than 4.5×. The surgical microscope guarantees a more ergonomic working posture (Zaugg *et al*. 2004), optimal lighting of the operation area, and freely selectable magnification levels. These advantages are countered by increased expenses of the equipment and an extended learning phase for the surgeon and his assistant. In order to visualize lingual or palatal sites that are difficult to access, the microscope must have sufficient maneuverability. Recent developments have enabled direct viewing of oral operation aspects. By means of these optical devices, it will be possible to perform all periodontal interventions with the surgical microscope.

Instruments

Proper instrumentation is fundamental for microsurgical intervention. While various manufacturers have sets of microsurgical instruments, they are generally conceived for vascular and nerve surgery and, therefore, inappropriate for the use in plastic periodontal surgery. As the instruments are primarily manipulated by the thumb, index and middle finger, their handles should be round, yet provide traction so that finely controlled rotating movements can be executed. The rotating movement of the hand from two o'clock to seven o'clock (for right-handed persons) is the most precise movement the human body is able to perform. The instruments should be approximately 18 cm long and lie on the saddle between the operator's thumb and the index finger; they should be slightly top-heavy to facilitate accurate handling (Fig. 45-8). In order to avoid an unfavorable metallic glare under the light of the microscope, the instruments often have a coloured coating surface. The weight of each instrument should not exceed 15–20 g (0.15–0.20 N) in order to avoid hand and arm muscle fatigue. The needle holder should be equipped with

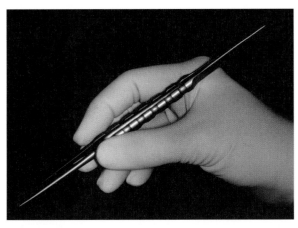

Fig. 45-8 Illustration demonstrating proper hand position for utilization of microsurgical instruments. Fine rotary movements which you get gripping the instrument like a pencil are needed for precise movements.

a precise working lock that should not exceed a locking force of 50 g (0.5–N). High locking forces generate tremor, and low locking forces reduce the feeling for movement.

Appropriate sets of steel or titanium instruments for periodontal surgery are available from different manufacturers. A basic set comprises a needle holder, micro scissors, micro scalpel holder, anatomic and surgical forceps, and a set of various elevators. In order to avoid sliding of the thread when tying the knot, the tips of the forceps have flat surfaces or can be finely coated with a diamond grain that improves the security by which the needle holder holds a surgical needle (Abidin *et al*. 1990). The configuration of the needle holder jaw has considerable influence on needle holding security. The presence of teeth in the tungsten carbide inserts provides the greatest deterrent to either twisting or rotating of the needle between the needle holder jaws. This benefit must be weighed against the potential damaging effects of the teeth on suture material. Smooth jaws without teeth cause no demonstrable damage to 6-0 monofilament nylon sutures, whereas needle holder jaws with teeth (7000/in^2) markedly reduce the suture breaking strength (Abidin *et al*. 1990). Additionally, the sharp outer edges of the needle holder jaws must be rounded to avoid breakage of fine suture materials (Abidin *et al*. 1989). When the needle holder jaws are closed, no light must pass through the tips. Locks aid in the execution of controlled rotation movements on the instrument handles without pressure. The tips of the forceps should be approximately 1–2 mm apart, when the instrument lies in the hand idly.

Various shapes and sizes of micro scalpels can be acquired from the discipline of ophthalmology or plastic surgery instrument sets and supplemented with fine instruments (fine chisels, raspatories, elevators, hooks, and suction) from conventional surgery.

In order to prevent damage, micro instruments are stored in a sterile container or tray. The tips of the instruments must not touch each other during sterilization procedures or transportation. The practice staff should be thoroughly instructed about the cleaning and maintenance of such instruments, as cleansing in a thermo disinfector without instrument fixation can irreparably damage the tip of these very expensive micro instruments.

Suture materials

Suture material and technique are essential factors to consider in microsurgery (Mackensen 1968). Wound closure is a key prerequisite for healing following surgical interventions and most important to avoid complications (Schreiber *et al*. 1975; Kamann *et al*. 1997). The most popular technique for wound closure is the use of sutures that stabilize the wound margins sufficiently and ensure proper closure over a defined period of time. However, the penetration of a needle through the soft tissue in itself causes a trauma, and the presence of foreign materials in a wound may significantly enhance the susceptibility to infection (Blomstedt *et al*. 1977; Österberg & Blomstedt 1979). Hence, it is obvious that needle and thread characteristics influence wound healing and surgical outcome.

Characteristics of the needle

The needle consists of a swage, body, and tip and differs concerning material, length, size, tip configuration, body diameter, and the nature of connection between needle and thread. In *atraumatic* sutures, the thread is firmly connected to the needle through a press-fit swage or stuck in a laser-drilled hole. There is no difference concerning stability between the two attachment modalities (Von Fraunhofer & Johnson 1992). The body of the needle should be flattened to prevent twisting or rotating in the needle holder. The needle tips differ widely depending on the specialty in which they are used. Tips of cutting needles are appropriate for coarse tissues or atraumatic penetration. In order to minimize tissue trauma in periodontal microsurgery, the sharpest needles, reverse cutting needles with precision tips or spatula needle with micro tips (Fig. 45-9), are preferred (Thacker *et al*. 1989).

The shape of the needle can be straight or bent to various degrees. For periodontal microsurgery, the 3/8″ circular needle generally ensures optimum results. There is a wide range of lengths, as measured along the needle curvature from the tip to the proximal end of the needle lock. For papillary sutures in the posterior area, needle lengths of 13–15 mm are appropriate. The same task in the front aspect requires needle lengths of 10–12 mm, and for closing a buccal releasing incision, needle lengths of 5–8 mm are adequate. To guarantee a perpendicular penetration through the soft tissues without tearing, an asymptotic curved needle is advantageous in areas where narrow penetrations are required (e.g. margins of gingivae, bases of papillae). To fulfil these prerequisites for ideal wound closure, at least two different

sutures are used in most surgical interventions. Table 45-2 serves as a basic guide to select the appropriate suture material.

Characteristics of the suture material

The suture material may be either *resorbable* or *non-resorbable* material. Within these two categories, the materials can be further divided into *monofilament* and *polyfilament* threads. The bacterial load of the oral cavity demands attention in the choice of the suture material. Generally, in the oral cavity the wound healing process is uneventful, hereby reducing the risk of infection caused by contamination of the thread. As polyfilament threads are characterized by a high capillarity, monofilament materials are to be preferred (Mouzas & Yeadon 1975). *Pseudomonofilaments* are coated polyfilament threads with the aim of reducing mechanical tissue trauma. During suturing the coating will break and the properties of the pseudomonofilament thread then corresponds to that of the polyfilament threads (Macht & Krizek 1978). Additionally, fragments of the coating may invade the surrounding tissues and elicit a foreign body reaction (Chu & Williams 1984).

Resorbable sutures
Resorbable threads may be categorized as *natural* or *synthetic*. Natural threads (i.e. surgical gut) are produced from intestinal mucosa of sheep or cattle. The twisted and polished thread loses its stability within 6–14 days by enzymatic breakdown (Meyer & Antonini 1989). Histologic examinations confirmed the inflammatory tissue reactions with a distinct infiltrate. For that reason, natural resorbable threads are generally obsolete (Bergenholtz & Isaksson 1967; Helpap *et al*. 1973; Levin 1980; Salthouse 1980).

Synthetic materials are advantageous due to their constant physical and biologic properties (Hansen 1986). The materials used belong to the polyamides, the polyolefines or the polyesters and disintegrate by hydration into alcohol and acid. Polyester threads are mechanically stable and, based on their different hydrolytic properties, lose their firmness in different,

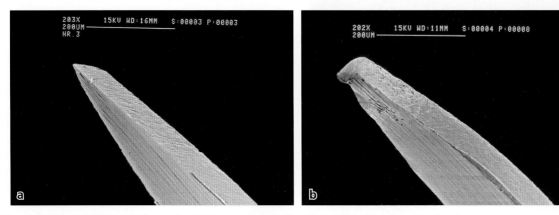

Fig. 45-9 (a) Intact sharp spatula needle. (b) Damaged needle tip after sticking into the enamel surface.

Table 45-2 Ideal needle–thread combinations (non-resorbable) for use in periodontal microsurgery

Indications	Suture gauge	Needle characteristics	Thread materials	Product name
Buccal releasing incisions	7-0	⅜ curvature, cutting needle with precision tip,	Polypropylene	Prolene®
	7-0	needle length 7.6 mm	Polypropylene	Prolene®
	9-0	asymptotic curved needle, cutting needle tip, round body, needle length 8.9 mm	Polyamide	Ethilon®
		⅜ curvature needle, spatula needle, needle length 5.2 mm		
Interdental sutures, front area	6-0	⅜ curvature, cutting needle with precision tip,	Polypropylene	Prolene®
	7-0	needle length 11.2 mm	Polyamide	Ethilon®
		⅜ curvature, cutting needle with precision tip, needle length 11.2 mm		
Interdental sutures, premolar area	6-0	⅜ curvature, cutting needle with precision tip,	Polyamide	Ethilon®
	6-0	needle length 12.9 mm	Polypropylene	Prolene®
		⅜ curvature, cutting needle with precision tip, needle length 12.9 mm		
Interdental suture, molar area	6-0	⅜ curvature, cutting needle, needle length 16.2 mm	Polyamide	Ethilon®
Crestal incisions	7-0	⅜ curvature, cutting needle with precision tip,	Polyamide	Ethilon®
	6-0	needle length 11.2 mm	Polypropylene	Prolene®
		⅜ curvature, cutting needle with precision tip, needle length 12.9 mm		
Papilla basis incisions	7-0	asymptotic curved needle, cutting needle tip,	Polypropylene	Prolene®
	9-0	round body, needle length 8.9 mm	Polyamide	Ethilon®
		½ curvature, cutting needle with micro tip, needle length 8.0 mm		

but constant times. A 50% reduction of breaking resistance can be expected after 2–3 weeks for polyglycolic acid and polyglactin threads, 4 weeks for polyglyconate, and 5 weeks for polydioxanone threads. The threads are available in twisted, polyfilament forms, and monofilament forms for finer suture materials. The capillary effect is limited and hardly exists for polyglactin sutures (Blomstedt & Österberg 1982).

Non-resorbable sutures

Polyamide is a commonly used material for fine monofilament threads (0.1–0.01 mm) that show adequate tissue properties. Tissue reactions seldom occur except after errors in the polymerization process (Nockemann 1981). Polyolefines, as a variation of choice, are inert materials that remain in the tissues without hydrolytic degradation (Salthouse 1980; Yu & Cavaliere 1983). Polypropylene and its newest development, polyhexafluoropropylene, are materials with excellent tissue properties. After suturing, the thread will be encapsulated in connective tissues and keep its stability for a longer period. In 5-0 and thicker gauges, the monofilament threads are relatively stiff and, for that reason, may impair patient comfort.

A substance with similar biologic, but improved handling properties, is polytetrafluoroethylene. Due to its porous surface structure, the monofilament

threads should only be used with restriction in the bacterially loaded oral cavity.

Intraoral tissue reactions around suture materials

The initial tissue reaction after suturing is a result of the penetration trauma, and reaches its culmination at the third post-operative day (Selvig et al. 1998). It is quite similar for resorbable and non-resorbable suture threads (Postlethwait & Smith 1975). Histologically, this early response is characterized by three zones of tissue alteration (Selvig et al. 1998): (1) an intensive cellular exudation in the immediate vicinity of the entry to the stitch canal, followed by (2) a concentric area, harboring damaged cells as well as intact tissue fragments, and (3) a wide zone of inflammatory cells in the surrounding connective tissues.

If a resorbable suture is left in situ for more than 2 weeks after wound closure, an acute inflammatory reaction still exists. This phenomenon is caused by bacteria entering the stitch canal and penetrating along the thread (Chu & Williams 1984; Selvig et al. 1998). The bacteriostatic effect of glycolic acid during the resorption process of polyglactin threads (Lilly et al. 1972) cannot be established (Thiede et al. 1980), and the resorption process of the polyglycolic thread is additionally inhibited by the acid environment caused by the infection (Postlethwait & Smith 1975).

Such studies confirm the increased risk for bacterial migration along the thread in the moist and bacterially loaded oral cavity. Experimental and clinical data indicate that most wound infections begin around suture material left within the wound (Edlich *et al.* 1974; Varma *et al.* 1974). Polyfilament threads additionally facilitate bacterial migration; bacteria can also penetrate into the inner compartment of the thread and evade the immunologic response of the host (Blomstedt *et al.* 1977; Haaf & Breuninger 1988). This is only one reason why monofilament, non-resorbable sutures should be preferred and removed at the earliest biologically acceptable time (Gutmann & Harrison 1991). The infectious potential can be further reduced by using an anti-infective therapy based on a daily rinsing or topical application of chlorhexidine (Leknes *et al.* 2005).

Another promising option to reduce bacterial migration along the suture is coating it with a bacteriostatic substance. Vicryl® Plus (Ethicon®, Norderstedt, Germany) is a resorbable suture material, coated with triclosan that inhibits bacterial growth for up to 6 days by damaging the membrane of the cells (Rothenburger *et al.* 2002; Storch *et al.* 2002).

Training concepts (surgeons and assistants)

The benefits of the operating microscope in periodontal surgery seem to be obvious. What then can be the reasons for the delay in taking advantage of periodontal surgery under the microscope? The main reason is that most surgeons do not adjust to the surgical microscope and those who have been using microscopes successfully, have not made adequate indepth practical recommendations to help other periodontal surgeons overcome their initial problems. Working with magnification changes the clinical settings as the visual direction during the surgical intervention does not meet the working ends of the instruments and the field of view has a smaller diameter. Additionally, the minimal size of tissue structures and suture threads requires a guidance of movement by visual rather than tactile control. This altered clinical situation requires an adjustment of the surgeon.

The three most common errors in the use of the surgical microscope are: (1) using magnification that is too high, (2) inadequate task sharing between surgeon and assistant, and (3) lack of practice.

High magnification

There is a tendency to use magnification which is too high. As described above, this is one of the fundamental optical principles: the higher the magnification, the narrower the field of vision and the smaller its depth. This concept is important because high magnification causes surgery to become more difficult, especially when it involves considerable movement. In these circumstances low magnification of 4–7× should be used. On the other hand, higher magnification of 10–15× may be useful when dissecting within a small area requiring less movement, e.g. in papilla preservation techniques. In general, the magnification should be that which allows the surgeons to operate with ease, and without increasing their usual operating time for a particular surgical procedure. Surgical time does not have to be increased once the surgeon has adapted fully to the microscope. The more experienced and skilled surgeons are with the microscope, the higher the magnification they can use with ease.

It may take 6 months or more for surgeons to be familiar with magnification of 10×, which usually is the maximum used in plastic periodontal surgery. A point of diminishing returns will eventually be reached where the advantages of increased magnification are outweighed by the disadvantages of a narrower field of vision.

Task sharing between surgeon and assistant (teamwork)

In microendodontics, during root canal treatment, the whole procedure is performed with a minimum amount of position changes of the operating persons. Focusing can easily be achieved by moving the mirror towards or away from the objective lenses. In periodontal surgery both hands are used to hold the instruments and position changes are more frequently required which increase the demands on the operating team and require for an ideal cooperation between surgeon and assistant.

In all surgeries at least two operating persons are involved: a surgeon and an assistant, who assists the surgeon in the most rudimentary tasks in the operation. However, the tasks that the assistant constantly repeats in almost all operations with varying levels of skill will be taken into consideration. These tasks include: flap retraction, suction, rinsing, and cutting the sutures. To guarantee a continuous work flow during the surgical intervention, a second assistant who organizes the instruments is frequently desirable.

In periodontal microsurgery, where there is inherently very little access enjoyed by the surgeon, retraction is absolutely vital. Retraction should be done in different positions and must be devoid of all tremor or movement. This is an exceptionally strenuous task as the human assistant is expected to maintain the same posture for up to 1 hour. This is extremely energy consuming and the fatigue experienced by the assistant increases the chances of tremor as time goes by.

For an optimal work flow, magnification is also required for the assistant. An assistant wearing loupes has the advantage of an open peripheral vision to arrange the instruments and to check the patient's facial expression during the operation. On the other hand, co-observer tubes allow the same view for surgeon and assistant, enabling the assistant to point the suction tube to the right place and keep the view clear. This also becomes an issue during suturing when the air intake of the suction tube can easily suck the fine threads.

Lack of practice

When working with high magnification, the surgeon has to adjust to being a prisoner within a narrow field of view. A new coordination has to be sought between the surgeon's eyes and hands – an adjustment which can come only after much regular practice with simple surgical procedures. The practice unit consists of a microscope, micro instruments, and different suitable models. To start training, a two-dimensional model, such as rubber dam, is appropriate to learn how to manipulate the instruments, how to pick up the needles, and tying knots. After the initial training, working with three-dimensional models (fruits, eggs, chicken) helps the surgeon to get used to the restricted depth of the field.

Another aim of training is the reduction of tremor. Its physiologic basis is uncertain, but it is important to be aware of the causes in order to prevent it. An important factor is the body posture, which must be natural, with the spinal column straight and the forearms and hands fully supported. An adjustable chair, preferably with wheels, is recommended for the surgeon who should place himself in the most comfortable position. Tremor varies with individuals and even in the same individual it varies under different conditions. In some people, intake of coffee, tea or alcohol may increase tremor; in others, emotions, physical exercise, or the carrying of heavy weights can cause it.

After the completion of appropriate training when instrument handling has become automatic, the surgeon has adjusted to the new conditions and can now fully concentrate on the surgical procedure in clinical practice without taking additional time.

Clinical indications and limitations

The clinical benefits of a microsurgical approach in periodontal practice are mainly evaluated by case reports (Shanelec & Tibbetts 1994, 1996; Michaelides 1996; de Campos *et al.* 2006) and case–cohort studies (Cortellini & Tonetti 2001; Wachtel *et al.* 2003; Francetti *et al.* 2004). The different procedures described apply to the surgical coverage of buccal root recessions and flap closure after regenerative interventions. In both interventions, delicate soft tissue structures have to be manipulated during the surgery, which could be refined by selecting a less traumatic surgical approach. All of the studies confirmed the beneficial effects of the microsurgical approach. When covering a root recession, the vascularization of the injured tissues becomes critical as there is no blood supply from the underlying root surface. Frequently, coverage is performed by a con-

nective tissue graft from the palate, which has different vascular characteristics compared to the supracrestal gingiva; supracrestal gingiva is the only tissue, naturally created and specifically designed, to survive and function over avascular root surfaces. As graft survival depends upon early plasmatic diffusion (Oliver *et al.* 1968; Nobutu *et al.* 1988), firm and stable flap or graft adaptation is of crucial importance to minimize the coagulum and facilitate the ingrowth of new vessels. A minimally traumatic approach allows more precise flap preparation and suturing with a reduction in tissue and vessel injuries, resulting in more rapid and more complete anastomosis of new capillary buds from the recipient bed with the existing, but severed, vessels of the graft or the flap.

The interdental gingiva is also a delicate tissue with a limited vascular network. As the gingival plexus does not extend interproximally, the central part of the interdental soft tissue is only supplied by vessels from the periodontal ligament space and arterioles that emerge from the crest of the interdental septa (Folke & Stallard 1967; Nuki & Hock 1974). These anatomic factors influence the wound-healing capacity of the tissues after surgical dissection and the small size of the structures (i.e. papilla or col) complicates a precise adaptation of the flap margins. Wound dehiscences, resulting in healing by secondary intention, are therefore a common finding after suturing the papilla in papilla-preservation techniques (Tonetti *et al.* 2004). Using microsurgery for a modified or simplified papilla preservation flap, primary wound closure could be noted in 92.3% of all treated sites 6 weeks after the intervention (Cortellini & Tonetti 2001).

Historic comparisons with studies performed by the same authors without the use of an operating microscope showed a clear advantage in the use of a microsurgical approach. Complete primary wound closure was observed in only 67% of the cases treated with a simplified (Cortellini *et al.* 1999), and in 73% of the cases treated with a modified papilla preservation flap (Cortellini *et al.* 1995). These results clearly demonstrated the improvement in tissue preservation and handling using a minimally invasive approach in order to achieve primary closure of the interdental space (Fig. 45-10).

A recently published case–cohort study, evaluating a new flap design for regeneration with enamel matrix derivates (MIST, *minimally invasive surgical technique*) combined with microsurgical techniques, confirmed the previous positive results, yielding a primary wound closure of the interdental tissues in all of the treated sites, 6 weeks post-operatively (Cortellini & Tonetti 2007) (Fig. 45-11).

Subjective observations of clinicians have found there is a less traumatic approach in periodontal surgery when magnification aids and fine suture materials are used. This ensures passive wound closure in most surgical interventions. This speculation was recently substantiated by an *in vitro* experiment, which evaluated the tearing characteristics of mucosal tissue samples for various suture sizes and needle characteristics in relation to the applied tension forces (Burkhardt *et al.* 2006). The pig jaw mucosal tissue samples were attached in a test-tearing apparatus of a Swiss textile company and the tension tearing diagrams were traced for 3-0, 5-0, 6-0, and 7-0 sutures with forces up to 20 N. While the 3-0 sutures almost exclusively led to tissue breakage at an average of 13.4 N, the 7-0 sutures broke before tissues were torn in every instance, at an applied mean force of 3.6 N. With 5-0 and 6-0 sutures both events occured at random, at a mean force of 10 N. This means that a clinician can influence the amount of damage to the tissue by selecting thicker or thinner suture material. Considering this fact, it may be speculated that wound dehiscence can be prevented and passive flap adaptation can be improved by the choice of thinner sutures; this inevitably requires magnification if its benefits are to be fully appreciated.

The opponents of periodontal microsurgery often mention the adverse effect of a prolonged duration of the intervention while working with microscopes.

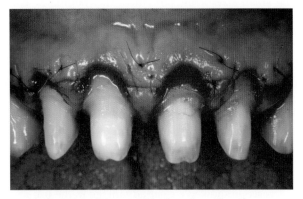

Fig. 45-10 Primary closure of the buccal papillae after a crown-lengthening procedure. Modified mattress sutures (vertically everting) with 7-0 polyamide thread (black) and two single-knot closures with 8-0 polypropylene threads (blue) in each interdental area.

It has been shown that the incidence and severity of complications and pain following periodontal surgery are correlated well with the duration of the surgical procedure (Curtis *et al.* 1985). It may be speculated that an extended operation time may compensate for the beneficial treatment effect of minimally invasive techniques. However, studies comparing micro- and macrosurgical approaches did not support such a hypothesis (Burkhardt & Lang 2005).

Considering all these facts there are no clinical contraindications for the use of magnification in periodontal surgery. From a user's point of view, only few areas in the oral cavity are difficult to access by an operating microscope which may limit its application. In these circumstances and in surgical interventions which require a frequent change of position, the use of loupes may be preferable.

Comparison to conventional mucogingival interventions

Today's *plastic periodontal surgery*, evolving from *mucogingival surgery*, includes all surgical procedures performed to prevent or correct anatomic, developmental, traumatic or disease-induced defects of the gingiva, alveolar mucosa or bone (Proceedings of the World Workshop in Periodontics 1996). To verify the beneficial effects of a microsurgical approach, the results after using a conventional technique in all the different indications have to be evaluated first. The variables to be used as descriptors of the therapeutic end-point of success may vary, depending on the specific goal of the mucogingival therapy. Some results, such as volume changes after ridge augmentation procedures, are clinically difficult to assess due to a lack of a defined end-point and are therefore documented in the literature by qualitative measurements only. Plastic surgical interventions with clearly defined landmarks for measurement, and thus well investigated in the literature, are the guided tissue regeneration procedures (Needleman *et al.* 2006) and the coverage of buccal root recessions (Roccuzzo

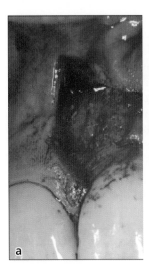
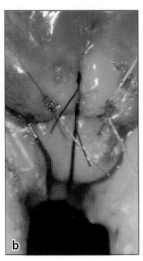
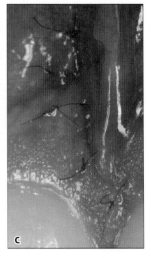

Fig. 45-11 Minimally invasive surgical technique (MIST) (Cortellini & Tonetti 2007). (a) Releasing incision, ending right-angled at the gingival margin. (b) Primary closure of the buccal papilla by a mattress suture (according to Laurell) with 7-0 polyamide thread (black) and two single-knot closures with 8-0 polypropylene threads (blue). (c) Clinical appearance of the releasing incision 4 days post-operatively.

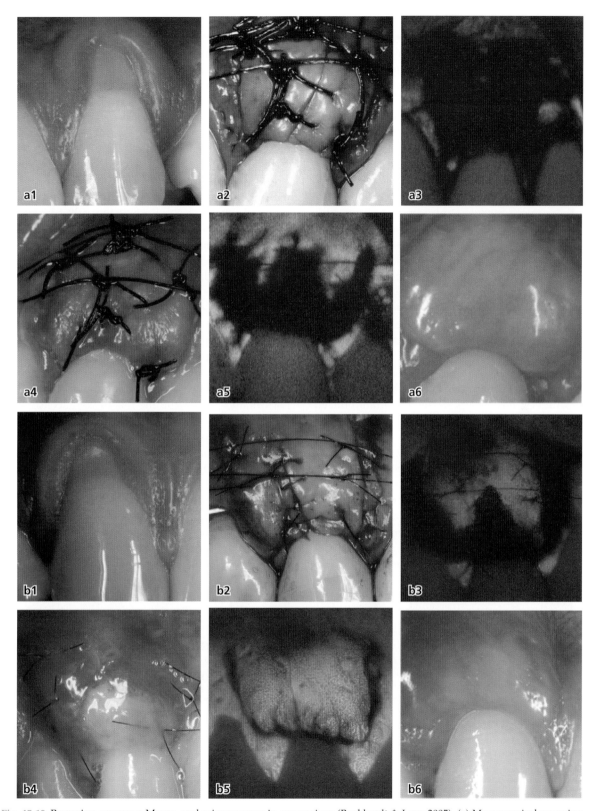

Fig. 45-12 Recession coverage: Macro- and microsurgery in comparison (Burkhardt & Lang 2005). (a) Macrosurgical recession coverage: (a1) pre-operative clinical situation; (a2) immediately after the surgical intervention; (a3) corresponding angiographic evaluation after the intervention; (a4) healing after 7 days; (a5) angiographic evaluation after 7 days; (a6) clinical situation after 3 months (visible contours of incision lines). (b) Microsurgical recession coverage: (b1) pre-operative clinical situation; (b2) immediately after the surgical intervention; (b3) corresponding angiographic evaluation after the intervention; (b4) healing after 7 days; (b5) angiographic evaluation after 7 days; (b6) clinical situation after 3 months (no traces of the intervention visible).

et al. 2002; Oates *et al.* 2003). While the former results in a reduction in probing measures, an improved attachment gain, and less increase in gingival recession compared to open flap debridement, the latter yields a significant reduction in recession depth and also an improvement in clinical attachment level measures. However there is a marked variability between the studies, indicating the influence of case selection, the materials used, the techniques applied, and the surgeons' dexterity. As a result, it is difficult to draw general conclusions because the factors affecting the outcomes are unclear from the literature and these might include study conduct issues such as bias. Among these factors, the dexterity of the surgeon ranks high and seems to influence the results strongly. It is a complicated, proprioceptive reflex involving eye, hand, and brain, and is therefore difficult to assess in clinical settings. To eliminate its influence and to estimate the magnitude of the real benefits of a microsurgical approach, micro- and macrosurgical techniques should be compared in controlled studies.

Concerning the coverage of mucosal recessions, a comparison between the two approaches (micro- and macrosurgery) has been performed in a randomized controlled clinical trial (Burkhardt & Lang 2005). The study population consisted of ten patients with bilateral class I and class II recessions at maxillary canines. In split-mouth design, the defects were randomly selected for recession coverage either by a microsurgical (test) or macrosurgical (control) approach. Immediately after the surgical procedures and after 3 and 7 days of healing, fluorescent angiograms were performed to evaluate graft vascularization. The results at test sites revealed a vascularization of 8.9 ± 1.9% immediately after the procedure. After 3 days and after 7 days, the vascularization rose to 53.3 ± 10.5% and 84.8 ± 13.5%, respectively. The corresponding vascularization at control sites were 7.95 ± 1.8%, 44. 5 ± 5.7%, and 64.0 ± 12.3%, respectively (Fig. 45-12). All the differences between test and control sites were statistically significant.

In addition, the clinical parameters were assessed before the surgical intervention, and 1, 3, 6, and 12 months post-operatively. The clinical measurement revealed a mean recession coverage of 99.4 ± 1.7% for the test and 90.8 ± 12.1% for the control sites after the first month of healing. Again, this difference was statistically significant. The percentage of root coverage in both test and control sites remained stable during the first year, at 98% and 90%, respectively.

The present clinical experiment has clearly demonstrated that mucogingival surgical procedures designed for the coverage of exposed root surfaces, performed using a microsurgical approach, improved the treatment outcomes substantially and to a clinically relevant level when compared with the clinical performance under routine macroscopic conditions. However, the choice of micro- and macrosurgical approaches must be seen in different lights, including treatment outcomes, logistics, cost, and patient-centered parameters. Future comparative studies will produce the evidence whether the use of the surgical microscope will further increase surgical effectiveness and thus become an indispensable part of periodontal surgical practice.

References

Abidin, M.R., Towler, M.A., Thacker, J.G., Nochimson, G.D, McGregor, W. & Edlich, R.F. (1989). New atraumatic rounded-edge surgical needle holder jaws. *American Journal of Surgery* **157**, 241–242.

Abidin, M.R., Dunlapp, J.A., Towler, M.A., Becker, D.G., Thacker, J.G., McGregor, W. & Edlich, R.F. (1990). Metallurgically bonded needle holder jaws. A technique to enhance needle holding security without sutural damage. *The American Surgeon* **56**, 643–647.

Apotheker, H. & Jako, G.J. (1981). Microscope for use in dentistry. *Journal of Microsurgery* **3**, 7–10.

Basset, S. (1983). Back problems amoung dentists. *Journal of the Canadian Dental Association* **49**, 251–256.

Baumann, R.R. (1977). How may the dentist benefit from the operating microscope? *Quintessence International* **5**, 17–18.

Bergenholtz, A. & Isaksson, B. (1967). Tissue reactions in the oral mucosa to catgut, silk and Mersilene sutures. *Odontologisk Revy* **18**, 237–250.

Blomstedt, B., Österberg, B. & Bergstrand, A. (1977). Suture material and bacterial transport. An experimental study. *Acta Chirurgica Scandinavica* **143**, 71–73.

Blomstedt, B. & Österberg, B. (1982). Physical properties of suture materials which influence wound infection. In: Thiede, A. & Hamelmann, H., eds. *Moderne Nahtmaterialien und Nahttechniken in der Chirurgie.* Berlin: Springer.

Buncke, H.J. & Schulz, W.P. (1965). Experimental digital amputation and reimplantation. *Journal of Plastic and Reconstructive Surgery* **36**, 62–70.

Buncke, H.J. & Rose, E.H. (1979). Free toe-to-fingertip neurovascular flap. *Plastic and Reconstructive Surgery* **63**, 607–612.

Burkhardt, R. & Hürzeler, M.B. (2000). Utilization of the surgical microscope for advanced plastic periodontal surgery. *Practical Periodontics and Aesthetic Dentistry* **12**, 171–180.

Burkhardt, R. & Lang, N.P. (2005). Coverage of localized gingival recessions: comparison of micro- and macrosurgical techniques. *Journal of Periodontology* **32**, 287–293.

Burkhardt, R., Preiss, A., Joss, A. & Lang, N.P. (2006). Influence of suture tension to the tearing characteristics of the soft tissues – an *in vitro* experiment. *Clinical Oral Implants Research*, accepted for publication.

Burton, J.F. & Bridgeman, G.F. (1990). Presbyopia and the dentist: the effect of age on clinical vision. *International Dental Journal* **40**, 303–311.

Burton, J.F. & Bridgeman, G.F. (1991). Eyeglasses to maintain flexibility of vision for the older dentist: the Otago dental lookover. *Quintessence International* **22**, 879–882.

Carr, G.B. (1992). Microscopes in endodontics. *Californian Dental Association Journal* **20**, 55–61.

Chu, C.C. & Williams, D.G. (1984). Effects of physical configuration and chemical structure of suture materials on bacterial adhesion. *American Journal of Surgery* **147**, 197–204.

Cobbett, J.R. (1969). Free digital transfer. *Journal of Bone and Joint Surgery* **51B**, 677–679.

Coburn, D.G. (1984). Vision, posture and productivity. *Oral Health* **74**, 13–15.

Cortellini, P., Pini Prato, G. & Tonetti, M. (1999). The modified papilla preservation technique. A new surgical approach for interproximal regenerative procedures. *Journal of Periodontology* **66**, 261–266.

Cortellini, P., Pini Prato, G. & Tonetti, M. (1999). The simplified papilla preservation flap. A novel surgical approach for the management of soft tissues in regenerative procedures. *International Journal of Periodontics and Restorative Dentistry* **19**, 589–599.

Cortellini, P. & Tonetti, M.S. (2001). Microsurgical approach to periodontal regeneration. Initial evaluation in a case cohort. *Journal of Periodontology* **72**, 559–569.

Cortellini, P. & Tonetti, M. (2007). A minimally invasive surgical technique with an enamel matrix derivate in regenerative treatment of intrabony defects: a novel approach to limit morbidity. *Journal of Clinical Periodontology* **34**, 87–93.

Curtis, J.W., McLain, J.B. & Hutchinson, R.A. (1985). The incidence and severity of complications and pain following periodontal surgery. *Journal of Periodontology* **56**, 597–601.

Diakkow, P.R. (1984). Back pain in dentists. *Journal of Manipulative and Physiological Therapeutics* **7**, 85–88.

De Campos, G.V., Bittencourt, S., Sallum, A.W., Nociti Jr., F.H., Sallum, E.A. & Casati, M.Z. (2006). Achieving primary closure and enhancing aesthetics with periodontal microsurgery. *Practical Procedures and Aesthetic Dentistry* **18**, 449–454.

Donaghy, R.M.P. & Yasargil, M.G. (1967). *Microvascular Surgery.* Stuttgart: Thieme, pp. 98–115.

Edlich, R.F., Panek, P.H., Rodeheaver, G.T., Kurtz, L.D. & Egerton, M.D. (1974). Surgical sutures and infection: a biomaterial evaluation. *Journal of Biomedical Materials Research* **8**, 115–126.

Folke, L.E.A. & Stallard, R.E. (1967). Periodontal microcirculation as revealed by plastic microspheres. *Journal of Periodontal Research* **2**, 53–63.

Foucher, G. (1991). Partial toe-to-hand transfer. In: Meyer, V.E. & Black, J.M., eds. *Hand and Upper Limb, Vol. 8: Microsurgical Procedures.* Edinburgh: Churchill Livingstone, pp. 45–67.

Francetti, L., Del Fabbro, M., Testori, T. & Weinstein, R.L. (2004). Periodontal microsurgery: report of 16 cases consecutively treated by the free rotated papilla autograft technique combined with the coronally advanced flap. *International Journal of Periodontics and Restorative Dentistry* **24**, 272–279.

Friedman, A., Lustmann, J. & Shaharabany, V. (1991). Treatment results of apical surgery in premolar and molar teeth. *Journal of Endodontics* **17**, 30–33.

Friedman, M.J. & Landesman, H.M. (1997). Microscope-assisted precision dentistry – advancing excellence in restorative dentistry. *Contemporary Esthetics and the Restorative Practice* **1**, 45–49.

Friedman, M.J. & Landesman, H.M. (1998). Microscope-assisted precision dentistry (MAP) – a challenge for new knowledge. *Californian Dental Association Journal* **26**, 900–905.

Gutmann, J.L. & Harrison, J.W. (1991). *Surgical Endodontics.* Boston: Blackwell Scientific, pp. 278–299.

Haaf, U. & Breuninger, H. (1988). Resorbierbares Nahtmaterial in der menschlichen Haut: Gewebereaktion und modifizierte Nahttechnik. *Der Hautarzt* **39**, 23–27.

Hansen, H. (1986). Nahtmaterialien. *Der Chirurg* **57**, 53–57.

Helpap, B., Staib, I., Seib, U., Osswald, J. & Hartung, H. (1973). Tissue reaction of parenchymatous organs following implantation of conventionally and radiation sterilized catgut. *Brun's Beiträge für Klinische Chirurgie* **220**, 323–333.

Jacobsen, J.H. & Suarez, E.L. (1960). Microsurgery in anastomosis of small vessels. *Surgical Forum* **11**, 243–245.

Kamann, W.A., Grimm, W.D., Schmitz, I. & Müller, K.M. (1997). Die chirurgische Naht in der Zahnheilkunde. *Parodontologie* **4**, 295–310.

Kanca, J. & Jordan, P.G. (1995). Magnification systems in clinical dentistry. *Journal of Dentistry* **61**, 851–856.

Kim, S., Pecora, G. & Rubinstein, R.A. (2001). Comparison of traditional and microsurgery in endodontics. In: *Color Atlas of Microsurgery in Endodontics.* Philadelphia: W.B. Saunders Company, pp. 1–12.

Komatsu, S. & Tamai, S. (1968). Successful replantation of a completely cut-off thumb. *Journal of Plastic and Reconstructive Surgery* **42**, 374–377.

Leknes, K.N., Selvig, K.A., Bøe, O.E. & Wikesjö, U.M.E. (2005). Tissue reactions to sutures in the presence and absence of anti-infective therapy. *Journal of Clinical Periodontology* **32**, 130–138.

Leknius, C. & Geissberger, M. (1995). The effect of magnification on the performance of fixed prosthodontic prcedures. *Californian Dental Association Journal* **23**, 66–70.

Levin, M.R. (1980). Periodontal suture materials and surgical dressings. *Dental Clinics of North America* **24**, 767–781.

Lilly, G.E., Cutcher, J.L., Jones, J.C. & Armstrong, J.H. (1972). Reaction of oral tissues to suture materials. *Oral Surgery Oral Medicine Oral Pathology* **33**, 152–157.

Macht, S.D. & Krizek, T.J. (1978). Sutures and suturing – current concepts. *Journal of Oral Surgery* **36**, 710–712.

Mackensen, G. (1968). Suture material and technique of suturing in microsurgery. *Bibliotheca Ophthalmologica* **77**, 88–95.

Meyer, R.D. & Antonini, C.J. (1989). A review of suture materials, Part I. *Compendium of Continuing Education in Dentistry* **10**, 260–265.

Michaelides, P.L. (1996). Use of the operating microscope in dentistry. *Journal of the Californian Dental Association* **24**, 45–50.

Millesi, H. (1979). Microsurgery of peripheral nerves. *World Journal of Surgery* **3**, 67–79.

Mora, A.F. (1998). Restorative microdentistry: A new standard for the twenty first century. *Prosthetic Dentistry Review* **1**, Issue 3.

Morrison, W.A., O'Brien, B.McC. & MacLeod, A.M. (1980). Thumb reconstruction with a free neurovascular wrap-around flap from the big toe. *Journal of Hand Surgery* **5**, 575–583.

Mounce, R. (1995). Surgical operating microscope in endodontics: The paradigm shift. *General Dentistry* **43**, 346–349.

Mouzas, G.L. & Yeadon, A. (1975). Does the choice of suture material affect the incidence of wound infection? *British Journal of Surgery* **62**, 952–955.

Needleman, I.G., Worthington, H.V., Giedrys-Leeper, E. & Tucker, R.J. (2006). Guided tissue regeneration for periodontal infrabony defects. *Cochrane Database of Systematic Reviews* **19**, CD001724.

Nobutu, T., Imai, H. & Yamaoka, A. (1988). Microvascularization of the free gingival autograft. *Journal of Periodontology* **59**, 639–646.

Nockemann, P.F. (1981). Wound healing and management of wounds from the point of view of plastic surgery operations in gynecology. *Gynäkologe* **14**, 2–13.

Nuki, K. & Hock, J. (1974). The organization of the gingival vasculature. *Journal of Periodontal Research* **9**, 305–313

Nylén, C.O. (1924). An oto-microscope. *Acta Otolaryngology* **5**, 414–416.

Oates, T.W., Robinson, M. & Gunsolley, J.C. (2003). Surgical therapies for the treatment of gingival recession. A systematic review. *Annals of Periodontology* **8**, 303–320.

Oliver, R.C., Löe, H. & Karring, T. (1968). Microscopic evaluation of the healing and revascularization of free gingival grafts. *Journal of Periodontal Research* **3**, 84–95.

Österberg, B. & Blomstedt, B. (1979). Effect of suture materials on bacterial survival in infected wounds. An experimental study. *Acta Chirurgica Scandinavica* **143**, 431–434.

Pecora, G. & Andreana, S. (1993). Use of dental operating microscope in endodontic surgery. *Oral Surgery, Oral Medicine, Oral Pathology* **75**, 751–758.

Postlethwait, R.W. & Smith, B. (1975). A new synthetic absorbable suture. *Surgery, Gynecology and Obstetrics* **140**, 377–380.

Proceedings of the World Workshop on Periodontics (1996). Consensus report on mucogingival therapy. *Annals of Periodontology* **1**, 702–706.

Roccuzzo, M., Bunino, M., Needleman, I. & Sanz, M. (2002). Periodontal plastic surgery for treatment of localized gingival recessions: a systematic review. *Journal of Clinical Periodontology* **29** (Suppl 3), 178–194.

Rothenburger, S., Spangler, D., Bhende, S. & Burkley, D. (2002). In vitro antimicrobial evaluation of coated VICRYL Plus antibacterial suture (coated polyglactin 910 with triclosan) using zone of inhibition assays. *Surgical Infections* **3** (Suppl 1), 79–87.

Rubinstein, R.A. (1997). The anatomy of the surgical operation microscope and operation positions. *Dental Clinics of North America* **41**, 391–413.

Rubinstein, R.A. & Kim, S. (1999). Short-term observation of the results of endodontic surgery with the use of a surgical operation microscope and Super EBA as root-end filling material. *Journal of Endodontics* **25**, 43–48.

Rubinstein, R.A. & Kim, S. (2002). Short-term follow-up of cases considered healed one year after microsurgery. *Journal of Endodontics* **28**, 378–383.

Ruddle, C.J. (1994). Endodontic perforation repair using the surgical operating microscope. *Dentistry Today* **5**, 49–53.

Salthouse, T.N. (1980). Biologic response to sutures. *Otolaryngological Head and Neck Surgery* **88**, 658–664.

Schreiber, H.W., Eichfuss, H.P. & Farthmann, E. (1975). Chirurgisches Nahtmaterial in der Bauchhöhle. *Der Chirurg* **46**, 437–443.

Seldon, H.S. (2002). The dental-operating microscope and its slow acceptance. *Journal of Endodontics* **28**, 206–207.

Selvig, K.A., Biagotti, G.R., Leknes, K.N. & Wikesjö, U.M. (1998). Oral tissue reactions to suture materials. *International Journal of Periodontics and Restorative Dentistry* **18**, 475–487.

Shanelec, D.A. (1991). Current trends in soft tissue. *Californian Dental Association Journal* **19**, 57–60.

Shanelec, D.A. (1992). Optical principles of loupes. *Californian Dental Association Journal* **20**, 25–32.

Shanelec, D.A. & Tibbetts, L.S. (1994). Periodontal microsurgery. *Periodontal Insights* **1**, 4–7.

Shanelec, D.A. & Tibbetts, L.S. (1996). A perspective on the future of periodontal microsurgery. *Periodontology 2000* **11**, 58–64.

Shugars, D., Miller, D. & Williams, D., Fishburne, C. & Strickland, D. (1987). Musculoskeletal pain among general dentists. *General Dentistry* **34**, 272–276.

Smith , J.W. (1964). Microsurgery of peripheral nerves. *Journal of Plastic and Reconstructive Surgery* **33**, 317–319.

Storch, M., Perry, L.C., Davidson, J.M. & Ward, J.J. (2002). A 28-day study of the effect of coated VICRYL Plus antibacterial suture (coated polyglactin 910 with triclosan) on wound healing in guinea pig linear incisional skin wounds. *Surgical Infections* **3** (Suppl 1), 89–98.

Strassler, H.E. (1989). Seeing the way to better care. *Dentist* **4**, 22–25.

Strassler, H.E., Syme, S.E., Serio, F. & Kaim, J.M. (1998). Enhanced visualization during dental practice using magnification systems. *Compendium of Continuing Education in Dentistry* **19**, 595–611.

Tamai, S. (1993). History of microsurgery – from the beginning until the end of the 1970s. *Microsurgery* **14**, 6–13.

Thacker, J.G., Rodeheaver, G.T. & Towler, M.A. (1989). Surgical needle sharpness. *American Journal of Surgery* **157**, 334–339.

Thiede, A., Jostarndt, L., Lünstedt, B. & Sonntag, H.G. (1980). Kontrollierte experimentelle, histologische und mikrobiologische Untersuchungen zur Hemmwirkung von Polyglykolsäurefäden bei Infektionen. *Der Chirurg* **51**, 35–38.

Tibbetts, L.S. & Shanelec, D.A. (1994). An overview of periodontal microsurgery. *Current Opinion in Periodontology* **2**, 187–193.

Tonetti, M.S., Fourmousis, I., Suvan, J., Cortellini, P., Brägger, U. & Lang, N.P. (2004). Healing, postoperative morbidity and patient perception of outcomes following regenerative therapy of deep intrabony defects. *Journal of Clinical Periodontology* **31**, 1092–1098.

Varma, S., Ferguson, H.L., Breen, H. & Lumb, W.V. (1974). Comparison of seven suture materials in infected wounds – an experimental study. *Journal of Surgical Research* **17**, 165–170.

Von Fraunhofer, J.A. & Johnson, J.D. (1992). A new surgical needle for periodontology. *General Dentistry* **5**, 418–420.

Wachtel, H., Schenk, G., Bohm, S., Weng, D., Zuhr, O. & Hürzeler, M.B. (2003). Microsurgical access flap and enamel matrix derivate for the treatment of periodontal intrabony defects: a controlled clinical study. *Journal of Clinical Periodontology* **30**, 496–504.

Yu, G.V. & Cavaliere, R. (1983). Suture materials, properties and uses. *Journal of the American Podiatry Association* **73**, 57–64.

Zaugg, B., Stassinakis, A. & Hotz, P. (2004). Influence of magnification tools on the recognition of artificial preparation and restoration defects. *Schweizerische Monatsschrift für Zahnmedizin* **114**, 890–896.

Zhong-Wei, C., Meyer, V.E., Kleinert, H.E. & Beasley, R.W. (1981). Present indications and contraindications for replantation as reflected by long-term functional results. *Orthopedic Clinics of North America* **12**, 849–870.

Chapter 46

Re-osseointegration

Tord Berglundh and Jan Lindhe

Introduction, 1045
Is it possible to resolve a marginal hard tissue defect adjacent to an oral implant?, 1045
   Non-contaminated, pristine implants at sites with a wide marginal gap (crater), 1045
   Contaminated implants and crater-shaped bone defects, 1046
Re-osseointegration, 1046

Is re-osseointegration a feasible outcome of regenerative therapy?, 1046
   Regeneration of bone from the walls of the defect, 1046
   "Rejuvenate" the contaminated implant surface, 1047
Is the quality of the implant surface important in a healing process that may lead to re-osseointegration?, 1048
   The surface of the metal device in the compromised implant site, 1048

Introduction

In Chapter 24 (Peri-implant Mucositis and Peri-implantitis) important features of inflammatory lesions in the peri-implant tissues were described. Peri-implantitis is defined as a progressive inflammatory process that involves the mucosa and the bone tissue at an osseointegrated implant in function, and that this process results in loss of osseointegration and supporting bone (Fig. 46-1).

In Chapter 41 (Treatment of Peri-implant Lesions) it is emphasized that peri-implantitis is associated with the presence of submarginal deposits of plaque and calculus and that the successful treatment of the condition must include (1) comprehensive debridement of the implant surface and (2) subsequent interceptive supportive therapy including professional and self-performed plaque removal measures.

An obvious, additional goal in the treatment of peri-implantitis is the regeneration and *de novo* bone formation, i.e. "re-osseointegration", at the portion of the implant that lost its "osseointegration" in the inflammatory process. Furthermore, since the level of the peri-implant mucosa is dependent on the level of the marginal bone, an increase of the height of the osseous tissue will result in a marginal shift of the mucosa. Soft tissue esthetics may also be enhanced, therefore, through re-osseointegration.

Is it possible to resolve a marginal hard tissue defect adjacent to an oral implant?

Non-contaminated, pristine implants at sites with a wide marginal gap (crater)

Peri-implantitis lesions are per definition associated with bone loss and loss of osseointegration. The pattern of bone loss is angular and the ensuing defect often has the shape of a marginally open crater.

Findings from animal experiments and fracture healing suggested that hard tissue bridging, through woven bone formation, may occur in a bone defect provided that the distance between the fracture lines was ≤1 mm (Schenk & Willenegger 1977). This concept was translated to implant dentistry. Thus, it was implied that if a large (>1 mm) marginal defect were present between a newly installed oral implant and the host bone of the alveolar process, osseointegration would become compromised (Wilson *et al.* 1998, 2003).

Results presented by Botticelli *et al.* (2004) challenged this hypothesis. In a human study that included implant placement in fresh extraction sockets, they were able to demonstrate that a large void (gap) between the newly installed implant and the socket walls could become completely resolved

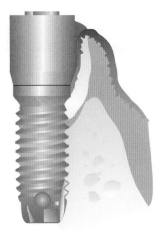

Fig. 46-1 Schematic drawing illustrating characteristics of peri-implantitis including the inflammatory lesion and the associated bone defect.

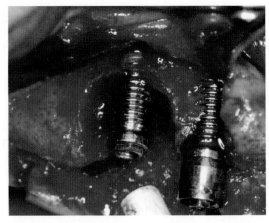

Fig. 46-2 Clinical photograph from a peri-implantitis site following flap elevation. Granulation tissue was removed and the implant surface was cleaned. The decision on whether a regenerative procedure may be considered is based on the morphology of the crater-like bone defect.

within a 4-month period. Furthermore, in animal experiments Botticelli *et al.* (2003a,b, 2005, 2006) produced – by mechanical means – large hard tissue defects in the marginal portion of edentulous sites prior to implant installation. The authors reported that (1) the presence of the wide marginal defect *per se* was not an impediment for osseointegration, (2) depending on the surface characteristics of the implant, complete resolution of the defect occurred within a 4-month period, and (3) bone fill in the defect was always the result of appositional osteogenesis.

Contaminated implants and crater-shaped bone defects

Experimental model

In order to study the ability of the tissues in the peri-implant defect to regenerate and to establish *de novo* bone tissue deposition on the contaminated implant surface, a research model was developed. The model was used to induce well defined peri-implantitis lesions in the dog (Lindhe *et al.* 1992) or in the monkey (Lang *et al.* 1993; Schou *et al.* 1993) and is described in detail in Chapter 24.

Re-osseointegration

"Re-osseointegration" can be defined as the establishment of *de novo* bone formation and *de novo* osseointegration to a portion of an implant that during the development of peri-implantitis suffered loss of bone-to-implant contact and became exposed to microbial colonization (alt. the oral environment) (Fig. 46-2). A treatment procedure that aims at re-osseointgration must (1) ensure that substantial regeneration of bone from the walls of the defect can occur and (2) "re-juvenate" the contaminated (exposed) implant surface.

Is re-osseointegration a feasible outcome of regenerative therapy?

Regeneration of bone from the walls of the defect

Persson *et al.* (1999) induced peri-implant tissue breakdown in beagle dogs according to the Lindhe model referred to above (Lindhe *et al.* 1992). Mandibular premolars were extracted, socket healing allowed, and fixtures (Brånemark System®) with a turned surface were placed and submerged. Abutment connection was performed after 3 months. When the mucosa surrounding all implants had attained a clinically normal appearance, plaque accumulation was allowed and ligatures (cotton floss) were placed around the neck of the implants and retained in a position close to the abutment/fixture junction. After 3 months when the soft tissue exhibited signs of severe inflammation and deep crater-like defects had formed in the peri-implant bone compartments, the ligatures were removed (Fig. 46-3a). Treatment was performed and included (1) systemic administration of antibiotics (amoxicillin and metronidazole for 3 weeks), (2) elevation of full-thickness flaps at the experimental sites and curettage of the hard tissue defect, (3) mechanical debridement of the exposed portion of the implants, (4) removal of the abutment portions of the implants and placement of pristine cover screws, and finally (5) flap management and closure of the soft tissue wound. Radiographs and biopsies were obtained after 7 months of submerged healing. The analysis of the radiographs indicated a complete bone fill in the hard tissue defects (Fig. 46-3b). The histologic analysis of the biopsy sections revealed that treatment had resulted in (1) a complete resolution of the soft tissue inflammation and (2) the formation of substantial

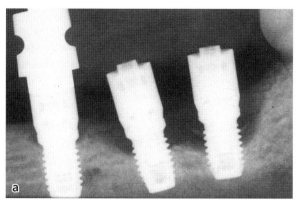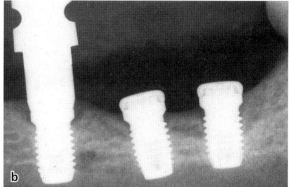

Fig. 46-3 (a) Radiographs obtained from two sites exposed to experimental peri-implantitis. (b) The sites in (a) at 7 months of submerged healing after treatment of peri-implantitis. Note the bone fill in the previous osseous defects.

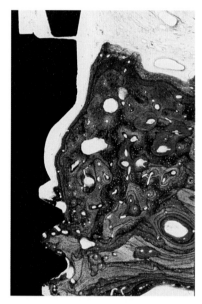

Fig. 46-4 Ground section representing 7 months of submerged healing after treatment of peri-implantitis. Note the newly formed bone in the hard tissue defects.

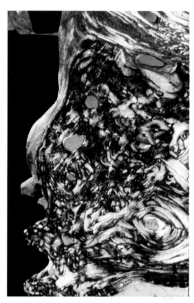

Fig. 46-5 The ground section in Fig. 46-4 in polarized light. Note the connective tissue capsule located between the newly formed bone and the implant surface.

amounts of new bone (appositional osteogenesis) in the previous hard tissue defects (Fig. 46-4). However, only small amounts of "re-osseointegration" to the decontaminated titanium surface could be observed and consistently only at the apical base of the defects. In most sites a thin connective tissue capsule separated the "exposed" implant surface from the newly formed bone (Fig. 46-5). Similar findings were reported by Wetzel *et al.* (1999) from another study in the beagle dog and the use of implants with various surface characteristics (turned, plasma sprayed, and sandblasted–etched surfaces).

Conclusion: Based on the outcome of the above studies it was concluded (1) that the inflammatory lesions in experimentally induced peri-implantitis can be resolved, (2) that *de novo* bone formation (appositional growth) predictably will occur from the hard tissue walls of the defect, and (3) that often the large defects may become more or less completely filled with new bone following a treatment that is

based on antimicrobial measures. Hence, the problem inherent in re-osseointegration appears to be the implant surface rather than the host tissues at the site.

"Rejuvenate" the contaminated implant surface

Different techniques have been proposed for a local therapy aimed at "rejuvenating" the once contaminated implant surface. Such techniques have included mechanical brushing of the surface, the use of air–powder abrasives, and the application of chemicals such as citric acid, hydrogen peroxide, chlorhexidine, and delmopinol (Persson *et al.* 1999; Wetzel *et al.* 1999; Kolonidis *et al.* 2003). These local therapies were effective in cleaning the titanium surface and allowing soft tissue healing and bone fill in the bone craters, but only limited amounts of re-osseointegration occurred.

Is the quality of the implant surface important in a healing process that may lead to re-osseointegration?

The surface of the metal device in the compromised implant site

It is well known that pristine implants made of commercially pure titanium are covered with a thin layer of titanium dioxide (Kasemo & Lausmaa 1985, 1986). This dioxide layer gives the implant a high surface energy that facilitates the interaction between the implant and the cells of the host tissues. Contamination of a titanium surface, however, alters its quality and an implant with a low surface energy results. Such a surface may not allow tissue integration to occur but may instead provoke a foreign body reaction (Baier & Meyer 1988; Sennerby & Lekholm 1993).

The problem regarding the implant surface was addressed a dog study (Persson *et al.* 2001a) in which pristine implant parts were placed in crater-like bone defects that had developed during "experimental peri-implantitis" (a.m. Lindhe *et al.* 1992). The test implants used were comprised of two separate parts, one 6 mm long apical and one 4 mm long marginal part, that were joined together via a connector. During surgical therapy following experimental peri-implantitis, the marginal portions of the implants were removed and replaced with pristine analogues. In biopsies obtained after 4 months of healing it was observed that new bone had formed in the crater-like defects and that "re-osseointegration" had occurred to a large area of the pristine implant components.

In an experiment in the dog, Persson *et al.* (2001b) evaluated the potential for "re-osseointegration" to implants designed with either smooth (polished) or roughened (SLA; sandblasted, large grit acid etched) surfaces. Custom-made solid screw implants were placed in the edentulous mandible; in the right side implants with a rough, SLA surface (Fig. 46-6) and in the left side implants with a smooth surface (Fig. 46-7). "Experimental peri-implantitis" was induced and then blocked when about 50% of the peri-implant bone support was lost (Fig. 46-8a). Treatment included (1) systemic antibiotics (amoxicillin and metronidazole for 17 days), (2) flap elevation and curettage of

the bone defect, and (3) mechanical debridement of the implant surface (cotton pellets soaked in saline). The implants were submerged and biopsies obtained after 6 months of healing. In all implant sites most of the crater-like defects had been filled with newly formed bone (Fig. 46-9b). However, at sites with smooth surface implants only small amounts of "re-osseointegration" (Fig. 46-10) had occurred. Examination of the histologic sections from sites with rough surface implants, however, revealed that >80% of the previously exposed rough surface exhibited "re-osseointegration" (Fig. 46-11).

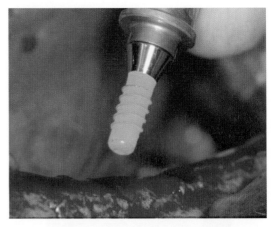

Fig. 46-6 Custom-made implant with a roughened (SLA) surface.

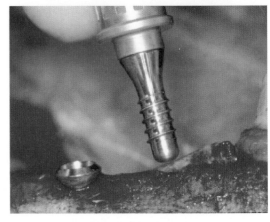

Fig. 46-7 Custom-made implant with a smooth (polished) surface.

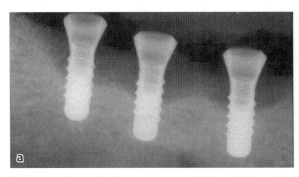
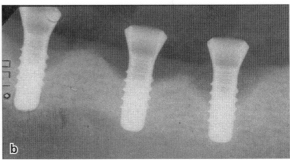

Fig. 46-8 Radiographs illustrating crater-like bone defects following experimental peri-implantitis at implants with a rough (a) and smooth (b) surface.

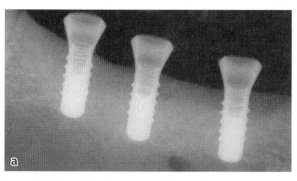
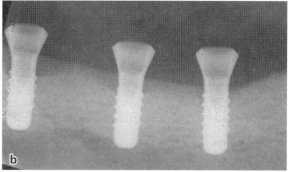

Fig. 46-9 Radiographs illustrating substantial bone-fill in bone defects at 6 months of healing after treatment of experimental peri-implantitis at implants with a rough (a) and smooth (b) surface.

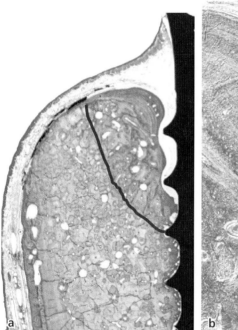
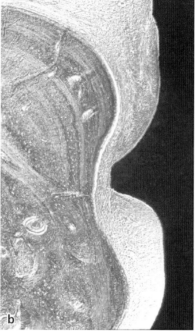

Fig. 46-10 (a) Ground section representing 6 months of healing after treatment of peri-implantitis at sites with smooth surface implants. The red line indicates the outline of the previous hard tissue defect. (b) Note the connective tissue capsule between the newly formed bone and the implant surface.

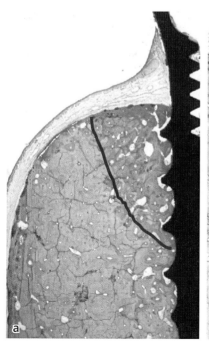
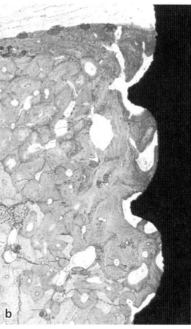

Fig. 46-11 (a) Ground section representing 6 months of healing after treatment of peri-implantitis at sites with rough surface implants. The red line indicates the outline of the previous hard tissue defect. (b) Note the high degree of re-osseointegration to the previously exposed rough implant surface.

Conclusion: Based on the above documentation it is proposed that the rough implant surface may have contributed to a better stability of the blood clot in the bone crater. In addition, during the phase of contraction of the coagulum and formation of granulation tissue, the rough surface may have ensured a continued contact between the newly formed immature tissue and the implant. This upheld contact relationship may, in turn, have facilitated the subsequent formation of a provisional matrix, an osteoid, and eventually woven bone (see Chapter 4). The maintained contact may thus have made possible the bridging of the gap between the walls of the hard tissue crater and the previously exposed implant surface.

In this context it is important to point out that the surface characteristics (smooth vs. rough) of the implant may also influence the risk for a rapid progression of peri-implantitis once initiated (see Chapter 24). Thus, in an experimental study in dogs Berglundh *et al.* (2007) demonstrated that progression of peri-implantitis was more pronounced at implants with a rough (SLA) than with a smooth (polished) surface.

References

Baier, R.E. & Meyer, A.E. (1988). Implant surface preparation. *International Journal of Oral and Maxillofacial Implants* **3**, 9–20.

Berglundh, T., Gotfredsen, K., Zitzmann, N., Lang, N.P. & Lindhe, J. (2007). Spontaneous progression of ligature induced periimplantatitis at implants with different surface roughness. An experimental study in dogs. *Clinical Oral Implants Research*, accepted for publication.

Botticelli, D., Berglundh, T., Buser, D. & Lindhe, J. (2003a). The jumping distance revisited. An experimental study in the dog. *Clinical Oral Implants Research* **14**, 35–42.

Botticelli, D., Berglundh T. & Lindhe, J. (2003b). Appositional bone growth in marginal defects at implants. *Clinical Oral Implants Research* **14**, 1–9.

Botticelli, D., Berglundh T. & Lindhe, J. (2004). Hard tissue alterations following immediate implant placement in extraction sites. *Journal of Clinical Periodontology* **31**, 820–828.

Botticelli, D., Berglundh, T. & Lindhe, J. (2005). Bone regeneration at implants with turned or rough surface in combination with submerged and non-submerged protocols. An experimental study in the dog. *Journal of Clinical Periodontology* **32**, 448–455.

Botticelli, D., Persson, L.P., Lindhe, J. & Berglundh, T. (2006). Bone tissue formation adjacent to implants placed in fresh extraction sockets. An experimental study in dogs. *Clinical Oral Implants Research* **17**, 351–358.

Kasemo, B. & Lausmaa, J. (1985). Metal skeleton and surface characteristics. In: Brånemark, P-I., Zarb, G.A. & Albrektsson, T., eds. *Tissue-Integrated Prosthesis*. Chicago: Quintessence Publishing Co Inc., pp. 99–116.

Kasemo, B. & Lausmaa, J. (1986). Surface science aspects on inorganic biomaterials. *CRC Critical Review of Biocompatibility* **2**, 235–338.

Kolonidis, S.G., Renvert, S., Hämmerle, C.H.F., Lang, N.P., Harris, D. & Claffey, N. (2003). Osseointegration on implant surfaces previously contaminated with plaque. An experimental study in the dog. *Clinical Oral Implants Research* **14**, 373–380.

Lang, N.P., Brägger, U., Walther, D., Beamer, B. & Kornman, K. (1993). Ligature-induced peri-implant infection in cynomolgus monkeys. *Clinical Oral Implants Research* **4**, 2–11.

Lindhe, J., Berglundh, T., Ericsson, I., Liljenberg, B. & Marinello, C.P. (1992). Experimental breakdown of periimplant and periodontal tissues. A study in the beagle dog. *Clinical Oral Implants Research* **3**, 9–16.

Persson, L.G., Araújo, M., Berglundh, T., Gröhndal, K. & Lindhe, J. (1999). Resolution of periimplantitis following treatment. An experimental study in the dog. *Clinical Oral Implants Research* **10**, 195–203.

Persson, L.G., Ericsson, I., Berglundh, T. & Lindhe, J. (2001a). Osseointegration following treatment of periimplantitis at different implant surfaces. An experimental study in the beagle dog. *Journal of Clinical Periodontology* **28**, 258–263.

Persson, L.G., Berglundh, T., Sennerby, L. & Lindhe, J. (2001b). Re-osseointegration after treatment of periimplantitis at different implant surfaces. An experimental study in the dog. *Clinical Oral Implants Research* **12**, 595–603.

Schenk, R. & Willenegger, H. (1977). Zur Histologie der primären Knochenheilung. Modifikationen une Grenzen der spaltheilung in Abhängigkeit von der defektgrösse. *Unfallheilkunde* **80**, 155–160.

Schou, S., Holmstrup, P., Stoltze, K., Hjørting-Hansen, E. & Kornman, K.S. (1993). Ligature-induced marginal inflammation around osseointegrated implants and anckylosed teeth. Clinical and radiographic observations in Cynomolgus monkeys. *Clinical Oral Implants Research* **4**, 12–22.

Sennerby, L. & Lekholm, U. (1993). The soft tissue response to titanium abutments retrieved from humans and reimplanted in rats. A light microscopic pilot study. *Clinical Oral Implants Research* **4**, 23–27.

Wetzel, A.C., Vlassis, J., Caffesse, R.G., Hämmerle, C.H.F. & Lang, N.P. (1999). Attempts to obtain re-osseointegration following experimental periimplantitis in dogs. *Clinical Oral Implants Research* **10**, 111–119.

Wilson, T.G. Jr., Schenk, R., Buser, D. & Cochran, D. (1998). Implants placed in immediate extraction sites: a report of histologic and histometric analyses of human biopsies. *International Journal of Oral and Maxillofacial Implants* **13**, 333–341.

Wilson, T.G. Jr., Carnio, J., Schenk, R. & Cochran, D. (2003). Immediate implants covered with connective tissue membranes: human biopsies. *Journal of Periodontology* **74**, 402–409.

Part 14: Surgery for Implant Installation

47 Timing of Implant Placement, 1053
Christoph H.F. Hämmerle, Maurício Araújo, and Jan Lindhe

48 The Surgical Site, 1068
Marc Quirynen and Ulf Lekholm

Chapter 47

Timing of Implant Placement

Christoph H.F. Hämmerle, Maurício Araújo, and Jan Lindhe

Introduction, 1053
Type 1: placement of an implant as part of the same surgical
   procedure and immediately following tooth extraction, 1055
   Ridge corrections in conjunction with implant placement, 1055
   Stability of implant, 1061
Type 2: completed soft tissue coverage of the tooth socket, 1061

Type 3: substantial bone fill has occurred in the extraction
   socket, 1062
Type 4: the alveolar ridge is healed following tooth loss, 1063
Clinical concepts, 1063
   Aim of therapy, 1063
   Success of treatment and long-term outcomes, 1065

Introduction

Restorative therapy performed on implant(s) placed in a fully healed and non-compromised alveolar ridge, has high clinical success and survival rates (Pjetursson *et al.* 2004). Currently, however, implants are also being placed in (1) sites with ridge defects of various dimensions, (2) fresh extraction sockets, (3) the area of the maxillary sinus, etc. Although some of these clinical procedures were first described many years ago, their application has only recently become common. Accordingly one issue of primary interest in current clinical and animal research in implant dentistry includes the study of tissue alterations that occur following tooth loss and the proper timing thereafter for implant placement.

In the optimal case, the clinician will have time to plan for the restorative therapy (including the use of implants) prior to the extraction of one or several teeth. In this planning, a decision must be made whether the implant(s) should be placed immediately after the tooth extraction(s) or if a certain number of weeks (or months) of healing of the soft and hard tissues of the alveolar ridge should be allowed prior to implant installation. The decision regarding the timing for implant placement, in relation to tooth extraction, must be based on a proper understanding of the structural changes that occur in the alveolar process following the loss of the tooth (teeth). Such adaptive processes were described in Chapter 2.

The removal of single or multiple teeth will result in a series of alterations within the edentulous segment of the alveolar ridge. Hence during socket

healing the hard tissue walls of the alveolus will resorb, the center of the socket will become filled with cancellous bone and the overall volume of the site will become markedly reduced. In particular, the buccal wall of the edentulous site will be diminished not only in the bucco-lingual/palatal direction but also with respect to its apico-coronal dimension (Pietrokovski & Massler 1967; Schropp *et al.* 2003). In addition to hard tissue alterations, the soft tissue in the extraction site will undergo marked adaptive changes. Immediately following tooth extraction, there is a lack of mucosa and the socket entrance is thus open. During the first weeks following the removal of a tooth, cell proliferation within the mucosa will result in an increase of its connective tissue volume. Eventually the soft tissue wound will become epithelialized and a keratinized mucosa will cover the extraction site. The contour of the mucosa will subsequently adapt to follow the changes that occur in the external profile of the hard tissue of the alveolar process. Thus, the contraction of the ridge is the net result of bone loss as well as loss of connective tissue. Figure 47-1 presents a schematic drawing illustrating the tissue alterations described above. It is obvious that no ideal time point exists following the removal of a tooth, at which the extraction site presents with (1) maximum bone fill in the socket and (2) voluminous mature covering mucosa.

A consensus report was published in 2004, describing issues related to the timing of implant placement in extraction (Hammerle *et al.* 2004). Attempts had previously been made to identify advantages and disadvantages with early, delayed, and late implant placements. Hämmerle and coworkers considered it necessary, however, to develop a new concept (classification) that incorporated the growing knowledge in this field of implant dentistry. This new classification took into consideration data describing structural alterations that occur following tooth extraction as well as knowledge derived from clinical observations.

The classification presented in Table 47-1 was introduced in the consensus report. Important aspects of this new classification included the following:

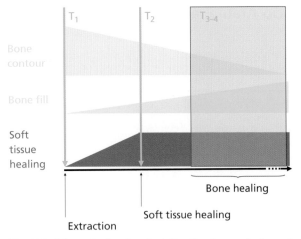

Fig. 47-1 Schematic drawing depicting the changes in the soft and hard tissues following tooth extraction over time. T_{1-4} represent the four different time points regarding timing for implant placement.

- In clinical practice the decision to place an implant following tooth extraction is usually determined by some soft and hard tissue characteristics of the healing socket. Healing does not necessarily follow rigid time frames, and may vary according to site and patient factors.
- To avoid temporal-based descriptions, this new classification used numerical descriptors – types 1, 2, 3, and 4 – that reflect the conditions of the hard and soft tissues:
  - ° Type 1 placement: the implant is placed immediately following the extraction of a tooth
  - ° Type 2 placement: the implant is placed in a site where the soft tissues have healed and a mucosa is covering the socket entrance
  - ° Type 3 placement: the implant is placed in an extraction site at which substantial amounts of new bone have formed in the socket
  - ° Type 4 placement: the implant is placed in a fully healed ridge
- It was further recognized that there is a clear separation between hard tissue healing and soft tissue healing within and around the extraction socket.

Advantages and disadvantages with the various timings are presented in Table 47-1.

Two methods for flap closure have been described at implant sites. One approach requires primary would closure, whereas the other one allows for a

Table 47-1 Classification types 1–4, descriptive definition as well as advantages and disadvantages of each type

Classification	Definition	Advantages	Disadvantages
Type 1	Implant placement as part of the same surgical procedure and immediately following tooth extraction	Reduced number of surgical procedures Reduce overall treatment time Optimal availability of existing bone	Site morphology may complicate optimal placement and anchorage Thin tissue biotype may compromise optimal outcome Potential lack of keratinized mucosa for flap adaptation Adjunctive surgical procedures may be required Technique-sensitive procedure
Type 2	Complete soft tissue coverage of the socket (typically 4–8 weeks)	Increased soft tissue area and volume facilitates soft tissue flap management Allows resolution of local pathology to be assessed	Site morphology may complicate optimal placement and anchorage Increased treatment time Varying amounts of resorption of the socket walls Adjunctive surgical procedures may be required Technique-sensitive procedure
Type 3	Substantial clinical and/or radiographic bone fill of the socket (typically 12–16 weeks)	Substantial bone fill of the socket facilitates implant placement Mature soft tissues facilitate flap management	Increased treatment time Adjunctive surgical procedures may be required Varying amounts of resorption of the socket walls
Type 4	Healed site (typically >16 weeks)	Clinically healed ridge Mature soft tissues facilitate flap management	Increased treatment time Adjunctive surgical procedures may be required Large variation in available bone volume

transmucosal position of the implant or the healing cap. No differences regarding survival rates and interproximal bone levels were found when these two methods were compared in a split-mouth design (Ericsson *et al.* 1997; Astrand *et al.* 2002; Cecchinato *et al.* 2004). These studies did, however, not analyze in detail the differences between submerged or transmucosal healing in sites of high esthetic importance. Hence, not only the width of the gap but also the width of the alveolar ridge are parameters to be considered during treatment planning.

Type 1: placement of an implant as part of the same surgical procedure and immediately following tooth extraction

Ridge corrections in conjunction with implant placement

It has become common to insert implants immediately after the removal of teeth that were scheduled for extraction for various reasons. Over the years, many claims have been made regarding advantages of immediate implant placement (Chen *et al.* 2004). These advantages include easier definition of the implant position, reduced number of visits in the dental office, reduced overall treatment time and costs, preservation of bone at the site of implantation, optimal soft tissue esthetics, and enhanced patient acceptance (Werbitt & Goldberg 1992; Barzilay 1993; Schwartz-Arad & Chaushu 1997a; Mayfield 1999; Hammerle *et al.* 2004).

It was proposed that placement of an implant in a fresh extraction socket may stimulate bone tissue formation and osseointegration and hence counteract the adaptive alterations that occur following tooth extraction. In other words, type 1 implant installation may allow the preservation of bone tissue of the socket and the surrounding jaw. It was in fact recommended (e.g. Denissen *et al.* 1993; Watzek *et al.* 1995; for review see Chen *et al.* 2004) that implant installation should be performed directly following tooth extraction as a means to avoid bone atrophy.

Clinical studies in man (Botticelli *et al.* 2004; Covani *et al.* 2004) and experiments in dogs (Araujo & Lindhe 2005; Araujo *et al.* 2006a,b) have examined the influence of implant installation in the fresh extraction socket on bone modeling and remodeling in the surgical site.

Botticelli *et al.* (2004) examined hard tissue alterations that occurred in the alveolar ridge during a 4-month period of healing following implant placement in fresh extraction sockets. Eighteen subjects (21 extraction sites) with moderate chronic periodontitis were studied. The treatment planning of all 18 subjects called for extraction of single teeth, and restoration by means of implants in the incisor, canine, and premolar regions of the dentition.

Following sulcus incisions, full-thickness mucosal flaps were raised and the tooth was carefully mobilized and removed with forceps. The site was prepared for implant installation with the use of pilot and twist drills. The apical portion of the socket was pre-tapped. A non-cutting solid screw implant (Straumann®; Basel, Switzerland) with a rough surface topography was installed. The implant was positioned in such a way that the marginal level of its rough surface portion was located apical of the marginal level of the buccal and lingual/palatal walls of the socket (Fig. 47-2a). After implant installation (1) the distance between the implant and the inner and outer surface of the buccal and/or lingual bone plates, and (2) the width of the marginal gap that was present between the implant and the buccal, lingual, mesial, and distal bone walls were determined with the use of sliding calipers.

The soft tissue flaps were replaced and the implants were "semi-submerged" during healing (Fig. 47-2b). After 4 months of healing a surgical re-entry procedure was performed (Fig. 47-2c). The clinical measurements were repeated so that alterations that had occurred during healing regarding (1) the thickness and height of the buccal and lingual/palatal socket walls and (2) the width of the marginal gap could be calculated.

Figure 47-3a presents a photograph of an extraction socket immediately after the removal of a maxillary canine tooth. At re-entry it was realized that the

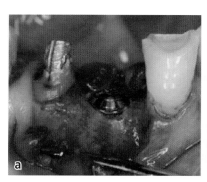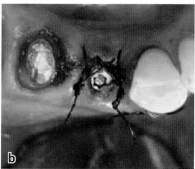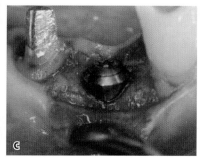

Fig. 47-2 (a) Clinical view of the implant position in the fresh extraction socket. (b) Clinical view of the flaps replaced and sutured. (c) Clinical buccal view of the implant site after 4 months of healing.

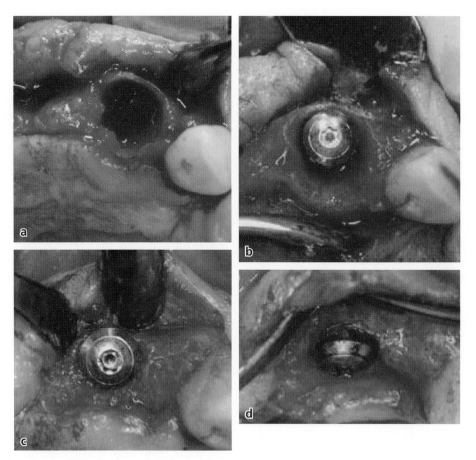

Fig. 47-3 (a) Clinical view of the alveolar socket of a maxillary canine. (b) Clinical view of the implant position in the fresh extraction socket. (c) Clinical occlusal view of the implant site after 4 months of healing. (d) Clinical buccal view of the implant site after 4 months of healing. Note the very thin bone covering the buccal aspect.

marginal gap had completely resolved. Furthermore, the thickness of the buccal as well as the palatal bone walls had become markedly reduced (Fig. 47-3c,d). In Fig. 47-3d the implant surface can be seen through the very thin remaining buccal bone wall.

Another site from this clinical study is presented in Fig. 47-4. The first maxillary premolar (tooth 14) was removed (Fig. 47-4a) and one implant was placed in the palatal socket of the fresh extraction site. A second implant was placed in the healed edentulous ridge and in position 25 (Fig. 47-4b). At re-entry, it was observed that (1) the marginal gap had been entirely resolved and (2) the distance between the implant and the outer surface of the buccal bone plate had become markedly reduced (Fig. 47-4c).

Botticelli et al. (2004) reported that during the 4 months of healing following tooth extraction and implant installation practically all marginal gaps had become resolved. At the time of implant placement, the mean distance (18 subjects, 21 sites) between the implant and the outer surface of the buccal bone wall was 3.4 mm while the matching dimension on the lingual/palatal aspect was 3.0 mm. At re-entry after 4 months, the corresponding dimensions were 1.5 mm (buccal) and 2.2 mm (lingual). In other words, the reduction of the buccal dimension was 1.9 mm (or

56%) while the equivalent reduction of the lingual dimension was 0.8 mm (or 27%).

The findings by Botticelli et al. (2004) strongly indicate that implant placement in a fresh extraction socket may, in fact, not prevent the physiologic modeling/remodeling that occurs in the ridge following tooth removal.

In order to study bone modeling/remodeling that occurs in the fresh extraction site following implant placement in more detail, Araújo and Lindhe (2005) performed an experiment in the dog. In this study the authors used histologic means to determine the magnitude of the dimensional alterations that occurred in the alveolar ridge following the placement of implants in fresh extraction sockets. Buccal and lingual full-thickness flaps were elevated in both quadrants of the mandible of beagle dogs. The distal roots of the 3rd and 4th premolars were removed (Fig. 47-5a). In the right jaw quadrants, implants (solid screw, Straumann®, Basel) with a rough surface were placed in the sockets so that the marginal border of the rough surface was below the buccal and lingual bone margin (Fig. 47-5b). The flaps were replaced to allow a "semi-submerged" healing (Fig. 47-5c). In the left jaws the corresponding sockets were left without implantation and the extraction sockets were fully submerged under the mobilized flaps (Fig. 47-5d).

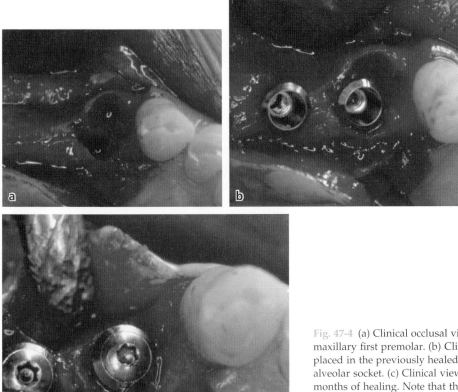

Fig. 47-4 (a) Clinical occlusal view of the alveolar socket of a maxillary first premolar. (b) Clinical view of the implants placed in the previously healed edentulous ridge and in the alveolar socket. (c) Clinical view of the implant sites after 4 months of healing. Note that the distance between the implant and the outer surface of the buccal bone plate had become markedly reduced.

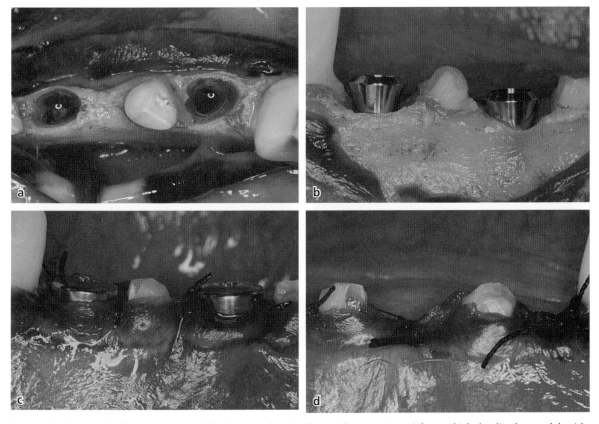

Fig. 47-5 (a) Photograph illustrating a mandibular premolar site (from a dog experiment) from which the distal root of the 4th premolar was removed. (b) In the test side of the mandible, the implant was placed in the socket in such way that the rough surface marginal limit was flush with the bone crest. (c) The mucosal, full-thickness flaps were replaced and sutured to allow a "semi-submerged" healing. (d) In the contralateral side of the mandible, the sockets were left without implantation.

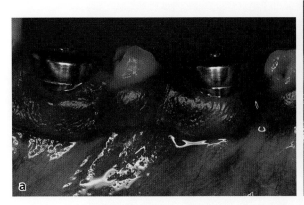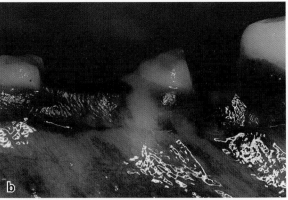

Fig. 47-6 Photograph illustrating the implant (a) and edentulous (b) sites after 6 months of healing.

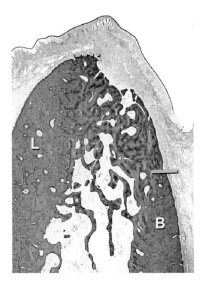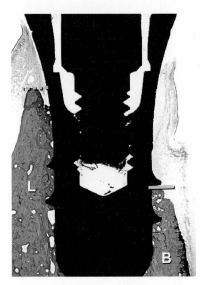

Fig. 47-7 Buccal–lingual section of the edentulous site. Note that the remaining buccal crest (continuous line) is located far below the lingual counterpart (dotted line). B = buccal aspect; L = lingual aspect.

Fig. 47-8 Buccal–lingual section of the implant site. Note that the remaining buccal crest (continuous line) is located far below the lingual counterpart (dotted line). B = buccal aspect; L = lingual aspect.

After 3 months, the mucosa at the experimental sites in the right and left jaw quadrants appeared properly healed (Fig. 47-6). The animals were sacrificed and tissue blocks containing the implant sites and the edentulous socket sites were dissected and prepared for histologic examination.

Figure 47-7 presents a buccal–lingual section of one edentulous site after 3 months of healing. Newly formed bone is covering the entrance of the socket. The lamellar bone of the buccal, cortical plate is located about 2.2 mm apical of its lingual counterpart. Figure 47-8a presents a similar section from an implant site in the same dog. The marginal termination of the buccal bone plate is located about 2.4 mm apical to the lingual crest. In other words, the placement of an implant in the fresh extraction socket failed to influence the process of modeling that occurred in the hard tissue walls of the socket following tooth removal. Thus, after 3 months of healing the amount of reduction of the height of the buccal bone wall (in comparison to lingual bone alteration)

was similar at the implant sites and the edentulous sites. At 3 months, the vertical discrepancy between the buccal and lingual bone margins was >2 mm in both categories of sites; edentulous sites = 2.2 mm and implant sites = 2.4 mm.

In a follow-up experiment in the dog, Araújo et al. (2006a,b) studied whether osseointegration, once established following implant placement in a fresh extraction socket, could be lost as a result of continued tissue modeling of the bone walls during healing. As was the case in their previous study the distal roots of the 3rd and 4th premolars in both quadrants of the mandible were removed following flap elevation. Implants were installed in the fresh extraction sockets, and initial stability of all implants was secured. The flaps were replaced and "semi-submerged" healing of the implant sites was allowed. Immediately following flap closure, biopsies were obtained from two dogs, while in five dogs healing periods of 1 month and 3 months were permitted prior to biopsy.

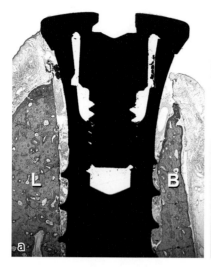
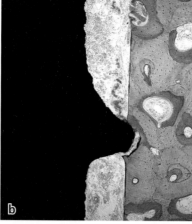

Fig. 47-9 (a) Buccal–lingual section of an extraction site immediately after implant installation. (b) Contact was established between the pitch on the surface of the implant body and the walls of the socket. B = buccal aspect; L = lingual aspect.

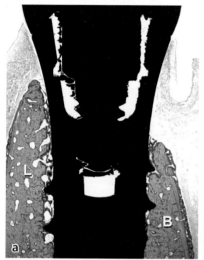
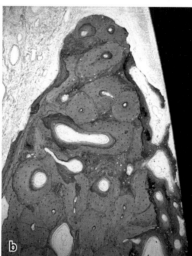
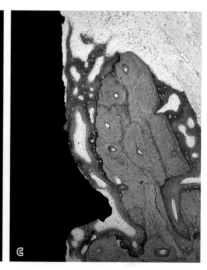

Fig. 47-10 (a) Buccal–lingual section 4 weeks after implant installation. The void between the implant surface and the bone wall was completely filled with newly formed bone in both lingual (b) and buccal (c) aspects. B = buccal aspect; L = lingual aspect.

Figure 47-9a presents a buccal–lingual aspect of an extraction site immediately after implant installation. Contact was established between the pitch on the surface of the implant body and the walls of the socket. A coagulum resided in the void between the contact regions (Fig. 47-9b) and also in the marginal gap. In sections representing 4 weeks of healing, it was observed that this void had become filled with woven bone that made contact with the rough surface part of the implant (Figs. Fig 47-10). In this 4-week interval, (1) the buccal and lingual bone walls had undergone marked surface resorption, and (2) the height of the thin buccal hard tissue wall had been reduced.

In the interval between 4 weeks and 12 weeks of healing the buccal bone crest shifted further in an apical direction (Fig. 47-11). The woven bone at the buccal aspect that in the 4-week sample made contact with the implant in the marginal gap region had modeled and only fragments of this bone remained (Fig. 47-11c). At the end of the study, the buccal bone crest was located >2 mm apical to the marginal border of the rough implant surface.

These findings demonstrate that the bone (woven bone)-to-implant contact that was established during the early phase of socket healing following implant installation, was in part lost when the buccal bone wall underwent continued atrophy.

It is obvious, therefore, that the alveolar process following tooth extraction (loss) will adapt to the altered functional demands by atrophy and that an implant, in this respect is unable to substitute for the tooth. The clinical problem with type 1 placement is that the bone loss will frequently cause the buccal portion of the implant to gradually lose its hard tissue coverage, and that the metal surface may become visible through a thin peri-implant mucosa and cause esthetic concerns (Fig. 47-12).

The question now arises whether it is possible to overcome this problem. This issue was studied in a beagle dog experiment by Araújo *et al.* (2006b). The distal root of the 3rd mandibular premolar and the

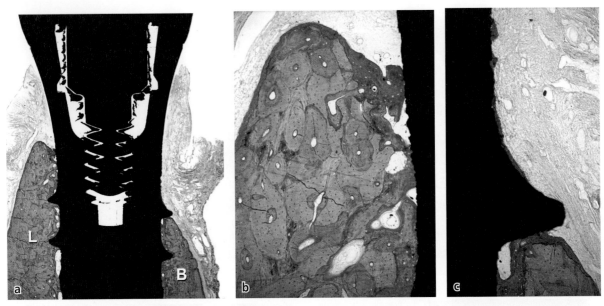

Fig. 47-11 (a) Buccal–lingual section 12 weeks after implant installation. Note that buccal bone crest shifted in an apical direction and fragments of it could be seen on the denuded implant surface (c). The lingual bone crest, however, remained stable (b). B = buccal aspect; L = lingual aspect.

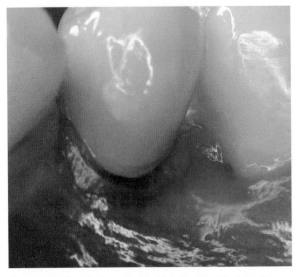

Fig. 47-12 Clincal view of an implant lacking the buccal bone. Note that the metal surface had become visible through the thin mucosa.

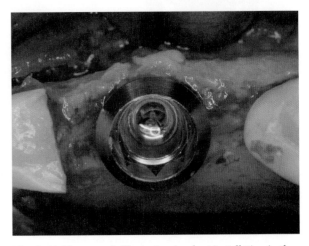

Fig. 47-13 Photograph illustrating implant installation in the narrow, 3rd premolar alveolar socket.

distal root of the 1st mandibular molar were removed and implants placed in the fresh extraction sockets. The 3rd premolar socket in this dog model is comparatively small, and hence the implant inserted (Straumann® Standard Implant, diameter 4.1 mm) occupied most of the hard tissue wound (Fig. 47-13). During healing resorption of the buccal bone wall occurred (Fig. 47-14) and >2 mm of the marginal portion of the implant became exposed to peri-implant mucosa.

The molar socket, on the other hand is very large (Fig. 47-15) and hence after implant (Straumann® Standard Implant, diameter 4.1 mm) placement a >1 mm wide marginal gap occurred between the metal body and the bone walls (Fig. 47-16b). Primary stability of the implant was achieved through contacts between the metal body and the bone in the apical (periapical) portions of the socket. During the early phase of healing this gap in the molar site became filled with woven bone. In the interval when the buccal bone wall underwent programmed atrophy, the newly formed bone in the gap region maintained osseointegration and continued to cover all surfaces of the implant (Fig. 47-16a,b).

Conclusion: The data reported illustrate an important biologic principle. Atrophy of the edentulous ridge will occur following tooth loss. This contraction of the ridge cannot be prevented by placing an implant in the fresh extraction socket. The atrophy includes a marked reduction of the width and the height of both the buccal and lingual bone plates; in particular the buccal bone plate will undergo marked change. To some extent the problem with buccal bone

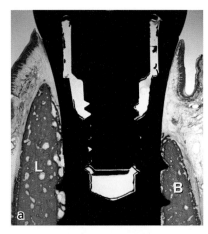
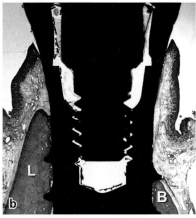

Fig. 47-14 Buccal–lingual section of the healed premolars sites representing (a) 4 and (b) 12 weeks after implant installation. B = buccal aspect; L = lingual aspect.

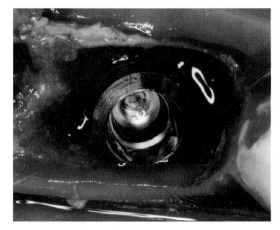

Fig. 47-15 Photograph illustrating implant installation in the wide, 1st molar alveolar socket.

resorption can be overcome by placing the implant deeper into the fresh socket and in the lingual/palatal portion of the socket.

As a consequence of the above described healing, bone regeneration procedures may be required to improve or retain bone volume and the buccal contour at a fresh extraction site. Such bone augmentation is sometimes mandatory in the esthetic area.

Stability of implant

Another issue with type 1 (and also type 2) placement is the anchorage of the implant to obtain primary stability in a position in the jaw that will enable the subsequent restoration to meet high demands regarding esthetics and function. In most cases of type 1 placement, the implants are fixed in native bone apical to the alveolus (Fig. 47-17). Additional retention may be achieved by anchoring the implant in the bony structures of the alveolar walls or inter-radicular septa.

In a recently presented controlled clinical trial (Siegenthaler *et al*. 2007) it was observed that primary stability for some implants in a type 1 procedure could not always be achieved. In this study implants were inserted to replace teeth either exhibiting peri-

apical pathology (test) or presenting healthy periapical conditions (control). In four implant sites in the test group and one in the control group no implants could be placed due to an unfavorable bone morphology, which precluded primary implant stability.

Type 2: completed soft tissue coverage of the tooth socket

There are several reasons why the type 2 approach is often recommended. At this stage of healing the socket entrance is covered with a mucosa. The soft tissue is (1) comparatively mature, (2) has proper volume, and (3) can be easily managed during flap elevation and replacement procedures. Furthermore, the type 2 timing permits an assessment of the resolution of periapical lesions that may have been associated with the extracted tooth. The disadvantages inherent in the type 2 approach include (1) resorption of the socket walls and (2) an extended treatment time (Table 47-1).

Following tooth extraction, the socket becomes filled with a coagulum that is replaced with granulation tissue within a few weeks. In the normal case it takes about 4–8 weeks before the soft tissue (granulation tissue, provisional connective tissue; see Chapter 2) fills the socket and its surface becomes covered with epithelium (Amler 1969; Zitzmann *et al*. 1999; Hämmerle & Lang 2001; Nemcovsky & Artzi 2002). The maturation of the soft tissue (further deposition and orientation of collagen fibers) that may facilitate flap management may require an even longer healing time.

The larger amount of soft tissue that is present at the site of implant placement when the type 2 approach is used will allow for precise management of the mucosal flap and hence optimal soft tissue healing (Fig. 47-18). This advantage with the type 2 timing must be matched against the hard tissue reduction and the change of the ridge contour that results from the resorption of the socket walls and of the buccal bone plate. It must be observed that at

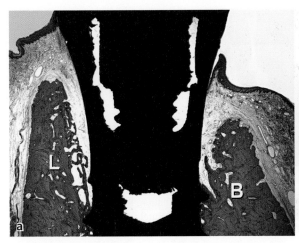
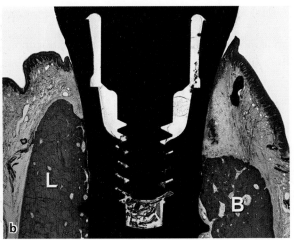

Fig. 47-16 Buccal–lingual section of the healed molars sites representing (a) 4 and (b) 12 weeks after implant installation. B = buccal aspect; L = lingual aspect.

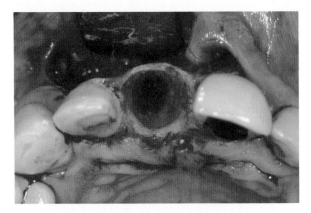

Fig. 47-17 Type 1 implant placement provides optimal availability of existing bone contours. Note the presence of a thin buccal bone plate. Anchorage of an implant can be achieved by engaging the bone apical to the apex of the extracted tooth and the palatal wall of the socket.

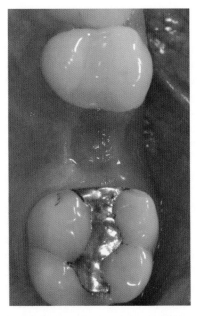

Fig. 47-18 The soft tissues have completely healed over the extraction socket 8 weeks after tooth removal (type 2).

some extraction sites the mucosa may remain adherent via scar tissue to the underlying bone or to the provisional connective tissue of the socket. In such cases it may be difficult to separate the soft tissue from the bone and to mobilize the flap. In such a situation, the trauma caused in conjunction with flap elevation may rupture the soft tissue and compromise healing. This in turn may result in soft tissue dehiscence, local infection, and inflammation (Zitzmann *et al*. 1997).

As described in the schematic drawing in Fig. 47-1 the initial gain in mucosa (area and volume) is later followed by an overall loss of soft tissue volume. This is evidenced by the fact that the volume of alveolar ridge – including the bone as well as the mucosal compartments – markedly decreased during the first 12 months following tooth extraction (Schropp *et al*. 2003).

During the 4–8 weeks between tooth extraction and type 2 implant placement only small amounts of new bone (woven bone) will form in the socket. This means that the risk of not achieving primary implant stability is similar in type 1 and type 2 approaches. Thus, in sites where the available bone height apical to the tip of the root is less than 3 mm, it is frequently impossible to obtain primary implant stability in the bone beyond the apex of the extracted tooth. When, in addition, a wide alveolus is precluding the engagement of its bony walls, the type 3 approach may be favored.

Type 3: substantial bone fill has occurred in the extraction socket

The type 3 time frame is chosen for implant installation at sites where, for various reasons, bone fill is required within the extraction socket. Newly formed woven bone will occupy the socket area after healing periods extending from 10–16 weeks (Evian *et al*. 1982). In this period, however, the walls of the socket are frequently completely resorbed and replaced with woven bone. The entrance to the socket is closed with a cap of woven bone that is in the process of remodeling. The mucosa that covers the extraction site is (1) residing on a mineralized ridge, and (2) mature and more easy to manage during surgical flap elevation and replacement procedures.

The type 3 approach often allows the clinician to place the implant in a position that facilitates the prosthetic phase of the treatment. The disadvantages with the type 3 approach encompass (1) a prolonged treatment time, (2) additional resorption and diminuton of the ridge including a substantial change of its contour, and (3) a concomitant loss of soft tissue volume.

Type 4: the alveolar ridge is healed following tooth loss

In the type 4 approach the implant is placed in a fully healed ridge. Such a ridge can be found after 4 but more likely after 6–12 months of healing following tooth extraction (loss). After 6–12 months of healing following tooth extraction, the clinician will find a ridge that is lined by a mature, often well keratinized mucosa that resides on dense cortical bone. Beneath the cortical bone plate, cancellous bone occupies a varying portion of the alveolar process (for detail see Chapter 2).

In a study including human volunteers it was observed that the rate of formation of new bone within the extraction site started to decrease after 3–4 months of healing. At this stage the newly formed bone and the remaining bone of the socket walls entered into a phase of remodeling (Evian *et al*. 1982). Concomitant with the remodeling of this centrally located bone tissue, extra-alveolar resorptive processes leading to a further contraction of the ridge and change of its contour continued for at least 12 months (Schropp *et al*. 2003).

The advantage of type 4 installation is that healing is more or less complete and that only minor additional change of the ridge may occur. The disadvantages include (1) increased treatment time and (2) further reduction of the overall volume of the ridge and change of its external contour. This pronounced additional loss of ridge volume may at times require complicated bone augmentation procedures (Fig. 47-19). As a consequence type 4 placement is avoided in most cases when the tooth (teeth) to be replaced is (are) present at the time of examination and treatment planning.

Clinical concepts

When implants are to be placed in the edentulous portion of the ridge, factors other than the tissue changes over time must be considered. Thus, in the treatment planning phase aspects, such as (1) the overall objective of the treatment, (2) the location of the tooth within the oral cavity – in the esthetic or

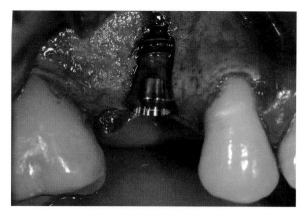

Fig. 47-19 A buccal dehiscence defect is present at an implant placed into a ridge, which has undergone substantial buccal bone resorption since tooth extraction several months ago (type 4).

non-esthetic zone – and (3) the anatomy of the bone and the soft tissue at the site(s) to be treated, must be evaluated.

Aim of therapy

Dental implants are most often used to restore health and function. During the surgical phase of therapy, therefore, ideal conditions must be established for successful bone and soft tissue integration to the implant. In a growing number of cases, however, treatment must also satisfy demands regarding the esthetic outcome. In such cases, the overall surgical and prosthetic treatment protocol may become more demanding, since factors other than osseointegration and soft tissue integration may play an important role.

Restoration of health and function

In cases where the restoration of health and function constitutes the primary goal of the treatment, the location and volume of available hard and soft tissues are the important factors to consider. In such cases the type 1 approach is usually selected (Wichmann 1990).

The replacement of a single-rooted tooth with an implant in a fully healed ridge will, in most cases, ensure proper primary stability with the implant in a correct position (Fig. 47-20). In addition, the soft tissues are sufficient in volume and area. The mucosal flap can be adapted to the neck (or the healing cap) of the implant (one-stage protocol). When primary wound closure is intended (two-stage protocol), mobilization of the soft tissue will allow tension-free adaptation and connection of the flap margins.

When an implant is placed in the fully healed site of a multi-rooted tooth, the surgical procedure becomes more demanding. Often the ideal position for the implant is in the area of the inter-radicular septum. If the septa are delicate, anchorage for

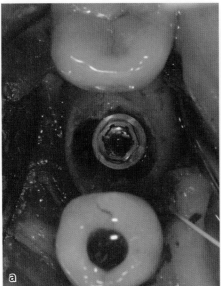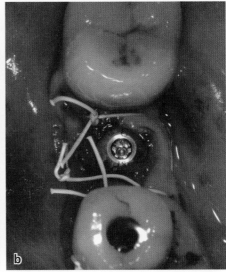

Fig. 47-20 (a) Immediate implant placement (type 1) in a mandibular premolar extraction socket. Note the buccal bone deficiency, where bone will be augmented by guided bone regeneration (GBR). (b) The same site as in (a) following adaptation of the flap around the neck of the implant obtaining a transmucosal mode of healing.

primary implant stability may become difficult to achieve. In addition, in molar sites there is often only a small amount of soft tissue present. This may create a problem with respect to wound closure with a mobilized, tension-free flap. In some molar sites, primary wound closure may not be possible at times following implant installation.

The presence of marginal defects (gaps) between the implant and the fully healed ridge following type 4 placement was regarded in the past as a significant problem that could compromise osseointegration. Recent studies in man and animals have demonstrated, however, that in such a horizontal marginal defect (gap) of ≤2 mm, new bone formation as well as defect resolution and osseointegration of the implant (with a rough titanium surface) will occur (Wilson *et al.* 1998; Botticelli *et al.* 2004; Cornelini *et al.* 2005).

Esthetic importance and tissue biotype

The replacement of missing teeth with implants in the esthetic zone is a demanding procedure. Deficiencies in the bone architecture and in the soft tissue volume and architecture may compromise the esthetic outcome of treatment (Grunder 2000). Hence, when an implant is to be placed in the esthetic zone, not only the anatomy of the hard tissues but also the texture and the appearance of the soft tissues must be considered.

Type 2 installation is often to be preferred when implants are placed in the esthetic zone (Fig. 47-21). The key advantage in type 2 (as opposed to type 1) is the increased amount of soft tissue that has formed during the first weeks of healing following tooth extraction. It must be emphasized, however, that comparative studies analyzing the treatment out-

comes in randomly selecting type 1 or type 2 placements have so far not been reported.

In a recent clinical study, implants were placed in fresh extraction sockets (Botticelli *et al.* 2004). During healing, the implants became clinically osseointegrated within the borders of the previous extraction socket. Significant loss of buccal bone height (contour) however also occurred. In esthetically critical situations this loss of contour may lead to a compromised outcome. Hence not infrequently, tissue augmentation procedures must be performed in the esthetic zone.

In this context it is important to realize that when a two-stage implant placement protocol is used, the labial mucosa will recede following abutment connection surgery. Mean values of recession between 0.5 mm and 1.5 mm with large variations have been reported in several clinical studies (Grunder 2000; Oates *et al.* 2002; Ekfeldt *et al.* 2003). These findings additionally stress the necessity for a careful treatment approach when implants are placed in the esthetic zone.

The biotype (see Chapter 3) of the soft and hard tissue tissues may play a role regarding the esthetic outcome of implant therapy. Characteristics of soft and hard tissues at teeth were described and classified into two biotypes: the flat thick or the pronounced scalloped thin biotype (Weisgold *et al.* 1997; Olsson & Lindhe 1991; Olsson *et al.* 1993). The thin tissues in the pronounced scalloped biotype include a thin free gingiva, a narrow zone of attached mucosa, and a pronounced "scalloped" contour of the gingival margin. In addition, the scalloped thin biotype is associated with a delicate bone housing. In a recent study it was found that buccal tissue recession at single-tooth implants was more pronounced in patients exhibiting a thin biotype compared to

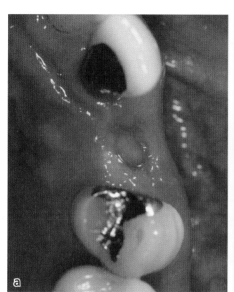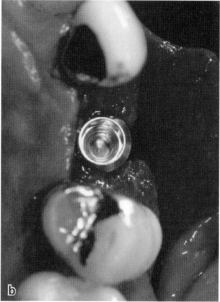

Fig. 47-21 (a) A single tooth gap 8 weeks following tooth extraction. The soft tissues have completely healed over the extraction socket. (b) The same site as in (a). An implant has been placed in the edentulous gap. The resulting buccal dehiscence defect will be augmented with bone by applying GBR.

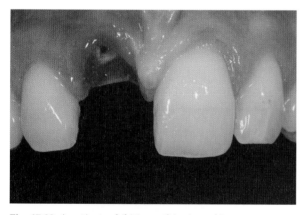

Fig. 47-22 A patient exhibiting a thin tissue biotype as characterized by a thin free gingiva, a narrow zone of keratinized and of attached mucosa, shallow probing depths, and a pronounced "scalloped" contour of the gingival margin including recessions at some maxillary anterior teeth. Tooth 11 is scheduled for extraction and replacement by an implant using a type 2 or 3 approach.

patients with a thick biotype (Evans & Chen 2007). Based on these findings and on clinical experience it was proposed that patients exhibiting a pronounced scalloped biotype should be treated with a type 2, 3, or 4 rather than with a type 1 implant installation approach (Fig. 47-22). Data collected from properly designed clinical studies regarding this issue are presently lacking.

Success of treatment and long-term outcomes

Numerous clinical studies have demonstrated that type 1 implant placement is a successful and predict-

able clinical method (Lang *et al.* 1994; Schwartz-Arad & Chaushu 1997b; Hämmerle *et al.* 1998; Covani *et al.* 2004). In addition, success and survival rates for type 1 implants have been reported to be of the same magnitude as implants placed in healed ridges (Gelb 1993; Grunder 2000; Gomez-Roman *et al.* 2001; Gotfredsen 2004; Schwartz-Arad *et al.* 2004). Histologic studies in animals confirmed the viability of type 1 placement. Unloaded titanium implants placed in extraction sockets showed a high degree of osseointegration (Anneroth *et al.* 1985), i.e. similar to the one at implants placed in healed sites. Furthermore, a few studies analyzing survival rates of type 2 and 3 placements have shown similar survival rates as the ones reported for types 1 and 4 (Watzek *et al.* 1995; Nir-Hadar *et al.* 1998; Polizzi *et al.* 2000).

Conclusions

In situations where teeth are to be replaced with implants, various factors govern the decision regarding the optimal time point for implantation following tooth extraction. Of special importance are the overall objective of the treatment, the location of the tooth within the oral cavity, the anatomy of the bone and the soft tissue at the site, and the adaptive changes of the alveolar ridge following tooth extraction. The decision regarding the timing for implant placement needs to be based on a thorough understanding of the structural changes that occur in the alveolar process following tooth extraction, with and without implant placement as presented in this chapter.

References

Amler, M.H. (1969). The time sequence of tissue regeneration in human extraction wounds. *Oral Surgery Oral Medicine & Oral Pathology* **27**, 309–318.

Anneroth, G., Hedstrom, K.G., Kjellman, O., Kondell, P.A. & Nordenram, A. (1985). Endosseus titanium implants in extraction sockets. An experimental study in monkeys. *International Journal of Oral Surgery* **14**, 50–54.

Araujo, M.G. & Lindhe, J. (2005). Dimensional ridge alterations following tooth extraction. An experimental study in the dog. *Journal of Clinical Periodontology* **32**, 212–218.

Araujo, M.G., Sukekava, F., Wennstrom, J.L. & Lindhe, J. (2006a). Tissue modeling following implant placement in fresh extraction sockets. *Clinical Oral Implants Research* **17**, 615–624.

Araujo, M.G., Wennstrom, J.L. & Lindhe, J. (2006b). Modeling of the buccal and lingual bone walls of fresh extraction sites following implant installation. *Clinical Oral Implants Research* **17**, 606–614.

Astrand, P., Engquist, B., Anzen, B., Bergendal, T., Hallman, M., Karlsson, U., Kvint, S., Lysell, L. & Rundcrantz, T. (2002). Nonsubmerged and submerged implants in the treatment of the partially edentulous maxilla. *Clinical Implant Dentistry and Related Research* **4**, 115–127.

Barzilay, I. (1993). Immediate implants: their current status. *International Journal of Prosthodontics* **6**, 169–175.

Botticelli, D., Berglundh, T. & Lindhe, J. (2004). Hard-tissue alterations following immediate implant placement in extraction sites. *Journal of Clinical Periodontology* **31**, 820–828.

Cecchinato, D., Olsson, C. & Lindhe, J. (2004). Submerged or non-submerged healing of endosseous implants to be used in the rehabilitation of partially dentate patients. *Journal of Clinical Periodontology* **31**, 299–308.

Chen, S.T., Wilson, T.G., Jr. & Hammerle, C.H. (2004). Immediate or early placement of implants following tooth extraction: review of biologic basis, clinical procedures, and outcomes. *International Journal of Oral and Maxillofacial Implants* **19** (Suppl), 12–25.

Cornelini, R., Cangini, F., Covani, U. & Wilson, T.G., Jr. (2005). Immediate restoration of implants placed into fresh extraction sockets for single-tooth replacement: a prospective clinical study. *International Journal of Periodontics and Restorative Dentistry* **25**, 439–447.

Covani, U., Crespi, R., Cornelini, R. & Barone, A. (2004). Immediate implants supporting single crown restoration: a 4-year prospective study. *Journal of Periodontology* **75**, 982–988.

Denissen, H.W., Kalk, W., Veldhuis, H.A. & van Waas, M.A. (1993). Anatomic consideration for preventive implantation. *International Journal of Oral and Maxillofacial Implants* **8**(2), 191–196.

Ekfeldt, A., Eriksson, A. & Johansson, L.A. (2003). Peri-implant mucosal level in patients treated with implant-supported fixed prostheses: a 1-year follow-up study. *International Journal of Prosthodontics* **16**, 529–532.

Ericsson, I., Randow, K., Nilner, K. & Petersson, A. (1997). Some clinical and radiographical features of submerged and non-submerged titanium implants. A 5-year follow-up study. *Clinical Oral Implants Research* **8**, 422–426.

Evans, C.D.J. & Chen, S.T. (2007). Esthetic outcome of immediate implant placements. *Clinical Oral Implants Research* (in press).

Evian, C.I., Rosenberg, E.S., Coslet, J.G. & Corn, H. (1982). The osteogenic activity of bone removed from healing extraction sockets in humans. *Journal of Periodontology* **53**, 81–85.

Gelb, D.A. (1993). Immediate implants surgery: three-year retrospective evaluation of 50 consecutive cases. *International Journal of Periodontics and Restorative Dentistry* **8**, 388–399.

Gomez-Roman, G., Kruppenbacher, M., Weber, H. & Schulte, W. (2001). Immediate postextraction implant placement with root-analog stepped implants: surgical procedure and statistical outcome after 6 years. *International Journal of Oral and Maxillofacial Implants* **16**, 503–513.

Gotfredsen, K. (2004). A 5-year prospective study of single-tooth replacements supported by the Astra Tech implant: a pilot study. *Clinical Implant Dentistry and Related Research* **6**, 1–8.

Grunder, U. (2000). Stability of the mucosal topography around single-tooth implants and adjacent teeth: 1-year results. *International Journal of Periodontics and Restorative Dentistry* **20**, 11–17.

Hammerle, C.H., Chen, S.T. & Wilson, T.G., Jr. (2004). Consensus statements and recommended clinical procedures regarding the placement of implants in extraction sockets. *International Journal of Oral and Maxillofacial Implants* **19** Suppl, 26–28.

Hämmerle, C.H.F., Brägger, U., Schmid, B. & Lang, N.P. (1998). Successful bone formation at immediate transmucosal implants. *International Journal of Oral and Maxillofacial Implants* **13**, 522–530.

Hämmerle, C.H.F. & Lang, N.P. (2001). Single stage surgery combining transmucosal implant placement with guided bone regeneration and bioresorbable materials. *Clinical Oral Implants Research* **12**, 9–18.

Lang, N.P., Brägger, U. & Hämmerle, C.H.F. (1994). Immediate transmucosal implants using the principle of guided tissue regeneration (GTR). I. Rationale, clinical procedures, and 2 1/2-year results. *Clinical Oral Implants Research* **5**, 154–163.

Mayfield, L. (1999). Immediate and delayed submerged and transmucosal implants. Paper presented at the 3rd European Workshop on Periodontology, Ittingen, Switzerland.

Nemcovsky, C.E. & Artzi, Z. (2002). Comparative study of buccal dehiscence defects in immediate, delayed, and late maxillary implant placement with collagen membranes: clinical healing between placement and second-stage surgery. *Journal of Periodontology* **73**, 754–761.

Nir-Hadar, O., Palmer, M. & Soskolne, W.A. (1998). Delayed immediate implants: alveolar bone changes during the healing period. *Clinical Oral Implants Research* **9**, 26–33.

Oates, T.W., West, J., Jones, J., Kaiser, D. & Cochran, D.L. (2002). Long-term changes in soft tissue height on the facial surface of dental implants. *Implant Dentistry* **11**, 272–279.

Olsson, M. & Lindhe, J. (1991). Periodontal characteristics in individuals with varying form of the upper central incisors. *Journal of Clinical Periodontology* **18**, 78–82.

Olsson, M., Lindhe, J. & Marinello, C.P. (1993). On the relationship between crown form and clinical features of the gingiva in adolescents. *Journal of Clinical Periodontology* **20**, 570–577.

Pietrokovski, J. & Massler, M. (1967). Alveolar ridge resorption following tooth extraction. *Journal of Prosthetic Dentistry* **17**, 21–27.

Pjetursson, B.E., Tan, K., Lang, N.P., Bragger, U., Egger, M. & Zwahlen, M. (2004). A systematic review of the survival and complication rates of fixed partial dentures (FPDs) after an observation period of at least 5 years. *Clinical Oral Implants Research* **15**, 625–642.

Polizzi, G., Grunder, U., Goene, R., Hatano, N., Henry, P., Jackson, W.J., Kawamura, K., Renouard, F., Rosenberg, R., Triplett, G., Werbitt, M. & Lithner, B. (2000). Immediate and delayed implant placement into extraction sockets: a 5-year report. *Clinical Implant Dentistry and Related Research* **2**, 93–99.

Schropp, L., Wenzel, A., Kostopoulos, L. & Karring, T. (2003). Bone healing and soft tissue contour changes following single-tooth extraction: a clinical and radiographic 12-month prospective study. *International Journal of Periodontics and Restorative Dentistry* **23**, 313–323.

Schwartz-Arad, D. & Chaushu, G. (1997a). The ways and wherefores of immediate placement of implants into fresh extraction sites: A literature review. *Journal of Periodontology* **68**, 915–923.

Schwartz-Arad, D. & Chaushu, G. (1997b). Placement of implants into fresh extraction sites: 4 to 7 years retrospective evaluation of 95 implants. *Journal of Periodontology* **68**, 1110–1116.

Schwartz-Arad, D., Yaniv, Y., Levin, L. & Kaffe, I. (2004). A radiographic evaluation of cervical bone loss associated with immediate and delayed implants placed for fixed restorations in edentulous jaws. *Journal of Periodontology* **75**, 652–657.

Siegenthaler, D., Jung, R., Holderegger, C., Roos, M. & Hämmerle, C. (2007). Replacement of teeth exhibiting periapical pathology by immediate implants. A prospective, controlled clinical trial. *Clinical Oral Implants Research*, accepted for publication.

Watzek, G., Haider, R., Mensdorff-Pouilly, N. & Haas, R. (1995). Immediate and delayed implantation for complete restoration of the jaw following extraction of all residual teeth: A retrospective study comparing different types of serial immediate implantation. *International Journal of Periodontics and Restorative Dentistry* **12**, 206–217.

Weisgold, A.S., Arnoux, J.P. & Lu, J. (1997). Single-tooth anterior implant: a world of caution. Part I. *Journal of Esthetic Dentistry* **9**, 225–233.

Werbitt, M.J. & Goldberg, P.V. (1992). The immediate implant: bone preservation and bone regeneration. *International Journal of Periodontics and Restorative Dentistry* **12**, 206–217.

Wichmann M. (1990). Visibility of front and side teeth. *ZWR* **99**, 623–626.

Wilson, T.G., Schenk, R., Buser, D. & Cochran, D. (1998). Implants placed in immediate extraction sites: A report of histologic and histometric analyses of human biopsies. *International Journal of Oral & Maxillofacial Implants* **13**, 333–341.

Zitzmann, N.U., Naef, R. & Schärer, P. (1997). Resorbable versus nonresorbable membranes in combination with Bio-Oss for guided bone regeneration. *International Journal of Oral & Maxillofacial Implants* **12**, 844–852.

Zitzmann, N.U., Schärer, P. & Marinello, C.P. (1999). Factors influencing the success of GBR. *Journal of Clinical Periodontology* **26**, 673–682.

Chapter 48

The Surgical Site

Marc Quirynen and Ulf Lekholm

Bone: shape and quality, 1068
  Clinical examination, 1068
  Radiographic examination, 1068
  Planning for implant placement, 1069
Implant placement, 1071
  Guiding concept, 1071
  Flap elevation, 1071
  Flapless implant insertion, 1071

Model-based guided surgery, 1071
  Bone preparation, 1071
Anatomic landmarks with potential risk, 1072
Implant position, 1073
  Number of implants, 1074
Implant direction, 1074
Healing time, 1076

Bone: shape and quality

It is imperative that the conditions of the soft and hard tissues as well as of the shape of the bone in the recipient sites intended for implants are carefully examined. Both clinical and radiographic parameters must be used in this examination.

Clinical examination

The clinical examination should include assessment of (1) colour and texture alterations of the mucosa (indicative of a lesion) and (2) the thickness of the soft tissues. The recipient site should also be palpated in order to estimate the volume of the tissues available in the edentulous region of the jaw. It must be realized, however, that both the mucosa and the bone of the edentulous region are included in this clinical measure. Hence, the clinician must realize that palpation may overestimate the volume of hard tissue present at the site.

The clinical examination must also determine the inter-arch gap and the dimensions of the edentulous area to ascertain that enough space is present (1) to allow optimal maneuvering (access of the hand piece together with the preparation drills) during surgical procedures, (2) to avoid damage of the periodontium of teeth adjacent to the edentulous area during implant insertion, and (3) to allow placement of the prosthetic device. As a rule of thumb, the inter-arch distance should be ≥5 mm, and the distance between a tooth and an implant should be ≥3 mm. If the size of the edentulous region is diminutive, implants with a small diameter must be selected, and eventually a surgical guide (stent) used to assist the surgeon during implant installation. This might help to avoid contact with the neighboring teeth.

The jaw relation (angle class) must also be determined, as this will have an influence on the direction of insertion of the implants (further discussed below). In the final step of the clinical examination impressions of the jaws (dentition) are obtained and stone cast models prepared. Such models can later be used during treatment planning and for the preparation of surgical position and direction stents.

Radiographic examination

The radiographic examination (see Chapter 28) will provide more detailed information on the amount and quality of the bone available at the recipient site. Lekholm and Zarb (1985) proposed that the edentulous jaw (segment of the jaw) should be classified regarding its shape and quality. Thus a grading into five groups was used to describe the shape of the jaw (Fig. 48-1a) while four groups were used to describe the quality of the bone tissue (Fig. 48-1b).

Panoramic and intraoral apical radiographic images give a first impression of the bone, as well as of important anatomic landmarks such as: the floor of sinusal and nasal cavities; the incisive nerve; the inferior alveolar nerve; the roots and apices of neighboring teeth; and the crest of the alveolar ridge. From the two-dimensional images it is also possible to obtain some information about the available height of the bone at the recipient site, while three-dimensional radiographs are essential to determine the width of the alveolar crest. It is important to realize that the definitive evaluation of the dimension

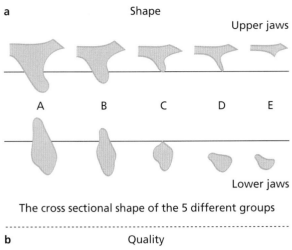

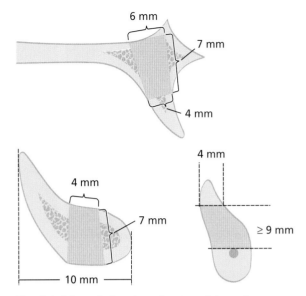

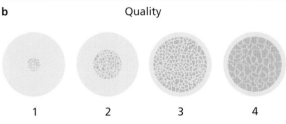

Fig. 48-2 Schematic drawings showing minimum bone volume needed for standard implants of the Brånemark System.

The cross sectional shape of the 5 different groups

b   Quality

1   2   3   4

The 4 different groups of bone quality

Fig. 48-1 Schematic drawings showing (a) residual jaw shape classification, and (b) jaw bone quality classification, according to Lekholm and Zarb (1985).

of the recipient site should not be based on observations made in intraoral radiographs or in orthopantomograms. This is especially true in cases where intraoral palpation indicated the presence of a narrow ridge (jaw). Indeed, the precise location of the inferior alveolar nerve must be identified via measurements made in images from conventional or computer-assisted tomography (CT). Correct identification of the mandibular canal may assist the clinician to avoid damaging the nerve during surgery and thereby preventing the occurrence of complications such as impaired sensory function and paresthesia of the lower lip and neighbouring soft tissues (Abarca et al. 2006).

The cylinder-shaped cavity prepared in the recipient site to house the endosseous part of the implant is, as a rule, 1–2 mm longer than the titanium device per se. Thus, for a 7-mm long implant, the required minimum height of the bone of the recipient site is 8–9 mm (Fig. 48-2). In cases where implants are to be installed in positions above the inferior alveolar nerve, a minimum height of 9–10 mm of bone is required for a 7-mm long implant.

Planning for implant placement

Radiographs are used to make preliminary decisions regarding the position(s) as well as the number and dimensions of implants to be used. The location of the most distal implant is determined first (Fig. 48-3). The number and the position of more mesially located implants are identified thereafter. In this treatment

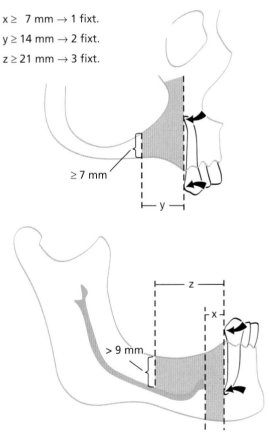

$x \geq$ 7 mm → 1 fixt.
$y \geq$ 14 mm → 2 fixt.
$z \geq$ 21 mm → 3 fixt.

Fig. 48-3 Schematic drawings indicating location of minimum bone volume areas in distal directions, and giving distances needed for various numbers of implants. Arrows indicate prominence and apex of the nearest tooth.

planning process it must be recognized that the inter-implant distance must be ≥3 mm.

The final decision regarding the number and dimension of implants to be inserted, however, is most often made during surgery, i.e. after the soft

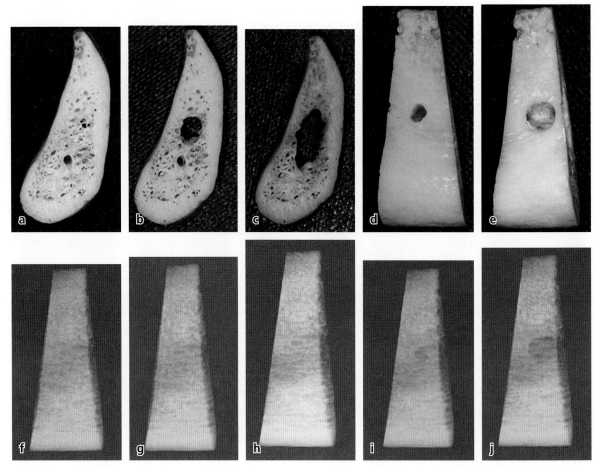

Fig. 48-4 An example (for this illustration without soft tissues) of part of a jawbone in which a progressively larger defect has been created, initially within the spongious bone (a–c), later (d,e) also perforating the cortex. The images (f–j) represent the corresponding radiographs.

tissue flaps have been elevated and the bone of the recipient sites has been exposed.

Defects in the jaw bone

Intraoral (conventional or digital) as well as extraoral radiographic images (conventional tomography, spiral CT) may not necessarily reveal all lesions and defects in the jawbone. In a recent *ex vivo* study (Van Assche *et al.* 2007), intraoral radiographs were taken of progressively larger, artificially created, defects in both the mandible and the maxilla. As illustrated in Fig. 48-4, a defect first became visible in the radiograph when the area (junction) including the cortical plate and cancellous bone was involved. This indicates that the clinician may overlook such intra-ridge lesions (Quirynen *et al.* 2005).

During implant installation surgery, minor fenestrations or marginal dehiscences sometimes occur. Hence some threads of the implants may be exposed (not covered by bone). In most cases such uncovered threads may be left unattended since no adverse reactions have been observed in the mucosa at such locations (Lekholm *et al.* 1996). On the other hand, if the jaws contain defects of such a magnitude that the

implants cannot be placed in proper positions without having major parts of their surfaces exposed, ridge augmentation is often recommended. This may include guided bone regeneration (Molly *et al.* 2006) and/or bone grafting (Buser *et al.* 1994; Deporter 2001). A recent systematic review on augmentation techniques (Chiapasco *et al.* 2006) indicated that several different procedures may enhance the bone volume in a predictable manner and establish better conditions for implant insertion. For further details regarding ridge augmentation see Chapter 49.

Summary: the local condition of edentulous areas considered for implants must be properly evaluated, and no pathology in the soft and/or hard tissues of the jaws should be accepted at the time of implant placement. Radiographic evaluations are necessary in order to identify important landmarks in the jaws as well as to study the shape and the quality of the bone tissue in areas considered for implants. Tomography is used when implants are to be placed above the inferior alveolar nerve, and/or when the clinical examination indicates that the recipient site harbors minute amounts of bone. The minimum amount of bone required for implant surgery is related to the size and surface of the implants to be used.

Implant placement

Guiding concept

The main purpose for the use of implants in dentistry is to establish a stable anchorage for a fixed or removable prosthesis (Brånemark *et al.* 1985). In order to allow osseointegration to occur and be maintained, the handling of the bone tissue during surgery must be diligent. It is important to recognize that bone is a living tissue that must not be exposed to undue trauma. The surgical procedure must be performed according to carefully established guidelines (e.g. Adell *et al.* 1985; Lekholm & Jemt 1989). Furthermore, the surgeon must pay maximum attention to basic rules of sterility and asepsis. It is often noticed that sterile drapes are used while the nose, the most infected site of the entire facial area, is left uncovered. The use of a sterile nose cap that allows the patient to breath freely but prevents the contamination of the sterile gloves and instruments (van Steenberghe *et al.* 1997) is recommended.

Flap elevation

The mucosa of the ridge can be incised using either a crestal or a vestibular approach. At present there is no information available to indicate that one of the two approaches is more advantageous than the other. Consequently, the clinician can select the method best suited for the individual situation. Crestal incisions may be preferred at sites where the crest of the ridge is wide. If the crest is high but narrow, a buccal approach might be preferred. Moreover, when ridge augmentation is to become part of the surgical procedure, incisions on top of the area to be augmented should be avoided (to prevent early exposure of bone substitute or membrane). In cases of so-called one-stage installation surgery, a crestal incision is, of course, mandatory.

Implants are often placed in edentulous sites that are bordered by teeth. Whenever possible, and in particular in the "esthetic zones", the gingiva (papillae) of the neighboring teeth should not be included in the flap. Shrinkage of the papillae during healing is therefore avoided and the occurrence of black triangles in the "tooth–implant" region prevented.

At narrow edentulous sites where implants must be placed close to teeth, it is often necessary to include the gingiva in the flap. In such cases, the crestal incision made in the edentulous area is continued mesially and/or distally into the pocket of the adjacent teeth and is sometimes combined with vertical releasing incisions in the gingiva. The flap is hereby increased in dimension, will receive a more adequate vascular support, and may be managed to allow full soft tissue coverage of the bone and the implant(s).

It is important to make sure that, during the soft tissue elevation procedure, the entire periosteum is properly released from the walls of the jaw and included in the flap (full-thickness flap). This is particularly important when a flap is released from the lingual side of the mandible. The exposure of the lingual hard tissue wall of the mandible allows the surgeon to detect an accidental perforation of the lingual cortex during drilling and implant installation. It is also important to release a full-thickness flap on the buccal side of both the maxilla and the mandible. This will make it possible to observe the presence of cavities and/or protrusions of the jaws, contours of tooth roots, and nerve entrances, i.e. structures that may influence the positioning of the implants. Finally flap elevation and exposure of the osseous tissue will facilitate irrigation (cooling) of the site during drilling.

Flapless implant insertion

Implant installation without flap elevation and exposure of the bone tissue was recently introduced. This approach is obviously supported by commercial pressure. Flapless surgery no doubt may offer some advantages including (1) reduction in complications for the patient (less pain and swelling), (2) reduced surgical time and no suturing, and (3) good fit between implant and soft tissues that facilitates the restorative phase of treatment. The success of this implant installation approach depends to a large extent on the quality of the surgical template (stent) that must be used.

The scientific data on flapless implant surgery is sparse (Becker *et al.* 2005; van Steenberghe *et al.* 2005; Fortin *et al.* 2006). Hence, the use of flapless implant insertion as "routine" procedure in daily practice is questioned, due to the absence of long-term data.

Model-based guided surgery

With the use of a plaster model that presents the edentulous area and with additional information on the thickness of the soft tissues, the dental technician can replicate the underlying jaw bone. The implant insertion can be planned and performed on the plaster model and the most convenient position for the permanent restoration can also be determined. In a next step, the model can be used to prepare a surgical template. The template can be fitted with sleeves (canals) to guide the drilling procedure. Since the model also reproduces the soft tissues of the recipient site, fabrication of a provisional restoration can be made even before the implants are actually inserted in the jaw of the patient.

Bone preparation

Bone tissue must not be exposed to adverse heat. Drilling in bone tissue may increase the temperature at the recipient site (Brånemark *et al.* 1985). The threshold level for osteocyte damage lies around 47°C, only about 10°C above body temperature

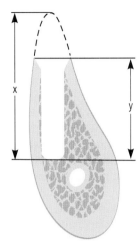

Fig. 48-5 Schematic drawing showing maximum drilling depth (x) without reaching the nerve, as measured from the top of the crest, and implant site length (y), as measured from the lowest bone level in the canal entrance.

(Eriksson & Adell 1986). Consequently, all mechanical preparation of the jaw must be performed with a minimum rise in temperature. This can be achieved via the use of an intermittent drilling technique, together with the use of sharp burs. The preparation of the implant bed should be performed in a sequence of steps, and consistently with profuse saline irrigation (Adell *et al.* 1985). In the presence of particularly dense bone, e.g. in the symphysis region of the mandible, it is also recommended to use an extra wide twist drill, prior to the pretapping procedure and/or insertion the implants (Friberg 1994). When implants are to be placed in soft bone, drilling must be performed with the greatest care, as there is a risk that the entrance of the implant site may be widened too much, and the inserted implant may become unstable. To minimize the risk of initial implant instability, an adjusted surgical technique using either thinner drills or wider diameter implants was recommended (Bahat 1993; Friberg 1994; Watzek & Ulm 2001).

The only structure that can clearly be identified both in radiographs and clinically is the top of the alveolar crest. Consequently, this configuration has to be used as reference for all measurements, both in radiographs and during surgery. During the preparation of the site it is also of particular importance to keep an eye on the depth indicators of the drills and how they relate to the top of the crest. It must be pointed out that during the preparation of the site, the reference point on the crest for the depth measurements may move in an apical direction, particularly if a narrow and drop-shaped alveolar crest is present in the recipient site (Fig. 48-5).

Anatomic landmarks with potential risk

Implant surgery is often regarded/promoted, especially by implant companies, as a safe and

minimally invasive procedure. This is not the case, however, especially when implants are placed in the lower jaw (Mraiwa *et al.* 2003a,b). Mechanical compression and/or direct injury during implant insertion may (1) disturb the nerve and initiate a neural degenerative process, or (2) disturb the microcirculation and cause edema and/or a local hematoma.

Neurosensory disorders of the inferior alveolar, mental, or incisive nerves have been reported to occur after implant surgery. Usually the resulting anesthesia, paresthesia, or even dysesthesia are transient phenomena, but certain long-lasting/permanent neuropathies have been reported. An optimal radiographic analysis of the lower jaw is mandatory when planning for implant placement in the neighborhood of the mental foramen or above the inferior alveolar nerve. It still remains a matter of discussion whether injury to the incisive canal in the lower jaw can cause neuropathy.

Several cases of severe hemorrhage in the floor of the mouth, with subsequent life-threatening upper airway obstruction, have been recorded in association with implant placement in both the anterior and posterior portions of the mandible (for review see Kalpidis & Setayesh 2004). Two arteries are responsible for the vascular supply to the mandible (Fig. 48-6a). At the anterior border of the hypoglossus muscle, the lingual artery gives rise to the sublingual artery. This important artery (2 mm in diameter) traverses the floor of the mouth in a frontal direction, near the medial and superior surface of the mylohyoid muscle, medially to the sublingual gland, and inferio-medially to the submandibular duct and the lingual nerve. The sublingual artery gives off several alveolar branches for complementary blood supply to the lingual anterior cortical plate of the mandible. A second small artery, the submental artery (2 mm in diameter), a branch of the facial artery, runs along the inferior plane of the mylohyoid muscle lateral to the anterior belly of the digastric muscle. As illustrated in Fig. 48–6b, the submental artery runs close to the lingual lower border of the mandible. The largest branches of this artery may be seen on a cone-beam or dental CT as they extend into the bone (Fig. 48-6c–e).

The intimate proximity of these arteries, or their vascular plexa, to the lingual cortical plate explains why a lingual perforation in the lower third of the mandible can result in a massive hematoma in the floor of the mouth. Due to the presence of the strong cervical fasciae in the neck region (the *superficial layer*, the *fasciae of the infra-hyoid muscles*, the *pretracheal layer*), the hematoma will displace the tongue and floor of the mouth superiorly and posteriorly, posing a potentially serious threat of obstruction of the upper airway (for review see Kalpidis & Setayesh 2004). Several reports have appeared in the literature describing massive hematoma in the floor of the mouth, where unfortunately a tracheostomy or

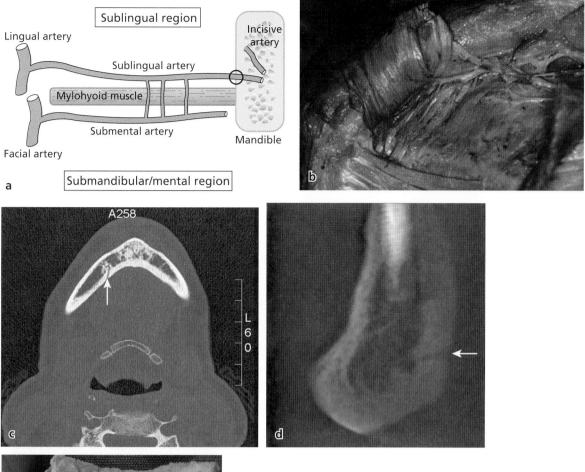

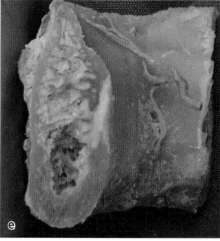

Fig. 48-6 (a) Schematic representation of the arterial anatomy in the floor of the mouth. The mandible is depicted in a midsagittal cross section. The sublingual and submental arteries follow almost parallel pathways, respectively superior and inferior to the mylohyoid muscle. The intimate proximity of these arteries (or their branches) to the lingual cortical plate of the mandible explains the risks for a hematoma after perforation of the latter. (b) Dissection, *ex vivo*, of submental artery illustrating its proximity with the lower lingual cortex of the mandible. (c) Axial slice with clear appearance of artery running into the bone at the canine position. (d) Reformatted cross section at canine position, fortunately the implant remained far away from the artery as well as from the lingual cortical plate. (e) Dissection of branches from sublingual artery running into the bone to make anastomosis with incisive artery.

intubation was the only option to save the life of the patient.

The shape of the lower jaw exhibits large individual variation. A small proportion of jaws (3%) (Quirynen *et al.* 2003) has a distinct lingual depression between lateral incisor and second premolar, superior to the mylohyoid muscle, to house the lingual gland (called the sublingual fovea). Perforation of the bone with a drill in this region must be avoided. As stated previously, deep dissection of the mucoperiosteal flap lingually is strongly recommended in implant installation surgery to expose the cortical plate of the mandible.

Implant position

If possible an implant should be placed in tooth position (Fig. 48-7), both in a mesio-distal and in a bucco-lingual direction. To achieve this, the starting point for the insertion in the bone must, in most instances, be located towards the buccal side of the crest in the mandible, and towards the palate in the maxilla. This is due to the presence of concavities that often exist in the jaws. Depending on the size of such concavities, the starting point (for the instertion) will be located either close to the top of the crest, as in the case of a wide alveolar process, or deeper down

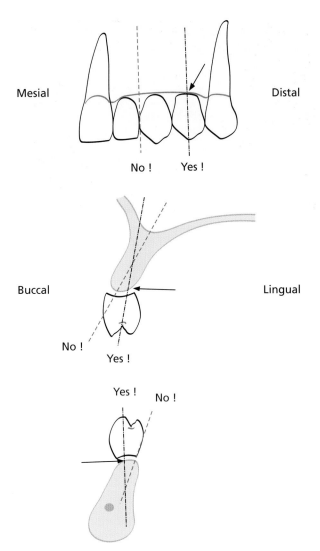

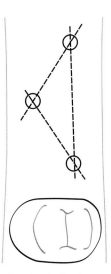

Fig. 48-8 Schematic drawing indicating a tripod placement of the implants in order to minimize individual load distribution onto each implant by creating several rotational axes.

Fig. 48-7 Schematic drawings showing implant positions in mesial–distal and buccal–lingual dimensions. Indicated starting points for drilling are marked with black arrows.

palatally or buccally (Fig. 48-7), if the jaw is thin in its coronal portion.

In cases of partial edentulism, the recipient site closest to a tooth must first be identified. The cylindrical canal in the recipient site is prepared approximately 3.5–4 mm away from the prominence of the tooth. The subsequent implant positions, in a distal direction, are then identified. The minimum amount of bone that must be present in a recipient site is dependent on the dimension of the implants used; as a rule of thumb: the bone tissue of the site should be about 4(5) mm (in a horizontal direction) and about 7(9) mm (in a vertical direction) (Figs. 48-2, 48-3).

In a fully edentulous jaw, it might be preferable to start by placing the most distal implants, so that the position of other implants can be selected accordingly. The longest distance that can be accepted between two implants has not yet been properly defined. As an alternative to a reduced inter-implant distance, and an increased number of implants, it is sometimes possible to use wider diameter implants, as discussed below.

Number of implants

In partially edentulous jaws preferably three implants should be inserted in order to avoid overloading of the anchorage units (Rangert *et al.* 1989). The failure rate has been reported to be higher for reconstorations placed on two than for those on three or more implants (Jemt & Lekholm 1993). Furthermore, the implants should be placed in a tripod position (Fig. 48-8) instead of being inserted in a straight line, thereby minimizing the transmission of bending forces on to each individual implant (Rangert *et al.* 1989). If only one implant can be inserted, then in most cases this anchorage should be used to support a single crown restoration. Implants should never be placed in the midline of the maxilla, not only because they might eventually expand the suture between the two maxillae, but such implants may eventually compromise the esthetics and phonetics after the prosthetic device has been inserted.

Implant direction

After the position of the implant has been identified, the direction/inclination of the implant in the jaw (bucco-lingual and mesio-distal) must be determined. If possible the implants should be placed in tooth position. This means that in the normal case the long axis of the implant should be directed through the occlusal surface of the final restoration. Regarding the bucco-lingual dimension (Fig. 48-9), the long axis of mandibular implants will mainly be directed towards the limbus part of the incisors or the palatal cusps of the teeth in the maxilla. For implants placed in the maxilla, the corresponding inclination should be towards the incisal edges of the frontal teeth or the buccal cusps of the premolars or molars of the mandible. If the starting point of the implant sites in the maxilla is located close to the top of the crest, and if

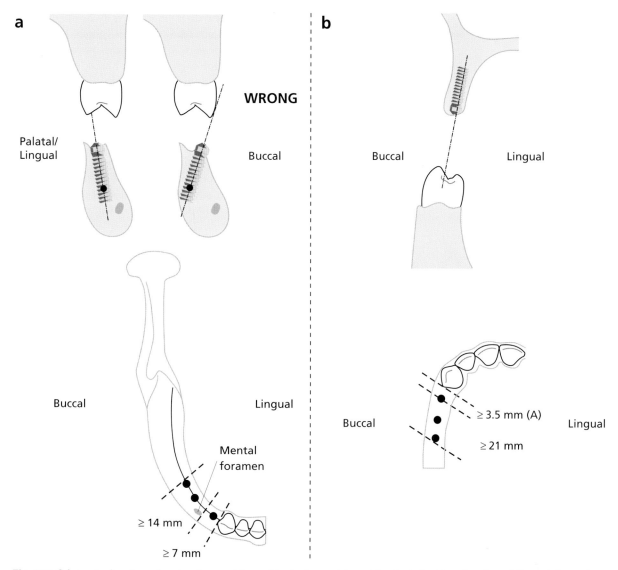

Fig. 48-9 Schematic drawings showing the most favorable starting points and implant directions in a buccal–lingual dimension within (a) the mandible and (b) the maxilla. A = closest distance of a site to a tooth.

a concavity on the buccal side of the ridge is present, there is a risk that the surgeon leans the long axis of the implants too far buccally. The equivalent for the mandible is an implant directed too far lingually owing to the presence of lingual concavities. Such adverse directions can impair the esthetics and function of the future restoration (Fig. 48-7), even though angulated abutments may to some extent compensate for such a surgical shortcoming.

In addition, the inclination of the implants to be inserted will depend on the existing jaw relation. In the case of angle class I jaw relation, the implants should be placed rather vertically in both jaws. In angle class II, the implants should often be placed vertically in the maxilla and slightly buccally in the mandible. In angle class III relations, the implants are inclined buccally in the maxilla and more lingually in the mandible. If the relation between the jaws is markedly adverse, orthognatic surgery may be considered (Clokie 2001) to correct the abnormal jaw relation. Another treatment option in such cases is an overdenture, retained by a bar construction on two implants in the mandible and/or on four implants in the maxilla. The overdenture often offers a favorable outcome to the patient with respect to esthetics, speech, lip and facial support, and function (Naert *et al.* 1998; van Steenberghe *et al.* 2001; Mericske-Stern *et al.* 2002; Eckert & Carr 2004; Kronstrom *et al.* 2006), even though the success rates of the supporting implants might be slightly lower than for implants that support fixed full bridges (Schwartz-Arad *et al.* 2005).

For the mesio-distal orientation of the implant (Fig. 48-10), the rule is that the implant closest to the last tooth is placed parallel with the long axis of the root of this tooth. The further distally the site is located into the molar region, on the other hand, the more inclined are the positions of the implants. In the mandible, for example, it is recommended that the most distal implants be placed in a slightly mesial direction to facilitate the connection of the abutments with the fixed bridge restoration.

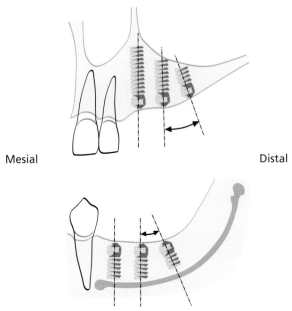

Mesial   Distal

Fig. 48-10 Drawings showing implant directions in the mesial–distal dimension of posterior parts of the jaws. In the maxilla, the most distal implant is directed distally due to the orientation of the sinus wall to engage more bone. In the mandible, the implant is tilted mesially to provide better access for instruments during abutment and prosthetic procedures.

In extremely resorbed mandibles, the most distal implant that is placed immediately in front of the mental foramen, can be tilted distally in order to achieve optimal spreading of the supporting units (Maló *et al.* 2005). Correspondingly, in the resorbed maxilla, the canal prepared for the most distal implant (lateral to the canine) can be directed slightly distally and follow the mesial wall of the maxillary sinus, thereby allowing a longer implant to be placed (Maló *et al.* 2005). An alternative to this procedure would be to use of sinus elevation and grafting techniques (Hochwald & Davis 1992; Neukam & Kloss 2001).

Healing time

According to early protocols the healing time following installation of implants with a turned surface was 3–4 months (Lekholm & Zarb 1985). For the maxilla and occasionally in the posterior areas of the mandible the healing time was 5–6 months, as the bone is normally more cancellous in these portions of the jaws (Adell *et al.* 1985; Watzek & Ulm 2001). Furthermore, for implants placed in quality 4 bone (Lekholm & Zarb 1985), it was recommended that the healing time in the mandible was also extended another 1 or 2 months (Friberg 1994). As variations may exist between different regions of the same jaw, e.g. between frontal and distal segments or even between different sites within the same region (Watzek & Ulm 2001), it is also important to individualize the healing time and to allow the softest bone site to decide the timing.

For implants with a (mechanically or chemically) modified surface, reduced healing times (6 weeks) have been advocated. Such implants have also been recommended for early or even immediate loading protocols (see also Chapter 47). Immediate loading of implants, both with the use of provisional (Balshi & Wolfinger 1997; Schnitman *et al.* 1997) and/or definite reconstructions has been proposed (Brånemark *et al.* 1999; Randow *et al.* 1995; Ericsson *et al.* 2000a; van Steenberghe *et al.* 2005). The current experience with immediate occlusal loading of oral implants was summarized in several consensus reports and systematic reviews (Aparicio *et al.* 2003; Cochran *et al.* 2004; Misch *et al.* 2004a,b; Nkenke & Fenner 2006). Thus, the outcomes of short-term randomized controlled trials have shown that survival and success rates of immediately loaded implants in fully edentulous jaws may be similar to those of conventionally loaded implants (Chiapasco *et al.* 2001; Romeo *et al.* 2002).

The survival rate of immediately restored single-tooth implants was similar to or slightly lower than that of conventionally loaded single-tooth implants (Ericsson *et al.* 2000b; Cannizzaro & Leone 2003). Ericsson *et al.* (2000b) had a restoration placed immediately on the implant, but occlusal contacts were avoided. Some clinicians try to protect "immediately loaded" implants from forces exerted by the tongue or during chewing by using occlusal splints (Lorenzoni *et al.* 2003). To date, there are no controlled studies that enable evidence-based decisions to be made as to whether single-tooth implants can be loaded immediately or should only be restored without occlusal contacts (Nkenke & Fenner 2006).

Currently, it is not possible to draw conclusions concerning exclusion and inclusion criteria for immediate loading, threshold values for implant stability that allow immediate loading, bone quality needed for immediate loading, and the relevance of immediate functional loading and immediate non-functional loading (Nkenke & Fenner 2006). In most of the studies on immediate loading, good bone quality has been mentioned as an important prognostic factor for the success of the procedure (Chiapasco *et al.* 2001; Romeo *et al.* 2002). Although this conclusion seems reasonable, the level of evidence that supports the assumption is low (Nkenke & Fenner 2006). There are, in fact, no controlled studies that have been especially designed to compare immediate loading of oral implants placed in bone of varying density (soft/hard). The same is true for the lengths and diameters of implants that should be used for immediate loading. In one controlled study, moderately rough implant surfaces appeared to improve the survival rate of immediately loaded implants (Rocci *et al.* 2003a,b). In this study, however, the difference between the moderately rough as opposed to the machined-surface implants was not significant.

Review papers on immediate loading have also addressed additional biomechanical aspects of this procedure (Szmukler-Moncler *et al.* 2000; Gapski *et al.* 2003; Chiapasco 2004; Nkenke & Fenner 2006). Based on different experimental studies, it was stated that a micromotion threshold should not be exceeded; otherwise, osseointegration would be hindered. The critical threshold seems to be 50–150 µm (Pilliar *et al.* 1986; Szmukler-Moncler *et al.* 1998). Therefore, it has been claimed that a high initial stability is necessary for immediate loading of dental implants (Chaushu *et al.* 2001; Calandriello & Tomatis 2005). For this purpose, these authors used modified drilling protocols combined with bone compaction with osteotomes to achieve increased primary stability. Some authors have chosen insertion torque as a measure of implant stability, and arbitrarily selected torque values of ≥32–40 Ncm as thresholds to allow immediate loading (Wöhrle 1998; Hui *et al.* 2001; Lorenzoni *et al.* 2003). With resonance frequency analysis (Meredith *et al.* 1996) it has become possible to measure initial implant stability, i.e. the density of the bone surrounding the implant. The bone quality can thereby be analyzed repeatedly over time and the healing period individualized without using any invasive technique for the tests. An implant stability quotient (ISQ) value of >60 was recommended (Sennerby & Meredith 2002) to allow oral implants to be loaded directly after their insertion. Until now, controlled studies that have compared the relationship between different levels of implant stability and implant survival rate have been lacking. Consequently, there is currently no proven threshold value that indicates that immediate loading will be successful. Besides high initial stability, it has been stressed that immediately loaded implants in multi-unit situations should be rigidly splinted by the use of superstructures (Nikellis *et al.* 2004; van Steenberghe *et al.* 2004). In order to optimize splinting, the use of metal-reinforced superstructures was advocated. High success rates have also been reported for immediate loading of implants connected with superstructures that were not reinforced with metal (Nikellis *et al.* 2004).

References

Abarca, M., van Steenberghe, D., Malevez, C., De Ridder, J. & Jacobs, R. (2006). Neurosensory disturbances after immediate loading of implants in the anterior mandible: an initial questionnaire approach followed by a psychophysical assessment. *Clinical Oral Investigations* **10**(4), 269–277.

Adell, R., Lekholm, U. & Brånemark, P-I. (1985). Surgical procedures. In: Brånemark, P-I., Zarb, G.A. & Albrektsson, T., eds. *Tissue-Integrated Prostheses. Osseointegration in Clinical Dentistry.* Chicago: Quintessence, pp. 211–232.

Aparicio, C., Rangert, B. & Sennerby, L. (2003). Immediate/ early loading of dental implants: a report from the Sociedad Espanola de Implantes World Congress consensus meeting in Barcelona, Spain, 2002. *Clinical Implant Dentistry and Related Research* **5**, 57–60.

Bahat, O. (1993). Treatment planning and placement of implants in the posterior maxillae: report of 732 consecutive Nobelpharma implants. *International Journal of Oral & Maxillofacial Implants* **8**, 151–161.

Bahlshi, T.J. & Wolfinger, G.J. (1997). Immediate loading of Brånemark implants in edentulous mandibles: a preliminary report. *Implant Dentistry* **6**, 83–88.

Becker, W., Goldstein, M., Becker, B.E. & Sennerby, L. (2005). Minimally invasive flapless implant surgery: a prospective multicenter study. *Clinical Implant Dentistry and Related Research* **7** (Suppl 1), S21–27.

Brånemark, P-I., Engstrand, P., Örnell, L-O., Gröndahl, K., Nilsson, P., Hagberg, K., Darle, C. & Lekholm, U. (1999). Brånemark Novum: A new treatment concept for rehabilitation of the edentulous mandible. Preliminary results from a prospective clinical follow-up study. *Clinical Implant Dentistry and Related Research* **1**, 2–16.

Brånemark, P-I., Zarb, G.A. & Albrektsson, T., eds. (1985). *Tissue-Integrated Prostheses. Osseointegration in Clinical Dentistry.* Chicago: Quintessence.

Buser, D., Dahlin, C. & Schenk, R.K., eds. (1994). *Guided Bone Regeneration in Implant Dentistry.* Chicago: Quintessence.

Calandriello, R. & Tomatis, M. (2005). Simplified treatment of the atrophic posterior maxilla via immediate/early function and tilted implants: a prospective 1-year clinical study. *Clinical Implant Dentistry and Related Research* **7** (Suppl 1), S1–S12.

Cannizzaro, G. & Leone, M. (2003). Restoration of partially edentulous patients using dental implants with a micro-

textured surface: a prospective comparison of delayed and immediate full occlusal loading. *International Journal of Oral & Maxillofacial Implants* **18**, 512–522.

Chaushu, G., Chaushu, S., Tzohar, A. & Dayan, D. (2001). Immediate loading of single-tooth implants: immediate versus non-immediate implantation. A clinical report. *International Journal of Oral & Maxillofacial Implants* **16**, 267–272.

Chiapasco, M. (2004). Early and immediate restoration and loading of implants in completely edentulous patients. *International Journal of Oral & Maxillofacial Implants* **19** (Suppl), 76–91.

Chiapasco, M., Abati, S., Romeo, E. & Vogel, G. (2001). Implant-retained mandibular overdentures with Brånemark system MKII implants: a prospective comparative study between delayed and immediate loading. *International Journal of Oral & Maxillofacial Implants* **16**, 537–546.

Chiapasco, M., Zaniboni, M. & Boisco, M. (2006). Augmentation procedures for the rehabilitation of deficient edentulous ridges with oral implants. *Clinical Oral Implants Research* **17** (Suppl 2), 136–159.

Clokie, C.M. (2001). Strategies for bone regeneration and osseointegration in completely edentulous patients. In: Zarb, G., Lekholm, U., Albrektsson, T. & Tenenbaum, H., eds. *Aging, Osteoporosis and Dental Implants.* Chicago: Quintessence, pp. 113–124.

Cochran, D.L., Morton, D. & Weber, H.P. (2004). Consensus statements and recommended clinical procedures regarding loading protocols for endosseous dental implants. *International Journal of Oral & Maxillofacial Implants* **19** (Suppl), 109–113.

Deporter, D. (2001). Surgical site development in the partially edentulous patient. In: Zarb, G., Lekholm, U., Albrektsson, T. & Tenenbaum, H., eds. *Aging, Osteoporosis and Dental Implants.* Chicago: Quintessence, pp. 99–112.

Eckert, S.E. & Carr, A.B. (2004). Implant-retained maxillary overdentures. *Dental Clinics of North America* **48**, 585–601.

Ericsson, I., Nilson, H., Lindh, T., Nilner, K. & Randow, K. (2000b). Immediate functional loading of Brånemark single tooth implants. An 18 months' clinical pilot follow-up study. *Clinical Oral Implants Research* **11**, 26–33.

Ericsson, I., Randow, K., Nilner, K. & Peterson, A. (2000a). Early functional loading of Brånemark dental implants:

5-year clinical follow-up study. *Clinical Implant Dentistry and Related Research* **2**, 70–77.

Eriksson, R.A. & Adell, R. (1986). Temperatures during drilling for the placement of implants using the osseointegration technique. *International Journal of Oral and Maxillofacial Surgery* **44**, 4–7.

Fortin, T., Bosson, J.L., Isidori, M. & Blanchet, E. (2006). Effect of flapless surgery on pain experienced in implant placement using an image-guided system. *International Journal of Oral & Maxillofacial Implants* **21**, 298–304.

Friberg, B. (1994). Bone quality evaluation during implant placement. Odont. lic. thesis. Göteborg: Faculty of Odontology, University of Göteborg.

Gapski, R., Wang, H.L., Mascarenhas, P. & Lang, N.P. (2003). Critical review of immediate implant loading. *Clinical Oral Implants Research* **14**, 515–527.

Hochwald, D.A. & Davis, W.H. (1992). Bone grafting in the maxillary sinus floor. In: Worthington, P. & Brånemark, P-I., eds. *Advanced Osseointegration Surgery*. Chicago: Quintessence, pp. 175–181.

Hui, E., Chow, J., Li, D., Liu, J., Wat, P. & Law, H. (2001). Immediate provisional for single-tooth implant replacement with Brånemark system: preliminary report. *Clinical Implant Dentistry and Related Research* **3**, 79–86.

Jemt, T. & Lekholm, U. (1993). Oral implant treatment in posterior partially edentulous jaws. A 5-year follow-up report. *International Journal of Oral & Maxillofacial Implants* **8**, 635–640.

Kalpidis, C.D. & Setayesh, R.M. (2004). Hemorrhaging associated with endosseous implant placement in the anterior mandible: a review of the literature. *Journal of Periodontology* **75**, 631–645.

Kronstrom, M., Widbom, C. & Soderfeldt, B. (2006). Patient evaluation after treatment with maxillary implant-supported overdentures. *Clinical Implant Dentistry and Related Research* **8**, 39–43.

Lekholm, U. & Jemt, T. (1989). Principles for single tooth replacement. In: Albrektsson, T. & Zarb, G.A., eds. *The Brånemark Osseointegrated Implant*. Chicago: Quintessence, pp. 117–126.

Lekholm, U., Sennerby, L., Roos, J. & Becker, W. (1996). Soft tissue and marginal bone conditions at osseointegrated implants with exposed threads. A 5-year retrospective study. *International Journal of Oral & Maxillofacial Implants* **11**, 599–604.

Lekholm, U. & Zarb, G.A. (1985). Patient selection. In: Brånemark, P-I., Zarb, G.A. & Albrektsson, T., eds. *Tissue Integrated Prostheses. Osseointegration in Clinical Dentistry*. Chicago: Quintessence, pp. 199–209.

Lorenzoni, M., Pertl, C., Zhang, K., Wimmer, G. & Wegscheider, W.A. (2003). Immediate loading of single-tooth implants in the anterior maxilla. Preliminary results after one year. *Clinical Oral Implants Research* **14**, 180–187.

Maló, P., Rangert, B. & Nobre, M. (2005). All-on-4 immediate-function concept with Brånemark System implants for completely edentulous maxillae: a 1-year retrospective clinical study. *Clinical Implant Dentistry and Related Research* **7** (Suppl 1), S88–94.

Meredith, N., Alleyne, D. & Cawley, P. (1996). Quantitative determination of the stability of the implant-tissue interface using resonance frequency analysis. *Clinical Oral Implants Research* **7**, 262–267.

Mericske-Stern, R., Oetterli, M., Kiener, P. & Mericske, E. (2002). A follow-up study of maxillary implants supporting an overdenture: clinical and radiographic results. *International Journal of Oral & Maxillofacial Implants* **17**, 678–686.

Misch, C.E., Hahn, J., Judy, K.W., Lemons, J.E., Linkow, L.I., Lozada, J.L., Mills, E., Misch, C.M., Salama, H., Sharawy, M., Testori, T. & Wang, H.L. (2004a). Immediate function consensus conference. workshop guidelines on immediate loading in implant dentistry. November 7, 2003. *Journal of Oral Implantology* **30**, 283–288.

Misch, C.E., Wang, H.L., Misch, C.M., Sharawy, M., Lemons, J. & Judy, K.W. (2004b). Rationale for the application of immediate load in implant dentistry: part II. *Implant Dentistry* **13**, 310–321.

Molly, L., Quirynen, M., Michiels, K. & van Steenberghe, D. (2006). Comparison between jaw bone augmentation by means of a stiff occlusive titanium membrane or an autologous hip graft: a retrospective clinical assessment. *Clinical Oral Implants Research* **17**, 481–487.

Mraiwa, N., Jacobs, R., Moerman, P., Lambrichts, I., van Steenberghe, D. & Quirynen, M. (2003b). Presence and course of the incisive canal in the human mandibular interforaminal region: two-dimensional imaging versus anatomical observations. *Surgical and Radiologic Anatomy* **25**, 416–423.

Mraiwa, N., Jacobs, R., van Steenberghe, D. & Quirynen, M. (2003a). Clinical assessment and surgical implications of anatomic challenges in the anterior mandible. *Clinical Implant Dentistry and Related Research* **5**, 219–225.

Naert, I., Gizani, S. & van Steenberghe, D. (1998). Rigidly splinted implants in the resorbed maxilla to retain a hinging overdenture: a series of clinical reports for up to 4 years. *Journal of Prosthetic Dentistry* **79**, 156–164.

Neukam, F.W. & Kloss, F.R. (2001). Compromised jawbone quantity and its influence on oral implant placement. In: Zarb, G., Lekholm, U., Albrektsson, T. & Tenenbaum, H., eds. *Aging, Osteoporosis and Dental Implants*. Chicago: Quintessence, pp. 85–97.

Nikellis, I., Levi, A. & Nicolopoulos, C. (2004). Immediate loading of 190 endosseous dental implants: a prospective observational study of 40 patient treatments with up to 2-year data. *International Journal of Oral & Maxillofacial Implants* **19**, 116–123.

Nkenke, E. & Fenner, M. (2006). Indications for immediate loading of implants and implant success. *Clinical Oral Implants Research* **17** (Suppl 2), 19–34.

Pilliar, R.M., Lee, J.M. & Maniatopoulos, C. (1986). Observations on the effect of movement on bone ingrowth into porous-surfaced implants. *Clinical Orthopedics and Related Research* **208**, 108–113.

Quirynen, M., Mraiwa, N., van Steenberghe, D. & Jacobs, R. (2003). Morphology and dimensions of the mandibular jaw bone in the interforaminal region in patients requiring implants in the distal areas. *Clinical Oral Implants Research* **14**, 280–285.

Quirynen, M., Vogels, R., Alsaadi, G., Naert, I., Jacobs, R. & van Steenberghe, D. (2005). Predisposing conditions for retrograde peri-implantitis, and treatment suggestions. *Clinical Oral Implants Research* **16**, 599–608.

Randow, K., Ericsson, I., Glantz, P.-O., Lindhe, J., Nilner, K. & Pettersson, A. (1995). *Influence of early functional contacts on fixture stability, soft tissue quality and bone level integrity. A clinical pilot study*. Presented at Brånemark System 30 Year Anniversary, Göteborg, Sweden.

Rangert, B., Jemt, T. & Jörneus, L. (1989). Forces and moments on Brånemark Implants. *International Journal of Oral & Maxillofacial Implants* **4**, 241–247.

Rocci, A., Martignoni, M., Burgos, P.M. & Gottlow, J. (2003a). Histology of retrieved immediately and early loaded oxidized implants: light microscopic observations after 5 to 9 months of loading in the posterior mandible. *Clinical Implant Dentistry and Related Research* **5** (Suppl 1), 88–98.

Rocci, A., Martignoni, M. & Gottlow, J. (2003b). Immediate loading of Brånemark System TiUnite and machined-surface implants in the posterior mandible: a randomized open-ended clinical trial. *Clinical Implant Dentistry and Related Research* **5** (Suppl 1), 57–63.

Romeo, E., Chiapasco, M., Lazza, A., Casentini, P., Ghisolfi, M., Iorio, M. & Vogel, G. (2002). Implant-retained mandibular overdentures with ITI implants. *Clinical Oral Implants Research* **13**, 495–501.

Schnitman, P.A., Wörle, P.S., Rubenstein, J.E., DaSilva, J.D. & Wang, N.H. (1997). Ten year results for Brånemark implants immediately loaded with fixed prostheses at implant placement. *International Journal of Oral & Maxillofacial Implants* **12**, 495–503.

Schwartz-Arad, D., Kidron, N. & Dolev, E. (2005). A long-term study of implants supporting overdentures as a model for implant success. *Journal of Periodontology* **76**, 1431–1435.

Sennerby, L. & Meredith, N. (2002). Analisi della Frequenza di Risonanza (RFA). Conoscenze attuali e implicazioni cliniche. In: Chiapasco, M. & Gatti, C., eds. *Osteointegrazione e Carico Immediato. Fondamenti biologici e applicazioni cliniche.* Milano: Masson, pp. 19–32.

Szmukler-Moncler, S., Piattelli, A., Favero, G.A. & Dubruille, J.H. (2000). Considerations preliminary to the application of early and immediate loading protocols in dental implantology. *Clinical Oral Implants Research* **11**, 12–25.

Szmukler-Moncler, S., Salama, H., Reingewirtz, Y. & Dubruille, J.H. (1998). Timing of loading and effect of micromotion on bone-dental implant interface: review of experimental literature. *Journal of Biomedical Materials Research* **43**, 192–203.

Van Assche, N., Jacobs, R., Coucke, W., van Steenberghe, D. & Quirynen, M. (2007). Critical size for radiographic detection of intra-bony defects. Submitted.

van Steenberghe, D., Glauser, R., Blomback, U., Andersson, M., Schutyser, F., Pettersson, A. & Wendelhag, I. (2005). A computed tomographic scan-derived customized surgical template and fixed prosthesis for flapless surgery and immediate loading of implants in fully edentulous maxillae: a prospective multicenter study. *Clinical Implant Dentistry and Related Research* **7** (Suppl 1), S111–120.

van Steenberghe, D., Molly, L., Jacobs, R., Vandekerckhove, B., Quirynen, M. & Naert, I. (2004). The immediate rehabilitation by means of a ready-made final fixed prosthesis in the edentulous mandible: a 1-year follow-up study on 50 consecutive patients. *Clinical Oral Implants Research* **15**, 360–365.

van Steenberghe, D., Quirynen, M., Naert, I., Maffei, G. & Jacobs, R. (2001). Marginal bone loss around implants retaining hinging mandibular overdentures, at 4-, 8- and 12-years follow-up. *Journal of Clinical Periodontology* **28**, 628–633.

van Steenberghe, D., Yoshida, K., Papaioannou, W., Bollen, C.M.L., Reybrouck, G. & Quirynen, M. (1997). Complete nose coverage to prevent airborne contamination via nostrils is unnecessary. *Clinical Oral Implants Research* **8**, 512–516.

Watzek, G. & Ulm, C. (2001). Compromised alveolar bone quality in edentulous jaws. In: Zarb, G., Lekholm, U., Albrektsson, T. & Tenenbaum, H., eds. *Aging, Osteoporosis and Dental Implants.* Chicago: Quintessence, pp. 67–84.

Wöhrle, P.S. (1998). Single-tooth replacement in the aesthetic zone with immediate provisionalization: fourteen consecutive case reports. *Practical Periodontics and Aesthetic Dentistry* **10**, 1107–1114.

Part 15: Reconstructive Ridge Therapy

49 Ridge Augmentation Procedures, 1083
Christoph H.F. Hämmerle and Ronald E. Jung

50 Elevation of the Maxillary Sinus Floor, 1099
Bjarni E. Pjetursson and Niklaus P. Lang

Chapter 49

Ridge Augmentation Procedures

Christoph H.F. Hämmerle and Ronald E. Jung

Introduction, 1083
Patient situation, 1084
Bone morphology, 1084
    Horizontal bone defects, 1084
    Vertical bone defects, 1084
Soft tissue morphology, 1085
Augmentation materials, 1085
    Membranes, 1085
    Bone grafts and bone graft substitutes, 1086
Long-term results, 1087
Clinical concepts, 1088

Ridge preservation, 1088
Extraction sockets (class I), 1089
Dehiscence defects (classes II and III), 1090
Horizontal defects (class IV), 1091
Vertical defects (class V), 1092
Future developments, 1093
    Growth and differentiation factors, 1093
    Delivery systems for growth and differentiation
      factors, 1093
    Membrane developments, 1093
    Future outlook, 1094

Introduction

Successful implant therapy is dependent upon an adequate volume of bone at the site of implant placement, since the long-term prognosis of dental implants is adversely affected by inadequate bone volume (Lekholm et al. 1986).

In principle, four methods have been described to increase the rate of bone formation and to augment bone volume: osteoinduction by the use of appropriate growth factors (Reddi 1981; Urist 1965); osteoconduction, where a grafting material serves as a scaffold for new bone growth (Buch et al. 1986; Reddi et al. 1987); distraction osteogenesis, by which a fracture is surgically induced and the two fragments are then slowly pulled apart (e.g. Ilizarov 1989a,b); and finally, guided tissue regeneration (GTR), which allows spaces maintained by barrier membranes to be filled with new bone (Dahlin et al. 1988, 1991a; Kostopoulos & Karring 1994; Nyman & Lang 1994).

Among these methods, guided bone regeneration (GBR) is the best documented for the treatment of localized bone defects in the jaws. GBR has allowed the use of endosseous implants in areas of the jaw with insufficient bone volume. Lack of bone volume may be due to congenital, post-traumatic, or post-surgical defects or result from disease processes. The predictability and success which can now be achieved with GBR procedures enable the clinician to obtain similar rates of treatment success at sites with bone defects compared to sites without defects (Hammerle et al. 2002).

Although bone augmentation procedures are an important part of contemporary implant therapy, other factors are also critical in order to obtain treatment success. In this respect a systematic approach to a given patient situation is key to achieving the desired aim. In complex cases with a multitude of problems, several aspects have to be taken into consideration. These include the patient's general health status, behavior of the patient, environmental factors, the presence of any oral diseases, and the situation at the site planned for implantation as well as the regions of the dentition adjacent to and opposing this site.

GBR is frequently part of complex treatments, but this chapter will focus only on the aspects of bone augmentation at localized defects in the alveolar process.

More than two decades have passed since the introduction of GBR into clinical practice. Today, general understanding of the mechanisms leading to regeneration of desired tissues still agrees with the initially published statements (Karring et al. 1980; Nyman et al. 1980, 1989). In brief, when a space is formed, cells from the adjacent tissues will grow into this space to form their parent tissue, i.e. the tissue they migrated in from. In order to give preference to cells from desired tissues, membranes are placed to prevent cells from undesired tissues having access to the space.

Patient situation

It is generally agreed that certain general health conditions represent a risk for successful GBR procedures. In a recent consensus conference one group examined the effect of systemic diseases on implant success (Mombelli & Cionca 2006). It was found that the scientific literature is inconclusive on these issues due to a lack of well performed clinical studies. Hence, it was concluded that neither the same rate of success nor an increased rate of failures have been documented in the presence of the specific systemic conditions under investigation. Furthermore, no conclusive data are available with respect to bone augmentation procedures in patients suffering from systemic diseases which cause impaired tissue healing. The same was found for patients who show behaviors (e.g. smoking, poor compliance) which lead to impaired tissue healing or to a higher susceptibility for disease development. Risk–benefit analysis should be performed with these uncertainties in mind, when planning implant therapy in the presence of bone defects.

It has been demonstrated that implant therapy in patients who have lost their teeth due to periodontal disease will be subject to more implant failures and complications regarding the supporting tissues than in patients who have lost their teeth due to other reasons (Mengel *et al.* 2001; Hardt *et al.* 2002; Karoussis *et al.* 2003; Wennstrom *et al.* 2004). Although, there are few well controlled studies available, it may be expected that these problems also exist when implants are supported by regenerated bone.

Bone morphology

Bone defects may be classified into intra-alveolar, horizontal, and vertical defects. Intra-alveolar defects are dealt with in Chapter 43.

When examining a clinical situation regarding bone morphology, the following aspects are of therapeutic importance: the presence of a bone defect; the size of the edentulous gap (single-tooth, double-tooth or multiple-tooth); and the bone level at the teeth adjacent to the defect.

Horizontal bone defects

Horizontal bone defects are the ones most frequently encountered. They include dehiscences and fenestrations.

The treatment of these types of defects has been shown to be highly successful in numerous studies (Balshi *et al.* 1991; Jung *et al.* 2003; Lundgren *et al.* 1994b; Mayfield *et al.* 1997; Simion *et al.* 1997). In addition, both bioresorbable and non-resorbable membranes have been successfully employed (Sandberg *et al.* 1993; Sevor *et al.* 1993; Schliephake *et al.* 1994; Crump *et al.* 1996; Chung *et al.* 1997; Hammerle *et al.* 1997, 1998; Lundgren *et al.* 1997). In a controlled clinical trial 18 implants with exposed surfaces were treated in nine patients (Simion *et al.* 1997). In the test sites bioresorbable membranes of polylactic and polyglycolic acid (PLA/PGA) were used, whereas non-resorbable membranes of expanded polytetrafluoroethylene (e-PTFE) were applied in the control sites. Autogenic bone was additionally placed to cover the exposed implant threads prior to membrane adaptation. The results at re-entry, 6–7 months later, revealed favorable healing and bone regeneration in both test and control sites, with the control sites demonstrating slightly higher amounts of bone regeneration.

In situations with a bone defect at a site where primary stability of an implant cannot be achieved, or when implant placement is not possible in the ideal location for subsequent prosthetic therapy, GBR prior to implantation represents the method of choice.

Experimental research on ridge augmentation using GBR was presented in the early 1990s (Seibert & Nyman 1990). In a dog model, large defects of the alveolar ridge were surgically prepared both in the mandible and in the maxilla. Morphologic and histologic analysis revealed that, in sites treated with membranes, with or without the addition of grafts, the entire space between the membrane and the jawbone was filled with bone. In the absence of membranes, bone formation was lacking.

The conclusions drawn from these and other pioneering experiments were that the method of GBR can indeed be successfully employed in the regeneration of alveolar ridge defects (Seibert & Nyman 1990; Schenk *et al.* 1994; Smukler *et al.* 1995).

Ridge augmentation in a lateral direction has been shown to be a method with predictable success (Nyman *et al.* 1990; Dahlin *et al.* 1991b; Becker *et al.* 1994b; Nevins & Mellonig 1994; Buser *et al.* 1996; von Arx *et al.* 1996). Successful methods regarding augmentation of the alveolar ridge in a vertical direction, however, are not well established.

Vertical bone defects

Data from animal experiments have clearly demonstrated that gain of bone above the external borders of the skeleton were possible using GBR (Lundgren *et al.* 1995; Hämmerle *et al.* 1996, 1997; Schliephake & Kracht 1997; Schmid *et al.* 1997; Lorenzoni *et al.* 1998).

Vertical ridge augmentation represents the most demanding indication in GBR therapy. Established techniques involve the placement of autogenous, particulated or block bone grafts, or bone substitute materials in combination with e-PTFE membranes of various configurations (Simion *et al.* 1994b, 1998;

Tinti *et al.* 1996; Tinti & Parma-Benfenati 1998; Chiapasco *et al.* 2004). The membranes were either supported by the graft alone or additionally supported by the implant protruding vertically from the host bone for various lengths. The results after submerged healing consistently showed bone formation reaching above the previous border of the alveolar crest. In some situations vertical bone formation reached up to 4 mm above the previous border of the alveolar crest. Within the area of the newly formed bone, osseointegration of the implants had occurred as demonstrated by histologic analysis of experimentally retrieved test implants. The amount of vertical bone formation, however, was not predictable and bone growth to the top of the membrane was not consistently reached when several millimeters of new bone formation were attempted. The remainder of the space between the newly formed bone and the membrane was occupied by non-mineralized tissue (Simion *et al.* 1994a).

Soft tissue morphology

The morphology of the soft tissues at the site of bone regeneration has a significant impact on the result of treatment. On the one hand, soft tissue coverage is a prerequisite for successful bone augmentation. On the other hand, in situations with high esthetic importance the soft tissues and the reconstruction determine whether or not a result is esthetically pleasing.

In many situations the availability of the soft tissues will limit the amount of bone formation possible. In other words a lack of soft tissues may prevent large amounts of bone volume gain because it is impossible to cover the area intended for regeneration. In such situations it may be advisable first to augment the volume of the soft tissues and then perform the bone augmentation procedure as a second step.

Critical aspects regarding the soft tissues include: vertical or horizontal soft tissue defects; level of the soft tissues at the teeth neighboring the gap; gingival biotype; and scars, pathologies or discolorations in the soft tissues lining the area of the bone defect.

Augmentation materials

Membranes

A wide range of membrane materials has been used in experimental and clinical studies to achieve GBR, including polytetrafluoroethylene (PTFE), expanded PTFE (e-PTFE), collagen, freeze-dried fascia lata, freeze-dried dura mater allografts, polyglactin 910, polylactic acid, polyglycolic acid, polyorthoester, polyurethane, polyhydroxybutyrate, calcium sulfate, micro titanium mesh, and titanium foils. Devices used for GBR in conjunction with endosseous implants should be safe and effective. Since no life-threatening diseases or deficiencies are treated, possible adverse effects emerging from the implanted devices should be kept to a minimum. At the same time, documentation of the effectiveness of the procedures and materials should be available. Certain critical criteria regarding membranes used for GTR have been formulated (Hardwick *et al.* 1994): biocompatibility, cell occlusiveness, integration by the host tissues, clinical manageability, and the space making function. For bioresorbable and biodegradable membranes additional criteria need to be fulfilled. Tissue reactions resulting from the resorption of the membrane should be minimal, these reactions should be reversible, and they should not negatively influence regeneration of the desired tissues (Gottlow 1993).

Although GBR is quite a successful procedure, a better understanding of the factors critical for success or failure is mandatory. This understanding will lead to more refined clinical protocols and will allow for the manufacturing of membrane materials with improved performance for a given indication. Some of these factors include membrane stability, duration of barrier function, enhanced access of bone and bone marrow-derived cells to the area for regeneration, ample blood fill of the space, prevention of soft tissue dehiscence, *in situ* forming, and delivery of factors influencing tissue formation beneficially.

Non-resorbable membranes

With the presentation of the first successful GBR procedures and the subsequent wide and successful application of e-PTFE membranes, this material soon became a standard for bone regeneration. Expanded PTFE is characterized as a polymer with high stability in biologic systems. It resists breakdown by host tissues and by microbes and does not elicit immunologic reactions.

A frequent complication with membrane application in conjunction with implants is membrane exposure and infection. Wound dehiscence and membrane exposure have been reported to impair the amount of bone regenerated in a number of experimental animal (Gotfredsen *et al.* 1993; Kohal *et al.* 1999a) and clinical investigations (Gher *et al.* 1994; Simion *et al.* 1994a; Hämmerle *et al.* 1998).

In situations where bone formation is desired in large defects or in supracrestal areas, conventional e-PTFE membranes do not adequately maintain space unless supported by grafting materials. The alternative approach involves the use of membranes with a stable form, such as titanium-reinforced membranes. Recent research has demonstrated the successful use of these membranes in vertical ridge augmentation and in the treatment of large defects in the alveolar process (Jovanovic & Nevins 1995; Tinti *et al.* 1996; Simion *et al.* 1998).

Many of the factors critical for successful bone formation were identified in experimental studies applying e-PTFE membranes. Furthermore, clinical protocols regarding surgical procedures, postoperative care, and healing times required were established using non-resorbable membranes. Today, as evidence of the effectiveness of bioresorbable membranes increases, non-resorbable membranes are losing importance in clinical practice and their use is increasingly limited to specific indications. Since e-PTFE membranes have been documented to allow successful GBR therapy, results obtained using new materials should always be compared with results of e-PTFE membranes.

Bioresorbable membranes

Non-resorbable membranes have to be removed during a second surgical intervention. The removal surgery will impose morbidity and psychologic stress on the patient and represents a risk for tissue damage. Since these disadvantages do not occur when working with bioresorbable membranes, they are increasingly applied in the clinic.

Apart from the fact that there is no need for surgical intervention for removal of the membrane, bioresorbable membranes offer some additional advantages. These include improved soft tissue healing (Lekovic et al. 1997, 1998; Zitzmann et al. 1997), the incorporation of the membranes by the host tissues (depending on material properties), and quick resorption in case of exposure, thus eliminating open microstructures prone to bacterial contamination (Zitzmann et al. 1997; Lorenzoni et al. 1998).

Bioresorbable materials that may be used for the fabrication of membranes all belong to the groups of natural or synthetic polymers. The best known groups of polymers used for medical purposes are collagen and aliphatic polyesters. Currently tested and used membranes are made of collagen, or of polyglycolide and/or polylactide or copolymers thereof (Hutmacher & Hürzeler 1995).

A wide range of bioresorbable membranes made of either collagen or polyglycolide and/or polylactic acid has been investigated in experimental and clinical studies (Lundgren et al. 1994a; Mayfield et al. 1997; Simion et al. 1997; Zitzmann et al. 1997). Results have generally been good, partly because of the low rate of complications, so bioresorbable membranes have become the standard for most clinical situations and have, thus, largely replaced the non-resorbable e-PTFE membranes.

It should be realized, however, that in a recent systematic review a reasonable comparison between bioresorbable and non-resorbable membranes could not be drawn due to a lack of well designed studies (Chiapasco et al. 2006). Only a few studies could be identified which compared the results of bioresorbable and non-resorbable membranes (Zitzmann et al. 1997, 2001b; Christensen et al. 2003). These studies did not find any difference between the two treatment modalities.

Obviously, choice of material is critical when it comes to bioresorbable membranes for GBR. Inflammatory reactions have been documented in the tissues adjacent to some bioresorbable membranes, ranging from mild (Sandberg et al. 1993; Piatelli et al. 1995; Aaboe et al. 1998; Kohal et al. 1999a,b) to severe (Gotfredsen et al. 1994). Another study reported on therapeutic failures using polylactic membranes for bone regeneration at peri-implant defects in dogs (Schliephake et al. 1997). Soft tissue complications were frequent, and the results did not reveal any improvement over control sites without the use of membranes.

Convincing results of bone regeneration in animal experiments have been reported for collagen membranes (Hürzeler et al. 1998; Zahedi et al. 1998). Furthermore, reports of human cases or case series (Hämmerle & Lang 2001) as well as controlled clinical studies (Zitzmann et al. 1997) have been presented describing the successful use of collagen membranes for GBR at exposed implant surfaces.

Bioresorbable membranes that are commercially available at present are not capable of maintaining adequate space unless the defect morphology is very favorable (Oh et al. 2003; Lundgren et al. 1994b). Even if the membranes seem able to maintain space initially, they generally lose their mechanical strength soon after implantation into the tissues. Favorable results have been reported only in situations where the bony borders of the defects adequately support the membrane. When defects do not maintain the space by themselves, failure of bone regeneration results (Zellin et al. 1995; Mellonig et al. 1998). Therefore, they need to be supported in some way.

In summary, animal experiments, human case reports, and initial controlled clinical studies demonstrate that bioresorbable and non-resorbable membranes can successfully be used for bone regeneration at implants with exposed surface areas. It appears, however, that bioresorbable membranes generally show better clinical performance compared with non-resorbable membranes. Hence, unless the defect morphology or other factors prevent the application of bioresorbable membranes their use is to be preferred. The choice of the best material has to be based on the individual patient situation.

Bone grafts and bone graft substitutes

Bone grafts have long been used in reconstructive surgery with the aim of increasing the bone volume in the previous defect area. Bone grafts and bone substitute materials may be classified into two main groups: autogenic and xenogenic materials. The term autogenic graft refers to tissues that are transplanted within one and the same organism. Xenogenic grafts encompass all materials of an origin other than the recipient organism and may further be divided into materials from the same species but different individuals, materials from other species, and finally products of non-organic origin.

Bone grafts or bone graft substitutes in conjunction with GBR need to fulfill a number of requirements. They should adequately support the membrane to provide a predefined volume of the regenerated bone. In addition, they should serve as a guiding structure into which the bone can grow or is even encouraged to grow. As a result capillaries and perivascular cells can easily form and migrate, respectively, within the voids provided by the supporting material. Later bone-forming cells can populate the spaces and produce new bone. Finally, the supporting material should be resorbed and replaced by the patient's own bone (Jensen *et al.* 1996; Fugazzotto 2003a,b).

The successful combination of autogenic corticocancellous bone grafts and GBR has been shown in a clinical study (Buser *et al.* 1990). A group of 40 patients, who had been treated with this method, demonstrated very low frequency of soft tissue complications and successful ridge augmentation in 66 sites. A mean gain in crest width of 3.5 mm was measured allowing implant placement in a proper position in all 66 sites. More recently, studies in humans and animals have lead to further development and refinement of this method with very good clinical success (Buser *et al.* 1996).

The necessity for membranes in conjunction with block grafts was tested in a prospective randomized clinical study involving 13 patients (Antoun *et al.* 2001). Patients were either treated with onlay bone grafts alone or additionally covered by e-PTFE membranes. The width of the ridges was evaluated clinically immediately following graft placement and at the time of membrane removal 6 months later. In the group with membranes significantly less resorption had occurred. This controlled clinical study confirms animal experimental data and is in accordance with case series reporting the occurrence of pronounced resorption of bone grafts (Jensen *et al.* 1995; Widmark *et al.* 1997; von Arx *et al.* 2001; Cochran *et al.* 2002).

Xenogenic bone substitutes have been developed and applied to GBR. Experimental studies have dealt with materials manufactured synthetically, derived from corals or algae, or originated from natural bone mineral (for review see Hammerle & Jung 2003). These materials are regarded to be biocompatible and osteoconductive. Nevertheless, considerable differences have been reported in their behavior based on material properties.

In a recent systematic review it was concluded that the paucity of available scientific data precludes clear recommendations regarding the choice of a specific supporting material for GBR procedures (Chiapasco *et al.* 2006). Comparative data were rarely found (Christensen *et al.* 2003) and no randomized controlled clinical trials were available as a basis for decision making.

The studies evaluating clinical outcomes of lateral ridge augmentation with GBR procedures in staged implantation commonly used autogenous bone as filler materials in combination with non-resorbable membranes (Nevins & Mellonig 1994; Buser *et al.* 1996). Limited data are available reporting on the application of bone substitutes in combination with bioresorbable membranes for ridge augmentation prior to implant placement (Zitzmann *et al.* 2001a; Friedmann *et al.* 2002; Hammerle *et al.* 2008).

In one of these studies 12 patients with 15 sites exhibiting lateral bone defects were treated using blocks of deproteinized bovine bone mineral and bioresorbable collagen membranes (Hammerle *et al.* 2008). The size of the defects precluded implant placement without prior bone augmentation. Initially the average ridge width amounted to 3.2 mm. At the re-entry operation 9–10 months later, the mean crestal bone width had increased to 6.9 mm. In all of the cases but one, the resulting bone volume was adequate to place the implant in a prosthetically optimal position. In one case, no gain of bone volume had occurred during the phase of regeneration for unknown reasons. While in previous clinical studies, small bone defects at implant sites had been augmented by use of DBBM (Hämmerle & Lang 2001; Zitzmann *et al.* 2001a; Friedmann *et al.* 2002; Hellem *et al.* 2003), larger bone defects were predictably augmented in this case series (Hammerle *et al.* 2008).

The technique of applying biomaterials to support bioresorbable membranes avoids the risks associated with harvesting autogenic bone (Nkenke *et al.* 2001; von Arx *et al.* 2005). This is a significant benefit to the patient and represents an important step in the development of GBR procedures. Future research should be focused on such patient-centered outcomes. The development of biomaterials, ideally coupled with the incorporation of bone growth factors and bioactive peptides, represents an important line of research in this direction (Jung *et al.* 2003).

Long-term results

Recent systematic reviews have compiled the literature regarding survival and success rates of implants partly or fully placed into regenerated bone (Hammerle *et al.* 2002; Fiorellini & Nevins 2003; Chiapasco *et al.* 2006). The survival rate of implants placed into sites with regenerated/augmented bone using barrier membranes varied between 79% and 100% with the majority of studies indicating more than 90% after at least 1 year of function. The survival rates obtained in the studies identified by these systematic reviews were similar to those generally reported for implants placed conventionally into sites without the need for bone augmentation. Two studies were identified that provided internal control data (Mayfield *et al.* 1998; Zitzmann *et al.* 2001b). In particular, the data from these two studies provided survival and success rates with no significant differences for implants in regenerated compared to non-regenerated bone. In addition, the loss of crestal bone was not different between test and control implants in one of these studies (Mayfield *et al.* 1998).

The long-term stability of vertically augmented bone was assessed in a multi-center study involving 123 patients (Simion *et al.* 2001). The results demonstrated marginal bone level changes to be within the range of variations reported for implants placed into intact bony beds.

Long-term analysis of the stability of the regenerated bone is almost exclusively focused on radiographic assessments of the interproximal bone and on implant survival. There is a need for studies to evaluate the fate of the buccal bone plate, regenerated or not, over time. As has been suggested in previous studies, the stability of the regenerated bone may be assessed using various clinical or radiographic measures (Chiapasco *et al.* 1999).

Clinical concepts

Analysis of the bony defect morphology is the basis for deciding which treatment strategy to follow and which materials to apply for GBR. Basically there are two procedures: a one-step (combined approach) and a two-step (staged approach) procedure. Whenever the bone morphology allows anchorage of the implant with primary stability in prosthetically correct position the one-step approach is preferred. In situations where the defect morphology precludes primary implant stability, the two-step procedure is performed, i.e. the bone volume is first augmented to a degree allowing implant placement in a second intervention. The classification of bone defects is intended as a guideline for choosing the best techniques and materials for GBR at implant sites (Fig. 49-1).

Ridge preservation

In situations where there is a substantial lack of soft and/or hard tissues it may be advisable to apply methods for improving hard tissue as well as soft tissue healing. Attempts have been made to maintain the contour of the ridge by placing non-resorbable materials into the fresh extraction socket. Cones of hydroxyapatite were placed into the socket (Denissen & de Groot 1979; Quinn & Kent 1984). Whereas the resorption of the ridge could be somewhat reduced the overall result was not satisfactory. A large number of soft tissue dehiscences occurred and in some situations the cones had to be removed (Kwon *et al.* 1986).

GBR has been used to preserve or augment the alveolar ridge at the time of tooth removal. Supporting materials were placed into fresh extraction sockets and subsequently covered by non-resorbable membranes (Nemcovsky & Serfaty 1996; Lekovic *et al.* 1997; Fowler *et al.* 2000). One of the problems encountered, as described above, is the lack of soft tissue to cover the GBR site completely. In order to solve this problem coronal and lateral sliding flaps or soft tissue grafts were employed. In some studies no attempt was made to contain the filler material with membranes nor was the soft tissue manipulated to allow for primary closure. In these situations and when necrosis of the covering soft tissues occurred, loss of grafting particles was a common finding (Nemcovsky & Serfaty 1996).

Histomorphometric analysis of biopsies revealed that more vital bone had formed at sites treated with GBR compared to sites that were left to spontaneous healing. The investigators attributed this positive finding to the characteristics of the filler materials.

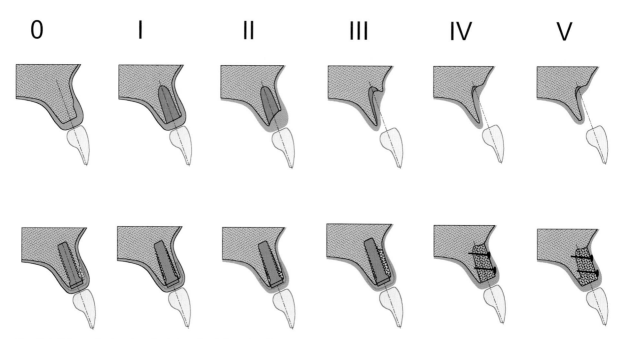

Fig. 49-1 Schematic drawing depicting the defect classification with classes 0–V.

Both osteoconductivity and resorbability of the materials apparently influenced new bone formation in a positive manner (Smukler *et al.* 1999; Artzi *et al.* 2000; Bolouri *et al.* 2001; Froum *et al.* 2002).

When applying GBR procedures it was clinically observed that the rate of resorption of the alveolar process could be reduced compared to untreated control sites (Lekovic *et al.* 1997, 1998; Yilmaz *et al.* 1998; Camargo *et al.* 2000). Complications with soft tissue dehiscences, however, frequently occurred in GBR-treated sites (Fowler *et al.* 2000; Yang *et al.* 2000). Although, the method of using GBR to reduce the loss of ridge volume has been well documented, it is not practical in many clinical situations due to the following shortcomings: it requires a long healing period before the implant therapy can be continued; the method is invasive and technique sensitive; soft tissue coverage is difficult to achieve and may lead a compromized esthetic result; and it is costly.

A different approach to provide optimal conditions for implant therapy regarding the profile of the alveolar ridge has led to the development of techniques aimed at improving the soft tissue conditions. Previous case reports described the use of autogenous soft tissue grafts to seal extraction sites before (Landsberg & Bichacho 1994) or at the time of implant placement (Evian & Cutler 1994; Landsberg 1997; Chen & Dahlin 1996; Tal 1999). Several problems exist with these procedures, including necrosis of the transplanted mucosa and poor color integration at the recipient site. In order to address this issue in a systematic way 20 patients in need of tooth extraction received soft tissue grafts to seal the entrance to the alveolus of the freshly extracted tooth (Jung *et al.* 2004) (Fig. 49-2a). First a grafting material was placed into the socket with the aim of maintaining the contour of the ridge. Subsequently, a soft tissue graft harvested from the palate was carefully sutured to cover the grafting material and thus seal off the alveolus from the oral cavity (Fig. 49-2b). Six weeks later, the vitality of the graft and the color match with respect to the surrounding mucosa were assessed. More than 99% of the grafted tissue area appeared vital. Digital measurement of the color difference between the grafted and the neighboring host tissues generated values below thresholds for normally detectable values in such situations (Fig. 49-2c). This technique, therefore, beneficially influenced the conditions at extraction sites for subsequent implant placement and soft tissue management in comparison to spontaneous healing (Fig. 49-3). Due to the effort and expense necessary to perform this treatment approach, it is primarily recommended for situations with high esthetic priority.

At times the implant is completely inserted into native bone but the buccal contour of the hard and soft tissues is insufficient for an optimal treatment outcome. This may be the case in esthetically highly demanding situations. In order to improve the esthetic result an augmentation procedure is con-

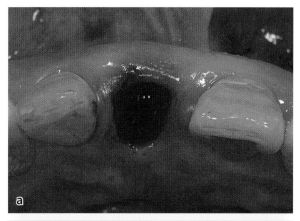

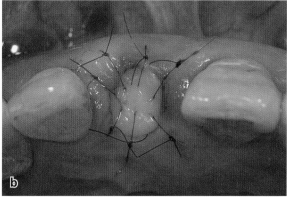

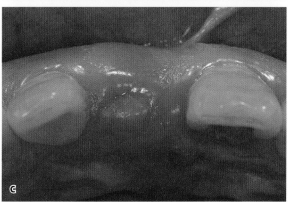

Fig. 49-2 (a) Occlusal view of an extraction site 11 immediately following removal of the tooth. Note the normal appearance of the external ridge contour and the soft tissue deficit over the extraction socket. (b) A soft tissue graft taken from the palate has been placed and sutured to seal the entrance of the alveolus. (c) After 6 weeks of healing, the soft tissue graft is completely integrated at the recipient site and a healthy soft tissue cover of the former entrance of the alveolus is present.

ducted (class 0). A membrane-supporting material and a membrane are placed to promote labial bone formation in order to obtain the desired tissue contours.

Extraction sockets (class I)

Currently implants are often placed in fresh extraction sockets. Although some of these clinical procedures were first described many years ago, their application has become more common in recent years.

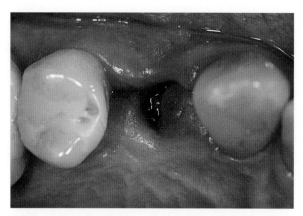

Fig. 49-3 An extraction site after 6 weeks of spontaneous healing. Note the incomplete healing rendering soft tissue management difficult.

In situations where teeth are to be replaced with implants, a decision must be taken during treatment planning whether the implant should be placed immediately after tooth extraction or if a certain number of weeks of healing of the soft and hard tissues of the alveolar ridge should be allowed prior to implant placement. For details regarding timing of implant placement into extraction sockets see Chapter 47.

If bone augmentation is required at implants immediately placed into extraction sockets, the following procedure is recommended. A flap is raised to allow easy access to the site and the implant is inserted. A membrane-supporting material is adapted to support the membrane. Depending on the defect morphology (for details see Chapter 47) this material is placed into the space between the walls of the socket and the implant surface. In addition, in some situations, especially in the esthetic zone, it may be necessary to augment the bone beyond the labial wall of the socket. Thus, the membrane-supporting material is also applied in order to correct the ridge profile to obtain a more prominent labial tissue contour. Subsequently, the membrane is adapted to cover the supporting material and a narrow zone of the adjacent bone and the flap is adapted and sutured. Whenever a partial or complete loss of the buccal wall of the socket is encountered the procedure described for dehiscence defects is applied.

Dehiscence defects (classes II and III)

Dehiscence defects may range from a very small lack of marginal bone to large areas of denuded implant surfaces. As long as the implant can be securely anchored in the existing bone, concomitant implantation and bone regeneration may be performed. When the defect is quite small, it may be questionable whether or not a regeneration procedure will improve the treatment outcome and its long-term stability (Hämmerle 1999). Often the esthetic result, as well as aspects of health and function, is important. In esthet-

ically demanding situations it is generally recommended to perform an augmentation procedure, whereas in other areas of the mouth recommendations are not as strict. It needs to be understood, however, that the presently available scientific data do not allow an evidence-based statement to be made regarding the borderline between a situation requiring bone augmentation and a situation without this requirement (Chiapasco et al. 2006).

In situations where it is decided to carry out a GBR procedure, the material of choice should fulfill the following requirements: it should have proven efficacy; be thoroughly researched and scientifically documented; and be re-evaluated at regular intervals. In recent clinical studies, it has been demonstrated that the application of bone substitutes in conjunction with the placement of implants lead to successful coverage of the previously exposed implant surfaces (Zitzmann et al. 1997; Hämmerle et al. 1998; Moses et al. 2005). Hence, harvesting of autogenous bone for the treatment of dehiscence defects may not always be necessary for a successful treatment outcome.

The grafting material should reliably support the area intended for bone augmentation, allow or preferably promote in-growth of bone forming cells, and support bone–implant contact formation. Among other materials deproteinized bovine bone mineral is very well researched and has consistently demonstrated excellent clinical results (Esposito et al. 2006).

When choosing an appropriate membrane the same basic documentation as required for the supporting materials needs to be available: i.e. it should have proven efficacy; be thoroughly researched and scientifically documented; and be re-evaluated at regular intervals. Additional parameters regarding selection of a suitable membrane include the mechanical properties, the risk for soft tissue dehiscence, and the ease of clinical handling. In most situations with dehiscence defects a bioresorbable collagen membrane will be optimal regarding the scientifically and clinically required characteristics. In contrast, in situations, where the defect morphology requires improved stability of the area to be regenerated, e-PTFE membranes are most suitable. Apart from the substantial risk for soft tissue dehiscence and subsequent infection of the area, the need for membrane-removal surgery represents the major disadvantage of non-resorbable membranes. As a consequence, bioresorbable membranes are preferred whenever possible for the treatment of small and larger dehiscence defects.

The clinical protocol to promote bone formation for successful coverage of exposed implant surfaces includes the following steps. After a flap is raised, the implant is inserted (Fig. 49-4a). A membrane-supporting material is placed in the area of the buccal dehiscence defect with the aim of promoting bone formation for bone integration of the implant and

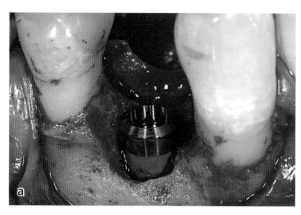 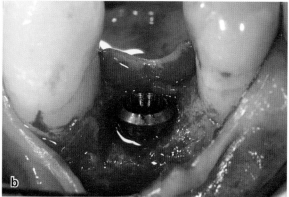

Fig. 49-4 (a) A small labial dehiscence defect at an implant in position of tooth 44. The defect is treated by GBR applying a bioresorbable membrane and a deproteinized bovine bone mineral for membrane support. (b) The same case as in (a) at re-entry surgery. New bone has formed within the previous defect area. A thin layer of non-mineralized tissue covers the regenerated bone.

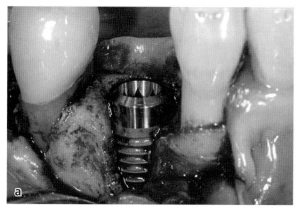 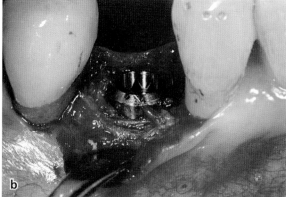

Fig. 49-5 (a) A large labial dehiscence defect at an implant in position of tooth 43. The defect is also treated by GBR applying a bioresorbable membrane and a deproteinized bovine bone mineral for membrane support. (b) The same case as in (a) at re-entry surgery. The dehiscence defect has been augmented with bone, which is covered by a thin layer of non-mineralized tissue.

obtaining a natural appearance of the bone and soft tissue contours of the alveolar ridge. Subsequently a membrane is adapted and placed to cover the supporting material and the defect. A decision has to be taken on how the membrane is fixed in place to provide the stability necessary for bone to form. This fixation may be obtained by simply adapting the membrane to the intact walls of the bone defect, by tacking it with pins, by suturing it to the soft tissues, or by adapting it to the implant. Thereafter, the flap is adapted and sutured to allow for submerged or transmucosal healing of the implant site. Following 4–6 months of healing the former defect is filled with new bone (Fig. 49-4b). The same clinical protocol is applied for the treatment of larger dehiscence defects (Fig. 49-5).

Horizontal defects (class IV)

The autogenous block transplant represents the gold standard for treatment of horizontal ridge defects (Becker *et al*. 1994a; Buser *et al*. 1996; von Arx *et al*. 2001). Both intraoral and extraoral harvesting procedures have been described. Intraoral sites have been preferred, especially for the treatment of localized bone defects in partially edentulous jaws (Joshi & Kostakis 2004). Intraorally, common donor sites include the chin and the area of the retromolar region in the mandible. Intraoral harvesting procedures also have disadvantages, such as limited availability of bone graft volume, complications including altered sensation of teeth, neurosensory disturbances, wound dehiscence, and infection (Nkenke *et al*. 2001; von Arx *et al*. 2005).

The advantages of autogenic block grafts include the large scientific and clinical documentation, handling properties, stabilization of the area intended for regeneration due to the possibility of securing the grafts in place by metal screws, and the optimal biologic properties. The disadvantages include donor site morbidity, technically difficult harvesting procedures, and the impossibility of using the graft as a carrier for growth factors.

Clinical procedures require harvesting of the graft, adaptation to the defect area, fixation by screws, coverage with a membrane, and primary closure with the soft tissue flap. During a second surgical intervention after 4–9 months of healing, the result of the

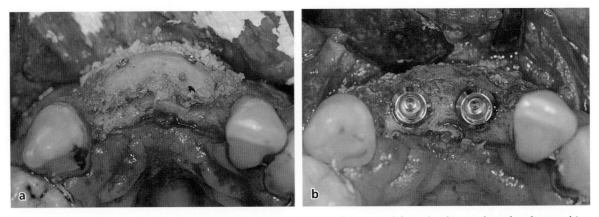

Fig. 49-6 (a) An extensive bone defect in the anterior maxilla. A bone graft harvested from the chin is adapted and secured in place by titanium screws. In the periphery bone chips and deproteinized bovine bone mineral are added to improve contouring of the area. Subsequently, a bioresorbable collagen membrane is placed to cover the area intended for bone augmentation and the flap is closed. (b) The same case as in (a) at the time of implant placement. Note the large volume of bone available for implant placement and as a basis for achieving an optimal esthetic result.

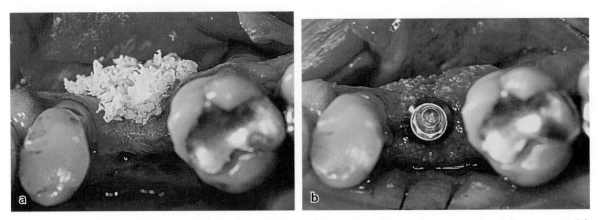

Fig. 49-7 (a) A lateral bone defect at a single tooth gap. A block of deproteinized bovine bone mineral and chips generated from this block are placed to support a bioresorbable collagen membrane before the flap is closed. (b) The same case as in (a) at the time of implant placement. Note the substantial volume of bone available for implant placement as a basis for achieving an optimal result.

augmentation procedure can be seen and implants can be placed (Fig. 49-6).

As described above recent case reports and case series have described the use of deproteinized bovine bone mineral in conjunction with bioresorbable collagen membranes and found successful bone augmentation at lateral ridge defects (Zitzmann *et al.* 2001a; Friedmann *et al.* 2002; Hammerle *et al.* 2008). During the second surgical intervention implants could be placed in a prosthetically optimal position in most situations (Fig. 49-7).

These newer studies indicate that, provided the appropriate protocols are developed, ridge augmentation without the use of autogenous block grafts could become a standard procedure.

Vertical defects (class V)

The indications for vertical ridge augmentation include situations where the remaining bone height is too small for proper anchorage of oral implants, where unfavorable crown:implant ratios will result, and where unfavorable esthetic outcomes are expected from the lack of remaining hard and soft tissues.

The same procedures are recommended for patient treatment as described for the class IV defects with the exception that the bone block is partially or fully placed on to the ridge in order to gain bone in a vertical direction. Other than that the materials and the techniques applied are identical to the ones for lateral bone augmentation using bone grafts. Obviously, flap adaptation is more difficult due to the increased volume intended for regeneration, which needs to be covered by the flap.

It appears that varying amounts of bone height may be gained, depending on the clinical treatment protocol. The factors critical for success or failure have not been elucidated. In addition, no data is presently available indicating whether there is a biologically limited maximum of bone gain, and if so, what parameters influence this maximum.

Future developments

Progress in every medical discipline is largely based on better understanding of the physiologic and pathologic mechanisms governing health, disease, and healing. This understanding is a key step to the development of new strategies and materials in medicine. The aim is to develop more effective techniques that predictably promote the body's natural ability to regenerate lost tissue instead of using external materials to repair lost tissue. The most intriguing method currently being investigated is the application of polypeptide or natural proteins that regulate wound and tissue regeneration.

Growth and differentiation factors

In the past decade a number of basic science experiments and clinical studies have clarified biologic mechanisms of several growth and differentiation factors on the regeneration of oral soft and hard tissue (Howell *et al.* 1997a). Growth and differentiation factors currently believed to contribute to periodontal and alveolar ridge augmentation include platelet-derived growth factor (PDGF), insulin-like growth factor (IGF-I and IGF-II), transforming growth factor beta (TGF-β), fibroblast growth factor (a-FGF and b-FGF), and bone morphogenetic proteins (BMPs 1–15). Among these bone morphogenetic protein is the most widely studied in the dental literature. BMP, by chemotaxis, triggers proliferation and differentiation of mesenchymal progenitor cells (Wozney *et al.* 1988). Recombinant biotechnology has enabled characterization of at least 15 BMPs and production of quantities of purified recombinant protein for therapeutic application (Groeneveld & Burger 2000). Recombinant human BMP-2 (rhBMP-2) has been found to exhibit very high osteogenic activity in experimental (Sigurdsson *et al.* 1996; Hanisch *et al.* 1997; Cochran *et al.* 1999; Higuchi *et al.* 1999; Jung *et al.* 2005) and in clinical studies (Boyne *et al.* 1997; Howell *et al.* 1997a; Jung *et al.* 2003, 2005).

Delivery systems for growth and differentiation factors

The regenerative potential of growth and differentiation factors depends upon the carrier material (Sigurdsson *et al.* 1996; Hunt *et al.* 2001). The effect of such proteins is dependent upon a carrier material, which serves as a delivery system and as a scaffold for cellular in-growth (Ripamonti & Reddi 1994).

Collagen has extensively been studied as a carrier material for growth factors applied to promote bone formation in different kinds of indications (Nevins *et al.* 1996; Boyne *et al.* 1997; Howell *et al.* 1997b). Different studies (Barboza *et al.* 2000) using rhBMP-2 in an absorbable collagen sponge (ACS) for alveolar ridge augmentation gained only small amounts of bone. The investigators concluded that the compro-

mised results were due to the failure of the ACS to adequately support the supra-alveolar wound space. In order to overcome this lack of structural strength rh-BMP-2/ACS has been combined with hydroxy-apatite (HA) in an experiment attempting lateral ridge augmentation (Barboza *et al.* 2000). In contrast to rhBMP-2/ACS alone, a significant clinical improvement in ridge width was observed with the addition of HA to rhBMP-2/ACS. However, the HA particles were largely encapsulated by fibrous tissue and they appeared partially to obstruct bone formation. The investigators concluded that space maintenance in BMP-induced bone formation is an important factor (Barboza *et al.* 2000). A recent study demonstrated that the results of GBR procedures in humans could be improved by the addition of rhBMP-2 to a xenogenic bone substitute mineral. This improvement was documented by a higher degree of bone maturation and an increased graft–bone contact fraction at the BMP-treated sites (Jung *et al.* 2003). Synthetic polymers, on the other hand, can reproducibly be fabricated and the growth factors can be incorporated under controlled manufacturing conditions (Weber *et al.* 2002).

In a recent study in dogs implants were placed in the mandible and peri-implant infra-osseous defects were prepared (Jung *et al.* 2007). The defects were grafted with a synthetic polyethylene glycol (PEG) matrix, which was either empty or contained a 35 amino acid peptide of parathyroid hormone (cys-PTH$_{1–34}$). Control defects were grafted with autogenous bone or left empty. One and three months later, the sites with PEG and PTH showed similar amounts of bone formation compared with the sites grafted with autogenous bone. In the two other groups less bone formation was observed. It was concluded that the synthetic PEG hydrogel containing PTH$_{1–34}$ was a suitable matrix-differentiation factor system to obtain bone regeneration.

However, the ideal carrier material, which is easy to apply, able to provide space for regeneration, bioresorbable, and allows controlled release of the bioactive molecules, has not yet been discovered. Further research is needed to determine the ideal combination of factors for regeneration, the best delivery system, and the optimum doses.

Membrane developments

The benefit of using both barrier membranes and BMP for bone augmentation remains controversial (Linde & Hedner 1995; Howell *et al.* 1997b; Cochran *et al.* 1999; Jung *et al.* 2003). It was found that the presence of a non-resorbable e-PTFE membrane initially (4 weeks) inhibited bone formation with rhBMP-2 but did no longer do so at later time points (12 weeks) (Cochran *et al.* 1999). It has been shown that bone induction by rhBMP-2 occurs at early time points and that rhBMP-2 undergoes rapid clearance. Hence, the use of a membrane may potentially reduce the bone-forming effect of rhBMP-2 due to limited availability of inducible cells. Another animal study in rats reported no difference in bone healing with the combination of rhBMP-2 and an e-PTFE membrane compared to rhBMP-2 alone (Linde & Hedner 1995). From a clinical point of view, the use of a membrane simplifies the handling and stabilization of the bone substitute mineral at the time of bone augmentation, but from a biologic point of view the use of a membrane may block the recruitment of cells from the environment.

The question whether or not bioactive molecules are best used in conjunction with membranes or in the absence of membranes has not yet been answered conclusively. On the one hand, it is reasonable to apply them as adjunctive agents to GBR therapy in order to accelerate membrane-guided bone regeneration. On the other hand, it may be hypothesized that their mode of action is best taken advantage of when membranes are not applied simultaneously, thus allowing all inducible cells from the wound environment access to the area to be regenerated.

Common to all presently used membranes is the fact that their fabrication is completed before they are delivered for patient use. Consequently, they are made available in standard sizes and forms and need to be adapted to the patient's individual situation. Alternatively, a membrane could be custom made directly for an individual defect intra-operatively, using a material different from the ones mentioned above.

Hydrogels made of PEG fulfill a number of criteria required to serve as synthetic membranes which form *in situ*. Polyethylene glycol has been shown to be highly biocompatible (Pang 1993; Working *et al*. 1997). It is presently approved for several pharmaceutical applications (Zalipsky & Harris 1997) and as medical devices, e.g. a sprayable adhesion barrier.

In a recent study in rabbits, four evenly distributed craniotomy defects, 6 mm in diameter, were prepared in the area of the right and left parietal and frontal bones (Jung *et al*. 2006). All sites were grafted with highly porous hydroxyapatite (HA)/tricalciumphosphate (TCP) granules. The sites were covered towards both the internal and external soft tissue either with e-PTFE or PEG membranes or left uncovered as control sites. A similar amount of newly formed bone was observed within the former defect space at e-PTFE- and PEG-treated sites. These findings demonstrated that the PEG membrane formed *in situ* could be successfully applied for bone regeneration.

Future outlook

Further developments in bone augmentation procedures can be related to either the simplification of clinical handling or influencing of biologic processes. In order to simplify clinical handling new materials should be comprised of a matrix with optimal cell in-growth capacities and with good mechanical properties providing space for tissue regeneration. No membrane and no specific procedures for mechanical fixation should be necessary. This would reduce the technique sensitivity and therefore increase the predictability of bone augmentation.

From a biologic point of view the growth and differentiation factors may induce earlier bone growth into the area to be regenerated. Thus, the area of regeneration would be stabilized earlier. Furthermore, the use of such materials would allow treatment of extensive bone defects. At present, large bone defects are regularly augmented with autogenous block grafts and membranes. The use of synthetic materials would result in lower surgical risks and lower morbidity in the augmentation procedure and would represent an important step forward in simplifying bone regeneration techniques.

Acknowledgments

The authors express their special thanks to Dr. Gianandrea Hälg and to Samantha Merki for valuable support in the preparation of this chapter.

References

Aaboe, M., Pinholt, E.M., Schou, S. & Hjørting-Hansen, E. (1998). Incomplete bone regeneration of rabbit calvarial defects using different membranes. *Clinical Oral Implants Research* **9**, 313–320.

Antoun, H., Sitbon, J.M., Martinez, H. & Missika, P. (2001). A prospective randomized study comparing two techniques of bone augmentation: onlay graft alone or associated with a membrane. *Clinical Oral Implants Research* **12**, 632–639.

Artzi, Z., Tal, H. & Dayan, D. (2000). Porous bovine bone mineral in healing of human extraction sockets. Part 1: histomorphometric evaluations at 9 months. *Journal of Periodontology* **71**, 1015–1023.

Balshi, T.J., Hernandez, R.E., Cutler, R.H. & Hertzog, C.F. (1991). Treatment of osseous defects using vicryl mesh (polyglactin 910) and the Brånemark implant: a case report. *International Journal of Oral & Maxillofacial Implants* **6**, 87–91.

Barboza, E.P., Leite Duarte, M.E., Geolas, L., Sorensen, R.G., Riedel, G.E. & Wikesjö, U.M.E. (2000). Ridge augmentation following implantation of recombinant human bone morphogenetic protein-2 in the dog. *Journal of Periodontology* **71**, 488–496.

Becker, W., Becker, B.E. & Caffesse, R. (1994a). A comparison of demineralized freeze-dried bone and autologous bone to induce bone formation in human extraction sockets. *Journal of Periodontology* **65**, 1128–1133.

Becker, W., Becker, B.E. & McGuire, M.K. (1994b). Localized ridge augmentation using absorbable pins and ePTFE barrier membranes: A new surgical approach. *International Journal of Periodontics and Restorative Dentistry* **14**, 48–61.

Bolouri, A., Haghighat, N. & Frederiksen, N. (2001). Evaluation of the effect of immediate grafting of mandibular postextraction sockets with synthetic bone. *Compendium of Continuing Education Dentistry* **22**, 955–958.

Boyne, P.J., Marx, R.E., Nevins, M., Triplett, G., Lazaro, E., Lilly, L.C., Alder, M. & Nummikoski, P. (1997). A feasibility study evaluating rhBMP-2/absorbable collagen sponge for maxillary sinus floor augmentation. *International Journal of Periodontics and Restorative Dentistry* **17**, 11–25.

Buch, F., Albrektsson, T. & Herbst, E. (1986). The bone growth chamber for quantification of electrically induced osteogenesis. *Journal of Orthopedic Research* **4**, 194–203.

Buser, D., Brägger, U., Lang, N.P. & Nyman, S. (1990). Regeneration and enlargement of jaw bone using guided tissue regeneration. *Clinical Oral Implants Research* **1**, 22–32.

Buser, D., Dula, K., Hirt, H.P. & Schenk, R.K. (1996). Lateral ridge augmentation using autografts and barrier membranes. A clinical study in 40 partially edentulous patients. *International Journal of Oral & Maxillofacial Surgery* **54**, 420–432.

Camargo, P., Lekovic, V., Weinlaender, M., Klokkevold, P., Kenney, E., Dimitrijevic, B., Nedic, M. & Jancovic, S.M.O. (2000). Influence of bioactive glass on changes in alveolar process dimensions after exodontia. *Oral Surgery Oral Medicine Oral Pathology Oral Radiology and Endodontics* **90**, 581–586.

Chen, S.T. & Dahlin, C. (1996). Connective tissue grafting for primary closure of extraction sockets treated with an osteopromotive membrane technique: surgical technique and clinical results. *International Journal of Periodontics and Restorative Dentistry* **16**, 348–355.

Chiapasco, M., Abati, S., Romeo, E. & Vogel, G. (1999). Clinical outcome of autogenous bone blocks or guided bone regeneration with e-PTFE membranes for the reconstruction of narrow edentulous ridges. *Clinical Oral Implants Research* **10**, 278–288.

Chiapasco, M., Romeo, E., Casentini, P. & Rimondini, L. (2004). Alveolar distraction osteogenesis vs. vertical guided bone regeneration for the correction of vertically deficient edentulous ridges: a 1–3-year prospective study on humans. *Clinical Oral Implants Research* **15**, 82–95.

Chiapasco, M., Zaniboni, M. & Boisco, M. (2006). Augmentation procedures for the rehabilitation of deficient edentulous ridges with oral implants. *Clinical Oral Implants Research* **17** (Suppl 2), 136–159.

Christensen, D.K., Karoussis, I.K., Joss, A., Hammerle, C.H. & Lang, N.P. (2003). Simultaneous or staged installation with guided bone augmentation of transmucosal titanium implants. A 3-year prospective cohort study. *Clinical Oral Implants Research* **14**, 680–686.

Chung, C.P., Kim, D.K., Park, Y.J., Nam, K.H. & Lee, S.J. (1997). Biological effects of drug-loadable biodegradable membranes for guided bone regeneration. *Journal of Periodontal Research* **32**, 172–175.

Cochran, D.L., Schenk, R.K., Buser, D., Wozney, J.M. & Jones, A. (1999). Recombinant human bone morphogenetic protein-2 stimulation of bone formation around endosseous dental implants. *Journal of Periodontology* **70**, 139–150.

Cochran, D.L., Buser, D., ten Bruggenkate, C.M., Weingart, D., Taylor T.M., Bernhard, J., Peters, F. & Simpson, J.P. (2002). The use of reduced healing times on ITI® implants with a sandblasted and acid-etched (SLA) surface: Early results from clinical trials on ITI® SLA implants. *Clinical Oral Implants Research* **13**, 144–153.

Crump, T.B., Rivera-Hidalgo, F., Harrison, J.W., Williams, F.E. & Guo, I.Y. (1996). Influence of three membrane types on healing of bone defects. *Oral Surgery Oral Medicine & Oral Pathology* **82**, 365–374.

Dahlin, C., Linde, A., Gottlow, J. & Nyman, S. (1988). Healing of bone defects by guided tissue regeneration. *Plastic and Reconstructive Surgery* **81**, 672–677.

Dahlin, C., Alberius, P. & Linde, A. (1991a). Osteopromotion for cranioplasty. An experimental study in rats using a membrane technique. *Journal of Neurosurgery* **74** (3), 487–491.

Dahlin, C., Andersson, L. & Linde, A. (1991b). Bone augmentation at fenestrated implants by an osteopromotive membrane technique. A controlled clinical study. *Clinical Oral Implants Research* **2**, 159–165.

Denissen, H. & de Groot, K. (1979). Immediate dental root implants from synthetic dense calcium hydroxylapatite. *Journal of Prosthetic Dentistry* **42**, 551–556.

Esposito, M., Grusovin, M.G., Coulthard, P. & Worthington, H.V. (2006). The efficacy of various bone augmentation procedures for dental implants: a Cochrane systematic review of randomized controlled clinical trials. *International Journal of Oral & Maxillofacial Implants* **21**, 696–710.

Evian, C. & Cutler, S. (1994). Autogenous gingival grafts as epithelial barriers for immediate implants: case reports. *Journal of Periodontology* **65**, 201–210.

Fiorellini, J.P. & Nevins, M.L. (2003). Localized ridge augmentation/preservation. A systematic review. *Annals of Periodontology* **8**, 321–327.

Fowler, E., Breault, L. & Rebitski, G. (2000). Ridge preservation utilizing an acellular dermal allograft and demineralized freeze-dried bone allograft: Part II. Immediate endosseous implant placement. *Journal of Periodontology* **71**, 1360–1364.

Friedmann, A., Strietzel, F., Maretzki, B., Pitaru, S. & Bernimoulin, J. (2002). Histological assessment of augmented jaw bone utilizing a new collagen barrier membrane compared to a standard barrier membrane to protect a granular bone substitute material. *Clinical Oral Implants Research* **13**, 587–594.

Froum, S., Wallace, S., Tarnow, D. & Cho, S. (2002). Effect of platelet-rich plasma on bone growth and osseointegration in human maxillary sinus grafts: three bilateral case reports. *International Journal of Periodontics and Restorative Dentistry* **22**, 45–53.

Fugazzotto, P. (2003a). GBR using bovine bone matrix and resorbable and nonresorbable membranes. Part 1: histologic results. *International Journal of Periodontics and Restorative Dentistry* **23**, 361–369.

Fugazzotto, P. (2003b). GBR using bovine bone matrix and resorbable and nonresorbable membranes. Part 2: Clinical results. *International Journal of Periodontics and Restorative Dentistry* **23**, 599–605.

Gher, M.E., Quintero, G., Assad, D., Monaco, E. & Richardson, A.C. (1994). Bone grafting and guided bone regeneration for immediate dental implants in humans. *Journal of Periodontology* **65**, 881–991.

Gotfredsen, K., Nimb, L., Buser, D. & Hjørting-Hansen, E. (1993). Evaluation of guided bone regeneration around implants placed into fresh extraction sockets. An experimental study in dogs. *Journal of Oral and Maxillofacial Surgery* **51**, 879–884.

Gotfredsen, K., Nimb, L. & Hjørting-Hansen, E. (1994). Immediate implant placement using a biodegradable barrier, polyhydroxybutyrate-hydroxyvalerate reinforced with polyglactin 910. *Clinical Oral Implants Research* **5**, 83–91.

Gottlow, J. (1993). Guided tissue regeneration using bioresorbable and non-resorbable devices: Initial healing and long-term results. *Journal of Periodontology* **64**, 1157–1165.

Groeneveld, E.H.J. & Burger, E.H. (2000). Bone morphogenetic proteins in human bone regenerations. *European Journal of Endocrinology* **142**, 9–21.

Hämmerle, C.H.F. (1999). Membranes and bone substitutes in guided bone regeneration. Paper presented at the 3rd European Workshop on Periodontology, Ittingen, Switzerland.

Hämmerle, C.H.F., Brägger, U., Schmid, B. & Lang, N.P. (1998). Successful bone formation at immediate transmucosal implants. *International Journal of Oral & Maxillofacial Implants* **13**, 522–530.

Hammerle, C. & Jung, R. (2003). Bone augmentation by means of barrier membrane. *Periodontology 2000* **33**, 36–53.

Hammerle, C.H., Jung, R.E. & Feloutzis, A. (2002). A systematic review of the survival of implants in bone sites augmented with barrier membranes (guided bone regeneration) in partially edentulous patients. *Journal of Clinical Periodontology* **29** (Suppl 3), 226–231; discussion 232–223.

Hammerle, C.H., Jung, R.E., Yaman, D. & Lang, N.P. (2008). Ridge augmentation by applying bio-resorbable membranes and deproteinized bovine bone mineral. A report of 12 consecutive cases. *Clinical Oral Implants Research* **19**(1) (in press).

Hämmerle, C.H.F. & Lang, N.P. (2001). Single stage surgery combining transmucosal implant placement with guided bone regeneration and bioresorbable materials. *Clinical Oral Implants Research* **12**, 9–18.

Hämmerle, C.H.F., Olah, A.J., Schmid, J., Flückiger, L., Winkler, J.R., Gogolowski, S. & Lang, N.P. (1997). The biological effect of deproteinized bovine bone on bone neoformation on the rabbit skull. *Clinical Oral Implants Research* **8**, 198–207.

Hämmerle, C.H.F., Schmid, J., Olah, A.J. & Lang, N.P. (1996). A novel model system for the study of experimental bone formation in humans. *Clinical Oral Implants Research* **7**, 38–47.

Hanisch, O., Tatakis, D.N., Boskovic, M.M., Rohrer, M.D. & Wikesjö, U.M.E. (1997). Bone formation and reosseointegration in peri-implantitis defects following surgical implantation of rhBMP-2. *International Journal of Oral & Maxillofacial Implants* **12**, 604–610.

Hardt, C.R., Grondahl, K., Lekholm, U. & Wennstrom, J.L. (2002). Outcome of implant therapy in relation to experienced loss of periodontal bone support: a retrospective 5-year study. *Clinical Oral Implants Research* **13**, 488–494.

Hardwick, R., Scantlebury, T.V., Sanchez, R., Whitley, N. & Ambruster, J. (1994). Membrane design criteria for guided bone regeneration of the alveolar ridge In: Buser, D., Dahlin, C. & Schenk, R.K., eds. *Guided Bone Regeneration in Implant Dentistry*. Chicago, Berlin: Quintessence, pp. 101–136.

Hellem, S., Astrand, P., Stenstrom, B., Engquist, B., Bengtsson, M. & Dahlgren, S. (2003). Implant treatment in combination with lateral augmentation of the alveolar process: a 3-year prospective study. *Clinical Implant Dentistry and Related Research* **5**, 233–240.

Higuchi, T., Kinoshita, A., Takahashi, K., Oda, S. & Ishikawa, I. (1999). Bone regeneration by recombinant human bone morphogenetic protein-2 in rat mandibular defects. An experimental model of defect filling. *Journal of Periodontology* **70**, 1026–1031.

Howell, T.H., Fiorellini, J.P., Jones, A., Alder, M., Nummikoski, P., Lazaro, E., Lilly, L.C. & Cochran, D.L. (1997a). A feasibility study evaluating rhBMP-2/absorbable collagen sponge device for local alveolar ridge preservation or augmentation. *International Journal of Periodontics and Restorative Dentistry* **17**, 125–139.

Howell, T.H., Fiorellini, J.P., Paquette, D.W., Offenbacher, S., Giannobile, W.V. & Lynch S.E. (1997b). A phase I/II clinical trial to evaluate a combination of recombinant human platelet-derived growth factor-BB and recombinant human insulin-like growth factor-I in patients with periodontal disease. *Journal of Periodontology* **68**, 1186–1193.

Hunt, D.R., Jovanovic, S.A., Wikesjö, U.M.E., Wozney, J.M. & Bernard, G.W. (2001). Hyaluronan supports recombinant human bone morphogenetic protein-2 induced bone reconstruction of advanced alveolar ridge defects in dogs. A pilot study. *Journal of Periodontology* **72**, 651–658.

Hürzeler, M.B., Kohal, R.J., Naghshbandi, J., Mota, L.F., Conradt, J., Hutmacher, D. & Caffesse, R.G. (1998). Evaluation of a new bioresorbable barrier to facilitate guided bone regeneration around exposed implant threads. An experimental study in the monkey. *International Journal of Oral & Maxillofacial Surgery* **27**, 315–320.

Hutmacher, D. & Hürzeler, M.B. (1995). Biologisch abbaubare Polymere und Membranen für die gesteurte Gewebe- und Knochenregeneration. *Implantologie* **1**, 21–37.

Ilizarov, G.A. (1989a). The tension-stress effect on the genesis and growth of tissues: Part I. The influence of stability of fixation and soft tissue preservation. *Clinical Orthopaedics* **238**, 249–281.

Ilizarov, G.A. (1989b). The tension-stress effect on the genesis and growth of tissues: Part II. The influence of the rate and frequency of distraction. *Clinical Orthopaedics* **239**, 263–285.

Jensen, O.T., Greer, R.O., Johnson, L. & Kassebaum, D. (1995). Vertical guided bone-graft augmentation in a new canine mandibular model. *International Journal of Oral & Maxillofacial Implants* **10**, 335–344.

Jensen, S.S., Aaboe, M., Pinholt, E.M., Hjorting-Hansen, E., Melsen, F. & Ruyter, I.E. (1996). Tissue reaction and material characteristics of four bone substitutes. *International Journal of Oral & Maxillofacial Implants* **11**, 55–66.

Joshi, A. & Kostakis, G. (2004). An investigation of postoperative morbidity following iliac crest graft harvesting. *British Dental Journal* **196**, 167–171.

Jovanovic, S.A. & Nevins, M. (1995). Bone formation utilizing titanium-reinforced barrier membranes. *International Journal of Periodontics and Restorative Dentistry* **15**, 57–69.

Jung, R., Cochran, D., Domken, O., Seibl, R., Jones, A., Buser, D. & Hammerle, C. (2007). The effect of matrix bound parathyroid hormone on bone regeneration. *Clinical Oral Implants Research* **18**, 319–325.

Jung, R.E., Glauser, R., Schärer, P., Hämmerle, C.H.F. & Weber, F.E. (2003). The effect of rhBMP-2 on guided bone regeneration in humans. A randomized, controlled clinical and histomorphometric study. *Clinical Oral Implants Research* **14**, 556–568.

Jung, R.E., Schmoekel, H.G., Zwahlen, R., Kokovic, V., Hammerle, C.H. & Weber, F.E. (2005). Platelet-rich plasma and fibrin as delivery systems for recombinant human bone morphogenetic protein-2. *Clinical Oral Implants Research* **16**, 676–682.

Jung, R., Siegenthaler, D. & Hammerle, C. (2004). Postextraction tissue management: a soft tissue punch technique. *International Journal of Periodontics and Restorative Dentistry* **24**, 545–553.

Jung, R., Zwahlen, R., Weber, F., Molenberg, A., van Lenthe, G. & Hämmerle, C. (2006). Evaluation of an in situ formed synthetic hydrogel as a biodegradable membrane for guided bone regeneration. *Clinical Oral Implants Research* **17**, 426–433.

Karoussis, I.K., Salvi, G.E., Heitz-Mayfield, L.J., Bragger, U., Hammerle, C.H. & Lang, N.P. (2003). Long-term implant prognosis in patients with and without a history of chronic periodontitis: a 10-year prospective cohort study of the ITI Dental Implant System. *Clinical Oral Implants Research* **14**, 329–339.

Karring, T., Nyman, S. & Lindhe, J. (1980). Healing following implantation of periodontitis affected roots into bone tissue. *Journal of Clinical Periodontology* **7**, 96–105.

Kohal, R.J., Trejo, P.M., Wirsching, C., Hürzeler, M.B. & Caffesse, R.G. (1999a). Comparison of bioabsorbable and bioinert membranes for guided bone regeneration around non-submerged implants. An experimental study in the mongrel dog. *Clinical Oral Implants Research* **10**, 226–237.

Kohal, R.J., Trejo, P.M., Wirsching, C., Hurzeler, M.B. & Caffesse, R.G. (1999b). Comparison of bioabsorbable and bioinert membranes for guided bone regeneration around non-submerged implants. An experimental study in the mongrel dog. *Clinical Oral Implants Research* **10**, 226–237.

Kostopoulos, L. & Karring, T. (1994). Augmentation of the rat mandible using guided tissue regeneration. *Clinical Oral Implants Research* **5**, 75–82.

Kwon, H., el Deeb, M., Morstad, T. & Waite, D. (1986). Alveolar ridge maintenance with hydroxylapatite ceramic cones in humans. *Journal of Oral and Maxillofacial Surgery* **44**, 503–508.

Landsberg, C. & Bichacho, N. (1994). A modified surgical/prosthetic approach for optimal single implant supported crown. Part I – The socket seal surgery. *Practical Periodontics and Aesthetic Dentistry* **6**, 11–17.

Landsberg, C. (1997). Socket seal surgery combined with immediate implant placement: a novel approach for single-tooth replacement. *International Journal of Periodontics and Restorative Dentistry* **17**, 140–149.

Lekholm, U., Adell, R. & Lindhe, J. (1986). Marginal tissue reactions at osseointegrated titanium fixtures. (II) A cross-sectional retrospective study. *International Journal of Oral & Maxillofacial Surgery* **15**, 53–61.

Lekovic, V., Kenney, E.B., Weinlaender, M., Han, T., Klokkevold, P.R., Nedic, M. & Orsini, M. (1997). A bone regenerative approach to alveolar ridge maintenance following tooth extraction. Report of 10 cases. *Journal of Periodontology* **68**, 563–570.

Lekovic, V., Camargo, P.M., Klokkevold, P.R., Weinlaender, M., Kenney, E.B., Dimitrijevic, B. & Nedic, M. (1998). Preservation of alveolar bone in extraction sockets using bioabsorbable membranes. *Journal of Periodontology* **69**, 1044–1049.

Linde, A. & Hedner, E. (1995). Recombinant bone morphogenetic protein-2 enhances bone healing, guided by osteopromotive e-PTFE membranes: An experimental study in rats. *Calcified Tissue International* **56**, 549–553.

Lorenzoni, M., Pertl, C., Keil, K. & Wegscheider, W.A. (1998). Treatment of peri-implant defects with guided bone regeneration: a comparative clinical study with various membranes and bone grafts. *International Journal of Oral & Maxillofacial Implants* **13**, 639–646.

Lundgren, A.K., Sennerby, L., Lundgren, D., Taylor, Å., Gottlow, J. & Nyman, S. (1997). Bone augmentation at titanium implants using autologous bone grafts and a bioresorbable barrier. *Clinical Oral Implants Research* **8**, 82–89.

Lundgren, D., Mathisen, T. & Gottlow, J. (1994a). The development of a bioresorbable barrier for guided tissue regeneration. *The Journal of the Swedish Dental Association* **86**, 741–756.

Lundgren, D., Sennerby, L., Falk, H., Friberg, B. & Nyman, S. (1994b). The use of a new bioresorbable barrier for guided bone regeneration in connection with implant installation. *Clinical Oral Implants Research* **5**, 177–184.

Lundgren, D., Lundgren, A.K., Sennerby, L. & Nyman, S. (1995). Augmentation of intramembranous bone beyond the skeletal envelope using an occlusive titanium barrier. An experimental study in the rabbit. *Clinical Oral Implants Research* **6**, 67–72.

Mayfield, L., Nobréus, N., Attström, R. & Linde, A. (1997). Guided bone regeneration in dental implant treatment using a bioabsorbable membrane. *Clinical Oral Implants Research* **8**, 10–17.

Mayfield, L., Skoglund, A., Nobreus, N. & Attström, R. (1998). Clinical and radiographic evaluation, following delivery of fixed reconstructions, at GBR treated titanium fixtures. *Clinical Oral Implants Research* **9**, 292–302.

Mellonig, J.T., Nevins, M. & Sanchez, R. (1998). Evaluation of a bioabsorbable physical barrier for guided bone regeneration. Part I. Material alone. *International Journal of Periodontics and Restorative Dentistry* **18**, 129–137.

Mengel, R., Schroder, T. & Flores-de-Jacoby, L. (2001). Osseointegrated implants in patients treated for generalized chronic periodontitis and generalized aggressive periodontitis: 3- and 5-year results of a prospective long-term study. *Journal of Periodontology* **72**, 977–989.

Mombelli, A. & Cionca, N. (2006). Systemic diseases affecting osseointegration therapy. *Clinical Oral Implants Research* **17** (Suppl 2), 97–103.

Moses, O., Pitaru, S., Artzi, Z. & Nemcovsky, C. (2005). Healing of dehiscence-type defects in implants placed together with different barrier membranes: a comparative clinical study. *Clinical Oral Implants Research* **16**, 210–219.

Nemcovsky, C. & Serfaty, V. (1996). Alveolar ridge preservation following extraction of maxillary anterior teeth. Report on 23 consecutive cases. *Journal of Periodontology* **67**, 390–395.

Nevins, M. & Mellonig, J.T. (1994). The advantages of localized ridge augmentation prior to implant placement. A staged event. *International Journal of Periodontics and Restorative Dentistry* **14**, 97–111.

Nevins, M., Kirker-Head, C., Nevins, M., Wozney, J.A., Palmer, R.M. & Graham, D. (1996). Bone formation in the goat maxillary sinus induced by absorbable collagen sponge implants impregnated with recombinant human bone morphogenetic protein-2. *International Journal of Periodontics and Restorative Dentistry* **16**, 9–19.

Nkenke, E., Schultze-Mosgau, S., Radespiel-Tröger, M., Kloss, F. & Neukam, F.W. (2001). Morbidity of harvesting of chin grafts: a prospective study. *Clinical Oral Implants Research* **12**, 495–502.

Nyman, S., Karring, T., Lindhe, J. & Planten, S. (1980). Healing following implantation of periodontitis affected roots into gingival connective tissue. *Journal of Clinical Periodontology* **7**, 394–401.

Nyman, S., Lindhe, J. & Karring, T. (1989). Reattachment – new attachment. In: Lindhe, J., ed. *Textbook of Clinical Periodontology*, 2nd edn. Copenhagen: Munksgaard, pp. 450–473.

Nyman, S., Lang, N.P., Buser, D. & Brägger, U. (1990). Bone regeneration adjacent to titanium dental implants using guided tissue regeneration. A report of 2 cases. *International Journal of Oral & Maxillofacial Implants* **5**, 9–14.

Nyman, S.R. & Lang, N.P. (1994). Guided tissue regeneration and dental implants. *Periodontology 2000* **4**, 109–118.

Oh, T.J., Meraw, S.J., Lee, E.J., Giannobile, W.V. & Wang, H.L. (2003). Comparative analysis of collagen membranes for the treatment of implant dehiscence defects. *Clinical Oral Implants Research* **14**, 80–90.

Pang, S.N.J. (1993). Final report on the safety assessment of polyethylene glycols (PEGs). *Journal of the American College of Toxicology* **12**, 429–456.

Piatelli, A., Scarano, A., Russo, P. & Matarasso, S. (1995). Evaluation of guided bone regeneration in rabbit tibia using bioresorbable and non-resorbable membranes. *Biomaterials* **17**, 791–796.

Quinn, J. & Kent, J. (1984). Alveolar ridge maintenance with solid nonporous hydroxylapatite root implants. *Oral Surgery Oral Medicine Oral Pathology* **58**, 511–521.

Reddi, A.H. (1981). Cell biology and biochemistry of endochondral bone development. *Collagen Related Research* **1**, 209–226.

Reddi, A.H., Weintroub, S. & Muthukumaran, N. (1987). Biologic principles of bone induction. *Orthopedic Clinics of North America* **18**, 207–212.

Ripamonti, U. & Reddi, A.H. (1994). Periodontal regeneration: potential role of bone morphogenetic proteins. *Journal of Periodontal Research* **29**(4), 225–235.

Sandberg, E., Dahlin, C. & Linde, A. (1993). Bone regeneration by the osteopromotion technique using bioabsorbable membranes. An experimental study in rats. *Journal of Oral and Maxillofacial Surgery* **51**, 1106–1114.

Schenk, R.K., Buser, D., Hardwick, W.R. & Dahlin, C. (1994). Healing pattern of bone regeneration in membrane-protected defects: a histologic study in the canine mandible. *International Journal of Oral and Maxillofacial Implants* **9**, 13–29.

Schliephake, H. & Kracht, D. (1997). Vertical ridge augmentation using polylactic membranes in conjunction with immediate implants in periodontally compromised extraction sites: an experimental study in dogs. *International Journal of Oral & Maxillofacial Implants* **12**, 325–334.

Schliephake, H., Neukam, F.W., Scheller, H. & Bothe, K.J. (1994). Local ridge augmentation using bone grafts and osseointegrated implants in the rehablilitation of partial edentulism: Preliminary results. *International Journal of Oral & Maxillofacial Implants* **9**, 557–564.

Schliephake, H., Neukam, F.W. & Wichmann, M. (1997). Survival analysis of endosseous implants in bone grafts used for the treatment of severe alveolar ridge atrophy. *Journal of Oral and Maxillofacial Surgery* **55**, 1227–1233.

Schmid, J., Hämmerle, C.H.F., Flückiger, L., Gogolewski, S., Winkler, J.R., Rahn, B. & Lang, N.P. (1997). Blood filled spaces with and without filler materials in guided bone regeneration. A comparative experimental study in the rabbit using bioresorbable membranes. *Clinical Oral Implants Research* **8**, 75–81.

Seibert, J. & Nyman, S. (1990). Localized ridge augmentation in dogs: a pilot study using membranes and hydroxyapatite. *Journal of Periodontology* **3**, 157–165.

Sevor, J.J., Meffert, R.M. & Cassingham, R.J. (1993). Regeneration of dehisced alveolar bone adjacent to endosseous dental implants utilizing a resorbable collagen membrane: clinical and histologic results. *International Journal of Periodontics and Restorative Dentistry* **13**, 71–83.

Sigurdsson, E.F., Tatakis, D.N., Fu, E., Turek, T.J., Jin, L., Wozney, J.A. & Wikesjö, U.M.E. (1996). Periodontal repair in dogs; Evaluation of rhBMP-2 carriers. *International Journal of Periodontics and Restorative Dentistry* **6**, 525–537.

Simion, M., Baldoni, M., Rossi, P. & Zaffe, D. (1994a). A comparative study of the effectiveness of e-PTFE membranes with and without early exposure during the healing period. *International Journal of Periodontics and Restorative Dentistry* **14**, 167–180.

Simion, M., Trisi, P. & Piattelli, A. (1994b). Vertical ridge augmentation using a membrane technique associated with osseointegrated implants. *International Journal of Periodontics and Restorative Dentistry* **14**, 497–511.

Simion, M., Misitano, U., Gionso, L. & Salvato, A. (1997). Treatment of dehiscences and fenestrations around dental implants using resorbable and nonresorbable membranes associated with bone autografts: a comparative clinical study. *International Journal of Oral & Maxillofacial Implants* **12**, 159–167.

Simion, M., Jovanovic, S.A., Trisi, P., Scarano, A. & Piattelli, A. (1998). Vertical ridge augmentation around dental implants using a membrane technique and autogenous bone or allografts in humans. *International Journal of Periodontics and Restorative Dentistry* **18**, 9–23.

Simion, M., Jovanovic, S.A., Tinti, C. & Benfenati, S.P. (2001). Long-term evaluation of osseointegrated implants inserted at the time or after vertical ridge augmentation. A retrospective study on 123 implants with 1–5 year follow-up. *Clinical Oral Implants Research* **12**, 35–45.

Smukler, H., Porto Barboza, E. & Burliss, C. (1995). A new approach to regeneration of surgically reduced alveolar ridges in dogs: a clinical and histologic study. *International Journal of Oral & Maxillofacial Implants* **10**, 537–551.

Smukler, H., Landi, L. & Setayesh, R. (1999). Histomorphometric evaluation of extraction sockets and deficient alveolar ridges treated with allograft and barrier membrane: a pilot study. *International Journal of Oral & Maxillofacial Implants* **14**, 407–416.

Tal, H. (1999). Autogenous masticatory mucosal grafts in extraction socket seal procedures: a comparison between sockets grafted with demineralized freeze-dried bone and deproteinized bovine bone mineral. *Clinical Oral Implants Research* **10**, 289–296.

Tinti, C., Parma-Benfenati, S. & Polizzi, G. (1996). Vertical ridge augmentation: what is the limit? *International Journal of Periodontics and Restorative Dentistry* **16**, 220–229.

Tinti, C. & Parma-Benfenati, S. (1998). Vertical ridge augmentation: surgical protocol and retrospective evaluation of 48 consecutively inserted implants. *International Journal of Periodontics and Restorative Dentistry* **18**, 445–443.

Urist, M.R. (1965). Bone: formation by autoinduction. *Science* **150**, 893–899.

von Arx, T., Hardt, N. & Wallkamm, B. (1996). The TIME technique: A new method for localized alveolar ridge augmentation prior to placement of dental implants. *International Journal of Oral & Maxillofacial Implants* **11**, 387–394.

von Arx, T., Cochran, D.L., Hermann, J.S., Schenk, R.K., Higginbottom, F.L. & Buser, D. (2001). Lateral ridge augmentation and implant placement: An experimental sutdy evaluating implant osseointegration in different augmentation materials in the canine mandible. *International Journal of Oral & Maxillofacial Implants* **16**, 343–354.

von Arx, T., Hafliger, J. & Chappuis, V. (2005). Neurosensory disturbances following bone harvesting in the symphysis: a prospective clinical study. *Clinical Oral Implants Research* **16**, 432–439.

Weber, F.E., Eyrich, G., Grätz, K.W., Maly, F.E. & Sailer, H.F. (2002). Slow and continuous application of human recombinant bone morphogenetic protein via biodegradable polylactide-co-glycolide foamspheres. *International Journal of Oral and Maxillofacial Surgery* **31**, 60–65.

Wennstrom, J.L., Ekestubbe, A., Grondahl, K., Karlsson, S. & Lindhe, J. (2004). Oral rehabilitation with implant-supported fixed partial dentures in periodontitis-susceptible subjects. A 5-year prospective study. *Journal of Clinical Periodontology* **31**, 713–724.

Widmark, G., Andersson, B., & Ivanoff, C.J. (1997). Mandibular bone graft in the anterior maxilla for single-tooth implants. Presentation of a surgical method. *International Journal of Oral & Maxillofacial Implants* **26**, 106–109.

Working, P.K., Newman, M.S., Johnson, J. & Cornacoff, J.B. (1997). Safety of poly(ethylene glycol) and poly(ethylene glycol) derivates. *Chemistry and Biological Applications* 45–57.

Wozney, J.M., Rosen, V., Celeste, A.J., Mitsock, L.M., Whitters, M.J., Kriz, R.W., Hewick, R.M. & Wang, E.A. (1988). Novel regulators of bone formation: Molecular clones and activities. *Science* **242**, 1528–1533.

Yang, J., Lee, H. & Vernino, A. (2000). Ridge preservation of dentition with severe periodontitis. *Compendium of Continuing Education Dentistry* **21**, 579–583.

Yilmaz, S., Efeoglu, E. & Kilic, A. (1998). Alveolar ridge reconstruction and/or preservation using root form bioglass cones. *Journal of Clinical Periodontology* **25**, 832–839.

Zahedi, S., Legrand, R., Brunel, G., Albert, A., Dewe, W., Coumans, B. & Bernard, J.-P. (1998). Evaluation of a diphenylphosphorylazide-crosslinked collagen membrane for guided bone regeneration in mandibular defects in rats. *Journal of Periodontology* **69**, 1238–1246.

Zalipsky, S. & Harris, J.M. (1997). Introduction to chemistry and biological applications of Poly(ethylene glycol). *Chemistry and Biological Applications* 1–13.

Zellin, G., Gritli-Linde, A. & Linde, A. (1995). Healing of mandibular defects with different biodegradable and non-degradable membranes: an experimental study in rats. *Biomaterials* **16**, 601–609.

Zitzmann, N.U., Naef, R. & Schärer, P. (1997). Resorbable versus nonresorbable membranes in combination with Bio-Oss for guided bone regeneration. *International Journal of Oral & Maxillofacial Implants* **12**, 844–852.

Zitzmann, N.U., Schärer, P., Marinello, C., Schüpbach, P. & Berglundh, T. (2001a). Alveolar ridge augmentation with Bio-Oss: a histologic study in humans. *International Journal of Periodontics and Restorative Dentistry* **21**, 289–295.

Zitzmann, N.U., Schärer, P. & Marinello, C.P. (2001b). Long-term results of implants treated with guided bone regeneration: A 5-year prospective study. *International Journal of Oral & Maxillofacial Surgery* **16**, 355–366.

Chapter 50

Elevation of the Maxillary Sinus Floor

Bjarni E. Pjetursson and Niklaus P. Lang

Introduction, 1099
Treatment options in the posterior maxilla, 1099
Sinus floor elevation with a lateral approach, 1100
  Anatomy of the maxillary sinus, 1100
  Pre-surgical examination, 1101
  Indications and contraindications, 1102
  Surgical techniques, 1102
  Post-surgical care, 1105
  Complications, 1106
  Grafting materials, 1107

Success and implant survival, 1108
Sinus floor elevation with the crestal approach (osteotome
  technique), 1110
  Indications and contraindications, 1111
  Surgical technique, 1111
  Post-surgical care, 1115
  Grafting material, 1115
  Success and implant survival, 1116
Short implants, 1117
Conclusions and clinical suggestions, 1118

Introduction

Elevation of the maxillary sinus floor was first reported by Boyne in the 1960s. Fifteen years later, Boyne and James (1980) reported on elevation of the maxillary sinus floor in patients with large, pneumatized sinus cavities as a preparation for the placement of blade implants. The authors described a two-stage procedure, where the maxillary sinus was grafted using autogenous particulate iliac bone at the first stage of surgery. In the second stage of surgery after approximately 3 months, the blade implants were placed and later used to support fixed or removable reconstructions (Boyne & James 1980).

As implant dentistry developed, it became more evident that the posterior maxillary region was often limited for standard implant placement, since the residual vertical bone height was reduced (Fig. 50-1). An elevation of the maxillary sinus floor was an option in solving this problem. Several surgical techniques have been presented for entering the sinus cavity, elevating the sinus membrane, and placing bone grafts.

A crestal approach for sinus floor elevation with subsequent placement of implants was first suggested (Tatum 1986). Utilizing this crestal approach, a "socket former" for the selected implant size was used to prepare the implant site. A "green-stick fracture" of the sinus floor was accomplished by hand tapping the "socket former" in a vertical direction.

After preparation of the implant site, a root-formed implant was placed and allowed to heal in a submerged way.

Summers (1994) later described another crestal approach, using tapered osteotomes with increasing diameters (Fig. 50-2). Bone was conserved by this osteotome technique because drilling was not performed. Adjacent bone was compressed by pushing and tapping as the sinus membrane was elevated. Then, autogenous, allogenic or xenogenic bone grafts were added to increase the volume below the elevated sinus membrane. A follow-up of 173 press-fit submerged implants, placed using this technique, reported a success rate of 96% at 18 months after loading (Rosen et al. 1999).

Today, two main procedures of sinus floor elevation for dental implant placement are in use: a two-stage technique using the lateral window approach, and a one-stage technique using a lateral or a crestal approach. The decision to use the one- or the two-stage technique is based on the amount of residual bone available and the possibility of achieving primary stability for the inserted implants.

Treatment options in the posterior maxilla

Implant placement in the posterior maxilla remains a challenge. Reduced bone volume due to alveolar

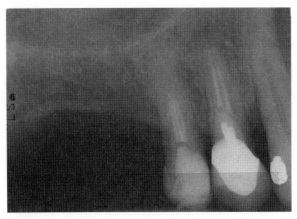

Fig. 50-1 Radiograph of a posterior maxilla, showing reduced residual bone height which will not allow standard implant placement.

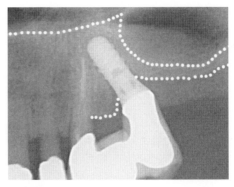

Fig. 50-3 Radiograph showing a tilted implant placed in the position of 25 to avoid entering the sinus cavity. After remodeling, the bone level on the distal aspect of the implant is more apical than at the time of implant placement. This may lead to increased probing pockets depths around tilted implants. (The dotted lines represent the outlines of the residual bone.)

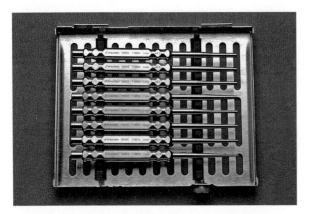

Fig. 50-2 In 1994, Summers introduced a set of tapered osteotomes with different diameters to compress and push the residual bone from the implant preparation into the sinus cavity and to elevate the sinus membrane.

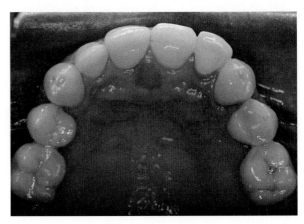

Fig. 50-4 Patient with a shortened dental arch. Three implants were placed in the positions of 15, 14, and 25 without elevating the maxillary sinus floor and, consequently, the patient was restored to the second premolar.

bone resorption and pneumatization of the sinus cavity makes it more difficult to place implants to support a dental prosthesis.

Several treatment options have been used in the posterior maxilla to overcome the problem of inadequate bone quantity. The most conservative treatment option would be to place short implants to avoid entering the sinus cavity. For placement of short implants, there is still a need for at least 6 mm of residual bone height, however. Another way of avoiding grafting the maxillary sinus would be to place tilted implants in a position mesial or distal to the sinus cavity if these areas have adequate bone (Fig. 50-3). Furthermore, extra-long zygomatic implants can be placed in the lateral part of the zygomatic bone.

However, in patients with appropriate residual bone height, minor augmentation of the sinus floor can be accomplished via the crestal approach using the osteotome technique (Summers 1994; Rosen *et al.* 1999; Ferrigno *et al.* 2006). The problem of inadequate bone height may be overcome by elevating the maxillary sinus floor via the closed technique to provide

sufficient quantity of bone for dental implant placement.

The most invasive treatment option in the posterior maxilla is the one- or two-stage sinus floor elevation with a lateral approach. By mastering these different methods, most edentulous areas in the maxilla can by restored with implant-supported reconstructions. The concept of a shortened dental arch must also be kept in mind. The work of Käyser (1981) has shown that patients maintained adequate (50–80%) chewing capacity with a premolar occlusion (Fig. 50-4).

Sinus floor elevation with a lateral approach

Anatomy of the maxillary sinus

The maxilla consists of a variety of anatomic structures, including the maxillary sinus, the lateral nasal walls, the pterygoid plates, associated vasculature structures, and teeth.

The maxillary sinus is pyramidal in shape. The base of the pyramid is the medial wall of the sinus that is also the lateral wall of the nasal cavity, and its apex is pointed towards the zygomatic bone. The roof of the sinus is also the floor of the orbit. The sinus has a non-physiologic drainage port high on the medial wall (maxillary ostium) that opens into the nasal cavity between the middle and lower nasal conchae.

The maxillary sinus maintains its overall size while the posterior teeth remain in function. It is, however, well known, that the sinus expands with age, and especially when posterior teeth are lost. The average volume of a fully developed sinus is about 15 ml but may range between 4.5 and 35.2 ml. The sinus cavity expands both inferiorly and laterally, potentially invading the canine region. This phenomenon is possibly the result of atrophy caused by reduced strain from occlusal function. One or more septa termed "Underwood's septa" may divide the maxillary sinus into several recesses.

The overall prevalence of one or more sinus septa is between 26.5% and 31% (Ulm *et al.* 1995; Kim *et al.* 2006) and is most common in the area between the second premolar and first molar. Edentulous segments have a higher prevalence of sinus septa than dentate maxillary segments.

The sinus is lined with respiratory epithelium (pseudo-stratified ciliated columnar epithelium) that covers a loose, highly vascular connective tissue (Fig. 50-5). Underneath the connective tissue, immediately next to the bony walls of the sinus, is the periosteum. These structures (epithelium, connective tissue, and periosteum) are collectively referred to as the Schneiderian membrane.

The blood supply to the maxillary sinus is derived primarily from the maxillary artery and, to a lesser degree, from the anterior ethmoidal and superior labial arteries. The sinus floor receives blood supply from the greater/lesser palatine and sphenopalatine arteries. These vessels penetrate the bony palate and ramify within the medial, lateral, and inferior walls of the sinus. The posterior superior alveolar artery has tributaries that perfuse the posterior and lateral

walls. The posterior superior alveolar and infraorbital arteries anastomose in the bony lateral wall, on average 19 mm from the alveolar bone crest (Solar *et al.* 1999). The dense vascular network of the maxilla reduces after tooth loss and with increased age. The vast majority of the blood vessels in the maxilla (70–100%) come from the periosteum (Chanavaz 1990, 1995). Venous drainage is into the sphenopalatine vein and pterygomaxillary plexus. Neural supply comes from branches of the maxillary nerve.

Non-hemolytic and alpha-hemolytic streptococci and *Neisseria* spp. are the normal commensal microbiota of the maxillary sinus. Staphylococci, diphtheroids, *Hemophilus* spp., pneumococci, *Mycoplasma* spp., and *Bacteroides* spp. are also found in varying amounts (Timmenga *et al.* 2003).

The healthy maxillary sinus is self-maintaining by postural drainage and actions of the ciliated epithelial lining, which propels bacteria toward the ostium. The maxillary sinus also produces mucus containing lysozymes and immunoglobulins. The significant vascularity of the Schneiderian membrane helps maintain its healthy state by allowing lymphocytic and immunoglobulin access to both the membrane and the sinus cavity.

The fact that the maxillary sinus opening to the nasal cavity is not in the lower part of the sinus (where a graft may be placed) is important and provides an anatomic rationale to sinus floor elevation, as the grafting procedure does not interfere with normal sinus function. In fact, a maxillary sinus floor elevation may improve symptoms of sinusitis/congestion by bringing the floor of the sinus closer to the drainage port.

Pre-surgical examination

Prior to planning complicated surgical procedures like elevation of the maxillary sinus floor, a thorough examination, including medical and dental history, should be obtained (see Chapters 27, 30, and 33).

The dental and periodontal status are evaluated using clinical and radiologic examination methods. The vitality of the neighbouring teeth has to be tested. The infraorbital, lateral nasal, and superior labial areas of the face must be examined regarding tenderness to palpation, swelling or asymmetry. The patient's history along with findings made during the clinical examination should provide sufficient information for diagnosing acute, allergic, and chronic sinusitis.

Pre-operative screening to assess a potential pathologic condition in the maxillary sinus should include radiographic examination, such as e.g. orthopantomography (OPT), tomography, computerized tomography (CT) scans or aquitomo-scans (see Chapter 28).

Before performing the sinus floor elevation surgery, all dentate patients should receive cause-related therapy (see Chapters 34–37).

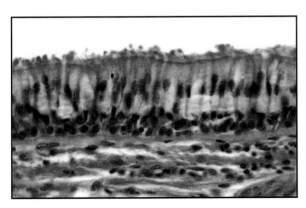

Fig. 50-5 Pseudostratified, ciliated columnar epithelium.

Medical or surgical therapy of sinusitis, and removal of polyps and tumors must be completed prior to sinus floor elevation.

Indications and contraindications

The main indication for maxillary sinus floor elevation utilizing a lateral approach is reduced residual bone height, which does not allow standard implant placement or placement of implants in combination with minor sinus floor elevation using the osteotome technique. In cases of reduced bone height due to alveolar bone resorption and pneumatization of the sinus cavity the so-called lateral approach, with or without horizontal bone augmentation, is indicated.

Contraindications for sinus floor elevation can by divided into three groups: intraoral contraindications, medical conditions, and local contraindications.

The *medical* contraindications include: chemotherapy or radiotherapy of the head and neck area at the time of sinus floor elevation or in the preceding 6 months depending on the field of radiation; immunocompromised patients; medical conditions affecting bone metabolism; uncontrolled diabetes; drug or alcohol abuse; patient non-compliance; and psychiatric conditions.

Whether or not smoking is an absolute contraindication for maxillary sinus floor elevation remains controversial. In a case series, Mayfield and coworkers (2001) evaluated survival of implants placed in combination with bone augmentations (horizontal, vertical, and sinus elevations). The survival rate of these implants was 100% for non-smokers compared to only 43% for smokers after 4–6.5 years of functional loading (Mayfield *et al.* 2001). This reduced survival rate has been corroborated by several other authors (Bain & Moy 1993; Jensen *et al.* 1996; Gruica *et al.* 2004). However, a large study evaluating 2132 implants after sinus floor elevation with simultaneous implant placement found conflicting results (Peleg *et al.* 2006). Two hundred and twenty-six sinus floor elevations (627 implants) were performed on smokers, and 505 sinus floor elevations (1505 implants) on non-smokers. After a follow-up time of up to 9 years, the survival rate of the implants was 97.9%, and there were no statistically significant differences between survival rates in smokers and in non-smokers.

Alteration of the nasal–maxillary complex that interferes with normal ventilation as well as the mucociliary clearance of the maxillary sinus, may be a contraindication for sinus floor elevation. However, such abnormal conditions may be clinically asymptomatic or only present with mild clinical symptoms. These conditions include viral, bacterial, and mycotic rhinosinusitis, allergic sinusitis, sinusitis caused by intra-sinus foreign bodies, and odontogenic sinusitis resulting from necrotic pulp tissue. All odontogenic,

periapical, and radicular cysts of the maxillary sinus should be treated prior to sinus floor elevation.

A sinus floor elevation under any of the above conditions may disturb the fine mucociliary balance, resulting in mucus stasis, suprainfection or a subacute sinusitis.

Absolute local contraindications for sinus floor elevation are: acute sinusitis; allergic rhinitis and chronic recurrent sinusitis; scarred and hypofunctional mucosae; local aggressive benign tumors; and malignant tumors.

Surgical techniques

The original Caldwell-Luc technique, commonly referred to as the lateral window or lateral approach, describes an osteotomy prepared in a superior position just anterior to the zygomatic buttress. Two other positions have also been described: a mid-maxillary position between the alveolar crest and zygomatic buttress area, and a low anterior position near the level of the existing alveolar ridge (Lazzara 1996; Zitzmann & Scharer 1998). The technique described in this chapter is a modification of these techniques:

- A presurgical rinse with chlorhexidine 0.1% is performed for a period of 1 minute.
- Local anesthesia is delivered buccal and palatal to the surgical area.
- The initial incision is midcrestal extending well beyond the planned extension of the osteotomy. The incision is carried on forward beyond the anterior border of the maxillary sinus. Releasing incisions are made anteriorly extending into the buccal vestibulum to facilitate reflection of a full-thickness mucoperiosteal flap.
- A mucoperiosteal flap is raised slightly superior to the anticipated height of the lateral window.
- After the lateral sinus wall has been exposed, a round carbide bur in a straight hand piece is used to mark the outline of the osteotomy (Fig. 50-6).

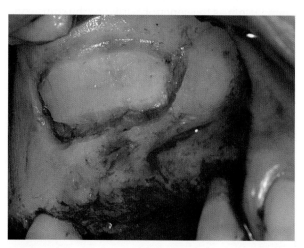

Fig. 50-6 The outline of the lateral window has been marked with a round bur.

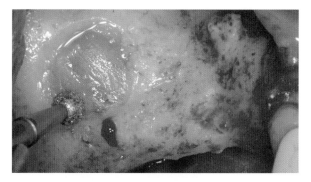

Fig. 50-7 The buccal bony plate is trimmed to a paper-thin lamella with a fine grit round diamond bur, avoiding the perforation of the sinus membrane.

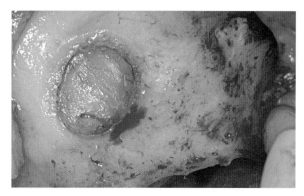

Fig. 50-9 Before elevating the sinus membrane the entire buccal bone is removed to gain access to the membrane.

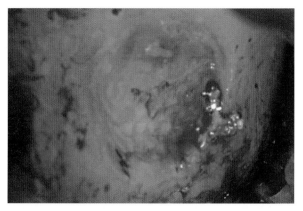

Fig. 50-8 After removing the buccal bony plate, the bluish hue of the sinus membrane becomes clearly visible.

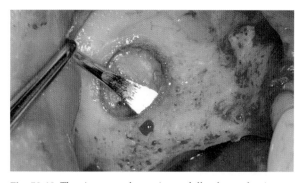

Fig. 50-10 The sinus membrane is carefully elevated using a blunt instrument. To avoid penetration, it is essential to keep contact with the underlying bone at all time during this procedure.

When the bone has been trimmed down to a thin bony plate, the preparation is continued with a round diamond bur (Fig. 50-7) in a straight hand piece until a bluish hue of the sinus membrane is observed (Fig. 50-8). Three methods for handling the buccal cortical bone plate have been proposed. The most common one is the thinning of the buccal bone to a paper-thin bone lamella using a round bur, and removing it prior to the elevation of the sinus membrane (Fig. 50-9). The second method is to fracture the cortical bony plate like a trap-door and use it as the superior border to the sinus compartment, leaving it attached to the underlying mucosa. Since the cortical bony plate is resistant to bone resorption this may protect the graft. The third method proposed is to remove the cortical bony plate during sinus floor elevation and replace it on the lateral aspect of the graft at the end of the grafting procedure. The rationale for this method was the notion that the lateral window would not completely heal without replacement of its cortical plate. However, healing of the lateral window by bone apposition has been demonstrated to occur without replacing the cortical bony plate (Boyne 1993).

- The next step will be chosen according to the technique used. If the buccal wall is eliminated, the sinus membrane is elevated directly with blunt

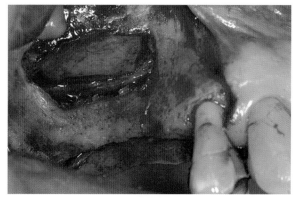

Fig. 50-11 The buccal cortical bony plate was fractured and moved upwards and inwards like a "trap-door". The cortical bony plate is delineating the superior border of the maxillary sinus compartment.

instruments (Fig. 50-10). On the other hand, gentle tapping is continued until movement of the bony plate is observed if the "trap-door" technique is used. Then, in combination with the elevation of the sinus membrane in the inferior part of the sinus, the bony plate is rotated inwards and upwards to provide adequate space for grafting material (Fig. 50-11). Care should be taken not to perforate the sinus membrane.

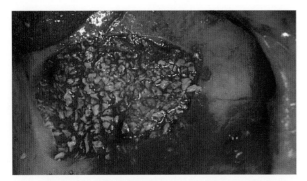

Fig. 50-12 The sinus compartment has been filled with a loosely packed 1 : 1 mixture of particulate autogenous bone and a xenograft.

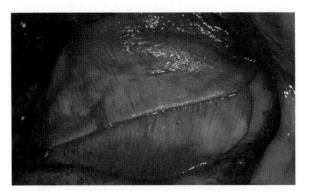

Fig. 50-13 The lateral window has been covered with single or double layer of resorbable barrier membrane.

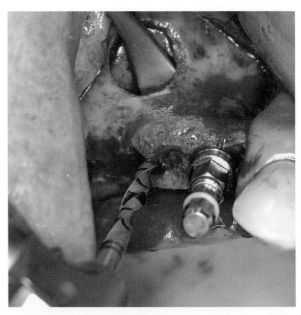

Fig. 50-14 If rotary instruments are used to prepare the implant site, the sinus membrane has to be protected with a periosteal elevator that is placed into the sinus compartment.

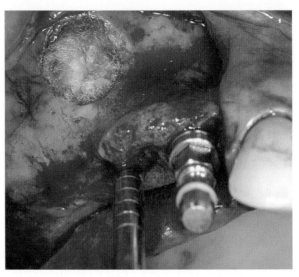

Fig. 50-15 If osteotomes are utilized to prepare the implant site, the sinus membrane can be protected by inserting sterile gauze into the sinus compartment.

Depending on the clinical condition and the surgeon's preference, a delayed (two-stage) or a one-stage sinus floor elevation simultaneously with the implant installation is chosen.

- Two-stage sinus elevation (delayed installation of the implant):
  - Grafting material is placed in the compartment made by the elevation of the sinus membrane. The grafting material should not be densely packed, because this reduces the space needed for ingrowth of newly forming bone. In addition, pressurizing the thin sinus membrane may result in a late perforation.
  - After the compartment has been filled with grafting material (Fig. 50-12), the lateral window is closed by covering it with a resorbable or a non-resorbable barrier membrane (Fig. 50-13). Subsequently, the flap is closed free of tension. In most conditions, there is a need for deep periosteal incisions to achieve tension-free closure.
- One-stage sinus floor elevation with simultaneous implant placement:
  - After the sinus membrane has been elevated, the implant sites are prepared. If rotary instruments are used, the sinus membrane has to be protected using a periosteal elevator (Fig. 50-14). Osteotomes of different diameters may

be used to prepare the implant site, and then the membrane can be protected by inserting sterile gauze into the sinus compartment (Fig. 50-15).

  - The appropriate implant length is measured with a blunt depth gauge (Fig. 50-16). Before placing the implant, the grafting material is inserted into the medial part of the sinus compartment (Fig. 50-17). After implant placement (Fig. 50-18), the lateral part of the compartment is filled with grafting material (Fig. 50-19).
  - The subsequent steps coincide with those described for the two-stage procedure.

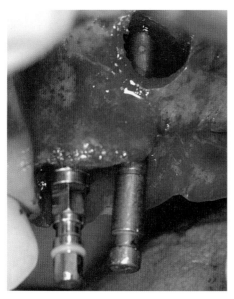

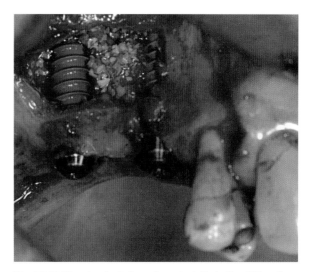

Fig. 50-18 Two implants have been installed after filling the medial part of the sinus compartment.

Fig. 50-16 If sinus floor elevation and simultaneous implant placement are performed, the height of the sinus compartment and implant length may be determined by inserting a blunt depth gauge into the implant site. Care must be taken not to apply too much pressure on the sinus membrane.

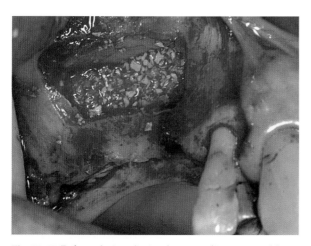

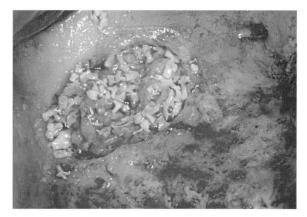

Fig. 50-19 After implant installation the lateral part of the sinus compartment is filled up with loosely packed grafting material.

Fig. 50-17 Before placing the implants, grafting material has to be inserted into the medial part of the sinus compartment, because access to the medial part of the sinus compartment is restricted after implant installation.

Similar results were obtained in a controlled clinical trial (Froum *et al.* 1998) measuring bone formation in 113 sinuses grafted either with xenograft alone or a composite of xenograft and autograft. The mean vital bone formation was 27.6% when a membrane was used compared to 16% without.

Post-surgical care

In order to minimize post-operative pain and discomfort for the patient, surgical handling should be as atraumatic as possible. Precautions must be taken to avoid perforation of the flap and the sinus membrane. The bone should be kept moist during the surgery, and a tension-free primary flap closure is essential. The pain experienced by patients is mostly limited to the first days after surgery. Swelling and bruising of the area are usually the chief post-operative sequelae. Often, swelling and bruising extend from the inferior border of the orbit to the lower border of the mandible or even to the neck. In order to reduce swelling, it is important to cool the area

The main differences between the methods used presently are the position and technique used to prepare the lateral window, the amount of sinus membrane elevation, the type of graft utilized, and the choice of one-stage or two-stage approaches.

Histomorphometric evidence of enhanced bone formation following membrane placement over the lateral window is available. In a randomized controlled clinical trial (Tarnow *et al.* 2000), a split mouth design with bilateral sinus grafts was performed for 12 patients with or without covering the lateral window using a membrane. After 12 months, histologic samples were taken through the lateral window. The mean percentage of vital bone formation was 25.5% with and 11.9% without a covering barrier.

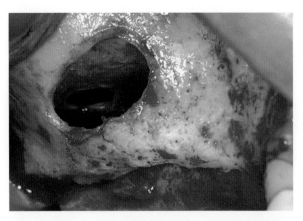

Fig. 50-20 The most frequent complication during maxillary sinus floor elevation is perforation of the sinus membrane. A medium-sized perforation can be detected after elevation of the membrane.

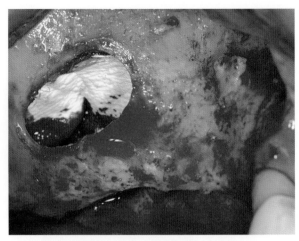

Fig. 50-21 Small- to medium-sized sinus membrane perforations may be closed by applying a resorbable barrier membrane.

with cooling pads at least for the first post-operative hours. Occasionally, minor bleeding may arise from the nose. It is important to inform the patients that some irritation in the nasal area may be expected. In the event of the need for sneezing, the nose should not be covered so that air pressure is allowed to escape. After the surgery, patients are placed on antibiotic therapy. Furthermore, antiseptic rinses with 0.1–0.2% chlorhexidine twice daily are indicated for the first 3 weeks after surgery.

Complications

When performing sinus floor elevation, the risk of complications must be considered and the appropriate treatment foreseen. The most common intra-operative complication is perforation of the sinus membrane (Fig. 50-20). Presence of maxillary sinus septa and root apices penetrating into the sinus may increase the risk of membrane perforation. The risk of perforation has been reported to be between 10 and 40% during surgery (Block & Kent 1997; Timmenga et al. 1997; Pikos 1999). In the event of a membrane perforation, it is recommended to elevate the membrane in the opposite direction to prevent further enlargement of the perforation. Smaller perforations (<5 mm) may be closed by using tissue fibrin glue, suturing or by covering them with a resorbable barrier membrane (Fig. 50-21). In cases of larger perforations, larger barrier membranes, lamellar bone plates or suturing may be used either alone or in combination with tissue fibrin glue to provide a superior border for the grafting material. In instances of larger perforations, where a stable superior border cannot be achieved the grafting of the maxillary sinus must by aborted and a second attempt at sinus floor elevation may be performed 6–9 months later (Tatum et al. 1993; van den Bergh et al. 2000).

Other complications that were reported during surgery included excessive bleeding from the bony window or the sinus membrane, and wound dehiscences. Iatrogenic complications include injury of the infraorbital neurovascular bundle from deep dissection to free the flap from tension or blunt trauma due to the compression of the neurovascular bundle during retraction. Implant migration, hematoma, and adjacent tooth sensitivity have also been reported.

Infection of the grafted sinuses is a rare complication. However, the risk for infection increases with a membrane perforation. Hence, it is recommended to avoid sinus grafting and simultaneous implant placement in situations of membrane perforation (Jensen et al. 1996). Infection of the grafted sinuses is usually seen 3–7 days post surgically and may lead to a failure of the graft. Possible complication secondary to infection may involve a parasinusitis with the spread of the infection to the orbita or even to the brain. For these reasons, infected sinus grafts must be treated immediately and aggressively. Surgical removal of the entire graft from the sinus cavity and administration of high doses of antibiotics are essential.

Sinusitis is another complication that may occur after sinus grafting. In a study (Timmenga et al. 1997) evaluating the function of the maxillary sinus after sinus floor elevation, 45 patients who had received 85 sinus grafts underwent endoscopic examination. Of these, five were diagnosed with sinusitis. In these five patients, the endoscopic examination revealed oversized turbinates and septal deviation. Hence, the result of this study showed that the incidence of sinusitis was low and mainly found in patients with an anatomic or functional disorder prior to the sinus grafting.

Late failure reports include chronic infection, graft exposure, loss of the entire bone graft, oro-antral fistula, ingrowth of soft tissue through the lateral window, granulation tissue replacing the graft, and sinus cysts.

Grafting materials

There are differences in opinion on the necessity of grafting material when elevating the maxillary sinus floor.

Sinus floor elevation without grafting material

Studies in monkeys (Boyne 1993) showed that implants protruding into the maxillary sinus following elevation of the sinus membrane without grafting material, exhibited spontaneous bone formation over more than half of the implant's height. Hence, protrusion of an implant into the maxillary sinus does not appear to be an indication for bone grafting. In the same study, it was also seen that the design of the implant influenced the amount of spontaneous bone formation. Implants with open apices or deep-threaded configurations did not reveal substantial amounts of new bone formation. On the other hand, implants with rounded apices tended to show spontaneous bone formation extending all around the implants if they only penetrated 2–3 mm into the maxillary sinus. However, when the same implants penetrated 5 mm into the maxillary sinus, only a partial (50%) growth of new bone was seen towards the apex of the implant.

In a clinical study (Ellegaard *et al.* 2006), 131 implants were placed using the lateral approach. The sinus membrane was elevated, implants were inserted and left to protrude into the sinus cavity. The sinus membrane was allowed to settle on to the apex of the implants, thus creating a space to be filled with a blood coagulum. After a mean follow-up time of 5 years, the survival rate of these implants was 90%. It must be kept in mind, however, that the residual bone height in this study was at least 3 mm.

Autogenous bone

Autogenous bone grafts are considered the gold standard for grafting due to their maintenance of cellular viability and presumptive osteogenic capacity. The use of autogenous grafts in sinus floor elevation was first reported by Boyne and James (1980) and Tatum (1986).

Grafts may be harvested intraorally or extraorally. Common intraoral donor sites are the maxillary tuberosity, the zygomatico-maxillary buttress, the zygoma, the mandibular symphysis and the mandibular body and ramus (Fig. 50-22). Bone may be harvested in block section or in particulate form. The extraoral donor sites that have been utilized are the anterior and posterior iliac crest, the tibial plateau, the rib, and the calvaria.

Autologous bone grafts contain bone morphogenic proteins (BMPs) that are capable of inducing osteogenic cells in the surrounding tissues. They also contain other growth factors essential for the process of graft incorporation. Processing of autograft, with

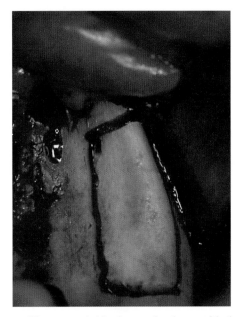

Fig. 50-22 The most suitable sites used to harvest block or particulate bone grafts intraorally are the mandibular body and the mandibular ramus.

grinding or morselizing, does not seem to disturb the viability of the osteogenic cells (Springer *et al.* 2004). The main source of osteogenic cells during graft consolidation is the periosteum that includes mesenchymal progenitor cells and provides a rich source of blood vessels. Osteoclasts are then required for remodeling of the graft–woven bone complex. The consolidation of the graft depends on the properties of the graft material and the osteogenic potential of the recipient bed. Initially, cortical bone grafts act as weight-bearing space fillers and remain a mixture of necrotic and viable bone for a prolonged period of time. The ideal graft material has to allow ingrowth of blood vessels and formation of bone on its surfaces for integration into the recipient bed (osteoconductivity).

In situations of sinus floor elevations that do not eventually receive dental implants, the bone grafts may resorb due to the lack of functional load and strain.

Bone substitutes

Loss of autografts during healing occurs when resorption of the autograft exceeds new bone formation during the consolidation phase. Thus, to overcome excessive resorption of autografts, bone substitutes that are known for their slow resorption process, are added to autografts to increase the stability of grafts during the consolidation phase.

Tricalcium phosphate was the first bone substitute to be applied successfully for sinus floor elevation (Tatum 1986). Over the years, allografts, alloplasts, and xenografts of various types have been used alone or in combination with autografts. Studies in animal models showed that the use of bone substitutes, such

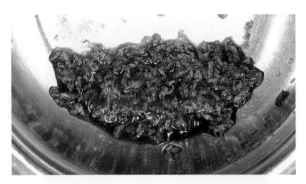

Fig. 50-23 A 1 : 1 mixture of particulate autologous bone and bone substitute. The autologous bone particles include viable osteogenic cells, bone morphogenic proteins, and other growth factors. The bone substitute is supposed to decrease the resorption of the grafting material.

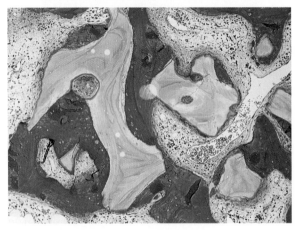

Fig. 50-24 The bovine bone mineral particles (xenograft) are mostly surrounded by new mature compact bone. No gaps can be seen at the interface between the xenograft particles and the newly formed bone. (Courtesy of Dr. Dieter D. Bosshardt, Berne.)

as bovine bone mineral, either alone or in combination with autografts, preserved the vertical height of the graft over time (Fig. 50-23). In a human study, sinus grafts consisting of autografts and demineralized allografts, were observed over a period of time. A graft resorption of up to 25% was seen. Furthermore, a more recent human study (Hatano *et al.* 2004) showed also significant reduction in graft volume, when either autogenous bone alone or a mixture of autogenous bone and xenografts were used. There is a definitive need for good long-term studies that address the stability of the different types of grafting materials in the maxillary sinuses over time.

Histologic analysis of human biopsy specimens from sinuses augmented with xenografts revealed that xenograft particles were mostly surrounded by mature compact bone (Fig. 50-24). In some Haversian canals, it was possible to observe small capillaries, mesenchymal cells, and osteoblasts in conjunction with new bone. No gaps were noted at the interface between the xenograft particles and the newly formed bone (Piattelli *et al.* 1999).

A human study (Froum *et al.* 1998) evaluating bone formation after sinus floor elevation using xenografts alone or in combination with autogenous bone and/or demineralized freeze-dried bone allografts reported statistically significant increase in vital bone formation, when as little as 20% of autologous bone was added to the bone substitutes. The mean vital bone formation was 27.1% after a healing period of 6–9 months. However, comparative studies (Hising *et al.* 2001; Hallman *et al.* 2002a,b; Valentini & Abensur 2003) reported higher survival rates for implants placed into sinuses grafted with 100% xenograft as compared to those placed in sinuses grafted with 100% autogenous bone or composite graft of xenograft and autogenous bone.

Another indication for using bone substitutes is to reduce the volume of bone that must be harvested. When a large sinus cavity is grafted with autologous bone alone, 5–6 ml of bone may be necessary. Using bone substitutes alone or in combination with autografts, the amount of autogenous bone to be harvested is greatly reduced.

Success and implant survival

Jensen and co-workers (1996) published the findings from the Consensus Conference of the Academy of Osseointegration. Retrospective data was collected from 38 clinicians who collectively performed 1007 sinus floor elevations and placed 2997 implants over a 10-year period. The majority of the implants had been followed for 3 years or more. Two hundred and twenty-nine implants were lost resulting in a overall survival rate of 90.0%. However, the database was so variable that no definitive conclusions regarding the grafting material, the type of implants, and the timing for implant placement could be drawn.

Survival of implants cannot be the sole criterion for success of maxillary sinus floor elevation. Factors, such as the pre-operative residual bone height, the long-term stability of the bone graft, and the incidence of failing two-stage sinus grafting due to graft resorption must also be considered.

Of the 900 patient records that were screened for the Consensus Conference in 1996, only 100 had radiographs of adequate quality for analysis of the residual bone height. In total, only 145 sinus grafts in 100 patients, with 349 implants, were analyzed. After a mean follow-up period of 3.2 years, 20 implants were lost. Of the implants lost, 13 were initially placed in residual bone with a height ≤4 mm, seven were placed in residual bone with a height of 5–8 mm. None of the implants placed in residual bone height of more than 8 mm was lost. There was a statistically significant difference in implant loss when residual bone height was 4 mm or less as compared to 5 mm or greater (Jensen *et al.* 1996).

A critical appraisal of the dental literature on maxillary sinus floor elevation shows that the two-stage approach (delayed implant installation) is more likely

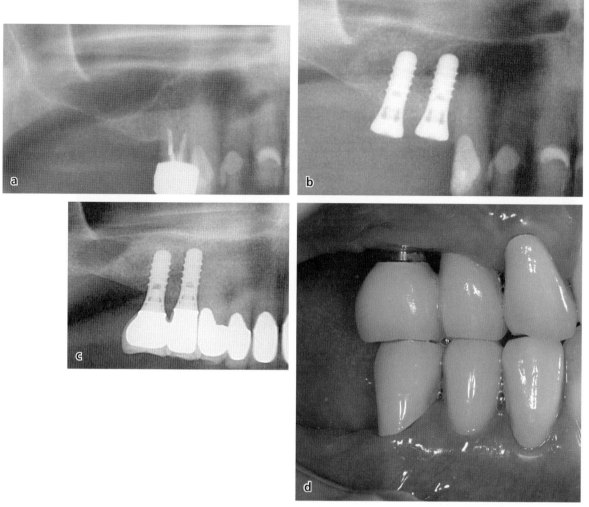

Fig. 50-25 One-stage sinus floor elevation. (a) A panoramic radiograph showing oblique inferior sinus borders and a residual bone height between 2 and 6 mm in the position of 25. (b) Two implants were placed, a standard implant placement in the position of 24 and an implant installed in combination with sinus floor elevation in the position of 25. A 1 : 1 mixture of particulate autologous bone harvested from the maxillary tuberosities and the zygomatic bone combined with bovine bone mineral was used as the grafting material. (c) OPT taken 1 year after functional loading. A new inferior border of the maxillary sinus and a stable graft volume was evident. (d) The clinical situation at the 1-year follow-up visit.

to be used in situations with less residual bone height compared to the one-stage approach (simultaneous implant placement).

The efficacy of performing a one-stage sinus floor elevation in patients whose residual alveolar bone height in the posterior maxilla was between 3 and 5 mm was assessed (Peleg *et al.* 1999). Using the modified Caldwell-Luc technique, the maxillary sinus was elevated with composite grafts of symphysal autograft and demineralized freeze-dried bone allograft in a 1 : 1 ratio. One hundred and sixty implants were placed in 63 elevated sinuses. A 100% survival rate of the implants was reported after 4 years. In a second study (Peleg *et al.* 1998) using a similar protocol on 55 implants placed into 20 elevated sinuses, the residual alveolar bone height was only 1–2 mm. All implants osseointegrated successfully, and no implants were lost after 2 years of functional loading.

Only one randomized controlled clinical trial (Wannfors *et al.* 2000) compared one- and two-stage

sinus floor elevation, in 40 patients divided into groups. The residual bone height ranged from 2 to 7 mm. The one-stage protocol (Fig. 50-25) with 75 implants placed reported a survival rate of 85.5% as compared to the two-stage protocol (Fig. 50-26) with 90.5% survival rate for 74 implants placed after 1 year in function. Apparently, the risk of implant failure in grafted areas for the one-stage procedure was greater than for two-stage procedure, although the results did not reach statistical significance.

The stability of the sinus graft height was evaluated on panoramic radiographs for 349 implants. After a mean follow-up period of 3.2 years, the reduction of the graft height varied between 0.8 mm (autograft and alloplast) and 2.1 mm (autograft). This indicated that all of the graft materials appeared to be stable, with only 1–2 mm of the graft height being lost over the 3-year period (Jensen *et al.* 1996). Further studies evaluating the long-term stability of sinus grafts (Block *et al.* 1998; Hatano *et al.* 2004) yielded similar results.

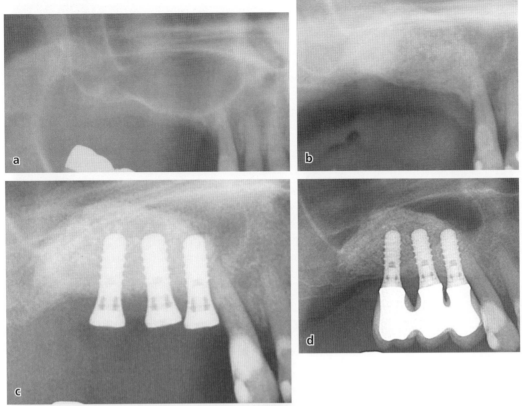

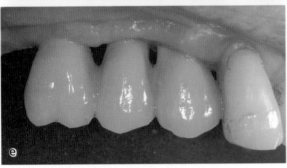

Fig. 50-26 Two-stage sinus floor elevation. (a) An OPT showing a large pneumatized maxillary sinus in the 1st quadrant and a residual bone height of only 1–2 mm. (b) The maxillary sinus floor was elevated with a 1 : 1 mixture of particulate autologous bone harvested from the mandibular ramus and bovine bone mineral. (c) Three 12 mm implants were inserted in a second-stage surgery 6 months after the elevation of the sinus floor. (d) OPT taken after 1 year of functional loading, indicating a stable situation. No changes in graft volume are visible. (e) The clinical situation at the 1-year follow-up visit.

In 2003, Wallace and Froum published a systematic review on the effect of maxillary sinus floor elevation on the survival of dental implants. The inclusion criteria were human studies with a minimum of 20 interventions, a follow-up time of 1 year of functional loading and with an outcome varied of implant survival. The main results indicated:

1. A survival rate of implants placed in conjunction with sinus floor elevation with the lateral approach varied between 61.7 and 100%, with an average of 91.8%.
2. Implant survival rates compared favorably to reported survival rates for implants placed in the non-grafted maxilla.
3. Rough-surfaced implants yielded higher survival rate than machined-surface implants when placed in grafted sinuses.
4. Implants placed into sinuses augmented with particulate autografts showed higher survival rates than those placed in sinuses that had been augmented with block grafts.
5. Implant survival rates were higher when barrier membranes were placed over the lateral window.
6. The utilization of grafts consisting of 100% autogenous bone or the inclusion of autogenous bone as a component of composite grafts did not affect implant survival.

Sinus floor elevation with the crestal approach (osteotome technique)

The osteotome technique was first developed to compress soft, type III and IV maxillary bone. The concept is intended to increase the density of bone in the maxilla leading to better primary stability of inserted dental implants.

In the maxilla, the bone crest in edentulous ridges is often narrow in the bucco-palatal dimension. This

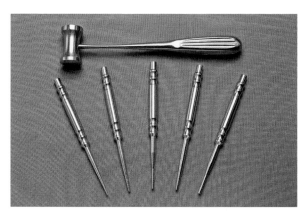

Fig. 50-27 Set of straight and tapered osteotomes used to prepare the implant site and to elevate the maxillary sinus floor.

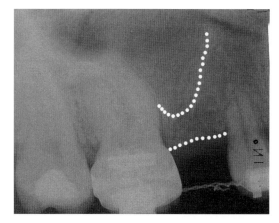

Fig. 50-28 Edentulous space in position 15. The oblique inferior border of the maxillary sinus lies at approximately 60° to the inferior border of the alveolar crest (the dotted lines represent the outlines of the residual bone). In a clinical situation like this, it is difficult to elevate the maxillary sinus floor with osteotomes. The osteotomes will first enter the sinus cavity distally at the lowest level of oblique sinus floor while still having bone resistance on the cranial level of the sinus floor. Hence, the risk of the sharp margin perforating the sinus membrane is high.

limits the possibility of standard drilling in preparing an implant site. Thus, to address this difficult situation, tapered round osteotomes of increasing diameters have been used to expand the compactible cancellous maxillary bone and gently move it in a lateral direction to increase crestal width. This procedure is known as "ridge expansion osteotome technique" and will not be addressed further in this chapter.

Tatum (1986) described the crestal approach to elevate the sinus floor. The osteotome technique for sinus floor elevation, using a set of osteotomes of varying diameters (Fig. 50-27) to prepare the implant site, was first presented by Summers (1994). The bone-added osteotome sinus floor elevation (BAOSFE), today referred to as the *Summers technique*, may be considered to be a more conservative and less invasive approach than the conventional lateral approach of sinus floor elevation. A small osteotomy is made through the crest of the edentulous ridge, at the inferior region of the maxillary sinus. This intrusion osteotomy procedure elevates the sinus membrane, thus creating a "tent". This creates space for bone graft placement. It should be noted that the bone grafts are placed blindly into the space below the sinus membrane. Hence, the main disadvantage of this technique is the uncertainty of possible perforation of the sinus membrane. However, an endoscopic study has shown that the sinus floor can be elevated up to 5 mm without perforating the membrane (Engelke & Deckwer 1997).

Indications and contraindications

Indications for the transalveolar osteotome technique (crestal approach) include a flat sinus floor with a residual bone height of at least 5 mm and adequate crestal bone width for implant installation.

The contraindications for the osteotome technique are similar to those previously described for the lateral approach. In addition, however, patients with

a history of inner ear complications and positional vertigo are not suitable for the osteotome technique. As for the local contraindications, an oblique sinus floor (>45° inclination) is not suitable for the osteotome technique either (Fig. 50-28). The reason is the fact that the osteotomes first enter the sinus cavity at the lower level of an oblique sinus floor, while still having bone resistance on the higher level. In this situation, there is a high risk of perforating the sinus membrane with the sharp margin of the osteotome (Fig. 50-29).

Surgical technique

Apart from the original technique (Summers 1994), only minor modifications have been presented (Rosen *et al.* 1999; Fugazotto 2001; Chen & Cha 2005). The technique described in this chapter represents a modification of the original technique:

- Pre-surgical patient preparation includes oral rinsing with 0.1% chlorhexidine for a period of 1 minute.
- Local anesthesia is administered into the buccal and palatal regions of the surgical area.
- A mid-crestal incision with or without releasing incision is made and a full-thickness mucoperiosteal flap is raised.
- With a surgical stent or a distance indicator, the implant positions are marked on the alveolar crest with a small round bur (#1). After exactly locating the implant positions, the opening of the preparations are widened with two sizes of round burs (#2 and #3) to a diameter about half a millimeter smaller than the implant diameter that is chosen (Fig. 50-30).

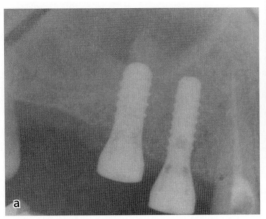 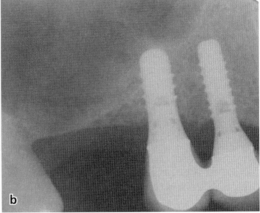

Fig. 50-29 (a) A sinus floor elevation was performed with the osteotome technique in a situation of an oblique sinus floor. The cortical bone of the sinus floor was in-fractured and rolled-up causing a perforation of the sinus membrane. Due to the membrane perforation no grafting material was utilized. (b) The same patient at the 5-year follow-up visit. The implant was stable, but only minor new bone formation is visible at the distal aspect of the implant.

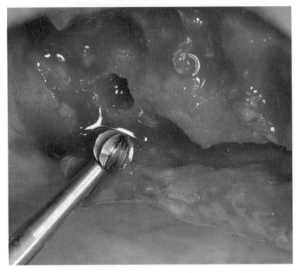

Fig. 50-30 The exact position of the implant site is first marked with a small round bur (#1) and then extended with two sizes of round burs (#2 and #3) to a diameter about 0.5–1 mm smaller than that of the implant to be installed.

- The distance from the crestal floor of the ridge to the floor of the maxillary sinus, measured prior to implant site preparation on the pre-operative radiograph, can in most cases, be confirmed at surgery by penetrating the opening of the preparation with a blunt periodontal probe through the soft trabecular bone (type III or IV bone) to the floor of the maxillary sinus.
- After confirming the distance to the sinus floor, pilot drills with small diameters (1–1.5 mm smaller than the implant diameter) are used to prepare the implant site to a distance of approximately 2 mm below from the sinus floor (Fig. 50-31a). In conditions of soft type IV bone and a residual bone height of 5–6 mm, there is usually no necessity to use the pilot drills. It is sufficient to perforate the cortical bone at the alveolar crest with the round burs.

- The first osteotome used in the implant site is a small diameter tapered osteotome (Fig. 50-32). With light malleting, the osteotome is pushed towards the compact bone of the sinus floor (Fig. 50-31b). After reaching the sinus floor, the osteotome is pushed about 1 mm further with light malleting in order to create a "greenstick" fracture on the compact bone of the sinus floor. A tapered osteotome with small diameter is chosen to minimize the force needed to fracture the compact bone.
- The second tapered osteotome, with a diameter slightly larger then the first one, is used to increase the fracture area of the sinus floor (Fig. 50-33). The second osteotome is applied to the same length as the first one.
- The third osteotome used is a straight osteotome with a diameter about 1–1.5 mm smaller than the implant to be placed (Fig. 50-34).

From this point onwards, the technique utilized in the surgical procedure depends on whether or not bone grafts or bone substitutes will be placed.

Implant placement without grafting material

- Without applying grafting material, the straight osteotome with a diameter about 1–1.5 mm smaller than that of the implant will be pushed further until it penetrates the sinus floor.
- The last osteotome to be used must have a form and diameter suitable for the implant to be placed. For example, for a cylindrical implant with a diameter of 4.1 mm, the last osteotome should be a straight osteotome with a diameter about 0.5 mm smaller than the implant diameter (3.5 mm). It is important that last osteotome only enters the preparation site once (Fig. 50-35). If several attempts have to be made in sites with soft bone (type III or IV), there is a risk of increasing the diameter of the

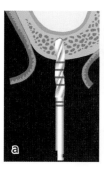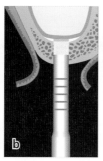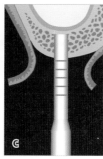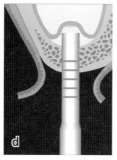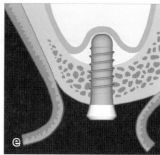

Fig. 50-31 (a) The implant site is prepared to a distance of approximately 2 mm below the sinus floor with a small diameter pilot drill. (b) After reaching the sinus floor, the osteotome is pushed approximately 1 mm further with light malleting in order to create a "greenstick" fracture on the compact bone of the sinus floor. (c) Grafting material is slowly pushed into the sinus cavity with a straight osteotome. This procedure is repeated several times. (d) The tip of the osteotome is only supposed to enter the sinus cavity after some grafting material has been pushed through the preparation site to elevate the sinus membrane. (e) The inserted implant and the grafting material maintain space below the sinus membrane.

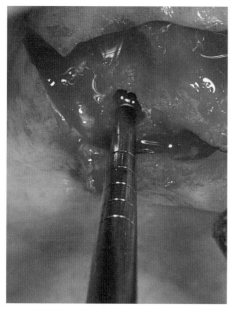

Fig. 50-32 The first osteotome used in the implant site is a small-diameter tapered osteotome. Such an osteotome is chosen to minimize the force needed to fracture the compact bone.

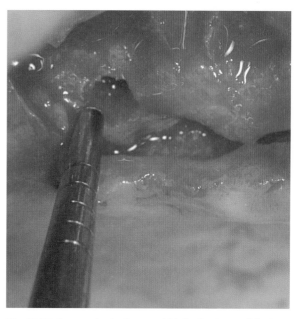

Fig. 50-33 A second osteotome, which is also tapered, but with a diameter slightly larger then the first one, is used to increase the fractured area of the sinus floor.

preparation that might jeopardize achieving good primary stability. On the other hand, if the last osteotome diameter is too small compared to the implant diameter, too much force must be used to insert the implant. By squeezing the bone, more bone trauma and, hence, greater bone resorption will occur, delaying the osseointegration process (Abrahamsson *et al.* 2004). It is thus important, especially when placing implants in sites with reduced bone volume, that the fine balance between good primary stability and traumatizing the bone is respected.

• During the entire preparation, it is crucial to maintain precise control of the penetration length. Regular osteotomes have sharp cutting edges, thus entry into the sinus cavity increases the risk of membrane perforation. The final step before placing the implant is to check that the preparation

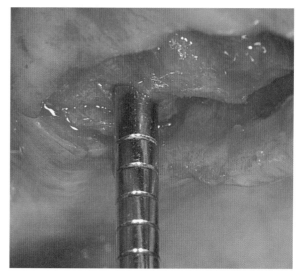

Fig. 50-34 The third osteotome utilized is a straight osteotome with a diameter about 1–1.5 mm smaller than that of the implant to be placed.

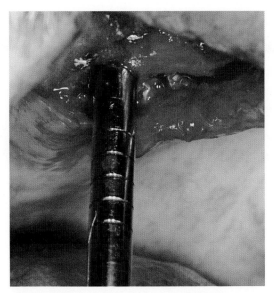

Fig. 50-35 The last osteotome to be used must have a form and diameter suitable for the implant to be placed. For example, for a cylindrical implant with a diameter of 4.1 mm, the last osteotome should be straight with a diameter approximately 0.5 mm smaller than that of the implant (3.5 mm). It is important that the last osteotome is allowed to enter the preparation site only once.

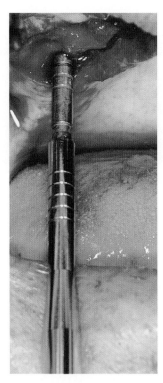

Fig. 50-36 The final step before placing the implant is to check that the preparation is patent to the planned insertion depth. An osteotome with a rounded tip or a depth gauge, for the relevant implant diameter, is pushed to the decided length.

is patent to the planned insertion depth. An osteotome with a rounded tip or a depth gauge, for the relevant implant diameter, is pushed to the decided length (Fig. 50-36).

Implant placement with grafting materials

- When performing the osteotome technique with grafting materials, the osteotomes are not supposed to enter the sinus cavity *per se*. Repositioned bone particles, grafting materials, and the trapped fluid will create a hydraulic effect moving the fractured sinus floor and the sinus membrane upwards. The sinus membrane is less likely to tear under this kind of pressure that has a fluid consistency.

- After pushing the third osteotome up to the sinus floor and before placement of any grafting material, the sinus membrane must by tested for any perforations. This is tested with the Valsalva maneuver (nose blowing). The nostrils of the patients are compressed (Fig. 50-37), and the patient blows against the resistance. If air leaks out of the implant site, the sinus membrane is perforated, and no grafting material should be placed into the sinus cavity.

- If the sinus membrane is judged to be intact, the preparation is filled with grafting material (Fig. 50-38). The grafting material is then slowly pushed into the sinus cavity with the same straight third osteotome (Fig. 50-39). This procedure is repeated four to five times (Fig. 50-31c) until about 0.2–0.3 g of grafting material has been pushed into the sinus cavity below the sinus membrane (Fig. 50-40). In the fourth and fifth time of applying

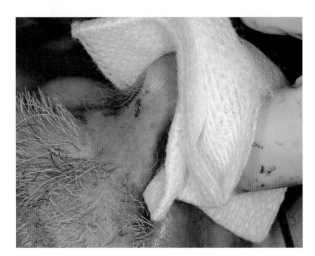

Fig. 50-37 To test the sinus membrane, the nostrils of the patients are compressed and the patient is asked to blow against the resistance. If air leaks out of the implant site, the sinus membrane is perforated, and no grafting material should be placed into the sinus cavity.

grafting material, the tip of the osteotome may enter about 1 mm into the maxillary sinus cavity to test if there is resistance in the preparation site (Fig. 50-31d).

- Finally, before implant placement (Fig. 50-41), the preparation is checked for patency, as mentioned before, and the Valsalva maneuver is repeated.

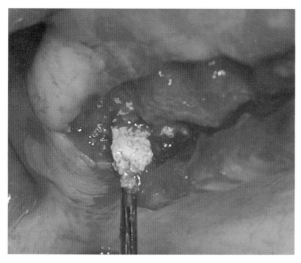

Fig. 50-38 If the sinus membrane is intact, the preparation site is filled four to five times with grafting material.

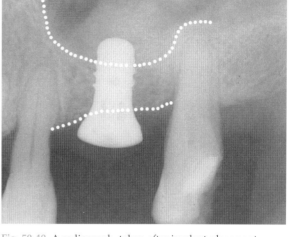

Fig. 50-40 A radiograph, taken after implant placement, showing a dome-shape configuration of the graft. In this instance, 0.25 g of grafting material (xenograft) was used to elevate the sinus membrane (the dotted lines represent the outlines of the residual bone).

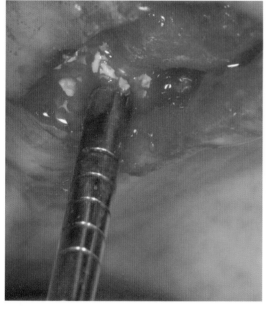

Fig. 50-39 The grafting material is then slowly pushed into the sinus cavity with a straight osteotome with a diameter about 1–1.5 mm smaller than that of the intended implant.

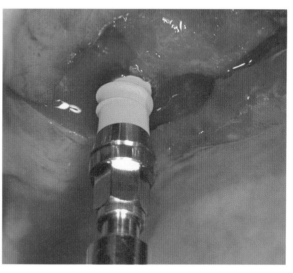

Fig. 50-41 A rough-textured implant was installed after preparing the implant site with the osteotome technique. Good primary stability was achieved.

Post-surgical care

The post-surgical care after placing implants with the osteotome technique is similar to that after standard implant placement. In addition to the standard oral home care, antiseptic rinsing with 0.1–0.2% chlorhexidine twice daily for the first 3 weeks after surgery is highly recommended. However, if bone substitutes were used, the patients are placed on antibiotic prophylaxis for a period of 1 week.

Grafting material

There is still controversy with regards to the necessity of a grafting material to maintain the space for new bone formation after elevating the sinus membrane utilizing the osteotome technique. Shortly after Summers introduced the BAOSFE, a multi-center retrospective study of eight centers was performed. Evaluation was carried out with 174 implants placed in 101 patients. The use of grafting material was decided by the individual clinician. Autografts, allografts, and xenografts were used, alone or in combinations. The authors concluded that the type of grafting material did not influence implant survival (Rosen *et al.* 1999).

When no grafting material is used, some dense structure is often visible apical to the implant, immediately after implant placement. However, after at least 1 year of remodeling, this structure may no longer be detectable and only a moderate amount of bone gain mesially and distally may persist

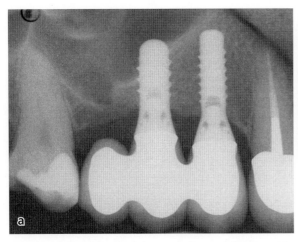 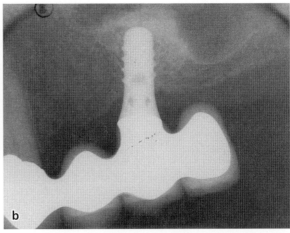

Fig. 50-42 (a) A radiograph, taken at the 5-year follow-up visit, of an implant placed in the 1st quadrant utilizing the osteotome technique without grafting material. A new cortical bony plate at the inferior border of the maxillary sinus is clearly visible, but no bony structure can be detected apical to the implant. (b) A radiograph (same patient) of an implant placed in the 2nd quadrant utilizing the osteotome technique with xenograft grafting material, taken after 5 years in function. A dome-shaped structure is clearly visible documenting a definite increase in bone volume compared to the initial situation. The "dome" is surrounded with a new cortical bony plate.

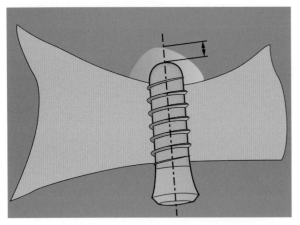

Fig. 50-43 Grafted area apical to the implants undergoes shrinkage and remodeling and the original border of the sinus is eventually consolidated and replaced by a new cortical plate (Brägger et al. 2004).

(Pjetursson et al. 2008a,b). When grafting material is used, a cloudy dome-shaped structure with a hazy demarcation may be visible after implant placement. The size of this dome is usually reduced after remodeling but still gives a definite increase in bone volume compared to the pre-operative situation (Pjetursson et al. 2008a,b) (Fig. 50-42).

Brägger and co-workers (2004) investigated the patterns of tissue remodeling after placement of 25 implants in 19 patients using the osteotome technique with composite xenografts and autografts. Intraoral radiographs were obtained pre-surgically and post-surgically at 3 and 12 months. The mean height of the new bone reaching apical and mesial to the implants was 1.52 mm at surgery, but was reduced significantly to 1.24 mm at 3 months and 0.29 mm after 12 months (Fig. 50-43). It was concluded that the grafted area apical to the implants underwent shrinkage and remodeling (Fig. 50-44) and the original

outline of the sinus was eventually consolidated and replaced by a new cortical plate.

Implants installed into the sinuses of 40 patients using an osteotome technique with no graft or cushion materials were recently evaluated (Leblebicioglu et al. 2005). The authors reported a mean gain of alveolar bone height in scanned panoramic radiographs of 3.9 ± 1.9 mm.

Success and implant survival

In a multi-center retrospective study (Rosen et al. 1999) evaluating the Summers technique applied to the placement of 174 implants in 101 patients, the survival rate was 96%, when residual bone height was 5 mm or more, but dropped down to 85.7% when residual bone height was 4 mm or less (Fig. 50-45).

Survival and success rates of 588 implants placed in 323 consecutive patients with a residual bone height ranging from 6–9 mm after a mean observation period of 5 years were 94.8% and 90.8%, respectively (Ferrigno et al. 2006). During the study period, only 13 perforations of the sinus membrane were detected, giving a perforation rate of only 2.2%. The authors also concluded that the installation of short implants in conjunction with osteotome sinus floor elevation is predictable and may reduce the indications for more invasive and complex procedures, such as the sinus floor elevation by the lateral approach.

Moreover, a systematic review (Emmerich et al. 2005) evaluated the effectiveness of sinus floor elevation using osteotomes. The inclusion criteria considered studies that had more than ten patients and at least 6 months of functional loading. Eight studies met these inclusion criteria. Within the limits of the small amount of long-term data, the reviewers con-

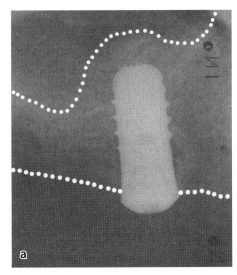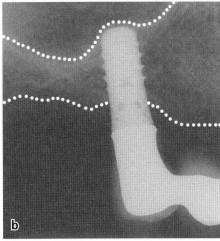

Fig. 50-44 (a) Radiograph taken immediately after implant insertion with the osteotome technique and grafting material, showing a cloudy dome-shaped structure extending 2–3 mm apical to the implant. (b) Radiograph of the same implant taken 1 year later showing significant reduction of the size of the "dome", but the new bony structure is clearly visible apical to the implant (the dotted lines represent the outlines of the grafting material and the residual bone).

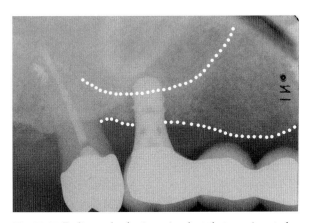

Fig. 50-45 Radiograph of a 6 mm implant that was inserted utilizing the osteotome technique without grafting material. The residual bone height was only 3 mm. After 6 months of functional loading, the implant became loose and had to be removed. After a healing time of 2 months, the maxillary sinus floor was elevated with the lateral approach and two new implants were placed simultaneously (the dotted lines represent the outlines of the residual bone).

cluded that the short-term success rates were similar to success rates of implants conventionally placed in partially edentulous patients (96.0% after 36 months). Long-term outcomes (>5 years) of implants placed with the osteotome technique are still scarse. The database was heterogenous regarding different surgical techniques, implant types, and grafting materials. Hence, no statistical analysis was performed on these parameters.

Short implants

In the light of sinus floor elevation techniques being indicated to facilitate the installation of dental implants in the maxillary posterior region without

adequate bone volume, treatment alternatives have to be discussed (see Chapter 31). Since patient-centered outcomes and morbidity associated with these procedures have not been addressed so far, it has to be anticipated that a great number of patients may not choose sinus floor elevation for their treatment. Hence, shortened dental arches (Käyser 1981) may have to be considered in treatment planning.

Another variation to conventional implant installation in the posterior maxilla is the choice of short implants to avoid penetration into the sinus cavity. Jemt and Lekholm (1995) reported that implant failure in edentulous maxilla correlated significantly with bone quality especially for short (7 mm) implants. Other studies (Friberg *et al.* 1991; Jaffin & Berman 1991) had also reported low survival rates of short implants. However, it must be kept in mind that all these studies reported on implants with machined surface geometries. Based on these studies and others, the clinical "dogma" has been followed, that generally only long implants should be inserted in type IV "poor-quality" bone in the posterior maxilla.

A targeted review (Hagi *et al.* 2004) of study outcomes with short (≤7 mm) implants placed in partially edentulous patients, concluded that machined-surface implants experienced greater failure rates than rough-textured implants. The implant surface geometry appeared to be a major determinant in the performance of these short implants.

In a multi-center study (ten Bruggenkate *et al.* 1998) evaluating 6-mm non-submerged rough-surface dental implants, only one of 208 short implants placed in the mandible was lost compared to six of 45 implants placed in the maxilla. Four of these implants were lost during the healing phase with three remaining in function. The survival rates were 99.5% and 86.7% respectively, after a follow-up time up to 7 years.

In contrast, recent clinical studies (Fugazotto *et al.* 2004; Renouard & Nisand 2005) on short implants with rough surfaces, designed for high initial stability, reported survival rates of about 95% which correlates with the survival rate reported for implants after 5 years in a systematic review (Berglundh *et al.* 2002). Two multi-center studies on rough-surface implants (Buser *et al.* 1997; Brocard *et al.* 2000) analyzed the survival and success rates of implants of different lengths. No significant difference was found between 8, 10, and 12 mm implants with rough-surface geometry after up to 8 years follow-up time.

The most recent review prepared for the Consensus Meeting of the European Association of Osseointegration (EAO) (Renouard & Nisand 2006) concluded on the basis of 12 studies on machined-surface implants meeting the inclusion criteria and 22 studies on rough-textured implants that the survival and success rates of short (<10 mm) implants was comparable to those obtained with longer implants, provided that surgical preparation was related to bone density, rough-textured implants were employed and operators' surgical skills were developed.

The use of short implants may be considered in sites thought unfavorable for implant placement, such as those associated with bone resorption or previous injury and trauma. While in these situations implant failure rates may be increased, outcomes should be compared with those associated with advanced surgical procedures such as bone grafting and sinus floor elevation.

Conclusions and clinical suggestions

In the posterior maxilla, implants with morphometry designed to achieve high initial stability and with rough surface geometry giving high percentage of bone-to-implant contact during initial healing phase (Abrahamsson *et al.* 2004), are to be preferred. Implants with slightly conical morphometry or implants with wider implant neck tend to give better primary stability in cases of reduced residual bone height and soft bone geometry.

The clinical decision on which method (short implants, osteotome technique or lateral approach) should be chosen, depends on the residual bone height of the alveolar crest and surgeons' preferences. The following recommendations are suggested:

1. Residual bone height of 8 mm or more and flat sinus floor: standard implant placement (Fig. 50-46).
2. Residual bone height of 8 mm or more and oblique sinus floor: standard implant placement using short implant or elevation of the maxillary sinus floor using the osteotome technique without grafting material (Fig. 50-47).

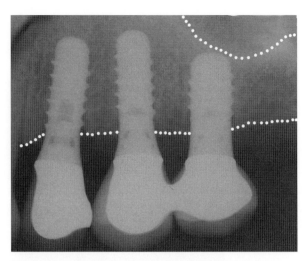

Fig. 50-46 Radiograph of a short (8 mm) implant in the posterior maxilla (the dotted lines represent the outlines of the residual bone).

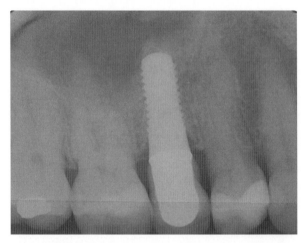

Fig. 50-47 Radiograph of an implant inserted in the posterior maxilla with an oblique sinus floor and a residual bone height of 8–10 mm. The osteotome technique without grafting material was used. The distal aspect of the apex of the implant extends into the sinus cavity, but the mesial aspect is covered with residual bone.

3. Residual bone height of 5–7 mm and flat sinus floor: elevation of the maxillary sinus floor using the osteotome technique with grafting material that is resistant to resorption (Fig. 50-48).
4. Residual bone height of 5–7 mm and oblique sinus floor: elevation of the maxillary sinus floor using lateral approach with grafting material, and simultaneous implant placement (one-stage) (Fig. 50-49).
5. Residual bone height of 3–4 mm and flat or oblique sinus floor: elevation of the maxillary sinus floor using lateral approach with grafting material, and simultaneous implant placement (one-stage) (Fig. 50-50).
6. Residual bone height of 1–2 mm and flat or oblique sinus floor: elevation of the maxillary sinus floor using lateral approach with grafting material and delayed implant placement 4–8 months later (two-stage) (Fig. 50-51).

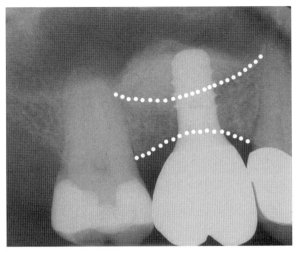

Fig. 50-48 Radiograph of an implant inserted in the posterior maxilla with a flat sinus floor and a residual bone height of 5–6 mm. The osteotome technique with grafting material was used. The radiograph shows a dome-shaped formation covering the entire apex of the implant (the dotted lines represent the outlines of the residual bone).

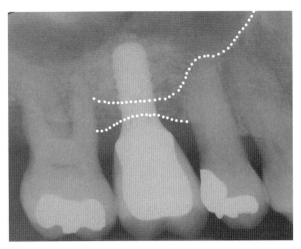

Fig. 50-50 Radiograph of an implant inserted in the posterior maxilla with a flat sinus floor and a residual bone height between 2 and 3 mm. The maxillary sinus floor was elevated using the lateral approach, and one implant was inserted simultaneously (the dotted lines represent the outlines of the residual bone).

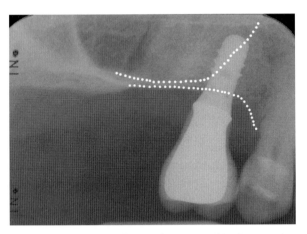

Fig. 50-49 Radiograph of an implant inserted in the posterior maxilla with a oblique sinus floor and a residual bone height between 2 and 8 mm. The maxillary sinus floor was elevated using the lateral approach, and one implant was inserted simultaneously (the dotted lines represent the outlines of the residual bone).

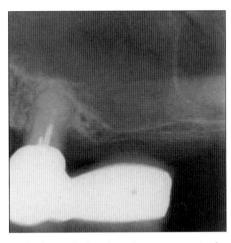

Fig. 50-51 Radiograph showing a large pneumatized maxillary sinus, where a two-stage sinus floor elevation with a delayed implant insertion has to be used.

References

Abrahamsson, I., Berglundh, T., Linder, E., Lang, N.P. & Lindhe, J. (2004). Early bone formation adjacent to rough and turned endosseous implant surfaces. An experimental study in the dog. *Clinical Oral Implants Research* **15**(4), 381–392.

Bain, C.A. & Moy, P.R. (1993). The association between the failure of dental implants and cigarette smoking. *International Journal of Oral and Maxillofacial Implants* **8**, 609–615.

Berglundh, T., Persson, L. & Klinge, B. (2002). A systematic review of the incidence of biological and technical complications in implant dentistry reported in prospective longitudinal studies of at least 5 years. *Journal of Clinical Periodontology* **29**, 197–212.

Block, M.S. & Kent, J.N. (1997). Sinus augmentation for dental implants: the use of autogenous bone. *Journal of Oral and Maxillofacial Surgery* **55**, 1281–1286.

Block, M.S., Kent, J.N., Kallukaran, F.U., Thunthy K. & Weinberg, R. (1998). Bone maintenance 5 to 10 years after sinus grafting. *Journal of Oral and Maxillofacial Surgery* **56**(6), 706–714.

Boyne, P.J. (1993). Analysis of performance of root-form endosseous implants placed in the maxillary sinus. *Journal of Long-Term Effects of Medical Implants* **3**, 143–159.

Boyne, P.J. & James, R. (1980). Grafting of the maxillary sinus floor with autogenous marrow and bone. *Journal of Oral Surgery* **38**, 613–618.

Brägger, U., Gerber, C., Joss, A., Haenni, S., Meier, A., Hashorva, E. & Lang, N.P. (2004). Patterns of tissue remodeling after placement of ITI dental implants using an osteotome technique: a longitudinal radiographic case cohort study. *Clinical Oral Implants Research* **15**(2), 158–166.

Brocard, D., Barthet, P., Baysse, E., Duffort, J.F., Eller, P., Justumus, P., Marin, P., Oscaby, F., Simonet, T., Benqué, E. & Brunel, G. (2000). A multicenter report on 1,022 consecutively placed ITI implants: A 7-year longitudinal study. *International Journal of Oral and Maxillofacial Implants* **15**, 691–700.

Buser, D., Mericske-Stern, R., Bernhard, J.P., Behneke, N., Hirt, H.P., Belser, U.C. & Lang, N.P. (1997). Long-term evaluation of non-submerged ITI implants. *Clinical Oral Implants Research* **8**, 161–172.

Chanavaz, M. (1995). Anatomy and histophysiology of the periosteum: quantification of the periosteal blood supply to the adjacent bone with 85 Sr and gamma spectrometry. *Journal of Oral Implantology* 21(3), 214–219.

Chanavaz, M. (1990). Maxillary sinus. Anatomy, physiology, surgery, and bone grafting relating to implantology – eleven years of clinical experience (1979–1990). *Journal of Oral Implantology* 16(3), 199–209.

Chen, L. & Cha, J. (2005). An 8-year retrospective study: 1,100 patients receiving 1,557 implants using the minimally invasive hydraulic sinus condensing technique. *Journal of Periodontology* 76(3), 482–491.

Ellegaard, B., Baelum, V. & Kølsen-Petersen, J. (2006). Nongrafted sinus implants in periodontally compromised patients: a time-to-event analysis *Clinical Oral Implants Research* 17, 156–164.

Emmerich, D., Att, W. & Stappert, C. (2005). Sinus floor elevation using osteotomes: a systematic review and meta-analysis. *Journal of Periodontology* 76 (8),1237–1251.

Engelke, W. & Deckwer, I. (1997). Endoscopically controlled sinus floor augmentation. A preliminary report. *Clinical Oral Implants Research* 8, 527–531.

Ferrigno, N., Laureti, M. & Fanali, S. (2006). Dental implants placement in conjunction with osteotome sinus floor elevation: 12-year life-table analysis from a prospective study on 588 ITI implants. *Clinical Oral Implants Research* 17(2), 194–205.

Friberg, B., Jemt, T. & Lekholm, U. (1991). Early failures in 4,641 consecutively placed Branmark dental implants: a study from stage 1 surgery to the connection of completed prostheses. *International Journal of Oral and Maxillofacial Implants* 6(2), 142–146.

Froum, S.J., Tarnow, D.P., Wallace, S.S., Rohrer, M.D. & Cho, S.C. (1998). Sinus floor elevation using anorganic bovine bone matrix (OsteoGraf/N) with and without autogenous bone: a clinical, histologic, radiographic, and histomorphometric analysis. Part 2 of an ongoing prospective study. *International Journal of Periodontics and Restorative Dentistry* 18(6), 528–543.

Fugazzotto, P.A. (2001). The modified trephine/osteotome sinus augmentation technique: technical considerations and discussion of indications. *Implant Dentistry* 10(4), 259–264.

Fugazzotto, P.A., Beagle, J.R., Ganeles, J., Jaffin, R., Vlassis, J. & Kumar, A. (2004). Success and failure rates of 9 mm or shorter implants in the replacement of missing maxillary molars when restored with individual crowns: preliminary results 0 to 84 months in function. A retrospective study. *Journal of Periodontology* 75(2), 327–332.

Gruica, B., Wang, H.Y., Lang, N.P. & Buser, D. (2004). Impact of IL-1 genotype and smoking status on the prognosis of osseointegrated implants. *Clinical Oral Implants Research* 15(4), 393–400.

Hagi, D., Deporter, D.A., Pilliar, R.M. & Aremovich, T. (2004). A targeted review of study outcomes with short (≤7 mm) endosseous dental implants placed in partially edentulous patients. *Journal of Periodontology* 75(6), 798–804.

Hallman, M., Hedin, M., Sennerby, L. & Lundgren, S. (2002). A prospective 1-year clinical and radiographic study of implants placed after maxillary sinus floor augmentation with bovine hydroxyapatite and autogenous bone. *Journal of Oral and Maxillofacial Surgery* 60, 277–284.

Hallman, M., Sennerby, L. & Lundgren, S. (2002). A clinical and histologic evaluation of implant integration in the posterior maxilla after sinus floor augmentation with autogenous bone, bovine hydroxyapatite, or a 20 : 80 mixture. *International Journal of Oral and Maxillofacial Implants* 17, 635–643.

Hatano, N., Shimizu, Y. & Ooya, K. (2004). A clinical long-term radiographic evaluation of graft height changes after maxillary sinus floor augmentation with a 2 : 1 autogenous bone/ xenograft mixture and simultaneous placement of dental implants. *Clinical Oral Implants Research* 15, 339–345.

Hising, P., Bolin, A. & Branting, C. (2001). Reconstruction of severely resorbed alveolarcrests with dental implants using a bovine mineral for augmentation. *International Journal of Oral and Maxillofacial Implants* 16, 90–97.

Jaffin, R.A. & Berman, C.L. (1991). The excessive loss of Branmerk fixtures in type IV bone: a 5-year analysis. *Journal of Periodontology* 62(1), 2–4.

Jemt, T. & Lekholm, U. (1995). Implant treatment in edentulous maxillae: a 5-year follow-up report on patients with different degrees of jaw resorption. *International Journal of Oral and Maxillofacial Implants* 10(3), 303–311.

Jensen, O.T., Shulman, L.B., Block, M.S. & Iavono, V.J. (1996). Report of the Sinus Consensus Conference of 1996. *International Journal of Oral and Maxillofacial Implants* 13 (Suppl), 11–45.

Kayser, A.F. (1981). Shortened dental arches and oral function. *Journal of Oral Rehabilitation* 8(5), 457–462.

Kim, M.J., Jung, U.W., Kim, C.S., Kim, K.D., Choi, S.H., Kim, C.K. & Cho, K.S. (2006). Maxillary sinus septa: prevalence, height, location, and morphology. A reformatted computed tomography scan analysis. *Journal of Periodontology* 77(5), 903–908.

Lazzara, R.J. (1996). The sinus elevation procedure in endosseous implant therapy. *Current Opinion in Periodontology* 3, 178–183.

Leblebicioglu, B., Ersanli, S., Karabuda, C., Tosun, T. & Gokdeniz, H. (2005). Radiographic evaluation of dental implants placed using an osteotome technique. *Journal of Periodontology* 76, 385–390.

Mayfield, L.J., Skoglund, A., Hising, P., Lang, N.P. & Attstrom, R. (2001). Evaluation following functional loading of titanium fixtures placed in ridges augmented by deproteinized bone mineral. A human case study. *Clinical Oral Implants Research* 12(5), 508–514.

Peleg, M., Garg, A.K. & Mazor, Z. (2006). Healing in smokers versus nonsmokers: survival rates for sinus floor augmentation with simultaneous implant placement. *International Journal of Oral and Maxillofacial Implants* 21(4), 551–559.

Peleg, M., Mazor, Z., Chaushu, G. & Garg, A.K. (1998). Sinus floor augmentation with simultaneous implant placement in the severely atrophic maxilla. *Journal of Periodontology* 69, 1397–1403.

Peleg, M., Mazor, Z. & Garg, A.K. (1999). Augmentation grafting of the maxillary sinus and simultaneous implant placement in patients with 3 to 5 mm of residual alveolar bone height. *International Journal of Oral and Maxillofacial Implants* 14, 549–556.

Piattelli, M., Favero, G.A., Scarano, A., Orsini, G. & Piattelli, A. (1999). Bone reactions to anorganic bovine bone (Bio-Oss) used in sinus augmentation procedures: a histologic long-term report of 20 cases in humans. *International Journal of Oral and Maxillofacial Implants* 14(6), 835–840.

Pikos, M.A. (1999). Maxillary sinus membrane repair: report of a technique for large perforations. *Implant Dentistry* 8, 29–33.

Pjetursson, B.E., Rast, C., Brägger, U., Zwahlen, M. & Lang, N.P. (2008). Maxillary sinus floor elevation using the osteome technique with or without grafting material. Part I – Implant survival and patient's perception. *Clinical Oral Implants Research* (in press).

Pjetursson, B.E., Ignjatovic, D., Matuliene, G., Brägger, U., Schmidlin, K. & Lang, N.P. (2008). Maxillary sinus floor elevation using the osteome technique with or without grafting material. Part II – Radiographic tissue remodelling. *Clinical Oral Implants Research* (in press).

Renouard, F. & Nisand, D. (2005). Short implants in the severely resorbed maxilla: A 2-year retrospective clinical study. *Clinical Implant Dentistry and Related Research* 7 (Suppl 1), 104–110.

Renouard, F. & Nisand, D. (2006). Impact of implant length and diameter on survival rates. *Clinical Oral Implants Research* **17** (Suppl 2), 35–51.

Rosen, P.D., Summers, R., Mellado, J.R., Salkin, L.M., Shanaman, R.H., Marks, M.H. & Fugazzotto, P.A. (1999). The bone-added osteotome sinus floor elevation technique: multicenter retrospective report of consecutively treated patients. *International Journal of Oral and Maxillofacial Implants* **14**(6), 853–858.

Solar, P., Geyerhofer, U., Traxler, H., Windisch, A., Ulm, C. & Watzek, G. (1999). Blood supply to the maxillary sinus relevant to sinus floor elevation procedures. *Clinical Oral Implants Research* **10**(1), 34–44.

Springer, I.N., Terheyden, H., Geiss, S., Harle, F., Hedderich, J. & Acil, Y. (2004), Particulated bone grafts – effectiveness of bone cell supply. *Clinical Oral Implants Research* **15**(2), 205–212.

Summers, R.B. (1994). A new concept in maxillary implant surgery: the osteotome technique. *The Compendium of Continuing Education in Dentistry* **15**(2), 152–162.

Tarnow, D.P., Wallace, S.S. & Froum, S.J. (2000). Histologic and clinical comparison of bilateral sinus floor elevations with and without barrier membrane placement in 12 patients: Part 3 an ongoing prospective study. *International Journal of Periodontics and Restorative Dentistry* **20**(2), 117–125.

Tatum, H. (1986). Maxillary and sinus implant reconstructions. *Dental Clinics of North America* **30**(2), 207–229.

Tatum, O.H., Lebowitz, M.S., Tatum, C.A. & Borgner, R.A. (1993). Sinus augmentation: rationale, development, long-term results. *New York State Dental Journal* **59**, 43–48.

ten Bruggenkate, C.M., Asikainen, P., Foitzik, C., Krekeler, G. & Sutter, F. (1998). Short (6 mm) nonsubmerged dental implants: results of a multicenter clinical trial of 1 to 7 years. *International Journal of Oral and Maxillofacial Implants* **13**(6), 791–798.

Timmenga, N.M., Raghoebar, G.M., Boering, G. & Van Weissenbruch, R. (1997). Maxillary sinus function after sinus lifts for insertion of dental implants. *Journal of Oral and Maxillofacial Implants* **55**, 936–939.

Timmenga, N.M., Raghoebar, G.M., van Weissenbruch, R. & Vissink, A. (2003). Maxillary sinus floor elevation surgery. A clinical radiographic and endoscopic evaluation. *Clinical Oral Implants Research* **14**, 322–328.

Ulm, C.W., Solar, P., Gsellmann, B., Matejka, M. & Watzek, G. (1995). The edentulous maxillary alveolar process in the region of the maxillary sinus – a study of physical dimension. *Journal of Oral and Maxillofacial Surgery* **24**, 279–282.

Valentini, P. & Abensur, D.J. (2003). Maxillary sinus grafting with anorganic bovine bone: A clinical report of long-term results. *International Journal of Oral and Maxillofacial Implants* **18**, 556–560.

Van den Bergh, J.P., ten Bruggenkate, C.M., Disch, F.J. & Tuinzing, D.B. (2000). Anatomical aspects of sinus floor elevations. *Clinical Oral Implants Research* **11**(3), 256–265.

Wallace, S.S. & Froum, S.J. (2003). Effect of maxillary sinus augmentation on the survival of endosseous dental implants. A systematic review. *Annals of Periodontology* **8**, 328–343.

Wannfors, K., Johansson, B., Hallman, M. & Strandkvist, T. (2000). A prospective randomized study of 1- and 2-stage sinus inlay bone grafts: 1 year follow up. *International Journal of Oral and Maxillofacial Implants* **15**, 625–632.

Zitzman, N. & Scharer, P. (1998). Sinus elevation procedures in the resorbed posterior maxilla: comparison of the crestal and lateral approaches. *Oral Surgery, Oral Medicine, Oral Pathology, Oral Radiology and Endodontics* **85**, 8–17.

Part 16: Occlusal and Prosthetic Therapy

51   Tooth-Supported Fixed Partial Dentures, 1125
Jan Lindhe and Sture Nyman

52   Implants in Restorative Dentistry, 1138
Niklaus P. Lang and Giovanni E. Salvi

53   Implants in the Esthetic Zone, 1146
Urs C. Belser, Jean-Pierre Bernard, and Daniel Buser

54   Implants in the Posterior Dentition, 1175
Urs C. Belser, Daniel Buser, and Jean-Pierre Bernard

55   Implant–Implant and Tooth–Implant Supported
Fixed Partial Dentures, 1208
Clark M. Stanford and Lyndon F. Cooper

56   Complications Related to Implant-Supported Restorations, 1222
Y. Joon Ko, Clark M. Stanford, and Lyndon F. Cooper

Chapter 51

Tooth-Supported Fixed Partial Dentures

Jan Lindhe and Sture Nyman

Clinical symptoms of trauma from occlusion, 1125
  Angular bony defects, 1125
  Increased tooth mobility, 1125
  Progressive (increasing) tooth mobility, 1125
Tooth mobility crown excursion/root displacement, 1125
  Initial and secondary tooth mobility, 1125
  Clinical assessment of tooth mobility (physiologic and pathologic tooth mobility), 1127

Treatment of increased tooth mobility, 1128
  Situation I, 1128
  Situation II, 1129
  Situation III, 1129
  Situation IV, 1132
  Situation V, 1134

Clinical symptoms of trauma from occlusion

Angular bony defects

It has been claimed that *angular bony defects* and *increased tooth mobility* are important symptoms of trauma from occlusion (Glickman 1965, 1967). The validity of this suggestion has, however, been questioned (see Chapter 14). Thus, angular bony defects have been found at teeth affected by *trauma from occlusion* as well as at teeth with normal occlusal function (Waerhaug 1979). *This means that the presence of angular bony defects cannot* per se *be regarded as an exclusive symptom of trauma from occlusion.*

Increased tooth mobility

Increased tooth mobility, determined clinically, is expressed in terms of amplitude of displacement of the crown of the tooth. Increased tooth mobility can, indeed, be observed in conjunction with *trauma from occlusion*. It may, however, also be the result of a reduction of the height of the alveolar bone with or without an accompanying angular bony defect caused by plaque-associated periodontal disease (see Chapter 14). Increased tooth mobility resulting from occlusal interferences may further indicate that the periodontal structures have become adapted to an altered functional demand, i.e. a widened periodontal ligament with a normal tissue composition has become the end result of a previous phase of progres-

sive tooth mobility (see Chapter 14) associated with trauma from occlusion.

Progressive (increasing) tooth mobility

In Chapter 14, it was concluded that the diagnosis trauma from occlusion should be used solely in situations where a progressive mobility could be observed. Progressive tooth mobility can be identified only through a series of repeated tooth mobility measurements carried out over a period of several days or weeks.

Tooth mobility crown excursion/root displacement

Initial and secondary tooth mobility

A tooth which is surrounded by a normal periodontium may be moved (displaced) in horizontal and vertical directions and may also be forced to perform limited rotational movements. Clinically, tooth mobility is usually assessed by exposing the crown of the tooth to a certain force and determining the distance the crown can be displaced in buccal and/or lingual direction. The mobility (= movability) of a tooth in a horizontal direction is closely dependent on the height of the surrounding supporting bone, the width of the periodontal ligament, and the shape and number of roots present (Fig. 51-1).

The mechanism of tooth mobility was studied in detail by Mühlemann (1954, 1960) who described a

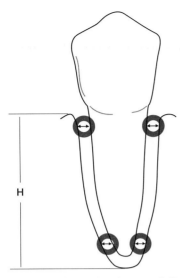

Fig. 51-1 The mobility of a tooth in horizontal direction is dependent on the height of the alveolar bone (H), the width of the periodontal ligament (encircled arrows), and the shape and number of roots.

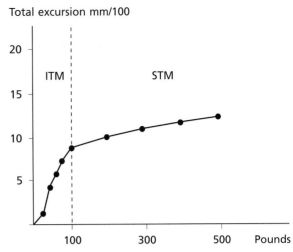

Fig. 51-3 Initial tooth mobility (ITM) means the excursion of the crown of a tooth when a force of 100 pounds is applied to the crown. Secondary tooth mobility (STM) means the excursion of the crown of the tooth when a force of 500 pounds is applied.

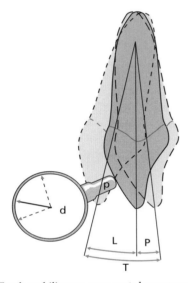

Fig. 51-2 Tooth mobility measurements by means of the Periodontometer. d = dial indicator; p = pointer; L = labial excursion of the crown; P = palatal excursion of the crown; T = L + P = total excursion of the crown.

standardized method for measuring even minor tooth displacements. By means of the "Periodontometer" a small force (~45 kg (100 pounds)) is applied to the crown of a tooth (Fig. 51-2). The crown starts to tip in the direction of the force. The resistance of the tooth-supporting structures against displacement of the root is low in the initial phase of force application and the crown is moved only 5/100–10/100 mm. This movement of the tooth was called *"initial tooth mobility"* (ITM) by Mühlemann (1954) and is the result of an *intra-alveolar* displacement of the root (Fig. 51-3). In the pressure zone (see Chapter 14) there is a 10% reduction in the width of the periodontal ligament and in the tension zone there is a corresponding increase. Mühlemann and Zander (1954)

stated that "there are good reasons to assume that the initial displacement of the root (ITM) corresponds to a reorientation of the periodontal membrane fibers into a position of functional readiness towards tensile strength". The magnitude of the ITM varies from individual to individual, from tooth to tooth, and is mainly dependent on the structure and organization of the periodontal ligament. The ITM value of ankylosed teeth is therefore zero.

When a larger force (~225 kg (500 pounds)) is applied to the crown, the fiber bundles on the tension side cannot offer sufficient resistance to further root displacement. The additional displacement of the crown that is observed in *"secondary tooth mobility"* (STM) (Fig. 51-3) is allowed by distortion and compression of the periodontium in the pressure side. According to Mühlemann (1960) the magnitude of STM, i.e. the excursion of the crown of the tooth when a force of 500 pounds is applied, (1) varies between different types of teeth (e.g. incisors 10–12/100 mm, canines 5–9/100 mm, premolars 8–10/100 mm and molars 4–8/100 mm), (2) is larger in children than in adults, and (3) is larger in females than males and increases during, for example, pregnancy. Furthermore, tooth mobility seems to vary during the course of the day; the lowest value is found in the evening and the largest in the morning.

A new method for determining tooth mobility was presented by Schulte and co-workers (Schulte 1987; Schulte *et al.* 1992) when the Periotest® (SiemensAG, Bensheim, Germany) system was introduced. The Periotest device measures the reaction of the periodontium to a defined percussion force which is applied to the tooth and delivered by a tapping instrument. A metal rod is accelerated to a speed of 0.2 m/s with the device and maintained at a constant velocity. Upon impact the tooth is deflected and the rod decelerated. The contact time between the tapping head and the tooth varies between 0.3 and 2 milliseconds and is shorter for stable than mobile teeth. The Periotest scale (the Periotest values) ranges from −8 to +50 and the following ranges should be considered:

- −8 to +9: clinically firm teeth
- 10–19: first distinguishable sign of movement
- 20–29: crown deviates within 1 mm of its normal position
- 30–50: mobility is readily observed.

The Periotest values correlate well with (1) tooth mobility assessed with a metric system, and (2) degree of periodontal disease and alveolar bone loss. The simple Periotest device is likely to be used in both the clinic and research settings in the future.

Clinical assessment of tooth mobility (physiologic and pathologic tooth mobility)

If, in the traditional clinical measurement of tooth mobility, a comparatively large force is exerted on the crown of a tooth which is surrounded by a normal periodontium, the tooth will tip within its alveolus until a closer contact has been established between the root and the marginal (or apical) bone tissue. The magnitude of this tipping movement, which is normally assessed using the tip of the crown as a reference point, is referred to as the *"physiologic"* tooth mobility. The term *"physiologic"* implies that *"pathologic"* tooth mobility may also occur.

What, then, is "pathologic" tooth mobility?

1. If a similar force is applied to a tooth which is surrounded by a periodontal ligament with an increased width, the excursion of the crown in horizontal direction will become increased; the clinical measurement consequently demonstrates that the tooth has an increased mobility. Should this increased mobility be regarded as *pathologic*?

2. An increased tooth mobility, i.e. an increased displacement of the crown of the tooth after force application, can also be found in situations where the height of the alveolar bone has been reduced but the remaining periodontal ligament has a normal width. At sites where this type of bone loss is extensive, the degree of tooth mobility (i.e. excursion of the crown) may be pronounced. Should this increased tooth mobility be regarded as "pathologic"?

Figure 51-4b illustrates a tooth which is surrounded by alveolar bone of reduced height. The width of the remaining periodontal ligament, however, is within normal limits. A horizontally directed force applied to the crown of the tooth in this case will result in a larger excursion of the crown than if a similar force is applied to a tooth with normal height of the alveolar bone and normal width of the periodontal ligament (Fig. 51-4a). There are reasons to suggest that the *so-called increased mobility* measured in the case of Fig. 51-4b is, indeed, *physiologic*. The validity of this statement can easily be demonstrated if the displacement of the two teeth is assessed not from the crown but from a point on the root at the level of the bone crest. If a horizontal force is directed to the teeth as indicated in Fig. 51-4 the reference points (*) on the root surfaces will be displaced a similar distance in both instances. *Obviously, it is not the length of the excursive movement of the crown that is important from a biologic point of view, but the displacement of the root within its remaining periodontal ligament.*

In plaque-associated periodontal disease, bone loss is a prominent feature. Another so-called classical symptom of periodontitis is "increased tooth mobility". It is important to realize, however, that in many situations with even or "horizontal" bone loss patterns, the increased crown displacement (tooth mobility) assessed in clinical measurements should, according to the above discussion, also be regarded as physiologic; the movement of the root within the space of its remaining "normal" periodontal ligament is normal.

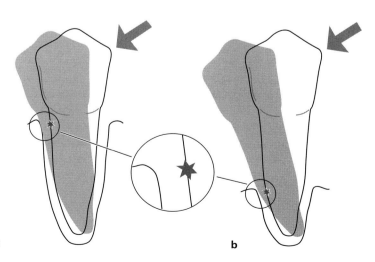

a   b

Fig. 51-4 (a) The normal "physiologic" mobility of a tooth with normal height of the alveolar bone and normal width of the periodontal ligament. (b) The mobility of a tooth with reduced height of the alveolar bone. The distance of the horizontal displacement of the reference point (*) on the roots is the same in the two situations (a,b).

3. Increased crown displacement (tooth mobility) may also be detected in a clinical measurement where a "horizontal" force is applied to teeth with angular bony defects and/or increased width of the periodontal ligament. If this mobility does not increase gradually – from one observation interval to the next – the root is surrounded by a periodontal ligament of increased width but normal composition. This mobility should also be considered *physiologic* since the movement is a function of the height of the alveolar bone and the width of the periodontal ligament.

4. Only *progressively increasing tooth mobility*, which may occur in conjunction with trauma from occlusion, is characterized by active bone resorption (see Chapter 14) and which indicates the presence of inflammatory alterations within the periodontal ligament tissue, may be considered *pathologic*.

Treatment of increased tooth mobility

A number of situations will be described below which may call for treatment aimed at reducing an increased tooth mobility.

Situation I

Increased mobility of a tooth with increased width of the periodontal ligament but normal height of the alveolar bone

If a tooth (for instance a maxillary premolar) is fitted with an improper filling or crown restoration, occlusal interferences develop and the surrounding periodontal tissues become the seat of inflammatory reactions, i.e. trauma from occlusion (Fig. 51-5). If the restoration is so designed that the crown of the tooth

in occlusion is subjected to undue forces directed in a buccal direction, bone resorption phenomena develop in the buccal–marginal and lingual–apical pressure zones with a resulting increase of the width of the periodontal ligament in these zones. The tooth becomes hypermobile or moves away from the "traumatizing" position. Since such traumatizing forces in teeth with normal periodontium or overt gingivitis cannot result in pocket formation or loss of connective tissue attachment, the resulting increased mobility of the tooth should be regarded as a physiologic adaptation of the periodontal tissues to the altered functional demands. A proper correction of the anatomy of the occlusal surface of such a tooth, i.e. occlusal adjustment, will normalize the relationship between the antagonizing teeth in occlusion, thereby eliminating the excessive forces. As a result, apposition of bone will occur in the zones previously exposed to resorption, the width of the periodontal ligament will become normalized and the tooth stabilized, i.e. it reassumes its normal mobility (Fig. 51-5). In other words, resorption of alveolar bone which is caused by trauma from occlusion is a reversible process which can be treated by the elimination of occlusal interferences.

The capacity for bone regeneration after resorption following trauma from occlusion has been documented in a number of animal experiments (Waerhaug & Randers-Hansen 1966; Polson *et al.* 1976a; Karring *et al.* 1982; Nyman *et al.* 1982). In such experiments, the induced bone resorption not only involved the bone within the alveolus but also the alveolar bone crest. When the traumatizing forces were removed, bone tissue was deposited not only in the walls of the alveolus, thereby normalizing the width of the periodontal ligament, but also on the bone crest area, whereby the height of the alveolar bone was normalized (Fig. 51-6) (Polson *et al.* 1976a). In the presence

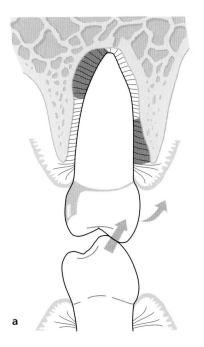
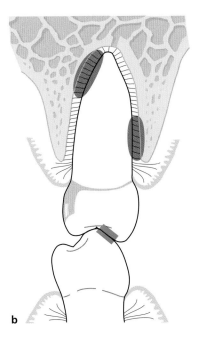

a   b

Fig. 51-5 (a) Contact relationship between a mandibular and a maxillary premolar in occlusion. The maxillary premolar is fitted with an artificial restoration with an improperly designed occlusal surface. Occlusion results in horizontally directed forces (arrows) which may produce an undue stress concentration within the "brown" areas of the periodontium of the maxillary tooth. Resorption of the alveolar bone occurs in these areas. A widening of the periodontal ligament can be detected as well as increased mobility of the tooth. (b) Following adjustment of the occlusion, the horizontal forces are reduced. This results in bone apposition ("red areas") and a normalization of the tooth mobility.

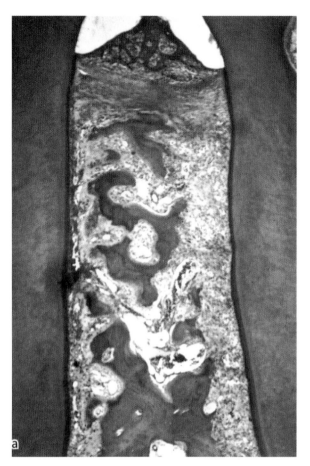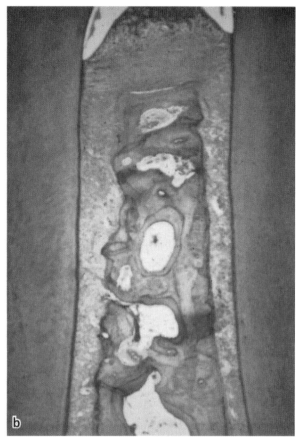

Fig. 51-6 Photomicrographs illustrating the interdental area between two mandibular premolars in the monkey. In (a) the two premolars are exposed to jiggling forces. Note the reduction of alveolar bone in the area and the location of the bone crest. Ten weeks after the elimination of the jiggling forces (b) a considerable regeneration of bone has occurred. Note the increase of the height of the interdental bone and the normalization of the width of the periodontal ligaments. The apical end of the junctional epithelium is located at the cemento-enamel junction. (Courtesy of Dr. A.M. Polson; from Polson *et al.* (1976a).)

of an untreated, plaque-associated lesion in the soft tissue, however, substantial bone regrowth did not always occur (Fig. 51-7) (Polson *et al.* 1976b).

Situation II

Increased mobility of a tooth with increased width of the periodontal ligament and reduced height of the alveolar bone

When a dentition has been properly treated for moderate to advanced periodontal disease, gingival health is established in areas of the dentition where teeth are surrounded by periodontal structures of reduced height. If a tooth with a reduced periodontal tissue support is exposed to excessive horizontal forces (trauma from occlusion), inflammatory reactions develop in the pressure zones of the periodontal ligament with accompanying bone resorption. These alterations are similar to those which occur around a tooth with supporting structures of a normal height; the alveolar bone is resorbed, the width of the periodontal ligament is increased in the pressure/tension zones and the tooth becomes hypermobile (Fig. 51-8a). If the excessive forces are reduced or eliminated

by occlusal adjustment, bone apposition to the "pre-trauma" level will occur, the periodontal ligament will regain its normal width and the tooth will become stabilized (Fig. 51-8b).

Conclusion: situations I and II

Occlusal adjustment is an effective therapy against increased tooth mobility when such mobility is caused by an *increased width* of the periodontal ligament.

Situation III

Increased mobility of a tooth with reduced height of the alveolar bone and normal width of the periodontal ligament

The increased tooth mobility which is the result of a reduction in height of the alveolar bone without a concomitant increase in width of the periodontal membrane cannot be reduced or eliminated by occlusal adjustment. In teeth with normal width of the periodontal ligament, no further bone apposition on the walls of the alveoli can occur. If such an increased

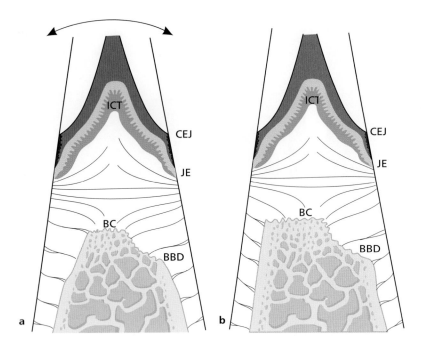

Fig. 51-7 In the presence of an existing marginal inflammation, alveolar bone, lost by jiggling trauma (a), will not always regenerate following elimination of the traumatic forces (b). ICT = infiltrated connective tissue; CEJ = cemento-enamel junction; JE = apical end of junctional epithelium; BC = alveolar bone crest; BBD = bottom of angular bony defect. From Polson *et al.* (1976b).

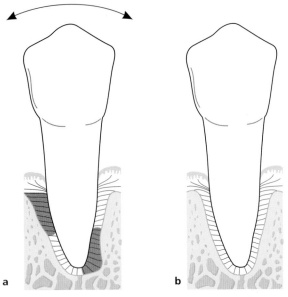

Fig. 51-8 If a tooth with reduced periodontal tissue support (a) has been exposed to excessive horizontal forces, a widened periodontal ligament space ("brown" areas) and increased mobility (arrow) result. (b) Following reduction or elimination of such forces, bone apposition will occur and the tooth will become stabilized.

tooth mobility does not interfere with the patient's chewing function or comfort, no treatment is required. If the patient experiences the tooth mobility as disturbing, however, the mobility can only be reduced in this situation by splinting, i.e. by joining the mobile tooth/teeth together with other teeth in the jaw into a fixed unit – a splint.

A splint, according to the Glossary of Periodontic Terms (1986) is "an appliance designed to stabilize mobile teeth". A splint can be fabricated in the form of joined composite fillings, fixed bridges, removable partial prostheses, etc.

Example: Case A, 64-year-old male

The periodontal condition of this patient is illustrated by the probing depth, furcation involvement and tooth mobility data as well as the radiographs from the initial examination in Fig. 51-9. Periodontal disease has progressed to a level where, around the maxillary teeth, only the apical third or less of the roots is invested in supporting alveolar bone. The following discussion is related to the treatment of the maxillary dentition.

In the treatment planning of this case it was decided that the first premolars (teeth 14 and 24) had to be extracted due to advanced periodontal disease and furcation involvement of degree III. For the same reasons, teeth 17 and 27 were scheduled for extraction. Teeth 16 and 26 were also found to have advanced loss of periodontal tissue support in combination with deep furcation involvements. The most likely *definitive* treatment should include periodontal and adjunctive therapy in the following parts of the dentition: 15 and 25, and 13, 12, 11, 21, 22, 23. For functional and esthetic reasons, 14 and 24 obviously had to be replaced. The question now arose as to whether these two premolars should be replaced by two separate unilateral bridges, using 13, 15 and 23, 25 as abutment teeth, or if the increased mobility of these teeth and also of the anterior teeth (12, 11, 21, 22) (Fig. 51-9) called for a bridge of cross-arch design, with the extension 15–25, to obtain a splinting effect. If 14 and 24 are replaced by two unilateral bridges, each one of these three-unit bridges will exhibit the same degree of mobility in a bucco-lingual direction as the individual abutment teeth (degree 2) (Fig. 51-9), since a unilateral straight bridge will not have a stabilizing effect on the abutment teeth in this force direction.

Periodontal chart

Tooth	Pocket depth M	B	D	L	Furcation involvement	Tooth mobility
18						
17	6	6	8	8	b2, m2, d1	
16	6	6	8	8	m1, d2	2
15	8	8	6	7		2
14	7	7	7	4	3	2
13	8	4	8	4		2
12	8	4	8	4		2
11	6	4	7	4		1
21	6	4	6	4		1
22	6	5	7			2
23	6		6	4		2
24	7		8		3	2
25	6	8	8	4		2
26	8		6		b2, m2, d2	
27	6	6	10	8	b2, d2	1
28						
48						
47						
46	8	6	6	7	b1, l2	
45	6		7	4		1
44	6		6	4		
43	7	7	6	4		
42	4		4	4		1
41	6	4				1
31	6					1
32	4		6	4		1
33	6		6	6		2
34	4		7	4		
35	7		4	6		2
36						
37	8	5	6	4	b2, l2	3
38						

a

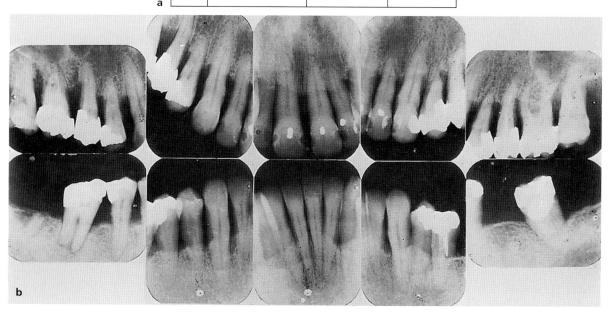

b

Fig. 51-9 Case A, 64-year-old male. Periodontal status (a) and radiographs (b) prior to therapy.

From the radiographs it can be seen that the increased mobility observed in the maxillary teeth of this patient is associated mainly with reduced height of the alveolar bone and not with increased width of the periodontal ligaments. This means that the mobility of the individual teeth should be regarded as normal or "physiologic" for teeth with such a reduced height of the supporting tissues. This in turn implies that the increased tooth mobility in the present case does not call for treatment unless it interferes with the chewing comfort or jeopardizes the position of the front teeth. This particular patient had not recognized any functional problems related to the increased mobility of his maxillary teeth. Consequently, there was no reason to install a cross-arch bridge in order to splint the teeth, i.e. to reduce tooth mobility.

Following proper treatment of the plaque-associated periodontal lesions, two separate provisional bridges of unilateral design were produced (15, 14, 13; 23, 24, 25, 26 palatal root). The provisional acrylic bridges were used for 6 months during which the occlusion, the mobility of the two bridges and the position of the front teeth were all carefully monitored. When, after 6 months, no change of position of the lateral and central incisors had occurred and no increase of the mobility of the two provisional bridges had been noted, the definitive restorative therapy was performed.

Figure 51-10 presents radiographs obtained 10 years after initial therapy. The position of the front teeth and the mobility of the incisors and the two bridges have not changed during the course of the maintenance period. There has been no further loss of periodontal tissue support during the 10 years of observation, no further spread of the front teeth and no widening of the periodontal ligaments around the individual teeth, including the abutment teeth for the bridgework.

Conclusion: situation III

Increased tooth mobility (or bridge mobility) as a result of reduced height of the alveolar bone can be accepted and splinting avoided, provided the occlusion is stable (no further migration or further increasing mobility of individual teeth), and provided the degree of existing mobility does not disturb the patient's chewing ability or comfort. Consequently, splinting is indicated when the mobility of a tooth or a group of teeth is so increased that chewing ability and/or comfort are disturbed.

Situation IV

Progressive (increasing) mobility of a tooth (teeth) as a result of gradually increasing width of the reduced periodontal ligament

Often in cases of advanced periodontal disease the tissue destruction may have reached a level where extraction of one or several teeth cannot be avoided. In such a dentition, teeth which are still available for periodontal treatment may, after therapy, exhibit such a high degree of mobility, or even signs of progressively increasing mobility, that there is an obvious risk that the forces elicited during function may mechanically disrupt the remaining periodontal ligament components and cause extraction of the teeth.

It will only be possible to maintain such teeth by means of a splint. In such cases a fixed splint has two objectives: (1) to stabilize hypermobile teeth and (2) to replace missing teeth.

Example: Case B, 26-year-old male

Figure 51-11 presents radiographs taken prior to therapy and Fig. 51-12 those obtained after periodon-

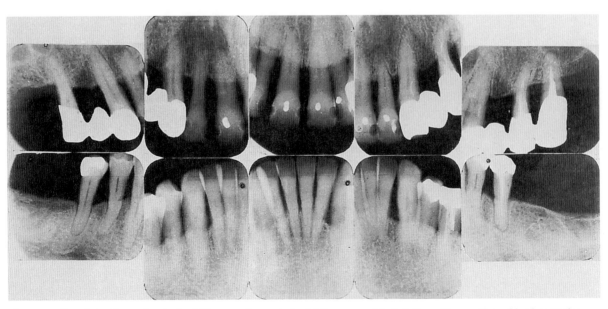

Fig. 51-10 Case A. Radiographs obtained 10 years after periodontal therapy and installation of two unilateral bridges in the maxilla.

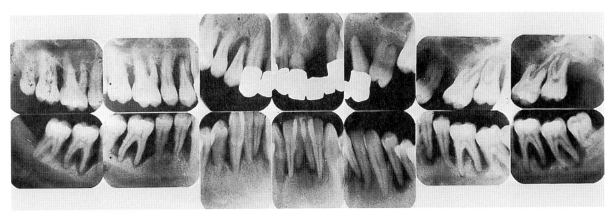

Fig. 51-11 Case B, 26-year-old male. Radiographs illustrating the periodontal conditions prior to therapy.

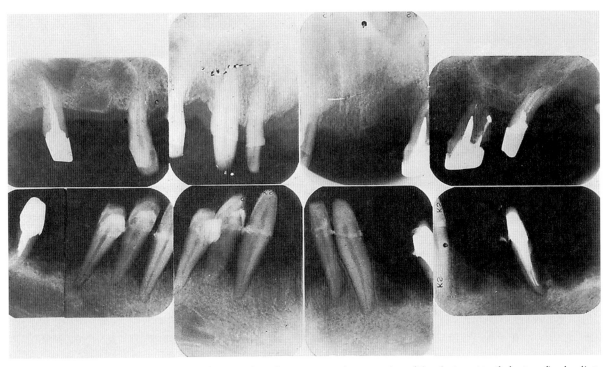

Fig. 51-12 Case B. Radiographs obtained after periodontal treatment and preparation of the abutment teeth for two fixed splints.

tal treatment and preparation of the remaining teeth as abutments for two fixed splints. All teeth except 13, 12, and 33 have lost around 75% or more of the alveolar bone and widened periodontal ligaments are a frequent finding. The four distal abutments for the two splints are root-separated molars, the maintained roots being the following: the palatal root of 17, the mesio-buccal root of 26, and the mesial roots of 36 and 47. It should be observed that tooth 24 is root-separated and the palatal root maintained with only minute amounts of periodontium left. Immediately prior to insertion of the two splints, all teeth except 13, 12, and 33 displayed a mobility varying between degrees 1 and 3. From the radiographs in Fig. 51-12 it can be noted that there is an obvious risk of extraction of a number of teeth such as 24, 26, 47, 45, 44, 43, and 36 if the patient is allowed to bite with a normal chewing force without the splints in position.

Despite the high degree of mobility of the individual teeth, the splints were entirely stable after insertion, and have maintained their stability during a maintenance period of more than 12 years. Figure 51-13 describes the clinical status and Fig. 51-14 presents the radiographs obtained 10 years after therapy. From these radiographs it can be observed (compare with Fig. 51-12) that during the maintenance period there has been no further loss of alveolar bone or widening of the various periodontal ligament spaces.

Conclusion: situation IV

Splinting is indicated when the periodontal support is so reduced that the mobility of the teeth is progressively increasing, i.e. when a tooth or a group of teeth are exposed to extraction forces during function.

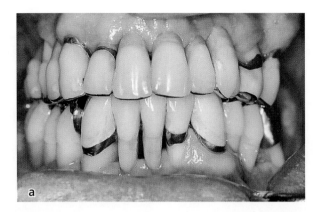

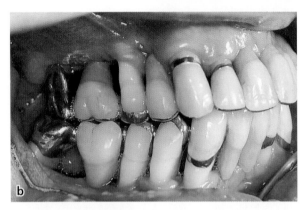

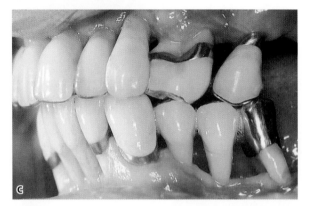

Fig. 51-13 Case B. Clinical status 9 years after therapy.

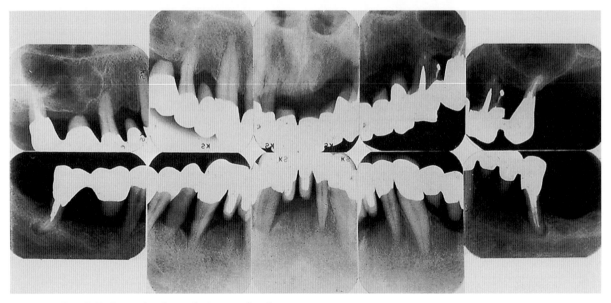

Fig. 51-14 Case B. Radiographs obtained 10 years after therapy.

Situation V

Increased bridge mobility despite splinting

In patients with advanced periodontal disease it can often be observed that the destruction of the periodontium has progressed to varying levels around different teeth and tooth surfaces in the dentition. Proper treatment of the plaque-associated lesions often includes multiple extractions. The remaining teeth may display an extreme reduction of the supporting tissues concomitant with increased or progressive tooth mobility. They may also be distributed in the jaw in such a way as to make it difficult, or impossible, to obtain a proper splinting effect even by means of a cross-arch bridge. The entire bridge/splint may exhibit mobility in frontal and/or lateral directions.

It was stated above (situation III) that a certain mobility of a tooth or a bridge of unilateral design can be accepted provided this mobility does not interfere with the patient's chewing ability or comfort. This is also valid for a cross-arch bridge/splint. From a biologic point of view there is no difference between increased tooth mobility on the one hand and increased bridge mobility on the other. However, neither progressive tooth mobility nor progressive bridge mobility are acceptable. In cases of extremely advanced periodontal disease, a cross-arch splint with an increased mobility may be regarded as an acceptable result of rehabilitation. The maintenance of status quo of the bridge/splint mobility and the prevention of tipping or orthodontic displacement of the total splint, however, requires particular attention regarding the design of the occlusion. Below, a case is reported which may serve as an interesting illustration of this particular clinical problem.

Example: Case C, 52-year-old female

Figure 51-15 shows radiographs obtained at the initial examination. A 12-unit maxillary bridge was installed 10–15 years prior to the present examination using 18, 15, 14, 13, 12, 11, 21, 22, 23, and 24 as abutments. After a detailed clinical examination it was obvious that 15, 14, 22, and 24 could not be maintained because of severe symptoms of caries and periodontal disease. The remaining teeth were subjected to periodontal therapy and maintained as abutments for a new bridge/splint in the maxilla extending from tooth 18 to the region of 26, i.e. a cross-arch splint was installed which carried three cantilever units, namely 24, 25, and 26. The mobility of the individual abutment teeth immediately prior to insertion of the splint was the following: degree 1 (tooth 18), degree 0 (tooth 13), degree 2 (teeth 12 and 11), degree 3 (tooth 21), and degree 2 (tooth 23).

Radiographs obtained 5 years after therapy are shown in Fig. 51-16. The bridge/splint had a mobility of degree 1 immediately after its insertion and this mobility was unchanged 5 years later. The radiographs demonstrate that no further widening of the periodontal ligament occurred around the individual teeth during the maintenance period.

When a cross-arch bridge/splint exhibits increased mobility, the center (fulcrum) of the movement must be identified. In order to prevent further increase in the mobility and/or to prevent displacement of the bridge, it is essential to design the occlusion in such a way that when the bridge/splint is in contact with the teeth of the opposing jaw, it is subjected to a balanced load, i.e. equal force on each side of the fulcrum. If this can be achieved, the force to which the bridge is exposed in occlusion can be used to retain the fixed prosthesis in proper balance (a further increase of mobility being thereby prevented).

Balanced loading of a mobile bridge/splint has to be established not only in the intercuspal position (IP) and centric occlusion (CP) but also in frontal and lateral excursive movements of the mandible if the bridge shows mobility or a tendency for tipping in the direction of such movements. In other words, a force which tends to displace the bridge in a certain direction has to be counteracted by the introduction of a balancing force on the opposite side of the fulcrum of the movement. If, for instance, a cross-arch splint in the maxilla exhibits mobility in frontal direction in conjunction with protrusive movements of the mandible, the load applied to the bridge in the frontal region has to be counterbalanced by a load in the distal portions of the splint; this means that there must be a simultaneous and equal contact relationship between the occluding teeth in both the frontal and the posterior regions of the splint. If the splint is mobile in a lateral direction, the force acting on the working side of the jaw must be counteracted by a force established by the introduction of balancing contacts in the non-working side of the jaw. The prin-

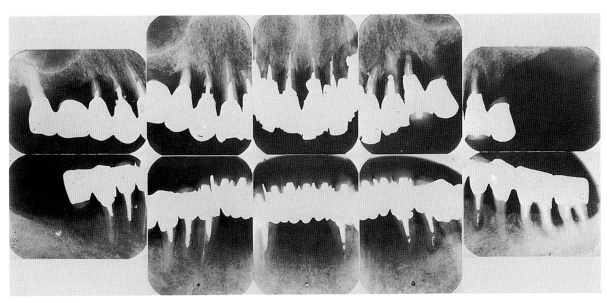

Fig. 51-15 Case C, 52-year-old female. Radiographs obtained at the initial examination.

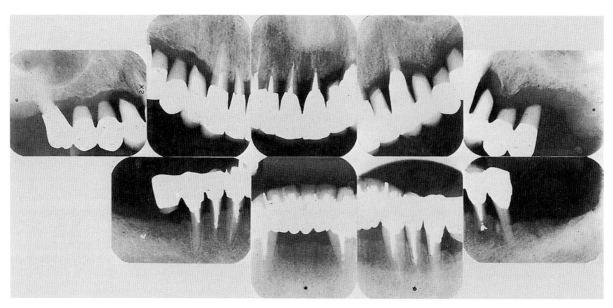

Fig. 51-16 Case C. Radiographs obtained 5 years after therapy.

ciple for establishing stability of a *mobile* cross-arch splint is consequently the same as that used to obtain stability in a complete denture. In situations where distal abutment teeth are missing in a cross-arch bridge/splint with increased mobility, balance and functional stability may be obtained by means of cantilever units. It is important in this context to point out that balancing contacts on the non-working side should not be introduced in a bridge/splint in which no increased mobility can be observed.

The maxillary splint in the patient described in Figs. 51-15 and 51-16 exhibited increased mobility in a frontal direction. Considering the small amount of periodontal support left around the anterior teeth, it is obvious that there would have been a risk of frontal displacement of the total bridge had the bridge terminated at the last abutment tooth (23) on the left side of the jaw. The installation of cantilever units in the 24 and 25 region prevented such a displacement of the bridge/splint by the introduction of a force counteracting frontally directed forces during protrusive movements of the mandible (Fig. 51-17). In addition, the cantilever units provide bilateral contact relationship towards the mandibular teeth in the intercuspal position, i.e. bilateral stability of the bridge.

In cases similar to the one described above, cantilever units can thus be used to prevent increasing mobility or displacement of a bridge/splint. It should, however, be pointed out that the insertion of cantilever units increases the risk of failures of a technical and biophysical character (fracture of the metal frame, fracture of abutment teeth, loss of retention, etc.).

In cases of severely advanced periodontal disease it is often impossible to anticipate in the planning phase whether a bridge/splint will show signs of instability and increasing (progressive) mobility after

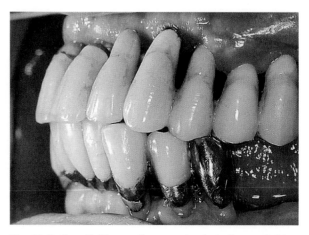

Fig. 51-17 Case C. The cantilever section including teeth 24, 25, and 26.

insertion. In such cases, a provisional splint should always be inserted. Any alterations of the mobility of the bridge/splint can be observed over a prolonged period of time and the occlusion continuously adjusted until, after 4–6 months, it is known whether stability (i.e. no further increase of the mobility) can be achieved. The design of the occlusion of the provisional acrylic bridge is then reproduced in the permanent bridge construction. If, on the other hand, stability cannot be obtained, the rehabilitation of the case cannot be achieved with a fixed splint. The alternative treatment then is a complete denture or an implant-supported restoration.

Conclusion: situation V

An increased mobility of a cross-arch bridge/splint can be accepted provided the mobility does not disturb chewing ability or comfort and the mobility of the splint is not progressively increasing.

References

Glickman, I. (1965). Clinical significance of trauma from occlusion. *Journal of the American Dental Association* **70**, 607–618.

Glickman, I. (1967). Occlusion and periodontium. *Journal of Dental Research* **46** (Suppl), 53.

Glossary of Periodontic Terms (1986). *Journal of Periodontology*. Supplement.

Karring, T., Nyman, S., Thilander, B. & Magnusson, I. (1982). Bone-regeneration in orthodontically produced alveolar bone dehiscences. *Journal of Periodontal Research* **17**, 309–315.

Mühlemann, H.R. (1954). Tooth mobility. The measuring method. Initial and secondary tooth mobility. *Journal of Periodontology* **25**, 22–29.

Mühlemann, H.R. (1960). Ten years of tooth mobility measurements. *Journal of Periodontology* **31**, 110–122.

Mühlemann, H.R. & Zander, H.A. (1954). Tooth mobility, III. The mechanism of tooth mobility. *Journal of Periodontology* **25**, 128.

Nyman, S., Karring, T. & Bergenholtz, G. (1982). Bone regeneration in alveolar bone dehiscences produced by jiggling forces. *Journal of Periodontal Research* **17**, 316–322.

Polson, A.M., Meitner, S.W. & Zander, H.A. (1976a). Trauma and progression of marginal periodontitis in squirrel monkeys. III. Adaptation of interproximal alveolar bone to repetitive injury. *Journal of Periodontal Research* **11**, 279–289.

Polson, A.M., Meitner, S.W. & Zander, H.A. (1976b). Trauma and progression of marginal periodontitis in squirrel monkeys. IV. Reversibility of bone loss due to trauma alone and trauma superimposed upon periodontitis. *Journal of Periodontal Research* **11**, 290–298.

Schulte, W. (1987). Der Periotest-Parodontalstatus. *Zahnärztliche Mitteilung* **76**, 1409–1414.

Schulte, W., Hoedt, B., Lukas, D., Maunz, M. & Steppeler, M. (1992). Periotest for measuring periodontal characteristics – correlation with periodontal bone loss. *Journal of Periodontal Research* **27**, 184–190.

Waerhaug, J. (1979). The infrabony pocket and its relationship to trauma from occlusion and subgingival plaque. *Journal of Periodontology* **50**, 355–365.

Waerhaug, J. & Randers-Hansen, E. (1966). Periodontal changes incident to prolonged occlusal overload in monkeys. *Acta Odontologica Scandinavica* **24**, 91–105.

Chapter 52

Implants in Restorative Dentistry

Niklaus P. Lang and Giovanni E. Salvi

Introduction, 1138
Treatment concepts, 1138
  Limited treatment goals, 1139
  Shortened dental arch concept, 1139
Indications for implants, 1139

Increase the subjective chewing comfort, 1141
Preservation of natural tooth substance and existing functional,
  satisfactory reconstructions, 1143
Replacement of strategically important missing
  teeth, 1144

Introduction

Ever since oral titanium implants were shown to yield high predicability (97–98%) for incorporation (Berglundh *et al*. 2002; Pjetursson *et al*. 2007) and satisfactory longevity (survival rates of approximately 89% after 10 years of service) (Pjetursson *et al*. 2007), the choice of oral implants as abutments for reconstructing the dentition has revolutionized restorative dentistry. Without adequate evidence, some clinicians trust an implant abutment even more than a natural tooth, and there is an erroneous belief that oral implants now solve most prosthetic problems with a lot more ease and less risk than traditional reconstructive dentistry did.

Even though there is an increasing body of evidence documenting that implant-supported reconstructions have a three-times higher incidence of technical complications than tooth-supported reconstructions (Lang *et al*. 2004; Pjetursson *et al*. 2004a,b; Tan *et al*. 2004) and that the incidence of biologic complications remains approximately the same for the two alternatives, the trend in dentistry, unfortunately, is to prefer the implant over the tooth abutment.

It has to be clearly stated that the decision to maintain and treat or to extract a compromised tooth has to precede the decision regarding the need for and the modalities of tooth replacement. In this sense, *"implants are here to replace missing teeth, they are not supposed to replace teeth"*.

If properly evaluated, the indication for oral implants as abutments in restorative dentistry is complementary to traditional approaches and helps to facilitate treatment planning in many instances.

Treatment concepts

When reconstructing a mutilated dentition, it has to be realized that teeth were usually lost due to the two most frequently encountered oral diseases, caries and periodontitis. Only a small proportion of teeth are lost due to trauma or are not present due to agenesis. Hence, the vast majority of patients in need of reconstructions present with an oral biofilm infection of variable severity and extent. It is evident that such patients need to be treated with a cause-related approach, i.e. systematic periodontal therapy has to precede any type of reconstructive therapy. It is of utmost importance that oral biofilm infections be under control prior to the placement of oral implants, since residual periodontal pockets or untreated ecologic niches within the oral cavity may serve as a source of infection and jeopardize the health of the peri-implant region (Mombelli *et al*. 1995). Hence, implant installation and prosthetic reconstruction is generally not a treatment in itself, but belongs to a systematic approach of comprehensively establishing esthetic and functional demands under healthy conditions (see Chapter 31).

It is obvious that chewing function is affected both by tooth loss and the type of prosthetic reconstruction chosen to replace missing teeth. A quantitative comparison by measuring bite force and chewing efficiency with identical methods in subjects with overdentures, complete full dentures, and natural dentitions was performed (Fontijn-Tekamp *et al*. 2000). In the latter group, chewing efficiency was significantly greater than that of patients with full dentures irrespective of the nature of their mandibular ridge. By installing implants, bite force and

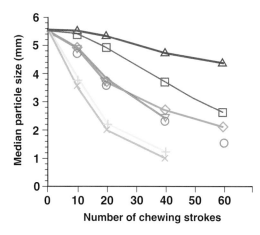

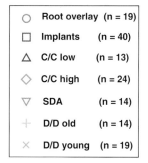

Fig. 52-1 Masticatory chewing efficiency. Number of chewing strokes needed to reach respective particle sizes of the same test food. From Fontijn-Tekamp *et al.* (2000).

chewing efficiency could be significantly improved, although it did not reach that of the dentate patients. Shortened dental arch patients exerted bite forces similar to those of patients with a complete natural dentition, but their chewing efficiency was slightly limited due to the reduced occlusal area. This, in turn, meant that patients with a shortened dental arch would have to perform approximately twice as many chewing strokes to reach the same efficiency as the fully dentate patient (Fig. 52-1).

Limited treatment goals

Generally, efforts are made to completely reconstruct a partially edentulous dentition. The question arises whether or not missing teeth have to be replaced at all and to the full extent. Usually, single teeth are replaced because of predominantly esthetic demands, while multiple missing teeth may also affect functionality and chewing capacity and, hence, are replaced to improve these aspects. However, it is evident from a number of cross-sectional and longitudinal studies (Käyser 1981; Battistuzzi *et al.* 1987; Witter *et al.* 1988, 1990a,b, 1991, 1994) that not all teeth lost are to be replaced. The loss of one or more molars has been thoroughly studied by the Nijmegen group of clinical researchers. No clinically significant differences were found in these studies between subjects with a complete dentition and those with reduced dental arches regarding masticatory capacity, signs and symptoms of temporomandibular disorders, migration of remaining teeth, periodontal support, and oral comfort.

Shortened dental arch concept

Studies on shortened dental arches (SDA) have shown that dentitions comprising anterior and premolar teeth generally fulfil the requirements of a functional dentition, including patient-assessed oral comfort and chewing ability. A review of the literature on SDA concluded that the concept deserves serious consideration in treatment planning for partially edentulous patients. However, with ongoing changes, e.g. in dental health and economy, the

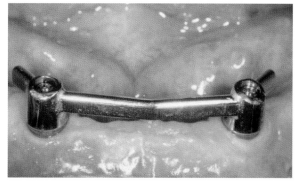

Fig. 52-2 Increasing subjective chewing comfort for completely edentulous patients. Two implants in the canine region united with a bar device (or solely with a retention element without the bar) can dramatically improve masticatory ability and efficacy.

concept requires continuing research, evaluation, and discussion (Kanno & Carlsson 2006).

Special attention has to be given to the patient's own needs and desires for increased chewing capacity when considering the SDA as a limited treatment goal. Clinical observation, as well as research findings, indicate that elderly patients can function at an acceptable level with a reduced dentition consisting of ten or even fewer occluding pairs of teeth (Käyser 1990). The WHO goal for the year 2020, namely to maintain a natural dentition of no less than 20 teeth throughout life, is also substantiated by a recent literature review as this proposed dentition will assure oral function (Gotfredsen & Walls 2007).

The choice of implants as abutments to fulfil individual needs may, therefore, become a welcome treatment option within the concept of a shortened dental arch.

Indications for implants

Three major indications can be defined for the use of oral implants:

- To increase subjective chewing comfort
- To preserve natural tooth substance and adequate, existing reconstructions
- To replace strategically important missing teeth.

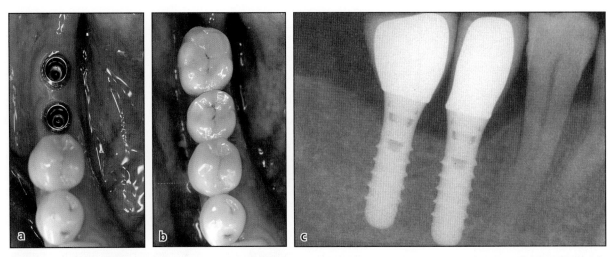

Fig. 52-3 Increasing subjective chewing comfort by replacing missing teeth in a free-end edentulous situation. (a) Installation of two standard size (4.1 mm diameter) Straumann® implants (10 mm), 5 and 11 mm distal to the distal aspect of tooth 45. (b) Chewing units are replaced as a premolar on implant in position 46 and a molar in position 46/47. (c) Radiographic view 5 years after the reconstruction.

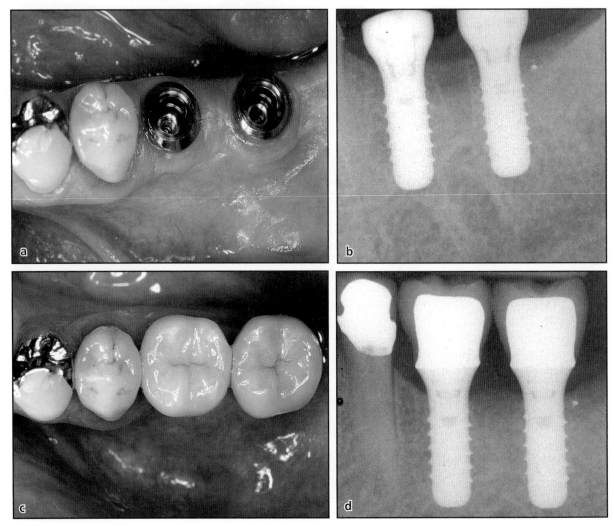

Fig. 52-4 Increasing subjective chewing comfort by replacing missing molars in a mandibular free-end situation. (a) Installation of two standard (4.1 mm diameter) Straumann® implants (8 mm), 6 and 14 mm distal to the distal aspect of tooth 35. (b) Radiographic view at the time of implant installation. (c) Two molar crowns on implants in position 36 and 37, 8 years after installation. (d) Radiographic view, 8 years after loading of the implants.

Increase the subjective chewing comfort

Studies have demonstrated that the installation of a small number of mandibular implants (two to four) may dramatically improve chewing function, especially if the edentulous mandibular ridge showed severe resorption (Fontijn-Tekamp *et al.* 2000, 2004a,b). Hence, it is evident that the completely edentulous patient will benefit from as few as two oral implants installed in the mandibular canine region (Fig. 52-2).

Likewise, subjective chewing comfort may be improved by supplementing single premolar chewing units in the posterior region in order to fulfill

individual demands for more chewing capacity under a shortened dental arch concept (Fig. 52-3). It is imperative that the implants be placed in the prosthetically correct location leaving enough space for an interdental (inter-implant) space and observing the dimensions of a premolar width (7 mm).

Instead of adding chewing comfort in premolar units, implant systems with wider necks or platforms may be installed in order to truly mimic the replacement of the missing molars. In these instances, an inter-implant distance of 8 mm has to be observed in order to create enough space for the molars and the inter-implant space (Fig. 52-4).

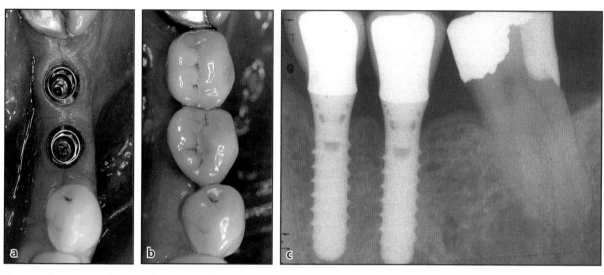

Fig. 52-5 Increasing subjective chewing comfort by closing a mandibular gap. (a) Installation of two standard (4.1 mm diameter) Straumann® implants (10 mm), 5 mm distal to the distal aspect of tooth 34 and 12 mm distal to tooth 34 (= 6 mm mesial to tooth 37). Total extension of the gap: 18 mm. (b) Reconstruction of the implants in premolar units to fit the size of the gap.
(c) Radiographic documentation, 6 years after loading. The filling on tooth 37 was satisfactory and did not need replacement.

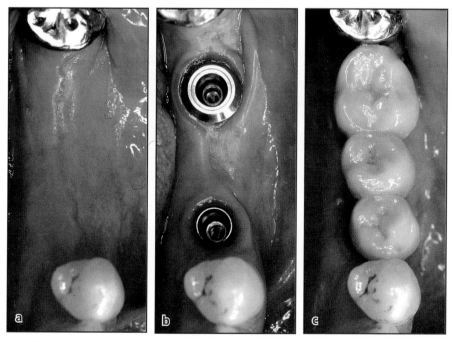

Fig. 52-6 Increasing subjective chewing comfort by filling a large mandibular gap. (a) Edentulous ridge between teeth 34 and 38 is 28 mm. (b) Installation of a standard (4.1 mm diameter) Straumann® implant, 5 mm distal to the distal aspect of tooth 34 and a wide-body (4.8 mm diameter), wide-neck Straumann® implant, 20 mm distal to the distal aspect of tooth 34 and 8 mm mesial to the mesial aspect of tooth 38. (c) Three-unit implant-supported fixed prosthesis filling the gap.

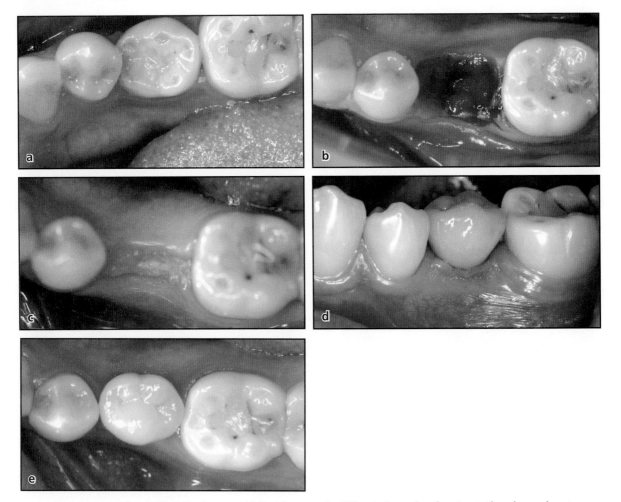

Fig. 52-7 Preservation of natural tooth substance. (a) Deciduous molar 75 has to be replaced owing to the advanced root resorption. (b) Following extraction of tooth 75, the site would be ideal for replacing the missing tooth with a three-unit bridge or a single implant. (c) The single implant is chosen to avoid jeopardizing the integrity and vitality of the two adjacent teeth, 34 and 36. Cutting preparations for full coverage of crowns will result in 10% of the prepared teeth loosing vitality after 10 years. (d) Single tooth replacement of 75, 5 years after reconstruction. (e) Occlusal view of the single implant-supported crown to replace a deciduous molar, 5 years after reconstruction. The adjacent teeth remain unsevered.

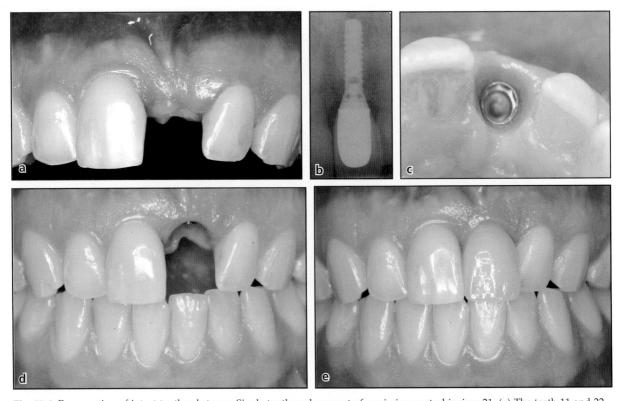

Fig. 52-8 Preservation of intact tooth substance. Single tooth replacement of a missing central incisor 21. (a) The teeth 11 and 22 adjacent to the edentulous space 21 are intact teeth with no fillings and with periodontally healthy conditions. Both mesial and distal papillae are intact and reach coronally to the contact area in this juvenile patient. (b) Following the installation of a Standard Plus (4.1 mm diameter) Straumann® implant with a length of 12 mm, the mucosal tissue is conditioned to achieve a perfect emergence profile. (c) Radiographic documentation 2 years after the prosthetic reconstruction of the implant. (d) Tissue conditioning due to a more apical insertion of the implant for esthetic sites. (e) Implant-supported single tooth replacement 21, 2 years after reconstruction.

Considering the dimensions of premolars (7 mm) and molars (8 mm) and adequate space for the interdental/inter-implant space (4–5 mm), edentulous ridges between existing teeth may be reconstructed and chewing comfort increased without involving adjacent teeth (Fig. 52-5). Obviously, risks can be minimized by reducing the length of bridge spans.

In combinations of molar and premolar reconstructions (Fig. 52-6), the surgical positioning of the implants has to be calculated in detail and restoration-driven stents may have to be used in order to create adequate conditions for prosthetic reconstruction.

Preservation of natural tooth substance and existing functional, satisfactory reconstructions

Oral implants are ideal abutments if natural tooth substance can be preserved. The preparation of a tooth to serve as an abutment for a crown or a bridge anchor opens about 40 000 to 70 000 dentinal tubules per mm². This, in turn, means that the integrity of a

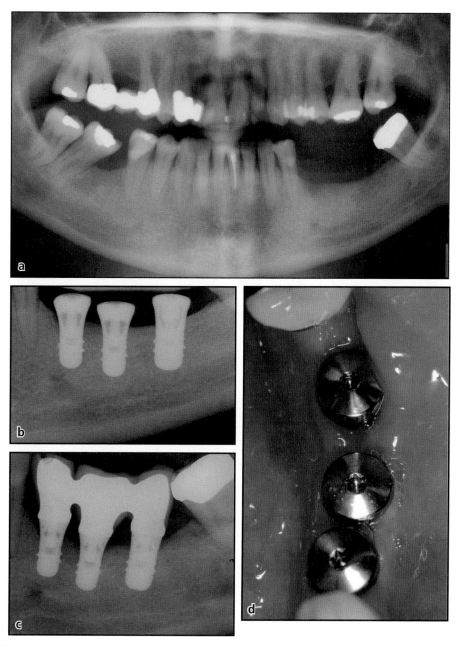

Fig. 52-9 Mandibular edentulous area after the extraction of teeth 35, 36 and 37. (a) Orthopantomogram revealing the neighboring anatomic structures (inferior mandibular nerve) and intact reconstructions on the teeth adjacent to the edentulous ridge. (b) Installation of two standard (4.1 mm diameter) and one wide-body (4.8 mm diameter) Straumann® implants at a distance of 5 mm, 11 mm and 20 mm distal to the distal aspect of tooth 34. (c) Transmucosal implant installation for two premolar and one molar unit. Implants covered with healing caps. The intact crown on tooth 38 is visible. (d) Radiographic documentation after 5 years. Implant crowns are splinted because of the short (6 mm) implants (in the neighborhood of the inferior mandibular nerve).

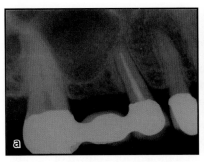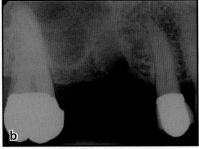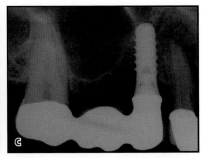

Fig. 52-10 Replacing strategically important teeth. (a) A fixed dental prosthesis is seated on two abutment teeth, 17 and 15. Tooth 15 was root canal treated and suffered from a root fracture jeopardizing the integrity of the entire reconstruction. (b) The bridge is separated between 17 and pontic 16. (c) A new fixed dental prosthesis was seated on the implant 15 and soldered to the existing, still satisfactory crown 17. In this manner, the implant helped to avoid a costly and extensive reconstruction.

vital tooth is severely compromized. Even though a small proportion of abutment teeth will lose their vitality immediately as a sequelae of the preparation procedure, it has been documented that approximately 10% of all vital abutments will have lost vitality after 10 years (Bergenholtz & Nyman 1984; Pjetursson *et al.* 2004b; Tan *et al.* 2004). Hence, it is obvious that an implant installation avoiding tooth preparation represents the most biologically sound way of replacing a missing tooth (Fig. 52-7).

In areas of esthetic priority, the replacement of a missing tooth with a single implant may, beyond any doubt, provide the best and most esthetic treatment option (Fig. 52-8). This is especially true in a periodontally healthy dentition and in situations where the papillae towards the adjacent teeth are still present. By placing the implant in a slightly (1–2 mm) submucosal location, an optimal emergence profile can be achieved.

Instead of preserving natural tooth substance, the clinician may choose to save existing, still satisfactory reconstructions, thereby simplifying the restoration of a mutilated dentition (Fig. 52-9). Occasionally, the reconstruction may have a smaller extent and, hence, have a reduced chance of encountering technical complications during the years of service.

Replacement of strategically important missing teeth

The loss of a strategically important tooth often creates a whole chain reaction of therapeutic measures to be taken. Treatment planning may become highly involved and extensive reconstructions may result from the loss of such a tooth. Especially in dentitions that have received multiple reconstructions, the loss of one strategic abutment may lead to time-consuming and costly therapy (Fig. 52-10). Oral implants provide valuable and indispensable treatment alternatives to redoing existing reconstructions. By the installation of oral implants in strategically correct locations, partial reconstruction of a dentition may be possible. Obviously, such implants have to be installed at locations that are restoration driven, at

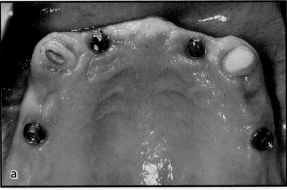
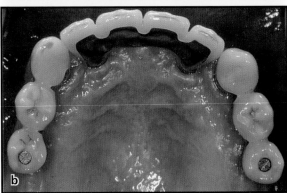

Fig. 52-11 Replacing strategically important abutments. (a) Only the two periodontally healthy maxillary canines 13 and 23 remain. To reconstruct this maxilla with a fixed dental prosthesis requires the installation of oral implants in strategically correct locations. An implant-supported maxillary front reconstruction and two mixed tooth–implant-supported reconstructions in the posterior segments are planned. (b) Eight years following implant installation. The maxillary front reconstruction is cemented on solid abutments that have been installed in the positions of 12 and 22, i.e. 5 mm mesial to the mesial aspects of the canines. The posterior segment reconstructions are cemented on the canines and screw-retained on two implants in the positions of 15 and 25, i.e. the implants are placed 11 mm distal to the distal aspects of the canines allowing the placement of three-unit reconstructions with minimal risks. A shortened dental arch as a limited treatment goal provides satisfactory chewing function.

the proper location for prosthetic reconstruction. In cases with bone dehiscence or lack of adequate bone volume, bone augmentation procedures may have to be performed (Fig. 52-11).

Conclusions

Oral implants are best used as abutments in restorative dentistry if subjective chewing comfort has to be increased, natural tooth substance or existing satisfactory reconstructions have to be preserved or strategically important missing teeth have to be replaced.

Hence, oral implants have become valuable, indispensable, and welcome treatment alternatives to traditional dental reconstructions. Obviously, oral implants should only be incorporated in oral cavities with healthy conditions, i.e. a thorough periodontal treatment has to precede restorative therapy.

References

Battistuzzi, P., Käyser, A. & Kanters, N. (1987). Partial edentulism, prosthetic treatment and oral function in a Dutch population. *Journal of Oral Rehabilitation* **14**, 549–555.

Bergenholtz, G. & Nyman, S. (1984). Endodontic complications following periodontal and prosthetic treatment of patients with advanced periodontal disease. *Journal of Periodontology* **55**, 63–68.

Berglundh, T., Persson, L. & Klinge, B. (2002). A systematic review of the incidence of biological and technical complications in implant dentistry reported in prospective longitudinal studies of at least 5 years. *Journal of Clinical Periodontology* **29** (Suppl 3), 197–212.

Fontijn-Tekamp, F.A., Slagter, A.P., van der Bilt, A., Van t'Hof, M.A., Kalk, W. & Jansen, J.A. (2004a). Swallowing thresholds of mandibular implant-retained overdentures with variable portion sizes. *Clinical Oral Implants Research* **15**, 375–380.

Fontijn-Tekamp, F.A., Slagter, A.P., van der Bilt, A., van t'Hof, M.A., Witter, D.J., Kalk, W. & Jansen, J.A. (2000). Biting and chewing in overdentures, full dentures and natural dentitions. *Journal of Dental Research* **79**, 1519–1524.

Fontijn-Tekamp, F.A., van der Bilt, A., Abbink, J.H. & Bosman, F. (2004b). Swallowing thresholds and masticatory performance in dentate adults. *Physiology and Behaviour* **83**, 431–436.

Gotfredsen, K. & Walls, A. (2007). What dentition assures oral function? *Clinical Oral Implants Research* **18** (Suppl 3), 34–45.

Kanno, T. & Carlsson, G.E. (2006). A review of the Shortened Dental Arch Concept focusing on the work by the Käyser/ Nijmegen group. *Journal of Oral Rehabilitation* **33**, 850–862.

Käyser, A.F. (1981). Shortened dental arches and oral function. *Journal of Oral Rehabilitation* **8**, 457–462.

Käyser, A.F. (1990). How much reduction of the dental arch is functionally acceptable for the aging patient? *International Dental Journal* **40**, 183–188.

Lang, N.P., Pjetursson, B.E., Tan, K., Brägger, U., Egger, M. & Zwahlen, M. (2004). A systematic review of the survival and complication rates of fixed partial dentures (FPDs) after an observation period of at least 5 years. II. Combined tooth-implant-supported FPDs. *Clinical Oral Implants Research* **15**, 643–653.

Mombelli, A., Marxer, M., Graberthüel, T., Grunder, U. & Lang, N.P. (1995). The microbiota of osseointegrated implants in patients with a history of periodontal disease. *Journal of Clinical Periodontology* **22**, 124–130.

Pjetursson, B.E., Brägger, U., Lang, N.P. & Zwahlen, M. (2007). Comparison of survival and complication rates of tooth-supported fixed dental prostheses (FDPs) and implant-supported FDPs and single crowns (SCs). *Clinical Oral Implants Research* **18** (Suppl 3), 97–113.

Pjetursson, B.E., Tan, K., Lang, N.P., Brägger, U., Egger, M. & Zwahlen, M. (2004a). A systematic review of the survival and complication rates of fixed partial dentures (FPDs) after an observation period of at least 5 years. I. Implant-supported FPDs. *Clinical Oral Implants Research* **15**, 625–642.

Pjetursson, B.E., Tan, K., Lang, N.P., Brägger, U., Egger, M. & Zwahlen, M. (2004b). A systematic review of the survival and complication rates of fixed partial dentures (FPDs) after an observation period of at least 5 years. IV. Cantilever or extension FPDs. *Clinical Oral Implants Research* **15**, 667–676.

Tan, K., Pjetursson, B.E., Lang, N.P. & Chan, E.S.Y. (2004). A systematic review of the survival and complication rates of fixed partial dentures (FPDs) after an observation period of at least 5 years. III. Conventional FPDs. *Clinical Oral Implants Research* **15**, 654–666.

Witter, D.J., Cramwinckel, A.B., van Rossum, G.M. & Käyser, A.F. (1990b). Shortened dental arches and masticatory ability. *Journal of Dentistry* **18**, 185–189.

Witter, D.J., de Haan, A.F., Käyser, A.F. & van Rossum, G.M. (1994). A 6-year follow-up study of oral function in shortened dental arches. Part II: Craniomandibular dysfunction and oral comfort. *Journal of Oral Rehabilitation* **21**, 353–366.

Witter, D.J., de Haan, A.F., Käyser, A.F. & van Rossum, G.M. (1991). Shortened dental arches and periodontal support. *Journal of Oral Rehabilitation* **18**, 203–212.

Witter, D.J., van Elteren, P. & Käyser, A.F. (1988). Signs and symptoms of mandibular dysfunction in shortened dental arches. *Journal of Oral Rehabilitation* **15**, 413–420.

Witter, D.J., van Elteren, P., Käyser, A.F. & van Rossum, G.M. (1990a). Oral comfort in shortened dental arches. *Journal of Oral Rehabilitation* **17**, 137–143.

Chapter 53

Implants in the Esthetic Zone

Urs C. Belser, Jean-Pierre Bernard, and Daniel Buser

Basic concepts, 1146
　General esthetic principles and related guidelines, 1147
　Esthetic considerations related to maxillary anterior implant
　　restorations, 1148
Anterior single-tooth replacement, 1149
　Sites without significant tissue deficiencies, 1152
　Sites with localized horizontal deficiencies, 1156
　Sites with extended horizontal deficiencies, 1156
　Sites with major vertical tissue loss, 1157

Multiple-unit anterior fixed implant restorations, 1161
　Sites without significant tissue deficiencies, 1163
　Sites with extended horizontal deficiencies, 1164
　Sites with major vertical tissue loss, 1165
Conclusions and perspectives, 1165
　Scalloped implant design, 1165
　Segmented fixed implant restorations in the
　　edentulous maxilla, 1166

Basic concepts

The clinical replacement of lost natural teeth by osseointegrated implants has represented one of the most significant advances in restorative dentistry. Numerous studies on various clinical indications have documented high implant survival and success rates with respect to specific application criteria (Ekfeldt et al. 1994; Laney et al. 1994; Andersson et al. 1995, 1998; Brånemark et al. 1995; Lewis 1995; Jemt et al. 1996; Lindqvist et al. 1996; Buser et al. 1997, 2002; Ellegaard et al. 1997a;b; Levine et al. 1997; Bryant & Zarb 1998; Eckert & Wollan 1998; Ellen 1998; Lindh et al. 1998; Mericske-Stern 1998; ten Bruggenkate et al. 1998; Wyatt & Zarb 1998; Gunne et al. 1999; Lekholm et al. 1999; Van Steenberghe et al. 1999; Wismeijer et al. 1999; Behneke et al. 2000; Hosny et al. 2000; Hultin et al. 2000; Weber et al. 2000; Boioli et al. 2001; Gomez-Roman et al. 2001; Kiener et al. 2001; Mengel et al. 2001; Oetterli et al. 2001; Zitzmann et al. 2001; Bernard & Belser 2002; Haas et al. 2002; Leonhardt et al. 2002; Romeo et al. 2002). Several recently published studies have focused on treatment outcome of implant therapy in partially edentulous patients in general, and related to maxillary anterior implant restorations in particular. Belser (1999) reviewed selected publications which appear to have impact when it comes to the discussion of esthetic aspects which will be addressed in this chapter. In a prospective longitudinal study involving a total of 94 implants (50 in the anterior maxilla) restored with fixed partial dentures (FPDs), Zarb and Schmitt (1993) published an average

success rate of 91.5% for an observation period up to 8 years. The respective data concerning the maxillary implants demonstrated a success rate of 94% (100% for the prosthesis success). It was concluded that implant therapy in anterior partial edentulism can replicate the data established in the literature for fully edentulous patients. The same authors (Schmitt & Zarb 1993) published an 8-year implant survival rate of 97.9% for single-tooth replacement in partially edentulous patients. These results were confirmed by Avivi-Arber and Zarb in 1996.

Andersson et al. (1998) published similarly favorable prospective 5-year data on single-tooth restorations, performed either in a specialist clinic or in general practices, while Eckert and Wollan (1998) presented a retrospective evaluation up to 11 years on a total of 1170 implants inserted in partially edentulous patients, and found no differences in survival rates with respect to the anatomic location of the implants. A meta-analysis concerning implants placed for the treatment of partial edentulism was carried out by Lindh et al. (1998). The 6–7-year survival rate for single implant crowns corresponded to 97.5%, while the survival rate of implant-supported FPDs was 93.6%. The influence of implant design and surface texture was investigated by Norton (1998) by means of a radiographic follow-up of 33 implants loaded for up to 4 years. A most favorable maintenance of marginal bone around the conical collar was revealed, with a mean marginal bone loss of 0.32 mm mesially and 0.34 mm distally for the whole group.

Soft tissue stability around implant restorations and adjacent teeth is of paramount importance within the appearance zone (Bengazi *et al.* 1996; Chang *et al.* 1999; Ericsson *et al.* 2000; Grunder 2000; Choquet *et al.* 2001; Cooper *et al.* 2001; Mericske-Stern *et al.* 2001; Bernard & Belser 2002; Engquist *et al.* 2002; Haas *et al.* 2002; Krenmair *et al.* 2002). Scheller *et al.* (1998) specifically addressed this parameter in their 5-year prospective multicenter study on 99 implant-supported single-crown restorations. The authors reported overall cumulative success rates of 95.9% for implants and 91.1% for implant crowns. Soft tissue levels around implant restorations and adjacent teeth remained stable over the entire evaluation period. Wyatt and Zarb (1998) published a longitudinal study on 77 partially edentulous patients, involving a total of 230 implants and 97 fixed partial dentures, with an observation period of up to 12 years (mean 5.41 years) after loading. The average implant success rate was 94%, while the continuous stability of the prostheses (fixed partial dentures) corresponded to 97%. This study comprised 70 anterior and 31 posterior maxillary implants. No significant differences with respect to longevity could be detected either between anterior and posterior locations or between maxillary and mandibular implant restorations.

Along with osseointegration and restoration of function, the patient's subjective satisfaction is a key element of the success of implant therapy. Especially when the implant is located in the anterior part of the oral cavity, an essential part of the therapy aims at creating appropriate conditions, so that the implant prosthesis cannot be distinguished from the adjacent natural teeth at the end of treatment. In this context, a variety of specific procedures have been developed, including novel bone augmentation protocols, connective tissue grafting and reconstruction of lost papillary tissue (Bahat *et al.* 1993; Salama & Salama 1993; Bahat & Daftary 1995; Salama *et al.* 1995; Price & Price 1999; Choquet *et al.* 2001).

Being part of a comprehensive textbook about clinical periodontology, this chapter will focus primarily on fixed implant restorations located in the esthetic zone.

General esthetic principles and related guidelines

The basic parameters related to dental and gingival esthetics in general and to the maxillary anterior segment in particular are well established in the dental literature (Goldstein 1976; Belser 1982; Schärer *et al.* 1982; Seibert & Lindhe 1989; Goodacre 1990; Rüfenacht 1990; Nathanson 1991; Magne *et al.* 1993a,b, 1994, 1996; Chiche & Pinault 1994; Kois 1996; Kokich 1996; Kokich & Spear 1997; Jensen *et al.* 1999) and have been recently summarized in the form of an updated integral check-list by Magne and Belser (2002). When it comes to the characteristics of the

Table 53-1 Fundamental objective esthetic criteria (Magne & Belser 2002, copyright © Quintessence Publishing Co, Inc)

1 Gingival health
2 Interdental closure
3 Tooth axis
4 Zenith of the gingival contour
5 Balance of the gingival levels
6 Level of the interdental contact
7 Relative tooth dimensions
8 Basic features of tooth form
9 Tooth characterization
10 Surface texture
11 Color
12 Incisal edge configuration
13 Lower lip line
14 Smile symmetry

Subjective criteria (esthetic integration)
Variations in tooth form
Tooth arrangement and positioning
Relative crown length
Negative space

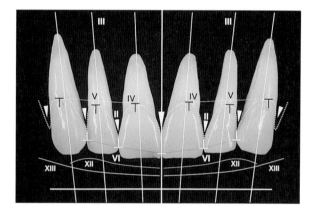

Fig. 53-1 The esthetic checklist, describing a number of respective fundamental objective criteria as they relate to the maxillary anterior segment (detailed description presented in Table 53-1). (Reprinted from Magne & Belser 2002, with permission, copyright © Quintessence Publishing Co, Inc.)

natural maxillary anterior dentition, a number of fundamental objective criteria, including gingival health and its normal morphology as well as dimension, form, specific structural composition, color, opalescence, translucency, transparency, and surface texture of incisors and canines, have been identified (Table 53-1, Fig. 53-1). This list is completed by an addition of subjective criteria associated with esthetic integration, such as variations in the arrangement and positioning of front teeth, relative crown length and negative space.

Depending on the type of a given initial clinical situation requiring the replacement of one or several teeth, the patient's expectations may vary from the achievement of an almost perfect illusion, i.e. that the untrained eye cannot easily distinguish the restoration from the surrounding natural dentition, to the

Table 53-2 Patient expectations related to maxillary anterior edentulous segments

- Long-lasting esthetic and functional result with a high degree of predictability
- Minimal invasiveness (preservation of tooth structure)
- Maximum subjective comfort
- Minimum risk for complications associated with surgery and healing phase
- Avoidance of removable prostheses
- Optimum cost effectiveness

Table 53-3 Therapeutic modalities for tooth replacement in the esthetic zone

- Conventional fixed partial dentures (FPDs), comprising cantilever units
- Resin-bonded ("adhesive") bridges
- Conventional removable partial dentures (RPDs)
- Tooth-supported overdentures
- Orthodontic therapy (closure of edentulous spaces)
- Implant-supported prostheses (fixed, retrievable or removable suprastructures)
- Combinations of the above

Table 53-4 Criteria favoring implant-borne restorations

- Normal wound healing capacity
- Intact neighboring teeth
- Unfavorable ("compromised") potential abutment teeth
- Extended edentulous segments
- Missing strategic abutment teeth
- Presence of diastemas

acceptance of various degrees of compromise from a purely esthetic point of view. The latter case is not infrequent after multiple anterior tooth loss in combination with significant hard and soft tissue deficiencies. In relation to maxillary anterior edentulous segments, patients generally expect a long-lasting functional and esthetic result with a high level of predictability (Table 53-2). To this primary objective are normally added a number of secondary goals which include parameters such as minimal invasiveness, low risk associated with eventual surgery, overall simplicity, and cost effectiveness.

Prior to selecting an implant-based solution, one should comprehensively review all of the possible treatment modalities available (Table 53-3) which have the potential to solve a given clinical problem, and carefully ponder their respective advantages and eventual shortcomings, and only then take the decision together with the adequately informed patient. Currently, the restorative spectrum in the case of missing maxillary anterior teeth comprises conventional FPDs, resin-bonded bridges, removable partial dentures (RPDs), tooth-supported overdentures and implant-supported fixed or removable prostheses. Furthermore, one should not forget that occasionally orthodontic therapy, e.g. closure of limited edentulous spaces, can represent an effective and elegant alternative or adjunct to a prosthetic treatment. However, the availability of scientific evidence – when possible at its highest level – for the planned treatment modality, should be the key parameter for the final choice.

In this clinical decision-making process certain criteria, for example the compromised structural, periodontal and/or endodontic status of potential natural abutments, or the extended dimension of the edentulous segment, are among the factors favoring an implant-borne restoration rather than a tooth-supported fixed prosthesis (Table 53-4).

Esthetic considerations related to maxillary anterior implant restorations

In the context of the natural dentition, long clinical crowns, the irregular contour of the gingival margin, i.e. any abrupt change in vertical tissue height between neighboring teeth, and the loss of papillary tissue often have an adverse influence on dental–facial esthetics (Seibert & Lindhe 1989). Furthermore, the same authors have underlined that in the case of a *high scalloped gingival morphotype* (in contrast to a rather *low scalloped gingival morphotype*) there is mostly an unpredictable relationship between the underlying bone and the gingival contour, often leading to so called "black hole cases" and presenting a high risk for losing soft tissue (e.g. gingival or mucosal recession at the labial aspect of teeth or implants), particularly in relation to restorative procedures, as for example insertion of retraction cords and impression taking.

Another esthetically relevant concern lies in the fact that under normal conditions a maxillary front tooth extraction leads on average to approximately 2 mm loss in vertical tissue height. The mean length of the clinical crown of a maxillary central incisor is 10.2 mm, the one of a lateral incisor 8.2 mm and that of a canine 10.4 mm. Consequently, any kind of maxillary anterior restoration should aim at staying within reasonable limits of these average morphologic dimensions, if a harmonious and esthetically pleasing result is to be achieved. Ultimately, an anterior implant restoration should correspond closely to an ovate pontic of a conventional FPD with respect to the relevant soft tissue parameters (Kois 1996).

Numerous publications, mostly in the form of textbooks, book chapters, reviews, case reports and descriptions of clinical and laboratory procedures and techniques, have addressed various aspects specifically related to esthetics and osseointegration (Parel & Sullivan 1989; Gelb & Lazzara 1993; Jaggers *et al.* 1993; Vlassis *et al.* 1993; Bichacho & Landsberg

Table 53-5 Evaluation of anterior tooth-bound edentulous sites prior to implant therapy

- Mesio-distal dimension of the edentulous segment, including its comparison with existing contralateral control teeth
- Three-dimensional analysis of the edentulous segment regarding soft tissue configuration and underlying alveolar bone crest (ref. "bone-mapping")
- Neighboring teeth:
  ° volume (relative tooth dimensions), basic features of tooth form and three-dimensional position and orientation of the clinical crowns
  ° structural integrity and condition
  ° surrounding gingival tissues (course/scalloping of the gingival line)
  ° periodontal and endodontic status/conditions
  ° crown-to-root ratio
  ° length of roots and respective inclinations in the frontal plane
  ° eventual presence of diastemata
- Interarch relationships:
  ° vertical dimension of occlusion
  ° anterior guidance
  ° interocclusal space
- Esthetic parameters:
  ° height of upper smile line ("high lip" versus "low lip")
  ° lower lip line
  ° course of the gingival-mucosa line
  ° orientation of the occlusal plane
  ° dental versus facial symmetry
  ° lip support

Table 53-6 Optimal three-dimensional implant positioning ("restoration-driven implant placement") in anterior maxillary sites

- Correct vertical position of implant shoulder (sink depth) using the cemento-enamel junction of adjacent teeth as reference:
  ° no visible metal
  ° gradually developed, flat axial profile
- Correct orofacial position of point of emergence for future suprastructure from the mucosa:
  ° similar to adjacent teeth
  ° flat emergence profile
- Implant axis compatible with available prosthetic treatment options (ideally: implant axis identical with "prosthetic axis")

Implant = apical extension of the ideal future restoration.

1994; Ghalili 1994; Landsberg & Bichacho 1994; Neale & Chee 1994; Studer *et al.* 1994; Carrick 1995; Corrente *et al.* 1995; De Lange 1995; Garber 1995; Garber & Belser 1995; Jansen & Weisgold 1995; Khayat *et al.* 1995; Touati 1995; Brugnolo *et al.* 1996; Davidoff 1996; Grunder *et al.* 1996; Hess *et al.* 1996; Marchack 1996; Mecall & Rosenfeld 1996; Bain & Weisgold 1997; Bichacho & Landsberg 1997; Chee *et al.* 1997; Garg *et al.* 1997; Spear *et al.* 1997; Salinas & Sadan 1998; Jemt 1999; Price & Price 1999; Belser *et al.* 2000; Tarnow *et al.* 2000).

In view of maxillary anterior implant restorations, the systematic and comprehensive evaluation of edentulous sites, including the surrounding natural dentition, is of paramount importance (Table 53-5). Key parameters comprise the mesio-distal dimension of the edentulous segment, the three-dimensional analysis of the underlying alveolar bone crest, the status of the neighboring teeth, and interarch relationships as well as specific esthetic parameters.

As one should consider the implant as the apical extension of the ideal future restoration and not the opposite, a respective optimal three-dimensional ("restoration-driven") implant position is mandatory (Table 53-6). Consequently, parameters addressing vertical (sink-depth) and oro-facial implant shoulder location, have been defined, as well as guidelines related to the long axis of the implant, as the latter

has a significant impact on the subsequent technical procedures during suprastructure conception and fabrication.

Recently, the ITI Consensus Conference has approved the distinctly submucosal implant shoulder location in the maxillary anterior segment in order to respond to natural esthetic demands (Buser & von Arx 2000). As the current implant design – in contrast to the scalloped cemento-enamel junction – features a straight horizontal, "rotation–symmetrical" restorative interface, interproximal implant crown margins are often located several millimeters submucosally, and are thus difficult to reach by the patient's routine oral hygiene efforts (Belser *et al.* 1998). Mainly for this reason a screw-retained implant suprastructure (Sutter *et al.* 1993; Hebel & Gajjar 1997; Keller *et al.* 1998) is preferred to a cemented one, as it benefits from the surface quality and marginal fidelity of prefabricated, machined components, and avoids potential problems associated with cement excess that may be difficult to reach and thoroughly eliminate.

Anterior single-tooth replacement

Favorable 5-year multicenter results for 71 single-tooth replacements in the anterior maxilla (implant success rate of 96.6%) were reported by Henry *et al.* (1996); however, this group mentioned an associated 10% esthetic failure rate. In a retrospective study on 236 patients treated with single-tooth implant restorations in the anterior maxilla (Walther *et al.* 1996), a Kaplan–Meier survival rate of 89% was found for an observation period of 10 years. The failure rate for lateral incisor replacement was lower than that for central incisors. Furthermore, 5% of the related prosthetic suprastructures had to be replaced during the 10 years of observation. Kemppainen *et al.* (1997) prospectively documented 102 implants (ASTRA/ITI) for single-tooth replacement in the anterior maxilla of 82 patients and found survival rates of 97.8% and 100%, respectively, after 1 year. Still related to single-tooth maxillary anterior implants, a prospective study on 15 patients revealed a 100% implant survival rate after 2 years of function (Palmer *et al.* 1997). At crown insertion (6 months after implant placement) the mean bone level was located 0.47 mm apically to the top of the implants. No significant additional changes in crestal bone level occurred during the remainder of the study.

Today, it is generally accepted that the final implant shoulder sink depth for esthetic fixed single-tooth restorations can be determined primarily by the location of the cemento-enamel junction (CEJ) of the neighboring teeth and by the level of the free gingival margin at the vestibular aspect of these same teeth. This means that the implant shoulder is positioned 1–2 mm more apically to the labial CEJ of the adjacent teeth (Belser *et al.* 1998, 2000). However, the noticeable esthetic progress made in this kind of implant restoration is the result of recent developments in the absence of extensive long-term documentation. Because the exclusive use of clinical signs for establishing peri-implant health or disease may not be sufficient, the evaluation of additional objective parameters is needed. A number of diagnostic tests have been utilized by clinicians to supplement clinical signs with objective methods. These tests include microbiologic monitoring, proteolytic bacterial enzyme markers, markers of tissue destruction, and finally, markers of tissue repair and regeneration. In this context peri-implant crevicular fluid (PICF) analysis has become the focus of intense investigation. It has been observed that the volume of crevicular fluid did not differ between implant sites and natural teeth and that the features of inflammation seem to be the same around teeth and implants. In addition, the histologic arrangement of peri-implant soft tissues resembles basically that observed around natural teeth, although there are also some aspects of scar tissue (Abrahamson *et al.* 1996, 1997; Berglundh & Lindhe 1996; Lindhe & Berglundh 1998).

Giannopoulou *et al.* (2003) investigated the effect of intracrevicular restoration margins on peri-implant health of 61 maxillary anterior implants – mainly single-tooth replacements – in 45 patients for up to 9 years. Results revealed that the only statistically significant differences between baseline and follow-up examination concerned pocket probing depth (PPD) and the distance between the implant shoulder and the mucosal margin (DIM measurements), which increased slightly over time. The remainder of the clinical measurements and almost all of the microbiologic and biochemical parameters analyzed did not change significantly. Probably the most critical parameter from a purely esthetic point of view is the DIM value, particularly on the labial aspect of the maxillary anterior implants investigated in this study. A mean value of -1.5 ± 1.1 mm was found at baseline examination, and a slight increase (-1.7 ± 1.1 mm) at the follow-up. This indicates that the risk for exposure of the implant-to-crown interface or margin can be considered low. These findings corroborate

recently published data addressing similar parameters (Grunder 2000). The consistently negative Periotest scores confirmed the stability and osseointegrated status of the implants examined. Furthermore, no associations were observed between the above results and the number of years that the implants had been in function. Based on these clinical, microbiologic, and biochemical data, and on an observation period of 4–9 years (mean 6.8 years), it was concluded that in patients with appropriate oral hygiene, implant-supported maxillary anterior crowns with distinctly intracrevicular margins did not predispose to unfavorable peri-implant host and microbial responses. In particular, overall healthy and stable peri-implant tissue conditions – a paramount criterion when it comes to esthetic implant crowns – were consistently encountered and maintained longitudinally. One of the patients participating in this study and who recently passed the 10-year clinical and radiographic follow-up control, is presented in Figs. 53-2 to 53-6. An adequate esthetic integration of the two single-tooth restorations, replacing the congenitally missing lateral incisors, could be achieved and maintained over time.

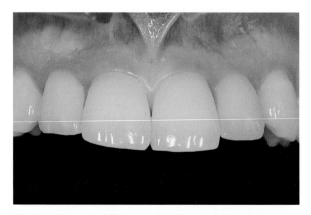

Fig. 53-2 Ten-year follow-up of a 28-year-old female patient. Both congenitally missing lateral incisors were replaced by implants, restored with screw-retained porcelain-fused-to-metal crowns.

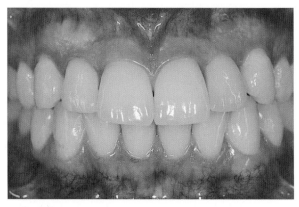

Fig. 53-3 The frontal view in centric occlusal position documents the harmonious integration of the two implant restorations after 10 years of clinical service.

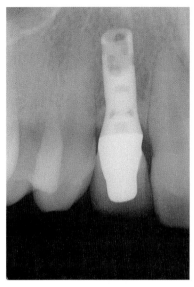

Fig. 53-4 Ten-year post operative radiograph of the maxillary right lateral single-tooth implant restoration.

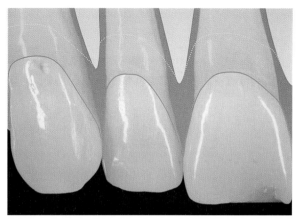

Fig. 53-7 Schematic representation of an intact maxillary right anterior segment. The alveolar bone follows the scalloped course of the cemento-enamel junction for a distance of approximately 2 mm (white dotted line), whereas, accordingly, the gingival tissue occupies the interdental area completely.

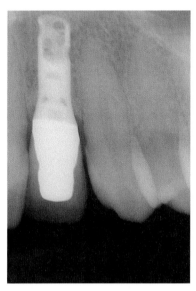

Fig. 53-5 Ten-year post-operative radiograph of the maxillary left lateral single-tooth implant restoration.

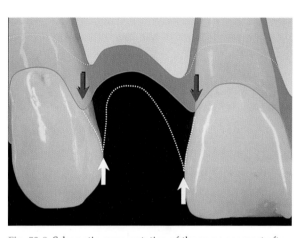

Fig. 53-8 Schematic representation of the same segment after loss of the lateral incisor. While the interproximal bone height has basically been maintained, the corresponding gingival tissue is flattened due to a lack of support originally provided by the now missing tooth.

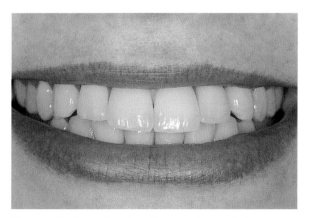

Fig. 53-6 During unforced smiling an adequate balance between implant-crowns and natural dentition can be noticed.

In a simplistic way, the morphologic and esthetic consequences in the frontal plane of the loss of a single maxillary incisor, when compared to the original intact situation, can be summarized as follows: maintenance of the tooth-sided interproximal bone height at the neighboring teeth, and vertical loss ("flattening") of the corresponding gingival tissue due to a lack of support originally provided by the now missing tooth (Figs. 53-7, 53-8). In case of an anterior single-tooth replacement, the related implant restoration should aim at replicating the clinical crown of the contralateral control tooth from the line of soft tissue emergence to the incisal border. Additionally, a gradually developed, flat emergence profile from the implant shoulder to the peri-implant mucosal margin is mandatory (Figs. 53-9, 53-10).

The basic considerations related to maxillary anterior single-tooth replacement, including the respective general achievements and limitations, and

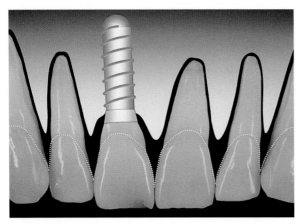

Fig. 53-9 The treatment objective in the case of an anterior single-tooth replacement is an implant restoration with a gradually developed, flat emergence profile from the implant shoulder to the peri-implant mucosal surface. Ideally, the clinical crown of the implant restoration should aim at replicating the clinical crown of the corresponding contralateral tooth.

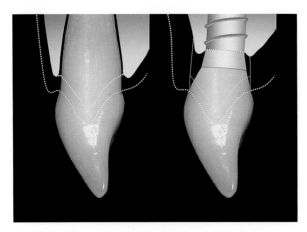

Fig. 53-10 Schematic comparison in the sagittal plane between a natural maxillary incisor and a respective implant borne single-tooth restoration. The decrease of alveolar bone height on the labial and palatal aspect following tooth loss leads to a more palatal implant position when compared to the original root position, which in turn influences the axial profile of the restoration.

addressing edentulous segments with different types of labial bone deficiencies, are presented in Table 53-7.

Sites without significant tissue deficiencies

An increasing body of evidence indicates that the most determinant parameter for achieving an esthetic single-tooth restoration is the interproximal bone height at the level of the teeth confining the edentulous gap. The related bone should be within a physiologic distance, i.e. approximately 2 mm, of the CEJ and thus provide the essential support for the overlaying soft tissue compartments. Consequently, preoperative diagnosis will include interproximal radiographic bone height assessment and periodontal probing of the soft tissue attachment level.

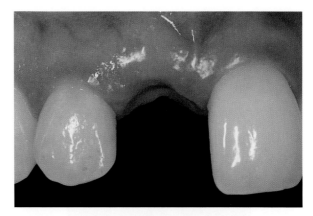

Fig. 53-11 Pre-operative close-up view of the upper right anterior region of a 22-year-old female patient with a missing right central incisor. The scalloped course of the gingiva is maintained, featuring interproximal soft tissue at the level of the cemento-enamel junction.

Table 53-7 Basic considerations related to anterior single-tooth replacement

Achievements	Predictable and reproducible results regarding both esthetic parameters and longevity in sites without significant vertical tissue deficiencies Well defined and well established surgical protocols: • *restoration-driven* implant placement Adequate and versatile restorative protocols and prosthetic components: • occlusal/transverse screw-retention • angulated abutments • high-strength ceramic components
Sites with buccal bone deficienies	Lateral bone augmentation using *autografts* and *barrier membranes*: • technique offers efficacy and predictability • *simultaneous* or *staged approach* depending on defect extension and defect morphology Lateral bone augmentation by means of *alveolar bone crest splitting* and/or various *osteotome techniques*: • limited clinical long-term documentation
Limitations	Combined vertical bone and soft tissue deficiencies: • following removal of ankylosed teeth or failing implants • advanced loss of periodontal tissues, including gingival recession, on neighboring teeth • limited scientific documentation related to *vertical bone augmentation* and *distraction osteogenesis*

If the comprehensive presurgical analysis of a given maxillary anterior single-tooth gap has confirmed a favorable vertical level of both soft tissue and underlying alveolar bone at the interproximal aspect of the two adjacent teeth on the one hand (Figs. 53-11 to 53-13), and no major vestibular bone deficiencies on the other hand, the site can be consid-

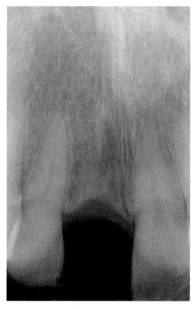

Fig. 53-12 The corresponding radiograph displays favorable bony conditions in view of implant therapy. Note in particular the interproximal bone height, following the cemento-enamel junction for a distance of less than 2 mm.

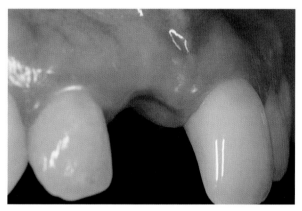

Fig. 53-13 The oblique close-up view confirms optimal conditions for the insertion of an implant, namely interproximal soft tissue height and no significant loss of the buccal bone plate.

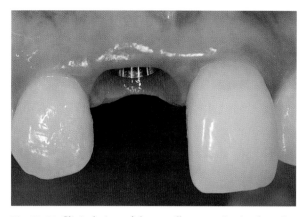

Fig. 53-14 Clinical view of the maxillary anterior implant site 8 weeks after insertion of a solid screw implant according to a one-stage transmucosal surgical protocol. A harmonious peri-implant soft tissue profile has been established by means of a titanium healing cap featuring a respective emergence profile and thus offering adequate interproximal soft tissue support.

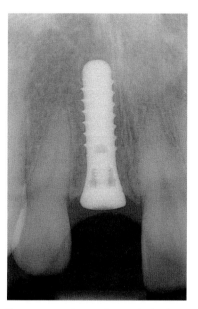

Fig. 53-15 The corresponding radiograph displays a continuous close contact between bone and implant and confirms that the vertical interproximal bone level has been maintained.

ered compatible with a straightforward implant surgical protocol. In order to ensure the best probability of a successful and long-lasting esthetic treatment outcome, the actual implant placement has to be carried out meticulously according to the surgical guidelines defined in Table 53-6. These guidelines include key parameters such as low-trauma surgical principles in general and precise three-dimensional ("restoration-driven") implant positioning in particular. In the case of standard single-tooth sites, most surgeons do not advocate the use of a surgical guide or stent, as the adjacent teeth and associated anatomic structures normally offer sufficient morphologic landmarks to reach the therapeutic objective safely. As far as the detailed surgical protocol is concerned, readers are referred to Chapter 48. Buser and von Arx (2000) have published the surgical step-by-step procedure related to maxillary anterior single-tooth implants, and insisted on a slightly palatal incision technique to preserve a maximum of keratinized mucosa on the labial aspect of the future implant restoration. Another crucial parameter is the maintenance of at least 1 mm of bone plate on the vestibular aspect of the implant in order to minimize the risk for peri-implant soft tissue recessions, a factor parameter when it comes to esthetics. Under such conditions one may consistently achieve post-surgical treatment outcomes featuring unaltered vertical soft tissue and underlying bone levels at the interproximal aspect of the adjacent natural teeth (Figs. 53-14 to 53-16).

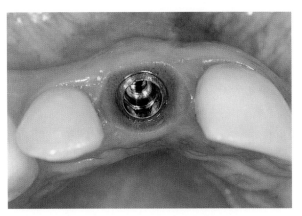

Fig. 53-16 The occlusal view reveals an implant position in the orofacial plane that is in accordance with the adjacent natural roots and thus permits development of a flat emergence profile.

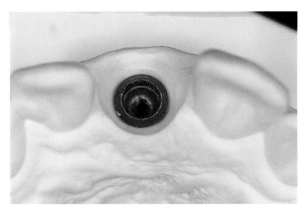

Fig. 53-18 The configuration of the peri-implant soft tissue is subsequently adapted on the stone model according to the diagnostic wax-up. Ultimately, it will be the restoration itself that completes the last phase of soft tissue conditioning by subtle respective physical displacement.

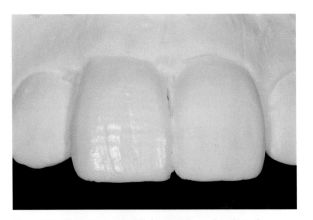

Fig. 53-17 On a stone model derived from the clinical situation, the laboratory technician defines the treatment objective in wax. At this stage priority is given to esthetic principles and maintenance of symmetry rather than to the actual position of the underlying implant.

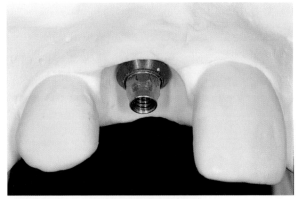

Fig. 53-19 An appropriate secondary titanium component (abutment) is selected as support for the planned screw-retained implant restoration.

Once osseointegration is confirmed radiologically and clinically, the clinical situation is transferred to the master model by means of an impression, normally assisted by auxiliary components in the form of prefabricated impression copings. On the master model, which in turn contains a replica (analogue) of the implant, the laboratory technician defines the final configuration of the single-tooth implant restoration by means of a diagnostic wax-up (Fig. 53-17). Under normal circumstances, i.e. when the natural contralateral control tooth corresponds mostly to the esthetic and functional requirements of an appropriate "target model", the technician basically copies the clinical crown of this control tooth in wax, regardless of the actual underlying implant position. At this stage a close-to-ideal restoration is planned, while its connection to the underlying implant will be addressed later. This approach comprises the minute shaping of the peri-implant soft tissue configuration (on the master model in the form of stone), in view of an identical emergence from the labial and interproximal soft tissue margin, to the one

observed on the natural tooth site (Fig. 53-18). Only after having completed this preparatory step, will the ceramist select the most adequate secondary component (i.e. abutment), depending on the three following cardinal criteria (Fig. 53-19):

1. Implant shoulder depth in relation to the labial mucosal margin
2. Oro-facial implant shoulder position with respect to the future line of emergence of the suprastructure
3. Long axis of the implant.

In most instances, preference will be given to a screw-retained implant suprastructure, unless a combination of mesiostructure and cemented restoration is chosen. Screw-retention is primarily preferred due to a marked submucosally located implant shoulder, in particular at the interproximal aspect, which may render the removal of excess cement difficult, and which is mostly not within reach of the patient's routine oral hygiene measures. In addition, screw-retained suprastructures benefit from the close-to-perfect surface quality characteristics and the

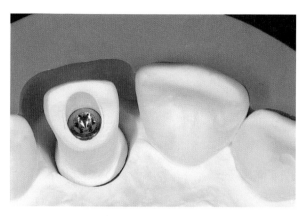

Fig. 53-20 Using a silicon template as guide, a prefabricated ceramic blank is inserted and subsequently reduced to provide adequate space for the external layers of cosmetic porcelain.

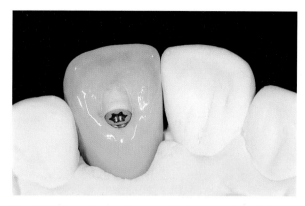

Fig. 53-22 In particular, the completed screw-retained all-ceramic restoration displays a high degree of translucency on its incisal third.

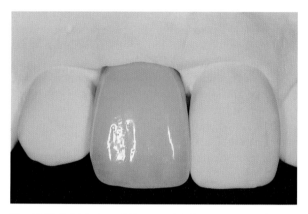

Fig. 53-21 Labial view of the completed ceramo-ceramic restoration on the master cast.

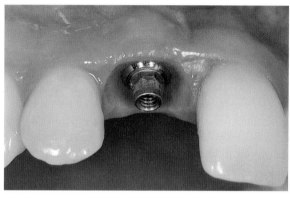

Fig. 53-23 A titanium abutment will serve as infrastructure for the transocclusally screw-retained high-strength all-ceramic restoration.

marginal precision of machined, prefabricated components. Nowadays several of the leading implant systems also offer high-strength ceramic tertiary components which may positively contribute to the esthetic treatment outcome, particularly in the case of a rather thin labial peri-implant mucosa (Fig. 53-20). Another parameter which is of primary importance when it comes to esthetic considerations relates to maxillary anterior implant restorations and is associated with the suprastructure design itself at the interproximal aspect. In order to provide optimal conditions for the related soft tissue, a long interdental contact line is established, located slightly more towards the palatal aspect of the restoration (Figs. 53-21, 53-22). This design offers optimal support for the interproximal soft tissue and thereby reduces the potential hazard of a so-called "black triangle" (Figs. 53-23 to 53-25). In this context some studies have indicated that there exists a predictable relationship between the location of the interdental contact point and the associated alveolar bone crest when it comes to presence or absence of interdental papillae fully occupying the interdental space of maxillary anterior teeth (Tarnow *et al.* 1992; Tarnow & Eskow 1995).

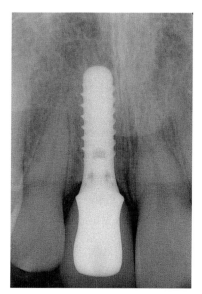

Fig. 53-24 The 1-year post-operative radiograph confirms favorable conditions at the bone-to-implant interface. Note a high degree of radio-opacity of the all-ceramic substrate, permitting the evaluation of the fidelity of the marginal adaptation.

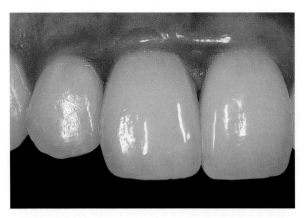

Fig. 53-25 An acceptable overall integration of the metal-free implant-borne restoration on site 11 can be noted.

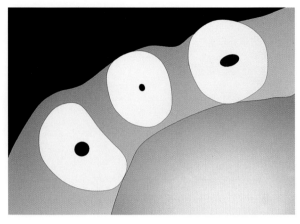

Fig. 53-26 Schematic representation of a horizontal section at the cemento-enamel junction level of the maxillary right anterior segment.

Sites with localized horizontal deficiencies

In a case of a localized (minor) horizontal deficiency, i.e. a confined vestibular alveolar bone crest defect at the vestibular aspect of a maxillary anterior single-tooth gap, one prefers to place the implant and simultaneously undertake a lateral bone augmentation procedure, on condition that several well defined prerequisites are fulfilled. These include an implant placement in accordance with the guidelines presented in Table 53-6 ("restoration-driven" implant placement), the achievement of an adequate primary stability and a resulting cervical dehiscence-type bony defect which is compatible with a predictable bone augmentation procedure. More specifically, the dehiscence should have the form of a two-wall bony defect, and the labial aspect of the inserted implant should not exceed the surrounding bone contours. Under such conditions, the treatment of choice consists of the application of autogenous bone chips, harvested at the site of the implant surgical intervention. The bone chips, which can be combined with one of the numerous available bone substitutes (e.g. BioOss®) if necessary, will provide adequate support for a subsequently adapted barrier membrane. The described grafting material is finally complemented with "bone slurry", constantly collected during the entire procedure. Subsequently, a bioabsorbable membrane is applied prior to repositioning and tension-free suturing of the mucoperiosteal flap. This implicates a rather extended flap design, comprising vertical releasing incisions.

In conclusion, a simultaneous lateral augmentation procedure is recommended if the three following conditions are present:

1. Ideal three-dimensional ("restoration-driven") implant position
2. Adequate primary implant stability
3. Localized two-wall bony defect, exceeding the labial contour of the implant and hereby assuring an appropriate bone regeneration potential and providing the necessary stability to the applied bone graft.

Under these specific conditions, the implant can be functionally loaded after 2–4 months, depending on size and configuration of the respective bone defect.

It is not infrequent in the anterior maxilla, due to its specific alveolar bone crest morphology, that "restoration-driven" rather than "bone-driven" implant positioning leads to a fenestration-type defect in the apical area of the implant. If adequate primary implant stability can be obtained, a similar simultaneous lateral bone augmentation procedure, as described for localized dehiscence-type defects, appears feasible. Under such circumstances the healing time prior to functional implant loading remains the same as advocated for standard implant protocols (i.e. 2 months for SLA-coated screw-type titanium implants).

Sites with extended horizontal deficiencies

In the case of more extended horizontal alveolar bone crest deficiencies, a simultaneous implant placement and lateral bone augmentation procedure becomes technically more difficult and less predictable, as the ultimate goal remains an optimal "restoration-driven" implant positioning (Figs. 53-26, 53-27). The described extended horizontal bone deficiency, on the one hand, may often not permit acceptable primary implant stability to be achieved, and, on the other hand, may lead to a vestibular bone dehiscence that does not have a distinct two-wall morphology. Furthermore, the labial implant contour would be more prominent than the respective surrounding bone (Fig. 53-28). Under these specific circumstances the principal prerequisites for a simultaneous approach are clearly not present, thus leading to the recommendation to proceed according to a staged surgical protocol, which will address the lateral bone augmentation first and the actual implant placement in a second stage.

This may represent a major problem for some patients, as two surgical interventions, normally

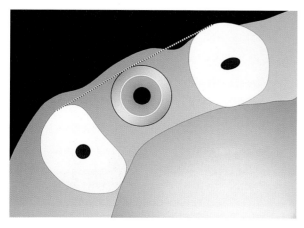

Fig. 53-27 "Restoration-driven" implant placement in the horizontal plane at the site of the maxillary right lateral incisor. In order to maintain at least 1 mm of alveolar bone also on the labial aspect, the implant has to be inserted approximately 1–2 mm more towards the palate when compared to the adjacent roots.

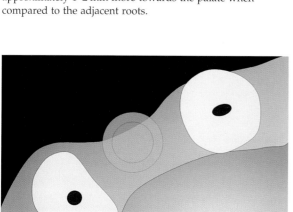

Fig. 53-28 In the case of an extended lateral bone deficiency, where an adequately placed implant would largely exceed the vestibular border of the alveolar bone crest, a lateral bone augmentation procedure (staged approach) is indicated.

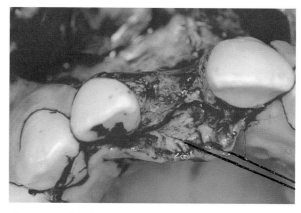

Fig. 53-29 After elevation of a mucoperiosteal flap a severe extended resorption on the vestibular aspect of the edentulous alveolar ridge becomes apparent. Such a morphology is hardly compatible with "restoration-driven" implant placement.

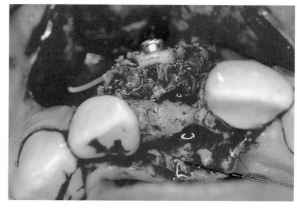

Fig. 53-30 An autogenous bone graft, harvested from the patient's chin region, has been secured with a fixation screw and its periphery filled in with additional bone chips prior to membrane placement.

separated by approximately 6 months, are necessary, leading to a total treatment time of 8 months or more. It is therefore indispensable to inform the patient thoroughly about both the reasons for the staged approach associated to implant therapy, and the possible conventional prosthodontic alternatives (e.g. a traditional tooth-borne FPD, eventually in combination with a connective tissue grafting procedure to optimize the deficient edentulous ridge in view of an optimal and esthetic pontic). The patient will then be in a position to give his or her informed consent to either of the two therapeutic modalities, according to individual preference.

In the case of implant therapy, the first step consists of the elevation of a rather extended mucoperiosteal flap featuring vertical releasing incisions, as the added site volume (due to the block graft and barrier membrane) will require subsequent splitting of the periosteum prior to flap repositioning and suturing (Fig. 53-29). Numerous studies reporting results of various bone augmentation techniques

and related materials have been published (Hürzeler *et al*. 1994; Buser *et al*. 1996; Ellegaard *et al*. 1997b; Chiapasco *et al*. 1999, 2001; von Arx *et al*. 2001a; Zitzmann *et al*. 2001). To date, autogenous bone block grafts, mostly harvested from the chin or the retromolar area, in combination with e-PTFE barrier membranes, still have the best clinical long-term documentation (Buser *et al*. 2002). These authors presented prospectively documented 5-year data of 40 consecutively treated patients, according to a staged protocol. Implants could subsequently be inserted on all laterally augmented sites. It was concluded that the clinical results of implants placed in regenerated bone were comparable to those reported for implants in non-regenerated bone. A clinical example of the described approach is presented in Figs. 53-29 to 53-37.

Sites with major vertical tissue loss

When it comes to maxillary anterior single-tooth gaps with significant vertical tissue loss, the predictable achievement of an esthetically pleasing

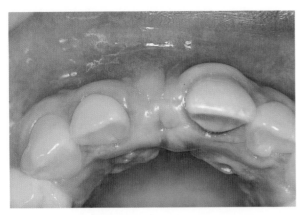

Fig. 53-31 Six months after the lateral ridge augmentation procedure the clinical occlusal view documents that uneventful healing has occurred and that the orofacial ridge profile has been improved.

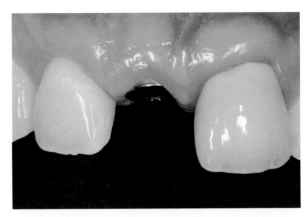

Fig. 53-34 Two weeks after mucosaplasty and exchange of healing caps the initiation of a harmoniously scalloped labial soft tissue course is apparent. Furthermore, the access from the surface to the underlying implant shoulder has been established.

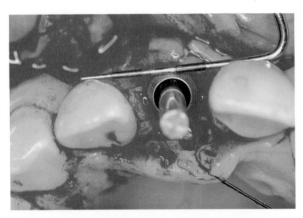

Fig. 53-32 During implant surgery. All key parameters characterizing an optimal implant position (shoulder sink depth, orofacial point of emergence, implant axis) could be satisfied.

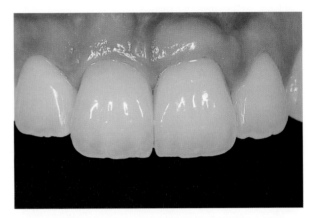

Fig. 53-35 The two ceramo-metal crown restorations – one tooth-borne (site 21) and one implant-borne (site 11) – display little difference in appearance since symmetry has been respected from the line of mucosal emergence to the incisal edge.

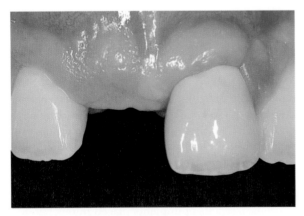

Fig. 53-33 After 3 months of healing the labial view documents a slight excess of keratinized peri-implant mucosa in a coronal direction, which is a prerequisite for the development of the final esthetic soft tissue contours. The first step of the subsequent procedure will consist of the insertion of a longer titanium healing cap, following a minor mucosaplasty.

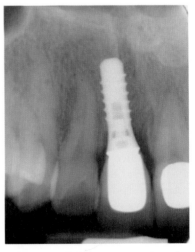

Fig. 53-36 The 1-year follow-up radiograph confirms the stability of the osseointegrated 10 mm titanium screw implant.

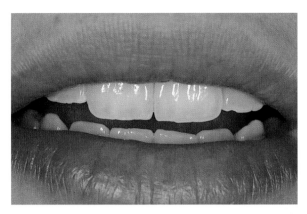

Fig. 53-37 An esthetically pleasing overall integration of the two maxillary anterior restorations is underlined by a close-up view of the patient's unforced smile.

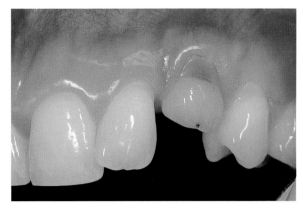

Fig. 53-38 Pre-operative view of a 35-year-old female patient consulting with a persistant primary tooth in the position of the maxillary left canine. Note the irregular course of the adjacent gingiva in general and the loss in vertical tissue height in particular.

treatment outcome, ideally providing a so-called perfect illusion with respect to its integration in the surrounding natural dentition, gets difficult. As pointed out earlier in this chapter, a close relationship exists between the interproximal bone height and the associated soft tissue level (Figs. 53-7, 53-8). If the coronal border of the alveolar bone is no longer within the physiologic distance of approximately 2 mm from the interproximal CEJ of the teeth confining the edentulous space, there is an increased risk of an altered respective soft tissue course (due to a lack of underlying bony support) and its adverse impact on the appearance. Such situations can be encountered following the removal of ankylosed teeth or failing implants, or in case of advanced periodontal tissue loss – including gingival recession – on neighboring teeth. Under these specific circumstances, the final decision whether or not to use implants will ultimately depend on (1) the careful and comprehensive evaluation of all of the therapeutic modalities available for anterior tooth replacement (Table 53-3), and (2) the patient's individual smile line and expectations. This process includes an objective analysis of the advantages and eventual shortcomings associated with each modality.

To illustrate these clinically relevant aspects, the initial situation and the subsequent implant treatment of a 35-year-old female patient consulting with an ankylosed maxillary deciduous left canine, are presented in Figs. 53-38 to 53-46. The preoperative analysis had led to the conclusion that the fabrication of a conventional tooth-borne three-unit FPD, using the intact lateral incisor and first premolar as abutments and featuring a canine pontic, was not opportune from several points of view. Among these should be particularly mentioned aspects related to the questionable mechanical resistance of the resulting conventional prosthesis, specific occlusal considerations (e.g. canine guidance in a pontic area), lack of esthetic superiority when compared to a virtual implant-borne fixed restoration, and, last but not least, the conflict with the general principle of

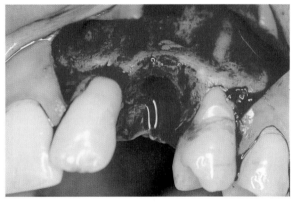

Fig. 53-39 One month after removal of the deciduous canine, the root of which was severely resorbed, a mucoperiosteal flap with vertical releasing incisions is elevated and the preparation of a calibrated implant bed performed. One can note an increased distance between the cemento-enamel junction and the coronal border of the alveolar bone and the left lateral incisor.

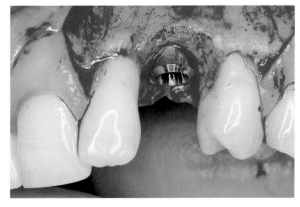

Fig. 53-40 Buccal view after insertion of the implant.

minimal invasiveness (maximum preservation of intact tooth structure).

Once the decision was made, both the implant surgical and the restorative strategies focused on improving or at least optimally exploiting the

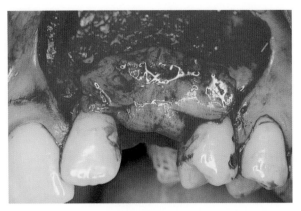

Fig. 53-41 In a case of rather thin mucosa, the utilization of a connective tissue graft, harvested from the palate, may be indicated to create a sufficient thickness of soft tissue at the implant site.

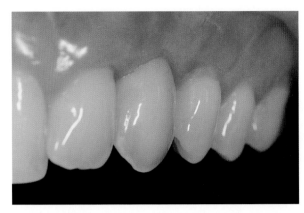

Fig. 53-44 The clinical aspect after insertion of the ceramo-metal implant crown reveals stable and esthetic peri-implant soft tissue contours.

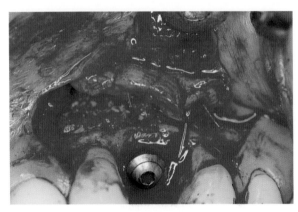

Fig. 53-42 Prior to flap closure, the connective tissue graft is secured to the flap with bioabsorbable sutures.

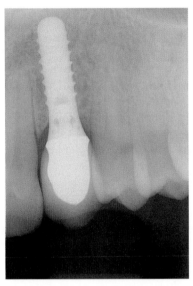

Fig. 53-45 The 2-year follow-up radiograph confirms the stability of the osseointegrated 10 mm solid screw titanium implant.

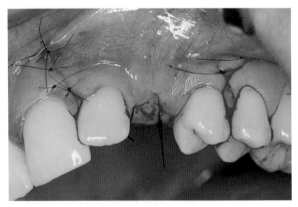

Fig. 53-43 Coverage of most of the healing cap during suturing is recommended, leading to a submerged or at least to a "semi-submerged" healing mode.

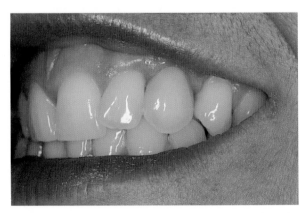

Fig. 53-46 On a left lateral view, during the patient's forced smiling, one can note that the lack of vertical soft tissue in the interproximal area has been compensated for with an apically extended interdental contact line.

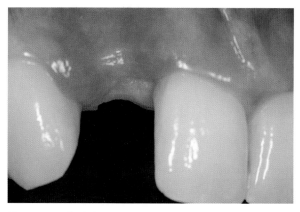

Fig. 53-47 Labial close-up view of the maxillary right anterior region of a 19-year-old female patient. The interdental soft tissue height distal to the central incisor and the corresponding underlying alveolar bone height are markedly reduced, leading to exposure of the cemento-enamel junction.

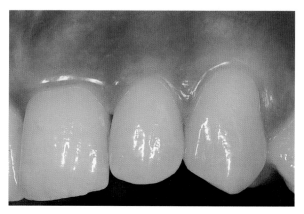

Fig. 53-48 The contralateral side of the dental arch shows perfectly intact and harmonious conditions with respect to the course of the gingiva.

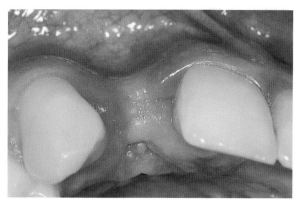

Fig. 53-49 On the occlusal view of the edentulous site a significant lateral crest deficiency becomes apparent, which calls for both a bone and soft tissue augmentation procedure, particularly if an implant solution is planned.

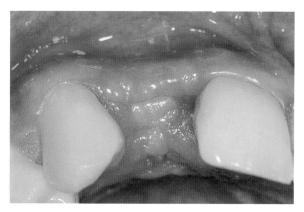

Fig. 53-50 Six months after combined lateral bone and soft tissue augmentation, the site appears to be compatible with "restoration-driven" implant placement.

pre-existing limited esthetic potential of the site. From the surgical side, this comprised a deeper than normal implant shoulder sink depth (Fig. 53-40), the use of a connective tissue graft on the vestibular aspect (Fig. 53-41), a localized lateral bone augmentation (simultaneous approach) procedure (Fig. 53-42) and a coronally repositioned flap (Fig. 53-43). The metal–ceramic implant restoration featured a transverse screw-retention to provide maximum space for esthetic porcelain stratification and a long contact line on the mesial aspect to compensate for the missing interdental soft tissue height (Figs. 53-44 to 53-46).

A more severe preoperative situation of vertical tissue deficiency, combined with a marked horizontal bone defect, is presented in Figs. 53-47 to 53-49. This 19-year-old female patient lost her maxillary right lateral incisor due to a localized periodontal problem. Again, the comprehensive site analysis concluded that a single-tooth implant restoration was the best compromise in view of major disadvantages associated with all of the conventional prosthodontic options. From a purely esthetic point of view, none

of the therapeutic modalities had the potential to predictably lead to a perfect re-establishment of a symmetrical, harmoniously scalloped soft tissue course at its original physiologic level. However, a rather low lip-line during the patient's normal communication and unforced smiling permitted the least invasive approach to be chosen. Following a lateral connective tissue and bone augmentation procedure (Fig. 53-50), an implant could be inserted in an acceptable position and subsequently restored with a screw-retained crown. The final frontal view, allowing a direct comparison between the intact (Fig. 53-51) and the restored side, clearly demonstrates the current esthetic limitations associated with implant therapy in sites with a marked vertical tissue deficiency (Fig. 53-52).

Multiple-unit anterior fixed implant restorations

The normal consequence following loss of two or more adjacent upper anterior teeth comprises a flattening of the edentulous segment. In particular one can observe the disappearance, in an apical direction, of the crestal bone originally located between the

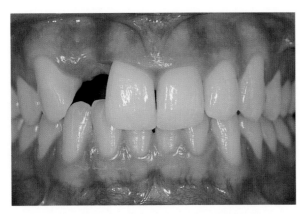

Fig. 53-51 The buccal view in centric occlusion position before therapy summarizes the problems associated with localized vertical tissue deficiencies: lack of a harmoniously scalloped soft tissue course in general and missing interdental papillae in particular.

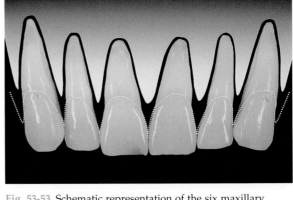

Fig. 53-53 Schematic representation of the six maxillary anterior teeth, including their bony support and the course of the marginal soft tissue, corresponding ideally approximately to the cemento-enamel junction (dotted line).

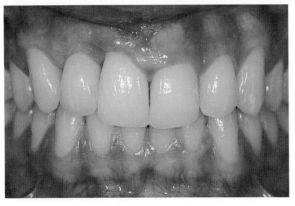

Fig. 53-52 The corresponding view after lateral bone and soft tissue augmentation and insertion of an implant-borne single-tooth restoration on the site of the right lateral incisor, underlines the resulting shortcomings with respect to esthetic parameters. Vertical tissue deficiencies – which at present cannot be predictably compensated for – clearly compromise the overall integration of an otherwise successful treatment.

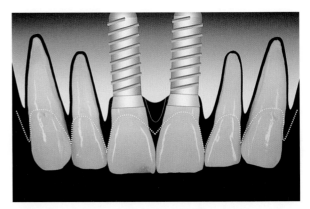

Fig. 53-54 Loss of the two central incisors and their subsequent replacement by implant restorations normally leads to well defined bone loss ("micro-gap", establishment of a "biologic width") around the implant sites. The main consequence from an esthetic point of view consists of vertical soft tissue deficiencies, namely between adjacent implants (dotted lines).

incisor teeth. This phenomenon is not, or only minimally, present at the interproximal aspect of the remaining anterior teeth and thus explains the fundamental difference between a maxillary anterior single-tooth gap and a multi-unit edentulous segment.

If two standard screw-type titanium implants are inserted to replace two missing maxillary central incisors (Figs. 53-53, 53-54), an additional peri-implant bone remodeling process will take place. In the frontal plane, two different characteristic processes, one between the natural tooth and the implant and the other between the two implants, can be distinguished. At the site between tooth and implant, the tooth-sided interproximal bone height should theoretically remain at its original location, i.e. within 2 mm from the CEJ, from where the implant-sided interproximal bone height drops in an oblique manner towards the first implant-to-bone contact, normally located approximately 2 mm apically of the

junction ("microgap") between the implant shoulder and the abutment or suprastructure. This phenomenon has been referred to in the literature as "saucerization" or establishment of a "biologic width" (Hermann *et al.* 1997, 2000, 2001a,b). In contrast, the inter-implant bone height normally decreases further in an apical direction, once the respective abutments or suprastructures are connected to the implant shoulder. This process is mostly accompanied by a loss of interimplant soft tissue height and hence may lead to unsightly, so-called "black interdental triangles". The schematic close-up views comparing the original dentate situation with the status after integration of two adjacent implant restorations, clearly demonstrate the negative consequences on the course of the marginal soft tissue line in a case of multiple adjacent maxillary anterior implants (Figs. 53-55, 53-56).

The basic considerations related to the current state of achievements and limitations of maxillary anterior fixed multiple-unit implant restorations in sites with and without horizontal and/or vertical soft

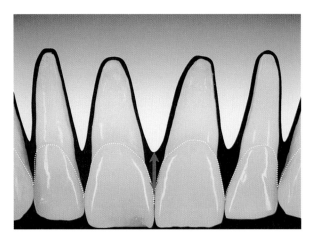

Fig. 53-55 Schematic close-up view of the relationship between cemento-enamel junction, alveolar bone, and course of the gingiva in the maxillary incisor area.

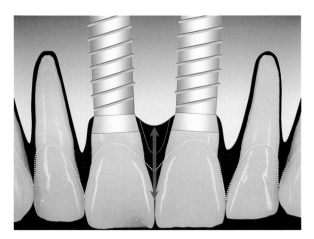

Fig. 53-56 Same area after implant therapy. The red arrow represents the distance between the inter-implant bone crest and the interdental contact point. The lack of bony support for the interdental soft tissue often causes the appearance of black triangles, compromising the esthetic treatment outcome.

and hard tissue deficiencies are summarized in Table 53-8.

Sites without significant tissue deficiencies

Due to the previously described shortcomings inherent in multiple adjacent implant restorations, the clinical decision-making process will thus address both the height of the patient's smile line (low, medium, high) and the individual gingival phenotype (thick and low scalloped or thin and high scalloped). In the presence of a favorable gingival morphotype, some restorative "tricks", including peri-implant soft tissue conditioning and particular interproximal crown design, need to be implemented to predictably achieve an acceptable esthetic compromise (Figs. 53-57 to 53-62). Peri-implant soft tissue conditioning is primarily achieved by using either healing caps featuring an appropriately shaped, continuously increasing (in a coronal direction) axial emergence profile, or by means of plastic compo-

Table 53-8 Basic considerations related to anterior fixed multiple-unit implant restorations in sites with horizontal and/or vertical soft and hard tissue deficiencies

Achievements	Predictable and reproducible results regarding lateral bone augmentation using barrier membranes supported by autografts: • allows implant placement in patients with a low lip line
Limitations	Vertical bone augmentation is difficult to achieve and related surgical techniques lack prospective clinical long-term documentation Inter-implant papillae cannot predictably be re-established as of yet

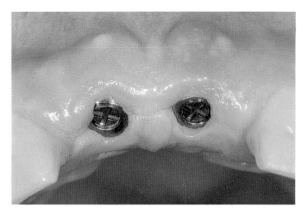

Fig. 53-57 Clinical close-up view of the maxillary anterior segment of a 32-year-old female patient following placement of two 12-mm solid screw implants according to a one-stage transmucosal surgical protocol.

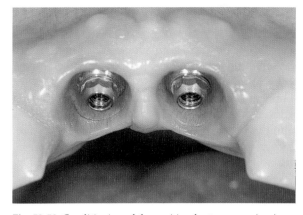

Fig. 53-58 Conditioning of the peri-implant mucosa, in view of the future restorations, has been performed by means of auxiliary plastic components with the possibility of individualizing the emergence profile.

nents permitting the customization of the best suited axial contour in the region from the implant shoulder or abutment to the mucosal margin (Fig. 53-58). The particular suprastructure design concerns the inter-implant aspect, where, instead of an interdental contact point, a long and slightly palatal contact line is developed in the form of two adjacent "wings",

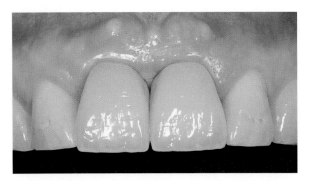

Fig. 53-59 The corresponding clinical close-up view, taken shortly after insertion of the two screw-retained ceramo-metal restorations, documents the effect of a long interdental contact line, the presence of pronounced mesial ridges, and a slight increase of color saturation in the cervico-interdental area. Such technical measures contribute to the compensation of a flat and more apically located labial mucosa line.

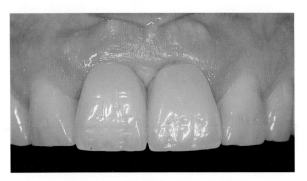

Fig. 53-60 Clinically, a slight fill-in of inter-implant mucosa and an overall stable soft tissue situation can be noted after 6 years of clinical service.

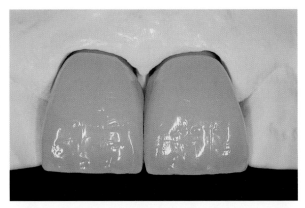

Fig. 53-61 In order to compensate for the reduced height of the inter-implant soft tissue, the ceramist has used an apically prolonged interdental contact line in the form of so-called "mini-wings". These interdental ceramic extensions are made of a more saturated root-like porcelain and are slightly displaced to the palatal aspects of the crowns. This approach results in restorations that integrate successfully, although they are physically larger than the original anatomic crowns.

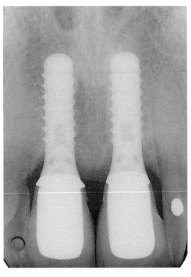

Fig. 53-62 Six years after placement of the 12 mm solid screw titanium implants, the respective radiographs reveal stable conditions at the osseointegrated interface and adequate marginal adaptation.

which are more color-saturated in order to create a discrete shade transition ("blending-in") at the mucosal margin. If the mesial oblique triangular ridges of the two adjacent implant restorations are located at their normal location, the ceramic crowns will not – despite their increased vestibular diameter – optically appear larger (Fig. 53-61). This design reduced the inter-implant cervical triangle to a minimum at the moment of the crown insertion (Fig. 53-59), and favored a coronal soft tissue increase, clearly visible at the 6-year clinical follow-up (Fig. 53-60).

Sites with extended horizontal deficiencies

If the absence of multiple adjacent teeth in the anterior maxilla is accompanied by a marked, but primarily horizontal, resorption of the edentulous alveolar bone crest towards the palate, one can adopt two different strategies. One consists of a so-called "bone-driven" implant placement which will lead to a distinct palatal implant position. In most instances this strategy calls for an implant assisted overdenture-type prosthesis which can more easily compensate for the discrepancy between the required position of the teeth to be replaced and the actual implant loca-

tion, when compared to a fixed implant prosthesis. Furthermore, the denture flange can quite efficiently solve shortcomings related to esthetics, phonetics, and/or insufficient labial and facial tissue support. Normally, denture stability and subjective comfort are excellent and – owing to its removable nature – access for oral hygiene is easy (Mericske-Stern 1998; Kiener et al. 2001). One should be aware, however, that this approach also has its inherent limits and has to take into account crucial parameters such as phonetics and minimal room required for the tongue. As this chapter focuses primarily on fixed maxillary anterior implant restorations, we refer to the relevant respective literature.

Another approach consists of one of the various lateral bone augmentation procedures reported in the literature (Buser *et al.* 1996, 1999, 2002; Chiapasco *et al.* 1999; von Arx *et al.* 2001a,b; Zitzmann *et al.* 2001), which ultimately should lead to a more "restoration-driven" implant placement, ideally compatible with a straightforward fixed implant prosthesis featuring a continuous, flat axial emergence profile. To date a scalloped course of the peri-implant mucosa cannot be predictably achieved around multiple adjacent maxillary anterior fixed implant restorations, and as an increased clinical crown length is normally inherent in this approach as well, the pre-operative assessment of the patient's lip line or smile line (Jensen *et al.* 1999) is of primary importance during the related decision-making process.

Sites with major vertical tissue loss

The replacement of multiple missing adjacent maxillary anterior teeth with a fixed implant prosthesis still represents a major therapeutic challenge in the presence of combined major horizontal and vertical alveolar ridge deficiencies. Vertical bone augmentation techniques, for example the distraction osteogenesis procedure (Chiapasco *et al.* 2001), hold promise for the future but lack clinical long-term documentation at present.

As a consequence, the treatment of choice consists in most instances of an implant-assisted (e.g. spherical attachments, bar devices) removable overdenture.

Conclusions and perspectives

When implants are to be inserted within the esthetic zone in view of a fixed restoration, deep placement – close to or at the alveolar bone crest level – of the shoulder of implants, often specifically designed for this indication, permits the suprastructure margin to be hidden below the mucosa, and the development of a gradual harmonious emergence profile from the implant shoulder to the surface. The resulting clinical crown replicates the profile of the natural control tooth despite a slightly more palatal implant position. This in turn leads to a secondary peri-implant bone loss or bone remodeling – particularly in a case of multiple adjacent implants – due to the reorganization of a biologic width (Hermann *et al.* 1997, 2000, 2001a,b). Under these particular circumstances, screw-retained restorations, based on prefabricated, machined components, will assure a maximum marginal adaptation, favoring the maintenance of the long-term stability of the esthetic result (Belser 1999; Belser *et al.* 1998, 2000). The currently flat, "rotation–symmetrical" design of standard screw-type titanium implants, leading to a marked submucosal implant shoulder position at the interproximal aspect, may not, however, represent the optimal design, in particular in the context of multiple adjacent implants.

Scalloped implant design

As pointed out earlier in this chapter, the traditional implant design may lead to esthetic shortcomings in a case of multiple adjacent maxillary anterior fixed implant restorations. One could hypothesize in this context whether a modified design at the coronal end of the implant, in the sense of a scalloped, more "CEJ-like" configuration, might lead to an improved preservation of peri-implant bone at the interproximal aspect in general, and between adjacent implants in particular. One of the possible design solutions and its anticipated theoretical impact on bone and esthetic parameters are presented in Figs. 53-63, 53-64, and 53-68. More specifically, this approach ultimately aims at creating an inter-implant bone height and resulting soft tissue level situation compatible with generally accepted esthetic criteria. Among these one should primarily mention the establishment and/or maintenance of a harmoniously scalloped course of the marginal peri-implant mucosa. At present, the combination of the following three elements appears important:

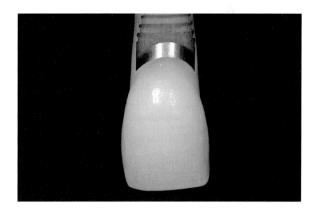

Fig. 53-63 Instead of the traditional implant design, featuring a flat rotation–symmetrical coronal aspect, a scalloped connection, inspired by the natural cemento-enamel junction, may lead to a more superficial implant insertion and by this to the preservation of more bone in the interproximal area.

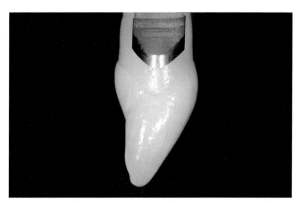

Fig. 53-64 Comparison in the sagittal plane of a natural maxillary central incisor and a titanium implant featuring a scalloped design at its coronal end. The radius corresponds to the amount of bone which might theoretically be preserved.

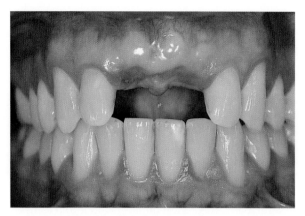

Fig. 53-65 Vestibular view in centric occlusion position of a 24-year-old male patient. The two maxillary central incisors have been lost due to a traumatic injury.

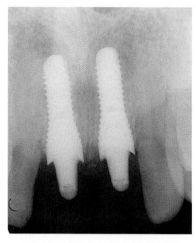

Fig. 53-67 The 1-year follow-up radiograph shows prototype of titanium implants featuring a scalloped design at their coronal end. This design permits a more superficial implant insertion, aiming at a better preservation of inter-implant alveolar bone.

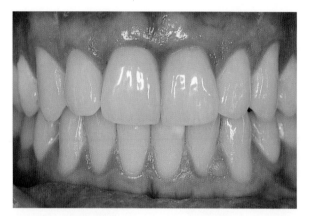

Fig. 53-66 After 1 year of clinical service, there is a harmoniously scalloped marginal soft tissue course, including the most critical inter-implant area.

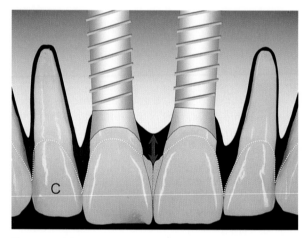

Fig. 53-68 Schematic representation of the theoretical advantages of a scalloped implant design: more superficial implant placement, increased bone and soft tissue preservation particularly in the inter-implant area, and improved esthetics (in combination with interdental "mini-wings").

1. Screw-type titanium implant body, featuring optimal surface characteristics
2. Tooth-colored transmucosal portion with adequate axial emergence profile and scalloped coronal end
3. Mechanically sound suprastructure connection, permitting both screw retention and cementation.

The clinical potential of such a novel, scalloped implant design is documented in Figs. 53-65 to 53-67, presenting a 24-year-old male patient who had lost his two maxillary central incisors in the course of an accident. The 1-year clinical and radiographic follow-up appears to support – at least short-term – the hypothesis that such an approach may preserve inter-implant crestal bone and overlying soft tissue to a certain extent.

Segmented fixed implant restorations in the edentulous maxilla

Another particular challenge from both a surgical and a prosthodontic point of view represents the implant-supported fixed prosthetic rehabilitation of the edentulous maxilla. Undoubtedly esthetic considerations and certain aspects associated with the patient's subjective comfort – both during the actual treatment phase and once the prosthesis is completed – also play a major role in this context. We will limit our reflections to (1) specific aspects of pre-implant diagnosis, (2) the importance of implant number, alignment and spatial distribution, and (3) conception of the suprastructure.

These elements are addressed in the form of a respective clinical case presentation, involving a 67-year-old female patient, edentulous in the maxilla (Figs. 53-69 to 53-89). Besides the traditional clinical and radiologic investigation, an in-mouth try-in of the envisioned treatment objective in the form of a

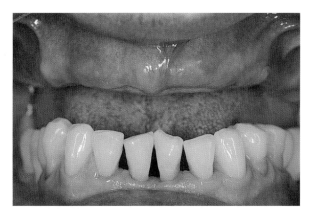

Fig. 53-69 Vestibular view of a 67-year-old female patient, edentulous in the maxilla for 18 months. The pre-existing fixed prosthetic rehabilitation had to be removed due to periodontal disease and was replaced by an immediate complete upper denture to which she never adapted. In the mandible a natural dentition is present to the premolar area.

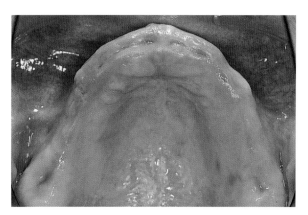

Fig. 53-72 On the occlusal view of the edentulous maxilla, one can note overall favorable conditions for implant therapy and the clinical signs of the recently performed tooth extractions.

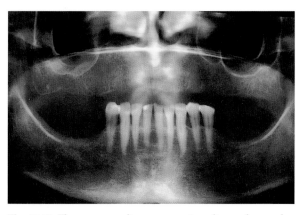

Fig. 53-70 The corresponding panoramic radiograph reveals – at least as far as the vertical bone volume is concerned – favorable conditions in view of implant therapy in both the upper and the lower posterior jaw.

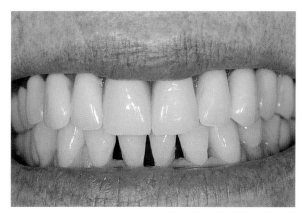

Fig. 53-73 During an unforced smile, the height of the smile line and the eventual need for additional lip support, are evaluated. Both parameters are decisive for the selection between a fixed implant prosthesis or an implant overdenture.

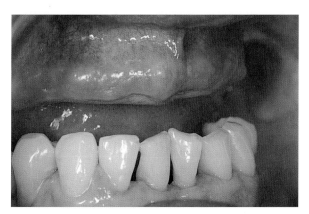

Fig. 53-71 The oblique view confirms the presence of an appropriate intermaxillary relationship which is essential for a fixed implant-supported prosthesis.

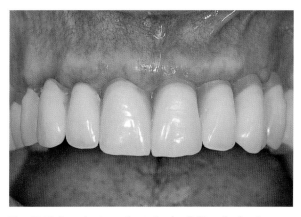

Fig. 53-74 In order to evaluate the feasibility of a fixed implant prosthesis, the clinical try-in of a diagnostic tooth set-up is of paramount importance. One should perform this tooth set-up without vestibular denture flange, so that the patient can realize how long the clinical crowns will be.

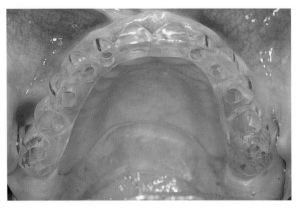

Fig. 53-75 A duplicate of the diagnostic tooth set-up in transparent acrylic will serve as a surgical guide. For optimal stability during surgery, the guide is extended to the posterior palate, an area which will not be concerned by the flap elevation.

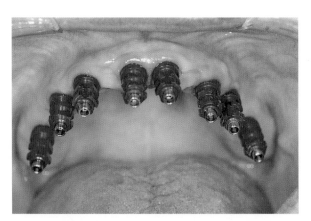

Fig. 53-78 Eight weeks after implant surgery, osseointegration is confirmed radiologically and clinically. Screw-retained impression copings are inserted to perform an implant-level impression.

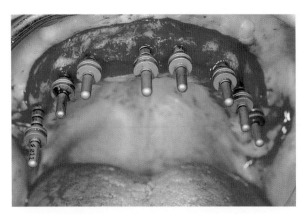

Fig. 53-76 Intrasurgical view of the edentulous maxilla, prepared for the insertion of eight implants to support a fixed prosthesis. Particular attention has been paid to achieving optimal parallelism of the implants by means of a respective surgical guide.

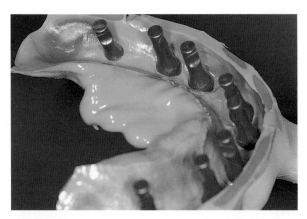

Fig. 53-79 Prior to the master cast fabrication, color-coded implant replicas (analogues) are secured to the respective impression copings.

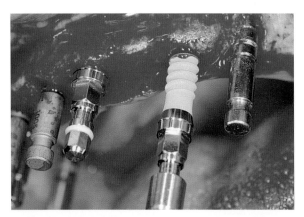

Fig. 53-77 Insertion of a titanium solid screw implant, featuring an SLA surface, in the area of the maxillary left canine.

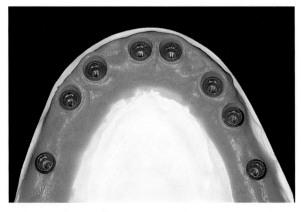

Fig. 53-80 The maxillary master cast features a removable silicon representation of the peri-implant soft tissues.

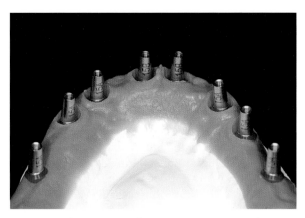

Fig. 53-81 After mounting the master cast in a second-generation, semi-adjustable articulator, the most suitable secondary components (abutments) in view of a cementable fixed implant prosthesis are selected.

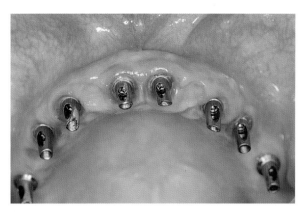

Fig. 53-84 Prior to cementation of the described ceramo-metal suprastructure, the secondary implant components (abutments) are tightened to 35 Ncm with a calibrated torque wrench.

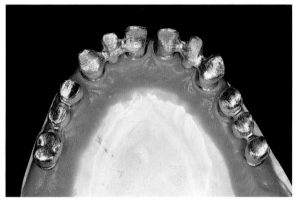

Fig. 53-82 Using a silicon key, derived from the diagnostic wax-up, as a guide, the laboratory technician has fabricated the cast metal framework in the form of four independent three-unit segments. Each segment will be supported by two implants.

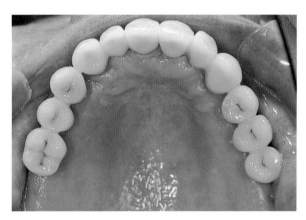

Fig. 53-85 The corresponding clinical view documents that a design similar to that applied in the natural dentition has been used.

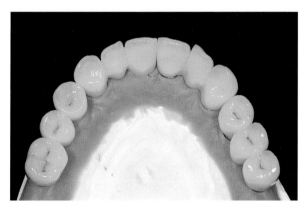

Fig. 53-83 The completed ceramo-metal implant prosthesis on the master cast, ready to be inserted in the patient's mouth.

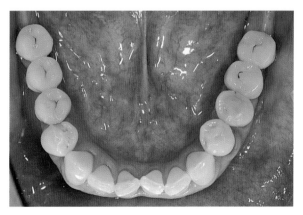

Fig. 53-86 In the mandible the bilaterally shortened arch has been prolonged to the first molar area by means of two fixed cemented ceramo-metal implant prostheses.

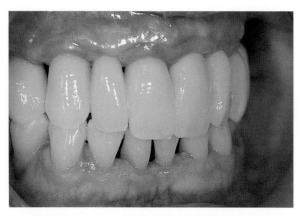

Fig. 53-87 The oblique clinical close-up view of the final implant restoration reveals an acceptable integration both from a functional and an esthetic point of view.

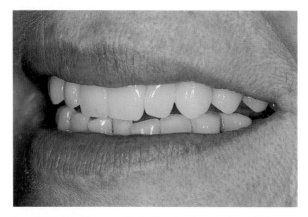

Fig. 53-88 Finally, an esthetically pleasing result could be achieved by means of a fixed implant-supported prosthesis.

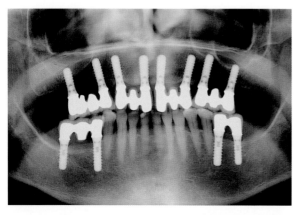

Fig. 53-89 The 1-year post-operative panoramic radiograph confirms osseointegration and documents that the maxillary prosthesis has been completed in four independent segments.

set-up of teeth without vestibular denture-type flange is of primary importance (Fig. 53-73). Among other aspects, this approach will allow the visualization of the length of the clinical crowns of the future fixed implant prosthesis, and the evaluation of whether a fixed prosthesis will provide sufficient lip and facial

support (Fig. 53-74). A surgical guide, derived from the described tooth set-up, will guarantee that the future implant positions are in accordance with the determined tooth positions. Whenever possible, parallelism of implants is recommended, as it permits an eventual early or immediate loading approach (Szmukler-Moncler *et al.* 2000; Cooper *et al.* 2001; Andersen *et al.* 2002; Cochran *et al.* 2002), and facilitates the subsequent clinical and laboratory procedures. Although little scientific evidence exists to indicate how many implants of which dimension and in what position are required for a predictable and long-lasting fixed implant rehabilitation of an edentulous maxilla, some clinical trends – mostly derived from traditional prosthodontic experience – do exist. If one plans to extend the prosthesis to the first molar area, and if the anatomic conditions allow the use of standard-size (length and diameter) implants, between six and eight implants seem reasonable. However, in order to increase the overall prosthetic versatility and to be able to apply the principle of segmenting, which includes the ease of eventual re-interventions in a case of localized complications (Priest 1996; Goodacre *et al.* 1999; Lang *et al.* 2000; Johnson & Persson 2001), eight implants may be considered adequate. The recommended respective positions are on both sides of the jaw: the sites of the central incisors, the canines, the first premolars, and the first molars (Fig. 53-76). This approach will ultimately allow the fabrication of four independent three-unit FPDs, with all the related technical and clinical advantages (Figs. 53-78 to 53-89). Some of the scientific data available to date and supporting the concept of smaller segments rather than full-arch splinting will be presented and discussed in Chapter 54.

In conclusion, the concepts and therapeutic modalities do exist nowadays to solve – by means of implants – elegantly as well as predictably a majority of clinical situations requiring the replacement of missing teeth in the esthetic zone, and the most promising novel approaches and perspectives can already be identified on a not too distant horizon.

Acknowledgments

The authors wish to acknowledge and thank Drs Jean-Paul Martinet, Nicholas Roehrich, and Dimitri Thiébaud (all of them clinicians at the School of Dental Medicine, University of Geneva, and involved in the treatment of some of the patients presented in this chapter) for their contributions. We would also like to thank the laboratory technicians and ceramists Michel Bertossa, Michel Magne, and Alwin Schönenberger, for their expertise and meticulous execution of the implant suprastructures presented in this chapter. Furthermore, our gratitude is extended to Dr. Pascal Magne (Senior Lecturer, University of Geneva) for his competent assistance in development of the schematic illustrations.

References

Abrahamson, I., Berglundh, T. & Lindhe, J. (1997). The mucosal barrier following abutment dis/reconnection. An experimental study in dogs. *Journal of Clinical Periodontology* **24**, 568–572.

Abrahamson, I., Berglundh, T., Wennström, J. & Lindhe, J. (1996). The peri-implant hard and soft tissues at different implant systems. *Clinical Oral Implants Research* **7**, 212–219.

Andersen, E., Haanæs, H.R. & Knutsen, B.M. (2002). Immediate loading of single-tooth ITI implants in the anterior maxilla: a prospective 5-year pilot study. *Clinical Oral Implants Research* **13**, 281–287.

Andersson, B., Ödman, P., Lindvall, A.M. & Brånemark, P.I. (1998). Five-year prospective study of prosthodontic and surgical single-tooth implant treatment in general practices and at a specialist clinic. *International Journal of Prosthodontics* **11**, 351–365.

Andersson, B., Ödman, P., Lindvall, A.M. & Lithner, B. (1995). Single-tooth restorations supported by osseointegrated implants: results and experiences from a prospective study after 2 to 3 years. *International Journal of Oral and Maxillofacial Implants* 10, 702–711.

Avivi-Arber, L. & Zarb, G.A. (1996). Clinical effectiveness of implant-supported single-tooth replacement: the Toronto study. *International Journal of Oral and Maxillofacial Implants* **11**, 311–321.

Bahat, O. & Daftary, F. (1995). Surgical reconstruction – a prerequisite for long-term implant success: a philosophic approach. *Practical Periodontics and Aesthetic Dentistry* **7**, 21–31.

Bahat, O., Fontanesi, R.V. & Preston, J. (1993). Reconstruction of the hard and soft tissues for optimal placement of osseointegrated implants. *International Journal of Periodontics and Restorative Dentistry* **13**, 255–275.

Bain, C.A. & Weisgold, A.S. (1997). Customized emergence profile in the implant crown – a new technique. *Compendium for Continuing Education in Dentistry* **18**, 41–46.

Behneke, A., Behneke, N. & d'Hoedt, B. (2000). The longitudinal clinical effectiveness of ITI solid screw implants in partially edentulous patients: A 5-year follow-up report. *International Journal of Oral and Maxillofacial Implants* **15**, 633–645.

Belser, U.C. (1982). Esthetics checklist for the fixed prosthesis. Part II: Biscuit-bake try-in. In: Schärer, P., Rinn, L.A., Kopp, F.R., eds. *Esthetic Guidelines for Restorative Dentistry*. Carol Stream, IL: Quintessence Publishing Co., pp. 188–192.

Belser, U.C. (1999). Esthetic implant restorations. In: Lang, N.P., Karring, T. & Lindhe, J., eds. *Proceedings of the 3rd European Workshop on Periodontology*. Berlin: Quintessence, pp. 304–332.

Belser, U.C., Buser, D., Hess, D., Schmid, B., Bernard, J.P. & Lang, N.P. (1998). Aesthetic implant restorations in partially edentulous patients – a critical appraisal. *Periodontology 2000* **17**, 132–150.

Belser, U.C., Mericske-Stern, R., Bernard, J.P. & Taylor, T.D. (2000). Prosthetic management of the partially dentate patient with fixed implant restorations. *Clinical Oral Implants Research* **11** (Suppl 1), 126–145.

Bengazi, F., Wennström, J.L. & Lekholm, U. (1996). Recession of the soft tissue margin at oral implants. A 2-year longitudinal prospective study. *Clinical Oral Implants Research* **7**, 303–310.

Berglundh, T. & Lindhe, J. (1996). Dimension of the periimplant mucosa. Biological width revisited. *Journal of Clinical Periodontology* **23**, 971–983.

Bernard, J.P. & Belser, U. (2002). Twelve years of clinical experience with the ITI Dental Implant System at the University of Geneva. *Journal de Parodontologie et d'Implantologie orale* **21**, 1–27.

Bichacho, N. & Landsberg, C.J. (1994). A modified surgical/prosthetic approach for an optimal single implant-supported crown. Part II. The cervical contouring concept. *Practical Periodontics and Aesthetic Dentistry* **6**, 35–41.

Bichacho, N. & Landsberg, C.J. (1997). Single implant restorations: prosthetically induced soft tissue topography. *Practical Periodontics and Aesthetic Dentistry* **9**, 745–754.

Boioli, L.T., Penaud, J. & Miller, N. (2001). A meta-analytic, quantitative assessment of osseointegration establishment and evolution of submerged and non-submerged endosseous titanium oral implants. *Clinical Oral Implants Research* **12**, 579–588.

Brånemark, P.I, Svensson, B. & van Steenberghe, D. (1995). Ten-year survival rates of fixed prostheses on four or six implants ad modum Brånemark in full edentulism. *Clinical Oral Implants Research* **6**, 227–231.

Brugnolo, E., Mazzocco, C., Cordioll, G. & Majzoub, Z. (1996). Clinical and radiographic findings following placement of single-tooth implants in young patients – case reports. *International Journal of Periodontics and Restorative Dentistry* **16**, 421–433.

Bryant, R.S. & Zarb, G.A. (1998). Osseointegration of oral implants in older and younger adults. *International Journal of Oral and Maxillofacial Implants* **13**, 492–499.

Buser, D., Dula, K., Hess, D., Hirt, H.P. & Belser, U.C. (1999). Localized ridge augmentation with autografts and barrier membranes. *Periodontology 2000* **19**, 151–163.

Buser, D., Dula, K., Hirt, H.P. & Schenk, R.K. (1996). Lateral ridge augmentation using autografts and barrier membranes: a clinical study with 40 partially edentulous patients. *Journal of Oral and Maxillofacial Surgery* **54**, 420–432.

Buser, D., Ingimarsson, S., Dula, K., Lussi, A., Hirt, H.P. & Belser, U.C. (2002). Long-term stability of osseointegrated implants in augmented bone: A 5-year prospective study in partially edentulous patients. *International Journal of Periodontics and Restorative Dentistry* **22**, 108–117.

Buser, D., Mericske-Stern, R., Bernard, J.P., Behneke, A., Behneke, N., Hirt, H.P., Belser, U.C. & Lang, N.P. (1997). Long-term evaluation of non-submerged ITI implants. Part I: 8-year life table analysis of a prospective multi-center study with 2359 implants. *Clinical Oral Implants Research* **8**, 161–172.

Buser, D. & von Arx, T. (2000). Surgical procedures in partially edentulous patients with ITI implants. *Clinical Oral Implants Research* **11** (Suppl I), 83–100.

Carrick, J.L. (1995). Post-trauma replacement of maxillary central incisors utilizing implants: a case report. *Practical Periodontics and Aesthetic Dentistry* **7**, 79–85.

Chang, M., Wennström, J.L., Oedman, P. & Andersson, B. (1999). Implant supported single-tooth replacements compared to contralateral natural teeth. Crown and soft tissue dimensions. *Clinical Oral Implants Research* **10**, 185–194.

Chee, W.W., Cho, G.C. & Ha, S. (1997). Replicating soft tissue contours on working casts for implant restorations. *Journal of Prosthodontics* **6**, 218–220.

Chiapasco, M., Abati, S., Romeo, E. & Vogel, G. (1999). Clinical outcome of autogenous bone blocks or guided regeneration with e-PTFE membranes for reconstruction of narrow edentulous ridges. *Clinical Oral Implants Research* **10**, 278–288.

Chiapasco, M., Romeo, E. & Vogel, G. (2001). Vertical distraction osteogenesis of edentulous ridges for improvement of oral implant positioning: A clinical report of preliminary results. *International Journal of Oral and Maxillofacial Implants* **16**, 43–51.

Chiche, G. & Pinault, A. (1994). *Esthetics of Anterior Fixed Prosthodontics*. Carol Stream, IL: Quintessence Publishing Co.

Choquet, V., Hermans, M., Adrienssens P., Daelemans, P., Tarnow, D.P. & Malevez, C. (2001). Clinical and radiographic evaluation of the papilla level adjacent to single-tooth dental implants. A retrospective study in the maxillary anterior region. *Journal of Periodontology* **72**, 1364–1371.

Cochran, D.L., Buser, D., ten Bruggenkate, C.M., Weingart, D., Taylor, T. M., Bernard, J.P., Peters, F. & Simpson, J.P. (2002). The use of shortened healing times on ITI implants with a sandblasted and acid-etched (SLA) surface. Early results from clinical trials on ITI SLA implants. *Clinical Oral Implants Research* **13**, 144–153.

Cooper, L., Felton, D.A., Kugelberg, C.F., Ellner, S., Chaffee, N., Molina, A.L., Moriarty, J.D., Paquette, D. & Palmqvist, U. (2001). A multicenter 12-months evaluation of single-tooth implants restored 3 weeks after 1-stage surgery. *International Journal of Oral and Maxillofacial Implants* **16**, 182–192.

Corrente, G., Vergnano, L., Pascetta, R. & Ramadori, G. (1995). A new custom-made abutment for dental implants: a technical note. *International Journal of Oral and Maxillofacial Implants* **10**, 604–608.

Davidoff, S.R. (1996). Late stage soft tissue modification for anatomically correct implant-supported restorations. *Journal of Prosthetic Dentistry* **76**, 334–338.

De Lange, G.L. (1995). Aesthetic and prosthetic principles for single tooth implant procedures: an overview. *Practical Periodontics and Aesthetic Dentistry* **7**, 51–62.

Eckert, S.E. & Wollan, P.C. (1998). Retrospective review of 1170 endosseous implants placed in partially edentulous jaws. *Journal of Prosthetic Dentistry* **79**, 415–421.

Ekfeldt, A., Carlsson, G.E. & Börjesson, G. (1994). Clinical evaluation of single-tooth restorations supported by osseointegrated implants: a retrospective study. *International Journal of Oral and Maxillofacial Implants* **9**, 179–183.

Ellegaard, B., Baelum, V. & Karring, T. (1997a). Implant therapy in periodontally compromised patients. *Clinical Oral Implants Research* **8**, 180–188.

Ellegaard, B., Kølsen-Petersen, J. & Baelum, V. (1997b). Implant therapy involving maxillary sinus lift in periodontally compromised patients. *Clinical Oral Implants Research* **8**, 305–315.

Ellen, R.P. (1998). Microbial colonization of the peri-implant environment and its relevance to long-term success of osseointegrated implants. *International Journal of Prosthodontics* **11**, 433–441.

Engquist, B, Åstrand, P., Dahlgren, S., Engquist, E., Feldman, H. & Gröndahl, K. (2002). Marginal bone reaction to oral implants: a prospective comparative study of Astra Tech and Brånemark System implants. *Clinical Oral Implants Research* **13**, 30–37.

Ericsson, I., Nilson, H., Nilner, K. & Randow, K. (2000). Immediate functional loading of Brånemark single tooth implants. An 18 months' clinical pilot follow-up study. *Clinical Oral Implants Research* **11**, 26–33.

Garber, D.A. (1995). The esthetic implant: letting restoration be the guide. *Journal of the American Dental Association* **126**, 319–325.

Garber, D.A. & Belser, U.C. (1995). Restoration-driven implant placement with restoration-generated site development. *Compendium of Continuing Education in Dentistry* **16**, 796–804.

Garg, A.K., Finley, J. & Dorado, L.S. (1997). Single-tooth implant-supported restorations in the anterior maxilla. *Practical Periodontics and Aesthetic Dentistry* **9**, 903–912.

Gelb, D.A. & Lazzara, R.J. (1993). Hierarchy of objectives in implant placement to maximize esthetics: use of pre-angulated abutments. *International Journal of Periodontics & Restorative Dentistry* **13**, 277–287.

Ghalili, K.M. (1994). A new approach to restoring single-tooth implants: report of a case. *International Journal of Oral and Maxillofacial Implants* **9**, 85–89.

Giannopoulou, C., Bernard, J.P., Buser, D., Carrel, A. & Belser, U.C. (2003). Effect of intracrevicular restoration margins on peri-implant health: Clinical, biochemical and microbiological findings around esthetic implants up to 9 years. *International Journal of Oral & Maxillofacial Implants* **18**(2), 173–181.

Goldstein, R. (1976). *Esthetics in Dentistry*. Philadelphia, PA: Lippincott Publishers.

Gomez-Roman, G., Kruppenbacher, M., Weber, H. & Schulte, W. (2001). Immediate postextraction implant placement with root-analog stepped implants: Surgical procedure and statistical outcome after 6 years. *International Journal of Oral and Maxillofacial Implants* **16**, 503–513.

Goodacre, C.A. (1990). Gingival esthetics. *Journal of Prosthetic Dentistry* **64**, 1–12.

Goodacre, C.J., Kan, J.I.K. & Rungcharassaeng, K. (1999). Clinical complications of osseointegrated implants. *Journal of Prosthetic Dentistry* **81**, 537–552.

Grunder, U. (2000). Stability of the mucosal topography around single-tooth implants and adjacent teeth: 1-year results. *International Journal of Periodontics and Restorative Dentistry* **20**, 11–17.

Grunder, U., Spielmann H.P. & Gaberthuel, T. (1996). Implant-supported single tooth replacement in the aesthetic region: a complex challenge. *Practical Periodontics and Aesthetic Dentistry* **8**, 835–842.

Gunne, J., Åstrand, P. Lindh, T., Borg, K. & Olsson, M. (1999). Tooth-implant and implant supported fixed partial dentures: A 10-year report. *International Journal of Prosthodontics* **12**, 216–221.

Haas, R., Polak C., Fürhauser, R., Mailath-Pokorny, G., Dörtbudak, O. & Watzek, G. (2002). A long-term follow-up of 76 Brånemark single-tooth implants. *Clinical Oral Implants Research* **13**, 38–43.

Hebel, K.S. & Gajjar, R.C. (1997). Cement-retained versus screw-retained implant restorations: achieving optimal occlusion and esthetics in implant dentistry. *Journal of Prosthetic Dentistry* **77**, 28–35.

Henry, P.J., Laney, W.R., Jemt, T., Harris, D., Krogh, P.H.J., Polizzi, G., Zarb, G.A. & Herrmann, I. (1996). Osseointegrated implants for single-tooth replacement: a prospective 5-year multicenter study. *International Journal of Oral and Maxillofacial Implants* **11**, 450–455.

Hermann, J.S., Buser, D., Schenk, R.K., Higginbottom, F.L. & Cochran, D.L. (2000). Biologic width around titanium implants. A physiologically formed and stable dimension over time. *Clinical Oral Implants Research* **11**, 1–11.

Hermann, J.S., Buser, D., Schenk, R.K., Schoolfield, J.D. & Cochran, D.L. (2001a). Biologic width around one- and two-piece titanium implants. A histometric evaluation of unloaded nonsubmerged and submerged implants in the canine mandible. *Clinical Oral Implants Research* **12**, 559–571.

Hermann, J.S., Cochran, D.L., Nummikoski, P.V. & Buser, D. (1997). Crestal bone changes around titanium implants. A radiographic evaluation of unloaded nonsubmerged and submerged implants in the canine mandible. *Journal of Periodontology* **68**, 1117–1130.

Hermann, J.S., Schoolfield, J.D., Nummikoski, P.V., Buser, D., Schenk, R.K & Cochran, D.L. (2001b). Crestal bone changes around titanium implants: A methodological study comparing linear radiographic with histometric measurements. *International Journal of Oral and Maxillofacial Implants* **16**, 475–485.

Hess, D., Buser, D., Dietschi, D., Grossen, G., Schönenberger, A. & Belser, U.C. (1996). Aesthetischer Einzelzahnersatz mit Implantaten – ein "Team-Approach". *Implantologie* **3**, 245–256.

Hosny, M., Duyck, J., van Steenberghe, D. & Naert, I. (2000). Within-subject comparison between connected and nonconnected tooth-to-implant fixed partial prostheses: Up to 14 year follow-up study. *International Journal of Prosthodontics* **13**, 340–346.

Hultin, M., Gustafsson, A. & Klinge, B. (2000). Long-term evaluation of osseointegrated dental implants in the treatment of partially edentulous patients. *Journal of Clinical Periodontology* **27**, 128–133.

Hürzeler, M.B., Quinones, C.R. & Strub, J.R. (1994). Advanced surgical and prosthetic management of the anterior single tooth osseointegrated implant: a case presentation. *Practical Periodontics and Aesthetic Dentistry* **6**, 13–21.

Jaggers, A., Simons, A.M. & Badr, S.E. (1993). Abutment selection for anterior single tooth replacement. A clinical report. *Journal of Prosthetic Dentistry* **69**, 133–135.

Jansen, C.E. & Weisgold, A. (1995). Presurgical treatment planning for the anterior single-tooth implant restoration. *Compendium of Continuing Education in Dentistry* **16**, 746–764.

Jemt, T. (1999). Restoring the gingival contour by means of provisional resin crowns after single-implant treatment. *International Journal of Periodontics and Restorative Dentistry* **19**, 21–29.

Jemt, T., Heath, M.R., Johns, R.B., McNamara, D.C., van Steenberghe, D. & Watson, R.M. (1996). A 5-year prospective multicenter follow-up report on overdentures supported by osseointegrated implants. *International Journal of Oral and Maxillofacial Implants* **11**, 291–298.

Jensen, J., Joss, A. & Lang, N.P. (1999). The smile line of different ethnic groups depending on age and gender. *Acta Medicinae Dentium Helvetica* **4**, 38–46.

Johnson, R.H. & Persson, G.R. (2001). A 3-year prospective study of a single-tooth implant – prosthodontic complications. *International Journal of Prosthodontics* **14**, 183–189.

Keller, W., Brägger, U. & Mombelli, A. (1998). Peri-implant microflora of implants with cemented and screw retained suprastructures. *Clinical Oral Implants Research* **9**, 209–217.

Kemppainen, P., Eskola, S. & Ylipaavalniemi, P. (1997). A comparative prospective clinical study of two single-tooth implants: a preliminary report of 102 implants. *Journal of Prosthetic Dentistry* **77**, 382–387.

Khayat, P., Nader, N. & Exbrayat, P. (1995). Single tooth replacement using a one-piece screw-retained restoration. *Practical Periodontics and Aesthetic Dentistry* **7**, 61–69.

Kiener, P., Oetterli, M., Mericske, E. & Mericske-Stern, R. (2001). Effectiveness of maxillary overdentures supported by implants: maintenance and prosthetic complications. *International Journal of Prosthodontics* **14**, 133–140.

Kois, J.C. (1996). The restorative-periodontal interface: biological parameters. *Periodontology 2000* **11**, 29–38.

Kokich, V.G. (1996). Esthetics: the orthodontic-periodontic restorative connection. *Seminars in Orthodontics* **2**, 21–30.

Kokich, V.G. & Spear, F.M. (1997). Guidelines for managing the orthodontic-restorative patient. *Seminars in Orthodontics* **3**, 3–20.

Krenmair, G., Schmidinger, S. & Waldenberger, O. (2002). Single-tooth replacement with the Frialit-2 System: A retrospective clinical analysis of 146 implants. *International Journal of Oral and Maxillofacial Implants* **17**, 78–85.

Landsberg, C.J. & Bichacho, N. (1994). A modified surgical/prosthetic approach for an optimal single implant supported crown. Part I: The socket seal surgery. *Practical Periodontics and Aesthetic Dentistry* **6**, 11–17.

Laney, W.R., Jemt, T., Harris, D., Henry, P.J., Krogh, P.H.J., Polizzi, G., Zarb, G.A. & Herrmann, I. (1994). Osseointegrated implants for single-tooth replacement: progress report from a multicenter prospective study after 3 years. *International Journal of Oral and Maxillofacial Implants* **9**, 49–54.

Lang, N.P., Wilson, T. & Corbet, E.F. (2000). Biological complications with dental implants: their prevention, diagnosis and treatment. *Clinical Oral Implants Research* **11** (Suppl I), 146–155.

Lekholm, U., Gunne, J., Henry, P., Higuchi, K., Linden, U., Bergstrom, C. & van Steenberghe, D. (1999). Survival of the Brånemark implant in partially edentulous jaws: a 10-year prospective multicenter study. *International Journal of Oral and Maxillofacial Implants* **14**, 639–645.

Leonhardt, Å., Gröndahl, K., Bergström, C. & Lekholm, U. (2002). Long-term follow-up of osseointegrated titanium implants using clinical, radiographic and microbiological parameters. *Clinical Oral Implants Research* **13**, 127–132.

Levine, R.A., Clem, D.S., Wilson, T.G., Higginbottom, F. & Saunders, S.L. (1997). A multicenter retrospective analysis of the ITI implant system used for single-tooth replacements: preliminary results at 6 or more months of loading. *International Journal of Oral and Maxillofacial Implants* **12**, 237–242.

Lewis, S. (1995). Anterior single-tooth implant restorations. *International Journal of Periodontics and Restorative Dentistry* **15**, 30–41.

Lindh, T., Gunne, J., Tillberg, A. & Molin, M. (1998). A meta-analysis of implants in partial edentulism. *Clinical Oral Implants Research* **9**, 80–90.

Lindhe, J. & Berglundh, T. (1998). The interface between the mucosa and the implant. *Periodontology 2000* **17**, 47–53.

Lindqvist, L.W., Carlsson, G.E. & Jemt, T. (1996). A prospective 15-year follow-up study of mandibular fixed prostheses supported by osseointegrated implants. Clinical results and marginal bone loss. *Clinical Oral Implants Research* **7**, 329–336.

Magne, P. & Belser, U.C. (2002). *Bonded Porcelain Restorations in the Anterior Dentition. A Biomimetic Approach.* Chicago/Berlin: Quintessence Books.

Magne, P., Magne, M. & Belser, U.C. (1993a). Natural and restorative oral esthetics. Part I: Rationale and basic strategies for successful esthetic rehabilitations. *Journal of Esthetic Dentistry* **5**, 161–173.

Magne, P., Magne, M. & Belser, U.C. (1993b). Natural and restorative oral esthetics. Part II: Esthetic treatment modalities. *Journal of Esthetic Dentistry* **5**, 239–246.

Magne, P., Magne, M. & Belser, U.C. (1994). Natural and restorative oral esthetics. Part III: Fixed partial dentures. *Journal of Esthetic Dentistry* **6**, 15–22.

Magne, P., Magne, M. & Belser, U.C. (1996). The diagnostic template: a key element to the comprehensive esthetic treatment concept. *International Journal of Periodontics and Restorative Dentistry* **16**, 561–569.

Marchack, C.B. (1996). A custom titanium abutment for the anterior single-tooth implant. *Journal of Prosthetic Dentistry* **76**, 288–291.

Mecall, R.A. & Rosenfeld, A.L. (1996). Influence of residual ridge resorption pattern on fixture placement and tooth position. Part III: Presurgical assessment of ridge augmentation requirements. *International Journal of Periodontics and Restorative Dentistry* **16**, 322–337.

Mengel, R., Schröder, T. & Flores-de-Jacoby, L. (2001). Osseointegrated implants in patients treated for generalized chronic periodontitis and generalized aggressive periodontitis: 3- and 5-year results of a prospective long-term study. *Journal of Periodontology* **72**, 977–989.

Mericske-Stern, R. (1998). Treatment outcomes with implant-supported overdentures: clinical considerations. *Journal of Prosthetic Dentistry* **79**, 66–73.

Mericske-Stern, R., Grütter, L., Rösch, R. & Mericske, E. (2001). Clinical evaluation and prosthetic complications of single tooth replacement by non submerged implants. *Clinical Oral Implants Research* **12**, 309–318.

Nathanson, D. (1991). Current developments in esthetic dentistry. *Current Opinions in Dentistry* **1**, 206–211.

Neale, D. & Chee, W.W. (1994). Development of implant soft tissue emergence profile: a technique. *Journal of Prosthetic Dentistry* **71**, 364–368.

Norton, M.R. (1998). Marginal bone levels at single tooth implants with a conical fixture design. The influence of surface macro- and microstructure. *Clinical Oral Implants Research* **9**, 91–99.

Oetterli, M., Kiener, P. & Mericske-Stern, R. (2001). A longitudinal study on mandibular implants supporting an overdenture: The influence of retention mechanism and anatomic-prosthetic variables on periimplant parameters. *International Journal of Prosthodontics* **14**, 536–542.

Palmer, R.M., Smith, B.J., Palmer, P.J. & Floyd, P.D. (1997). A prospective study of Astra single tooth implants. *Clinical Oral Implants Research* **8**, 173–179.

Parel, S.M. & Sullivan, D.Y. (1989). *Esthetics and Osseointegration*. Dallas, TX: Taylor Publishing.

Price, R.B.T. & Price, D.E. (1999). Esthetic restoration of a single-tooth dental implant using a subepithelial connective tissue graft: a case report with 3-year follow-up. *International Journal of Periodontics and Restorative Dentistry* **19**, 93–101.

Priest, G.F. (1996). Failure rates of restorations for single-tooth replacement. *International Journal of Prosthodontics* **9**, 38–45.

Romeo, E., Chiapasco, M., Ghisolfi, M. & Vogel, G. (2002). Long-term clinical effectiveness of oral implants in the treatment of partial edentulism. Seven-year life table analysis of a prospective study with ITI® Dental Implant System used for single-tooth restorations. *Clinical Oral Implants Research* **13**, 133–143.

Rüfenacht, C.R. (1990). *Fundamentals of Esthetics*. Carol Stream, IL: Quintessence Publishing Co.

Salama, H. & Salama, M. (1993). The role of orthodontic extrusive modeling in the enhancement of soft and hard tissue profiles prior to implant placement: a systematic approach to the management of extraction site defects. *International Journal of Periodontics and Restorative Dentistry* **13**, 312–334.

Salama, H., Salama, M. & Garber, D.A. (1995). Techniques for developing optimal peri-implant papillae within the esthetic zone. Part I, guided soft tissue augmentation: the three-stage approach. *Journal of Esthetic Dentistry* **7**, 3–9.

Salinas, T.J. & Sadan, A. (1998). Establishing soft tissue integration with natural tooth-shaped abutments. *Practical Periodontics and Aesthetic Dentistry* **10**, 35–42.

Schärer, P., Rinn, L.A. & Kopp, F.R. (eds). (1982). *Esthetic Guidelines for Restorative Dentistry*. Carol Stream, IL: Quintessence Publishing Co., Inc.

Scheller, H., Urgell, J.P., Kultje, C., Klineberg, I., Goldberg, P.V., Stevenson-Moore, P., Alonso, J.M., Schaller, M., Corria, R.M., Engquist, B., Toreskog, S., Kastenbaum, F. & Smith, C.R. (1998). A 5-year multicenter study on implant-supported single crown restorations. *International Journal of Oral and Maxillofacial Implants* **13**, 212–218.

Schmitt, A. & Zarb, G.A. (1993). The longitudinal clinical effectiveness of osseointegrated implants for single-tooth replacement. *International Journal of Prosthodontics* **6**, 197–202.

Seibert, J. & Lindhe, J. (1989). Esthetics and periodontal therapy. In: Lindhe, J., ed. *Textbook of Clinical Periodontology*, 2nd edn. Copenhagen: Munksgaard, pp. 477–514.

Spear, F.M., Mathews, D.M. & Kokich, V.G. (1997). Interdisciplinary management of single-tooth implants. *Seminars in Orthodontics* **3**, 45–72.

Studer, S., Pietrobon, N. & Wohlwend, A. (1994). Maxillary anterior single-tooth replacement: comparison of three treatment modalities. *Practical Periodontics and Aesthetic Dentistry* **6**, 51–62.

Sutter, F., Weber, H.P., Sorensen, J. & Belser, U.C. (1993). The new restorative concept of the ITI Dental Implant System: Design and engineering. *International Journal of Periodontics and Restorative Dentistry* **13**, 409–431.

Szmukler-Moncler, S., Piatelli, J.A., Favero, J.H. & Dubruille, J.H. (2000). Considerations preliminary to the application of early and immediate loading protocols in dental implantology. *Clinical Oral Implants Research* **11**, 12–25.

Tarnow, D.P., Cho, S.C. & Wallace, S.S. (2000). The effect of inter-implant distance on the height of inter-implant bone crest. *Journal of Periodontology* **71**, 546–549.

Tarnow, D.P. & Eskow, R.N. (1995). Considerations for single-unit esthetic implant restorations. *Compendium of Continuing Education in Dentistry* **16**, 778–788.

Tarnow, D.P., Magner, A.W. & Fletcher, P. (1992). The effect of the distance from the contact point to the crest of bone on the presence or absence of the interproximal dental papilla. *Journal of Periodontology* **63**, 995–996.

ten Bruggenkate, C.M., Asikainen, P., Foitzik, C., Krekeler, G. & Sutter, F. (1998). Short (6 mm) non-submerged dental implants: results of a multicenter clinical trial of 1–7 years. *International Journal of Oral and Maxillofacial Implants* **13**, 791–798.

Touati, B. (1995). Improving aesthetics of implant-supported restorations. *Practical Periodontics and Aesthetic Dentistry* **7**, 81–92.

Van Steenberghe, D., Quirynen, M. & Wallace, S.S. (1999). Survival and success rates with oral endosseous implants. In: Lang, N.P., Karring, T. & Lindhe, J., eds. *Proceedings of the 3rd European Workshop on Periodontology*. Berlin: Quintessence, pp. 242–254.

Vlassis, J.M., Lyzak, W.A. & Senn, C. (1993). Anterior aesthetic considerations for the placement and restoration of nonsubmerged endosseous implants. *Practical Periodontics and Aesthetic Dentistry* **5**, 19–27.

von Arx, T., Cochran, D.L., Hermann, J.S., Schenk, R.K. & Buser, D. (2001b). Lateral ridge augmentation using different bone fillers and barrier membrane application. A histologic and histomorphometric pilot study in the canine mandible. *Clinical Oral Implants Research* **12**, 260–269.

von Arx, T., Cochran, D.L., Hermann, J., Schenk, R.K., Higginbottom, F. & Buser, D. (2001a). Lateral ridge augmentation and implant placement: An experimental study evaluating implant osseointegration in different augmentation materials in the canine mandible. *International Journal of Oral and Maxillofacial Implants* **16**, 343–354.

Walther, W., Klemke, J., Wörle, M. & Heners, M. (1996). Implant-supported single-tooth replacements: risk of implant and prosthesis failure. *Journal of Oral Implantology* **22**, 236–239.

Weber, H.P., Crohin, C.C. & Fiorellini, J.P. (2000). A 5-year prospective clinical and radiographic study of non-submerged dental implants. *Clinical Oral Implants Research* **11**, 144–153.

Wismeijer, D., van Waas, M.A.J., Mulder, J., Vermeeren, I.J.F. & Kalk, W. (1999). Clinical and radiological results of patients treated with three treatment modalities for overdentures on implants of the ITI dental implant system. A randomised controlled clinical trial. *Clinical Oral Implants Research* **10**, 297–306.

Wyatt, C.L. & Zarb, G.A. (1998). Treatment outcomes of patients with implant-supported fixed partial prostheses. *International Journal of Oral and Maxillofacial Implants* **13**, 204–211.

Zarb, G.A. & Schmitt, A. (1993). The longitudinal clinical effectiveness of osseointegrated dental implants in anterior partially edentulous patients. *International Journal of Prosthodontics* **6**, 180–188.

Zitzmann, N.U., Schärer, P. & Marinello, C.P. (2001). Long-term results of implants treated with guided bone regeneration: A 5-year prospective study. *International Journal of Oral and Maxillofacial Implants* **16**, 355–366.

Chapter 54

Implants in the Posterior Dentition

Urs C. Belser, Daniel Buser, and Jean-Pierre Bernard

Basic concepts, 1175
  General considerations, 1175
  Indications for implant restorations in the load carrying part of the dentition, 1177
  Controversial issues, 1180
Restoration of the distally shortened arch with fixed implant-supported prostheses, 1180
  Number, size, and distribution of implants, 1180
  Implant restorations with cantilever units, 1182
  Combination of implant and natural tooth support, 1183
  Sites with extended horizontal bone volume deficiencies and/or anterior sinus floor proximity, 1184
Multiple-unit tooth-bound posterior implant restorations, 1187
  Number, size, and distribution of implants, 1187
  Splinted versus single-unit restorations of multiple adjacent posterior implants, 1189

Posterior single-tooth replacement, 1191
  Premolar-size single-tooth restorations, 1191
  Molar-size single-tooth restorations, 1191
  Sites with limited vertical bone volume, 1192
Clinical applications, 1193
  Screw-retained implant restorations, 1193
  Abutment-level impression versus implant shoulder-level impression, 1196
  Cemented multiple-unit posterior implant prostheses, 1197
  Angulated abutments, 1198
  High-strength all-ceramic implant restorations, 1199
  Orthodontic and occlusal considerations related to posterior implant therapy, 1200
Concluding remarks and perspectives, 1203
  Early and immediate fixed implant restorations, 1203

Basic concepts

General considerations

The overall favorable long-term survival and success rates reported in the recent literature for osseointegrated implants in the treatment of various types of edentulism (Brånemark *et al.* 1995; Jemt *et al.* 1996; Lindqvist *et al.* 1996; Buser *et al.* 1997, 1998b, 2002; Andersson *et al.* 1998; Eckert & Wollan 1998; Lindh *et al.* 1998; Mericske-Stern 1998; ten Bruggenkate *et al.* 1998; Wyatt & Zarb 1998; Gunne *et al.* 1999; Lekholm *et al.* 1999; Van Steenberghe *et al.* 1999; Wismeijer *et al.* 1999; Behneke *et al.* 2000; Hosny *et al.* 2000; Hultin *et al.* 2000; Weber *et al.* 2000; Boioli *et al.* 2001; Gomez-Roman *et al.* 2001; Kiener *et al.* 2001; Mengel *et al.* 2001; Oetterli *et al.* 2001; Zitzmann *et al.* 2001; Bernard & Belser 2002; Haas *et al.* 2002; Leonhardt *et al.* 2002; Romeo *et al.* 2002) permit consideration of dental implants as one of the reliable therapeutic modalities during the establishment of any prosthetic treatment plan. In numerous clinical situations implants can clearly contribute to a notable simplification of therapy, frequently enabling removable prostheses to be avoided, keeping it less invasive with respect to remaining tooth structure or rendering the treatment both more elegant and versatile as well as more predictable (Belser *et al.* 2000).

As part of a textbook focusing essentially on clinical periodontics, this chapter will address primarily implant therapy performed in the posterior segments of partially edentulous patients. In this context, the use of implants may often significantly reduce the inherent risk of a "borderline" conventional tooth-borne fixed prosthesis (e.g. compromised or missing "strategic" abutment teeth, long-span fixed partial dentures, cantilevers) by implementing the principle of segmentation. It is currently widely accepted that – in comparison with extended splinted prosthetic segments – small ones are preferable as they are easier to fabricate, generally provide improved "passive fit" and marginal fidelity, offer better access for the patient's oral hygiene, and ultimately are less complicated to handle where there is need for re-intervention. When it comes to treatment planning in general, and to the choice *implant versus tooth-borne fixed partial denture (FPD) versus tooth* in particular, the related decision-making criteria should be essentially derived from scientific evidence and objective prosthetically oriented risk assessment in the broad

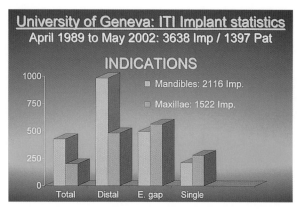

Fig. 54-1 University of Geneva implant statistics, 1989–2002. Indications.

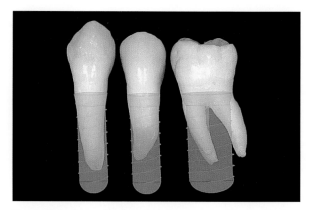

Fig. 54-3 Different implant diameters are available for the replacement of posterior teeth.

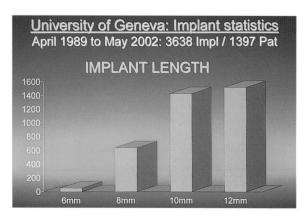

Fig. 54-2 University of Geneva implant statistics, 1989–2002. Implant length distribution.

sense, including additional parameters such as simplicity, cost effectiveness, and quality of life. Beyond any doubt, the advent of osseointegration has had a fundamental impact on the therapeutic approach and strategies implemented today in the field of prosthetic rehabilitation of the compromised posterior dentition. The implant statistics of the University of Geneva School of Dental Medicine, for example, reveal that from April 1989 until May 2002 more than 3600 implants of 6–12 mm length were inserted in about 1400 patients presenting with different types of edentulism (Figs. 54-1, 54-2). This treatment method is increasingly applied worldwide and has had a tremendous influence on traditional prosthodontic attitudes (Beumer *et al.* 1993; Zarb & Schmitt 1995; Tarnow *et al.* 1997; Zitzmann & Marinello 1999; Belser *et al.* 2000; Schwarz-Arad & Dolev 2000; Brägger *et al.* 2001; Deporter *et al.* 2001; Zitzmann & Marinello 2002). Since most of the established dental implant systems today comprise a wide range of mostly screw-type implants with different diameters and dimensions to replace missing premolars and molars (Fig. 54-3), the versatility of implant therapy in the load-carrying part of the dentition of partially edentulous patients has been significantly enhanced.

Numerous other indications have been added to the so-called classical indications for the use of implants, i.e. severely atrophied edentulous jaws, missing teeth in otherwise intact dentitions (congenitally missing teeth; tooth loss due to trauma or due to a localized endodontic/restorative/periodontal complication or failure), and the distally shortened dental arch (particularly when premolars are missing). Among these other indications one should mention all the strategies aiming at either reducing the prosthodontic risk in general or rendering the treatment simpler and more cost effective. Virtually no limits for the placement of implants seem to exist any more owing, for example, to advanced bone augmentation techniques, comprising anterior sinus floor elevation and distraction osteogenesis (Buser *et al.* 1993, 1995, 1996, 1998a, 2002; Chiapasco *et al.* 1999, 2001a; Buser & von Arx 2000; Simion *et al.* 2001; von Arx *et al.* 2001a,b).

When it comes to the technique of placing implants in the posterior segments of the jaws, a one-step non-submerged surgical protocol can be associated with notable advantages. On the one hand, healing of the peri-implant soft tissues occurs simultaneously with osseointegration, and on the other hand the location of the junction between the implant shoulder and the secondary components is normally positioned close to the mucosal surface. It is ultimately the position of this junction which determines the apical migration of the peri-implant epithelium and the crestal bone level, once the so-called biologic width has been established (Abrahamson *et al.* 1997; Hermann *et al.* 1997, 2000, 2001a,b; Lindhe & Berglundh 1998; Engquist *et al.* 2002; Wyatt & Zarb 2002). Positioning of the transition between implant shoulder and secondary components at the level of the mucosa rather than at the crestal bone also represents a biomechanical advantage, as it contributes to the reduction of the lever effect and resulting bending moments acting on the junction between implant and suprastructure. This is clinically relevant, as one should be aware of the existence of an increasing body of evidence reporting technical complications, such as loosening/fracture of screws or fracture of components/veneers, related to implant-supported prosthetic suprastructures (Lundgren & Laurell 1994; Wie 1995;

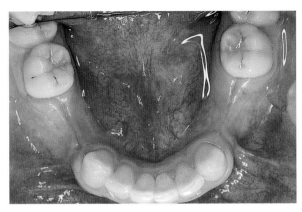

Fig. 54-4 Occlusal view of the mandible of a 22-year-old male patient. All premolars are congenitally missing, the remainder of the dentition is intact.

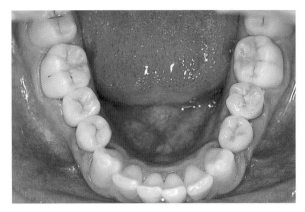

Fig. 54-5 Final view after insertion of four implants, restored with cemented metal–ceramic suprastructures.

Hebel & Gajjar 1997; Rangert *et al.* 1997; Bosse & Taylor 1998; Glantz & Nilner 1998; Taylor 1998; Brägger 1999; Goodacre *et al.* 1999; Isidor 1999; Keith 1999; Schwarz 2000; Johnson & Persson 2001). Besides mechanical types of complications, a number of other conditions that are rather biologic in nature, for example peri-implantitis, are reported in the recent literature (Ellegaard *et al.* 1997a,b; Ellen 1998; Lang *et al.* 2000; Brägger *et al.* 2001; Quirynen *et al.* 2001, 2002). As these are addressed in detail in another chapter, we will only focus on aspects related to fixed posterior implant restoration design and maintenance.

It is the aim of this chapter to present clinically oriented guidelines and procedures for implant therapy of various types of edentulism located in the load-carrying part of the dentition, addressing primarily the partially dentate patient and mainly focusing on fixed implant-supported prostheses.

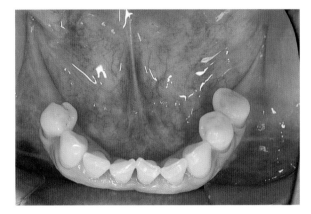

Fig. 54-6 Bilaterally distally shortened dental arch in the mandible of a 66-year-old female patient.

Indications for implant restorations in the load carrying part of the dentition

When it comes to partial edentulism in the posterior segments of the jaws, implants are increasingly used either to preserve sound mineralized tooth structure or to avoid removable partial dentures (RPDs) and high-risk conventional fixed partial dentures (FPDs). This includes situations with missing teeth in otherwise intact dentitions (Figs. 54-4, 54-5), the distally shortened dental arch (Figs. 54-6 to 54-8), extended edentulous segments, missing "strategic" tooth abutments, and structurally, endodontically or periodontally compromised potential abutment teeth (Table 54-1).

The rapid advance in terms of the broad utilization of dental implants is not exclusively based on the associated favorable long-term reports for this treatment modality. Other parameters such as purely "mechanical" advantages and the availability of prefabricated components and auxiliary parts, which in turn contribute notably to the simplification of the treatment, had a significant impact on current con-

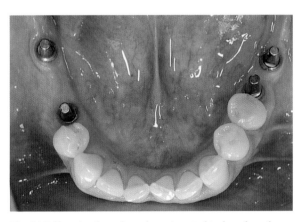

Fig. 54-7 Four implants have been inserted to lengthen the arch bilaterally to the region of the first molars.

cepts and strategies as well (Table 54-2). Furthermore, clinical decision making based on prosthetically oriented risk assessment (Table 54-3), frequently leads to the need for an increased number of abutments. The objective is to reduce the overall risk associated with a given prosthetic solution on the one hand, and to implement the principle of segmenting on the other.

A representative clinical example is given in Figs. 54-9 and 54-10. Instead of a conventional five-unit

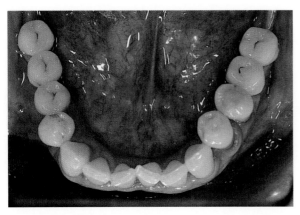

Fig. 54-8 Five premolar-sized metal–ceramic elements were used to restore the four implants.

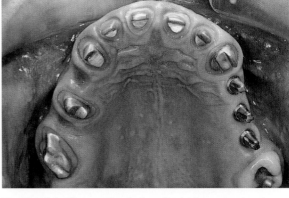

Fig. 54-9 Maxillary occlusal view displaying natural and implant abutments prior to the insertion of an extended porcelain-fused-to-metal restoration. In order to avoid a high-risk long-span FPD, three implants have been added in the left posterior segment.

Table 54-1 Indications for posterior implants

- Replacement of missing teeth in intact dentitions (e.g. congenitally missing premolars), i.e. preservation of tooth structure
- Avoidance of removable partial dentures (RPDs)
- Increase of the number of abutments:
  ° Reduction of the prosthetic risk
  ° Application of the principle of segmenting
  ° Ease of eventual reinterventions
- Maintenance of pre-existing crowns and FPDs
- Following prosthetic complications and failures

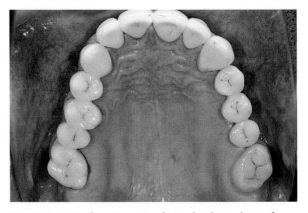

Fig. 54-10 A similar restorative design has been chosen for both natural and implant-supported metal–ceramic suprastructures.

Table 54-2 Impact of dental implants related to the treatment of posterior partial edentulism

- Favorable overall long-term results
- Preservation of mineralized tooth structure
- "Mechanical" advantages:
  ° Commercially pure (c.p.) titanium (biocompatibility, mechanical properties, no risk for caries)
  ° Reproducible, prefabricated ("machined") primary, secondary and tertiary components and auxiliary parts
- Simplified clinical and laboratory protocols

Table 54-3 "High risk" conventional fixed partial dentures (FPDs)

- Long-span fixed partial bridges
- Cantilever units (mainly distal extensions)
- Missing "strategic" tooth abutments
- Structurally/periodontally/endodontically compromised tooth abutments
- Reduced interarch distance
- Presence of occlusal parafunctions/bruxism

FPD, replacing the missing maxillary left first and second premolars as well as the absent first molar, three implants have been inserted. This approach allowed the avoidance of a long-span bridge, a full coverage preparation of the second molar, and an associated surgical crown-lengthening procedure. The additional cost related to the three implants was justified by an overall reduced prosthodontic risk. The question about adequate number, size, and distribution of implants will be addressed later in this chapter. Prosthetically oriented risk assessment comprises the comprehensive evaluation of potential natural abutment teeth, including their structural, restorative, periodontal, and endodontic status. Several well documented treatment modalities are often possible to replace missing posterior teeth, so this objective evaluation is of primary importance and represents an ever increasing challenge to the clinician. This is illustrated by a maxillary posterior segment where both the first premolar and the first molar were missing (Figs. 54-11 to 54-14). The insertion of a five-unit tooth-borne FPD was discarded because of its too invasive nature related to the intact canine, and owing to a slightly questionable status of

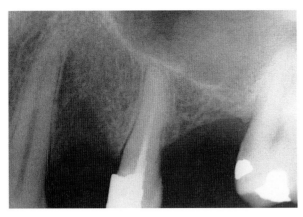

Fig. 54-11 Pre-operative radiograph of the left maxilla, revealing two missing dental elements. One should note in particular an intact canine, a structurally reduced second premolar, and an extended recessus of the sinus in the area of the missing first molar.

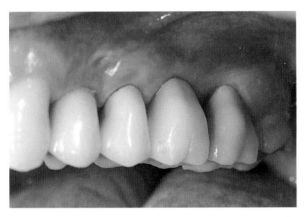

Fig. 54-12 Vestibular view of the prosthetic rehabilitation of the maxillary left quadrant: an implant-supported single-tooth restoration on the site of the first premolar, and a three-unit tooth-borne FPD to replace the missing first molar.

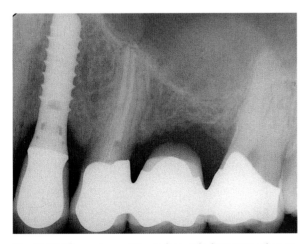

Fig. 54-13 The post-operative radiograph documents that an endodontic revision has been performed on the second premolar prior to its restoration with an adhesive carbon-fibre-post based build-up and a metal–ceramic crown (bridge retainer).

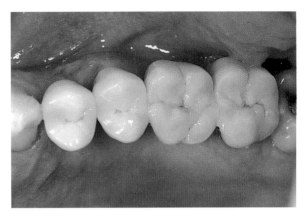

Fig. 54-14 An identical prosthetic design has been applied for both the implant-supported and the tooth-supported restoration.

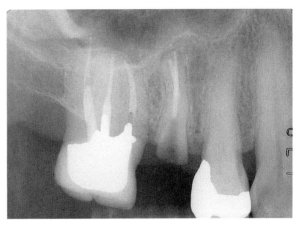

Fig. 54-15 Ad hoc radiograph of the upper right posterior sextant. One notes the presence of a structurally compromised second premolar. The treatment of that particular root would require build-up and crown lengthening (margin exposure, creation of an adequate ferrule) which in turn would negatively affect the adjacent teeth.

the endodontically treated second premolar in view of its eventual use as so-called "peer-abutment". Finally, an implant has been placed at the site of the missing first premolar and subsequently restored with a single-unit restoration. As the proximity of the maxillary sinus at the location of the missing first molar would have required a grafting procedure to make an implant installation possible, a three-unit tooth-supported FPD was ultimately chosen, after having duly discussed the respective advantages and shortcomings with the patient. Having attributed a "strategic value" to the moderately compromised second premolar by using it as abutment of a short-span bridge, there was still a difficulty in consistently establishing clinical treatment plans that were fully based on scientific evidence.

Still under the influence of the high level of predictability and longevity reported for implant therapy, the clinician is currently not only pondering implant-borne restorations versus conventional FPDs, but increasingly implant versus maintaining a compromised tooth (Figs. 54-15, 54-16). In this

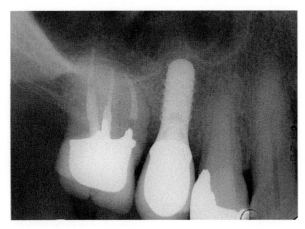

Fig. 54-16 The post-operative radiograph documents that the root of the second premolar has been replaced by a single-tooth implant restoration. In particular, the pre-existing metal–ceramic crown on the first molar could be maintained by this approach.

Table 54-4 Controversial issues related to posterior implant restorations

- Adequate number, size (length/diameter), configuration and distribution of implants
- Cemented versus screw-retained (transocclusal/transverse screw retention)
- Single units versus splinted adjacent implant restorations
- Longest possible versus shorter implants
- Impact of implant axis
- Optimal implant shoulder sink depth
- Minimal ratio between implant length and suprastructure height
- Combination of natural teeth and implants in the same restoration
- Design of the optimal abutment-to-implant connection
- Implant-specific occlusal concepts, including occluding restorative materials, non-axial loading, type of guidance during mandibular excursions
- Healing times prior to functional loading (immediate/early/delayed)
- Significance of offset/staggered implant positioning

particular clinical case, the evaluation focused on whether or not it was objectively opportune to restore the structurally compromised root of a maxillary second premolar. This would have required – after elimination of the decayed dentin – a surgical crown-lengthening procedure to create access to the margin, which in turn would have included the risk for an adverse effect (furcation proximity of the adjacent first molar) on the neighboring teeth. Furthermore, a three-unit FPD was out of the question for obvious reasons. Based on this rationale and in the context of a more comprehensive analysis of the situation, it was finally decided to extract a *per se* treatable root and to replace it by an implant. One should never forget, however, that this trend to consider, under certain circumstances, an implant as a better solution than "acrobatically" treating a severely compromised tooth, calls for well defined evidence-based respective criteria and represents a non-negligible ethical responsibility for the clinician.

Controversial issues

Despite the ever-growing body of scientific evidence indicating that implant therapy in the partially eden-tulous patient is an overall highly predictable treatment modality, several conceptional issues remain controversial to date (Table 54-4). These controversial issues include open questions addressing adequate number, size, and distribution of implants for optimal therapy of a given type and configuration of partial edentulism, as well as parameters related to occlusion and occlusal materials, to implant axis, to the minimal acceptable ratio between suprastructure height and implant length, and – last but not least – related to questions focusing more specifically on the mechanical aspects and requirements of posterior implant prosthodontics. Among these, the kinds of connection between implant and abutment have to be mentioned in particular. Most of these questions

will be discussed in the remainder of this chapter, at length where possible and appropriate, or more superficially when solid information is missing or when the topic is more adequately covered by other authors in this book.

Restoration of the distally shortened arch with fixed implant-supported prostheses

As pointed out earlier in this chapter, from 1989–2002 the distally shortened arch represented the most frequent indication for the use of implants at the University of Geneva School of Dental Medicine. In fact, out of a total of 3638 implants, almost 1500 were placed in distally shortened arches, with close to 1000 implants inserted in the mandible and about 500 in the posterior maxilla (Fig. 54-1). Implants were primarily used when premolars were also missing. Whenever possible, the adopted treatment strategy consisted of restoring the shortened dental arch to the region of the first molars. Occasionally, implant therapy was restricted to the premolar area, according to the principles of the well established premolar occlusion concept, or extended to the second molar area if an antagonistic contact had to be established for an opposing natural second molar.

Number, size, and distribution of implants

It is still unclear to date how many implants of which dimension at which location are required to optimally rehabilitate a given edentulous segment in the load-carrying part of the dentition. Several different respective recommendations and related strategies are currently in use, mostly derived from traditional prosthodontic experience and attitudes, and based on so-called clinical experience and common sense

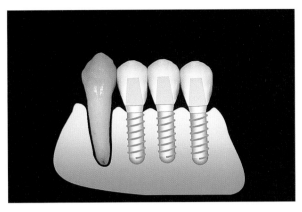

Fig. 54-17 Schematic representation of the distally shortened dental arch. One therapeutic option consists of replacing each missing occlusal unit up to the first molar area with an implant.

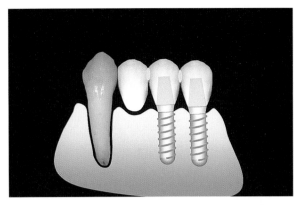

Fig. 54-19 In a case of an inadequate bone volume in the area of the missing first premolar, the placement of two distal implants may be considered, leading to a three-unit suprastructure with a mesial cantilever.

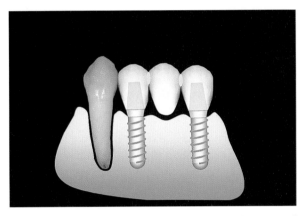

Fig. 54-18 An alternative option would be the replacement of the three missing occlusal units by two implants to support a three-unit suprastructure with a central pontic.

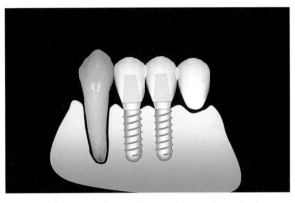

Fig. 54-20 In a case of an inadequate bone volume in the area of the missing first molar, the placement of two mesial implants may be considered, leading to a three-unit suprastructure with a distal cantilever.

rather than on solid scientific evidence. In defense of the situation one should be aware, however, that it is often difficult to design and carry out randomized clinical trials evaluating exclusively and without interference one specific parameter of conceptual relevance.

In a situation where the canine is the most distal remaining tooth of a dental arch, at least five different options can be taken into consideration if one plans to replace the missing teeth up to the first molar area (Figs. 54-17 to 54-21). These include the replacement of each missing occlusal unit by one implant (Fig. 54-17), a mesial and a distal implant to support a three-unit FPD with a central pontic (Fig. 54-18), two distal implants to permit the insertion of a three-unit FPD with a mesial cantilever (Fig. 54-19), two mesial implants to sustain a three-unit FPD with a distal cantilever (Fig. 54-20) and, finally, only one distally inserted implant in view of a four-unit FPD combining implant and natural tooth support (Fig. 54-21).

As far as the recommendation to use premolar-sized units for implant-borne posterior FPDs is concerned, it has proven its practical validity in more than 10 years of clinical experience (Buser *et al*. 1997;

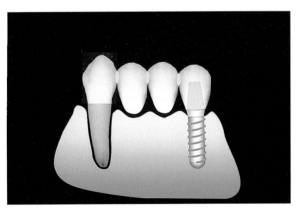

Fig. 54-21 In a case of inadequate bone volume in the area of the two missing premolars, the placement of a distal implant may be considered, leading to a four-unit suprastructure with a mixed (tooth and implant) support.

Bernard & Belser 2002). In fact, a crown featuring a mesio-distal diameter of 7–8 mm at its occlusal surface allows the optimal generation of a harmonious axial profile, gradually emerging from the standard implant shoulder (diameter 4–5 mm on average) to the maximum circumference. In addition, the

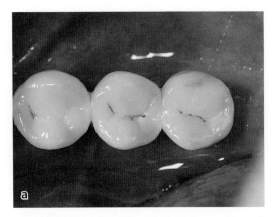 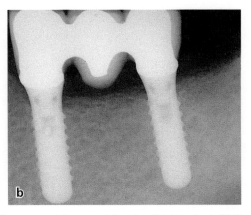

Fig. 54-22 (a) Occlusal view of a cemented three-unit metal–ceramic FPD, supported by a mesial and a distal implant. (b) The corresponding 3-year follow-up radiograph confirms stable conditions at the implant to bone interface of the two 12 mm solid screw implants.

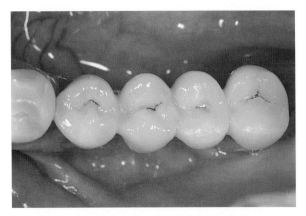 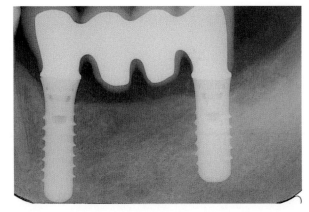

Fig. 54-23 Occlusal view of a cemented four-unit metal–ceramic FPD supported by a mesial and a distal implant.

Fig. 54-24 The related 2-year follow-up radiograph documents that at the distal site a 10 mm solid screw implant with an increased diameter ("wide-body implant") has been used.

width of the occlusal table is confined, thereby limiting the risk for unfavorable bending moments to the implant–abutment–suprastructure complex (Belser *et al*. 2000).

Based on an increasing body of scientific evidence, most clinicians' first choice represents the mesial and distal implant and the respective FPD with the central pontic (Fig. 54-22). Prospective long-term multicenter data (Buser *et al*. 1997; Bernard & Belser 2002) have confirmed the efficacy and predictability of this specific modality. In fact, it permits the defined treatment objective with a minimal number of implants and associated costs. Although presently still lacking formal evidence at the level of prospectively documented, randomized clinical trials, it appears from clinical experience that the use of two implants to support a four-unit FPD with two central pontics (Figs. 54-23, 54-24) may be adequate in certain clinical situations. Clinicians tend to use this approach in the presence of favorable bone conditions, permitting standard-size or wide-diameter implants with appropriate length (i.e. 8 mm or more).

If the alveolar bone crest dimension is also sufficient in an oro-facial direction, the utilization of wide-diameter/wide-platform implants is preferred. Due to their increased dimensions a more adapted

suprastructure volume and improved axial emergence profile of the implant restoration – when compared to a so-called premolar unit – can be achieved in the molar area (Figs. 54-25 to 54-28). By this token the intercuspation with an opposing natural molar is also facilitated.

Implant restorations with cantilever units

There is strong evidence in the relevant dental literature that cantilever units – in particular distal extensions – of conventional tooth-borne FPDs are associated with a significantly higher complication rate when compared to FPDs featuring a mesial and a distal abutment and a central pontic. Respective failure rates could be attributed to decisive factors such as non-vital abutment teeth as well as specific occlusal conditions such as a reduced interarch distance and/or occlusal parafunctions (Glantz & Nilner 1998). These authors concluded in their review of the current relevant literature that risks were lower for mechanical failures with cantilevered implant-borne reconstructions than with comparable conventional fixed situations. Risks, however, do exist. As loss of

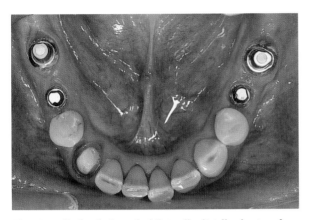

Fig. 54-25 Occlusal view of a bilaterally distally shortened mandibular arch. Two implants have been placed on either side to restore the arch to the area of the first molars. The two distal implants feature an increased diameter, better suited for the replacement of a missing molar.

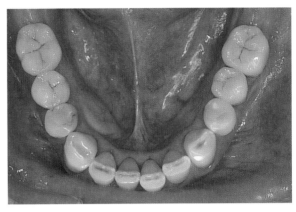

Fig. 54-28 The respective clinical view confirms an acceptable integration of the four implant restorations in the existing natural dentition.

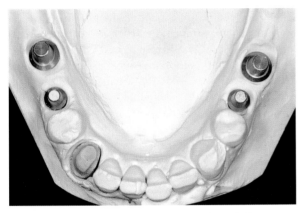

Fig. 54-26 The master model comprises color-coded aluminum laboratory analogues at the implant sites, facilitating the technician's work in view of the suprastructure fabrication. This is in contrast to the site of the prepared natural abutment.

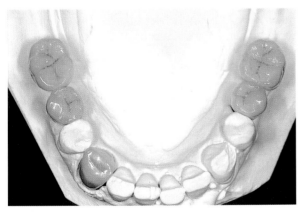

Fig. 54-27 Once the metal–ceramic restorations are completed, no noticeable design difference between implant-supported and tooth-supported suprastructures is apparent.

retention, which was one of the frequent complications encountered on conventional cantilevered prostheses, can easily be prevented when it comes to implant-supported restorations of this type, the latter seem to be a viable alternative in cases where the local alveolar bone crest conditions do not allow the insertion of an implant at the most favorable location. In such situations the clinician has to ponder whether a bone augmentation procedure can be objectively justified or if the risk for complications of a more simple, straightforward approach can be considered low.

The 6-year clinical and radiographic follow-up of a three-unit FPD featuring a mesial cantilever is presented in Figs. 54-29 and 54-30.

Combination of implant and natural tooth support

There is general agreement that, from a purely scientific point of view, the combination of implants and natural teeth to support a common FPD is feasible. Clinical studies reporting prospectively documented long-term data did not show adverse effects of splinting teeth to implants (Olsson *et al*. 1995; Gunne *et al*. 1997, 1999; Hosny *et al*. 2000; Lindh *et al*. 2001; Naert *et al*. 2001a,b; Tangerud *et al*. 2002). The issue of connecting implants and teeth by means of rigid or non-rigid connectors, however, remains controversial to date, but intrusion of natural roots has been reported in the literature as a potential hazard of non-rigid connection (Sheets & Earthman 1993). Most of the recently published respective literature reviews conclude with the general clinical recommendation that one should avoid, whenever possible, the direct combination of implants and teeth as it may frequently lead to a more complicated type of prosthesis. If there is no viable alternative available, a rigid type of connection is preferred to prevent an eventual intrusion of the involved abutment teeth (Lundgren & Laurell 1994; Gross & Laufer 1997).

Furthermore, it has been demonstrated that despite the fundamental difference between an osseointe-

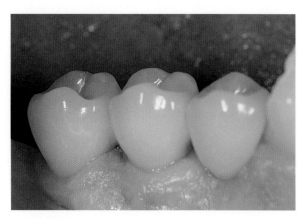

Fig. 54-29 Six-year clinical follow-up view of a mandibular three-unit FPD supported by two distal implants.

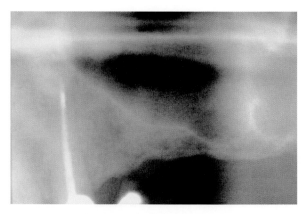

Fig. 54-31 Initial radiograph of the maxillary left posterior segment of a 67-year-old male patient. The canine represents the most distal remaining tooth element. Note the marked extension of the anterior recessus of the sinus.

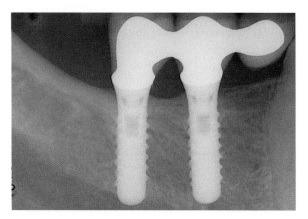

Fig. 54-30 The 6-year radiograph displays stable bony conditions around the two implants supporting a cemented suprastructure with a premolar-sized mesial cantilever unit.

grated implant and a tooth surrounded by a periodontal ligament, the assumption that when these two structures are combined, the entire occlusal load will ultimately go to the implant and hence create an unfavorable "cantilever-type" situation, is not valid from a scientific point of view (Richter, Isidor, Brägger). In fact, under normal function, such as during mastication, the tooth abutment is similarly load-bearing. This may change, however, during severe occlusal parafunctions, like nocturnal bruxism.

Sites with extended horizontal bone volume deficiencies and/or anterior sinus floor proximity

It is not infrequent that distally shortened dental arches do not feature an adequate local bone volume at the prospective implant sites. This may refer to bone height, bone width, alveolar bone crest axis or to the vicinity of noble structures such as the mandibular alveolar nerve canal or the anterior part of the maxillary sinus. Often a combination of several of the mentioned limitations is encountered. As implant insertion is clearly a three-dimensional

surgical and restorative procedure on the one hand, and as "restoration-driven" rather than "bone-driven" implant placement is widely recommended on the other hand, a meticulous presurgical site analysis – based on the envisioned treatment objective – is of primary importance. In order to keep the treatment as easy and finally also as cost-effective as possible, one should comprehensively evaluate whether a minor deviation from the ideal implant position could be considered acceptable, i.e. not leading to a compromise which might adversely affect predictability, longevity, and/or subjective comfort. This approach may still permit a professionally defendable result in some cases, but without a complexity of treatment that would be difficult to bear by some patients.

Advanced invasive procedures like lateral bone augmentation, anterior sinus floor elevation, alveolar ridge splitting or distraction osteogenesis, require a high level of skills and respective experience and hence should only be deployed if the relation between benefit and risk/cost is soundly balanced (Buser *et al.* 1993, 1995, 1996, 1999, 2002; Chiapasco *et al.* 1999, 2001a; Simion *et al.* 2001; von Arx *et al.* 2001a,b; Zitzmann *et al.* 2001).

In this specific context, a complex implant treatment of a 67-year-old male patient whose most distal remaining tooth in the left maxilla was an endodontically treated canine, is shown in Figs. 54-31 to 54-44. Pre-operative diagnosis revealed the necessity to perform – according to a staged approach – first a combined lateral bone augmentation procedure and anterior sinus floor elevation and, after a 6 month healing period, the insertion of implants. For the sinus floor elevation the so-called "trap-door" technique was used and the created space grafted with autogenous bone chips and BioOss®. The lateral bone augmentation comprised the fixation of a large block graft in the area of the first premolar. After application of an e-PTFE barrier membrane, primary wound closure was achieved by sectioning of the periosteum of the respective mucoperiosteal flap. This often leads

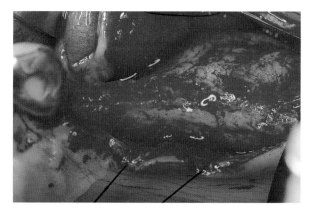

Fig. 54-32 After elevation of a mucoperiosteal flap, an insufficient horizontal bone volume in the region of the premolars becomes apparent.

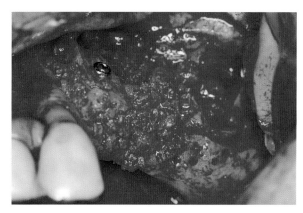

Fig. 54-35 The lateral bone augmentation procedure is completed by adding a combination of autogenous bone chips, bone slurry, and BioOss®.

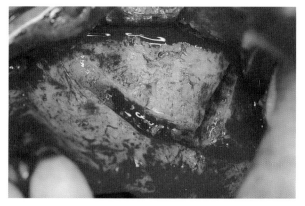

Fig. 54-33 In view of an anterior sinus floor elevation procedure, the first step for a respective osteotomy is performed. Attention is given not to perforate the Schneiderian membrane.

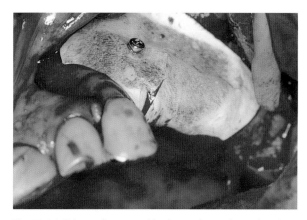

Fig. 54-36 Prior to flap repositioning and suturing, a barrier membrane is applied.

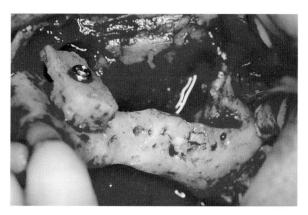

Fig. 54-34 After the so-called "trap-door" procedure in the region of the maxillary sinus, an autogenous bone block graft, harvested from the patient's retromolar area, is positioned and then immobilized by a fixation screw at the location of the missing first premolar.

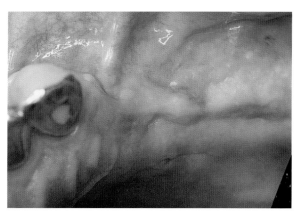

Fig. 54-37 One month after primary wound closure and uneventful healing, the involved soft tissues have recovered their normal appearance.

to a lack of attached keratinized mucosa on the vestibular aspect of the surgical site, which has to be subsequently corrected, most conveniently at the moment of implant placement. When it comes to sites that have been previously grafted, the majority of surgeons advocate inserting one implant per missing occlusal unit. This attitude appears to be based more on the reflection that the overall heaviness of the approach would largely justify this additional security and/or on the hypothesis that augmented bone may not have exactly the same "load-bearing" capacity as the pre-existing bone, than on irrefutable scientific evidence. Accordingly, three adjacent screw-type

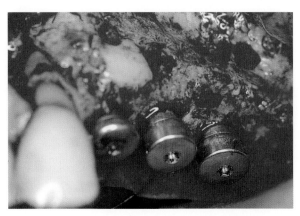

Fig. 54-38 Eight months following the combined anterior sinus floor elevation and lateral bone augmentation procedure, the site is reopened and three implants are inserted.

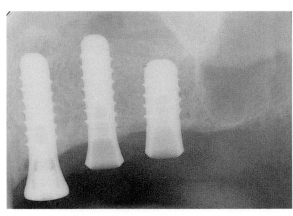

Fig. 54-41 The corresponding radiograph confirms successful osseointegration of the three implants that are mostly located in augmented bone.

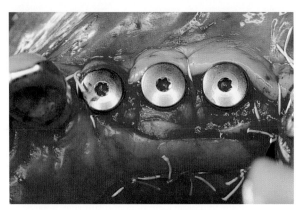

Fig. 54-39 In order to increase the amount of keratinized mucosa on the vestibular aspect of the implants, the flap is repositioned accordingly. The resulting deficiency on the palatal aspect is compensated for by means of a connective tissue being part of the partial-thickness flap.

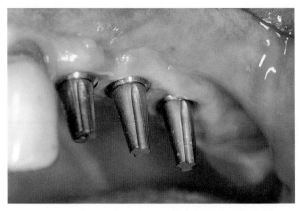

Fig. 54-42 In a case of implant shoulder location compatible with cementation, respective solid abutments are selected and tightened to 35 Ncm with a calibrated torque wrench.

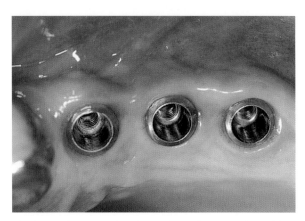

Fig. 54-40 Three months after implant placement, favorable peri-implant soft tissue conditions have been re-established.

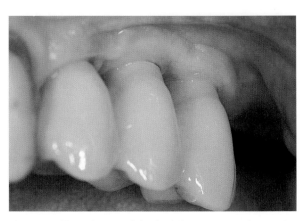

Fig. 54-43 Clinical view of the final three-unit metal–ceramic implant suprastructure, featuring a flat and continuous emergence profile and adequate access for inter-implant oral hygiene.

implants – the most distal one an increased-diameter titanium screw – had been placed and subsequently restored by a three-unit splinted metal-ceramic FPD (Figs. 54-38 to 54-44).

Results from a recently published longitudinal clinical study (Buser *et al.* 2002) on 40 consecutively enrolled patients, who were first treated with a lateral bone augmentation procedure and subsequently, in a second stage, received implants inserted in the previously augmented area. Implants could finally be placed as planned in all the treated sites, and a 97% success rate was revealed at the 5-year clinical and

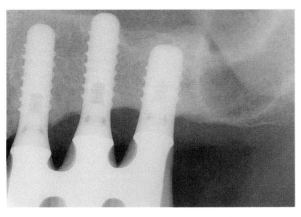

Fig. 54-44 The 4-year follow-up radiograph confirms stable conditions at the osseointegrated interface.

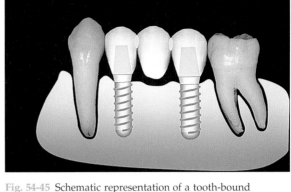

Fig. 54-45 Schematic representation of a tooth-bound posterior edentulous segment, restored by two implants and a three-unit FPD with a central pontic.

radiographic follow-up examination. It was thus concluded that lateral bone augmentation is indeed a predictable procedure and that implants subsequently inserted in augmented sites do have similar success rates to implants placed in comparable non-augmented sites.

Multiple-unit tooth-bound posterior implant restorations

Number, size, and distribution of implants

When it comes to implant therapy in extended posterior edentulous segments confined mesially and distally by remaining teeth, the question about optimal number, size, and distribution of implants has to be raised again. Among the key parameters to be addressed during the decision-making process are the mesio-distal dimension of the edentulous segment, the precise alveolar bone crest volume (including bone height and crest width in an orofacial direction), the opposing dentition (premolars or molars), interarch distance and specific occlusal parameters, as well as the periodontal, endodontic, and structural conditions of the neighboring teeth.

One feasible approach consists of segmenting the edentulous space in premolar-size units of approximately 7 mm of mesio-distal diameter at the level of the occlusal plane, and of approximately 5 mm at the prospective implant shoulder. On posterior locations, clinicians increasingly prefer a rather superficial implant shoulder location or in many instances even a supramucosal one, so the respective measurements can be carried out at the crest level of study casts. It is important during this process to anticipate a minimal distance between implant shoulders of approximately 2 mm, and between a natural tooth and an implant of about 1.5 mm (to be measured at the interproximal soft tissue level). Again, the treatment objective, i.e. a long-lasting implant-supported FPD, should be predictably reached (1) with optimal efficacy and (2) with a minimum of invasiveness and

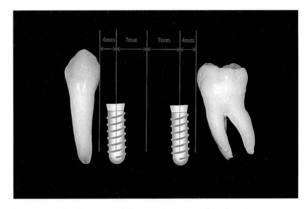

Fig. 54-46 In the case of three missing occlusal units, an implant-supported FPD with a central pontic (approximately 7 mm in width) may be considered as a viable solution.

cost. The still existing controversy of whether each missing occlusal unit should be replaced by one implant or whether a minimal number of implants should be used, has already been addressed earlier in this chapter.

In the case of three missing occlusal units and in the absence of other particular restrictive conditions such as limited local bone volume, the authors recommend the insertion of a mesial and a distal implant to support a three-unit FPD with a central pontic (Fig. 54-45). This approach permits the fabrication of three metal–ceramic elements featuring a mesio-distal diameter of about 7 mm each. Based on an average implant shoulder dimension of approximately 5 mm, one can anticipate a gradually increasing, harmonious emergence profile from the implant shoulder to the occlusal surface. In order to satisfy the remaining important dimensional conditions, i.e. respecting the minimal distance between adjacent implants and in between teeth and implants, one needs to dispose of a minimal total mesio-distal gap distance of 21–22 mm (Fig. 54-46).

In the case of two missing occlusal units, one should try as a general rule to select the largest possible implant diameters with respect to the total mesio-distal distance of the given tooth-bound

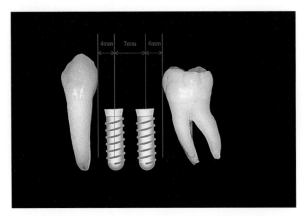

Fig. 54-47 If a given tooth-bound edentulous space only permits the insertion of two adjacent implants, a minimal interimplant distance of 2 mm and a minimal implant-to-tooth distance of 1.5 mm (at the interproximal soft tissue level) should be respected.

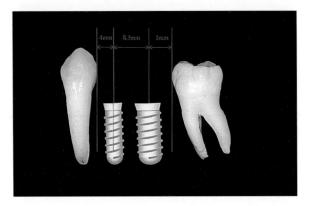

Fig. 54-48 In the presence of a mesio-distal gap width of approximately 17 mm, one may consider the combination of a standard and an increased-diameter ("wide-neck") implant. The same minimal inter-implant and implant-to-tooth distances have to be respected.

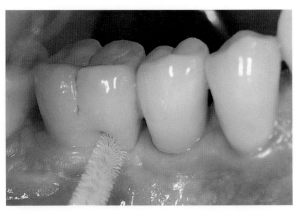

Fig. 54-49 Vestibular aspect of a metal–ceramic restoration supported by two screw-type implants. Due to an excess of mesio-distal space, the implants have been separated by approximately 4 mm. Instead of a traditional pontic, a root imitation has been performed close to the distal implant, providing an adequate guide for an interdental brush in view of an efficient plaque control at the marginal area of the implant restoration.

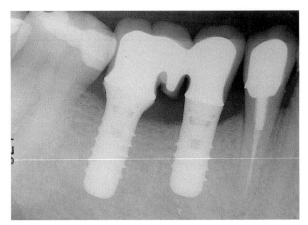

Fig. 54-50 With respect to cleanability, the respective prosthesis design is clearly visible on the post-operative radiograph.

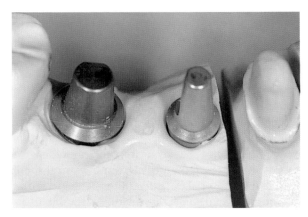

Fig. 54-51 The corresponding master model visualizes the different dimensions and distances involved in this individual case.

edentulous segment. Decisive parameters are again interimplant distance and space between implants and adjacent teeth, as well as oro-facial crest width at the two prospective implant sites. For a total gap diameter of about 14–15 mm, two standard-size implants are most suitable (Fig. 54-47), while for one of 17 to 18 mm the combination of one standard and one wide-diameter/wide-platform implant is considered adequate (Fig. 54-48). It goes without saying that the latter choice also requires the respective oro-facial bone volume.

These are just frequently encountered clinical examples, but in the function of other morphology and dimensions of edentulous tooth-bound segments, additional approaches and implant combinations may be envisioned. Two such clinical situations are presented in Figs. 54-49 to 54-52 and Figs. 54-53 to 54-55. In the first case, the gap diameter required the two adjacent implants to be spaced wider than the normally advocated interproximal 2 mm. The laboratory technician compensated for this excess of space with a root-imitation pontic which in turn

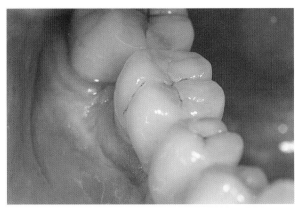

Fig. 54-52 On an oblique view the vestibular axial profile of the implant restoration becomes visible. Soft tissue (cheek and tongue) support and harmony with adjacent teeth are of paramount importance.

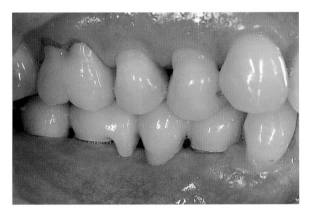

Fig. 54-53 Buccal view of an extended edentulous right mandibular tooth-bound gap treated with an implant restoration. In the pontic area a design favoring the efficacy of an interdental brush close to the implant margins has been applied.

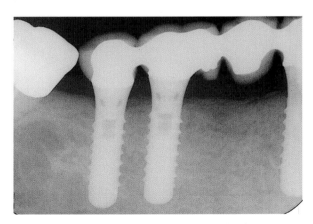

Fig. 54-54 The related radiograph illustrates the chosen design in the pontic area in terms of access to and efficacy of interproximal plaque control.

provided an excellent guide facilitating the use of an interdental brush (Fig. 54-49). In the second case, only the placement of three standard-size implants was possible due to a restricted bone volume in orofacial direction. Again, the technician could optimally distribute the different restoration volumes but still

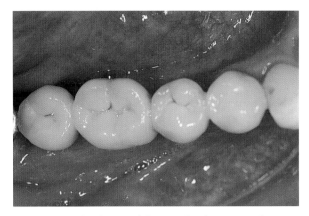

Fig. 54-55 Occlusal view of the completed 4-unit implant-borne fixed porcelain-fused-to-metal prosthesis.

Table 54-5 Splinting of multiple adjacent posterior implants

Parameters to consider:
- Access for oral hygiene
- Marginal adaptation/"passive fit"
- Technical simplicity/ease of eventual reinterventions
- "Overload" of the osseointegrated interface
- "Rotational forces" on implant components
- Screw-loosening/fatigue fractures

comply with basic prerequisites such as a flat axial emergence profile and optimal access for the patient's oral hygiene (Figs. 54-53, 54-54).

Splinted versus single-unit restorations of multiple adjacent posterior implants

Another persisting controversial issue relates to the question whether multiple adjacent implants in the load-carrying part of the dentition should support splinted or segmented single-unit restorations (Table 54-5). There still appears to be a confrontation between rather "biological" considerations versus more "mechanical" thinking.

Generally speaking, the biologically oriented considerations, insisting on easy access for oral hygiene and optimal marginal adaptation, represent probably the more scientifically-based point of view. Clinicians advocating splinting of multiple adjacent implants do so primarily for mechanical reasons. They hypothesize that this approach decreases forces and force moments at the level of the suprastructures and the various underlying implant components, and that relatively frequent mechanical complications such as screw-loosening and fractures may be significantly reduced or prevented by this measure. The related literature does not at present provide a clear answer, as randomized long-term clinical trials addressing this particular parameter are still scarce. Some more general reports do exist, however, addressing mainly type and frequency of mechanical complications (Goodacre *et al.* 1999).

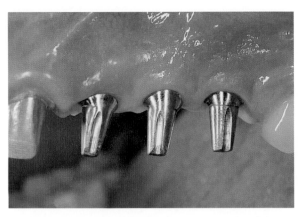

Fig. 54-56 The implant shoulder-abutment complex of the three left maxillary posterior implants has been prepared with fine-grain diamond burrs under abundant water cooling in order to facilitate the configuration of the related suprastructure. Particular emphasis was given to margins following closely the scalloped course of the soft tissue.

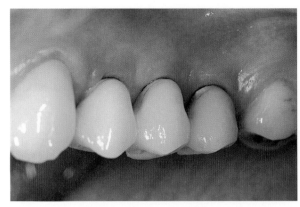

Fig. 54-58 The vestibular view of the final metal–ceramic restoration illustrates the impact on esthetics of a metal margin. This aspect should be discussed with the patient before treatment. In case of a high smile line, one may consider an increased sink depth during implant surgery.

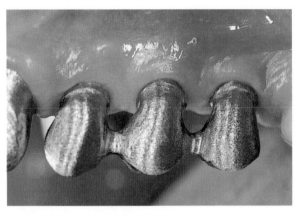

Fig. 54-57 In a case of reduced-diameter implants, splinting of adjacent units may reduce the risk for technical complications. A metal framework try-in prior to the application of the ceramic veneering may help to detect and eliminate an eventual non-passive fit at an early stage.

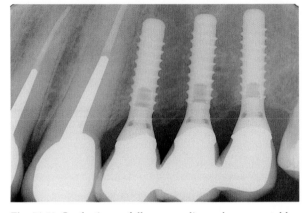

Fig. 54-59 On the 1-year follow-up radiograph an acceptable marginal fidelity can be assessed.

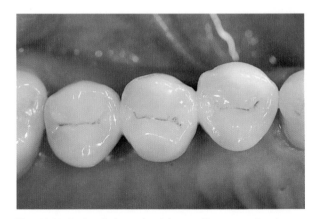

Fig. 54-60 Occlusal view of a right maxillary posterior three-unit implant restoration featuring premolar-sized segments.

Among the frequently forwarded arguments to plead the case of splinting are reduced-diameter (Figs. 54-56 to 54-59) or short (i.e. less than 8 mm) implants, implants inserted in low-density bone, implants placed in augmented or grafted (e.g. after anterior sinus floor elevation) bone, or implant restorations in the posterior segments of patients with verified notable occlusal parafunctions or bruxism. One should be aware, however, that the majority of these arguments are primarily based on clinical opinions and eventually common sense, and that to date they lack formal scientific evidence. In fact, there is increased indication, derived from prospective multicenter studies (although not addressing this parameter in particular), that splinting does not appear to be a prerequisite for preventing excessive crestal bone resorption or even loss of osseointegration. Nowadays, the authors would seriously reconsider their respective choice related to the suprastructure design presented in Figs. 54-60 and 54-61. In the presence of standard-size (i.e. addressing both diameter

and length) implants, which are placed in normal density, original (non-augmented or grafted) bone, single-unit restorations are definitely recommended as they comply better with the various parameters that are important from a more biologic point of view, as demonstrated by the clinical example presented in Figs. 54-62 and 54-63.

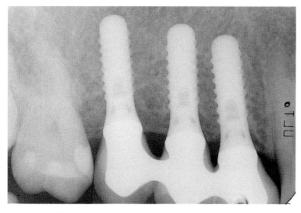

Fig. 54-61 The corresponding follow-up radiograph confirms acceptable peri-implant conditions.

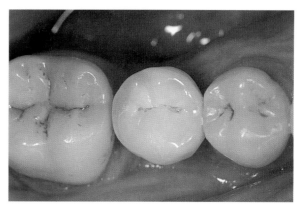

Fig. 54-64 Occlusal view of a single-tooth implant restoration replacing a missing mandibular right second premolar.

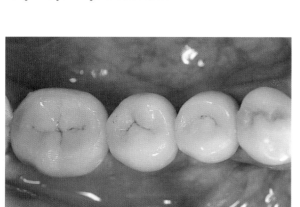

Fig. 54-62 Occlusal view of three independent, implant-supported fixed metal–ceramic restorations in the right posterior mandible.

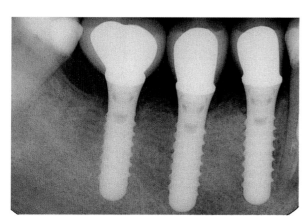

Fig. 54-63 As confirmed by the follow-up radiograph, an increased (more molar-like) dimension has been given to the most distal restoration, despite the fact that a standard-sized implant had to be used for restricted bone volume reasons.

Posterior single-tooth replacement

At the time when most implant systems had basically only one "standard" dimension at disposition, this corresponded to approximately 4–5 mm at the implant shoulder and thus was optimally suited for premolar-size restorations, featuring a continuously increasing (towards coronally) flat axial emergence profile and a mesio-distal diameter of about 7–8 mm at the occlusal surface. Clinicians were not infrequently faced with posterior single-tooth sites, however, that did not comply with these dimensions, for example in the case of missing first molars or after the loss of persisting deciduous (primary) second molars. As a consequence, the resulting implant restorations featured either unfavorable excessive interproximal overcontour or wide open embrasures. The first situation was difficult to clean, while the second led to undesired food retention (impaction). Nowadays most of the leading implant manufacturers offer wide-body/wide-platform implants designed for the replacement of multi-rooted teeth (Fig. 54-3).

Premolar-size single-tooth restorations

When it comes to posterior single-tooth gaps that correspond dimensionally to an average premolar, standard-size screw-form implants are well suited. The respective implant dimensions which include both the intrabony part and the implant shoulder, offer the additional advantage of being mostly compatible with a limited bone volume in an oro-facial direction. Whenever feasible, a straightforward low-maintenance restorative design is advocated, which normally consists of a cementable porcelain-fused-to-metal crown with vestibular and oral axial contours that are in harmony with the adjacent teeth and thus provide adequate guidance for cheek and tongue (Figs. 54-64 to 54-66).

Molar-size single-tooth restorations

If a given posterior single-tooth gap corresponds rather to the mesio-distal dimension of a molar, it is recommended, for the reasons quoted in the previous paragraph, that the insertion of a wide-neck implant is planned (Bahat & Handelsman 1996). This approach, however, also requires the respective bone volume in an oro-facial direction. If this is not the case, presurgical site analysis, eventually in the form

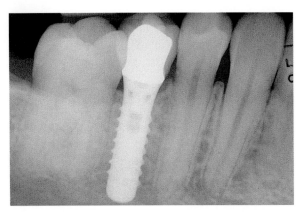

Fig. 54-65 The 5-year radiographic follow-up displays favorable bony conditions around this 12 mm solid screw implant.

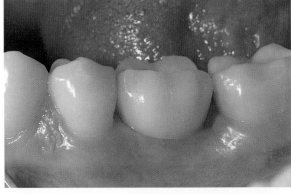

Fig. 54-67 In a case of the replacement of a single missing molar, ideally the use of an implant with corresponding dimensions is recommended to permit a restoration featuring optimal subjective comfort and cleansibility.

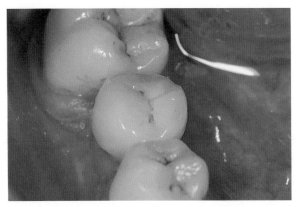

Fig. 54-66 On the oblique view one can notice that an axial contour similar to that present on the adjacent natural teeth has been applied to facilitate oral hygiene and to assure adequate soft tissue (cheek and tongue) guidance and support.

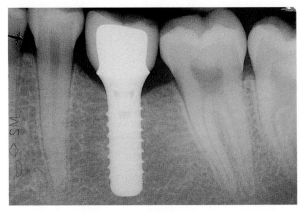

Fig. 54-68 On the 1-year radiographic follow-up a diameter-increased ("wide-neck") implant can be noted which is essential for a suprastructure design without extremely open interdental embrasures, which would be prone to food retention and oral parafunctions.

of a bone-mapping, should identify whether it is possible to have an implant placement in combination with a lateral bone augmentation procedure using a simultaneous approach. If the local bone anatomy requires a bone augmentation according to a staged protocol, one has to carefully ponder and discuss with the patient if this additional effort, risk, and ultimately also cost can be justified by an anticipated implant restoration featuring close-to-ideal axial contours and embrasures.

A clinical example demonstrating the potential of increased-diameter implants for the optimal replacement of a single missing mandibular molar is given in Figs. 54-67 and 54-68.

Sites with limited vertical bone volume

The clinician is quite frequently confronted with posterior single-tooth gaps that present all of the major prerequisites for successful implant therapy listed earlier in this chapter, with the exception of sufficient vertical bone height for the insertion of an implant featuring what is broadly accepted as an adequate length of the implant itself and in relation to the

prospective length of the suprastructure. The question that arises is whether there is a minimal implant length required in the context of posterior single-tooth restorations and whether the ratio between implant length and suprastructure length has an influence on crestal bone resorption and ultimately on the longevity of the entire implant–suprastructure complex. The analysis of the respective implant data collected at the University of Geneva School of Dental Medicine in the frame of a prospective multicenter study from 1989 to 2002, permitted the conclusion that shorter implants (6–8 mm) did not show more average crestal bone resorption than longer implants (10–12 mm), and that a so-called unfavorable ratio between implant length and suprastructure height did not lead to more pronounced crestal bone resorption (Bernard *et al.* 1995a; Bernard & Belser 2002). This data is corroborated by other recently published reports (ten Bruggenkate *et al.* 1998; Bischof *et al.* 2001; Deporter *et al.* 2001).

Two examples of respective clinical anecdotal-type evidence, one premolar-size and one molar-size single-tooth restoration, are presented in Figs. 54-69 and 54-70, and Figs. 54-71 and 54-72, respectively.

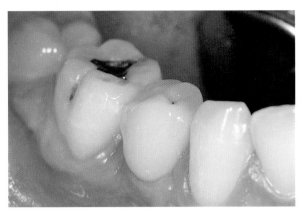

Fig. 54-69 Clinical aspect of a single-tooth implant restoration in the mandibular right premolar area.

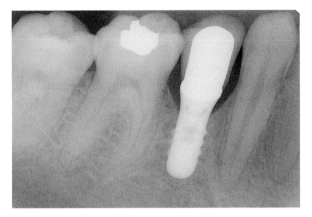

Fig. 54-70 The related 2-year follow-up radiograph shows a so-called unfavorable relationship between the height of the suprastructure and the length of the supporting implant. The placement of a longer implant was not possible due to the limited local bone conditions.

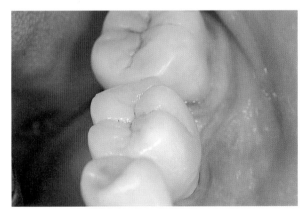

Fig. 54-71 Oblique view of a molar single-tooth implant restoration in the left mandible.

Clinical applications

Screw-retained implant restorations

For many years there was a strong tendency to design most of the fixed implant restorations as screw-retained suprastructures. Retrievability, and by this

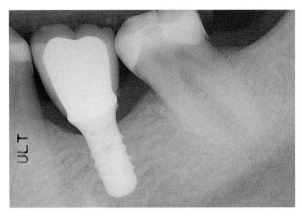

Fig. 54-72 A short diameter-increased screw implant supporting a long molar-sized suprastructure is displayed on the 1-year follow-up radiograph. Note that a normal level of the first bone-to-implant contact has been maintained.

Table 54-6 Indications for screw-retained posterior fixed implant restorations

Parameters to consider:
- Implant shoulder location incompatible with a cemented suprastructure, i.e. inaccessible for meticulous excess cement removal (>2 mm submucosally)
- Reduced intermaxillary distance (<5 mm)
- Foreseeable need for reintervention at the respective implant site
- Extended implant-supported rehabilitations, involving numerous implants
- High overall level of complexity (e.g. non-parallel implants)

maintaining the possibility for modification, extension or eventually repair of the prosthesis, was the main rationale for this strategy. One should be aware, however, that this approach also encompasses notable specific inconveniences: colonization of the inner compartments of the implant–abutment–suprastructure complex with mostly anaerobic microorganisms, risk for loosening or fracture of screws, increased technical complexity and related costs, possible interference with structural parameters (weakening of the metal-ceramic design) and esthetics, as well as a "higher maintenance profile" (Sutter et al. 1993; Wie 1995; Hebel & Gajjar 1997; Keller et al. 1998). As far as the microbial colonization is concerned, it remains unknown to date whether and under which conditions this may have an adverse effect on the longevity of osseointegrated implants.

For these reasons there is currently a distinct trend towards cementable fixed implant restorations in the load-carrying part of the dentition.

The main indications for screw-retention are listed in Table 54-6.

Transocclusal screw retention

If for one of the aforementioned reasons a transocclusally screw-retained suprastructure is adopted,

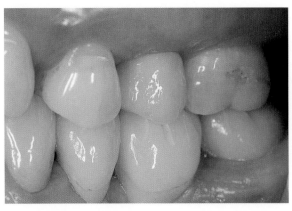

Fig. 54-73 Left lateral view showing the intermaxillary relationship of a young patient in centric occlusion. The missing maxillary second premolar has been replaced by a single-tooth, screw-retained implant restoration. Screw retention was chosen for two reasons: limited interocclusal distance and implant shoulder location incompatible with cementation.

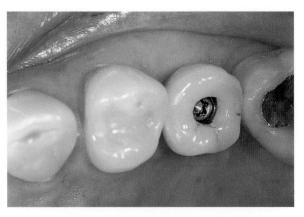

Fig. 54-75 Ideally, the screw-access channel should be located in the center of the occlusal surface. This reduces both the risk for interference with an appropriate metal–ceramic design in general, and the risk for porcelain fractures in particular.

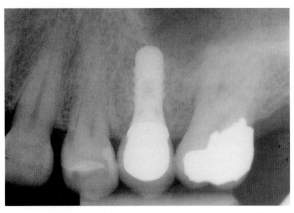

Fig. 54-74 One-year follow-up radiograph of the described 8 mm solid screw implant.

several parameters should be taken into consideration. First, the screw-access channel should be centered on the occlusal surface in order not to interfere too much with the area to be occupied by the cuspids.

A typical clinical example documenting an indication for a screw-retained posterior single-tooth restoration is given in Figs. 54-73 to 54-75. A reduced interarch distance has led to a deeper than usual implant shoulder location which in turn is neither accessible for well controlled excess cement removal nor in reach for the patient's routine oral hygiene. In order to benefit from their superior surface quality characteristics and marginal precision, prefabricated machined cast-on components have been used for the respective suprastructure fabrication. Ideally, the screw-access channel occupies a restricted area in the centre of the occlusal table, and the distance from the head of the screw to the occlusal surface should be sufficient for a subsequent composite cover-restoration (Fig. 54-75).

Furthermore, the principles of the metal–ceramic technology require a well defined space for develop-

ing an adequate metal support for a uniform thickness of the overlaying stratification of porcelain. Even in a case of a well centered occlusal perforation, the latter occupies close to half of the mesio-distal and oro-facial diameter of the occlusal table, and thereby significantly weakens the overall mechanical resistance of the structure. If the screw-access channel is not centered, however, additional problems are created in the sense of both weakening the restoration and interfering with esthetic criteria. Under such circumstances one should consider, for example, the use of angled abutments as currently offered by most of the leading implant systems.

Another key parameter represents the interarch distance, or more specifically, the distance between the implant shoulder and the plane of occlusion. According to our experience this distance should be at least equal to 5 mm. This is minimal and does not permit – for esthetic reasons – the occlusal screw to be subsequently covered with a composite resin restoration. In this context 6–7 mm are clearly more adequate.

A combination of several well known problems, which are frequently encountered after implant placement in the posterior mandible, are shown in Figs. 54-76 to 54-78. Two implants have been inserted to restore a distally shortened arch with a three-unit FPD. Owing to the local bone anatomy, the implants were placed in a more lingual position than the original teeth (Fig. 54-76). The implant shoulder location was too superficial for these particular circumstances and did not provide sufficient distance to gradually correct the discrepancy between the actual implant shoulder position and the ideal occlusal location. Furthermore, the necessity of keeping the screw access in the center of the occlusal table, and the insufficient room for composite screw-head coverage, ultimately led to a considerable compromise (Fig. 54-77). The final radiograph (Fig. 54-78) clearly shows that the presurgical bone volume would have permitted a vertical reduction of the edentulous bone

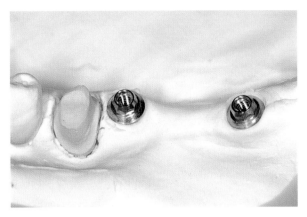

Fig. 54-76 Occlusal view of a mandibular master model comprising two posterior implant analogues and a prepared natural second premolar abutment. Note the proximity of the mesial implant and the second premolar on the one hand, and the distinct lingual position of the two implants on the other.

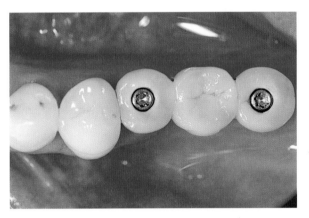

Fig. 54-77 The clinical view of the completed transocclusally screw-retained three-unit implant-supported FPD demonstrates that the lingual implant position did not allow for a suprastructure that is in line with the adjacent teeth. Furthermore, the screws are reaching the occlusal surface, leaving no space for an esthetic coverage with composite resin.

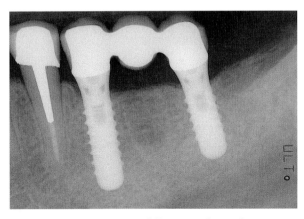

Fig. 54-78 The related 3-year follow-up radiograph documents an only minimal distance between implant shoulder and occlusal surface. Under such conditions, a slight reduction of the alveolar ridge prior to implant placement would have provided more vertical leeway for compensating the lingual implant position and ultimately for covering the occlusal screw.

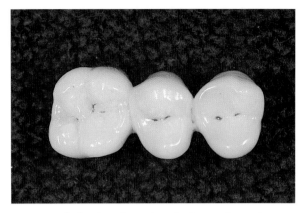

Fig. 54-79 Occlusal configuration of a three-unit metal–ceramic implant restoration designed for transverse screw retention. Note the absence of any interference due to screws on the occlusal aspect of the restoration.

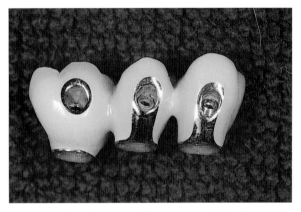

Fig. 54-80 The oral aspect of that same prosthesis features the decisive elements related to the transverse screw retention: improved esthetics, no weakening of the ceramo-metal design. The screw-access channels are completely protected by the metal framework.

crest to be performed prior to implant insertion. By this token the suboptimal implant position could have been partially corrected by the implant restoration, and the occlusal screw covered by composite resin, or a screw-retained restoration eventually avoided as there would be adequate conditions for a cemented suprastructure.

Transverse screw retention

When it comes to screw-retained posterior implant restorations one should not forget the option of transverse screw retention (Figs. 54-79 to 54-84). This specific technical approach leaves the occlusal surface of the restoration free from any screw and permits the design of a screw-access channel on the oral aspect, featuring a metal protection on the entire circumference of the perforation (Fig. 54-80). These two factors significantly improve both the overall mechanical resistance and the esthetic appearance. Furthermore, the metal protects the surrounding porcelain during removal and tightening of the transverse screw and

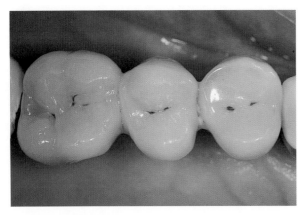

Fig. 54-81 Clinical 5-year follow-up of this three-unit implant restoration. No significant changes can be noticed on the occlusal surface.

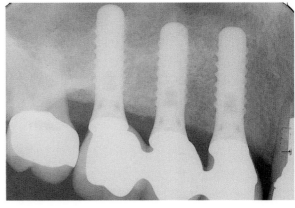

Fig. 54-84 Five-year follow-up radiograph of the same quadrant, now restored with a three-unit transverse screw-retained metal–ceramic implant suprastructure. Note that the distal retainer of the original tooth-borne FPD could be maintained.

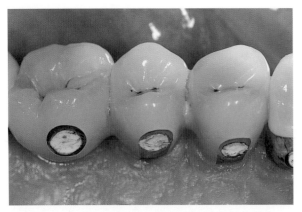

Fig. 54-82 Palatal view of the transverse screw-retained implant prosthesis after 5 years of clinical service. The screw-access channels are blocked by a temporary material.

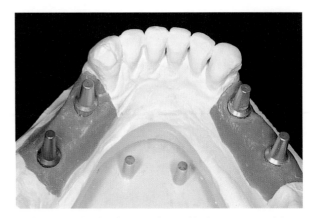

Fig. 54-85 Example of a typical mandibular master model, derived from an impression at the abutment level, comprising four colour-coded implant–abutment analogues.

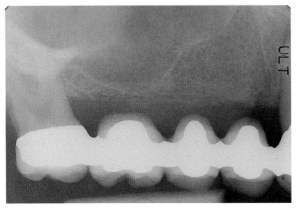

Fig. 54-83 Pre-operative radiograph of the patient's maxillary right posterior segment, revealing a tooth-borne long-span FPD which had failed after 4 years of function due to loss of retention and subsequent damage on the mesial abutment.

thereby prevents the induction of fissures prone to subsequent propagation and ultimately leading to ceramic fractures. One has to be aware, however, that from a purely technical and economic point of view, transverse screw-retained restorations require additional, more complex components and advanced technical skills, and are more expensive. In the long-term, on the other hand, the distinct advantages should clearly outweigh these inconveniences in numerous clinical situations.

Abutment-level impression versus implant shoulder-level impression

Most of the leading implant systems currently offer the possibility of taking impressions either at the level of a previously inserted abutment or at the level of the implant shoulder itself (Figs. 54-85 and 54-86). The former approach is mostly indicated if the patient does not wear a removable temporary prosthesis and in the case of optimally placed, "restoration-driven" implants, comprising accessibility of the implant shoulder, point of emergence from the soft tissue, implant axis, interarch distance, and overall easy access for use of simple "pop-on" plastic transfer copings. As shown later, a clear preference is given to cemented suprastructures under such simple, straightforward conditions. In fact, the clinician is only required to keep a limited stock of components, i.e. cementable titanium abutments of various heights

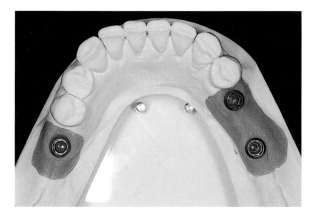

Fig. 54-86 Example of a typical mandibular master model, derived from an impression at the implant shoulder level, comprizing three colour-coded implant analogues.

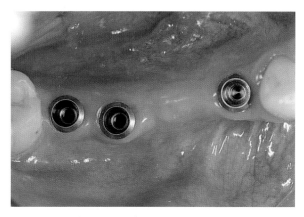

Fig. 54-87 Occlusal view of the mandibular right posterior quadrant with three implants that had been placed according to a single-step transmucosal surgical protocol.

and injection-molded impression copings, in his office. Whenever the clinical situation deviates notably from the previously described conditions, one may consider taking an impression directly at the level of the implant shoulder. For that approach, only transfer copings have to be available in the dental practice. In fact, the patient is leaving the office after the impression session exactly as he came in, i.e. with the same cover screw and with the same unaltered temporary prosthesis. After master model fabrication and articulator mounting, the technician will then select the most appropriate secondary components in the laboratory and ultimately deliver the finished restoration together with the respective supporting abutments.

Cemented multiple-unit posterior implant prostheses

In recent years, an increasing trend towards cemented posterior implant restorations, using either temporary or permanent luting agents, could be observed. The associated original paradigm, indicating that maintaining "retrievability" was one of the fundamental advantages of implant-borne suprastructures, permitting re-intervention, modification, and/or extension at any time, has been lately challenged by parameters such as increased clinical and technical simplicity, low-maintenance design of the restorations, and superior cost effectiveness. As more implants are utilized in clinical situations where conventional FPDs would also be easily possible, but where the latter have become second choice, the sites are more favorable for this type of therapy and these implants come closer to the characteristics currently termed as "restoration-driven". Parallel to this improved mastering of three-dimensional implant positioning, secondary components such as abutments that are optimally designed for subsequent cemented restorations have been developed, in combination with auxiliary parts such as simplified impression copings, laboratory analogues, and burn-

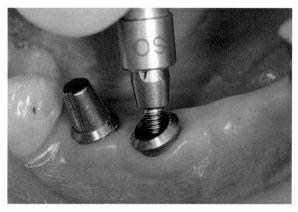

Fig. 54-88 In accordance with the available interocclusal space, adequately dimensioned solid abutments are selected, inserted and subsequently tightened to 35 Ncm in view of a cemented suprastructure.

out patterns. A typical clinical example of the treatment of an extended tooth-bound posterior segment by means of implants and a subsequently cemented suprastructure is presented in Figs. 54-87 to 54-94. Three screw-type implants have been inserted according to a single-step transmucosal (non-submerged) surgical protocol, leading 8 weeks after implant installation to a clinical situation which is well suited for a restorative procedure similar to the one traditionally used in the context of natural tooth abutments. More particularly, all of the involved implant shoulders are easily accessible (Figs. 54-87 to 54-90) for restorative procedures and later for maintenance, and the surrounding peri-implant mucosa healing and tissue maturation has occurred simultaneously with implant osseointegration, both being key factors in facilitating prosthetic procedures. Furthermore, the superficially located interface between implant shoulder and suprastructure or abutment will reduce the length of suprastructure leverage and by this the resulting bending moments. Under the assumption that presurgical site analysis and, derived from that, prosthetic treatment planning has predictably led to optimal implant positioning, the resulting implant

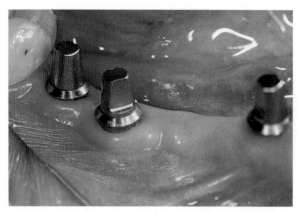

Fig. 54-89 With the solid abutments in place, the inter-implant parallelism is confirmed. Note the easily accessible implant shoulders which will facilitate the following impression and restorative procedures.

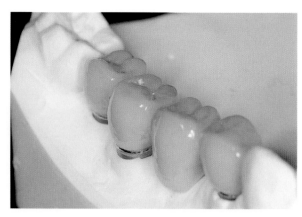

Fig. 54-92 Based on prefabricated burn-out patterns, the final metal–ceramic restoration has been completed. Note the continuous flat axial emergence profile of the individual elements.

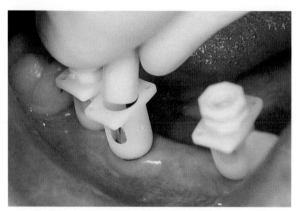

Fig. 54-90 Prefabricated injection-molded, self-centering impression copings and related color-coded positioning cylinders are inserted prior to impression taking with a stock tray.

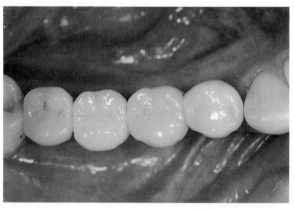

Fig. 54-93 The clinical occlusal view of the cemented four-unit implant prosthesis composed of premolar-sized segments.

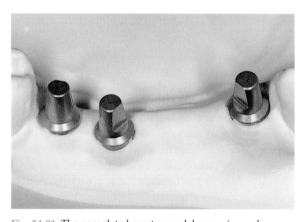

Fig. 54-91 The completed master model comprises color-coded aluminum implant analogues.

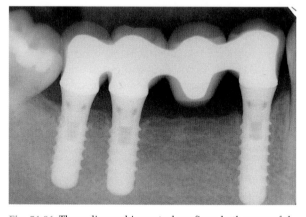

Fig. 54-94 The radiographic control confirms both successful osseointegration of the involved implants and accurate marginal adaptation of the suprastructure.

prosthesis should almost by definition feature a gradually increasing, flat axial emergence profile, adequate embrasures and overall design, and occlusal characteristics similar to those advocated for tooth-borne FPDs (Figs. 54-92 to 54-94).

Angulated abutments

It is not infrequent that all of the parameters defining an optimal three-dimensional implant position cannot be readily reached. Under such conditions the clini-

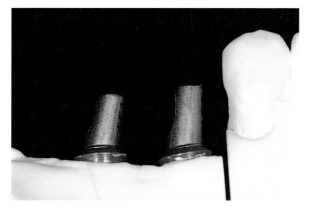

Fig. 54-95 Lateral view of a master model comprising implant level analogues in the right mandibular posterior sextant. Angulated abutments have been selected to correct a too distal implant axis.

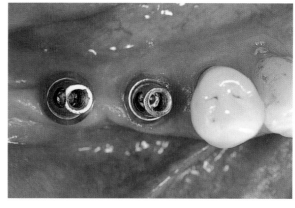

Fig. 54-97 Using an appropriate index, the two angulated abutments are transferred intraorally and subsequently tightened to 35 Ncm with a torque wrench.

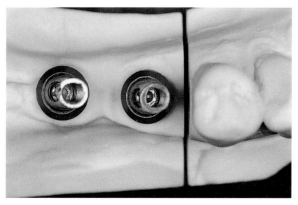

Fig. 54-96 The corresponding occlusal aspect visualizes the amount of axis correction achieved.

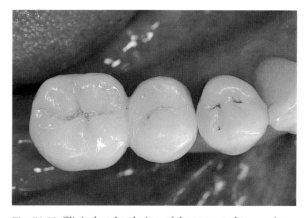

Fig. 54-98 Clinical occlusal view of the cemented two-unit metal–ceramic implant restoration.

cian basically has three options. Either a bone augmentation procedure is undertaken, or a conventional tooth-borne prosthesis is chosen, or one evaluates carefully whether a minor positional compromise can be considered acceptable. The related parameters have to be objectively pondered prior to taking the respective decision together with the duly informed patient. The heaviness of a so-called "site-development" procedure (e.g. lateral or vertical bone augmentation or anterior sinus floor elevation) should definitely be put in direct relation with the expected benefit. In some instances this approach allows significantly invasive procedures to be avoided. Particularly in situations where only the implant axis interferes with an otherwise optimal implant positioning, the subsequent use of angled abutments may still lead to a largely acceptable treatment outcome (Figs. 54-95 to 54-98). In other word, there appears to exist limited room for sometimes considering a slightly "bone-driven" instead of a purely "restoration-driven" implant placement in order to render implant therapy bearable for a given individual patient.

Angled abutments, encompassing various inclinations and dimensions, are currently part of the armamentarium of most of the leading implant systems.

They are frequently used and compatible with both a cementable or a screw-retained suprastructure design.

High-strength all-ceramic implant restorations

Additional options, such as milled titanium frameworks as infrastructures for metal–ceramic prostheses or high-strength all-ceramic restorations, have also become recently available in the context of posterior implant restorations. Some of these approaches are based on computer-assisted design and computer-assisted machining (CAD/CAM) technology. As implants and their secondary components are mostly industrially produced or machined, and as their related dimensions and tolerances are well defined, they appear particularly well suited to this kind of technology. In this context, and in order to explain the particular interest associated with this type of technology, it has to be underlined that using either the same metal (i.e. c.p. titanium) or no metal at all for the suprastructure fabrication, would be highly preferable. Porcelain-fused-to-metal alloys with high gold content are primarily utilized due to their superior casting ability.

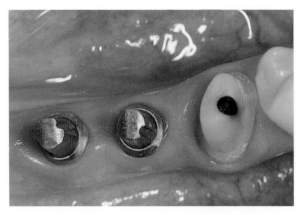

Fig. 54-99 Mandibular right posterior segment, featuring a full-coverage preparation on the non-vital second premolar and two implants equipped with solid abutments in the area of the missing first molar.

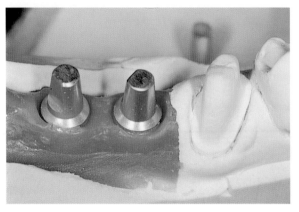

Fig. 54-100 Master model including the stone die of the prepared premolar and the two implant analogues.

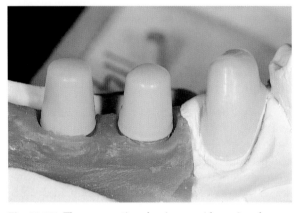

Fig. 54-101 Three respective aluminous oxide copings have been fabricated according to the PROCERA® technique.

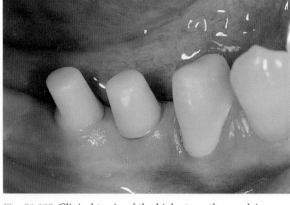

Fig. 54-102 Clinical try-in of the high-strength porcelain infrastructures.

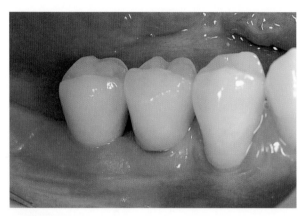

Fig. 54-103 Vestibular view of the cemented final all-ceramic restorations.

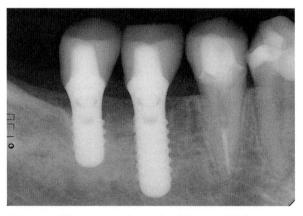

Fig. 54-104 The 1-year radiographic follow-up displays sufficient radio-opacity of the all-ceramic substrate to evaluate the marginal adaptation of the three single-unit restorations.

It would go beyond the scope of this textbook to describe in detail the current evolution in the field of CAD/CAM systems in general and to their impact on implant dentistry in particular. A representative clinical example, however, is given in Figs. 54-99 to 54-105.

All-ceramic implant suprastructures are still preferred as single-unit restorations, primarily for purely technical reasons.

Orthodontic and occlusal considerations related to posterior implant therapy

As one increasingly strives for the best possible biologic, functional and esthetic integration of a given implant restoration in the pre-existing dentition, three-dimensional pre-operative site analysis is of paramount importance. It is not infrequent that this subsequently calls for a pluridisciplinary approach

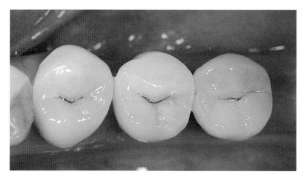

Fig. 54-105 Occlusal view of the two posterior implant-borne premolar-sized suprastructures and the tooth-supported ceramic restoration on the second premolar.

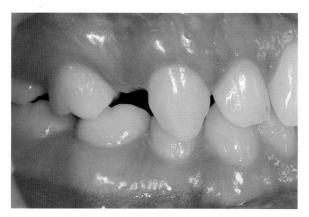

Fig. 54-106 Right lateral view of a 19-year-old female patient, congenitally missing all four permanent maxillary premolars. One can note both an inadequate mesio-distal gap width and a reduced interarch distance.

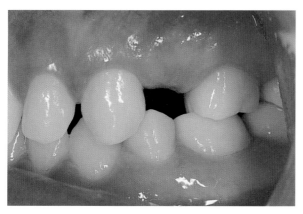

Fig. 54-107 A similar situation regarding interarch distance is present on the patient's left side.

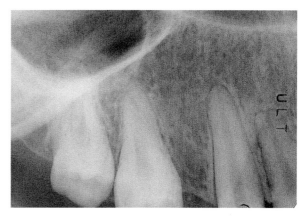

Fig. 54-108 The corresponding radiograph underlines the need for additional orthodontic therapy prior to the insertion of an implant in order to optimize the gap width and the inter-radicular distance.

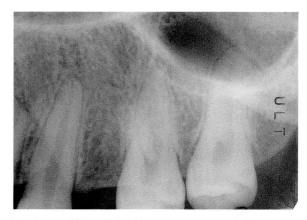

Fig. 54-109 Although to a lesser degree, presurgical orthodontic therapy is also indicated on the maxillary left posterior segment.

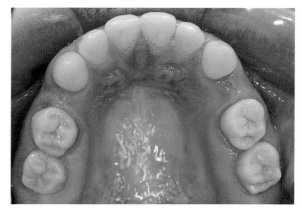

Fig. 54-110 The clinical occlusal view displays the bilateral edentulous spaces in the premolar area. Despite previously performed orthodontic therapy, aiming at reducing the edentulous spaces to the size of one premolar, the mesio-distal gap width on the right side is insufficient for the insertion of an implant.

termed "site development", which may also include presurgical orthodontic therapy (Figs. 54-106 to 54-119). The objective is clearly to create local conditions that are best suited for the type of therapy chosen. If implants are to be involved, the local bone and soft tissue anatomy, as well as the mesio-distal and oro-facial distances of a given edentulous segment, have to comply optimally with the respective most appropriate implant dimensions. Quite often mesio-distal gap dimensions have to be optimized orthodontically and neighboring roots aligned, so that they will not interfere with "restoration-driven" implant positioning. Site development in the broad sense of the term

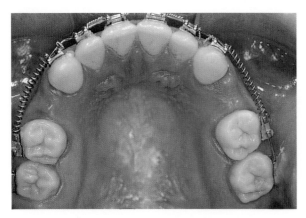

Fig. 54-111 After six months of additional orthodontic treatment using an upper fixed full-arch appliance, the dimensions of the two prospective implant sites appear compatible with this kind of therapy.

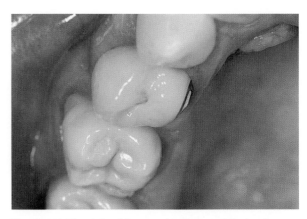

Fig. 54-114 The right oblique occlusal view of the implant restoration clearly demonstrates the advantage of the transverse screw-retention design: no occlusal screw access channel interfering with the functional occclusal morphology and esthetics or with structural requirements inherent to the metal–ceramic technology.

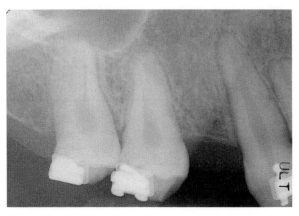

Fig. 54-112 The respective radiograph confirms adequate space in the upper right premolar region for the placement of a standard single-tooth implant.

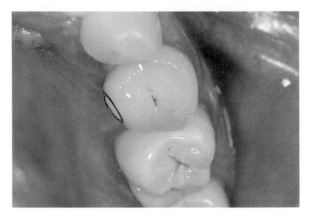

Fig. 54-115 As described for the patient's right side, the left maxillary fixed single-tooth implant restoration integrates appropriately the existing natural dentition.

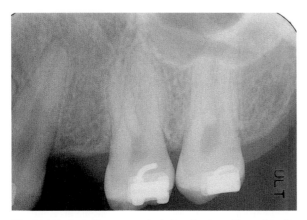

Fig. 54-113 A similar presurgical situation is radiographically confirmed for the upper left premolar site.

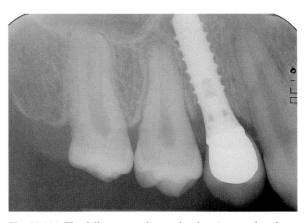

Fig. 54-116 The follow-up radiograph taken 1 year after the insertion of the 12 mm solid screw implant, shows adequate marginal fidelity and stable conditions at the bone-to-implant interface.

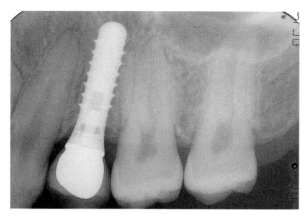

Fig. 54-117 Similar findings are present in the corresponding left-sided follow-up radiograph.

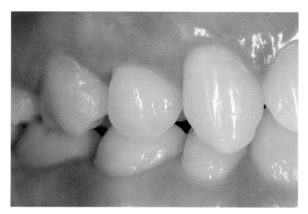

Fig. 54-118 The final right lateral view in centric occlusion features acceptable general interarch conditions and related intercuspation.

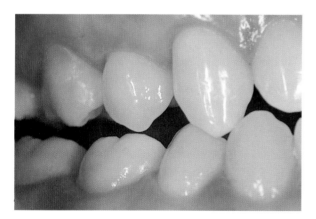

Fig. 54-119 During the right lateral excursion of the mandible (working-side movement), a canine guidance could be established.

also comprises parameters associated with intermaxillary relationships such as occlusal plane, interarch space, and occlusal guidance during mandibular excursions. As osseointegrated implants do provide excellent anchorage for orthodontic appliances (Melsen & Lang 2001), and thus can significantly contribute to the efficacy and simplicity of such a treatment, one may also consider implant insertion prior to orthodontic therapy. This, however, requires meticulous pre-operative analysis and precise three-

Table 54-7 Hypothetical implant-specific occlusal concept

- "Light infraocclusion" in centric occlusion position (CO) on posterior implant restorations
- "Narrow" occlusal table
- Only "axial" loading on implant restorations
- No or only "minimal contacts" on implant restorations during "mandibular excursions"
  - ° No canine guidance on implants
  - ° Eventually "minimal" group function on the working side

dimensional implant positioning, anticipating perfectly the ideal location with respect to the final treatment objective.

When it comes to occlusal considerations related to posterior implant restorations, one should note that most of the relevant literature available to date addresses eventual effects of occlusal loading on the various components of the implant–abutment–suprastructure complex (Brägger 1999, 2001; Bassit et al. 2002; Wiskott et al. 2002). In fact, various recommendations are derived from such studies, including various occlusal restorative materials, type and mechanical characteristics of different abutment to implant connections, as well as general guidelines for optimal suprastructure design.

Little information is presently available regarding an eventual direct relationship between occlusal loading and maintenance of osseointegration in general and occurrence of peri-implant crestal bone resorption in particular (Wiskott & Belser 1999; Duyck et al. 2001; Engel et al. 2001; Gotfredsen et al. 2001a,b,c; O'Mahony et al. 2001; Engquist et al. 2002; Wright et al. 2002). Attempts have been made to take into account the fundamental differences between a tooth surrounded by a periodontal ligament and an "ankylosed" osseointegrated implant, the latter disposing neither of local mechanoreceptors nor of a so-called "damping" capacity. This led to a hypothetical implant-specific occlusal concept (Table 54-7), featuring parameters such as lighter contacts in centric occlusion when compared with the surrounding natural dentition, and no or only minimal contacts on implant restorations during mandibular excursions. One should clearly note, however, that these guidelines are primarily derived from clinical experience, subjective opinions and eventually common sense, and that there is little or no solid scientific evidence available to date which would support such a concept (Taylor et al. 2000).

Concluding remarks and perspectives

Early and immediate fixed implant restorations

Currently, one can observe a strong tendency towards shortened healing delays and ultimately towards immediate loading or at least "immediate restoration" protocols in association with dental implants (Tarnow *et al.* 1997; Ericsson *et al.* 2000; Gatti *et al.* 2000; Szmuk-ler-Moncler *et al.* 2000; Bernard *et al.* 2001; Chiapasco *et al.* 2001b; Ganeles *et al.* 2001; Gomez-Roman *et al.* 2001; Roccuzzo *et al.* 2001; Romanos *et al.* 2002). Improved implant surface characteristics have contributed to this evolution (Buser *et al.* 1998a; Deporter *et al.* 2001; Gotfredsen *et al.* 2001b; Roccuzzo *et al.* 2001; Cochran *et al.* 2002). Numerous studies have reported that such an approach can be considered predictable under certain well defined conditions. These conditions include four to six implants inserted in the interforaminal part of the edentulous mandible and which are subsequently splinted with a bar device (Gatti *et al.* 2000), as well as multiple implants evenly distributed around an edentulous arch and then immediately restored – according to the principle of "cross-arch stabilization" – with a splinted full-arch FPD (Tarnow *et al.* 1997). Achieving adequate primary stability at the moment of implant installation, and confining, during the crucial first healing period, an eventual mobility below the threshold of approximately 50 microns, appear to be among the decisive parameters for predictably achieving osseointegration (Szmukler *et al.* 2000). With regard to the routine application of immediate loading protocols for posterior single-tooth restorations, it appears advisable to wait for scientific confirmation of its respective potential in the form of randomized controlled clinical trials.

In conclusion, the possibility of performing highly predictable treatments which are more simple, require less time and which can be conducted in a standard dental practice set-up, as well as the associated quality of treatment outcomes, have nowadays made implant therapy in the load-carrying part of the dentition an integral part of the restorative spectrum for any kind of edentulism. This evolution is most dynamic and holds promise for further significant developments.

Acknowledgments

The authors wish to acknowledge and thank Drs Viviana Coto-Hunziker, Stephan Dieth, Thierry Doumas, German Gallucci, Robin Jaquet, Nikolaos Perakis, and Valérie Wouters (all of them clinicians at the School of Dental Medicine, University of Geneva, and involved in the treatment of some of the patients presented in this chapter) for their contributions. We would also like to thank the laboratory technicians and ceramists, Michel Bertossa, Cédric Bertsch, Pierre Martini, Roger Renevey, Alwin Schönenberger, and Gérard Verdel, for their expertise and meticulous execution of the implant suprastructures presented in this chapter. Furthermore, our gratitude is extended to Dr. Pascal Magne (Senior Lecturer, University of Geneva) for his competent assistance in development of the schematic illustrations.

References

Abrahamson, I., Berglundh, T. & Lindhe, J. (1997). The mucosal barrier following abutment dis/reconnection. An experimental study in dogs. *Journal of Clinical Periodontology* **24**, 568–572.

Andersson, B., Ödman, P., Lindvall, A.M. & Brånemark, P.I. (1998). Five-year prospective study of prosthodontic and surgical single-tooth implant treatment in general practices and at a specialist clinic. *International Journal of Prosthodontics* **11**, 351–365.

Bahat, O. & Handelsman, M. (1996). Use of wide implants and double implants in the posterior jaw: a clinical report. *International Journal of Oral and Maxillofacial Implants* **11**, 379–386.

Bassit, R., Lindström, H. & Rangert, B. (2002). In vivo registration of force development with ceramic and acrylic resin occlusal materials on implant-supported prostheses. *International Journal of Oral and Maxillofacial Implants* **17**, 17–23.

Behneke, A., Behneke, N. & d'Hoedt, B. (2000). The longitudinal clinical effectiveness of ITI solid screw implants in partially edentulous patients: A 5-year follow-up report. *International Journal of Oral and Maxillofacial Implants* **15**, 633–645.

Belser, U.C., Mericske-Stern, R., Bernard, J.P. & Taylor, T.D. (2000). Prosthetic management of the partially dentate patient with fixed implant restorations. *Clinical Oral Implants Research* **11** (Suppl I), 126–145.

Bernard, J.P. & Belser, U. (2002). Twelve years of clinical experience with the ITI Dental Implant System at the University of Geneva. *Journal de Parodontologie et d'Implantologie orale* **21**, 1–27.

Bernard, J.P., Belser, U.C., Smukler-Moncler, S., Martinet, J.P., Attieh, A. & Schaad, P.J. (1995a). Intérêt de l'utilisation d'im-plants ITI de faible longueur dans les secteurs postérieurs: resultats d'une etude clinique à trois ans. *Médecine Buccale & Chirurgie Buccale* **1**, 11–18.

Bernard, J.P., Szmukler-Moncler, S. & Samson, J. (2001). A 10-year life-table-analysis on TPS coated implants inserted in type IV bone. *Clinical Oral Implants Research* **12**, 395 (abstract no. 10).

Beumer III, J., Hamada, M.O. & Lewis, S. (1993). A prosthodontic overview. *International Journal of Prosthodontics* **6**, 126–130.

Bischof, M., Nedir, R., Smukler-Moncler, S. & Bernard, J.P. (2001). A 5-year life-table-analysis of ITI implants. Results from a private practice with emphasis on the use of short implants. *Clinical Oral Implants Research* **12**, 396 (abstract no. 13).

Boioli, L.T., Penaud, J. & Miller, N. (2001). A meta-analytic, quantitative assessment of osseointegration establishment and evolution of submerged and non-submerged endosseous titanium oral implants. *Clinical Oral Implants Research* **12**, 579–588.

Bosse, L.P. & Taylor, T.D. (1998). Problems associated with implant rehabilitation of the edentulous maxilla. *Dental Clinics of North America* **42**, 117–127.

Brägger, U. (1999). Technical failures and complications related to prosthetic components of implant systems and different types of suprastructures. In: Lang, N.P., Karring, T. & Lindhe, J., eds. *Proceedings of the 3rd European Workshop on Periodontology*. Berlin: Quintessence, pp. 304–332.

Brägger, U., Aeschlimann, S., Bürgin, W., Hämmerle, C.H.F. & Lang, N.P. (2001). Biological and technical complications and failures with fixed partial dentures (FPD) on implants and teeth after 4–5 years of function. *Clinical Oral Implants Research* **12**, 26–34.

Brägger, U., Bürgin, W.B., Hämmerle, C.H.F. & Lang, N.P. (1997). Associations between clinical parameters assessed around implants and teeth. *Clinical Oral Implants Research* **8**, 412–421.

Brånemark, P.I, Svensson, B. & van Steenberghe, D. (1995). Ten-year survival rates of fixed prostheses on four or six implants ad modum Brånemark in full edentulism. *Clinical Oral Implants Research* **6**, 227–231.

Buser, D., Belser, U.C. & Lang, N.P. (1998b). The original one-stage dental implant system and its clinical applications. *Periodontology 2000* **17**, 106–118.

Buser, D., Dula, K., Belser, U.C., Hirt, H.P. & Berthold, H. (1993). Localized ridge augmentation using guided bone regeneration. I. Surgical procedure in the maxilla. *International Journal of Periodontics and Restorative Dentistry* **13**, 29–45.

Buser, D., Dula, K., Belser, U.C., Hirt, H.P. & Berthold, H. (1995). Localized ridge augmentation using guided bone regeneration. II. Surgical procedure in the mandible. *International Journal of Periodontics and Restorative Dentistry* **15**, 13–29.

Buser, D., Dula, K., Hess, D., Hirt, H.P. & Belser U.C. (1999). Localized ridge augmentation with autografts and barrier membranes. *Periodontology 2000* **19**, 151–163.

Buser, D., Dula, K., Hirt, H.P. & Schenk, R.K. (1996). Lateral ridge augmentation using autografts and barrier membranes: a clinical study with 40 partially edentulous patients. *Journal of Oral and Maxillofacial Surgery* **54**, 420–432.

Buser, D., Ingimarsson, S., Dula, K., Lussi, A., Hirt, H.P. & Belser, U.C. (2002). Long-term stability of osseointegrated implants in augmented bone: A 5-year prospective study in partially edentulous patients. *International Journal of Periodontics and Restorative Dentistry* **22**, 108–117.

Buser, D., Mericske-Stern, R., Bernard, J.P., Behneke, A., Behneke, N., Hirt, H.P., Belser, U.C. & Lang, N.P. (1997). Long-term evaluation of non-submerged ITI implants. Part I: 8-year life table analysis of a prospective multi-center study with 2359 implants. *Clinical Oral Implants Research* **8**, 161–172.

Buser, D., Nydegger, T., Oxland, T., Schenk, R.K., Hirt, H.P., Cochran, D.L., Snétivy, D. & Nolte, L.P. (1998a). Influence of surface characteristics on the interface shear strength between titanium implants and bone. A biomechanical study in the maxilla of miniature pigs. *Journal of Biomedical Materials Research* **45**, 75–83.

Buser, D. & von Arx, T. (2000). Surgical procedures in partially edentulous patients with ITI implants. *Clinical Oral Implants Research* **11** (Suppl I), 83–100.

Chiapasco, M., Abati, S., Romeo, E. & Vogel, G. (1999). Clinical outcome of autogenous bone blocks or guided regeneration with e-PTFE membranes for reconstruction of narrow edentulous ridges. *Clinical Oral Implants Research* **10**, 278–288.

Chiapasco, M., Abati, S., Romeo, E. & Vogel, G. (2001b). Implant-retained mandibular overdentures with Brånemark System MKII implants: A prospective study between delayed and immediate loading. *International Journal of Oral and Maxillofacial Implants* **16**, 537–546.

Chiapasco, M., Romeo, E. & Vogel, G. (2001a). Vertical distraction osteogenesis of edentulous ridges for improvement of oral implant positioning: A clinical report of preliminary results. *International Journal of Oral and Maxillofacial Implants* **16**, 43–51.

Cochran, D.L., Buser, D., ten Bruggenkate, C.M., Weingart, D., Taylor, T.M., Bernard, J.P., Peters, F. & Simpson, J.P. (2002). The use of shortened healing times on ITI implants with a sandblasted and acid-etched (SLA) surface. Early results from clinical trials on ITI SLA implants. *Clinical Oral Implants Research* **13**, 144–153.

Deporter, D., Pilliar, R.M., Todescan, R., Watson, P. & Pharoah, M. (2001). Managing the posterior mandible of partially edentulous patients with short, porous-surfaced dental implants: Early data from a clinical trial. *International Journal of Oral and Maxillofacial Implants* **16**, 653–658.

Duyck, J., Rønold, H.J., Van Oosterwyck, H., Naert, I., Vander Sloten, J. & Ellingsen, J.E. (2001). The influence of static and dynamic loading on marginal bone reactions around osseointegrated implants: an animal experimental study. *Clinical Oral Implants Research* **12**, 207–218.

Eckert, S.E. & Wollan, P.C. (1998). Retrospective review of 1170 endosseous implants placed in partially edentulous jaws. *Journal of Prosthetic Dentistry* **79**, 415–421.

Ellegaard, B., Baelum, V. & Karring, T. (1997a). Implant therapy in periodontally compromised patients. *Clinical Oral Implants Research* **8**, 180–188.

Ellegaard, B., Kolsen-Petersen, J. & Baelum, V. (1997b). Implant therapy involving maxillary sinus lift in periodontally compromised patients. *Clinical Oral Implants Research* **8**, 305–315.

Ellen, R.P. (1998). Microbial colonization of the peri-implant environment and its relevance to long-term success of osseointegrated implants. *International Journal of Prosthodontics* **11**, 433–441.

Engel, E., Gomez-Roman, G. & Axmann-Krcmar, D. (2001). Effect of occlusal wear on bone loss and periotest values of dental implants. *International Journal of Prosthodontics* **14**, 444–450.

Engquist, B, Åstrand, P., Dahlgren, S., Engquist, E., Feldman, H. & Gröndahl, K. (2002). Marginal bone reaction to oral implants: a prospective comparative study of Astra Tech and Brånemark System implants. *Clinical Oral Implants Research* **13**, 30–37.

Ericsson, I., Nilson, H., Nilner, K. & Randow, K. (2000). Immediate functional loading of Brånemark single tooth implants. An 18 months' clinical pilot follow-up study. *Clinical Oral Implants Research* **11**, 26–33.

Ganeles, J., Rosenberg, M.M., Holt, R.L. & Reichman, L.H. (2001). Immediate loading of implants with fixed restorations in the completely edentulous mandible: Report of 27 patients from a private practice. *International Journal of Oral and Maxillofacial Implants* **16**, 418–426.

Gatti, C., Haefliger, W. & Chiapasco, M. (2000). Implant-retained mandibular overdentures with immediate loading: a prospective study of ITI implants. *International Journal of Oral and Maxillofacial Implants* **15**, 383–388.

Glantz, P.O. & Nilner, K. (1998). Biomechanical aspects of prosthetic implant-borne reconstructions. *Periodontology 2000* **17**, 119–124.

Gomez-Roman, G., Kruppenbacher, M., Weber, H. & Schulte, W. (2001). Immediate postextraction implant placement with root-analog stepped implants: Surgical procedure and statistical outcome after 6 years. *International Journal of Oral and Maxillofacial Implants* **16**, 503–513.

Goodacre, C.J., Kan, J.I.K. & Rungcharassaeng, K. (1999). Clinical complications of osseointegrated implants. *Journal of Prosthetic Dentistry* **81**, 537–552.

Gotfredsen, K., Berglundh, T. & Lindhe, J. (2001a). Bone reactions adjacent to titanium implants subjected to static load. A study in the dog (I). *Clinical Oral Implants Research* **12**, 1–8.

Gotfredsen, K., Berglundh, T. & Lindhe, J. (2001b). Bone reactions adjacent to titanium implants with different surface characteristics subjected to static load. A study in the dog (II). *Clinical Oral Implants Research* **12**, 196–201.

Gotfredsen, K., Berglundh, T. & Lindhe, J. (2001c). Bone reactions adjacent to titanium implants subjected to static load of different duration. A study in the dog (III). *Clinical Oral Implants Research* **12**, 552–558.

Gross, M. & Laufer, B.Z. (1997). Splinting osseointegrated implants and natural teeth in rehabilitation of partially edentulous patients. Part I: Laboratory and clinical studies. *Journal of Oral Rehabilitation* **24**, 863–870.

Gunne, J., Åstrand, P., Lindh, T., Borg, K. & Olsson, M. (1999). Tooth-implant and implant supported fixed partial dentures: A 10-year report. *International Journal of Prosthodontics* **12**, 216–221.

Gunne, J., Rangert, B., Glantz, P-O. & Svensson, A. (1997). Functional load on freestanding and connected implants in three-unit mandibular prostheses opposing complete dentures: An in vivo study. *International Journal of Oral and Maxillofacial Implants* **12**, 335–341.

Haas, R., Polak, C., Fürhauser, R., Mailath-Pokorny, G., Dörtbudak, O. & Watzek, G. (2002). A long-term follow-up of 76 Brånemark single-tooth implants. *Clinical Oral Implants Research* **13**, 38–43.

Hebel, K.S. & Gajjar, R.C. (1997). Cement-retained versus screw-retained implant restorations: achieving optimal occlusion and esthetics in implant dentistry. *Journal of Prosthetic Dentistry* **77**, 28–35.

Hermann, J.S., Buser, D., Schenk, R.K., Higginbottom, F.L. & Cochran, D.L. (2000). Biologic width around titanium implants. A physiologically formed and stable dimension over time. *Clinical Oral Implants Research* **11**, 1–11.

Hermann, J.S., Buser, D., Schenk, R.K., Schoolfield, J.D. & Cochran, D.L. (2001a). Biologic width around one-and two-piece titanium implants. A histometric evaluation of unloaded nonsubmerged and submerged implants in the canine mandible. *Clinical Oral Implants Research* **12**, 559–571.

Hermann, J.S., Cochran, D.L., Nummikoski, P.V. & Buser, D. (1997). Crestal bone changes around titanium implants. A radiographic evaluation of unloaded nonsubmerged and submerged implants in the canine mandible. *Journal of Periodontology* **68**, 1117–1130.

Hermann, J.S., Schoolfield, J.D., Nummikoski, P.V., Buser, D., Schenk, R.K & Cochran, D.L. (2001b). Crestal bone changes around titanium implants: A methodological study comparing linear radiographic with histometric measurements. *International Journal of Oral and Maxillofacial Implants* **16**, 475–485.

Hosny, M., Duyck, J., van Steenberghe, D. & Naert, I. (2000). Within-subject comparison between connected and nonconnected tooth-to-implant fixed partial prostheses: up to 14 year follow-up study. *International Journal of Prosthodontics* **13**, 340–346.

Hultin, M., Gustafsson, A. & Klinge, B. (2000). Long-term evaluation of osseointegrated dental implants in the treatment of partially edentulous patients. *Journal of Clinical Periodontology* **27**, 128–133.

Isidor, F. (1999). Occlusal loading in implant dentistry. In: Lang, N.P., Karring, T. & Lindhe, J., eds. *Proceedings of the 3rd European Workshop on Periodontology.* Berlin: Quintessence, pp. 358–375.

Jemt, T., Heath, M.R., Johns, R.B., McNamara, D.C., van Steenberghe, D. & Watson, R.M. (1996). A 5-year prospective multicenter follow-up report on overdentures supported by osseointegrated implants. *International Journal of Oral and Maxillofacial Implants* **11**, 291–298.

Johnson, R.H. & Persson, G.R. (2001). A 3-year prospective study of a single-tooth implant – Prosthodontic complications. *International Journal of Prosthodontics* **14**, 183–189.

Keith, S.E., Miller, B.H., Woody, R.D. & Higginbottom, F.L. (1999). Marginal discrepancy of screw-retained and cemented metal-ceramic crowns on implant abutments. *International Journal of Oral and Maxillofacial Implants* **14**, 369–378.

Keller, W., Brägger, U. & Mombelli, A. (1998). Peri-implant microflora of implants with cemented and screw retained suprastructures. *Clinical Oral Implants Research* **9**, 209–217.

Kiener, P., Oetterli, M., Mericske, E. & Mericske-Stern, R. (2001). Effectiveness of maxillary overdentures supported by implants: maintenance and prosthetic complications. *International Journal of Prosthodontics* **14**, 133–140.

Lang, N.P., Wilson, T. & Corbet, E.F. (2000). Biological complications with dental implants: their prevention, diagnosis and treatment. *Clinical Oral Implants Research* **11** (Suppl I), 146–155.

Lekholm, U., Gunne, J., Henry, P., Higuchi, K., Linden, U., Bergstrøm, C. & van Steenberghe, D. (1999). Survival of the Brånemark implant in partially edentulous jaws: a 10-year prospective multicenter study. *International Journal of Oral and Maxillofacial Implants* **14**, 639–645.

Leonhardt, Å., Gröndahl, K., Bergström, C. & Lekholm, U. (2002). Long-term follow-up of osseointegrated titanium implants using clinical, radiographic and microbiological parameters. *Clinical Oral Implants Research* **13**, 127–132.

Lindh, T., Bäck, T., Nyström, E. & Gunne, J. (2001). Implant versus tooth-implant supported prostheses in the posterior maxilla: a 2-year report. *Clinical Oral Implants Research* **12**, 441–449.

Lindh, T., Gunne, J., Tillberg, A. & Molin, M. (1998). A meta-analysis of implants in partial edentulism. *Clinical Oral Implants Research* **9**, 80–90.

Lindhe, J. & Berglundh, T. (1998). The interface between the mucosa and the implant. *Periodontology 2000* **17**, 47–53.

Lindqvist, L.W., Carlsson, G.E. & Jemt, T. (1996). A prospective 15-year follow-up study of mandibular fixed prostheses supported by osseointegrated implants. Clinical results and marginal bone loss. *Clinical Oral Implants Research* **7**, 329–336.

Lundgren, D. & Laurell, L. (1994). Biomechanical aspects of fixed bridgework supported by natural teeth and endosseous implants. *Periodontology 2000* **4**, 23–40.

Melsen, B. & Lang, N.P. (2001). Biological reactions of alveolar bone to orthodontic loading of oral implants. *Clinical Oral Implants Research* **12**, 144–152.

Mengel, R., Schröder, T. & Flores-de-Jacoby, L. (2001). Osseointegrated implants in patients treated for generalized chronic periodontitis and generalized aggressive periodontitis: 3- and 5-year results of a prospective long-term study. *Journal of Periodontology* **72**, 977–989.

Mericske-Stern, R. (1998). Treatment outcomes with implant-supported overdentures: clinical considerations. *Journal of Prosthetic Dentistry* **79**, 66–73.

Merz, B.R., Hunenbart, S. & Belser, U.C. (2000). Mechanics of the connection between implant and abutment – an 8γ morse taper compared to a butt joint connection. *International Journal of Oral and Maxillofacial Implants* **15**, 519–526.

Morneburg, T.R. & Pröschel, P.A. (2002). Measurement of masticatory forces and implant loads: A methodological clinical study. *International Journal of Prosthodontics* **15**, 20–27.

Naert, I.E., Duyck, J.A.J., Hosny, M.M.F., Quirynen, M. & van Steenberghe, D. (2001b). Freestanding and tooth-implant connected prostheses in the treatment of partially edentulous patients. Part II: An up to 15-years radiographic evaluation. *Clinical Oral Implants Research* **12**, 245–251.

Naert, I.E., Duyck, J.A.J., Hosny, M.M.F. & van Steenberghe, D. (2001a). Freestanding and tooth-implant connected prostheses in the treatment of partially edentulous patients. Part I: An up to 15-years clinical evaluation. *Clinical Oral Implants Research* **12**, 237–244.

Oetterli, M., Kiener, P. & Mericske-Stern, R. (2001). A longitudinal study on mandibular implants supporting an overdenture: The influence of retention mechanism and anatomic-prosthetic variables on periimplant parameters. *International Journal of Prosthodontics* **14**, 536–542.

Olsson, M., Gunne, J., Åstrand, P. & Borg, K. (1995). Bridges supported by free standing implants vs. bridges supported by tooth and implants. A five-year prospective study. *Clinical Oral Implants Research* **6**, 114–121.

O'Mahony, A.M., Williams, J.L. & Spencer, P. (2001). Anisotropic elasticity of cortical and cancellous bone in the posterior mandible increases peri-implant stress and strain under oblique loading. *Clinical Oral Implants Research* **12**, 648–657.

Quirynen, M., De Soete, M. & van Steenberghe, D. (2002). Infectious risks for oral implants: a review of the literature. *Clinical Oral Implants Research* **13**, 1–19.

Quirynen, M., Peeters, W., Naert, I., Coucke, W. & van Steenberghe, D. (2001). Peri-implant health around screw-shaped c.p. titanium machined implants in partially edentulous patients with or without ongoing periodontitis. *Clinical Oral Implants Research* **12**, 589–594.

Rangert, B., Sullivan, R.M. & Jemt, T.M. (1997). Load factor control for implants in the posterior partially edentulous segment. *International Journal of Oral and Maxillofacial Implants* **12**, 360–370.

Roccuzzo, M., Bunino, M., Prioglio, F. & Bianchi, S.D. (2001). Early loading of sandblasted and acid-etched (SLA) implants: a prospective split-mouth comparative study. *Clinical Oral Implants Research* **12**, 572–578.

Romanos, G.E., Toh, C.G., Siar, C.H., Swaminathan, D. & Ong, A.H. (2002). Histologic and histomorphometric evaluation of peri-implant bone subjected to immediate loading: An experimental study with macaca fascicularis. *International Journal of Oral and Maxillofacial Implants* **17**, 44–51.

Romeo, E., Chiapasco, M., Ghisolfi, M. & Vogel, G. (2002). Long-term clinical effectiveness of oral implants in the treatment of partial edentulism. Seven-year life table analysis of a prospective study with ITI® Dental Implant System used for single-tooth restorations. *Clinical Oral Implants Research* **13**, 133–143.

Schwarz, M.S. (2000). Mechanical complications of dental implants. *Clinical Oral Implants Research* **11** (Suppl I), 261–264.

Schwartz-Arad, D. & Dolev, E. (2000). The challenge of endosseous implants placed in the posterior partially edentulous maxilla: a clinical report. *International Journal of Oral and Maxillofacial Implants* **15**, 261–264.

Sheets, C.G. & Earthman, J.C. (1993). Natural tooth intrusion and reversal in implant-assisted prosthesis: evidence of and a hypothesis for the occurrence. *Journal of Prosthetic Dentistry* **70**, 513–522.

Simion, M., Jovanovic, S.A., Tinti, C. & Parma Benfenati, S. (2001). Long-term evaluation of osseointegrated implants inserted at the time of or after vertical ridge augmentation. A retrospective study on 123 implants with 1–5 year follow-up. *Clinical Oral Implants Research* **12**, 35–45.

Sutter, F., Weber, H.P., Sørensen, J. & Belser, U.C. (1993). The new restorative concept of the ITI Dental Implant System: Design and engineering. *International Journal of Periodontics and Restorative Dentistry* **13**, 409–431.

Szmukler-Moncler, S., Piatelli, J.A., Favero, J.H. & Dubruille, J.H. (2000). Considerations preliminary to the application of early and immediate loading protocols in dental implantology. *Clinical Oral Implants Research* **11**, 12–25.

Tangerud, T., Grønningsæter, A.G. & Taylor, Å. (2002). Fixed partial dentures supported by natural teeth and Brånemark System implants: A 3-year report. *International Journal of Oral and Maxillofacial Implants* **17**, 212–219.

Tarnow, D.P., Emtiaz, S. & Classi, A. (1997). Immediate loading of threaded implants at stage 1 surgery in edentulous arches: ten consecutive case reports with 1- to 5-year data. *International Journal of Oral and Maxillofacial Implants* **12**, 319–324.

Taylor, T.D. (1998). Prosthodontic problems and limitations associated with osseointegration. *Journal of Prosthetic Dentistry* **79**, 74–78.

Taylor, T.D., Belser, U.C. & Mericske-Stern, R. (2000). Prosthodontic considerations. *Clinical Oral Implants Research* **11** (Suppl I), 101–107.

ten Bruggenkate, C.M., Asikainen, P., Foitzik, C., Krekeler, G. & Sutter, F. (1998). Short (6 mm) non-submerged dental implants: results of a multicenter clinical trial of 1–7 years. *International Journal of Oral and Maxillofacial Implants* **13**, 791–798.

Van Steenberghe, D., Quirynen, M. & Wallace, S.S. (1999). Survival and success rates with oral endosseous implants. In: Lang, N.P., Karring, T. & Lindhe, J., eds. *Proceedings of the 3rd European Workshop on Periodontology*. Berlin: Quintessence, pp. 242–254.

von Arx, T., Cochran, D.L., Hermann, J., Schenk, R.K., Higginbottom, F. & Buser, D. (2001a). Lateral ridge augmentation and implant placement: an experimental study evaluating implant osseointegration in different augmentation materials in the canine mandible. *International Journal of Oral and Maxillofacial Implants* **16**, 343–354.

von Arx, T., Cochran, D.L., Hermann, J.S., Schenk, R.K. & Buser, D. (2001b). Lateral ridge augmentation using different bone fillers and barrier membrane application. A histologic and histomorphometric pilot study in the canine mandible. *Clinical Oral Implants Research* **12**, 260–269.

Weber, H.P., Crohin, C.C. & Fiorellini, J.P. (2000). A 5-year prospective clinical and radiographic study of non-submerged dental implants. *Clinical Oral Implants Research* **11**, 144–153.

Wie, H. (1995). Registration of localization, occlusion and occluding materials for failing screw joints in the Brånemark implant system. *Clinical Oral Implants Research* **6**, 47–63.

Wiskott, A.H.W. & Belser, U.C. (1999). Lack of integration of smooth titanium surfaces: a working hypothesis based on strains generated in the surrounding bone. *Clinical Oral Implants Research* **10**, 429–444.

Wiskott, A.H.W., Perriard, J, Scherrer, S.S., Dieth, S. & Belser, U.C. (2002). In vivo wear of three types of veneering materials using implant-supported restorations. A method evaluation. *European Journal of Oral Sciences* **110**, 61–67.

Wismeijer, D., van Waas, M.A.J., Mulder J., Vermeeren I.J.F. & Kalk, W. (1999). Clinical and radiological results of patients treated with three treatment modalities for overdentures on implants of the ITI dental implant system. A randomised controlled clinical trial. *Clinical Oral Implants Research* **10**, 297–306.

Wright, P.S., Glantz, P-O., Randow, K. & Watson, R.M. (2002). The effects of fixed and removable implant-stabilised prostheses on posterior mandibular residual ridge resorption. *Clinical Oral Implants Research* **13**, 1169–1174.

Wyatt, C.L. & Zarb, G.A. (1998). Treatment outcomes of patients with implant-supported fixed partial prostheses. *International Journal of Oral and Maxillofacial Implants* **13**, 204–211.

Wyatt, C.L. & Zarb, G.A. (2002). Bone level changes proximal to oral implants supporting fixed partial prostheses. *Clinical Oral Implants Research* **13**, 162–168.

Zarb, G.A. & Schmitt, A. (1995). Implant prosthodontic treatment options for the edentulous patient. *Journal of Oral Rehabilitation* **22**, 661–671.

Zitzmann, N.U. & Marinello, C.P. (1999). Treatment plan for restoring the edentulous maxilla with implant supported restorations: removable overdenture versus fixed partial denture design. *Journal of Prosthetic Dentistry* **82**, 188–196.

Zitzmann, N.U. & Marinello, C.P. (2002). A review of clinical and technical considerations for fixed and removable implant prostheses in the edentulous mandible. *International Journal of Prosthodontics* **15**, 65–67.

Zitzmann, N.U., Schärer, P. & Marinello, C.P. (2001). Long-term results of implants treated with guided bone regeneration: A 5-year prospective study. *International Journal of Oral and Maxillofacial Implants* **16**, 355–366.

Chapter 55

Implant–Implant and Tooth–Implant Supported Fixed Partial Dentures

Clark M. Stanford and Lyndon F. Cooper

Introduction, 1208
Initial patient assessment, 1208
Implant treatment planning for the edentulous arch, 1209
  Prosthesis design and full-arch tooth replacement therapy, 1210
  Complete-arch fixed complete dentures, 1211
Prosthesis design and partially edentulous tooth replacement
  therapy, 1211

Implant per tooth versus an implant-to-implant
  FPD?, 1212
Cantilever pontics, 1213
Immediate provisionalization, 1215
Disadvantages of implant–implant fixed partial
  dentures, 1215
Tooth–implant fixed partial dentures, 1216

Introduction

The restoration of the fully and partially edentulous situation involves a combination of systematic diagnosis, treatment planning, and careful assessment of the therapy choices and the outcomes. The replacement of a continuous span of teeth creates challenges involving assessment of anatomic, physiologic, cost, time, impact on quality of life (QOL), and patient desires. The clinician is faced with balancing each of these aspects when developing a treatment plan for the patient. Modern dental care assures that tooth replacement therapy is provided in an economical and expedient manner. To this end, dental implants offer advantages for many clinical situations. In certain situations, the restoration of missing teeth using individual free-standing implant-supported crowns is a logical and satisfactory treatment option. At other times use of an implant-supported fixed partial denture (FPD) is a satisfactory approach (Fig. 55-1). Because of functional and esthetic priorities, anterior and posterior multi-tooth implant restorations can present different clinical challenges. This chapter will consider implant-to-implant supported FPD (bridges) separately from tooth-to-implant supported prosthesis since there are unique issues with each type of prosthesis. The use of a fixed complete denture to replace all of the teeth in an arch will be considered as a form of a fixed partial denture.

Initial patient assessment

The predictable esthetic and functional outcomes of implant treatment require comprehensive diagnostic and treatment planning (Stanford 2005a). As a member of the implant team, the prosthodontist needs to collaborate with the surgical specialist, laboratory technician, and allied team members such as radiologists, and dental and surgical assistants. The initial assessment of the patient's medical and dental history assists in the determination of the implant system and devices that will meet the patient's therapeutic needs. The initial patient interview should establish the patient's individual esthetic requirements. This assessment should determine a patient's history of bruxism, periodontal disease, tobacco use, uncontrolled diabetes mellitus, and metabolic bone diseases (Moy et al. 2005). Recent literature suggests implant therapy in patients with advanced chronic periodontitis may have an altered prognosis, although stabilized with maintenance therapy (Nevins & Langer 1995; Ellegaard et al. 1997; Brocard et al. 2000; Pjetursson et al. 2004; Wennstrom et al. 2004a). Maintenance therapy is vital since longitudinal implant bone loss occurs and can be observed after many years of asymptomatic clinical service (Hardt et al. 2002; Fransson et al. 2005). In addition, the assessment should educate patients about the etiology of tooth loss, reveal their attitudes about treatment as well as the ability to tolerate it,

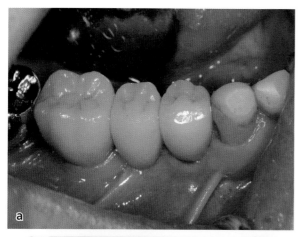

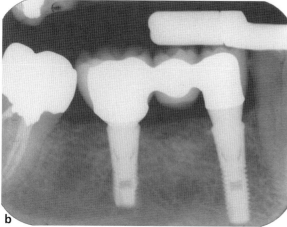

Fig. 55-1 Implant-supported fixed partial denture (FPD). (a) Patient restored with two implants (44 and 46) and three-unit FPD. (b) Five-year recall radiograph demonstrates stability of osseous tissues around the implants.

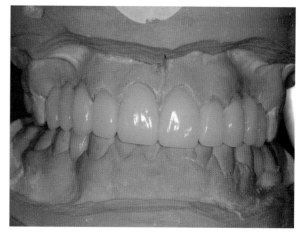

Fig. 55-2 Diagnostic wax-up for implant therapy demonstrating desired contours for the planned definitive restorations.

and inform them of estimated treatment costs (Pjetursson *et al.* 2005; Stanford 2005a). Throughout the surgical and prosthetic phases of the implant reconstruction, the dental practitioner should obtain comprehensive written and verbal informed consent for patient treatment. The consent form should document the risks, benefits, and alternatives discussed with the patient. The option for and consequences of no treatment should be included. This initial assessment phase should provide the clinical team with sufficient information to characterize the patient-related risk factors that will influence treatment.

To assure the implant location, number, and implant dimension are congruent with the anticipated prosthesis, it is essential the dentist design and compose the proposed prosthesis during the diagnostic phase. Pre-operative planning gives insights into both technical aspects (number, implant dimension, position, and angulation) as well as potential surgical site development needed prior to or at the time of implant placement. The complete treatment plan then assimilates clinical, radiographic, and psychologic information gathered using the patient interview, clinical examination, and radiographic survey. During the clinical examination, the dentist carefully evaluates the residual ridge for shape and

contour, and evaluates alternative intraoral sites for mucosal recession. A careful evaluation of patient's risk factors for soft and hard tissue changes, whatever final restoration is planned, should be made to comply with the informed consent process and encourage realistic patient expectations. However, to move beyond assessing the feasibility of implant treatment, it is essential to utilize articulated diagnostic study casts to fully assess the tissue architecture and relationship of teeth and mucosa with existing edentulous areas.

Thus, the initial clinical examination should conclude only when sufficient materials are available to accurately mount diagnostic casts and interpret the study casts and screening radiographs using recorded clinical information. Based on this diagnostic information, a surgical guide or denture is fabricated using a process of diagnostic waxing of the planned prostheses, evaluation of the desired implant position, angulation, probable abutment dimension and angulation, and, finally, the need for hard or soft tissue augmentation as supportive therapy to implant placement (Fig. 55-2). The diagnostic waxing process is a key step in the assessment of local risk factors affecting fixed partial dentures supported by dental implants and is critical to the process of strategically planning implant placement to limit these risks.

Implant treatment planning for the edentulous arch

The edentulous mandibular arch can be restored using a fixed complete denture, fixed partial dentures or an overdenture. The fixed complete denture can be a gold casting or CAD/CAM milled titanium framework, either with prosthetic acrylic resin teeth or teeth veneered with porcelain (Adell *et al.* 1990) The edentulous arch can also be restored with a series of FPDs that allows the clinic to manage multiple implants without seeking the precision fit of a full-arch prosthesis (Fig. 55-3). This approach also pro-

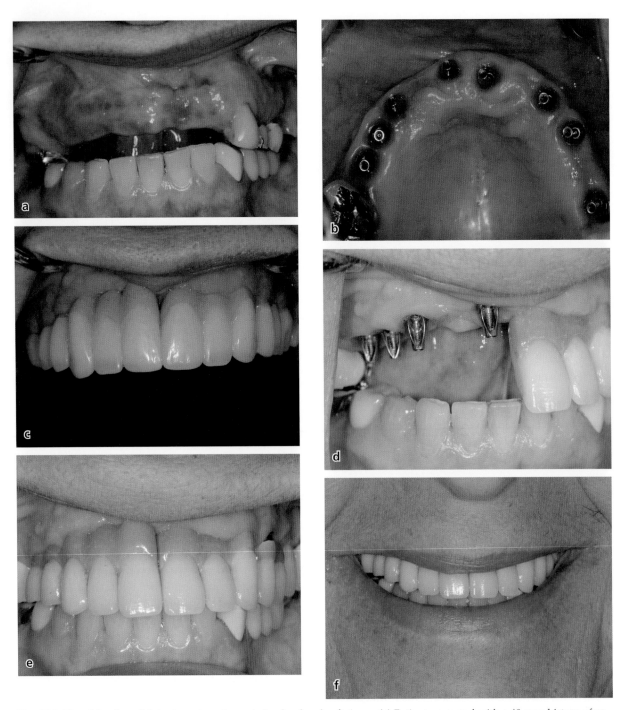

Fig. 55-3 Use of fixed partial dentures to restore missing hard and soft tissue. (a) Patient presented with a 40-year history of an edentulous space in the maxilla. Following placement of eight implants (b), a long-term acrylic resin provisional was fabricated simulating desired tooth and soft tissue dimensions (c). (d) Based on the long-term provisional, a ceramometal fixed prosthesis was fabricated using mucosa-colored ceramic materials on a metal framework. (e,f) Five-year recall demonstrating fixed prosthetic outcomes and anterior esthetics.

vides for greater flexibility in case of complications related to porcelain fracture, recession, wear, etc., and has demonstrated successful long-term outcomes (Bragger *et al.* 2001). An overdenture with attachment to the implant can be fully implant supported and retained or a combination mucosa/implant-borne prosthesis. Clinical studies indicate high patient acceptance of this form of therapy (Feine *et al.* 1994, 2002; Duyck *et al.* 2004; Naert *et al.* 2004a,b; Zitzmann *et al.* 2005).

Prosthesis design and full-arch tooth replacement therapy

If minimal bone resorption exists, restoring the edentulous maxillae with a porcelain-fused-to-metal restoration has a reasonable outcome (Stanford 2005a). The restorative dentist must perform a diagnostic work-up including impressions, jaw relationship records, and an esthetic try-in using prosthetic denture teeth on a trial denture base. The degree of lip support and smile line (i.e. anterior and posterior occlusal planes) of the diagnostic denture set-up should be evaluated intraorally. It is also useful to evaluate the patient's lip support with and without the anterior facial denture flange (Lewis *et al.* 1992; Stanford 2002). The amount of tooth exposure of the anterior smile line (relaxed and exaggerated), provides clues about the expected crown length, gingival display, and potential need to use gingival tone porcelain for appropriate tooth length and esthetics in a full-arch reconstruction. Communication and discussion with the dental laboratory technician is very helpful at this point prior to finalizing the treatment plan. A fixed maxillary prosthesis has greater incidence of esthetic, phonetic, and oral hygiene problems compared with an overdenture prosthesis, in part associated with excessively long anterior teeth, excessive facial cantilever pontics, and mesial–distal complications with embrasure forms (Lewis *et al.* 1992). Given the clinical and laboratory complexity of these prostheses, a maxillary overdenture on four to six implants may be an alternative (Phillips & Wong 2001; Anon. 2003; Naert *et al.* 2004b).

Complete-arch fixed complete dentures

A complete-arch fixed complete denture (FCD) provides excellent function and patient acceptance (Lewis *et al.* 1992; Feine *et al.* 1994). During the diagnostic phases, the advantages and disadvantages of the FCD compared with those of an overdenture should be discussed with the patient. If using a ceramometal full-arch fixed reconstruction, consider replacing every three teeth with a three-unit fixed partial denture on two implants (e.g. #13–11) using the pontic contours to adjust for implant alignment and esthetic demands (Fig. 55-3) (Stanford 2002). A fixed maxillary reconstruction entails between six and eight implants (first molar, first premolar, canine, and central incisor) with four independent fixed partial dentures (molar to premolar, canine to central incisor, bilaterally) (Stanford 2005a). With care made to limit loading, six implants may be used with distal cantilevers on two fixed partial dentures (cantilever pontics limited to one premolar sized tooth). An overdenture should use a sufficient number of implants for long-term stability, typically four in the maxilla (canine and second premolar region) and two in the lower canine or first premolar region (Mericske-Stern *et al.* 2000). Using the denture set-up, a radiographic guide is fabricated with radio-opaque markers (e.g. gutta-percha or bur shanks) within the denture at the sites of interest. An alternative approach involves duplicating the denture set-up with teeth made using 5% medical grade barium sulfate mixed with clear autopolymerizing resin. This approach allows easy visualization of tooth size, angle, and position on conventional and/or CT-aided treatment planning. In the mandible, the trial set-up evaluates the height and position of the prosthetic

teeth relative to the symphyseal cross-sectional anatomy. A conventional fixed complete denture with acrylic teeth requires a minimum of 15 mm from the alveolar crest to the planned incisal edge (Stanford 2005a). If the vertical dimension of occlusion and jaw anatomy is insufficient, one alternative is to perform an aggressive alveoectomy or to rehabilitate with ceramometal restorations (along with treatment planning for the additional cost).

Radiographic information and diagnostic set-up will help determine the type of definitive prosthesis design. Skeletal class I and II relationships with minimal resorption may allow normal contours and lip support with a fixed complete denture. Prognathic class III relationship can increase prosthetic problems, especially if implants cannot be placed distal to the mental foramens. In such cases, an overdenture approach yields a more predictable result (Naert *et al.* 1997).

Prosthesis design and partially edentulous tooth replacement therapy

Clinician or patient preferences for the use of implants for restoration of partial edentulism using FPDs must be carefully weighed against the potential limitations associated with this therapy. Technical complications related to implant components and the suprastructure are more frequently reported than complications related to peri-implant tissues (Berglundh *et al.*, 2002). Also, these complications for implant-supported fixed partial dentures are together more frequent than implant loss or implant fracture. For example, Bragger *et al.* (2001) reported for a 10-year follow-up period that the percentage of reconstructions without any biologic nor technical failure/complication was 66.5% for single-crown implant restorations, 54.4% for implant-supported FPD, and 50% for tooth–implant-supported FPD. Importantly, the authors concluded that prostheses with history of complications were at greater risk of implant failure. It may be possible to infer that complications reflect the functional features of the prosthesis or the patient and, furthermore, that some of these complications are due to limitations in implant and prosthesis planning, placement, construction or the innate limitations of implant components. Complications most frequently observed for FPDs include veneer fracture, opposing restoration fracture, bridge screw loosening or fracture, abutment screw loosening or fracture, and metal framework fractures (Goodacre *et al.* 2003a). The considerations for treatment planning of implant-supported FPDs must include features that affect not only implant success, but also abutment and bridge screw performance, and prosthesis esthetics and longevity.

Primary among clinical considerations for any implant prosthesis is some estimation of the potential forces that will be exerted during function. It is well

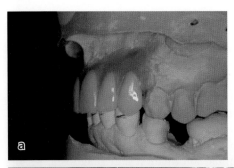

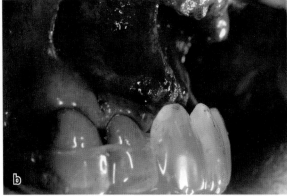

Fig. 55-4 (a) Diagnostic wax-up demonstrating desired tooth position and wax used to demonstrate the amount of planned augmentation needed. (b) At the time of site development, the surgical guide demonstrates the difference between the desired tooth position and the residual ridge.

recognized that masticatory forces increase as the point of interaction moves posterior in the arch. Additionally, damaging bending moments are increased with the acting lever arm length. Greater concern is warranted when implants are planned to support prostheses with large occluso-gingival dimension (extensive resorption) or for prostheses with extensive mesial, buccal or lingual cantilevers or any substantial distal cantilever. Additional immediate considerations typically address the esthetic potential of the prosthesis. This is clearly most relevant for anterior FPDs. Tooth-like restorations are dependent on proper dimensions and, again, greater concern is raised with increasing residual ridge resorption. However, basic features of implant placement such as avoiding encroachment of embrasures are critically important for anterior FPDs. These matters are revealed through the process of evaluating the diagnostic waxing (Fig. 55-4).

The current absence of discrete rules governing the number and dimension of implants (or a particular implant) needed to support a given masticatory function is acknowledged. Krekmanov *et al.* (2002) proposed that support factors can be attributed to implants and that relative risk can be assigned to various clinical scenarios. This approach of recognizing relative risk factors and modifying the clinical approach to therapy – even in a subjective way – merits consideration. At the very least, each clinical scenario should be considered in terms of prosthetic and implant risk both biologically and biomechani-

cally and treatment should be adapted to recognize these risks if possible. Obvious examples would include the use of additional or larger implants to support molar function as opposed to premolar function and the avoidance of distal cantilevers in bruxing patients.

A simple strategy for reducing the biomechanical risks to implants and prostheses of implant-supported FPDs is to plan for implants located beneath the cervical aspect of the terminal mesial and distal FPD retainers whenever possible. This approach reduces the length of bending moments, irrespective of the imposed load, and also assures that the implant and abutment do not encroach on the embrasures to limit oral hygiene or esthetic potential of the restoration (Fig. 55-1).

When multiple implants are placed in an edentulous span, careful treatment planning will indicate mesial and distal width of desired restorative teeth. This plan will in turn indicate proposed sites where implants (e.g. every other tooth) may be placed for stability of the prosthesis. Choice of implant location may depend on available osseous tissues, soft tissue thickness, esthetics, phonetics, and need for ridge development.

Implant per tooth versus an implant-to-implant FPD?

In having a dialog with patients about the desired tooth replacement therapy, clinicians often recommend an implant per tooth approach when replacing multiple contiguous teeth. When this approach is done with individual free-standing crowns, the approach provides potential for a natural tooth-by-tooth replacement. On the other hand, it can create significant issues for the prosthetic restoration if the implants are not placed in exactly the desired location. The use of short-span FPDs therefore has certain general advantages. First, the use of two implants to replace three teeth allows the technician to judiciously use the pontic contours to alter the shape and contour of the prosthesis, compensating for implants that are not optimally positioned. For instance, implants that emerge at the interproximal area can be compensated by the use of angled abutments or custom abutments facilitating the use of the connector dimensions to create an illusion of natural teeth. Another advantage cited by some is the establishment of interproximal contacts between the prosthesis and adjacent teeth.

In order to assess the predictability of these types of restorations, clinical research studies need to be assessed. Randomized, controlled clinical trials of partially edentulous patients with a previous history of periodontal bone loss were evaluated in a 5-year trial by Wennström *et al.* (2004a). This study reported on 149 self-tapping implants (Astra Tech AB, Mölndal, Sweden) placed in the maxilla (n = 83) and mandible (n = 66) in the premolar and molar area. Each patient received two implants (machined surface versus grit blasted with Ti dioxide) that were allowed to heal for 6 months prior to loading. Screw-retained FPDs were completed and maintenance therapy provided following the CIST program (Lang *et al.* 2004). Implant loss was 5.9% at the subject level. FPDs demonstrated a total 5-year bone loss from implant placement of 0.41 ± 0.78 mm (subject level) (Wennstrom *et al.* 2004a). There was a statistical difference in the frequency of bone loss between those placed in the upper versus those in the lower jaw: 38% of the maxillary implants demonstrated >1 mm bone loss while 9% of the FPD in the lower arch had >1 mm bone loss at 5 years.

Previous studies evaluating bone loss with the implant system used in this study have reported mean marginal bone loss from implant placement to be an average of −0.46 ± 0.38 mm (Olsson *et al.* 1995; Yusuf & Ratra 1996; Karlsson *et al.* 1997, 1998; Makkonen *et al.* 1997; Norton 1997, 2001; Arvidson *et al.* 1998; Astrand *et al.* 1999; Cooper *et al.* 1999, 2001; Palmer *et al.* 2000, 2005; Puchades-Roman *et al.* 2000; van Steenberghe *et al.* 2000; Gotfredsen & Karlsson 2001; Steveling *et al.* 2001; Weibrich *et al.* 2001; Engquist *et al.* 2002; Wennstrom *et al.* 2004a,b, 2005; Rasmusson *et al.* 2005). When implants were placed in the posterior maxilla with the indirect sinus lift technique and restored with FPDs at 6 weeks using a fluoride-modified implant, outcomes demonstrated bone loss −0.19 to −0.4 mm (sd = 0.73) from implant placement with a 98.3% cumulative implant survival rate (CISR) (Stanford 2006). These data support the concept that partially edentulous patients can be restored with FPDs (Gotfredsen & Karlsson 2001). However, post-insertion maintenance is critical. Hardt *et al.* (2002) observed in a population with a history of bone loss associated with periodontitis, that poor oral hygiene and compliance with maintenance therapy resulted in an elevated failure rate of 8% at 5 years; 62% of the implants in patients susceptible to periodontitis vs. 44% in non-perio groups demonstrated more than 2 mm bone loss (Hardt *et al.* 2002). This emphasizes the need for ongoing supportive care for patients undergoing tooth replacement therapy (Lang *et al.* 2004a; Schou *et al.* 2004).

Cantilever pontics

In managing tooth replacement therapy there are times when a mesial or distal extension is needed to the FPD. The use of cantilever extensions increases the mechanical angular moment on the prosthesis and increases the potential for early fatigue and prosthetic complications (Brunski 2003). The use of cantilever extensions were first advocated as a routine prosthetic approach in the Toronto mandibular fixed complete denture designed for the edentulous arch (Zarb 1988; Zarb and Schmitt 1990a,b, 1991). Clinical studies on the use of cantilever extensions suggest greater complications with longer extensions beyond

15 mm, although there are many opinion-based recommendations that range from 10–20 mm (Shackleton *et al.* 1994). Cantilever extensions increase the angular moment on the most distal implant and abutment connection and the complications such as loosening screws, fractured components, etc. are related to a combination of factors including cantilever design, composition, occlusion, jaw relationships, and implant/abutment design (Brunski *et al.* 1986). In a survival analysis though 80 months of fixed complete dentures with an acrylic resin tooth replacement and the external hex Branemark system, Shackleton *et al.* (1994) observed a 100% survival rate for cantilever extension <15 mm but a decline to <30% survival for extension >15 mm.

In the anterior quadrant where esthetics are desired, there are often missing lateral incisors that leave only minimal mesial–distal space for implant placement. One option may be to use narrow diameter implants in such sites but control of occlusion is important (Stanford 2005b). An alternative, especially when there are missing adjacent teeth, is to use cantilever pontics of minimal dimension to replace the missing teeth (Fig. 55-5). This has the potential for more predictable esthetics without excessive site development, expense, and time. The use of cantilever pontics in the posterior quadrants is more controversial. Cantilever pontics in ceramometal FPDs create larger moment arms on the prosthesis and have the potential for increase mechanical complications with the implant–abutment stack (Stanford 1999; Brunski 2000, 2003; Brunski *et al.* 2000; Gratton *et al.* 2001). There are times where posterior cantilever pontics are useful but the clinician should consider these for areas of controlled occlusal forces and primarily for esthetics. Further, in use with ceramometal FPD, their use should be limited with no more than a premolar size pontic (~7 mm mesial-distal dimension) with only light centric occlusal contacts on the pontic (Stanford 2005b).

There are ongoing issues regarding cemented relative to screw-retained FPDs. While the choice of prosthesis is dependent on multiple factors (clinician preference, flexibility, passivity of fit, cost, etc.) there are times when one approach is preferable. For instance, in situations where the patient has multiple clinical signs of recession (thin tissue biotype, recession, lack of keratinized mucosa, etc.) a screw-retained fixed prosthesis may be preferable (Stanford 2005a). This approach will allow the clinician to remove the prosthesis at a later point in time and make repairs which may salvage the prosthesis. Patients with a history of implant loss in the area, difficult implant placement or elevated medical risk are other indications to consider a screw-retained fixed prosthesis. Further, if the prosthesis needs to be routinely removed (e.g. in a research protocol) for accurate measurements of pocket probing depths (PPD) and bleeding on probing (BOP), the clinician may want to chose a screw-retained prosthesis. At times there

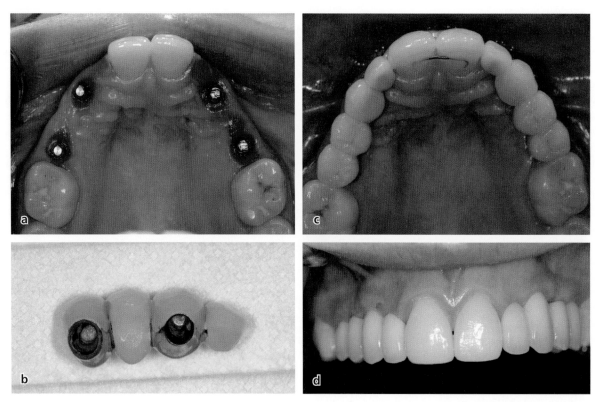

Fig. 55-5 Use of cantilever pontics to replace missing lateral incisors as a part of fixed partial denture (FPD) therapy. (a) Four implants were placed in the maxilla in the second premolar and canine region. (b) A four-unit FPD with cantilever pontics (12 and 22) was fabricated. (c) Restoration of eight missing teeth with four implants allowing establishment of an acceptable esthetic result (d).

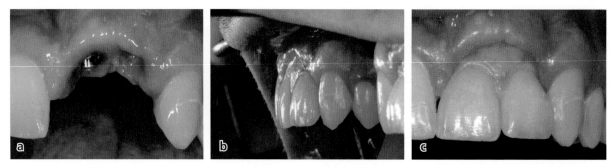

Fig. 55-6 Soft and hard tissue prosthetic replacement. (a) Patient presented with soft tissue loss in the area of 21 and 22. (b) Missing mucosal and hard tissue contours were replaced with a combination of gingival and tooth-colored ceramic materials. (c) A prosthetic solution to a difficult esthetic situation. Ceramic reconstruction by Henry Husemann CDT (University of Iowa).

are indications for fabricating a fixed prosthesis that replaces both hard and soft tissues (Garcia & Verrett 2004). In sites where there has been considerable loss of supporting structures, common following trauma or long-term chronic bone loss such as periodontal disease, it may be necessary to replace both dental and osseous supporting structures (Fig. 55-3). If this cannot be accomplished with biological site development, the clinicians may need to reconstruct this area with a combination of porcelain teeth developed with the appropriate mesial-distal and inciso-gingival dimensions to match the adjacent teeth and blend into the esthetic contours of the dentition and face. In doing so, it may become obvious that the gingival tissues need to be replicated in "mucosal" colored

porcelain or acrylic. The development of tissue-matched mucosal shades takes significant laboratory skill and dexterity and often means the patient needs to be seen directly by the technician along with the restorative dentist (Malament 2000; Malament & Neeser 2004). Custom mucosal shades often need to be developed and matched chairside. While these approaches can be quite time consuming the end results can be quite satisfactory and surpass what can be accomplished by repeated soft tissue procedures (Fig. 55-6). The restorative dentist needs carefully to assess the patient early in the diagnostic process for implant therapy and determine if they are at elevated risk for unpredictable loss of soft tissue. Key factors to assess are thin tissue biotype, previous history of recession, mucosal inflammation, tooth loss due to trauma or chronic progressive osseous disease (e.g. periodontitis). All of these conditions influence the stability and position of the mucosal tissues following implant tooth replacement therapy.

Immediate provisionalization

The application of implant-supported FPDs has a unique role especially in early and immediate loading procedures. While the splinting of implants for long-term osseointegration is not considered routinely necessary, the early splinting of multiple implants during the osseous healing process is considered important (Cooper *et al.* 2002, 2005, 2006; Slaets *et al.* 2005; De Kok *et al.* 2006; Duyck *et al.* 2006). Immediate provisionalization procedures have the potential to provide rapid function, esthetics, and patient satisfaction, and the use of implant-supported FPD prosthetic designs plays an intimate role in controlling micromotion and allowing successful outcomes similar to conventional loading procedures (De Kok *et al.* 2006; Duyck *et al.* 2006; Hall *et al.* 2006; Peleg *et al.* 2006).

The immediate provisionalization of implant-supported fixed dentures has a unique role in the retreatment of failing fixed prostheses. When large fixed prostheses are present with only one or two failing abutments, further tooth-supported restoration often requires extensive restoration. This is particularly true if strategic abutments such as a canine or terminal abutment tooth are not salvageable due to caries, fracture or localized periodontitis. In such cases, segmental resection of the failed tooth and supported pontic teeth can be replaced by dental implants. The advantages are obvious in terms of preventing the retreatment of a much larger FPD and providing an esthetic and functional treatment option for an anterior restoration.

Disadvantages of implant–implant fixed partial dentures

The disadvantages of FPDs on implants are associated with increased difficulty of cleaning and maintaining the prosthesis along with the prosthesis complications associated with conventional tooth-supported FPDs. Based on patient expectations, there is the potential that the patient isn't satisfied with the inability to clean between the retainers and pontic contours. FPDs on implants can also be more difficult to fabricate in the laboratory. In this case there may be issues with the path of insertion on the abutments (necessitating customized abutment) or difficulties in obtaining draw and passive fit between multiple abutments. There is also the danger of mechanical wear and material failure with the completed prosthesis such as abutment loosening, prosthesis fracture or veneer material failure. The use of screw-retained prosthesis may be helpful if retriev-

ability is critical but the screw access hole itself may weaken the strength of the veneering material. Lastly, there is the danger that if one of the supporting implants are lost or the abutment demonstrates recession exposing the transmucosal titanium surface, the entire prosthesis may have to be replaced increasing time and expense to the patient.

In assessing the clinical success of implant-supported FPDs, it is difficult to determine outcomes due to incomplete reporting of the specific types of prosthesis in a range of dental implant studies and yet the primary measure of evidence-based care is the systematic assessment of the clinical question of interest. The literature supporting the use of this type of prosthesis is often retrospective in nature with different outcome measures, end points, duration of recall, etc. This makes comparisons between studies difficult and limited. In the assessment of prosthodontic mechanical complications, the pattern of defects often will vary with a time-dependent pattern. In implant-supported FPDs, early failures (before loading) are often associated with implant loss (Goodacre *et al.* 2003b). As discussed by Pjetursson *et al.* (2004), implant loss prior to restoration can be expected on average to be 2.5% of all implants placed with an additional 2–3% lost over the first 5 years of function. In this systematic assessment of the more recent literature from the 1990s though 2004, 21 studies of 176 reviews were considered based on the inclusion and exclusion criteria. The authors summarized the current literature of five implant systems with 1123 patients, 1336 FPDs on 3578 implants followed for at least 5 years. Implant survival, FPD survival, success, and complications were reported (Table 55-1). The authors outlined that this type of assessment has limitations based on the quality of the studies, their duration, drop-outs, and reliability but in this instance, with the limited dataset, the authors outlined that the most common complication was

Table 55-1 Implant supported fixed partial dentures (FPDs) with an average of 5 years' follow-up (Pjetursson *et al.* 2004: in this review, 90% of the FPDs were screw-retained)

	Average	**95% confidence interval**
Implant survival	95.6%	93.3–97.2%
FPD prosthesis survival*	95%	92.2–96.8%
FPD success†	61.3%	55.3–66.8%
Complications	38.7%	
• Veneer fracture	13.2%	8.3–20.6%
• Lost occlusal restorations	8.2%	
• Loose screws	5.8%	3.8–8.7%
• Fractured abutments/ occlusal screws	1.5%	0.8–2.8%
• Fractured implants	0.4%	0.1–1.2%

* Survival was defined as retained in function within the mouth. Prosthesis may have had multiple repairs.
† Success was defined as in function with no clinical complications.

Table 55-2 Local features considered in risk assessment for implant-supported fixed partial dentures (FPDs)

FPD location	Anterior locations possess higher esthetic risk Posterior locations may possess higher functional risk
Length of span	Long span increases complexity of prosthesis, mechanical loads and prosthetic complications Short span may increase abutment crowding and restrict hygiene
Occluso-gingival dimension	Increased occluso-gingival dimension results in lower bending moments at abutment and bridge screw connections Reduced occluso-gingival dimension (<6 mm) may limit prosthesis construction and integrity
Excessive vertical residual ridge resorption	Excessive vertical residual ridge resorption results in increased occluso-gingival dimensions of the restoration
Implant malposition	Buccal or lingual malposition creates unintended buccal or lingual cantilever of prosthesis Mesial or distal malposition encroaches on embrasure and hygiene access; both reduce esthetic potential Excessive deep placement increases bending moment at abutment screw, may create anaerobic environment, can lead to bone resorption and esthetic complications
Thin mucosal biotype	Risk of mucosal resorption and unesthetic display of abutment material
History of periodontitis	Elevated risk for peri-implantitis if control is absent. May need multiple staged procedures to replace hard and soft tissue contours

loss of veneering material (often acrylic facings) followed by other mechanical complications inherent in screw-retained style prosthesis. Biologic complications such as peri-implantitis (probing pocket depth >5 mm) with bleeding on probing (BOP) have been reported in one study to average 10% of patients (Pjetursson *et al.* 2004). Pjetursson *et al.* (2004) used a random-effects Poisson modeling approach to determine a pooled cumulative rate of 8.6% for biologic complications (95% CI: 5.1–14.1%) based on a assessment of nine studies providing sufficient information for analysis.

A FPD supported by two or more implants provides a valuable treatment option. It has a role in providing rehabilitation for patients with challenging implant positions and angulation, lost hard and soft tissues, reduced cost, and may allow avoidance of some grafting procedures (e.g. sinus grafting). The selection of a FPD supported by implants often represents the alternative to selecting a much larger FPD supported by many teeth (Table 55-2). While recent reviews suggest there may be little difference in the long-term complication rates for FPDs supported by teeth and implants, it is of practical importance that implant-supported FPDs often are smaller prostheses. On balance, the use of FPDs plays a valuable role in providing multiple tooth replacement therapy.

Tooth–implant fixed partial dentures

The use of dental implants combined with teeth as retainers for FPDs has been advocated by a number of clinicians to restore multiple missing teeth. There are multiple case reports in the literature of prosthe-

sis designs that have either a rigid connection between the natural tooth and implant retainers and or that utilize a non-rigid connection to ostensibly allow individual movement of the implant(s) relative to the greater mobility of the natural teeth (Stanford & Brand 1999). The difference in mobility can be of the order of about one magnitude with mobility on teeth with a healthy PDL being 50–200 μm while an integrated implant will have mobility of <10 μm (Brunski & Hipp 1984; Brunski 1988a,b, 1999, 2003; Rangert *et al.* 1997). The use of implant–tooth FPD does have the potential to reduce costs, time, and morbidity especially if the outcome provides a service to the patient that would be equivalent to implant–implant FPD or single-tooth implant restorations (Fig. 55-7). The advantages must be balanced with the potential complication of pathology associated with the dental retainers or the implant(s). The fate of both is tied together.

Lang *et al.* (2004b) performed a systematic review of the clinical studies that evaluated tooth–implant FPDs over at least 5 years and were able to identify 13 studies using the inclusion/exclusion criteria. Of these, nine were prospective and four retrospective in nature addressing outcomes with five different implant systems in 555 patients (538 FPDs on 1002 implants); the majority (91%) were reported as being screw-retained. The authors assessed the thirteen studies by evaluating those with follow-up from 5–6.5 years. In this group, of the 932 implants installed, 25 were lost prior to restoration and 65 during the recall period. This resulted in a 5-year implant survival proportion of 90.1% (CI: 82.4–94.5%) (Lang *et al.* 2004b). In the second group, followed though 10 years, implant survival was estimated at 82.1% (CI: 55.8–93.6%). Following the same theme, a systematic

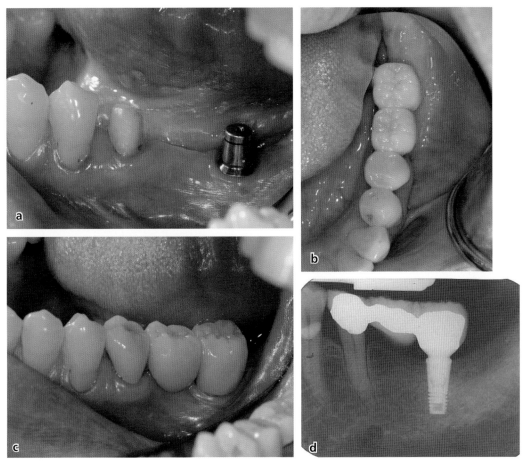

Fig. 55-7 Implant–tooth fixed partial denture. (a) Example demonstrates use of a rigid fixed partial denture (FPD) framework on a three-unit FPD (35–37). (b) A metal–ceramic prosthesis was cemented which has been monitored with frequent recall over 5 years (c). (d) Five-year recall radiograph indicates healthy peri-apical and peri-implant osseous tissues.

review of biologic and technical complications (Berglundh *et al.* 2002) indicated that tooth–implant-borne FPDs were at greater risk for implant loss (irrespective of complications leading to abutment tooth loss) than implant–implant FPDs. In regards to the prosthesis survival, estimates of 94.1% (CI: 90.2–96.5%) at 5 years and 77.8% (CI: 66.4–85.7%) at 10 years were determined (Lang *et al.* 2004). Assessment of dental abutment survival indicated 3.2% were lost by 5 years due to fracture, caries, or endodontic or periodontal complications (Lang 2004) If the patient has the option to restore missing teeth with a conventional removable partial denture combined with implant-fixed prosthodontics it is interesting to assess the long-term outcomes.

There has been a number of concerns raised with connecting teeth to implants with FPDs. Some of these complications are associated with technical complications of the prosthesis. For instance, the prognosis of the FPD can be shortened by veneer fractures and other esthetic issues (Kindberg *et al.* 2001). Loss of retention through fracture of the abutment/prosthetic screws or loss of cement retention are possible. Lang *et al.* (2004b) reported in a systematic review of two studies that assessed lost retention

and described an average of 6.2% (CI: 3.7–10.4%) at 5 years (Hosny *et al.* 2000; Naert *et al.* 2001; Lang *et al.* 2004b). Endodontic complications on the abutment teeth can also be a significant concern with a range of 3–28% of teeth needing post-insertion root canal therapy (RCT) (average of 11%) (Goodacre *et al.*). Naert *et al.* (2001) reported on the complications after a mean period of 6.5 (1.5–15) years in a retrospective comparison study of implant–implant to tooth–implant FPDs on 123 patients in each group with tooth-implant FPDs. The authors reported a history of chronic apical periodontitis (3.5%), tooth fracture (0.6%) along with a tooth intrusion (3.4%), and cement failure (8%) (Naert *et al.* 2001).

An interesting and unusual observation is the issue of natural tooth intrusion that has been observed (Pesun 1997). Earlier use of implants combined with teeth advocated the use of non-rigid attachments within the prosthetic design to allow differential movement between the implant and tooth. In some cases, the natural tooth appears to retract away from the prosthesis. This phenomenon has been suggested to be due to the interplay of disuse atrophy, food impaction, rebound memory of the PDL, and/or mechanical binding (Rieder & Parel 1993;

Schlumberger *et al.* 1998; Cordaro *et al.* 2005; Palmer *et al.* 2005). In a multicenter study, Block *et al.* (2002) assessed posterior FPD connected either rigidly or non-rigidly with one type of attachment. Of the 30 subjects followed though 5 years, there was no difference in bone loss between the two types of connections but there was a 66% incidence of measurable intrusion in the non-rigid group versus 44% for the rigid group. The authors concluded that tooth–implant FPD had a higher level of maintenance and post-operative complications. Fugazzotto *et al.* (1999) retrospectively assessed a multi-group practice outcome of 843 patients (1206 implants, 3096 attachments) over a period of 3–14 years and observed nine instances of intrusion (0.3%) associated with fractured or lost lateral set screws (rigid-retention). In a prospective study through 3 years, Palmer *et al.* (2005) evaluated 19 subjects with rigid cemented prostheses between natural teeth and implants. These short-term outcomes at 3 years indicated no greater implant bone loss than would be expected (0.78 ± 0.64 mm) with no signs of intrusion with the rigid tooth–implant FPD designs. These results have led to the clinical recommendation that if the clinician needs to join natural teeth with implants, a rigid connection is advocated with close monitoring for clinical signs of complications (Naert *et al.* 2001; Palmer *et al.* 2005; Stanford 2005a).

Fixed partial dentures joining teeth to implants is a controversial issue. There are times when an assessment of clinical needs, patient desires, costs, time, and risk provide support for the clinician to consider this treatment option. It is critical that the patient be informed of the relative risks associated with this type of prosthesis, the implant, and the abutment tooth in the process of informed consent.

Conclusion

Fixed partial denture therapy for the restoration of multiple missing teeth has a long track record in dental implant care. Connecting two or more implants, or in selected cases, teeth with implants, can provide a stable, esthetic, and predictable outcome. All treatment options need to start with a careful assessment of anatomic, clinical, and patient needs and desires. The patient needs to be informed of the assumptions made and the relative costs and benefits that this treatment approach can provide.

References

Adell, R., Eriksson, B., Lekholm, U., Branemark, P.I. & Jemt, T. (1990). Long-term follow-up study of osseointegrated implants in the treatment of totally edentulous jaws. *International Journal of Oral & Maxillofacial Implants* **5**(4), 347–359.

Anon. (2003). The McGill consensus statement on overdentures. *Quintessence International* **34**(1), 78–79.

Arvidson, K., Bystedt, H., Frykholm, A., von Konow, L. & Lothigius, E. (1998). Five-year prospective follow-up report of the Astra Tech Dental Implant System in the treatment of edentulous mandibles. *Clinical Oral Implants Research* **9**(4), 225–234.

Astrand, P., Engquist, B., Dahlgren, S., Engquist, E., Feldmann, H. & Grondahl, K. (1999). Astra Tech and Branemark System implants: a prospective 5-year comparative study. Results after one year. *Clinical Implant Dentistry & Related Research* **1**(1), 17–26.

Berglundh, T., Persson, L. & Klinge, B. (2002). A systematic review of the incidence of biological and technical complications in implant dentistry reported in prospective longitudinal studies of at least 5 years. *Journal of Clinical Periodontology* **29** (Suppl 3), 197–212; discussion 232–233.

Block, M.S., Lirette, D., Gardiner, D. *et al.* (2002). Prospective evaluation of implants connected to teeth. *International Journal of Oral & Maxillofacial Implants* **17**(4), 473–487.

Bragger, U., Aeschlimann, S., Burgin, W., Hammerle, C.H. & Lang, N.P. (2001). Biological and technical complications and failures with fixed partial dentures (FPD) on implants and teeth after four to five years of function. *Clinical Oral Implants Research* **12**(1), 26–34.

Brocard, D., Barthet, P., Baysse, E. *et al.* (2000). A multicenter report on 1,022 consecutively placed ITI implants: a 7-year longitudinal study. *International Journal of Oral & Maxillofacial Implants* **15**(5), 691–700.

Brunski, J., Hipp, J.A. & El-Wakad, M. (1986). Dental implant design: biomechanics and interfacial tissue. *Journal of Oral Implantology* **12**(3), 365–377.

Brunski, J.B. (1988a). Biomechanical considerations in dental implant design. *International Journal of Oral Implantology* **5**(1), 31–34.

Brunski, J.B. (1988b). Implants. Biomaterials and biomechanics. *CDA Journal* **16**(1), 66–77.

Brunski, J.B. (1999). In vivo bone response to biomechanical loading at the bone/dental-implant interface. *Advances in Dental Research* **13**, 99–119.

Brunski, J.B. (2000). The new millennium in biomaterials and biomechanics. *International Journal of Oral & Maxillofacial Implants* **15**(3), 327–328.

Brunski, J.B. (2003). Biomechanical aspects of oral/maxillofacial implants. *International Journal of Prosthodontics* **16** (Suppl), 30–32; discussion 47–51.

Brunski, J.B. & Hipp, J.A. (1984). In vivo forces on dental implants: hard-wiring and telemetry methods. *Journal of Biomechanics* **17**(11), 855–860.

Brunski, J.B., Puleo, D.A. & Nanci, A. (2000). Biomaterials and biomechanics of oral and maxillofacial implants: Current status and future developments (Review). *International Journal of Oral & Maxillofacial Implants* **15**(1), 15–46.

Cooper, L., De Kok, I.J., Reside, G.J., Pungpapong, P. & Rojas-Vizcaya, F. (2005). Immediate fixed restoration of the edentulous maxilla after implant placement. *Journal of Oral & Maxillofacial Surgery* **63**(9 Suppl 2), 97–110.

Cooper, L., Felton, D.A., Kugelberg, C.F. *et al.* (2001). A multicenter 12-month evaluation of single-tooth implants restored 3 weeks after 1-stage surgery. *International Journal of Oral & Maxillofacial Implants* **16**(2), 182–192.

Cooper, L.F., Rahman, A., Moriarty, J., Chaffee, N. & Sacco, D. (2002). Immediate mandibular rehabilitation with endosseous implants: simultaneous extraction, implant placement, and loading. *International Journal of Oral & Maxillofacial Implants* **17**(4), 517–525.

Cooper, L.F., Scurria, M.S., Lang, L.A., Guckes, A.D., Moriarty, J.D. & Felton, D.A. (1999). Treatment of edentulism using

Astra Tech implants and ball abutments to retain mandibular overdentures. *International Journal of Oral & Maxillofacial Implants* **14**(5), 646–653.

Cooper, L.F., Zhou, Y., Takebe, J., Guo, J., Abron, A., Holmen, A. & Ellingsen, J.E. (2006). Fluoride modification effects on osteoblast behavior and bone formation at TiO2 grit-blasted c.p. titanium endosseous implants. *Biomaterials* **27**(6), 926–936.

Cordaro, L., Ercoli, C., Rossini, C., Torsello, F. & Feng, C. (2005). Retrospective evaluation of complete-arch fixed partial dentures connecting teeth and implant abutments in patients with normal and reduced periodontal support. *Journal of Prosthetic Dentistry* **94**(4), 313–320.

De Kok, I.J., Chang, S.S., Moriarty, J.D. & Cooper, L.F. (2006). A retrospective analysis of peri-implant tissue responses at immediate load/provisionalized microthreaded implants. *International Journal of Oral & Maxillofacial Implants* **21**(3), 405–412.

Duyck, J., Cooman, M.D., Puers, R., Van Oosterwyck, H., Sloten, J.V. & Naert, I. (2004). A repeated sampling bone chamber methodology for the evaluation of tissue differentiation and bone adaptation around titanium implants under controlled mechanical conditions. *Journal of Biomechanics* **37**(12), 1819–1822.

Duyck, J., Vandamme, K., Geris, L. *et al.* (2006). The influence of micro-motion on the tissue differentiation around immediately loaded cylindrical turned titanium implants. *Archives of Oral Biology* **51**(1), 1–9.

Ellegaard, B., Baelum, V. & Karring, T. (1997). Implant therapy in periodontally compromised patients. *Clinical Oral Implants Research* **8**(3), 180–188.

Engquist, B., Astrand, P., Dahlgren, S., Engquist, E., Feldmann, H. & Grondahl, K. (2002). Marginal bone reaction to oral implants: a prospective comparative study of Astra Tech and Branemark System implants. *Clinical Oral Implants Research* **13**(1), 30–37.

Feine, J.S., Carlsson, G.E., Awad, M.A. *et al.* (2002). The McGill consensus statement on overdentures. Mandibular two-implant overdentures as first choice standard of care for edentulous patients. Montreal, Quebec, May 24–25, 2002. *International Journal of Oral & Maxillofacial Implants* **17**(4), 601–602.

Feine, J.S., de Grandmont, P., Boudrias, P., Brien, N., LaMarche, C., Tache. R. & Lund, J.P. (1994). Within-subject comparisons of implant-supported mandibular prostheses: choice of prosthesis. *Journal of Dental Research* **73**(5), 1105–1111.

Fransson, C., Lekholm, U., Jemt, T. & Berglundh, T. (2005). Prevalence of subjects with progressive bone loss at implants. *Clinical Oral Implants Research* **16**(4), 440–446.

Fugazzotto, P.A., Kirsch, A., Ackermann, K.L. & Neuendorff, G. (1999). Implant/tooth-connected restorations utilizing screw-fixed attachments: a survey of 3,096 sites in function for 3 to 14 years. *International Journal of Oral & Maxillofacial Implants* **14**(6), 819–823.

Garcia, L.T. & Verrett, R.G. (2004). Metal-ceramic restorations – custom characterization with pink porcelain. *Compendium of Continuing Education Dentistry* **25**(4), 242, 244, 246.

Goodacre, C.J., Bernal, G., Rungcharassaeng, K. & Kan, J.Y. (2003a). Clinical complications in fixed prosthodontics. *Journal of Prosthetic Dentistry* **90**(1), 31–41.

Goodacre, C.J., Bernal, G., Rungcharassaeng, K. & Kan, J.Y. (2003b). Clinical complications with implants and implant prostheses. *Journal of Prosthetic Dentistry* **90**(2), 121–132.

Gotfredsen, K. & Karlsson, U. (2001). A prospective 5-year study of fixed partial prostheses supported by implants with machined and TiO2-blasted surface. *Journal of Prosthodontics* **10**(1), 2–7.

Gratton, D.G., Aquilino, S.A. & Stanford, C.M. (2001). Micro-motion and dynamic fatigue properties of the denial implant-abutment interface. *Journal of Prosthetic Dentistry* **85**(1), 47–52.

Hall, J.A., Payne, A.G., Purton, D.G. & Torr, B. (2006). A randomized controlled clinical trial of conventional and immediately loaded tapered implants with screw-retained crowns. *International Journal of Prosthodontics* **19**(1), 17–19.

Hardt, C.R., Grondahl, K., Lekholm, U. & Wennström, J.L. (2002). Outcome of implant therapy in relation to experienced loss of periodontal bone support: a retrospective 5-year study. *Clinical Oral Implants Research* **13**(5), 488–494.

Hosny, M., Duyck, J., van Steenberghe, D. & Naert, I. (2000). Within-subject comparison between connected and nonconnected tooth-to-implant fixed partial prostheses: up to 14-year follow-up study. *International Journal of Prosthodontics* **13**(4), 340–346.

Karlsson, U., Gotfredsen, K. & Olsson, C. (1997). Single-tooth replacement by osseointegrated Astra Tech dental implants: a 2-year report. *International Journal of Prosthodontics* **10**(4), 318–324.

Karlsson, U., Gotfredsen, K. & Olsson, C. (1998). A 2-year report on maxillary and mandibular fixed partial dentures supported by Astra Tech dental implants. A comparison of 2 implants with different surface textures. *Clinical Oral Implants Research* **9**(4), 235–242.

Kindberg, H., Gunne, J. & Kronstrom, M. (2001). Tooth- and implant-supported prostheses: a retrospective clinical follow-up up to 8 years. *International Journal of Prosthodontics* **14**(6), 575–581.

Krekmanov, L., Kahn, M., Rangert, B. & Lindstrom, H. (2000). Tilting of posterior mandibular and maxillary implants for improved prosthesis support. *International Journal of Oral & Maxillofacial Implants* **15**(3), 405–414.

Lang, N.P., Berglundh, T., Heitz-Mayfield, L.J., Pjetursson, B.E., Salvi, G.E. & Sanz, M. (2004a). Consensus statements and recommended clinical procedures regarding implant survival and complications. *International Journal of Oral & Maxillofacial Implants* **19** (Suppl), 150–154.

Lang, N.P., Pjetursson, B.E., Tan, K., Bragger, U., Egger, M. & Zwahlen, M. (2004b). A systematic review of the survival and complication rates of fixed partial dentures (FPDs) after an observation period of at least 5 years. II. Combined tooth–implant-supported FPDs. *Clinical Oral Implants Research* **15**(6), 643–653.

Lewis, S., Sharma, A. & Nishimura, R. (1992). Treatment of edentulous maxillae with osseointegrated implants. *Journal of Prosthetic Dentistry* **68**(3), 503–508.

Makkonen, T.A., Holmberg, S., Niemi, L., Olsson, C., Tammisalo, T. & Peltola, J. (1997). A 5-year prospective clinical study of Astra Tech dental implants supporting fixed bridges or overdentures in the edentulous mandible. *Clinical Oral Implants Research* **8**(6), 469–475.

Malament, K.A. (2000). Prosthodontics: achieving quality esthetic dentistry and integrated comprehensive care. *Journal of the American Dental Association* **131**(12), 1742–1749.

Malament, K.A. & Neeser, S. (2004). Prosthodontic management of ridge deficiencies. *Dental Clinics of North America* **48**(3), 735–744, vii.

Mericske-Stern, R.D., Taylor, T.D. & Belser, U. (2000). Management of the edentulous patient. *Clinical Oral Implants Research* **11** (Suppl 1), 108–125.

Moy, P.K., Medina, D., Shetty, V. & Aghaloo, T.L. (2005). Dental implant failure rates and associated risk factors. *International Journal of Oral & Maxillofacial Implants* **20**(4), 569–577.

Naert, I., Alsaadi, G. & Quirynen, M. (2004a). Prosthetic aspects and patient satisfaction with two-implant-retained mandibular overdentures: a 10-year randomized clinical study. *International Journal of Prosthodontics* **17**(4), 401–410.

Naert, I., Alsaadi, G., van Steenberghe, D. & Quirynen, M. (2004b). A 10-year randomized clinical trial on the influence of splinted and unsplinted oral implants retaining mandibular overdentures: peri-implant outcome. *International Journal of Oral & Maxillofacial Implants* **19**(5), 695–702.

Naert, I.E., Duyck, J.A., Hosny, M.M. & Van Steenberghe, D. (2001). Freestanding and tooth-implant connected prostheses in the treatment of partially edentulous patients. Part I: An up to 15-years clinical evaluation. *Clinical Oral Implants Research* **12**(3), 237–244.

Naert, I.E., Hooghe, M., Quirynen, M. & van Steenberghe, D. (1997). The reliability of implant-retained hinging overdentures for the fully edentulous mandible. An up to 9-year longitudinal study. *Clinical Oral Investigations* **1**(3), 119–124.

Nevins, M. & Langer, B. (1995). The successful use of osseointegrated implants for the treatment of the recalcitrant periodontal patient. *Journal of Periodontology* **66**(2), 150–157.

Norton, M.R. (1997). The Astra Tech Single-Tooth Implant System: a report on 27 consecutively placed and restored implants. *International Journal of Periodontics & Restorative Dentistry* **17**(6), 574–583.

Norton, M.R. (2001). Biologic and mechanical stability of single-tooth implants: 4- to 7-year follow-up. *Clinical Implant Dentistry & Related Research* **3**(4), 214–220.

Olsson, M., Gunne, J., Astrand, P. & Borg, K. (1995). Bridges supported by free-standing implants versus bridges supported by tooth and implant. A five-year prospective study. *Clinical Oral Implants Research* **6**(2), 114–121.

Palmer, R.M., Howe, L.C. & Palmer, P.J. (2005). A prospective 3-year study of fixed bridges linking Astra Tech ST implants to natural teeth. *Clinical Oral Implants Research* **16**(3), 302–307.

Palmer, R.M., Palmer, P.J. & Smith, B.J. (2000). A 5-year prospective study of Astra single tooth implants. *Clinical Oral Implants Research* **11**(2), 179–182.

Peleg, M., Garg, A.K. & Mazor, Z. (2006). Predictability of simultaneous implant placement in the severely atrophic posterior maxilla: A 9-year longitudinal experience study of 2132 implants placed into 731 human sinus grafts. *International Journal of Oral & Maxillofacial Implants* **21**(1), 94–102.

Pesun, I.J. (1997). Intrusion of teeth in the combination implant-to-natural-tooth fixed partial denture: a review of the theories. *Journal of Prosthodontics* **6**(4), 268–277.

Phillips, K. & Wong, K.M. (2001). Space requirements for implant-retained bar-and-clip overdentures. *Compendium of Continuing Education in Dentistry* **22**(6), 516–518.

Pjetursson, B.E., Karoussis, I., Burgin, W., Bragger, U. & Lang, N.P. (2005). Patients' satisfaction following implant therapy. A 10-year prospective cohort study. *Clinical Oral Implants Research* **16**(2), 185–193.

Pjetursson, B.E., Tan, K., Lang, N.P., Bragger, U., Egger, M. & Zwahlen, M. (2004). A systematic review of the survival and complication rates of fixed partial dentures (FPDs) after an observation period of at least 5 years. *Clinical Oral Implants Research* **15**(6), 625–642.

Puchades-Roman, L., Palmer, R.M., Palmer, P.J., Howe, L.C., Ide, M. & Wilson, R.F. (2000). A clinical, radiographic, and microbiologic comparison of Astra Tech and Branemark single tooth implants. *Clinical Implant Dentistry & Related Research* **2**(2), 78–84.

Rangert, B., Sennerby, L., Meredith, N. & Brunski, J. (1997). Design, maintenance and biomechanical considerations in implant placement. *Dental Update* **24**(10), 416–420.

Rasmusson, L., Roos, J. & Bystedt, H. (2005). A 10-year follow-up study of titanium dioxide-blasted implants. *Clinical Implant Dentistry & Related Research* **7**(1), 36–42.

Rieder, C.E. & Parel, S.M. (1993). A survey of natural tooth abutment intrusion with implant-connected fixed partial dentures. *International Journal of Periodontics and Restorative Dentistry* **13**(4), 334–347.

Schlumberger, T.L., Bowley, J.F. & Maze, G.I. (1998). Intrusion phenomenon in combination tooth-implant restorations: a review of the literature. *Journal of Prosthetic Dentistry* **80**(2), 199–203.

Schou, S., Berglundh, T. & Lang, N.P. (2004). Surgical treatment of peri-implantitis. *International Journal of Oral & Maxillofacial Implants* **19** (Suppl), 140–149.

Shackleton, J.L., Carr, L., Slabbert, J.C. & Becker, P.J. (1994). Survival of fixed implant-supported prostheses related to cantilever lengths. *Journal of Prosthetic Dentistry* **71**(1), 23–26.

Slaets, E., Duyck, J. et al. (2005). Time course of the effect of immediate loading on titanium implants. *Computer Methods in Biomechanics and Biomedical Engineering* **8**, 257–258.

Stanford, C. (2006). Outcomes of a fluoride modified implant one year after loading in the posterior-maxilla when placed with the osteotome surgical technique. *Applied Osseointegration Research* **5**, 50–55.

Stanford, C.M. (1999). Biomechanical and functional behavior of implants. *Advances in Dental Research* **13**, 88–92.

Stanford, C.M. (2002). Achieving and maintaining predictable implant esthetics through the maintenance of bone around dental implants. *Compendium of Continuing Education in Dentistry* **23**(9 Suppl 2), 13–20.

Stanford, C.M. (2005a). Application of oral implants to the general dental practice. *Journal of the American Dental Association* **136**(8), 1092–1100; quiz 1165–1166.

Stanford, C.M. (2005b). Issues and considerations in dental implant occlusion: what do we know, and what do we need to find out? *Journal of the California Dental Association* **33**(4), 329–336.

Stanford, C.M. & Brand, R.A. (1999). Toward an understanding of implant occlusion and strain adaptive bone modeling and remodeling. *Journal of Prosthetic Dentistry* **81**(5), 553–561.

Steveling, H., Roos, J. & Rasmusson, L. (2001). Maxillary implants loaded at 3 months after insertion: results with Astra Tech implants after up to 5 years. *Clinical Implant Dentistry & Related Research* **3**(3), 120–124.

van Steenberghe, D., De Mars, G., Quirynen, M., Jacobs, R. & Naert, I. (2000). A prospective split-mouth comparative study of two screw-shaped self-tapping pure titanium implant systems. *Clinical Oral Implants Research* **11**(3), 202–209.

Weibrich, G., Buch, R.S., Wegener, J. & Wagner, W. (2001). Five-year prospective follow-up report of the Astra tech standard dental implant in clinical treatment. *International Journal of Oral & Maxillofacial Implants* **16**(4), 557–562.

Wennstrom, J., Zurdo, J., Karlsson, S., Ekestubbe, A., Grondahl, K. & Lindhe, J. (2004b). Bone level change at implant-supported fixed partial dentures with and without cantilever extension after 5 years in function. *Journal of Clinical Periodontology* **31**(12), 1077–1083.

Wennstrom, J.L., Ekestubbe, A., Grondahl, K., Karlsson, S. & Lindhe, J. (2004a). Oral rehabilitation with implant-supported fixed partial dentures in periodontitis-susceptible subjects. A 5-year prospective study. *Journal of Clinical Periodontology* **31**(9), 713–724.

Wennstrom, J.L., Ekestubbe, A., Grondahl, K., Karlsson, S. & Lindhe, J. (2005). Implant-supported single-tooth restorations: a 5-year prospective study. *Journal of Clinical Periodontology* **32**(6), 567–574.

Yusuf, H. & Ratra, N. (1996). Observations on 25 patients treated with ball-retained overdentures using the Astra Tech implant system. *European Journal of Prosthodontics & Restorative Dentistry* **4**(4), 181–183.

Zarb, G.A. (1988). Implants for edentulous patients. *International Journal of Oral Implantology* **5**(2), 53–54.

Zarb, G.A. & Schmitt, A. (1990a). The longitudinal clinical effectiveness of osseointegrated dental implants: the Toronto

Study. Part II: The prosthetic results. *Journal of Prosthetic Dentistry* **64**(1), 53–61.

Zarb, G.A. & Schmitt, A. (1990b). The longitudinal clinical effectiveness of osseointegrated dental implants: the Toronto study. Part III: Problems and complications encountered. *Journal of Prosthetic Dentistry* **64**(2), 185–194.

Zarb, G.A. & Schmitt, A. (1991). Osseointegration and the edentulous predicament. The 10-year-old Toronto study. *British Dental Journal* **170**(12), 439–444.

Zitzmann, N.U., Sendi, P. & Marinello, C.P. (2005). An economic evaluation of implant treatment in edentulous patients – preliminary results. *International Journal of Prosthodontics* **18**(1), 20–27.

Chapter 56

Complications Related to Implant-Supported Restorations

Y. Joon Ko, Clark M. Stanford, and Lyndon F. Cooper

Introduction, 1222
Clinical complications in conventional fixed restorations, 1222
Clinical complications in implant-supported restorations, 1224
  Biologic complications, 1224
  Mechanical complications, 1226
Other issues related to prosthetic complications, 1231
  Implant angulation and prosthetic complications, 1231
  Screw-retained vs. cement-retained restorations, 1233
  Ceramic abutments, 1233
  Esthetic complications, 1233
  Success/survival rate of implant-supported prostheses, 1234

Introduction

The quality of dental implants and prosthetic outcomes has significantly improved since their introduction. This has been coupled with the steady increase in the clinical success and/or survival rate (Cochran 1996; Esposito et al. 1998; Lindh et al., 1998; Jokstad et al. 2003). The biologic aspect, namely osseointegration, has been the particular target of intensive investigation and there have been conspicuous advances. As a part of these developments there have been continuous efforts to improve the characteristics, microtopographies and chemistries of the implant surface. A major change in surface topography can be summarized by the evolution from machined surfaces to a production-based moderately roughened surface. Superior biologic response, or osseointegration, to roughened implant surfaces has been widely documented in the literature (Astrand et al. 1999; Rocci et al. 2003; Schneider et al. 2003). The cumulative effect of all these efforts is reflected in the extremely high biologic success rate of dental implants. With the enhanced predictability of the integration process of implants becoming well documented, an ongoing issue is related to restorative complications of therapy. These complications can be related to both biologic and prosthetic issues. This chapter discusses potential complications of dental implant-supported restorations, particularly focusing on complications related to the prosthetic aspects of therapy.

Clinical complications in conventional fixed restorations

Implant dentistry shares many of the long-term mechanical complications shared with conventional dental restorative therapy. Goodacre et al. (2003b) presented data regarding the incidence of clinical complications associated with conventional dental fixed restorations/prostheses including single crowns (all-metal, metal ceramic, resin veneered metal) and fixed partial dentures (all-metal, metal ceramic, resin-veneered metal); all-ceramic crowns; resin-bonded prostheses; and posts and cores. Regarding single crowns, the most common complication was post-cementation endodontic therapy (3%), followed by porcelain fracture (3%), loss of retention (2%), periodontal disease (0.6%), and caries (0.4%). Regarding fixed partial dentures, the most common complications were: caries (18% abutments; 8% prostheses), need for endodontic treatment (11% abutments; 7% prostheses), loss of retention (7%), esthetics (6%), periodontal disease (4%), tooth fracture (3%), prosthesis fracture (2%), and porcelain veneer fracture (2%). In this narrative review, the authors concluded that complication incidence with conventional dental fixed partial dentures was significantly higher than single crowns. In addressing issues related to implant restorations, material failure and wear are common occurrences with both dental and implant-supported restorations (Fig. 56-1). It is likely that the higher

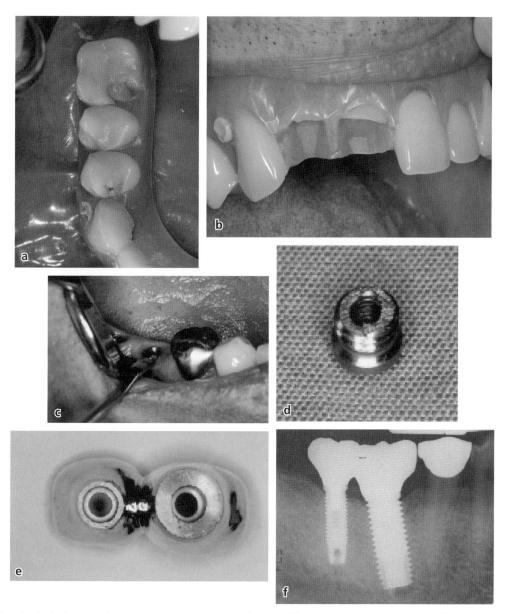

Fig. 56-1 Prosthetic challenges related to wear and component fracture. Wear, fracture, and change in esthetics is a common occurrence with acrylic resin teeth (a) as are fractures of acrylic resin prosthetic teeth on fixed complete denture (b). While implant fractures are rare, the consequences are challenging. (c) Case example of implant that was mobile 2 years after delivery; (d) the prosthesis was removed and the head of the implant was fractured. (e) The implant was replaced with a wide diameter implant in order to increase the wall thickness and provide a greater abutment-to-implant interface. (f) Recall at 10 years.

biomechanical complexity of the design of the prosthesis contributes to higher complication incidence. Among these complications, pulpal complications, periodontal disease, and caries will apply to only tooth-supported restorations.

Tan *et al.* (2004) assessed the long-term success/survival rate of conventional fixed partial dentures (FPDs) and evaluated the failure rates of FPDs due to specific biologic and technical complications. The result of the systematic review based meta-analysis indicated a 10-year survival rate of FPDs was 89.1%. The 10-year success rate of FPDs declined to 71.1%. Success suggests no intervention was needed over the recall period, relative to survival which suggests retention with or without intervention during the recall period. In general in the literature, the mean 10-year survival rate of conventional FPDs was 90%,

and success rate 80%. In this study, the most common reasons for dental FPD failure include periodontal disease and secondary caries. Regarding the complications related to caries, the 10-year risk for decay on abutments was 9.5%, but only 2.6% of FPDs were lost as a result of this disease process. In this study, it was clear that loss of vitality of abutment teeth occurred at a later date and so could not be attributed to the trauma from the preparation of the teeth. This may either indicate a slow progressive tissue degeneration induced by the procedure or reflect the increased susceptibility of pulpal infection by dentinal tubules in advanced periodontitis (Bergenholtz & Nyman 1984). The presence of cast post and dowels and non-vital abutments, especially in distal abutments, has been shown to be associated with increased loss of retention and fracture of teeth and cores. This cautions against over-dependence on non-vital teeth as strategic abutments.

The 10-year risk of loss of FPDs due to recurrent periodontitis was only 0.5%. Overall, there seemed to be no adverse changes in FPDs incorporated into periodontally well-maintained patients even if they presented with a history of advanced periodontal disease. Where the recall or maintenance is less stringent, periodontal breakdown may occur, and may be more pronounced when margins were subgingivally located (Valderhaug & Karlsen 1976). Secondary use of the bridge for removable prosthesis has a detrimental effect on the gingival tissue (Libby et al. 1997). The 10-year risk for technical complications, such as loss of retention, loss due to abutment fracture and the occurrence of material complications, were also calculated in this study. An issue in any of these studies is the multifactorial nature of the causes of failure. The highest 10-year risk was for loss of retention, amounting to 6.4%. Far lower was the 10-year risk for the loss of FPD due to abutment tooth fracture. Relatively low 10-year risks were obtained for material complications. These included fractures of the framework, veneers and/or cores and amounted to a 10-year risk of 3.2%. A comparison of the difference in survival between FPDs with acrylic facings and metal–ceramic FPDs showed that over an 18-year period, 38% of FPDs with acrylic facings and 4% with metal ceramic FPDs were replaced (Sundh & Odman 1997). Reasons cited for the increase in failures were the greater incidence of discoloration and fracture after extensive wear of the acrylic resin material.

Clinical complications in implant-supported restorations

Biologic complications

Surgical complications

Surgical complications directly related to implant placement are generally rare. However, due to the surgical nature of implant therapy, it is impossible to avoid surgical sequelae. Recent surgical methods propose excluding tissue flap openings (so called "flapless approaches") which seek to minimize surgical trauma but carry their own risks as well. Goodacre et al. (2003a) provided data regarding the types of complications that have been reported in conjunction with endosseous root form implants. The most common surgical complications associated with implant surgery were hemorrhage-related complications (24%), neurosensory disturbance (7%), and mandibular fracture (0.3%).

Implant loss

To date, there is no known single factor that contributes to an implant loss. Some of the factors that are generally accepted as the etiology include infection and/or contamination, patients' physical status, trauma from surgical procedure, excessive and/or premature occlusal loading, unfavorable axial loading, etc. Most of the surgery-related implant losses can be managed by maintaining a strict infection control protocol, meticulous patient screening prior to the surgery, and reducing the amount of time/trauma during surgery. Occlusal loading is a more challenging factor since the operator has more limited control. Premature occlusal loading can be detrimental to the osseointegration when it is combined with excessive load and/or off-axis force. This can happen during the stage of early or immediate provisionalization and illustrates that the patient should be closely monitored during this initial healing period. In the literature, it has been stated that overloading at any stage of osseointegration can lead to bone loss or even complete disintegration of the implant (Isidor 1996, 1997; Brunski et al. 2000; Steigenga et al. 2003). However, the concept of implant "overload" has recently been questioned with a series of studies indicating bone is highly responsive to dynamic loads and is resistant to bone loss even with high levels of occlusal function (Stanford & Brand 1999; Duyck et al. 2000, 2001; Stanford 2005b).

According to the literature, implant loss ranges from a high of 19% with maxillary overdentures to a low of 3% that occurred with both mandibular fixed complete dentures and single crowns (Goodacre et al. 2003a). Implant loss is greater with implants 10 mm or less in length compared with implants greater than 10 mm long (ten Bruggenkate et al. 1998; Lekholm et al. 1999; Friberg et al. 2000; Palmer et al. 2000). The implant loss is more likely to occur in the presence of type IV bone compared with more favorable typed bones (Stanford, 1999, 2005b; Stanford & Brand, 1999). Other risk factors that have been suggested include smoking and a previous history of radiation therapy (Moy et al. 2005). If indeed a loss of implant occurs, approximately half or more of the lost implants were lost prior to functional loading. This result is in agreement with the result from a previous systematic review (Berglundh et al. 2002).

Peri-implant complications

Possible peri-implant complications include marginal bone loss, peri-implant mucosal inflammation/proliferation, soft/hard tissue fenestration/dehiscence, fistula, etc. It is widely accepted that continuous marginal bone loss around established implants over time jeopardizes the potential success and/or survival of the implant therapy. Factors that potentially induce marginal bone loss include surgical trauma during implant placement, trauma during repeated abutment insertions and removal, functional load transfer and concentration, micromotion at the implant–abutment junction, and peri-implant gingival inflammation. According to the literature, the mean bone loss occurring during the first year is, on average, around 0.9–1.5 mm, and the subsequent loss per year after the first year is around 0.1 mm (Albrektsson *et al.* 1986).

Peri-implantitis is defined as an inflammatory reaction associated with the loss of supporting bone in the tissues around a functioning implant (Albrektsson *et al.* 1994). Peri-implantitis could be asymptomatic but it often accompanies bleeding and/or suppuration. Clinically, bony defects are detected by increased probing depth. Radiographically, a saucer-shaped radiolucent lesion may be observed around the implant. From a prosthetic perspective, the onset of peri-mucositis or peri-implantitis (associated with bone loss) can lead to soft tissue recession and unesthetic show of abutment or prosthetic components.

Marginal defects on the facial aspect of the implant complex are not only esthetically compromising, but can jeopardize the stability and long-term success of the implant. These defects, dehiscence or fenestration, are typically caused by the resorption of the buccal/labial plate of the alveolar bone. In order to prevent this type of defect it is important to maintain a minimum of 1 mm thickness of buccal/labial plate (Stanford 2005a). However, in certain areas, this may be difficult to achieve. To reduce the risks of facial marginal defects one can utilize bone augmentation procedures, mainly autogenous, around the marginal alveolar bone in order to maintain the thickness around the implants. In this case, autogenous bone particles derived from the drilling of the osteotomy may be enough for the purpose. In terms of the timing of implant placement after tooth extraction, it is generally accepted that immediate placement has a greater risk of facial marginal defects compared to delayed placement (Nemcovsky *et al.* 2002).

Malpositioned implants

The definition of a 'malpositioned implant' is an implant placed in a position that created restorative and biomechanical challenges for an optimal result. A malpositioned implant could be caused by numerous factors, the most common being deficiency of the osseous housing around the proposed implant site. Bone resorption is observed in osseous remodeling following tooth loss, osteoporosis, orthopedic revisions, craniofacial defects, or post oral cancer ablation associated with surgery/radiation. For the best biologic, biomechanical, and esthetic result of implant rehabilitations, proper implant placement is essential. The placement of an implant into a defective osseous site not only prevents adequate positioning of the final prosthetic restoration, but also results in compromised integration and subsequently a poor prognosis for the therapeutic outcome. In order to place an implant in the optimal prosthetic position for a restoration, augmentation procedures are often necessary. Current approaches in bone reconstruction use biomaterials, autografts or allografts, although restrictions on all these techniques exist. Restrictions include donor site morbidity and donor

shortage for autografts (Damien & Parson 1991), as well as immunologic barriers for allografts and the risk of transmitting infectious diseases (Meyer *et al.* 2004). Numerous artificial bone substitutes containing metals, ceramics, and polymers have been introduced to maintain bone function. However, each material has specific disadvantages, and none of these can perfectly substitute for autografts in current clinical dentistry.

If the status of the existing, deficient bone were addressed prior to the surgery and the restorative dentist confirms it will be possible to fabricate the final prosthesis with the implant(s) in the proposed location, generally implant placement can be a straightforward procedure. It is a significant complication for the implant team and the patient when the implants are placed only in the available bone ignoring the optimal desired prosthetic position (Fig. 56-2). Communication between the surgical and restorative team is vital. The best way of communication between the two parties is through use of comprehensive treatment planning, diagnostic wax-up on mounted casts, and fabrication of a surgical guide. The standard protocol for placing implants will start with a treatment plan developed by the restorative dentist. The surgical guide represents the ideal position and angle of the implant determined by a series of diagnostic procedures. The surgical guide should ideally indicate the three dimensions of the proposed implant position – horizontal position, vertical position, and angle (Fig. 56-3). Horizontally, the surgical guide should clearly indicate the bucco-lingual and mesio-distal location of the proposed site. In most cases, this is determined by the morphology and location of the diagnostic wax-up of the missing tooth. Vertically, the surgical guide should indicate how deep the surgeon should place the implant relative to the planned cemento-enamel junction (CEJ). This is particularly important for implants placed in the esthetic zone. As a general rule, the restorative margin for an implant-supported restoration should be located at the vertical height slightly deeper than that of the CEJ of the adjacent teeth. Thus, when an implant system in which the head of the implant represents the restorative margin, the implant should be placed 2–3 mm below the planned CEJ or occasionally on a line connecting the CEJ of adjacent teeth. When an implant system is used which is capable of adjusting the height of the restorative margin through a separate abutment(s), the depth of the implant may be more flexible (Fig. 56-4). Whichever system is used, the surgical guide should have a component that could notify the surgeon of the proposed depth of the implant. The angle of the implant should also be correct to prevent facial or lingual fenestration of the implant as well as penetration into the radicular portions of adjacent teeth or other structures. The angle should be correct for the prosthesis as well. Should the angle of the implant be too facial, the restorative dentist could face significant esthetic challenges, for example, screw access hole position, necessity of the

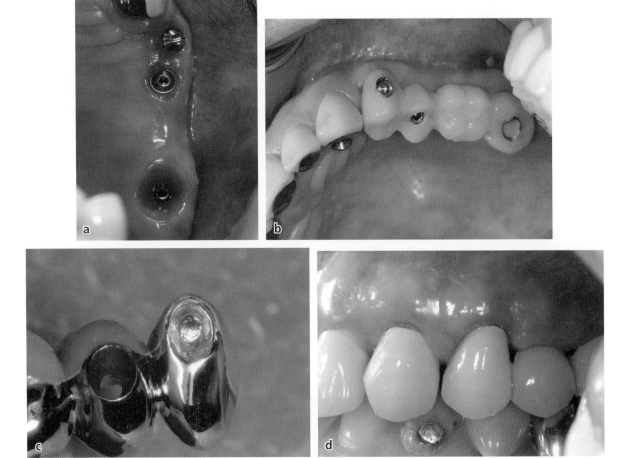

Fig. 56-2 Prosthetic complications with malpositioned implants. (a) Patient had an implant placed in area of 24 with facial angulation. (b) The provisional fixed bridge demonstrated the facial position. Due to the depth and position of the implant, a fixed prosthesis was made that rested on the implant abutment (c) allowing a satisfactory esthetic and functional restoration (d).

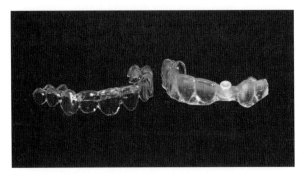

Fig. 56-3 Surgical guides for implant placement. Using a guide with a restrictive channel allows for evaluation in diagnostic imaging studies and during the surgical placement phase.

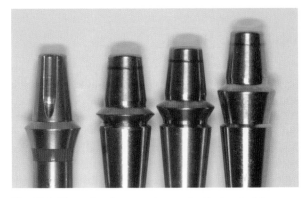

Fig. 56-4 The restorative margin may be the head of the implant with certain implant designs necessitating the surgeon placing the implant to have a clear idea of where the final margin will be. Other systems use an abutment for cemented restorations that allows variation in the vertical position of the restorative margin.

use of angled abutments, expensive custom abutments, etc. (Fig. 56-5).

Mechanical complications

Overdenture complications

Numerous studies indicate that the use of an acrylic-based implant overdenture has the highest number of post-operative complications (complication being defined as a need for some form of intervention, the degree of which is not necessarily defined). Complications include loss of attachment retention or fracture of the attachment system, fracture of components of the denture, prosthesis-related adjustments, etc.

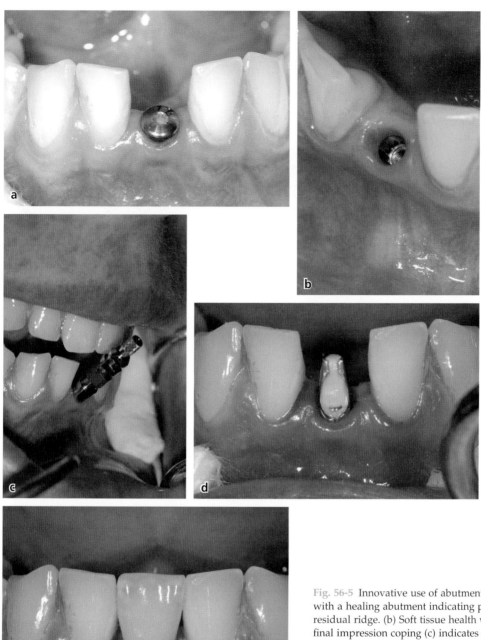

Fig. 56-5 Innovative use of abutments. (a) Patient presented with a healing abutment indicating placement within the residual ridge. (b) Soft tissue health was adequate though final impression coping (c) indicates angled position relative to remaining teeth. Patient was restored with a cement retained restoration but using a low profile abutment designed for a conventional screw-retained crown (d,e). (Courtesy of Dr. Michael Scalia DDS, and Mr. Henry Husemann CDT (University of Iowa).)

Goodacre *et al.* (2003a) suggested the most common complication in this category was the need for adjustments due to loss of retention and/or attachment system fracture. O-ring systems, Hader-bar and clip-, IMZ-, Ceka-, ERA-, ZAAG-, Locator-attachments all use various forms of plastic components within the anchorage system. Over time, the plastic component tends to wear and distort. Traditional ball attachment systems utilize metal spring matrices and these, too, tend to deform and lose retention with time. Studies that assessed the difference in frequency of maintenance requirement between bar/clip systems and individual attachment systems indicated that individual attachment systems require more frequent adjustments mainly due to loss of retention of the matrix or patrix (van Kampen *et al.* 2003; Walton 2003; MacEntee *et al.* 2005). However, the simplicity and ease of the repair procedure in some individual attachment systems may reduce frequent maintenance and have lead to increasing popularity of these abutment designs. Systems with exchangeable plastic components have especially become popular due to easy maintenance procedures. Further, the conversion of a complete denture patient who rarely returns for maintenance therapy to a routine recall patient (valuable for early

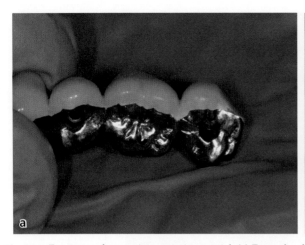 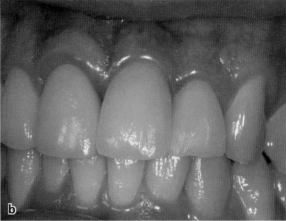

Fig. 56-6 Fractures of veneering ceramic material. (a) Example of facial shear fracture of porcelain on posterior unit. (b) Ceramic shear fracture on facial surface of 22 all-ceramic restoration.

caries detection, oral cancer exams, etc.) by way of their desire to have the attachment system serviced provides a valuable ethical service for the patient.

Because of the housing and attachment components, overdentures typically have a reduced thickness of acrylic resin base in certain areas compared to conventional dentures. It is these thin areas that have a higher risk of fracture. In addition, patients with implant-supported overdentures have a tendency to generate higher masticatory force compared to patients with conventional dentures. The incidence of acrylic base fracture may increase depending on the opposing occlusion. For example, an overdenture opposing an implant-supported fixed complete denture will be at a greater risk of fracture, accelerated wear or prosthetic tooth fracture than one opposing a conventional denture. Overdenture fracture is a relatively common problem according to some studies, and could be as high as 7% of all the mechanical complications related to implant-supported restorations (Carlson & Carlsson 1994; Goodacre *et al.* 2003a).

Prosthesis-related adjustments include reline/rebase of the overdenture, occlusal adjustments, denture adjustment due to soft tissue complications, etc. Normally the hard and soft tissue under the overdenture will remodel with time. Additionally, overdentures only allow limited rotational movements between the abutment and the anchorage system. This means there will be positive vertical and horizontal load on the edentulous ridge, in the area away from the anchorage system. This may increase the rate of resorption and induce the need for denture relines. The change in mucosal adaptation of the prostheses will induce subsequent problems like occlusion changes and soft tissue trauma.

Fracture of fixed restoration veneers/fixed restorations

Without the periodontal ligament (PDL) to provide shock absorption and proprioceptive reflex, dental implants are essentially ankylosed to the surrounding bone. Further, patients tend to generate higher masticatory forces on implant-supported restorations relative to the natural dentition. It has been reported that the maximum bite force generated with conventional dentures is around 50–60 N, whereas implant-supported restorations can generate above 200 N (Carr & Laney 1987; Mericske-Stern *et al.* 1996; Fontijn-Tekamp *et al.* 1998; Morneburg & Proschel 2002; Steigenga *et al.* 2003). As a result, an implant-supported prosthesis is exposed to a risk of higher restorative material failure. Of prosthetic failures, studies suggest the fracture of the restorative veneer material is the most common type of mechanical complication (Fig. 56-6). It includes fracture of the veneering porcelain or resin. Veneer fracture can happen anywhere in the mouth; restorations in the areas of heavy functional forces and higher non-axial forces, such as the occlusal surfaces of mandibular posterior restorations, facial cusps of maxillary posterior restorations, and maxillary anterior restorations, have a greater tendency to shear. To reduce or avoid material failure, especially veneer material fracture, the restoration should have sound supporting structures. The framework that supports the restorative veneer should have sufficient strength and stability to safely support the overlying veneer material. The framework should have minimal flexure even under functional loading – veneer materials usually lack tensile strength and as a result are weak under flexural stress. The framework should be carefully designed so that it will provide maximum support with no unsupported areas of the veneer material (Fig. 56-7). Another important approach to reduce the complication of veneering materials is through control of the occlusion. To reduce or eliminate excessive stress on one particular tooth or restoration, wide distribution of the occlusal force will be better than loads concentrated on a localized area. Also limiting the main occlusal force on to the restoration directly supported by implants may be beneficial: cantilevered restorations may be at higher risk

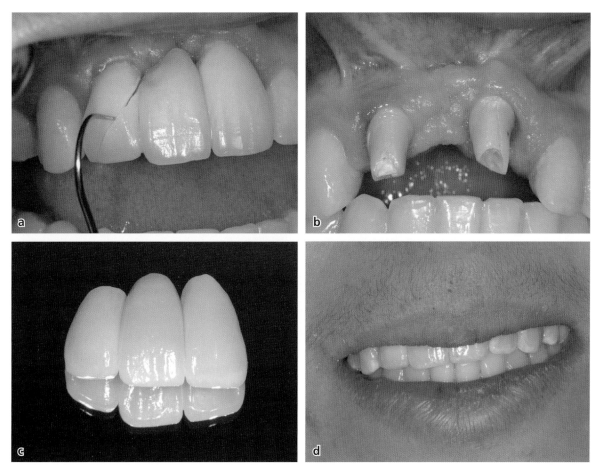

Fig. 56-7 Fractured all-ceramic implant restoration. Patient had a three-unit fixed partial denture (FPD) (12 to 21) with glass-infused ceramic structure. (a) Restoration demonstrated catastrophic rupture 2 years after delivery. Restoration was removed (b), zirconia abutments cleaned and a new Zirconia reinforced FPD fabricated for enhanced strength (c). (d) Final esthetic appearance for the FPD.

of fracture than those supported by the implant/abutment under an identical amount of occlusal load (Becker 2004; Pjetursson *et al.* 2004).

Occlusal wear is more evident in implant-supported restorations for the same reason. When there is a mismatch of opposing restorative materials, the wear could be especially dramatic. Thus one must be prudent in not only selecting the material for the occlusal surface of the restoration but also the status of polishing to avoid serious maintenance issues. It is known that porcelain can be abrasive when opposed with enamel, metal, resin, or even porcelain, especially when it lacks a highly polished surface (Monasky & Taylor 1971). Exposed opaque layer and use of external characterizations with metal oxides all add to the abrasiveness of porcelain and should be used with care.

A rare but possible complication related to prosthesis fracture is the fracture of mandibular implant-supported fixed complete denture at the midline (Fig. 56-8). It is speculated that the flexure of the mandible during function can cause this type of complication. Repeated extreme mouth opening can accumulate fatigue in the metal framework, and once this accumulated fatigue exceeds the fatigue strength of the material, the prosthesis may facture or veneering

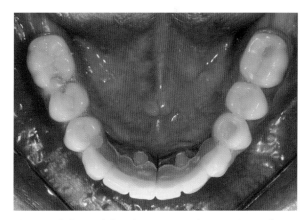

Fig. 56-8 Splitting full-arch ceramometal restoration at the midline to reduce impact of mandibular flexure.

material delaminate from the framework. Clinically, patients with this type of restoration may feel tightness of the mandible especially during function, and once the restoration fails, they express "relief" from the tightness. To avoid this problem, fabricating a two-piece fixed restoration has been advocated by some, although this has generated its own problem: because of the lack of the bracing effect and rigidity of the framework, these restorations may tend to have a higher incidence of screw-related problems.

Implant screw-related complications

Numerous studies indicate that complications related to the screw components of the implant system are very common and require clinical intervention, which could range from simple retightening of the screw(s) to total replacement of the abutment and screw(s). This requires additional time and cost for both dentists and patients. Jemt and Linden (1992) observed with earlier screw abutment designs that screw loosening occurred in 49% of maxillary implant-supported restorations and 20.8% of prostheses in the mandible. They also observed that 57% of the abutment screw loosening occurred within the first year of service and only 37% remained stable over a 3-year period. Goodacre *et al.* (2003a) observed that the frequency of complications related to implant screws like screw loosening or fracture of abutment or prosthetic screws could be as high as 19% of all the potential mechanical complications in implant restorations. Ding *et al.* (2003) reported that the incidence of screw loosening for an external hex system could be as high as 38%. In their systematic review, Pjetursson *et al.* (2004) found that abutment or occlusal screw loosening/fracture was the third most common technical complication, only after restoration veneer fracture and loss of occlusal screw access hole restoration. Its cumulative incidence after 5 years of follow-up was 7.3%.

Theoretically, the lifespan of an abutment or prosthetic screw in an implant restoration needs to last greater than 10^8 cycles of loading or approximately 20 years under the assumption that the system is accurately constructed and the loading conditions are simulating the natural oral environment (Patterson & Johns 1992). However, there are several factors that could drastically reduce the predicted service life resulting in screw loosening and/or fracture. For example, the abutment/implant interface geometry, precision of fit and/or passivity of components, and the amount of preload may lead to reduced service life. In external hexagonal implant system studies, it has been shown that larger implant/abutment contact area provides superior stability of the system and resistance to screw complications and has been one driving force for the use of wider-diameter implant devices (Binon 2000). Additionally, precise anti-rotational features should be present for the joint components to withstand rotational movements that could potentially cause screw loosening (Khraisat 2005). Precise fit of the abutment to the implant interface is highly important. In a study on machining accuracy of several different external hex implant systems, all systems demonstrated rotational movement in excess of four degrees (Binon 1995). Systems that have such "slip-joint" figures such as external hex implant systems are naturally vulnerable to vibration and micromotion during functional loading (Schwarz 2000; Hoyer *et al.* 2001). In the absence of passivity between the implant components, it has been shown that screws accumulate internal stress and this eventually results in metal fatigue failure and screw loosening/fracture (Kano *et al.* 2006). The resulting clamping force exhibited between the abutment and implant generated by the screw is called *preload*. In an external hex system, the preload, along with the frictional force of the abutment/implant joint wall, is the major force resisting functional loads. In most implant systems, a tightening torque is applied and the preload stress in the interface is increased, where this stress should be within the elastic range of the screw material. The screw tightening should result in optimum preload level for the maximum outcome of the implant complex after dynamic loading. Literature indicates that as long as the external loading stress does not exceed the preload stress, the abutment/implant connection can be regarded as safe (Patterson & Johns 1992; Lang *et al.* 2003). Insufficient or excessive preload stress could result in compromised lifespan of the abutment/implant connection.

Chronic problems associated with the external hex or butt-joint interface implant systems have been documented. Because of these inherent problems with external hex design, investigators have presented new concepts in implant design, which aim to improve support and reduce the complications associated with external hex design, by means of additional frictional force between the internal wall of the implant and the external wall of a 1-piece abutment/abutment screw. Sutter and colleagues proposed an 8-degree internal-taper connection between the implant and abutment (ten Bruggenkate *et al.* 1998). The original concept of Morse taper comes from engineering, particularly from the area of machine taper. When connecting exchangeable working bits into the work piece, a popular and very effective method is to use frictional forces between the two components, where the pressure of the spindle against the work-piece drives the tapered shank tightly into the tapered hole. The friction across the entire interface surface area provides a surprisingly large amount of torque transmission. The abutment/implant junction can be designed such that an internal connection is utilized with minimal taper (2–15°), while the screw base portion of the abutment will be connected into the receiving portion of the implant. There are numerous studies reporting on the higher mechanical and enhanced clinical behavior of these internal connection designed implants (Binon 2000). Norton (1997, 1999) verified that the internal conical designed systems significantly enhanced the resistance of connection system against external bending forces. Levine *et al.* (1999) found that the internal connection showed significantly lower incidence (3.6–5.3%) of screw-related complications compared to external hex designed systems. The use of the internal interference fit abutment designs has simplified the

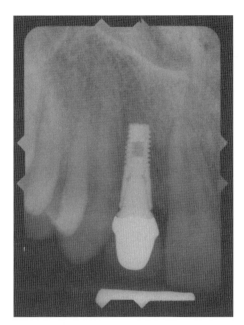

Fig. 56-9 Incomplete seating of abutment in a two-piece implant system. Implant abutment was incompletely seated in implant due to contact on the adjacent osseous contours.

prosthetic phase of therapy and has increased the long-term stability of the screw–joint connections (Stanford & Brand 1999; Brunski 2000, 2003; Jokstad *et al.* 2003).

Abutment-related complications

In positioning an abutment into the implant, there are potential mechanical complications that can arise. One common issue is incomplete seating of the abutment to the implant body (Fig. 56-9). Depending on the implant position and depth, it is also possible that the peri-implant bone may inhibit complete seating of the abutment (giving the dentist the impression that the abutment is fully seated when in fact it is resting on adjacent bone). This may or may not be evident on a radiograph depending on the implant abutment angulation relative to the central beam of the radiographic unit.

Since most prefabricated abutments are produced in standard size and shape, it can be challenging to customize them to individual patients. The modification procedures to a prefabricated abutment may in turn compromise the biomechanical properties of the abutment to achieve an esthetic result. Some systems provide a stock titanium abutment that can be modified by conventional laboratory reshaping or though use of CAD/CAM milling approaches. Depending on the angulation of the implant relative to the prosthesis, the presence of a central abutment screw can sometimes become a complication. This is especially true for narrow-diameter abutments which generally lack sufficient wall thickness for an ideal preparation.

When the head of the implant is placed below the adjacent bone, the architecture of the bone can develop sloped architecture extending from the PDL support of the adjacent teeth down and across to the implant. This often happens in the maxilla area where implants are generally placed deeper to avoid esthetic issues. Periodically this scalloped osseous architecture necessitates the prosthodontist to assess and then modify the abutment and occasionally the implant body in this area (Fig. 56-10). In this case, the mucosal transition zone of the abutment is modified to avoid placing pressure on the bone and soft tissues. It is also helpful to develop a flat or even concave emergence profile of the final restoration to maintain soft tissue dimensions around the restoration (Stanford 2005a).

Other issues related to prosthetic complications

Implant angulation and prosthetic complications

The role of angled implants on clinical outcomes is often of significant concern. Clelland *et al.* (1995) evaluated the stresses and strains generated by an abutment system capable of three angulations (0°, 15°, and 20°). In this study, they observed peak stresses were located in the cortical bone, and the magnitude of these stresses increased with an increase in the abutment angulation. The maximum stress values were generally within the physiologic parameters described for animals, but in one case, the peak compressive stress for the 20° abutment was slightly above this physiologic zone. Peak tensile strains also increased with abutment angulation, but maximum compressive strain values were the same for all three angles. This study suggested that angled abutments were safe to use relative to the bone stability around the implant body.

One approach advocated by some has been to use multiple implants and place a facial–lingual offset between them to enhance the mechanical stability of a connected FPD. Sutpideler *et al.* (2004) evaluated the effect of an offset on the force transmission to bone-supporting implants aligned in either a straight-line configuration or an offset configuration. Also, they addressed the effect of different prosthesis heights and different directions of force application. They observed vertical loading of an implant-supported prosthesis produced the lowest stress to the supporting bone and increasing the angle resulted in greater stress that theoretically simulated surrounding bone. They also observed reducing the height of the prosthesis from 12 mm to 6 mm (crown to implant ratio) or establishing an offset implant location for the middle of three implants can reduce stress, but this reduction did not compensate for the increase in stress found with non-axial loading. This concept has been extended with the recent advocacy for intentionally placing implants at significant

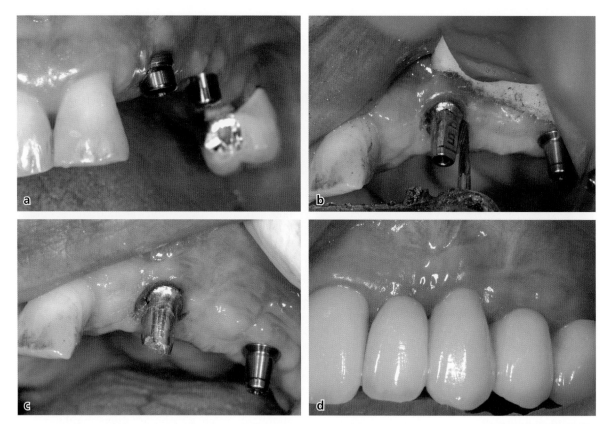

Fig. 56-10 Implant and abutment modification. (a) Patient presented with soft tissue dehiscence on an integrated implant, necessitating placement of an abutment and preparation of the abutment and implant body (b). A fixed partial denture was fabricated using the modified abutment (c) that achieved a reasonable esthetic and functional outcome for this compromised situation (d). Restorative work accomplished by Dr. Manuel Romo DDS (University of Iowa).

angulation relative to each other to avoid vital structures and sinus cavities, and to improve the putative biomechanical position of the implants (Krennmair et al. 2005).

Chun et al. (2006) investigated the effect of three different abutment types (one-piece, internal-hex, and external-hex) on stress distribution in bone under vertical and inclined loads by finite element analysis. With one-piece implant designs, they observed that the load was transferred evenly into bone as well as within the implant system. However, the maximum stress generated in bone with the one-piece system was always higher than that generated with the internal-hex implant, regardless of load angle inclination. In the case of the internal-hex implant, the contact condition with friction between abutment and implant in the tapered joints and at abutment neck reduced the effect of bending caused by horizontal component of inclined load. The maximum stress in bone was the highest for the external-hex implants.

Erneklint et al. (2006) evaluated the load resistance in a conical implant system with two different screw-retained abutment angled designs (20° and 45°) and three different retaining screw materials. They observed that the 20° abutment withstood non-axial forces to a greater extent than a 45° abutment, regardless of retaining screw material. The 45° abutment failed under oblique loads between 450 and 530 N

while the 20° abutment failed at 1280–1570 N. Regarding the retaining screw materials, differences were more obvious in a 20° abutment, but not insignificant in the 45° abutment as well. In general, they concluded that abutment taper angles were more important than retaining screw material in determining the assembly strength.

The angulation of the implants can also influence the outcomes of implant overdenture therapy. Gulizio et al. (2005) evaluated the retentive capacity of gold and titanium overdenture attachments placed on implants positioned at 0°, 10°, 20°, and 30° from a vertical reference axis. They observed that significant differences in retention of gold matrices were noticed when ball abutments were positioned at 20° and 30°, but not at 0° and 10°. Also they noticed significantly higher variance in retention among the titanium matrices, despite the finding that angle was not a factor affecting retention for titanium matrices. In other words, angle of the implants had an effect on the retention of gold matrices, but not for titanium matrices. This study supports the clinical observation that implant-supported overdentures have higher maintenance needs and may have higher long-term ongoing costs relative to conventional tooth replacement therapies (Naert et al. 2004a,b; Krennmair et al. 2005; Zitzmann et al. 2005; Trakas et al. 2006; Visser et al. 2006).

Screw-retained vs. cement-retained restorations

The method of attachment of the prosthesis to the implant/abutment can create prosthetic complications. The major advantages of screw-retained implant-supported restorations include their retrievability and freedom from residual cement problems. Thus this type of restoration scheme can be applied when there is a need for future removal, e.g. necessary hygiene maintenance procedures or questionable prognosis of the restoration. It could also be applied when the restorative margin is located too deep for removal of excess cement at the time of restoration delivery. The same advantage applies to provisional restorations as well. However, this type of restoration has inherent disadvantages. Because of the required screw access hole, it not only compromises the esthetics and occlusion, but also has the potential to undermine the strength of the restoration due to the lack of material. The presence of the prosthetic screw also bears the potential of screw complications. Additionally, this type of restoration is more sensitive to the passive fit of the restoration to the supporting implants.

Regarding the clinical performance of each type of restoration, the literature indicates that screw-retained restorations may present more postoperative complications compared to cement-retained restorations. Duncan *et al.* (2003) reported that patients restored with screw-retained restorations had problems with prosthetic screws and screw access hole filling material while no complications were encountered with patients restored with cement-retained restorations after 3 years. Karl *et al.* (2006) found that cement-retained FPDs may result in lower strain levels compared to conventional screw-retained FPDs at the time of either the cementation or screw-tightening procedure. Higher strain level at the time of delivery may reduce the passivity of the fit of the restoration and increase potential future complications. This result is in accordance with other *in vitro* studies (Guichet *et al.* 2000; Taylor *et al.* 2000). However, this study carefully suggests that regardless of the type of restoration, no true passive fit can be achieved. Skalak (1983) theorized that a nonpassive fit of the restoration can induce biologic and prosthetic complications. However, Jemt and Book (1996) reported that they could not find a direct association between implant prosthesis misfits with marginal bone loss over 5 years. Vigolo *et al.* (2004) found no evidence of different behavior of the peri-implant marginal bone and soft tissue response around screw-retained or cement-retained single-tooth implant restorations.

Overall, there is no consensus of the superiority of one type over the other – it may be determined by the clinical situation and the operator's preference.

Ceramic abutments

Ceramic implant abutments have recently gained in popularity due to superior esthetic results compared to conventional titanium abutments, especially in thin tissue biotypes (Stanford 2005a). Because of the strength concerns, the current material of choice for ceramic abutments is reinforced ceramic abutment, e.g. alumina (Al_2O_3) or yettria-stabilized Zirconia (ZrO_2) (Fig. 56-7). These abutments were introduced during the 1990s and the first of these abutments consisted of densely sintered aluminum oxide (alumina). Andersson *et al.* (2003) conducted a 5-year multi-center prospective study evaluating the clinical outcome of alumina ceramic abutments. According to this study, the cumulative success rate for alumina ceramic abutments was 98.1% at 5 years compared to 100% for conventional titanium abutments. More recently, zirconia has become popular for ceramic implant abutments. Because ceramic materials are vulnerable to tensile stress, especially around defects or cracks, a ceramic material with higher fracture toughness will be a good material for ceramic abutments. Zirconia is generally known to have higher range of fracture toughness (K_{IC}, ~7–15 $MPam^{-1}$) than that of alumina (K_{IC}, ~4–4.5 $MPam^{-1}$). Its fracture toughness is comparable to that of metal alloys (K_{IC}, ≥20 $MPam^{-1}$) (Piconi & Maccauro 1999; Kelly 2004). Zirconia is known to have the relatively unique property of transformation toughening, where the metastable tetragonal phase can be converted into monoclinic phase with the associated volume expansion (Chevalier 2006). This phenomenon is induced by stress concentration at defect or crack tips, through which the crack is put into compression and its growth retarded. This is the main mechanism for its higher fracture toughness, and it could significantly extend the reliability and lifetime of the restoration. However, there is little evidence if the abutment will still retain this property after being reduced down to less than 1 mm during clinical usage. Further, the hydrolytic properties of water interacting with the material during ageing (hydrolytic ageing) is still an active area of laboratory investigation (Rekow & Thompson 2005). There are outstanding questions relative to the use of this material including long-term fatigue strength, degree of preparation/wall thickness needed, intraoral sites, clinical long-term prognosis, etc. Due to the relatively short period after its introduction, there are few studies that assess the clinical performance of these abutments (Att *et al.* 2006; Denry & Holloway 2006; Deville *et al.* 2006; Itinoche *et al.* 2006; Studart *et al.* 2006).

Esthetic complications

The most frustrating and challenging complication is unacceptable esthetic outcome either at the time of restoration or during long-term follow up. With

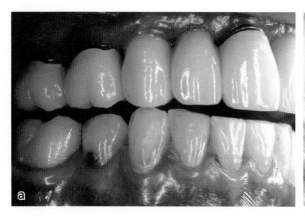
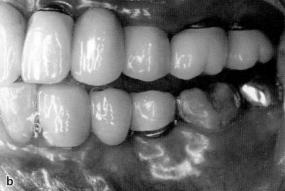

Fig. 56-11 Soft tissue recession on facial aspect of implant supported restoration.

the growing population of esthetically concerned patients, esthetic complications are a serious matter even if the implant team has done its best throughout the procedure. This is an important issue that the implant team and the patient need to be aware of and endeavor to find solutions to prevent or overcome. Common esthetic complications include complications due to malpositioned implants, thin tissue biotypes, and unfavorable soft tissue responses.

The potential cause and impact of malpositioned implants was previously described. A very difficult aspect of implant rehabilitation is that sometimes a slight malpositioning can induce dramatic esthetic compromises which do not become evident until the technician is working with the case. A facially mal-positioned implant can become a major challenge for the restorative team (Fig. 56-11). In this case, the restorative dentist may have to address a variety of potential problems, including excessive inciso-gingival dimensions of the crown, exposed head of the implant, unequal gingival margins, etc. Usually, facially malpositioned implants create greater prob-lems than other malpositioned implants. A 1 mm lingual position to the implant in the maxillary esthetic zone can create a prosthetic challenge to have the final restoration appear even and uniform with the natural dentition. Mesially, or distally malposi-tioned implants can induce improper anatomy of the restoration as the technician attempts to compensate for implant components in the interproximal space (Fig. 56-12).

Unfavorable soft tissue response can also make the treatment very difficult. It is generally accepted that individuals that have relatively thin attached gingiva, or thin tissue biotype, are more vulnerable to gingi-val/periodontal disease and subsequent sequelae including gingival recession. Similar findings are reported for the tissue response around implant res-torations (Kan *et al.* 2003). Thin biotype tissues tend to show more recessive response to trauma. Restorative procedures, like preparation, impression, repeated abutment/provisional removal, or even toothbrushing, can sometimes cause enough trauma

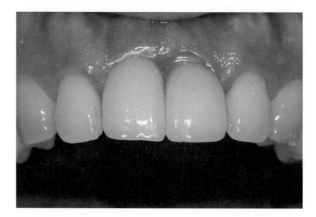

Fig. 56-12 Challenges in creating esthetic outcomes when implants are insufficiently placed. Example demonstrates teeth 11 and 21 with compromised contours due to close proximity of the implants.

to these thin biotype tissues to result in significant recession and compromise the treatment outcome. It is very important to identify the tissue type early at the treatment planning stage to prevent unfavorable treatment outcome.

Success/survival rate of implant-supported prostheses

As previously described, the biologic success/sur-vival rate is extremely high and has become more predictable even in areas that were considered of high risk (e.g. maxillary posterior region). It may be beneficial to know what the literature indicates regarding the success/survival rate of restorations fabricated on the osseointegrated implants. Pjeturs-son *et al.* (2004) obtained estimates of the long-term survival/success rates of implant-supported FPDs and of the incidence of technical complications in partially edentulous patients with an observation period of more than 5 years. "FPD survival" was defined as "the FPD remaining *in situ* with or without modification for the observation period", as com-pared to the definition of "FPD success" being "FPD being free of all complications over the entire observation period" in this study. The cumulative FPD survival rate was 95% after 5 years and 86.7% after 10 years, respectively. In this study, the authors noted an important fact that most of the prosthetic complications occur after 5 years of clinical service. The underlying issue this illustrates is the problem associated with the rapid rate of manufacturing market changes in implant products and components. By the time the restoration needs repair or replacement, the required components may be difficult if not impossible to obtain. Regarding comparison of different implant systems, there is little evidence of superiority of one system over another in terms of mechanical failure. Implant–abutment joint geometry, design of the restoration, and patient factors like parafunctional habits or heavy occlusal forces tend to have more impact on the outcome of implant-supported restoration than implant surface material or topography (Rangert *et al.* 1995; Astrand *et al.* 1999; Naert *et al.* 2002a,b). Some studies indicate that the cumulative complication rate of prosthetic problems can be as high as 43.1% after 5 years (Jemt *et al.* 2003), compared to other studies finding it to be as low as 19.3% after 5 years (Bragger *et al.* 2001; Pjetursson *et al.* 2004). A summary of these studies indicates that one may expect one out of four implant-supported restorations will require some type of repair whether it be minor, such as screw or abutment tightening, or major, such as entire restoration replacement, after 5 years. This implies that significant chair time may be necessary for the maintenance of these restorations (Pjetursson *et al.* 2004).

Berglundh *et al.* (2002) also noticed the higher mechanical/technical complication rate compared to the lower biologic complication rate. This study observed interesting aspects: the incidence of implant loss prior to functional loading was higher by three-fold when multiple implants are placed for larger restorations like overdentures or fixed complete restorations than that of single-tooth restorations; implant loss during function occurred in 2–3% of implants supporting fixed reconstructions, while twice as many implants were lost in overdenture therapy during a 5-year period. In this case, the highest frequencies of implant loss during function occurred in the maxilla.

Conclusions

Implant therapy provides many benefits as a form of tooth replacement therapy. As with any form of prosthetic rehabilitation it has limitations including wear, material fatigue and fracture, soft tissue recession and subsequent complications, increased maintenance and costs. The benefits, though, can be enormous with the enhanced patient quality of life that comes with a definitive replacement of teeth. Patients need to be aware during the treatment planning process that the treatment provided may need to be replaced periodically as normal ageing and wear occurs. Specific patient-based risk factors such as parafunctional habits should be discussed and the patient made aware of the risks to the prosthetic reconstructions.

References

Albrektsson, T., Zarb, G., Worthington, P. & Eriksson, A.R. (1986). The long-term efficacy of currently used dental implants: a review and proposed criteria of success. *International Journal of Oral & Maxillofacial Implants* 1(1), 11–25.

Albrektsson, T.O., Johansson, C.B. & Sennerby, L. (1994). Biological aspects of implant dentistry: osseointegration. *Periodontology 2000* 4, 58–73.

Andersson, B., Glauser, R., Maglione, M. & Taylor, A. (2003). Ceramic implant abutments for short-span FPDs: a prospective 5-year multicenter study. *International Journal of Prosthodontics* 16(6), 640–646.

Antoun, H., Sitbon, J.M., Martinez, H. & Missika, P. (2001). A prospective randomized study comparing two techniques of bone augmentation: onlay graft alone or associated with a membrane. *Clinical Oral Implants Research* 12(6), 632–639.

Astrand, P., Engquist, B., Dahlgren, S., Engquist, E., Feldmann, H. & Grondahl, K. (1999). Astra Tech and Branemark System implants: a prospective 5-year comparative study. Results after one year. *Clinical Implant Dentistry & Related Research* 1(1), 17–26.

Att, W., Kurun, S., Gerds, T. & Strub, J.R. (2006). Fracture resistance of single-tooth implant-supported all-ceramic restorations after exposure to the artificial mouth. *Journal of Oral Rehabilitation* 33(5), 380–386.

Becker, C.M. (2004). Cantilever fixed prostheses utilizing dental implants: a 10-year retrospective analysis. *Quintessence International* 35(6), 437–441.

Bergenholtz, G. & Nyman, S. (1984). Endodontic complications following periodontal and prosthetic treatment of patients with advanced periodontal disease. *Journal of Periodontology* 55(2), 63–68.

Berglundh, T., Persson, L. & Klinge, B. (2002). A systematic review of the incidence of biological and technical complications in implant dentistry reported in prospective longitudinal studies of at least 5 years. *Journal of Clinical Periodontology* 29 (Suppl 3), 197–212; discussion 232–233.

Binon, P.P. (1995). Evaluation of machining accuracy and consistency of selected implants, standard abutments, and laboratory analogs. *International Journal of Prosthodontics* 8(2), 162–178.

Binon, P.P. (2000). Implants and components: entering the new millennium. *International Journal of Oral & Maxillofacial Implants* 15(1), 76–94.

Bragger, U., Aeschlimann, S., Burgin, W., Hammerle, C.H. & Lang, N.P. (2001). Biological and technical complications and failures with fixed partial dentures (FPD) on implants and teeth after four to five years of function. *Clinical Oral Implants Research* 12(1), 26–34.

Brunski, J.B. (2000). The new millennium in biomaterials and biomechanics. *International Journal of Oral & Maxillofacial Implants* 15(3), 327–328.

Brunski, J.B. (2003). Biomechanical aspects of oral/maxillofacial implants. *International Journal of Prosthodontics* 16 (Suppl), 30–32; discussion 47–51.

Brunski, J.B., Puleo, D.A. & Nanci, A. (2000). Biomaterials and biomechanics of oral and maxillofacial implants: current status and future developments. *International Journal of Oral & Maxillofacial Implants* 15(1), 15–46.

Carlson, B. & Carlsson, G.E. (1994). Prosthodontic complications in osseointegrated dental implant treatment. *International Journal of Oral & Maxillofacial Implants* **9**(1), 90–94.

Carr, A.B. & Laney, W.R. (1987). Maximum occlusal force levels in patients with osseointegrated oral implant prostheses and patients with complete dentures. *International Journal of Oral & Maxillofacial Implants* **2**(2), 101–108.

Chevalier, J. (2006). What future for zirconia as a biomaterial? *Biomaterials* **27**(4), 535–543.

Chun, H.J., Shin, H.S., Han, C.H. & Lee, S.H. (2006). Influence of implant abutment type on stress distribution in bone under various loading conditions using finite element analysis. *International Journal of Oral & Maxillofacial Implants* **21**(2), 195–202.

Clelland, N.L., Lee, J.K., Bimbenet, O.C. & Brantley, W.A. (1995). A three-dimensional finite element stress analysis of angled abutments for an implant placed in the anterior maxilla. *Journal of Prosthodontics* **4**(2), 95–100.

Cochran, D. (1996). Implant therapy I. *Annals of Periodontology* **1**(1), 707–791.

Dahlin, C., Andersson, L. & Linde, A. (1991). Bone augmentation at fenestrated implants by an osteopromotive membrane technique. A controlled clinical study. *Clinical Oral Implants Research* **2**(4), 159–165.

Damien, J. & Parson, J. (1991). Bone graft and bone graft substitutes: A review of current technology and applications. *Journal of Applied Biomaterials* **2**, 187–208.

Denry, I.L. & Holloway, J.A. (2006). Microstructural and crystallographic surface changes after grinding zirconia-based dental ceramics. *Journal of Biomedical Materials Research. Part B, Applied Biomaterials* **76**(2), 440–448.

Deville, S., Chevalier, J. & Gremillard, L. (2006). Influence of surface finish and residual stresses on the ageing sensitivity of biomedical grade zirconia. *Biomaterials* **27**(10), 2186–2192.

Ding, T.A., Woody, R.D., Higginbottom, F.L. & Miller, B.H. (2003). Evaluation of the ITI Morse taper implant/abutment design with an internal modification. *International Journal of Oral & Maxillofacial Implants* **18**(6), 865–872.

Duncan, J.P., Nazarova, E., Vogiatzi, T. & Taylor, T.D. (2003). Prosthodontic complications in a prospective clinical trial of single-stage implants at 36 months. *International Journal of Oral & Maxillofacial Implants* **18**(4), 561–565.

Duyck, J., Ronold, H.J., Van Oosterwyck, H., Naert, I., Vander Sloten, J. & Ellingsen, J.E. (2001). The influence of static and dynamic loading on marginal bone reactions around osseointegrated implants: an animal experimental study. *Clinical Oral Implants Research* **12**(3), 207–218.

Duyck, J., Van Oosterwyck, H., Vander Sloten, J., De Cooman, M., Puers, R. & Naert, I. (2000). Magnitude and distribution of occlusal forces on oral implants supporting fixed prostheses: an in vivo study. *Clinical Oral Implants Research* **11**(5), 465–475.

Erneklint, C., Odman, P., Ortengren, U. & Karlsson, S. (2006). An in vitro load evaluation of a conical implant system with 2 abutment designs and 3 different retaining-screw alloys. *International Journal of Oral & Maxillofacial Implants* **21**(5), 733–737.

Esposito, M., Hirsch, J.M., Lekholm, U. & Thomsen, P. (1998). Biological factors contributing to failures of osseointegrated oral implants. (II). Etiopathogenesis. *European Journal of Oral Science* **106**(3), 721–764.

Fontijn-Tekamp, F.A., Slagter, A.P., van't Hof, M.A., Geertman, M.E. & Kalk, W. (1998). Bite forces with mandibular implant-retained overdentures. *Journal of Dental Research* **77**(10), 1832–1839.

Friberg, B., Grondahl, K., Lekholm, U. & Branemark, P.I. (2000). Long-term follow-up of severely atrophic edentulous mandibles reconstructed with short Branemark implants. *Clinical Implant Dentistry & Related Research* **2**(4), 184–189.

Goodacre, C.J., Bernal, G., Rungcharassaeng, K. & Kan, J.Y. (2003a). Clinical complications with implants and implant prostheses. *Journal of Prosthetic Dentistry* **90**(2), 121–132.

Goodacre, C.J., Bernal, G., Rungcharassaeng, K. & Kan, J.Y. (2003b). Clinical complications in fixed prosthodontics. *Journal of Prosthetic Dentistry* **90**(1), 31–41.

Guichet, D.L., Caputo, A.A., Choi, H. & Sorensen, J.A. (2000). Passivity of fit and marginal opening in screw- or cement-retained implant fixed partial denture designs. *International Journal of Oral & Maxillofacial Implants* **15**(2), 239–246.

Gulizio, M.P., Agar, J.R., Kelly, J.R. & Taylor, T.D. (2005). Effect of implant angulation upon retention of overdenture attachments. *Journal of Prosthodontics* **14**(1), 3–11.

Hoyer, S.A., Stanford, C.M., Buranadham, S., Fridrich, T., Wagner, J. & Gratton, D. (2001). Dynamic fatigue properties of the dental implant-abutment interface: joint opening in wide-diameter versus standard-diameter hex-type implants. *Journal of Prosthetic Dentistry* **85**(6), 599–607.

Isidor, F. (1996). Loss of osseointegration caused by occlusal load of oral implants. A clinical and radiographic study in monkeys. *Clinical Oral Implants Research* **7**(2), 143–152.

Isidor, F. (1997). Histological evaluation of peri-implant bone at implants subjected to occlusal overload or plaque accumulation. *Clinical Oral Implants Research* **8**(1), 1–9.

Itinoche, K.M., Ozcan, M., Bottino, M.A. & Oyafuso, D. (2006). Effect of mechanical cycling on the flexural strength of densely sintered ceramics. *Dental Materials* **22**(11), 1029–1034.

Jemt, T. & Book, K. (1996). Prosthesis misfit and marginal bone loss in edentulous implant patients. *International Journal of Oral & Maxillofacial Implants* **11**(5), 620–625.

Jemt, T., Henry, P., Linden, B., Naert, I., Weber, H. & Wendelhag, I. (2003). Implant-supported laser-welded titanium and conventional cast frameworks in the partially edentulous law: a 5-year prospective multicenter study. *International Journal of Prosthodontics* **16**(4), 415–421.

Jemt, T. & Linden, B. (1992). Fixed implant-supported prostheses with welded titanium frameworks. *International Journal of Periodontics and Restorative Dentistry* **12**(3), 177–184.

Jokstad, A., Braegger, U., Brunski, J.B., Carr, A.B., Naert, I. & Wennerberg, A. (2003). Quality of dental implants. *International Dental Journal* **53** (6 Suppl 2), 409–443.

Kan, J.Y., Rungcharassaeng, K., Umezu, K. & Kois, J.C. (2003). Dimensions of peri-implant mucosa: an evaluation of maxillary anterior single implants in humans. *Journal of Periodontology* **74**(4), 557–562.

Kano, S.C., Binon, P., Bonfante, G. & Curtis, D.A. (2006). Effect of casting procedures on screw loosening in UCLA-type abutments. *Journal of Prosthodontics* **15**(2), 77–81.

Karl, M., Taylor, T.D., Wichmann, M.G. & Heckmann, S.M. (2006). In vivo stress behavior in cemented and screw-retained five-unit implant FPDs. *Journal of Prosthodontics* **15**(1), 20–24.

Kelly, J.R. (2004). Dental ceramics: current thinking and trends. *Dental Clinics of North America* **48**(2), viii, 513–530.

Khraisat, A. (2005). Stability of implant-abutment interface with a hexagon-mediated butt joint: failure mode and bending resistance. *Clinical Implant Dentistry & Related Research* **7**(4), 221–228.

Krennmair, G., Furhauser, R., Krainhofner, M., Weinlander, M. & Piehslinger, E. (2005). Clinical outcome and prosthodontic compensation of tilted interforaminal implants for mandibular overdentures. *International Journal of Oral & Maxillofacial Implants* **20**(6), 923–929.

Lang, L.A., Kang, B., Wang, R.F. & Lang, B.R. (2003). Finite element analysis to determine implant preload. *Journal of Prosthetic Dentistry* **90**(6), 539–546.

Lekholm, U., Gunne, J., Henry, P., Higuchi, K., Linden, U., Bergstrom, C. *et al.* (1999). Survival of the Branemark implant in partially edentulous jaws: a 10-year prospective multicenter study. *International Journal of Oral & Maxillofacial Implants* **14**(5), 639–645.

Levine, R.A., Clem, D.S., 3rd, Wilson, T.G., Jr., Higginbottom, F. & Solnit, G. (1999). Multicenter retrospective analysis of the ITI implant system used for single-tooth replacements: results of loading for 2 or more years. *International Journal of Oral & Maxillofacial Implants* 14(4), 516–520.

Libby, G., Arcuri, M.R., LaVelle, W.E. & Hebl, L. (1997). Longevity of fixed partial dentures. *Journal of Prosthetic Dentistry* 78(2), 127–131.

Lindh, T., Gunne, J., Tillberg, A. & Molin, M. (1998). A meta-analysis of implants in partial edentulism. *Clinical Oral Implants Research* 9(2), 80–90.

MacEntee, M.I., Walton, J.N. & Glick, N. (2005). A clinical trial of patient satisfaction and prosthodontic needs with ball and bar attachments for implant-retained complete overdentures: three-year results. *Journal of Prosthetic Dentistry* 93(1), 28–37.

Mericske-Stern, R., Piotti, M. & Sirtes, G. (1996). 3-D in vivo force measurements on mandibular implants supporting overdentures. A comparative study. *Clinical Oral Implants Research* 7(4), 387–396.

Meyer, U., Joos, U. & Wiesmann, H.P. (2004). Biological and biophysical principles in extracorporal bone tissue engineering. Part I. *International Journal of Oral & Maxillofacial Surgery* 33(4), 325–332.

Monasky, G.E. & Taylor, D.F. (1971). Studies on the wear of porcelain, enamel, and gold. *Journal of Prosthetic Dentistry* 25(3), 299–306.

Morneburg, T.R. & Proschel, P.A. (2002). Measurement of masticatory forces and implant loads: a methodologic clinical study. *International Journal of Prosthodontics* 15(1), 20–27.

Moy, P.K., Medina, D., Shetty, V. & Aghaloo, T.L. (2005). Dental implant failure rates and associated risk factors. *International Journal of Oral & Maxillofacial Implants* 20(4), 569–577.

Naert, I., Alsaadi, G. & Quirynen, M. (2004a). Prosthetic aspects and patient satisfaction with two-implant-retained mandibular overdentures: a 10-year randomized clinical study. *International Journal of Prosthodontics* 17(4), 401–410.

Naert, I., Alsaadi, G., van Steenberghe, D. & Quirynen, M. (2004b). A 10-year randomized clinical trial on the influence of splinted and unsplinted oral implants retaining mandibular overdentures: peri-implant outcome. *International Journal of Oral & Maxillofacial Implants* 19(5), 695–702.

Naert, I., Koutsikakis, G., Duyck, J., Quirynen, M., Jacobs, R. & van Steenberghe, D. (2002a). Biologic outcome of implant-supported restorations in the treatment of partial edentulism. part I: a longitudinal clinical evaluation. *Clinical Oral Implants Research* 13(4), 381–389.

Naert, I., Koutsikakis, G., Quirynen, M., Duyck, J., van Steenberghe, D. & Jacobs, R. (2002b). Biologic outcome of implant-supported restorations in the treatment of partial edentulism. Part 2: a longitudinal radiographic study. *Clinical Oral Implants Research* 13(4), 390–395.

Nemcovsky, C.E., Artzi, Z., Moses, O. & Gelernter, I. (2002). Healing of marginal defects at implants placed in fresh extraction sockets or after 4–6 weeks of healing. A comparative study. *Clinical Oral Implants Research* 13(4), 410–419.

Norton, M.R. (1997). An in vitro evaluation of the strength of an internal conical interface compared to a butt joint interface in implant design. *Clinical Oral Implants Research* 8(4), 290–298.

Norton, M.R. (1999). Assessment of cold welding properties of the internal conical interface of two commercially available implant systems. *Journal of Prosthetic Dentistry* 81(2), 159–166.

Palmer, R.M., Palmer, P.J. & Smith, B.J. (2000). A 5-year prospective study of Astra single tooth implants. *Clinical Oral Implants Research* 11(2), 179–182.

Patterson, E.A. & Johns, R.B. (1992). Theoretical analysis of the fatigue life of fixture screws in osseointegrated dental implants. *International Journal of Oral & Maxillofacial Implants* 7(1), 26–33.

Piconi, C. & Maccauro, G. (1999). Zirconia as a ceramic biomaterial. *Biomaterials* 20(1), 1–25.

Pjetursson, B.E., Tan, K., Lang, N.P., Bragger, U., Egger, M. & Zwahlen, M. (2004). A systematic review of the survival and complication rates of fixed partial dentures (FPDs) after an observation period of at least 5 years. *Clinical Oral Implants Research* 15(6), 667–676.

Rangert, B., Krogh, P.H., Langer, B. & Van Roekel, N. (1995). Bending overload and implant fracture: a retrospective clinical analysis. *International Journal of Oral & Maxillofacial Implants* 10(3), 326–334.

Rekow, D. & Thompson, V.P. (2005). Near-surface damage – a persistent problem in crowns obtained by computer-aided design and manufacturing. *Proceedings of the Institution of Mechanical Engineers. Part H, Journal of Engineering in Medicine* 219(4), 233–243.

Rocci, A., Martignoni, M. & Gottlow, J. (2003). Immediate loading of Branemark System TiUnite and machined-surface implants in the posterior mandible: a randomized open-ended clinical trial. *Clinical Implant Dentistry & Related Research* 5 (Suppl 1), 57–63.

Schneider, G.B., Perinpanayagam, H., Clegg, M., Zaharias, R., Seabold, D., Keller, J. *et al.* (2003). Implant surface roughness affects osteoblast gene expression. *Journal of Dental Research* 82(5), 372–376.

Schwarz, M.S. (2000). Mechanical complications of dental implants. *Clinical Oral Implants Research* 11 (Suppl 1), 156–158.

Skalak, R. (1983). Biomechanical considerations in osseointegrated prostheses. *Journal of Prosthetic Dentistry* 49(6), 843–848.

Stanford, C.M. (1999). Biomechanical and functional behavior of implants. *Advances in Dental Research* 13, 88–92.

Stanford, C.M. (2005a). Application of oral implants to the general dental practice. *Journal of the American Dental Association* 136(8), 1092–1100; quiz 1165–1166.

Stanford, C.M. (2005b). Issues and considerations in dental implant occlusion: what do we know, and what do we need to find out? *Journal of the California Dental Association* 33(4), 329–336.

Stanford, C.M. & Brand, R.A. (1999). Toward an understanding of implant occlusion and strain adaptive bone modeling and remodeling. *Journal of Prosthetic Dentistry* 81(5), 553–561.

Steigenga, J.T., al-Shammari, K.F., Nociti, F.H., Misch, C.E. & Wang, H.L. (2003). Dental implant design and its relationship to long-term implant success. *Implant Dentistry* 12(4), 306–317.

Studart, A.R., Filser, F., Kocher, P. & Gauckler, L.J. (2006). Fatigue of zirconia under cyclic loading in water and its implications for the design of dental bridges. *Dental Materials* 23(1), 106–114.

Sundh, B. & Odman, P. (1997). A study of fixed prosthodontics performed at a university clinic 18 years after insertion. *International Journal of Prosthodontics* 10(6), 513–519.

Sutpideler, M., Eckert, S.E., Zobitz, M. & An, K.N. (2004). Finite element analysis of effect of prosthesis height, angle of force application, and implant offset on supporting bone. *International Journal of Oral & Maxillofacial Implants* 19(6), 819–825.

Tan, K., Pjetursson, B.E., Lang, N.P. & Chan, E.S. (2004). A systematic review of the survival and complication rates of fixed partial dentures (FPDs) after an observation period of at least 5 years. *Clinical Oral Implants Research* 15(6), 654–666.

Taylor, T.D., Agar, J.R. & Vogiatzi, T. (2000). Implant prosthodontics: current perspective and future directions. *International Journal of Oral & Maxillofacial Implants* 15(1), 66–75.

ten Bruggenkate, C.M., Asikainen, P., Foitzik, C., Krekeler, G. & Sutter, F. (1998). Short (6-mm) nonsubmerged dental implants: results of a Multicenter clinical trial of 1 to 7 years. *International Journal of Oral & Maxillofacial Implants* 13(6), 791–798.

Trakas, T., Michalakis, K., Kang, K. & Hirayama, H. (2006). Attachment systems for implant retained overdentures: a literature review. *Implant Dentistry* **15**(1), 24–34.

Valderhaug, J. & Karlsen, K. (1976). Frequency and location of artificial crowns and fixed partial dentures constructed at a dental school. *Journal of Oral Rehabilitation* **3**(1), 75–81.

van Kampen, F., Cune, M., van der Bilt, A. & Bosman, F. (2003). Retention and postinsertion maintenance of bar-clip, ball and magnet attachments in mandibular implant overdenture treatment: an in vivo comparison after 3 months of function. *Clinical Oral Implants Research* **14**(6), 720–726.

Vigolo, P., Givani, A., Majzoub, Z. & Cordioli, G. (2004). Cemented versus screw-retained implant-supported single-tooth crowns: a 4-year prospective clinical study. *International Journal of Oral & Maxillofacial Implants* **19**(2), 260–265.

Visser, A., Meijer, H.J., Raghoebar, G.M. & Vissink, A. (2006). Implant-retained mandibular overdentures versus conventional dentures: 10 years of care and aftercare. *International Journal of Prosthodontics* **19**(3), 271–278.

Walton, J.N. (2003). A randomized clinical trial comparing two mandibular implant overdenture designs: 3-year prosthetic outcomes using a six-field protocol. *International Journal of Prosthodontics* **16**(3), 255–260.

Zitzmann, N.U., Sendi, P. & Marinello, C.P. (2005). An economic evaluation of implant treatment in edentulous patients-preliminary results. *International Journal of Prosthodontics* **18**(1), 20–27.

Part 17: Orthodontics and Periodontics

57 Tooth Movements in the Periodontally Compromised Patient, 1241
Björn U. Zachrisson

58 Implants Used for Orthodontic Anchorage, 1280
Marc A. Schätzle and Niklaus P. Lang

Chapter 57

Tooth Movements in the Periodontally Compromised Patient

Björn U. Zachrisson

Orthodontic tooth movement in adults with periodontal tissue
  breakdown, 1241
  Orthodontic treatment considerations, 1243
  Esthetic finishing of treatment results, 1248
  Retention – problems and solutions; long-term follow-up, 1248
  Possibilities and limitations; legal aspects, 1249
Specific factors associated with orthodontic tooth movement in
  adults, 1252
  Tooth movement into infrabony pockets, 1252
  Tooth movement into compromised bone areas, 1253
  Tooth movement through cortical bone, 1253
  Extrusion and intrusion of single teeth – effects on periodontium,
    clinical crown length, and esthetics, 1255

Regenerative procedures and orthodontic tooth
  movement, 1261
Traumatic occlusion (jiggling) and orthodontic treatment, 1262
Molar uprighting, furcation involvement, 1262
Tooth movement and implant esthetics, 1263
Gingival recession, 1267
  Labial recession, 1267
  Interdental recession, 1271
Minor surgery associated with orthodontic therapy, 1274
  Fiberotomy, 1274
  Frenotomy, 1274
  Removal of gingival invaginations (clefts), 1275
  Gingivectomy, 1275

Orthodontic treatment may be adjunctive to periodontal therapy. The loss of periodontal support or teeth may result in elongation, spacing, and proclination of incisors, rotation, and tipping of premolars and molars with collapse of the posterior occlusion, and decreasing vertical dimension. But orthodontic tooth movement can also facilitate the management of several restorative and esthetic problems in adults. Such difficulties may be related to subgingivally fractured or lost teeth, tipped abutment teeth, excess spacing, inadequate implant or pontic space, supra-erupted teeth, narrow alveolar ridges that prevent implant placement, and other conditions (Ong *et al.* 1998). The purpose of this chapter is to discuss how recent basic and clinical information may be used to improve treatment planning, clinical management, and retention for patients in whom different malocclusions are caused or complicated by moderate to advanced periodontal destruction.

Orthodontic tooth movement in adults with periodontal tissue breakdown

Poorly executed orthodontic treatment in periodontal patients can certainly contribute to further periodontal tissue breakdown. In particular, the combination of inflammation, orthodontic forces, and occlusal trauma may produce a more rapid destruction than would occur with inflammation alone (Kessler 1976). However, with properly performed treatment, extensive orthodontic tooth movement can be made in adults with a reduced but healthy periodontium without further periodontal deterioration. Figures 57-1 to 57-6 show the pretreatment and post-treatment conditions in four different adult orthodontic patients with advanced periodontitis. The findings of no significant further periodontal tissue breakdown in these patients were the result of carefully controlled treatment planning considerations.

Only a few well controlled studies have been published on groups of adults with advanced periodontitis, who have received comprehensive orthodontic fixed-appliance treatment. Boyd *et al.* (1989) described ten adults with generalized periodontitis who received pre-orthodontic periodontal treatment including surgery, and then regular maintenance at 3-month intervals during a 2-year orthodontic treatment period. They were compared with ten control adults who had normal periodontal tissues, and 20 adolescent orthodontic patients. The results demonstrated that:

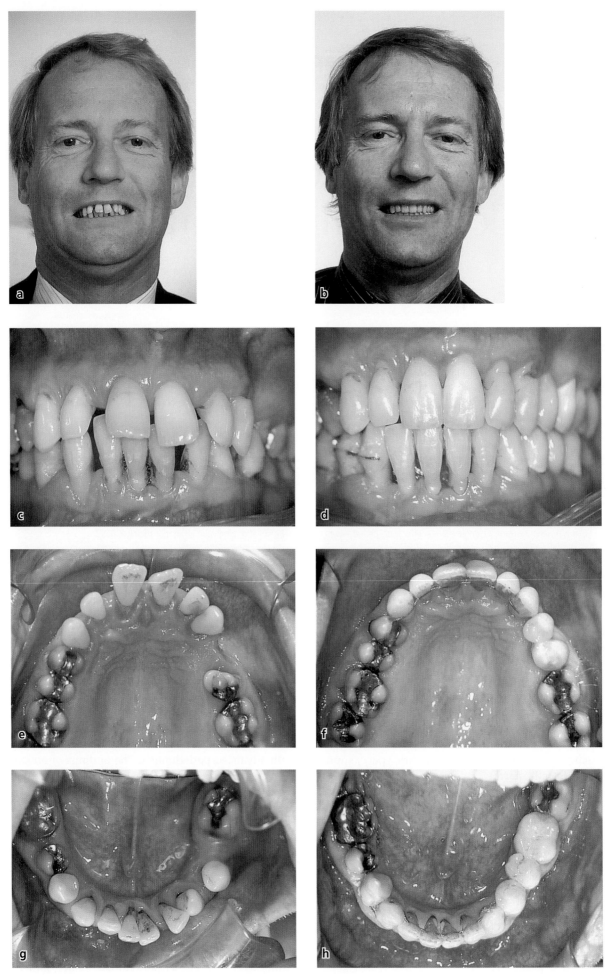

Fig. 57-1 Adult male patient with advanced periodontitis and marked pathologic migration of the anterior teeth before (left column) and after (right column) periodontal and orthodontic fixed-appliance treatment for 2 years. Clinical appearance of the face and dentition are dramatically improved after the combined periodontic/orthodontic treatment. The dental result is maintained by means of bonded lingual retainer wires. A maxillary two-unit and a mandibular three-unit bridge were constructed. Some interdental recession was unavoidable in the mandibular anterior region (d), but it does not show much clinically (b).

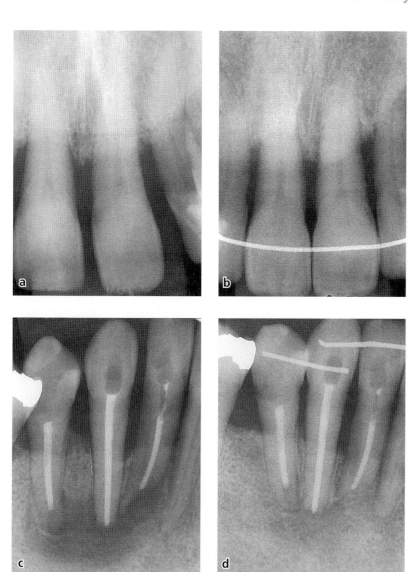

Fig. 57-2 Long-term radiographic follow-up of the same patient as in Fig. 57-1. Radiographs of maxillary and mandibular anterior regions 7 years after the completion of orthodontic therapy (b,d) show reduced but healthy periodontium, with no progression of periodontal tissue destruction compared with the initial situation (a,c).

- Adults were more effective than adolescents in removing plaque, especially late in the orthodontic treatment period.
- Tooth movement in adults with reduced, but healthy, periodontium did not result in significant further loss of attachment (none of the adults had additional mean loss of attachment of more than 0.3 mm).
- Adults with teeth that did *not* have healthy periodontal tissues may experience further breakdown and tooth loss due to abscesses during orthodontic treatment.

In another study by Årtun and Urbye (1988), 24 patients with advanced loss of marginal bone and pathologic tooth migration received active appliance therapy for an average of 7 months, following periodontal treatment. Bone level measurements on radiographs indicated that the majority of sites showed little or no additional loss of bone support. However, a few sites demonstrated pronounced additional bone loss.

More recent studies on much larger groups (350–400 patients) of consecutively treated adult patients from different practices (Nelson & Årtun 1997; Re *et al.* 2000) have confirmed that: (1) pretreatment evidence of periodontal tissue destruction is no contraindication for orthodontics, (2) orthodontic therapy improves the possibilities of saving and restoring a deteriorated dentition, and (3) the risk of recurrence of an active disease process is not increased during appliance therapy. However, these larger samples have indicated that adult orthodontic patients are at a somewhat higher risk than adolescents for tissue breakdown. The mean bone loss on radiographs of the six anterior teeth in the study of Nelson and Årtun (1997) was 0.54 mm (SD 0.62). Only 2.5% of the patients had average bone loss of 2 mm or more, but as many as 36% of these patients had one or more surfaces with bone loss exceeding 2 mm.

Orthodontic treatment considerations

The key element in the orthodontic management of adult patients with periodontal disease is to eliminate, or reduce, plaque accumulation and gingival inflammation. This implies much emphasis on oral hygiene instruction, appliance construction,

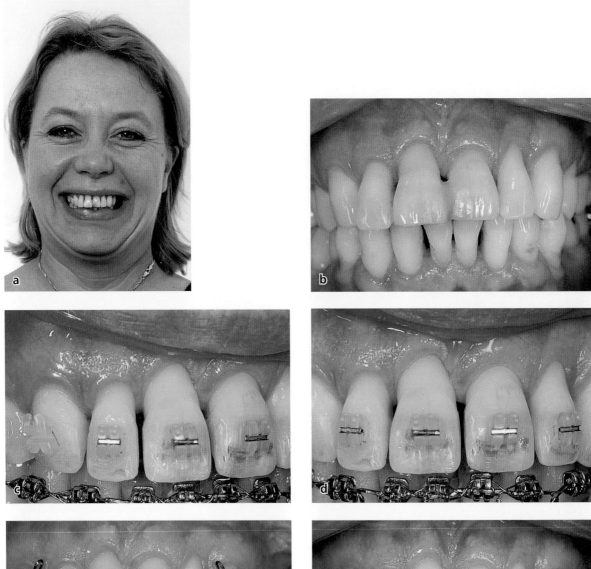

Fig. 57-3 Adult female periodontitis patient with pathologic migration of the maxillary incisors before (a,b), during (c–e), and after (f) periodontal and orthodontic treatment. An attempt had been made by the periodontist to grind and splint the overextruded right central incisor with composite resin (b) before orthodontic treatment was started. Due to extensive mesial and distal recontouring of the incisors (stripping) during the treatment (c,d), it was possible to obtain an esthetic final result with almost intact gingival papillae between the incisors in both the maxilla and in the mandible (f).

and periodic check-ups throughout treatment (Zachrisson 1996).

The most appropriate method for tooth movement must be determined in each particular case. Although minor or partial orthodontic treatment with sectional or removable appliances may be possible in some instances, in the majority of cases a fully controlled technique with fixed appliances in both dental arches

is preferred in order to carefully control the movement of teeth in three planes.

The orthodontic appliance has to be properly designed. It must provide stable anchorage without causing tissue irritation, and must be esthetically acceptable. For psychologic reasons bonded ceramic brackets are preferred in the most visible regions (Figs. 57-3 to 57-6), generally for the maxillary teeth,

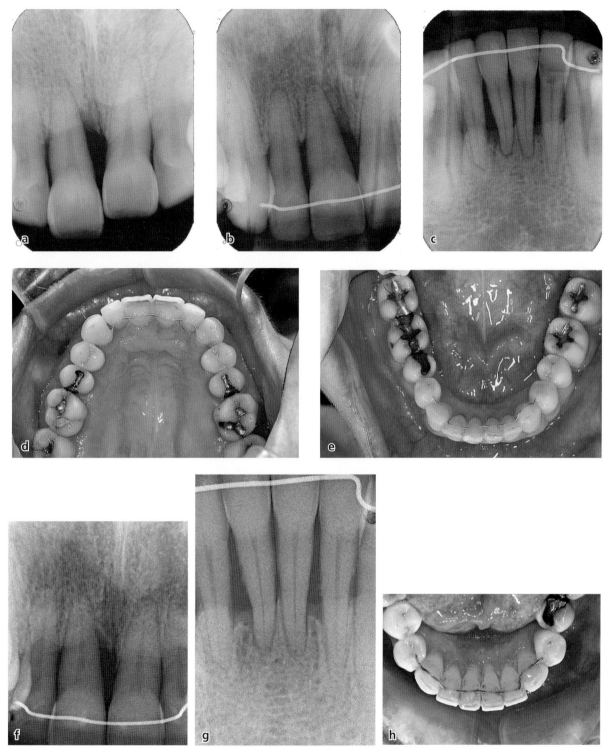

Fig. 57-4 Radiographic and clinical occlusal appearance of the same patient as in Fig. 57-3. No noticeable progression of the periodontal tissue destruction has occurred (compare a and b), and although markedly reduced the periodontium is healthy after the orthodontic therapy (b,c). The treatment result is maintained by means of gold-coated lingual retainers over six maxillary and eight mandibular anterior teeth (d,e).These bonded retainers act as effective orthodontic retainers as well as neat and hygienic periodontal splints. Despite the unfavorable crown–root ratios of particularly the mandibular incisors, the situation is largely unchanged 6 years later (f,g), and the gingival papillae fill in the spaces between the lower anterior teeth nicely (h).

whereas stainless steel or gold-coated attachments are commonly used elsewhere in the mouth (Figs. 57-3, 57-5).

To counteract the tendency of orthodontic appliances to increase the accumulation of plaque on the teeth, attempts should be made to keep the appliances and mechanics simple, and avoid hooks, elastomeric rings, and excess bonding resin outside the bracket bases. The use of steel ligatures is recommended on all brackets (Figs. 57-3 to 57-6), since elastomeric rings have been shown to be significantly more plaque attractive than steel ties (Forsberg *et al.*

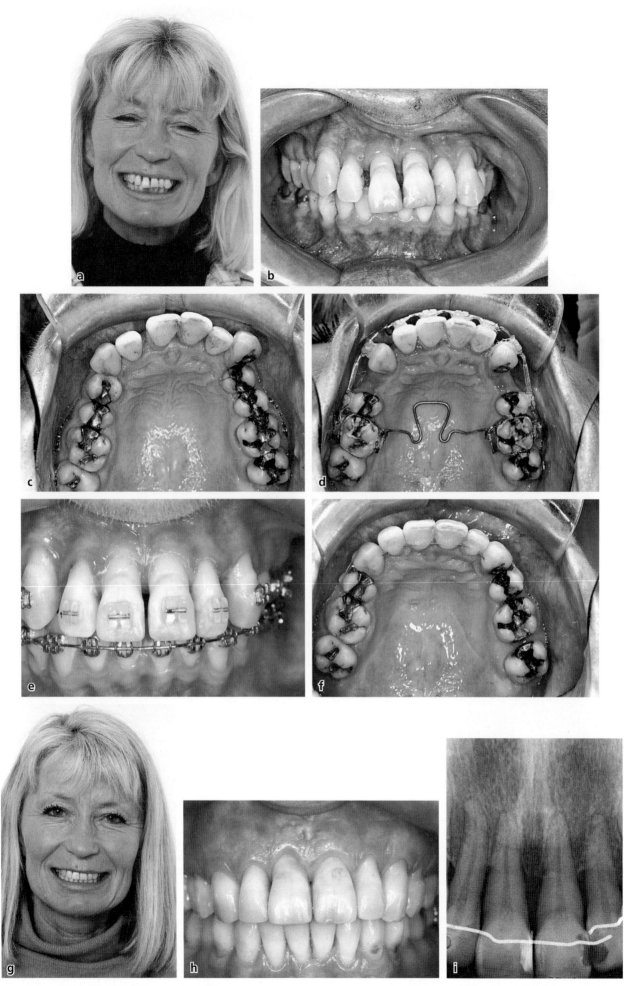

Fig. 57-5 Another adult female periodontitis patient with pathologic migration of the maxillary incisors before (a–c), during (d,e), and after (f) periodontal and orthodontic treatment. Despite the advanced periodontal tissue break-down, the case was treated with extraction of two upper first premolars (d). Due to the extensive mesial and distal recontouring of the incisors (stripping) during the treatment (e), it was also possible in this case to obtain an esthetic final result with almost intact gingival papillae between the incisors (h). The clinical and radiographic situation 1.5 years after treatment is shown in g–i. Note gold-coated short labial retainer wires about the closed extraction sites to prevent space reopening (f).

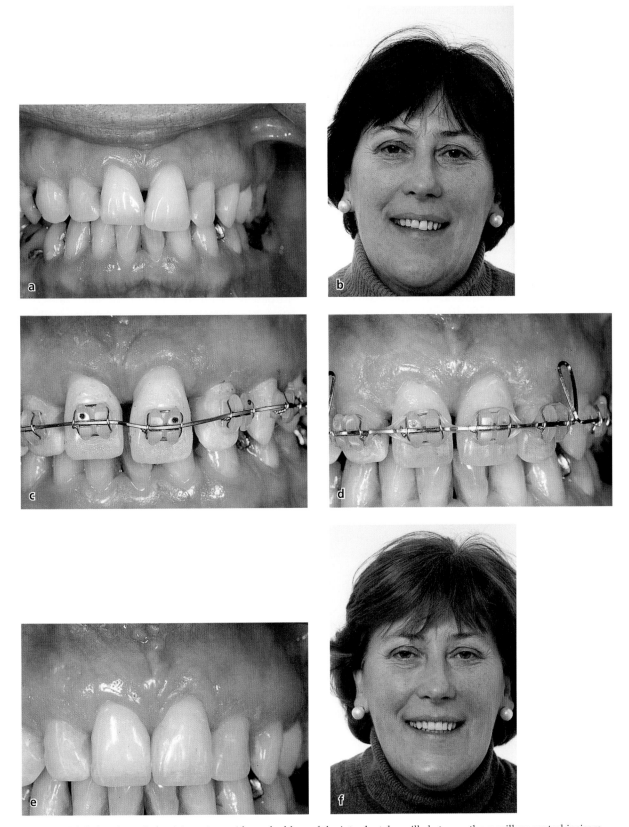

Fig. 57-6 Adult female periodontitis patient with marked loss of the interdental papilla between the maxillary central incisors (a,b). This gap is caused by the "fan-shaped" morphology of the central incisors, which places the interproximal contact too near the incisal edge. To eliminate the unesthetic soft tissue gap, the mesial surfaces of the central incisors were reshaped (c) to lengthen their connector area and move the contact point gingivally (d). After continued orthodontic space closure, a more esthetic final result was achieved (e,f).

1991). Bonds are preferable to bands (Boyd & Baumrind 1992). Bonded molars show less plaque accumulation, gingivitis, and loss of attachment interproximally than banded molars during orthodontic treatment of adults. However, bonding is more complicated in adult patients than in adolescents. Many adults have amalgam restorations and crown-and-bridge restorations made of porcelain or precious metals. Thanks to the introduction of new techniques and materials, it is feasible to bond orthodontic brackets, buccal tubes, and retainer wires to artificial surfaces. Clinical experience with bonding to different artificial tooth surfaces, except gold, is excellent (Zachrisson 2000a,b).

Renewed oral hygiene instruction and motivation is made after placement of the orthodontic appliances. During the treatment period professional tooth cleaning by a dental hygienist or periodontist may be performed at 3-month intervals (Boyd *et al.* 1989; Boyd & Baumrind 1992), or after regular examination updates at 6- and 12-month intervals, depending on the situation. The re-examinations should include recordings of probing depths, mobility, bleeding on probing, suppuration, gingival recessions, bone levels, etc. Professional scaling may be indicated during *active intrusion* of elongated maxillary incisors, since orthodontic intrusion may shift supragingival plaque to a subgingival location (Ericsson *et al.* 1977, 1978). If efforts at maintaining excellent-to-good oral hygiene are unsuccessful, orthodontic treatment should be terminated (Machen 1990).

After appliance removal, reinstruction in oral hygiene measures should be given. Otherwise, subsequent labial gingival recession may be risked due to overzealous toothbrushing, since cleaning is now easier to perform.

Esthetic finishing of treatment results

Adults with a reduced periodontium represent different challenges for orthodontists than adolescents. Worn or abraded teeth, missing papillae and uneven crown lengths are common problems, and it is therefore more difficult to obtain an esthetically optimal appearance of the teeth and gingiva after bracket removal.

Most incisor teeth in adults with malocclusions have more or less worn incisal edges, which represent an adaptation to functional demands. When the axial inclinations and rotations of such incisors are corrected, there is frequently a need for incisal grinding towards a more normal contour. Such grinding can be performed safely as long as the wear is limited, the overbite is adequate, and the patients display enough tooth material in conversation and on smiling. When the abrasion is more significant, however, cooperation with a restorative dentist is generally indicated.

The presence of papillae between the maxillary incisors is a key esthetic factor after orthodontic treat-

ment. Normally, when long-standing crowding with incisor overlap is corrected orthodontically in adults, it is generally not possible to have an intact papilla. This is because the contact point becomes located too far incisally on the triangular crowns that have not had a normal interdental wear pattern. Similarly, in patients with advanced periodontal disease and destruction of the crestal bone between the incisors, the papillae may be absent. This produces unesthetic gaps between the teeth after orthodontics. The best method of correcting this problem is to recontour the mesiodistal surfaces of the incisors during the orthodontic finishing stage (Tuverson 1980). When the diastemata thus created are closed, the roots of the teeth can come closer together. The contact point is lengthened and moved apically, and the papilla can fill out the interdental space more easily (Figs. 57-3, 57-5, 57-6; also see Fig. 57-28).

In patients with high or normal smile lines, the relationship of the gingival margins of the maxillary anterior teeth may be another important factor in the esthetic appearance of the crowns (Kokich 1996a,b). When adult patients have gingival margin discrepancies between adjacent teeth, the orthodontist must determine the proper solution for the problem: orthodontic movement to reposition the gingival margin (see Fig. 57-17) or surgical correction (gingivectomy) to increase the crown length of single or several teeth (see Fig. 57-29).

Retention – problems and solutions; long-term follow-up

Due to the anatomic and biologic differences in tissue reaction between adults and children (Melsen 1991), adults undergoing extensive orthodontic treatment will generally need, at least, a longer period of retention than would an adolescent patient. Also, growth and development no longer take place and cannot aid in changing occlusal levels or in space closure by the eruption of posterior teeth with mesial drift. The space reopening tendency of closed extraction sites in adults can be mitigated by use of labially bonded retainers (Figs. 57-1, 57-5).

The migration of teeth associated with periodontal tissue breakdown around the incisors in adults is usually blamed on inflammatory swelling or the tongue thrust. However, according to Proffit (1978), two major primary factors are involved in the equilibrium which determines the final position of teeth. These are the resting pressures of lip or cheek and tongue, and forces produced by metabolic activity within the periodontal membrane. With an intact periodontium, unbalanced tongue–lip forces are normally counteracted by forces from the periodontal membrane. However, when the periodontium breaks down, its stabilizing function no longer exists and the incisors begin to move. A consequence of this concept would be that persons with advanced periodontal disease and tooth migration would need permanent retention after the orthodontic correction. For patients with minimum-to-moderate loss of periodontal tissue support, more "normal" retention periods may be sufficient.

The optimal long-term retainer for adults with reduced periodontium is the flexible spiral wire (FSW) retainer bonded lingually on each tooth in a segment. The bonded retainer in the anterior region is generally used together with a maxillary removable plate. The fabrication and long-term evaluation of bonded retainers is described by Dahl and Zachrisson (1991). Figures 57-3, 57-4, 57-5 and 57-20 demonstrate different designs of FSW retainers in the maxilla and the mandible in several patients. At the same time as the FSW retainer works as a reliable, invisible orthodontic retainer, it concomitantly acts as a periodontal splint, which allows the individual teeth within the splint to exert physiologic mobility. As long as the retainer remains intact, small spaces might open up distal to, but not within, the retainer.

Splinting may not be needed for most teeth with increased mobility after periodontal therapy (Ramfjord 1984). However, reduced mobility of teeth after combined periodontal and orthodontic treatment by using a bonded retainer would seem to be of considerable benefit. If a bonded retainer is not used, and instead a removable plate or spring retainer is used at night on a long-term basis, there is a risk for ongoing jiggling of the teeth because of the relapse tendency during the day. Experimental studies in animals indicate that jiggling forces may facilitate the progress of attachment loss in periodontitis, or at least result in more bone resorption. Also, more connective tissue reattachment and bone regeneration may occur around non-jiggled teeth. Monkey experiments have shown that when experimental jiggling of teeth was stopped, a significant gain of alveolar bone occurred (Nyman et al. 1982). Similarly, Burgett et al. (1992) demonstrated that healing following periodontal therapy may be more advantageous in patients who received occlusal adjustment than in non-adjusted patients.

Long-term follow-up of patients who have received combined periodontal and orthodontic treatment, and have used bonded retainers for several years, demonstrates excellent stability and apparently unchanged, or even improved, periodontal condition (Figs. 57-4, 57-7, 57-8). It should be pointed out, however, that a bonded maxillary retainer must be placed out of occlusion with the mandibular incisors, because biting on a retainer wire will lead to unacceptably high bond failure rates (Årtun & Urbye 1988).

Possibilities and limitations; legal aspects

Adult orthodontic patients with marked periodontal destruction may represent potential problems even when optimal treatment is provided. There are,

however, no definite metric limits in terms of probing depths or loss of attachment when orthodontic tooth movement can no longer be performed (Diedrich 1999). Each individual treatment plan may depend on a variety of factors and can be limited by biomechanical considerations (force systems, limited anchorage), by periodontal risk factors (tooth/alveolar bone topography, sinus recesses, activity and prognosis of the periodontitis), and by limited patient motivation and poor oral hygiene cooperation.

Single case reports have documented successful periodontal–orthodontic treatment with localized juvenile periodontitis (LJP) after conventional periodontal therapy (Harpenau & Boyd 2000), or with continous antiseptic and short-term systemic (Folio et al. 1985) or local (Hoerman et al. 1985) antibiotic applications, and microbiologic testing during the orthodontic treatment period to reduce the risk of recurrent disease. However, until more evidence is accumulated, it may seem wise to avoid orthodontic treatment in patients with particularly aggressive forms of periodontal disease. Similarly, multi-rooted teeth with questionable prognosis should be moved orthodontically only in exceptional situations.

"Hopeless teeth": According to old concepts, the retention of teeth diagnosed as periodontally "hopeless" would accelerate the destruction of the adjacent interproximal periodontium. Such teeth were therefore frequently extracted in the past. However, the theoretic rationale for such extractions would seem unsupported, and recent follow-up studies have demonstrated that retained periodontally "hopeless" teeth do not significantly affect the interproximal periodontium of adjacent teeth following periodontal therapy (Chace & Low 1993). The clinical implication is that these teeth can be useful for orthodontic anchorage, if the periodontal inflammation can be controlled (Fig. 57-9). Occasionally, the hopeless tooth may be so improved after orthodontic treatment that it is retained (Mathews & Kokich 1997). Alternatively, a hopeless molar may be hemisectioned after the orthodontic treatment, and the best root may be used as a bridge abutment (Fig. 57-10). Most of the time, however, the hopeless tooth will be extracted, especially if other restorations are planned in the segment.

For improved patient care, stress reduction, and reduction or elimination of law suits, careful examination protocols, documentation and correspondence techniques, and regular progress evaluations are important. The legal implications of orthodontic risk management concepts may be that it is preferable to terminate treatment for patients who fail to improve oral hygiene care, despite the orthodontist's efforts. In the long term, this will be better for both patient and orthodontist, since termination, if properly handled, will be more easily defended than permitting the condition to worsen (Machen 1990). However, if proper procedures are followed, termination of

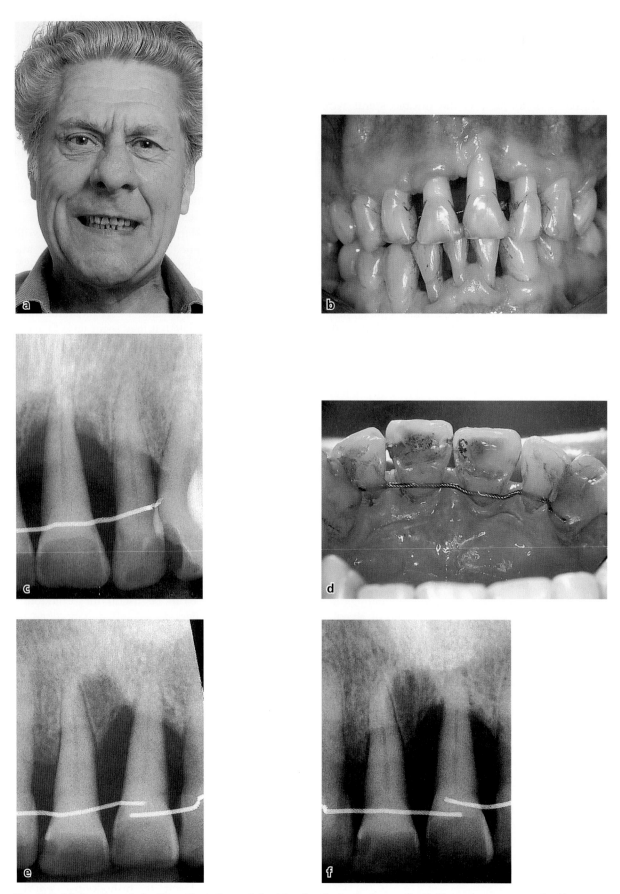

Fig. 57-7 Adult male periodontitis patient after periodontal and orthodontic therapy (a–d). The patient was treated with generalized gingivectomies according to concepts aiming at pocket elimination. The orthodontic result is maintained with a six-unit lingually bonded retainer (d). The bonded wire will act both as an orthodontic retainer and as a periodontal splint, which would appear advantageous in cases where the tissue destruction is as advanced as in this patient. (e) and (f) show the radiographic appearances 7 and 9 years, respectively, after removal of the orthodontic appliances. The left central incisor had so little bone support that if the bonded retainer had not been used, the tooth would probably had been lost over time (see also Fig. 57-8).

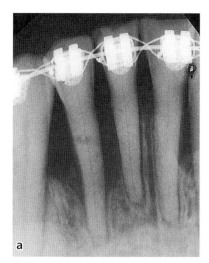
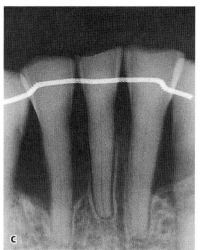
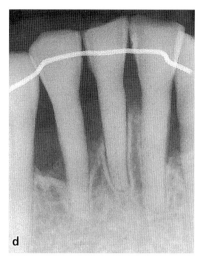
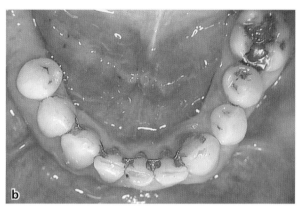

Fig. 57-8 Post-treatment radiographic (a) and clinical (b) appearance of the mandibular dentition in the same patient as in Fig. 57-7 after periodontal and orthodontic treatment. The mandibular six-unit retainer bonded lingual retainer (b) concomitantly acts as a periodontal splint. Note signs of improvement of periodontal condition 7 and 9 years, respectively, after the orthodontic treatment (c,d), with marked crestal lamina dura contours.

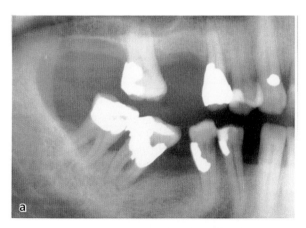
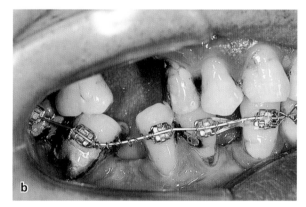
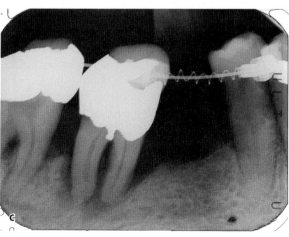
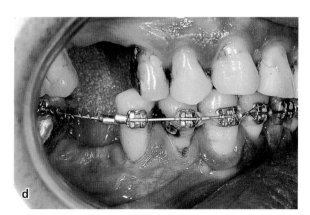

Fig. 57-9 "Hopeless" mandibular right first molar (a) can be used as part of anchorage to move the premolars mesially and upright the second molar (b–d). The first molar may be kept, or extracted, after the orthodontic treatment period.

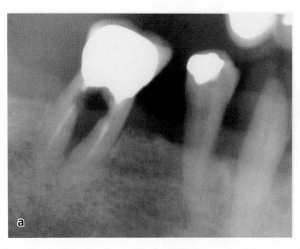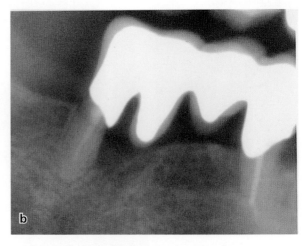

Fig. 57-10 "Hopeless" mandibular right first molar (a) was used as anchorage during orthodontic treatment to close spaces anteriorly, before it was hemisectioned and the distal root employed as a bridge abutment (b).

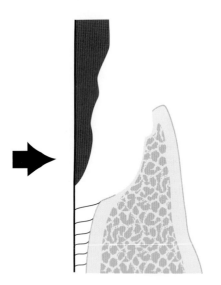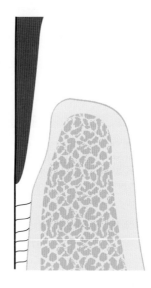

Fig. 57-11 Schematic illustration of persisting junctional epithelium subsequent to orthodontic tooth movement (direction of arrow) into an infrabony pocket.

orthodontic care for periodontal patients will very rarely be needed.

Specific factors associated with orthodontic tooth movement in adults

Tooth movement into infrabony pockets

Orthodontic forces *per se* are unlikely to convert gingivitis into destructive periodontitis. The plaque-induced lesion in gingivitis is confined to the supra-alveolar connective tissue, whereas tissue reactions to orthodontic forces occur in the connective tissue between the root and the alveolar bone. However, infrabony pockets, i.e. angular bony defects with inflamed connective tissue and epithelium apical to the bone crest, may develop as a result of destructive periodontitis. Infrabony pockets may also be created by orthodontic tipping and/or intruding movements of teeth harboring plaque (Ericsson *et al.*

1977). The effect of bodily tooth movement into infrabony defects has been evaluated experimentally in monkeys (Polson *et al.* 1984) and in dogs (Wennström *et al.* 1993). Provided elimination of the subgingival infection was performed before the orthodontic tooth movement was started, no detrimental effects on the attachment level were observed. The angular bony defect was eliminated by the orthodontic treatment, but no coronal gain of attachment was found and a thin epithelial lining covered the root surface corresponding to its pretreatment position (Fig. 57-11). It was therefore concluded that orthodontic tooth movement into infrabony periodontal defects had no favorable effects on the level of connective tissue attachment. However, it was possible to move teeth with reduced *healthy* periodontium without additional attachment loss. If, on the other hand, the orthodontic treatment involved movement of teeth into and through a site with inflammation and angular bone loss, an enhanced rate of periodontal destruction was noted.

Conclusion

Since orthodontic movement of teeth into inflamed infrabony pockets may create a high risk for additional periodontal destruction, and because infrabony pockets are frequently found at teeth that have been tipped and/or elongated as a result of periodontal disease, it is clinically essential that periodontal treatment with elimination of the plaque-induced lesion is performed before orthodontic therapy is begun. It is equally important that excellent oral hygiene is maintained throughout the course of the orthodontic treatment. Following these principles, clinical and radiographic observations confirm that orthodontic treatment can be successfully performed in patients with infrabony pockets resulting from periodontal disease.

Tooth movement into compromised bone areas

Orthodontic tooth movement may sometimes be performed in adults with partially edentulous dentitions (due to agenesis or previous extractions of teeth) and such patients may have a more or less compromised alveolar process. Experimental reports (Lindskog-Stokland et al. 1993) and clinical studies (Stepovich 1979; Hom & Turley 1984; Goldberg & Turley 1989; Thilander 1996) have shown that a reduction in vertical bone height is not a contraindication for orthodontic tooth movement towards, or into, the constricted area. Mandibular second molars can be moved mesially through remodeled edentulous first molar areas in adults (Fig. 57-12), with only a limited reduction in vertical bone height, averaging −1.3 mm (Hom & Turley 1984). Space closure is possible also in edentulous maxillary first molar areas, although vertical bone loss and some space reopening can be a complication.

Histologic observations in animal experiments have confirmed that when light forces were applied to move teeth bodily into an area with reduced bone height, a thin bone plate was recreated ahead of the moving tooth (Fig. 57-13) (Lindskog-Stokland et al. 1993). The key to moving teeth with bone is direct resorption in the direction of tooth movement, and avoiding hyalinization. Teeth can also be moved with bone into the maxillary sinus (Melsen 1991).

Conclusion

Although the results of clinical experiments and follow-ups are encouraging, provided light forces are used and excellent oral hygiene is maintained, it is probably wise not to stretch the indications for tooth movement into constricted bone areas too far. Marked gingival invaginations are sometimes seen in such areas (Fig. 57-12), and computer tomography analysis and human histologic findings indicate that buccal or lingual bone dehiscences may occur (Diedrich 1996). Such defects are not revealed by conventional radiography. The clinical significance of the gingival clefts and bone dehiscences with regard to relapse tendency and periodontal status is not known. For orthodontic tooth movement into markedly atrophied alveolar ridges, the possibility to acquire new bone by, for example, guided bone regeneration (GBR) procedures should be considered.

Tooth movement through cortical bone

Experimental studies in animals have demonstrated that when a tooth is moved bodily in a labial direction towards and through the cortical plate of the alveolar bone, no bone formation will take place in front of the tooth (Steiner et al. 1981; Karring et al. 1982). After initial thinning of the bone plate, a labial bone dehiscence is therefore created (Fig. 57-14). Such perforation of the cortical plate can occur during orthodontic treatment either accidentally or because it was considered unavoidable. It may happen, for example, (1) in the mandibular anterior region due to frontal expansion of incisors (Wehrbein et al. 1994), (2) in the maxillary posterior region during lateral expansion of cross-bites (Greenbaum & Zachrisson 1982), (3) lingually in the maxilla associated with retraction and lingual root torque of maxillary incisors in patients with large overjets (Ten Hoeve & Mulie 1976), and (4) by pronounced traumatic jiggling of teeth (Nyman et al. 1982). The soft tissue reactions accompanying such tooth movements are discussed later in this chapter and in Chapter 51.

Interestingly, however, there is potential for repair when malpositioned teeth are moved back toward their original positions, and bone apposition may take place (Fig. 57-14). Evidently, the soft tissue facial to an orthodontically produced bone dehiscence may contain soft tissue components (vital osteogenic cells) with a capacity for forming bone following repositioning of the tooth into the alveolar process (Nyman et al. 1982).

Conclusion

The clinical implication of these observations is encouraging. Bone dehiscences which may occur due to uncontrolled expansion of teeth through the cortical plate may be repaired when the teeth are brought back, or relapse, towards a proper position within the alveolar process, even if this occurs several months later. Similar repair mechanisms may be expected to occur when marked jiggling of teeth is brought under control and stabilized. In the case of buccal cross-bites, the initial discrepancy can apparently be overcorrected with both slow and rapid expansion treatment approaches without causing permanent periodontal injury to the settled occlusion.

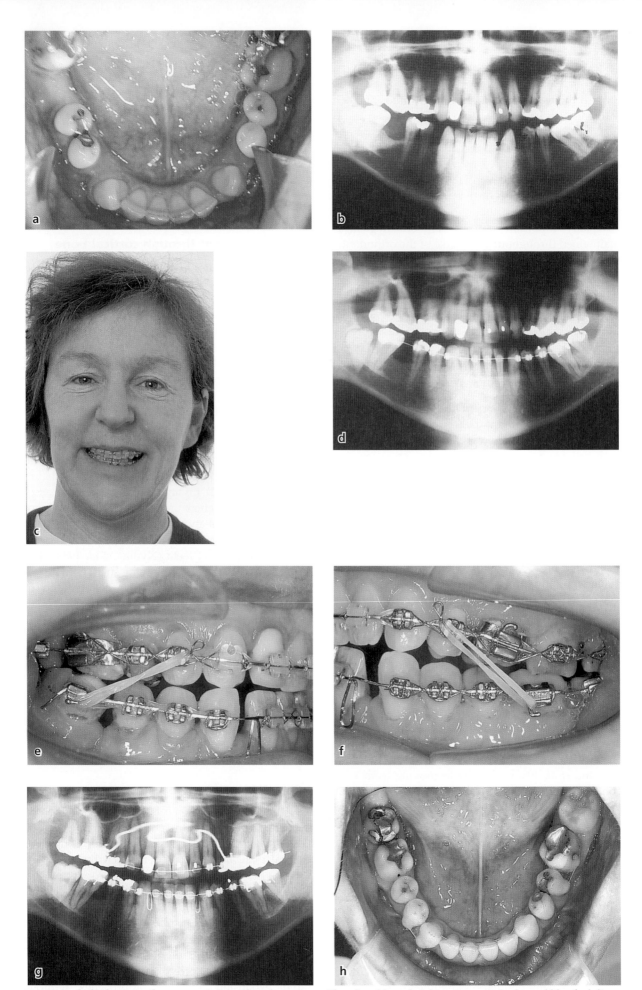

Fig. 57-12 Orthodontic tooth movements into edentulous areas with reduced bone height in compromised mandible of adult female patient. During the orthodontic treatment (c–g), the teeth were moved to close three areas of marked alveolar bone constriction (a,b), most notably in the right first molar area. Note that the impacted third molar erupted spontaneously as the second molar was moved mesially (g). (h) Final result with bonded six-unit lingual and two-unit labial retainers.

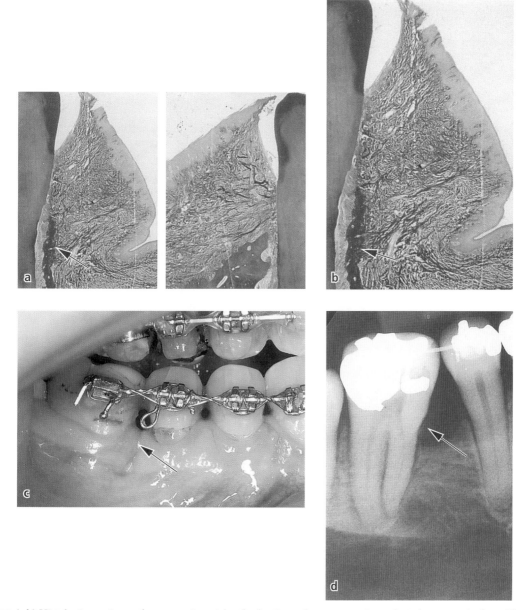

Fig. 57-13 (a,b) Histologic specimens from experimental orthodontic tooth movement into edentulous areas in dogs. The thin bone spicule along the pressure side of the test tooth (b) indicates tooth movement with, and not through, bone. (c,d) The same patient as in Fig. 57-12. Note radiographic visualization of the thin bone spicule on the mesial side of the second molar (arrow in d). Although the molar is moved to contact the second premolar, a marked gingival invagination is present in the area (arrow in c). (a) and (b) from Lindskog-Stokland *et al.* (1993).

Extrusion and intrusion of single teeth – effects on periodontium, clinical crown length, and esthetics

Extrusion

Orthodontic extrusion of teeth, or so-called "forced eruption", may be indicated for (1) shallowing out intraosseous defects and (2) for increasing clinical crown length of single teeth. The forced eruption technique was originally described by Ingber (1974) for treatment of one-wall and two-wall bony pockets that were difficult to handle by conventional therapy alone. The extrusive tooth movement leads to a

coronal positioning of intact connective tissue attachment, and the bony defect is shallowed out. This was confirmed in animal experiments (van Venroy & Yukna 1985) and clinical trials. Because of the orthodontic extrusion, the tooth will be in supra-occlusion. Hence, the crown of the tooth will need to be shortened, in some cases followed by endodontic treatment.

During the elimination of an intraosseous pocket by means of orthodontic extrusion, the relationship between the CEJ and the bone crest is maintained. This means that the bone follows the tooth during the extrusive movement. This may or may not be beneficial depending on the clinical situation. In other

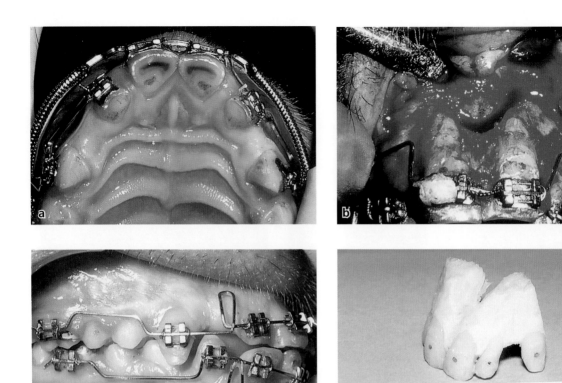

Fig. 57-14 Techniques used by Steiner *et al.* (1981) to advance incisors bodily through the labial bone plate in monkeys (a,b) and by Engelking and Zachrisson (1982) to retract the incisors to their original position (after the teeth had remained in extreme labioversion for 8 months) in a study of periodontal regeneration to such tooth movement. (d) Tissue blocks after tooth repositioning show evident bone regeneration.

words, it is sometimes desirable to have the periodontium follow the tooth and in other situations it is desirable to move a tooth out of the periodontal support. This is further discussed under slow versus rapid eruption of teeth in Chapter 51.

Extrusion with periodontium

Orthodontic extrusion of a single tooth that needs to be extracted is an excellent method for improvement of the marginal bone level before the surgical placement of single implants (Figs. 57-15, 57-21, 57-22). Not only the bone, but also the soft supporting tissues will move vertically with the teeth during orthodontic extrusion. Using tattoo marks in monkeys to indicate the mucogingival junction and clinical sulcus bottom, Kajiyama *et al.* (1993) made a metric evaluation of the gingival movement associated with vertical extrusion of incisors. The results indicated that the free gingiva moved about 90% and the attached gingiva about 80% of the extruded distance. The width of the attached gingiva and the clinical crown length increased significantly, whereas the position of the mucogingival junction was unchanged. Orthodontic extrusion of a "hopeless" incisor is also, therefore, a useful method for esthetic improvement of the marginal gingival level associated with the placement of implants (Fig. 57-22).

Extrusion out of periodontium

In teeth with crown–root fracture, or other subgingival fractures, the goal of treatment may be to extrude the root out of the periodontium (Figs. 57-16, 57-17), and then provide it with an artificial crown. When an increased distance between the CEJ and the alveolar bone crest is aimed at, the forced eruption should be combined with gingival fiberotomy (Pontoriero *et al.* 1987; Kozlowsky *et al.* 1988). In animal experiments, Berglundh *et al.* (1991) showed that when the fiberotomy (i.e. excision of the coronal portion of the fiber attachment around the tooth) was performed frequently (every 2 weeks), the tooth was virtually moved out of the bony periodontium, without affecting the bone heights or level of the marginal gingiva of the neighboring teeth. This procedure is illustrated in Fig. 57-17.

Intrusion

Similar to the indications for extrusion, the orthodontic intrusion of teeth has been recommended (1) for teeth with horizontal bone loss or infrabony pockets, and (2) for increasing the clinical crown length of single teeth. However, the benefits of intrusion for improvement of the periodontal condition around teeth are controversial.

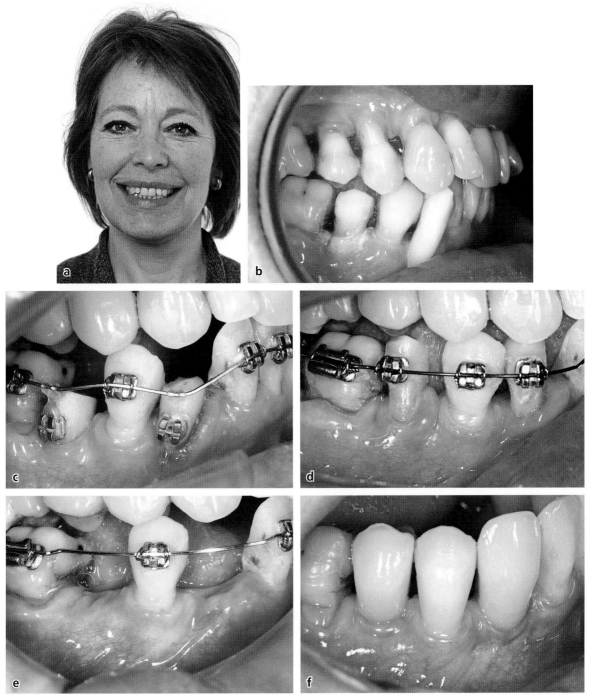

Fig. 57-15 (a,b) Adult female patient with evidence of local severe periodontal tissue breakdown before treatment. The bone loss is particularly pronounced on the mandibular right second premolar (g) and canine (j), whereas the bone support for the first premolar is much better (g,j). The treatment plan included slow orthodontic extrusion of the second premolar and canine to regenerate an improved vertical alveolar bone height prior to the placement of implant-supported restorations. Brackets were placed in a gingival location on the teeth to be extruded (c) and leveling was started with super-elastic rectangular arch-wires. After removal of the pulp, the crowns of the teeth to be extruded were ground with diamond instruments to avoid jiggling with the teeth in the opposing arch (c). A cantilever spring was added for the canine. After 10 months, the leveling was completed (d) and the extruded teeth were extracted with forceps (e). Note the even bone levels (e) and compare with the initial situation (b). A remarkable amount of bone build-up is seen on the radiographs at 10 months of leveling (h,k) before insertion of the implants. A comparison of the final bone heights relative to the cemento-enamel junctions of the neighboring teeth with the initial situation reveals that a significant portion of the bone support for the well integrated implants has been created by the slow vertical tooth movements. The clinical and radiographic situation at the 3-year follow-up is shown in f, i and l.

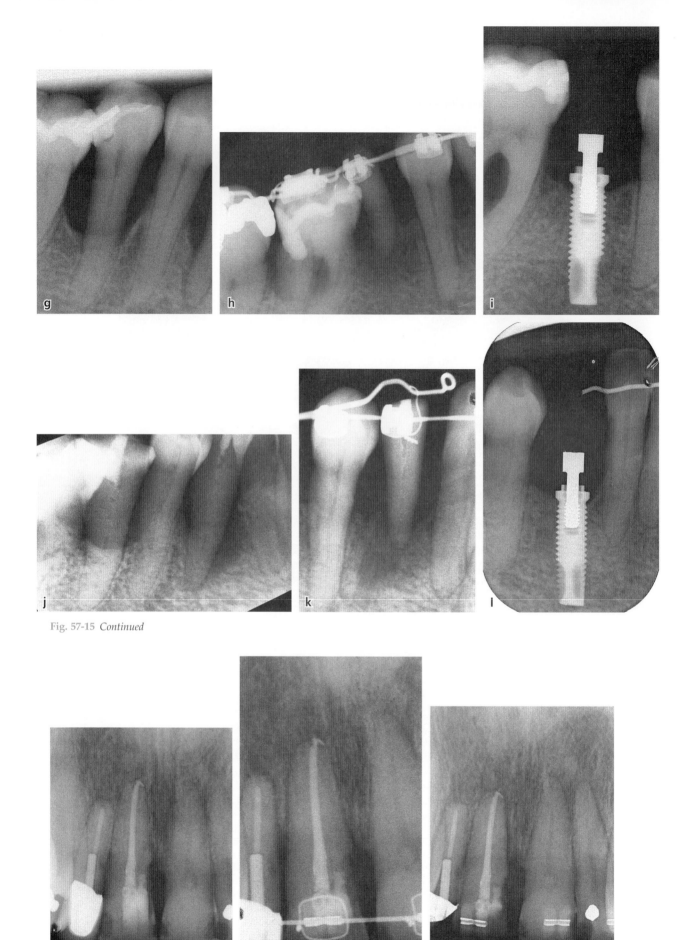

Fig. 57-15 *Continued*

Fig. 57-16 (a) Extrusion out of the periodontium of central incisor with deep crown-root fracture. Rapid extrusion with continuous orthodontic force combined with fiberotomy every 2 weeks. The amount of extrusion can be evaluated by comparing the root ends of the incisors in a–c. (b) The situation after 1.5 months of extrusion. (c) After 4 months, the fracture line was moved from a location below the bone level (a) to a position well above it (c), and the incisor could now be properly restored.

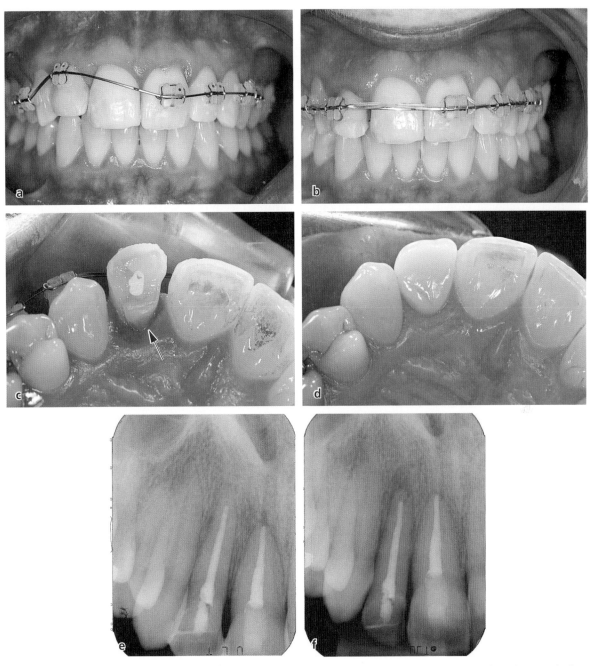

Fig. 57-17 Extrusion out of periodontium. Due to subgingival crown-root fracture on the maxillary right lateral incisor (a,d), this tooth was extruded out of the periodontium with continuous force (a,b) and fiberotomy was performed with 2-week intervals. The amount of extrusion is evident by comparison of the relationship between lateral and central incisor root ends in (e) and (f). Having moved the fracture line to a supragingival position (arrow in c), the tooth could be safely restored. (d) The clinical situation 4 years after treatment.

As mentioned, the intrusion of plaque-infected teeth may lead to the formation of angular bony defects and increased loss of attachment. When oral hygiene is inadequate, tipping and intrusion of the teeth may shift supragingivally located plaque into a subgingival position, resulting in periodontal destruction (Ericsson *et al.* 1977, 1978). This explains why professional subgingival scaling is particularly important during the phase of active intrusion of elongated, tipped, and migrated maxillary incisors commonly occurring in association with advanced periodontal disease. Even in a healthy periodontal environment the question remains as to whether the orthodontic tooth movement intrudes a long epithelial attachment beneath the margin of the alveolar bone or whether the alveolar crest is continuously resorbed in front of the intruding tooth.

Histologic (Melsen 1986; Melsen *et al.* 1988) and clinical (Melsen *et al.* 1989) studies indicate that new attachment is possible associated with orthodontic intrusion of teeth. In monkey experiments, periodontal tissue breakdown was induced and intrusion along the axis of the incisors with light forces was initiated following flap surgery. Histologic analysis showed new cementum formation and connective tissue attachment on the intruded teeth, by an average of 1.5 mm, provided a healthy gingival environment was maintained throughout the tooth movement. The increased activity of periodontal ligament cells and the approximation of formative cells to the tooth surface was suggested to contribute to the new attachment. In the clinical study, the periodontal condition was evaluated following the intrusion of extruded and spaced incisors in patients who had advanced periodontal disease. Judging from clinical probing depths and radiography, there was a beneficial effect on clinical crown lengths and marginal bone levels in many cases, despite large individual variation.

However, the reported clinical and histologic findings associated with a combined orthodontic–periodontal approach must be assessed with great caution, and these findings have not been confirmed by others. Furthermore, new techniques like guided tissue regeneration (GTR) and other regenerative procedures (see below) would appear to be more promising when it comes to creation of new attachment.

Similar to the case with extrusion, metric and histologic studies have been made after experimental intrusion of teeth in monkeys. According to Murakami *et al.* (1989), the gingiva moved only about 60% of the distance when the teeth were intruded with a continuous force of 80–100 g. However, Kokich *et al.* (1984) recommended an interrupted, continuous force for levelling of gingival margins on supra-erupted teeth (Fig. 57-18).

The key to understanding why intrusion can be used to increase clinical crown length is related to the subsequent restorative treatment. When orthodontic intrusion is used for levelling of the gingival margins to desired heights, such teeth must then be provided with porcelain laminate veneers or crowns (Fig. 57-18).

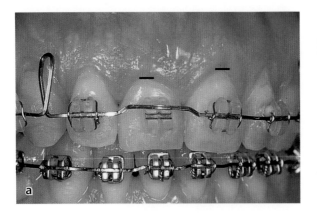
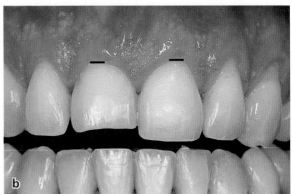
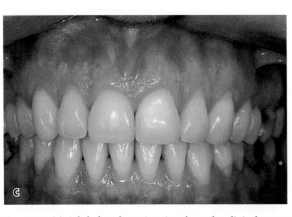
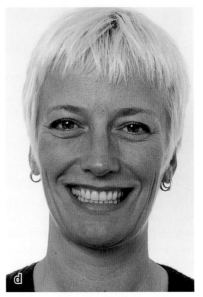

Fig. 57-18 (a) Adult female patient in whom the clinical crown length of the maxillary right central incisor was shorter than that of the left central incisor. Because the sulcular depths were normal, the crown lengths were corrected by orthodontic intrusion of the right central incisor (b) and restoring the incisal edge (b) with enamel-bonded ultrathin porcelain laminate veneer (c,d). The alignment and correction of the crown length discrepancy has improved the esthetic appearance of the dentition. Restoration courtesy of Dr. S. Toreskog.

Regenerative procedures and orthodontic tooth movement

The development of barrier membranes to prevent cells of the epithelium and gingival connective tissue from colonizing the decontaminated root surface, as well as the use of Emdogain®, would appear to provide a distinct improvement in orthodontic therapy in the periodontally compromised patient. New supracrestal and periodontal ligament collagen fibers may be gained on the tension side, which can transfer the orthodontic force stimulus to the alveolar bone (Diedrich 1996). In theory, the regenerative techniques would be advantageous associated with both extrusion and intrusion of teeth with infrabony defects, and for uprighting of tipped molars with mesial angular lesions. Moreover, if the epithelium can be prevented from proliferating apically, a bodily tooth movement into or through an intraosseous defect could eliminate the bony pocket more effectively than in the past (Fig. 57-11).

So far, however, relatively little clinical information is available about the use of different regenerative procedures in connection with orthodontic treatment. Diedrich (1996) reported an experiment in dogs in which orthodontic intrusion with flap surgery and GTR were compared with flap surgery alone on periodontally affected teeth. In the presence of minimal or no round cell infiltration, the marking notch was located beneath the alveolar margin indicating that new attachment had formed. The potential of the intrusive/regenerative mechanism was most impressive within the inter-radicular area. Some clinical observations (Nemcovsky *et al.* 1996; Stelzel & Flores-de-Jacoby 1998; Rabie *et al.* 2001) confirm that different regenerative procedures may enrich the therapeutic spectrum in combined periodontal/ orthodontic approaches (Fig. 57-19). The combined regenerative and periodontal surgical treatments used together with orthodontic tooth movements create new perspectives and should be an interesting field for further experiments on adults with severe loss of periodontal tissues.

However, other clinical trials have demonstrated that treatment results with barrier membranes in the GTR technique may vary between different patients and that the method is operator and technique sensitive (Leknes 1995). The patient's oral hygiene during the healing phase is critical, and inflammation around the membrane, particularly if it becomes exposed and contaminated, may lead to discouraging clinical results with marked gingival retraction.

Since the membrane is covered in the GBR technique, the risk for inflammation is reduced. The possibility for orthodontic movement of teeth into alveolar processes with deficient bone volume may

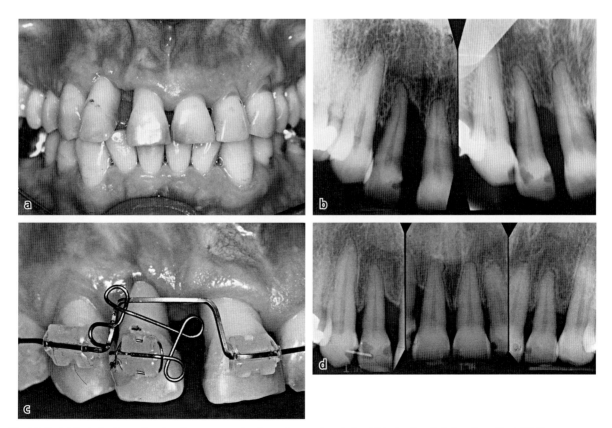

Fig. 57-19 (a) Pathologic tooth migration as a result of an advanced periodontal lesion in adult female patient. (b) Severe intraosseous defect between the right central and lateral incisors. (c) Three months after GTR treatment (GoreTex membrane) partial reossification is evident, possibly with new attachment. (d) Orthodontic leveling with controlled space closure and intrusion of the lateral incisor. (e) Result 6 months after orthodontic tooth movements shows no root resorption and a consolidated alveolar crest. From Diedrich (1996).

thus be improved (Basdra *et al.* 1995). Preorthodontic GBR of markedly constricted alveolar ridges also has the advantage that tooth movement through cancellous bone is easier, and the formation of interfering gingival invaginations can be reduced.

Traumatic occlusion (jiggling) and orthodontic treatment

As discussed in Chapter 14, the role of occlusal trauma in periodontal treatment has not been determined. From an orthodontic perspective, it is of interest that several studies indicate that traumatic occlusion forces (1) do not produce gingival inflammation or loss of attachment in teeth with healthy periodontium, (2) do not aggravate and cause spread of gingivitis or cause loss of attachment in teeth with established gingivitis, (3) may aggravate an active periodontitis lesion, i.e. be a co-destructive factor in an ongoing process of periodontal tissue breakdown (in one way or another favor the apical proliferation of plaque-induced destruction), and (4) may lead to less gain of attachment after periodontal treatment – non-surgical or surgical.

A major problem in this regard is the lack of established and reliable criteria to identify and quantitate different degrees of traumatic occlusion. Various clinical and radiographic indications, such as unfavorable crown/root ratio, increased tooth mobility, widened periodontal ligament space, angular bone loss, alterations in root morphology, etc. are uncertain and insufficient in diagnosis of occlusal trauma, and there have been few scientific clinical reports to evaluate these signs (Jin & Cao 1992).

The extent to which it is necessary to avoid, or reduce, occlusal trauma during orthodontic treatment is controversial and unsupported by scientific evidence. Some orthodontists use bite-planes in virtually every periodontal case with bone deformities, to reduce occlusal trauma and for the purpose of shallowing the bony defects, as teeth supra-erupt. However, independent studies have shown that surgical pocket elimination including bone sculpturing offers no advantage compared with more conservative periodontal treatment (Ramfjord 1984), and apparently there is little need to shallow or eliminate bony deformities. It would still appear sensible to avoid gross interferences, like raising the bite when a maxillary incisor in lingual inversion is moved over the mandibular teeth, and to mitigate evident occlusal interferences on single teeth with markedly increased mobility. However, it may be a futile exercise to try and eliminate all occlusal trauma during active tooth movement, and a more practical solution is to concentrate on controlling the inflammation. After appliance removal, however, occlusal adjustment by selective grinding may be required. Even though good occlusal function is part of the orthodontic treatment goal, correct cusp–fossa relationships cannot always be achieved in adults with

orthodontic therapy alone. In general terms, the adjustment should be directed toward obtaining even and stable tooth contacts in centric relation, a straight forward slide from centric relation to centric occlusion without any side shifts or lateral deviation, freedom in centric, smooth gliding contacts in centric and eccentric mandibular motion, and elimination of balancing side interferences (Burgett *et al.* 1992).

The importance of reducing jiggling of teeth *after* orthodontic treatment of patients with moderate to advanced periodontitis may be significant: (1) tooth mobility generally increases with loss of support for the teeth, (2) animal experiments have shown that bone dehiscences produced by jiggling forces will regenerate after elimination of the jiggling trauma, and (3) occlusal adjustment may be a factor in the healing of periodontal defects, especially bony defects, after periodontal treatment. Therefore, the bonded orthodontic retainers, which stabilize the teeth, may secure optimal conditions for improved periodontal healing and bone regeneration after the orthodontic treatment period (Figs. 57-5, 57-7, 57-8). In fact, long-term follow-ups of orthodontic patients with advanced periodontal tissue breakdown may demonstrate better periodontal conditions, with marked crestal lamina dura contours, many years after appliance removal than at the end of the orthodontic treatment (Figs. 57-7, 57-8). If bonded retainers had not been used in many such cases, the most affected teeth would probably have been lost with time.

Molar uprighting, furcation involvement

The problem of mesially tipped mandibular molars because of non-replacement of missing first molars has been the subject of many anecdotal reports over the past 30 years. Tipped molars have been considered a causative or at least an aggravating factor for future periodontal tissue breakdown. However, Lundgren *et al.* (1992) recently observed that 73 molars that had remained in a markedly tipped position for at least 10 years, with most molars having been tipped for as long as 20–30 years, did not constitute an increased risk for initiation or aggravation of moderate periodontal disease at their mesial surface. The study did not consider the potential risk for aggravation of already established advanced periodontitis lesions. This lack of correlation may not exclude other indications for molar uprighting, such as functionally disturbing interferences, paralleling or space problems associated with prosthetic rehabilitation, or traumatic occlusion.

In this context it must be emphasized that the apparent angular bone loss along the mesial surface of tipped molars may be illusive and solely represent an anatomic variation, since lines drawn from the adjacent cemento-enamel junctions appear to parallel the alveolar crest (Ritchey & Orban 1954). While uprighting such a tooth appears to cause a shallowing-out of the angular defect, with new bone forming at the mesial alveolar crest, it may merely reflect the inclination of the molar relative to the alveolar bone, and the attachment level remains unchanged. When there is a definite osseous defect caused by periodontitis on the mesial surface of the inclined molar, uprighting the tooth and tipping it distally will widen the osseous defect. Any coronal position of bone may be due to the extrusion component of the mechanotherapy.

Furcation defects generally remain the same or get worse during orthodontic treatment. For example, if tipped molars have furcation involvement before orthodontic uprighting, simultaneous extrusion may increase the severity of the furcation defects, especially in the presence of inflammation (Burch *et al.* 1992). Hence, initial periodontal therapy and maintenance is essential. The mandibular molar can be split into two roots, one or both of which may be kept and moved orthodontically into new positions. However, this is difficult treatment (Müller *et al.* 1995).

In a thorough study of periodontal conditions around tipped mandibular molars before prosthetic replacement, Lang (1977) reported that after completion of the hygiene phase, significant pocket reduction (mean 1.0 mm) was noted on all surfaces. In addition, a further significant reduction in pocket depth (mean 0.6 mm), associated with a gain of clinical attachment (mean 0.4 mm), was found on the mesial and lingual aspects of the molars as a result of the orthodontic uprighting. He concluded that uprighting of tipped molars is a simple and predictable procedure, provided excellent plaque control is maintained.

Kessler (1976), on the other hand, stated that uprighting of mesially inclined molars is not a panacea, and showed some cases in which evident bone loss and furcation involvement developed during the orthodontic uprighting procedure. Because of the furcation involvement and increased mobility, these teeth were no longer considered suitable as abutments, although they were properly uprighted. Radiographic indications that furcation involvement may develop between the roots at the end of orthodontic molar uprighting is evident also in other studies, even when extrusive movement of the tipped molars has been avoided (Diedrich 1989). However, it is not unlikely that this radiolucent area reflects immature bone.

Conclusion

As risks may be involved in orthodontic uprighting of mesially tipped molars in cases with periodontal lesions along their mesial surface, or with furcation involvement, the indications for molar uprighting must be apparent. Excellent oral hygiene is required during the orthodontic treatment, with careful consideration of the force distribution, and avoiding extrusion as much as possible. The developments of regenerative techniques may make it possible in the future to obtain better outcomes in orthodontic therapy of periodontally compromised patients.

Tooth movement and implant esthetics

Osseointegrated implants may be used (1) to provide anchorage for orthodontic tooth movement and later serve as abutments for restorative treatment, and (2) to replace single missing teeth. The use of implants as anchors for orthodontic treatment is discussed in Chapter 58, and will not be dealt with here.

It is difficult to achieve esthetically satisfactory results with artificial crowns on single-tooth implants, and the orthodontist may play a role in the interdisciplinary treatment planning team of specialists. There are at least three areas where orthodontics may be considered:

- Redistribution of the available space in the dental arch when tooth positions for implant placement are not optimal
- Orthodontic ridge augmentation by vertical tooth movement
- Orthodontic ridge augmentation by horizontal tooth movement.

Redistribution of space

Orthodontic movement of neighboring teeth to optimal positions is often required in association with placement of implants substituting missing maxillary central or lateral incisors (Spear *et al.* 1997). Another common indication is a lack of adequate space for the implant. Figure 57-20 illustrates a typical case with small spaces between the teeth and not enough room to place implants in the maxillary and mandibular first premolar regions.

Ridge augmentation – vertical movement

During selective orthodontic extrusion of one single tooth, both the alveolar bone and the soft periodontal tissues will follow the extruded tooth in an incisal direction, as discussed under forced eruption earlier in this chapter. By this means, it is possible to significantly improve the periodontal tissue esthetics associated with fabrication of prosthetic crowns on single implants (Figs. 57-21, 57-22). The technique of "orthodontic extraction" of a hopeless incisor or molar (Salama & Salama 1993; Zuccati & Bocchieri 2003) may be useful to improve the results for single-tooth implants in patients in whom one or more teeth are to be extracted. Following progressive grinding of the extruded tooth to prevent it from jiggling (Figs. 57-21, 57-22), new periodontal tissues are generated that provide improved conditions for the implant, after extraction of the extruded tooth (Fig. 57-21). Upon extruding a tooth, the periodontal ligaments are pulled away from the bone and thus transfer

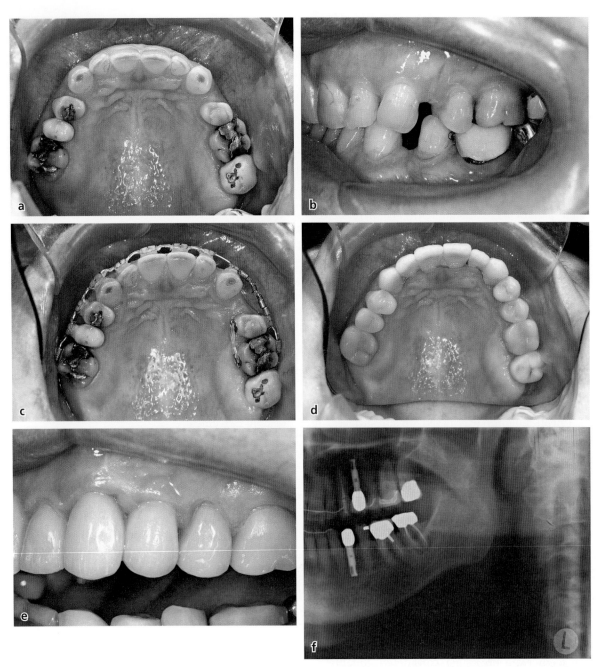

Fig. 57-20 Typical orthodontic space reopening before insertion of two implants in the second and third quadrant in an adult female patient (a–f). Note the lingually tipped maxillary and mandibular incisors and the small spaces before treatment (a,b). Continuous force from push-coils (c) was used to open adequate space for the implants in the first premolar regions in both dental arches (d–f).

mechanical strain to cells in the bone. A series of mechano-transduction mediators (Indian hedgehog), are expressed and lead to bone formation (Tang *et al.* 2004). The type of bone formed initially is the "emergency type of bone" with type III collagen (Chayanupatkul *et al.* 2003; Tang *et al.* 2004). This bone is somewhat weak because the cross-links between the collagen fiber matrix are weak. It takes about 6 months to mature to the more stable type I collagen (Chayanupatkul *et al.* 2003). The stable type of bone may accept an implant without showing relapse. The stability of the newly formed bone can thus be influenced by whether the clinician allows the newly formed bone to remodel to the more stable

bone. It is conceivable that the time periods for the extrusion and the observation time before implant insertion should be at least 6 months for the newly formed bone to mature into more stable bone (Figs. 57-21, 57-22). To allow for rest periods in between the activations, an interrupted continuous force is recommended, by using small step bends in the arch-wires (Figs. 57-21b,c, 57-22d).

Ridge augmentation – horizontal movement

If an implant cannot be placed because of reduced bucco-lingual ridge thickness after a previous extraction, one option is to move a premolar into the eden-

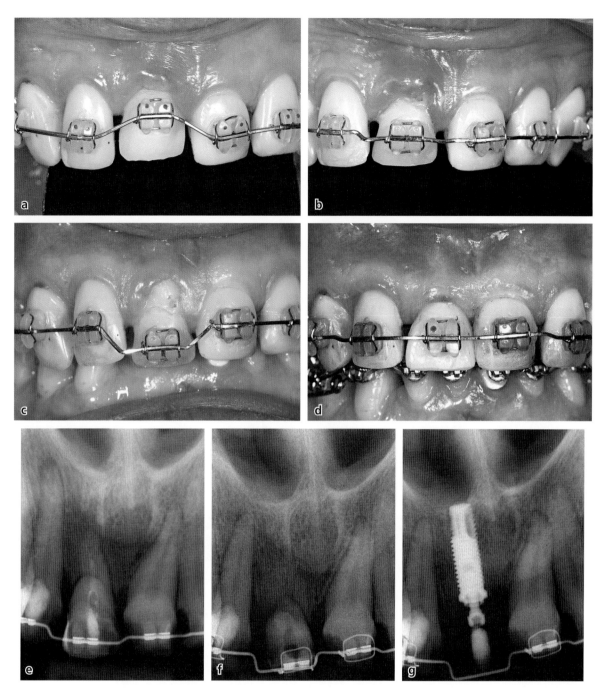

Fig. 57-21 Implant site development by "orthodontic extraction" of maxillary right central incisor with poor prognosis (a,e). The ceramic bracket was positioned in a gingival location on the incisor to be extruded (a), and initial leveling was started with continuous force from a rectangular super-elastic leveling wire. After 1 month, this arch-wire was replaced with a thin rectangular stainless steel wire, using small step-bends for the extrusion (b,e). Such step-bends create an interrupted continuous force which is active for about 2 weeks and then allows 2 weeks of rest before the re-activation at the monthly visits (b,c). The temporary crown on the implant in (d) shows the clinical status at 6 months after implant insertion. The radiographs demonstrate the extensive bone build-up at 10 months (f) and the implant in the regenerated bone at 6 months (g). Note the organization of the bony lamellae reflecting the direction of pull in (f).

tulous space and to place the implant in the position previously occupied by the premolar (Spear *et al.* 1997). The bucco-lingual volume of the new bone on the tension side will be markedly greater than that on the pressure side (Figs. 57-23, 57-24). This is an alternative to surgical ridge augmentation (GBR or bone graft). The situation is similar to that of when a canine is moved distally to open the space for a maxillary lateral incisor implant (Spear *et al.* 1997;

Beyer *et al.* 2007). The root of the canine creates an adequate ridge through stretching of the periodontal ligament.

It should be emphasized that there is much less shrinkage of the alveolar bone after horizontal tooth movements than after extractions of teeth. Spear *et al.* (1997) used cast measurements and tomograms through the edentulous ridge to measure the amount of bone loss with time in cases with orthodontic space

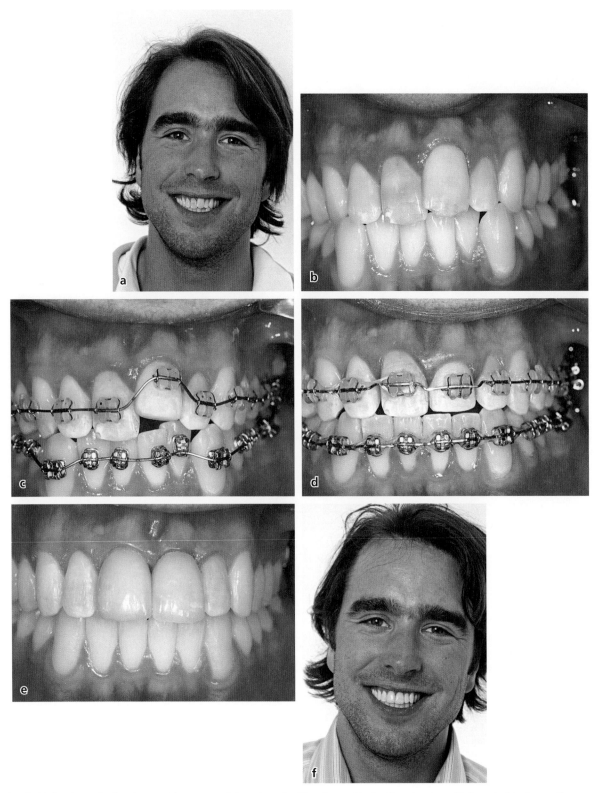

Fig. 57-22 Implant site development in young adult male patient by slow orthodontic extrusion of left central incisor with poor prognosis (a,b). Same procedure as in Fig. 57-21. The ceramic bracket was bonded in a gingival location on the tooth to be extracted. After 1 month of leveling with super-elastic wire, the remaining extrusion for 7 months was made with interrupted continuous force from stainless steel arch-wire, using small step-bends that were reinforced at monthly visits (d). The implant was inserted 4 months after the incisor was extracted. Note the improved gingival margin contour after the orthodontic extrusion (b,d), which permitted an optimal emergence profile of the implant crown (e,f).

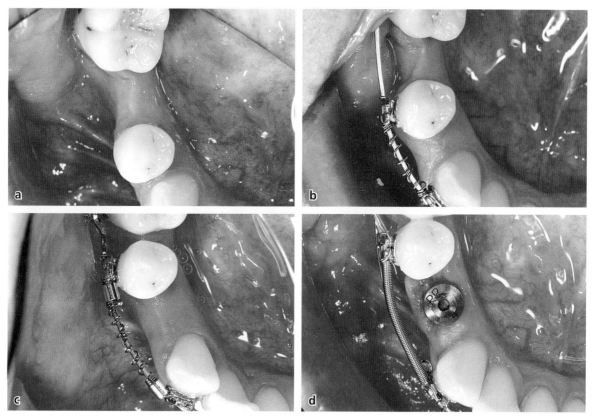

Fig. 57-23 Ridge augmentation by horizontal tooth movement before implant insertion in adult female patient, in whom the alveolar bone in the second premolar area was insufficient to accommodate an implant (a). The first premolar was moved distally with continuous force from a push-coil (b,c). Note wide area of bone regenerated on the tension side of the premolar (b,d) which provided optimal conditions for insertion of the implant (d).

opening for maxillary lateral incisor implants. They found less than 1% alveolar bone shrinkage from the end of treatment up to 4 years later. This contrasts with previous studies showing about 34% reduction of the alveolar ridge over 5 years when anterior teeth are extracted (Carlson 1967).

Figure 57-23 shows a case in which the distal movement of a mandibular first premolar provided new bone of adequate width for implant placement in a previously atrophied alveolar bone area. Similar generation of bone can be obtained in patients who have no molars by moving a terminal premolar distally in the dental arch. Autotransplantation of teeth also represents inherent potential for bone induction and re-establishment of a normal alveolar process after traumatic bone loss (Zachrisson *et al.* 2004).

Gingival recession

Labial recession

"Normal" age changes

Gingival recession, with exposure of cementum on facial surfaces of teeth, may occur on single or multiple teeth. Many factors have been implicated in the etiology, including plaque, position of the tooth in the arch, faulty toothbrushing, traumatic occlusion, high frenum or muscle attachments, lack in dimension of gingiva, lip pressure, etc. (Baker & Seymor 1976). It is difficult to see a single cause of, or a solitary mechanism in the development of, labial gingival recession. Two basic types of recession may occur, one related to periodontal disease, or to factors associated with periodontal disease, and the other relating to mechanical factors, including toothbrushing.

Labial gingival recessions are always accompanied by alveolar bone dehiscences, and there is a direct correlation between the millimetric extension of labial bone dehiscences and the corresponding gingival recessions (Bernimoulin & Curilovic 1977). It has been postulated that a root dehiscence may establish an environment which, for one reason or another, may predispose to gingival recession (Wennström 1990). The position in which a tooth erupts through the alveolar process has a profound influence on the amount of gingiva that will be established around the tooth. When a tooth erupts close to the mucogingival line, only a minimal width, or complete lack, of gingiva may be observed labially, and localized gingival recessions may occur in patients at a young age. Thus the "normal" age changes that will then take place are important. Longitudinal monitoring of labial gingival dimensions during the development of the dentition has shown that provided

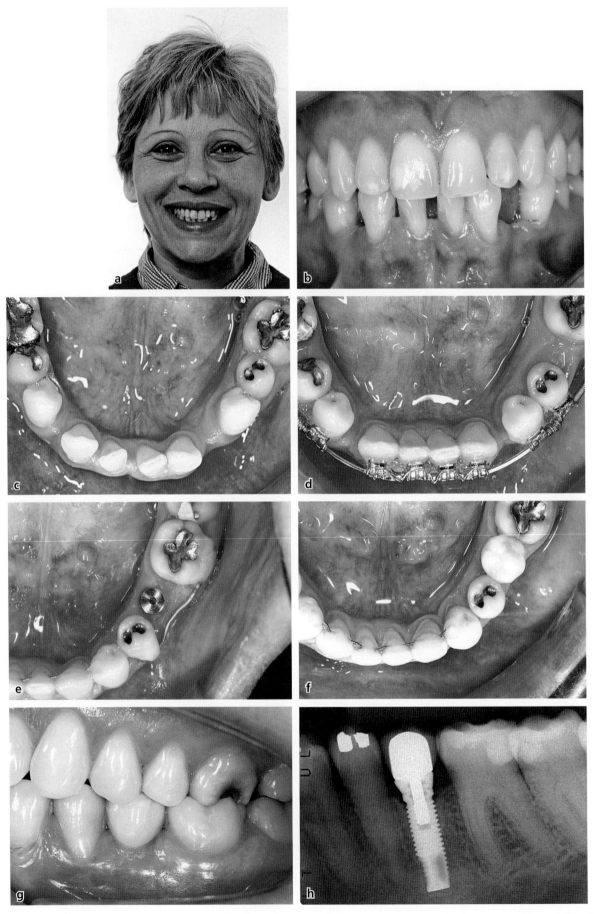

Fig. 57-24 Female patient, 41 years of age, with agenesis of both mandibular central incisors, multiple spacings, thin periodontal tissues, and prominent root topography (a–c). The alveolar bone is too thin labio-lingually to accommodate a titanium implant in the anterior regions (c). The treatment principle was, therefore, to close spaces anteriorly by moving the left first and second premolars mesially (d), and to open up space posteriorly for an implant (e). Note the wide area of alveolar bone on the tension side (d,e), providing ample bucco-lingual space for implant insertion. Permanent implant-supported crown at 3.5 years after treatment (courtesy of Dr. Roy Samuelsson, Oslo, Norway) is shown in f–h.

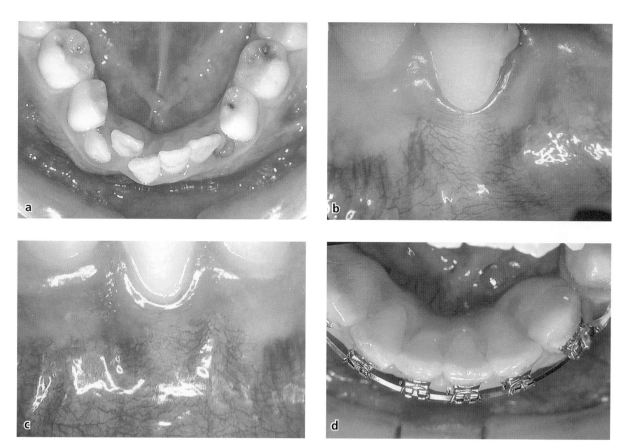

Fig. 57-25 Thin labial gingiva on prominent mandibular right central incisor (a,b) spontaneously became thicker when the incisor was orthodontically moved lingually and aligned (c) after premolar extractions. (d) Condition after appliance removal.

adequate plaque control is established and maintained, a significant increase of the gingival height will generally occur. Spontaneous improvement of localized mandibular labial recessions is the rule rather than the exception, and in some teeth the recessions were totally eliminated during a 3-year observation period (Andlin-Sobocki *et al.* 1991). Also, spontaneous changes of tooth positions in a bucco-lingual direction will affect the gingival dimension. These alterations in gingival dimensions are similar to, albeit less pronounced than, those observed during orthodontic treatment (see below).

Favorable tooth movements, and tissue factors

Alterations of mucogingival dimensions may occur during orthodontic treatment. Contrary to beliefs in the past, these changes are independent of the apico-coronal width of the keratinized and attached gingiva. Wennström *et al.* (1987) found no relationship between the initial width of keratinized gingiva and the tendency for development of gingival recession during orthodontic tooth movements in monkeys. Instead, it is the bucco-lingual thickness (volume), which may be the determining factor for the development of gingival recession and attachment loss at sites with gingivitis during orthodontic treatment.

A tooth that is positioned facially within the alveolar process may show an alveolar bone dehiscence with a thin covering soft tissue. When such a tooth is moved lingually during orthodontic treatment, the gingival dimensions on the labial aspects will increase in thickness (Figs. 57-25, 57-26). Furthermore, because the mucogingival junction is a stable anatomic landmark and the gingiva is anchored to the supracrestal portion of the root, it will follow the tooth during the movement lingually and will consequently get an increase in gingival height (decreased clinical crown height).

Conclusion: It follows that in cases with a thin (delicate) gingiva caused by a prominent position of the teeth, there is no need for a preorthodontic gingival augmentation procedure. In the case of labial gingival recessions a mucogingival surgical procedure should not be performed before orthodontic therapy, when the position of the tooth is improved by the treatment. The recession, as well as the bone dehiscence, will decrease as a consequence of the lingual movement of the tooth into a more proper position within the alveolar bone. If still indicated at the end of orthodontic therapy, the surgical procedure will have a higher predictability of success than if it had been performed before the tooth movement (Wennström 1996).

Unfavorable tooth movements, and tissue factors

Orthodontic movements of teeth *away* from the genetically determined envelope of the alveolar

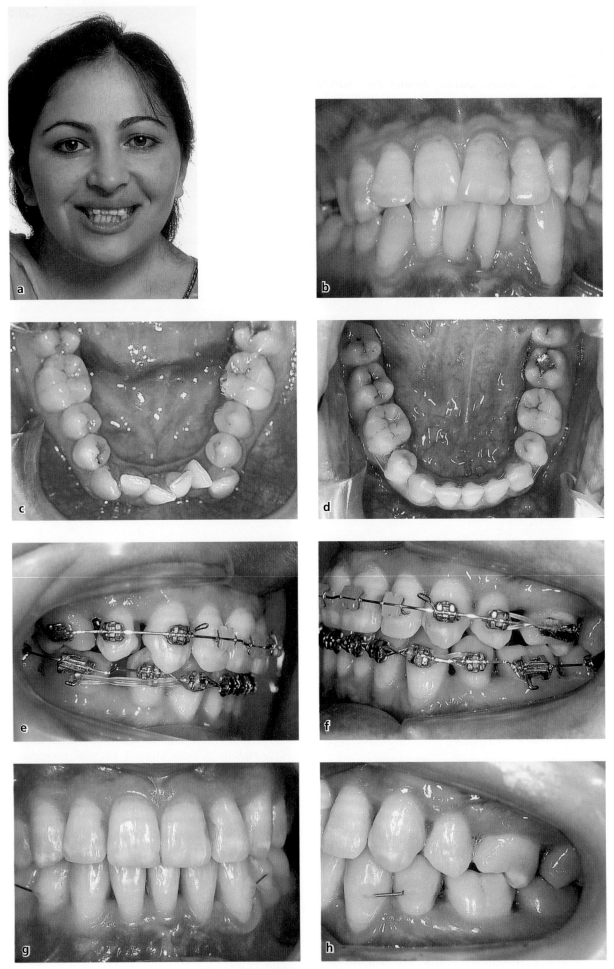

Fig. 57-26 Marked labial gingival recession on prominent left mandibular canine in female young adult patient (a–c). (d) After extraction of two premolars and the left central incisor (sic!), the mandibular arch was leveled orthodontically. (e) and (f) show the clinical condition towards end of orthodontic therapy, and (g,h) at follow-up 1 year after appliance removal. Note spontaneous improvement of gingival recession (f–h).

process are risk movements for development of mucogingival problems, particularly in thin bone and gingival tissues. During frontal and lateral expansion of teeth, tension may develop in the marginal tissues due to the forces applied to the teeth. This stretching may result in thinning of the soft tissues. However, recession-type defects will not develop as long as the tooth is moved within the alveolar bone. If, however, the expansion results in the establishment of a bone dehiscence, the volume (thickness) of the covering soft tissue must be considered as a factor that may influence the development of soft tissue recessions. This may be true both during and after the active orthodontic treatment period. The labial orthodontic tooth movement *per se* will not cause soft tissue recession. However, the thin gingiva that will be the consequence of such movement may serve as a *locus minoris resistentia* to developing soft tissue defects in the presence of bacterial plaque and/or mechanical trauma caused by improper toothbrushing techniques, or orthodontic correction of marked rotations of the incisors.

For stability reasons as well, expansion in the mandibular arch should normally be avoided, if possible. If frontal expansion is still performed in association with orthodontic therapy, the bucco-lingual thickness of the hard and soft tissues should be evaluated. If surgical intervention is considered necessary in order to reduce the risk for development of soft tissue recessions, this should aim at increasing the thickness of the covering tissue (e.g. grafts), and not the apico-coronal width of the gingiva.

Conclusion: Before any kind of orthodontic therapy is started, it is important to check the bucco-lingual thickness of the bone and soft tissues on the pressure side of all teeth, which are to be moved. When tissues are delicate and thin, careful instructions in adequate plaque control measures should be provided, and controlled before and during treatment as well as after removal of the fixed appliances, in order to reduce the risk for development of labial gingival recession.

Interdental recession

Esthetic considerations with regard to defect papillae

Until recently, most clinical emphasis with regard to gingival recession was given to labial defects. If left untreated, most labial gingival recessions will not progress significantly with time, at least if oral hygiene is good, and the main indication for treatment is the esthetic implication for the patient. From an esthetic point of view, however, it would appear that interdental recession, manifest as more or less pronounced empty spaces ("dark triangles") between the teeth, would be equally or more important. Compared with a labial recession, in most patients the loss

of interdental papillae would be more visible, both in normal conversation and upon smiling.

Since quality of life (esthetics and lack of pain) has become increasingly important in recent years in selection of periodontal therapies, disfigurement of the gingival papillae during orthodontic treatment of periodontal patients must be avoided, if possible. The development of interdental recession during orthodontic treatment in adults may be caused by one of three factors: (1) advanced periodontal disease, by the tissue destruction or due to pocket elimination by surgery, (2) triangular tooth shape due to abnormal interproximal wear of teeth in crowded positions before the orthodontic treatment, and (3) diverging roots of teeth due to improper bracket placement. To begin with, there is an obvious difference in dental esthetics between patients with advanced periodontitis who have been treated according to "old" and "new" concepts for periodontal therapy. In the past, pocket elimination by gingivectomies frequently resulted in advanced root exposure and complete loss of interdental papillae. However, even with careful non-surgical periodontal therapy in the preparation of patients with advanced periodontal disease for orthodontic treatment, the clinical outcome of the interdisciplinary treatment will normally result in marked interdental recessions, if special precautions are not taken (see below).

Clinical options for treatment

There are only a few options available for the treatment of interdental gingival recession associated with orthodontic treatment in the periodontal patient:

1. Mucogingival surgery, using coronally positioned flaps and GTR techniques (Pini Prato *et al.* 1992)
2. The provision of a gingival prosthesis
3. Orthodontic paralleling of the roots of neighboring teeth
4. Mesio-distal enamel reduction ("stripping").

Of these techniques, the mucogingival surgery aspects are discussed in Chapter 44, and will not be commented on here. A gingival prosthesis may be useful in cases of markedly compromised dentitions, where the psychologic implications of having pronounced retractions are serious. It may be regarded as a last resort. In contrast, the mesio-distal contouring of teeth is a very useful technique to routinely improve the esthetic results achieved by orthodontic treatment in most adult and adolescent patients (Figs. 57-3, 57-5, 57-6, 57-27, 57-28).

Benefits of mesio-distal enamel reduction ("stripping")

Introduced by Tuverson in 1980, mesio-distal recontouring of teeth has now become a routine procedure in orthodontics. It is generally performed on three

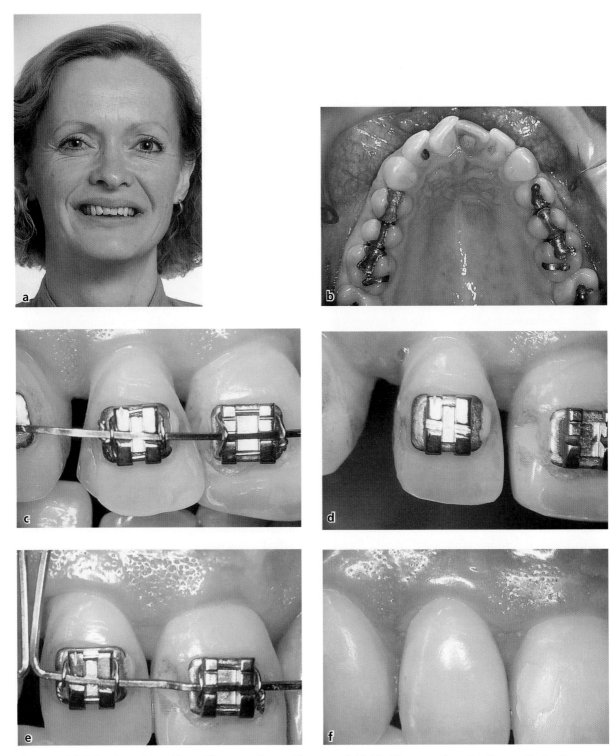

Fig. 57-27 Adult female patient with maxillary crowding and large overjet (a,b). After premolar extractions, orthodontic distalization of canines resulted in the development of marked interdental recessions in the anterior region (c). Marked triangular incisor morphology and uneven incisal edges necessitated extensive recontouring (c,d) to allow gingival fill-in after treatment (e,f).

indications: (1) treatment of slight-to-moderate crowding without arch expansion, (2) correction of width discrepancies (so-called TSD, tooth size discrepancies) between maxillary and mandibular teeth, and (3) to prevent interdental recession from developing during orthodontic treatment. The principle involved in stripping is to recontour those teeth which for one reason or another have abnormal

morphology, towards an ideal anatomic shape (Figs. 57-6, 57-25). In doing so, the contact points between teeth will be relocated in an apical direction and reduce the contact-to-bone distances (Tarnow *et al.* 1992), and the connector areas (the zone in which two adjacent teeth appear to touch) can be restored towards the optimal 50-40-30 relationships (Morley & Eubank 2001). By this means, normal interdental

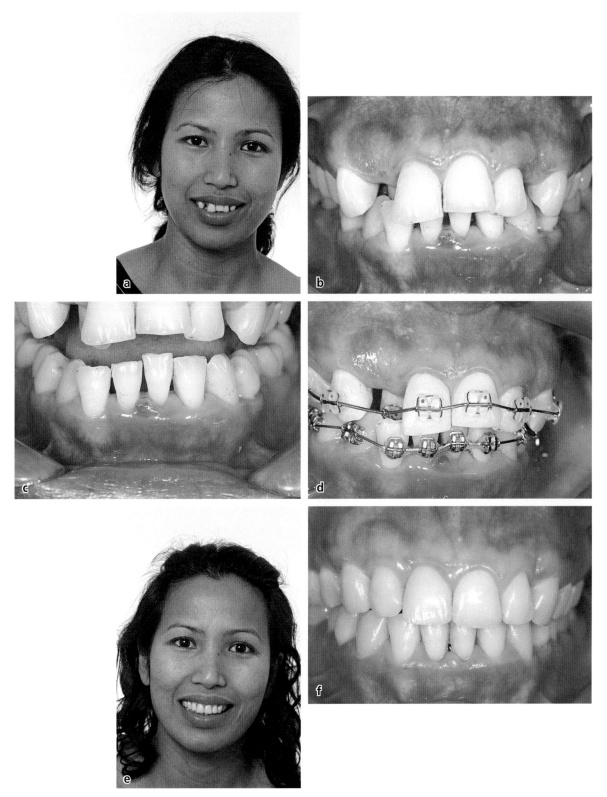

Fig. 57-28 Young adult female patient with moderate periodontal tissue breakdown in the anterior region, extruded and irregular maxillary incisors with triangular crown form and incisal wear, and marked interdental gingival recession in the mandibular anterior region (a–c). After 1 month of leveling, the maxillary and mandibular incisors were recontoured by stripping to a more optimal tooth morphology (d). The "new" tooth shapes allowed space closure and leveling and aligning to an esthetic final result (e,f).

gingival papillary contours will be achievable (Figs. 57-3, 57-6, 57-27, 57-28).

In many adult patients with malocclusion, particularly in cases with crowded and overlapping incisors, the crowns of the incisors are much wider at their incisal edges than at the cervical region. As the crowding is unraveled by orthodontic leveling in these instances, the contact point between the incisors will become located in the incisal 1 mm, and a more or less evident space develops above the interproximal contacts of the incisors. Similar, or even more pronounced, loss of the interdental papillae between the maxillary and mandibular incisors, is commonly seen after orthodontic treatment in patients with advanced periodontal destruction.

Short-term (Zachrisson & Mjör 1975) and long-term (>10 years) (Thordarson *et al.* 1991; Zachrisson *et al.* 2007) follow-up studies after extensive grinding of teeth have demonstrated that no harmful side effects are observed subsequent to the procedure, provided adequate cooling is used during the grinding and the prepared surfaces are made smooth and self-cleansing. After the diastema is created, the space between the teeth is closed orthodontically. As this occurs, the roots of neighboring teeth come closer together, the contact area is lengthened, and the reduced papilla can fill out the small space between the teeth (Tarnow *et al.* 1992). In patients with advanced periodontal disease, it is not always possible to restore all papillae in the dentition. Even if it is not possible to eliminate the interdental recession completely after the orthodontic treatment, the esthetic appearance is in most patients substantially improved by stripping, even in cases with extensive periodontal tissue breakdown, such as those in Figs. 57-3 and 57-5.

Minor surgery associated with orthodontic therapy

Several forms of minor periodontal surgery may be used to improve or stabilize the results achieved by orthodontic treatment of malocclusion. More than 30 years ago, Edwards (1970) described clinical techniques to help prevent rotational relapse, reopening of closed extraction spaces (Edwards 1971), and a simple yet effective technique for frenotomy (Edwards 1977). At about the same time, a gingivectomy technique to increase clinical crown length for esthetic improvement of orthodontic results in specific situations was reported (Monefeldt & Zachrisson 1977). Removal of gingival invaginations in extraction sites following orthodontic space closure has also been a subject of considerable interest to orthodontists.

Fiberotomy

The problem of relapse of orthodontically treated teeth in general, and rotated teeth in particular, has been well recognized for years. Methods to reduce the occurrence of rotational relapse may include (1) complete correction, or overcorrection, of rotated teeth, (2) long-term retention with bonded lingual retainers, and (3) the use of fiberotomy.

Two soft-tissue periodontal entities may influence the stability: the principal fibers of the periodontal ligament, and the supra-alveolar fibers. Whereas the fibers of the periodontal ligament and trans-septal groups remodel efficiently and histologically completely in only 2–3 months after orthodontic rotation of teeth, the supra-alveolar fibers are apparently more stable, with a slow turnover. Since the gingival soft tissues are composed primarily of non-elastic collagenous fibers, the exact mechanism by which the gingival soft tissues may apply a force capable of moving the teeth is as yet unknown. From a practical and clinical point of view, however, the supracrestal gingival tissues seemingly do contribute to rotational relapse, as evidenced by the effect of the circumferential supracrestal fiberotomy (CSF) technique.

Basically this technique consists of inserting a scalpel into the gingival sulcus and severing the epithelial attachment surrounding the involved teeth. The blade also transects the trans-septal fibers by interdentally entering the periodontal ligament space. Various modifications of the original CSF technique have been described, in which the scalpel is inserted below the gingival margin, or the cut is reduced to interdental vertical incisions buccally and lingually. In neither case are surgical dressings indicated, and clinical healing is usually complete in 7–10 days. The fiberotomy procedure is not recommended during active tooth movement, or in the presence of gingival inflammation. When performed in healthy tissues after orthodontic therapy, there is negligible loss of attachment (Edwards 1988).

The long-term effectiveness of fiberotomy was evaluated in a prospective follow-up study over a period of 15 years by Edwards (1988). The degree of crowding was examined for CSF and control cases at 4–6 years and at 12–14 years after treatment. A significant effect of the fiberotomy was observed at both time intervals. The surgical procedure was more successful in the maxillary than in the mandibular anterior region; more effective in alleviating rotational than labiolingual relapse; and more useful in reducing relapse in cases with severe rather than mild irregularity of teeth. There was no clinically significant increase in sulcus depth, nor signs of gingival labial recession.

Frenotomy

The contribution of the maxillary labial frenum to the etiology of a persisting midline diastema, and to reopening of diastemas after orthodontic closure, is controversial. The probability for diastema closure in the long run is the same whether or not frenectomy is performed. However, very hyperplastic types of frenum, with a fan-like attachment, may obstruct diastema closure and should be relocated.

In the past, the most common surgical procedure was *frenectomy*, an excision-type operation, which was often carried over to the palatal aspects. However, a frequently observed complication may be an undesirable loss of the interdental papilla between the maxillary central incisors. For this reason, the *frenotomy*, which represents a more gentle operation, will produce esthetically preferable results. With frenotomy, the attachment of the frenum to gingiva and periosteum is severed, and the insertion of the frenum is relocated several millimeters up on to the alveolar mucosa. If a marked sutural bone cleft is observed in the pretreatment radiographs, the cut is extended to sever the fibers within the coronal part of the mid-palatal suture. Tissue healing after a frenotomy procedure is usually uneventful. To further reduce the relapse tendency and/or to increase clinical crown height of single or several teeth, the frenotomy may be combined with fiberotomy and gingivectomy.

Removal of gingival invaginations (clefts)

Incomplete adaptation of supporting structures during orthodontic closure of extraction spaces in adults may result in infolding or invagination of the gingiva. The clinical appearance of such invaginations may range from a minor one-surface crease to deep clefts that extend across the interdental papilla from the buccal to the lingual gingivae. Although gingival invaginations are quite common, the precise cause of the infolding as teeth are moved through an extraction area remains unclear. Since approximated teeth appear to displace the gingival tissue more than move through it, a "piling-up" of gingival tissue is conceivable. There is some resolution of these defects with time, but many invaginations persist for 5 years or more after completion of orthodontic therapy.

Several authors have suggested that compression of trans-septal fibers and alterations of gingival tissue will contribute to extraction-space reopening, but no correlation was found between space reopening and presence and severity of invaginations by Rivera Circuns and Tulloch (1983). They still felt the damage to the gingiva was severe enough to warrant the surgical removal of these defects in selected patients. Edwards (1971) suggested that simple removal of only the excess gingiva in the buccal and lingual area of approximated teeth would be sufficient to alleviate the tendency for the teeth to separate after orthodontic movement. The removal of the gingival papillae in closure sites may enhance the restitution of a more normal connective tissue, although the epithelial hyperplasia, invaginations, and loss of collagen in the underlying gingiva are surprisingly long-standing.

Gingivectomy

The relationship of the gingival margins of the six maxillary anterior teeth plays an important role in the esthetic appearance of the crowns (Kokich 1996a,b). In some instances, it may be necessary to increase clinical crown length of one or several teeth during or after orthodontic treatment. If a gingival margin discrepancy is present, but the patient's lip does not move upward to expose the discrepancy upon smiling, it does not require correction. If the gingival discrepancy is apparent, however, one of four different techniques may be used:

1. Gingivectomy
2. Intrusion + incisal restoration or porcelain laminate veneer (Fig. 57-18)
3. Extrusion + fiberotomy + porcelain crown (Fig. 57-17)
4. Surgical crown lengthening, by flap procedure and ostectomy/ostoplasty of bone (Brägger *et al.* 1992).

Each of these techniques has its specific indications, and whenever gingival margin discrepancies are present, the clinician must determine the proper solution (see also Chapter 44). For example, gingivectomy is not indicated when there is a risk for root exposure, such as when one single incisor has supra-erupted (Fig. 57-18).

The gingivectomy technique has proven to be useful in improving orthodontic results, particularly in difficult cases with missing maxillary central or lateral incisors (Fig. 57-29); after premolar autotransplantation to the anterior region; and in some "gummy" smiles. Clinical and histologic examination demonstrated that it was possible to permanently increase clinical crown length after orthodontic treatment by making a labial gingivectomy to the bottom of the clinical pocket. The healing and regeneration of the gingiva was uneventful, provided excellent oral hygiene was maintained in the wound area for 2 months. The result may be explained by one or more of three factors: (1) the effect of the gingivectomy itself, (2) elimination of accumulated hyperplastic gingiva often seen associated with fixed appliance therapy (Fig. 57-29), and (3) elimination of a normally occurring deep pocket. Whatever the reason, the net gain in crown length was close to half the probing depth in all instances (Monefeldt & Zachrisson 1977). The increase in crown length of 1–2 mm may be important to improve the clinical outcome, as shown in Fig. 57-29. Similar long-term results on the position of the marginal soft tissue following periodontal surgery have been reported by others (Lindhe & Nyman 1980). Interestingly, Wennström (1983) demonstrated that even if the gingivectomy is extended into the alveolar mucosa, the regenerated tissue will still be normal gingiva with keratinized epithelium. Thus the human periodontal membrane tissue has the capacity to form a granulation tissue which will prevent the alveolar mucosa from becoming the border tissue against the tooth. When local labial gingivectomies are made in adults, the cut is reduced mesio-distally in order to eliminate the risk for developing interdental recession. Then the incision should not follow the gingival contour all the way, but should be limited by two small vertical cuts towards the interdental papillae.

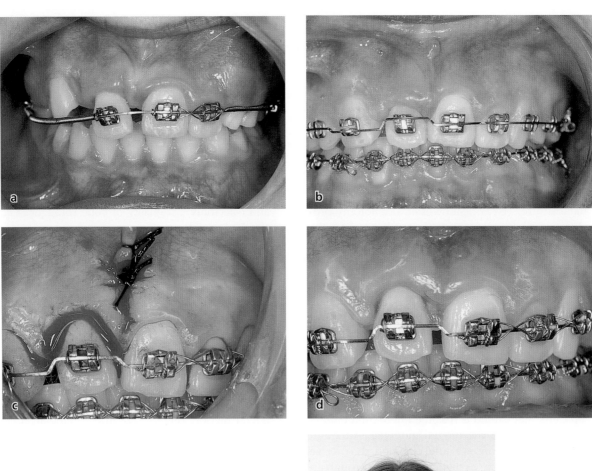

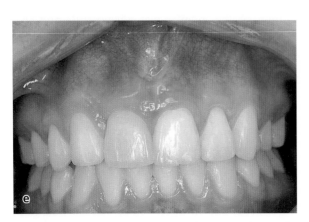

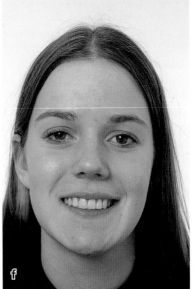

Fig. 57-29 Orthodontic space closure substitution after accidental loss of maxillary right central incisor in young female patient (a). The marginal gingival level on the "new" central incisor was corrected by selective intrusion bends in the arch-wire (b–d) and local gingivectomy and frenotomy (c,d). Local gingivectomies were also performed on the right first premolar in the canine position, and on the left lateral incisor (e). Enamel-bonded ultrathin porcelain veneer on lateral incisor, and vital bleaching of right canine, courtesy of Dr. S. Toreskog. By these means, it was possible to obtain an optimally esthetic result (e,f).

References

Andlin-Sobocki, A., Marcusson, A. & Persson, M. (1991). 3-year observation on gingival recession in mandibular incisors in children. *Journal of Clinical Periodontology* **18**, 155–159.

Årtun, J. & Urbye, K.S. (1988). The effect of orthodontic treatment on periodontal bone support in patients with advanced loss of marginal periodontium. *American Journal of Orthodontics* **93**, 143–148.

Baker, D.L. & Seymor, G.J. (1976). The possible pathogenesis of gingival recession. *Journal of Clinical Periodontology* **3**, 208–219.

Basdra, E.K., Mayer, T. & Komposch, G. (1995). Guided tissue regeneration precedes tooth movement and crossbite correction. *The Angle Orthodontist* **65**, 307–310.

Berglundh, T., Marinello, C.P., Lindhe, J., Thilander, B. & Liljenberg, B. (1991). Periodontal tissue reactions to orthodontic extrusion. An experimental study in the dog. *Journal of Clinical Periodontology* **18**, 330–336.

Bernimoulin, J.P. & Curilovic, Z. (1977). Gingival recession and tooth mobility. *Journal of Clinical Periodontology* **4**, 107–114.

Beyer, A., Tausche, E., Boening, K. & Harzer,W. (2007). Orthodontic space opening in patients with congenitally missing lateral incisors. *The Angle Orthodontist* **77**, 404–409.

Boyd, R.L. & Baumrind, S. (1992). Periodontal considerations in the use of bonds or bands on molars in adolescents and adults. *The Angle Orthodontist* **62**, 117–126.

Boyd, R.L., Leggott, P.J., Quinn, R.S., Eakle, W.S. & Chambers, D. (1989). Periodontal implications of orthodontic treatment in adults with reduced or normal periodontal tissues versus those of adolescents. *American Journal of Orthodontics and Dentofacial Orthopedics* **96**, 191–199.

Brägger, U., Lauchenauer, D. & Lang, N.P. (1992). Surgical lengthening of the clinical crown. *Journal of Clinical Periodontology* **19**, 58–63.

Burch, J.G., Bagci, B., Sabulski, D. & Landrum, C. (1992). Periodontal changes in furcations resulting from orthodontic uprighting of mandibular molars. *Quintessence International* **23**, 509–513.

Burgett, F.G., Ramfjord, S.P., Nissle, R.R., Morrison, E.C., Charbeneau, T.D. & Caffesse, R.G. (1992). A randomized trial of occlusal adjustment in the treatment of periodontitis patients. *Journal of Clinical Periodontology* **19**, 381–387.

Carlson, G. (1967). Changes in contour of the maxillary alveolar process under immediate dentures. *Acta Odontologica Scandinavia* **25**, 1–31.

Chace, R. & Low, S.B. (1993). Survival characteristics of periodontally-involved teeth: A 40-year study. *Journal of Periodontology* **64**, 701–705.

Chayanuupatkul, A., Rabie, A.B.M. & Hägg, U. (2003). Temporomandibular response to early and late removal of bite-jumping devices. *European Journal of Orthodontics* **25**, 465–470.

Dahl, E.H. & Zachrisson, B.U. (1991). Long-term experiences with direct-bonded lingual retainers. *Journal of Clinical Orthodontics* **25**, 619–630.

Diedrich, P. (1989). Wechselbeziehungen zwischen Kieferorthopädie und Parodontologie. *Fortschritte der Kieferorthopädie* **50**, 347–364.

Diedrich, P. (1996). Guided tissue regeneration associated with orthodontic therapy. *Seminars in Orthodontics* **2**, 39–45.

Diedrich, P. (1999). The eleventh hour or where are our orthodontic limits? *Journal of Orofacial Orthopedics/Fortschritte der Kieferorthopädie* **60**, 60–65.

Edwards, J.G. (1970). A surgical procedure to eliminate rotational relapse. *American Journal of Orthodontics* **57**, 33–46.

Edwards, J.G. (1971). The reduction of relapse in extraction cases. *American Journal of Orthodontics* **60**, 128–141.

Edwards, J.G. (1977). The diastema, the frenum, the frenectomy: A clinical study. *American Journal of Orthodontics* **71**, 489–508.

Edwards, J.G. (1988). A long-term prospective evaluation of the circumferential supracrestal fiberotomy in alleviating orthodontic relapse. *American Journal of Orthodontics and Dentofacial Orthopedics* **93**, 380–387.

Engelking, G. & Zachrisson, B.U. (1982). Effects of incisor repositioning on monkey periodontium after expansion through the cortical plate. *American Journal of Orthodontics* **83**, 23–32.

Ericsson, I., Thilander, B. & Lindhe, J. (1978). Periodontal condition after orthodontic tooth movements in the dog. *The Angle Orthodontist* **48**, 210–218.

Ericsson, I., Thilander, B., Lindhe, J. & Okamoto, H. (1977). The effect of orthodontic tilting movements on the periodontal tissues of infected and non-infected dentitions in the dog. *Journal of Clinical Periodontology* **4**, 78–293.

Folio, J., Rams, T.E. & Keyes, P.H. (1985). Orthodontic therapy in patients with juvenile periodontitis. Clinical and micro-

biologic effects. *American Journal of Orthodontics* **87**, 421–431.

Forsberg, C.M., Brattstrom, V., Malmberg, E. & Nord, C.E. (1991). Ligature wires and elastomeric rings: Two methods of ligation, and their association with microbial colonization of *Streptococcus mutans* and lactobacilli. *European Journal of Orthodontics* **13**, 416–420.

Goldberg, D. & Turley, P. (1989). Orthodontic space closure of edentulous maxillary first molar area in adults. *International Journal of Orthodontics and Orthognathic Surgery* **4**, 255–266.

Greenbaum, K.R. & Zachrisson, B.U. (1982). The effect of palatal expansion therapy on the periodontal supporting tissues. *American Journal of Orthodontics* **81**, 12–21.

Harpenau, L.A. & Boyd, R.L. (2000). Long-term follow-up of successful orthodontic-periodontal treatment of localized aggressive periodontitis: a case report. *Clinical Orthodontics and Research* **3**, 220–229.

Hoerman, K.C., Lang, R.L., Klapper, L. & Beery, J. (1985). Local tetracycline therapy of the periodontium during orthodontic treatment. *Quintessence International* **16**, 161–166.

Hom, B.M. & Turley, P.K. (1984). The effects of space closure on the mandibular first molar area in adults. *American Journal of Orthodontics* **85**, 457–469.

Ingber, J. (1974). Forced eruption. Part I. A method of treating isolated one and two wall infrabony osseous defects – rationale and case report. *Journal of Periodontology* **45**, 199–206.

Jin, L.J. & Cao, C.F. (1992). Clinical diagnosis of trauma from occlusion and its relation with severity of periodontitis. *Journal of Clinical Periodontology* **19**, 92–97.

Kajiyama, K., Murakami, T. & Yokota, S. (1993). Gingival reactions after experimentally induced extrusion of the upper incisors in monkeys. *American Journal of Orthodontics and Dentofacial Orthopedics* **104**, 36–47.

Karring, T., Nyman, S., Thilander, B. & Magnusson, B. (1982). Bone regeneration in orthodontically produced alveolar bone dehiscences. *Journal of Periodontal Research* **17**, 309–315.

Kessler, M. (1976). Interrelationships between orthodontics and periodontics. *American Journal of Orthodontics* **70**, 154–172.

Kokich, V. (1996a). Managing complex orthodontic problems: the use of implants for anchorage. *Seminars in Orthodontics* **2**, 153–160.

Kokich,V. (1996b). Esthetics: the ortho-perio restorative connection. *Seminars in Orthodontics* **2**, 21–30.

Kokich, V., Nappen, D. & Shapiro, P. (1984). Gingival contour and clinical crown length: their effect on the esthetic appearance of maxillary anterior teeth. *American Journal of Orthodontics* **86**, 89–94.

Kozlowsky, A., Tal, H. & Lieberman, M. (1988). Forced eruption combined with gingival fiberotomy. A technique for clinical crown lengthening. *Journal of Clinical Periodontology* **15**, 534–538.

Lang, N.P. (1977). Das präprotetische Aufrichten von gekippten unteren Molaren im Hinblick auf den parodontalen Zustand. *Schweizerische Monatschrift für Zahnheilkunde* **87**, 560–569.

Leknes, K.N. (1995). Membrane surgery – possibilities and limitations. *Den Norske Tannlegeforenings Tidende* **105**, 352–359.

Lindhe, J. & Nyman, S. (1980). Alterations of the position of the marginal soft tissue following periodontal surgery. *Journal of Clinical Periodontology* **7**, 525–530.

Lindskog-Stokland, B., Wennström, J.L., Nyman, S. & Thilander, B. (1993). Orthodontic tooth movement into edentulous areas with reduced bone height. An experimental study in the dog. *European Journal of Orthodontics* **15**, 89–96.

Lundgren, D., Kurol, J., Thorstensson, B. & Hugoson, A. (1992). Periodontal conditions around tipped and upright molars in adults. An intra-individual retrospective study. *European Journal of Orthodontics* **14**, 449–455.

Machen, D.E. (1990). Periodontal evaluation and updates: don't abdicate your duty to diagnose and supervise. *American Journal of Orthodontics and Dentofacial Orthopedics* **98**, 84–85.

Mathews, D.P. & Kokich, V.G. (1997). Managing treatment for the orthodontic patient with periodontal problems. *Seminars in Orthodontics* **3**, 21–38.

Melsen, B. (1986). Tissue reaction following application of extrusive and intrusive forces to teeth in adult monkeys. *American Journal of Orthodontics* **89**, 469–475.

Melsen, B. (1991). Limitations in adult orthodontics. In: Melsen, B., ed. *Current Controversies in Orthodontics*. Chicago: Quintessence, pp. 147–180.

Melsen, B., Agerbæk, N., Eriksen, J. & Terp, S. (1988) New attachment through periodontal treatment and orthodontic intrusion. *American Journal of Orthodontics and Dentofacial Orthopedics* **94**,104–116.

Melsen, B., Agerbæk, N. & Markenstam, G. (1989). Intrusion of incisors in adult patients with marginal bone loss. *American Journal of Orthodontics and Dentofacial Orthopedics* **96**, 232–241.

Monefeldt, I. & Zachrisson, B.U. (1977). Adjustment of clinical crown height by gingivectomy following orthodontic space closure. *The Angle Orthodontist* **47**, 256–264.

Morley, J. & Eubank, J. (2001). Macroesthetic elements of smile design. *Journal of the American Dental Association* **132**, 39–45.

Müller, H-P, Eger, T. & Lange, D.E. (1995). Management of furcation-involved teeth. A retrospective analysis. *Journal of Clinical Periodontology* **22**, 911–917.

Murakami, T., Yokota, S., & Takahama, Y. (1989). Periodontal changes after experimentally induced intrusion of the upper incisors in Macaca fuscata monkeys. *American Journal of Orthodontics and Dentofacial Orthopedics* **95**, 115–126.

Nelson, P.A. & Årtun, J. (1997). Alveolar bone loss of maxillary anterior teeth in adult orthodontic patients. *American Journal of Orthodontics and Dentofacial Orthopedics* **111**, 328–334.

Nemcovsky, C.E., Zubery, Y., Artzi, Z. & Lieberman, M.A. (1996). Orthodontic tooth movement following guided tissue regeneration: report of three cases. *International Journal of Adult Orthodontics and Orthognathic Surgery* **11**, 347–355.

Nyman, S., Karring, T. & Bergenholz, G. (1982). Bone regeneration in alveolar bone dehiscences produced by jiggling forces. *Journal of Periodontal Research* **17**, 316–322.

Ong, M.A., Wang, H-L. & Smith, F.N. (1998). Interrelationship between periodontics and adult orthodontics. *Journal of Clinical Periodontology* **25**, 271–277.

Pini Prato, G., Tenti, C., Vincenzi, G., Magnani, C., Cortellini, P. & Clauser, C. (1992). Guided tissue regeneration versus mucogingival surgery in the treatment of human buccal gingival recession. *Journal of Periodontology* **63**, 919–928.

Polson, A., Caton, J., Polson, A.P., Nyman, S., Novak, J. & Reed, B. (1984). Periodontal response after tooth movement into intrabony defects. *Journal of Periodontology* **55**, 197–202.

Pontoriero, R., Celenza, F., Ricci, G. & Carnevale, G. (1987). Rapid extrusion with fiber resection: a combined orthodon-tic-periodontic treatment modality. *International Journal of Periodontics and Restorative Dentistry* **7**, 31–43.

Proffit, W.R. (1978). Equilibrium theory revisited: Factors influencing position of the teeth. *The Angle Orthodontist* **48**, 175–186.

Rabie, A.B.M., Gildenhuys, R. & Boisson, M. (2001). Management of patients with severe bone loss: bone induction and orthodontics. *World Journal of Orthodontics* **2**, 142–153.

Ramfjord, S.P. (1984). Changing concepts in periodontics. *Journal of Prosthetic Dentistry* **52**, 781–785.

Re, S., Corrente, G., Abundo, R. & Cardaropoli, D. (2000). Orthodontic treatment in periodontally compromised patients: 12 year report. *International Journal of Periodontics and Restorative Dentistry* **20**, 31–39.

Ritchey, B. & Orban, B. (1954). Crests of the interdental alveola septa. *Dental Radiography and Photography* **27**, 37–56.

Rivera Circuns, A.L. & Tulloch, J.F.C. (1983). Gingival invagination in extraction sites of orthodontic patients: Their incidence, effects on periodontal health, and orthodontic treatment. *American Journal of Orthodontics* **83**, 469–476.

Salama, H. & Salama, M. (1993). The role of orthodontic extrusive remodeling in the enhancement of soft and hard tissue profiles prior to implant placement: a systematic approach to the management of extraction site defects. *International Journal of Periodontics and Restorative Dentistry* **13**, 312–333.

Spear, F.M., Mathews, D.M. & Kokich, V.G. (1997). Interdisciplinary management of single-tooth implants. *Seminars in Orthodontics* **3**, 45–72.

Steiner, G.G., Pearson, J.K. & Ainamo, J. (1981). Changes of the marginal periodontium as a result of labial tooth movement in monkeys. *Journal of Periodontology* **52**, 314–320.

Stelzel, M.J. & Flores-de-Jacoby, L. (1998). Guided tissue regeneration in a combined periodontal and orthodontic treatment: a case report. *International Journal of Periodontics and Restorative Dentistry* **18**, 189–195.

Stepovich, M.L. (1979). A clinical study on closing edentulous spaces in the mandible. *The Angle Orthodontist* **49**, 227–233.

Tarnow, D.P., Magner, A.W. & Fletcher, P. (1992). The effect of the distance from the contact point to the crest of bone on the presence or absence of the interproximal papilla. *Journal of Periodontology* **63**, 995–996.

Ten Hoeve, A. & Mulie, R.M. (1976). The effect of antero-posterior incisor repositioning on the palatal cortex as studied with laminography. *Journal of Clinical Orthodontics* **6**, 804–822.

Thilander, B. (1996). Infrabony pockets and reduced alveolar bone height in relation to orthodontic therapy. *Seminars in Orthodontics* **2**, 55–61.

Thilander, B., Nyman, S., Karring, T. & Magnusson, I. (1983). Bone regeneration in alveolar bone dehiscences related to orthodontic tooth movements. *European Journal of Orthodontics* **5**, 105–114.

Thordarson, A., Zachrisson, B.U. & Mjör, I.A. (1991). Remodeling of canines to the shape of lateral incisors by grinding: a long-term clinical and radiographic evaluation. *American Journal of Orthodontics and Dentofacial Orthopedics* **100**, 123–132.

Tuverson, D.L. (1980). Anterior interocclusal relations. *American Journal of Orthodontics* **78**, 361–393.

van Venroy, J.R. & Yukna, R.A. (1985). Orthodontic extrusion of single-rooted teeth affected with advanced periodontal disease. *American Journal of Orthodontics* **87**, 67–73.

Wehrbein, H., Fuhrmann, R.A.W. & Diedrich, P.R. (1994). Periodontal conditions after facial root tipping and palatal root torque of incisors. *American Journal of Orthodontics and Dentofacial Orthopedics* **106**, 455–462.

Wennström, J.L. (1983). Regeneration of gingiva following surgical excision. A clinical study. *Journal of Clinical Periodontology* **10**, 287–297.

Wennström, J.L. (1990). The significance of the width and thickness of the gingiva in orthodontic treatment. *Deutsche Zahnärztliche Zeitschrift* **45**, 136–141.

Wennström, J.L. (1996). Mucogingival considerations in orthodontic treatment. *Seminars in Orthodontics* **2**, 46–54.

Wennström, J.L., Lindhe, J., Sinclair, F. & Thilander, B. (1987). Some periodontal tissue reactions to orthodontic tooth movement in monkeys. *Journal of Clinical Periodontology* **14**, 121–129.

Wennström, J.L., Lindskog Stokland, B., Nyman, S. & Thilander, B. (1993). Periodontal tissue response to orthodontic movement of teeth with infrabony pockets. *American Journal of Orthodontics and Dentofacial Orthopedics* **103**, 313–319.

Zachrisson, B.U. (1996). Clinical implications of recent orthodontic-periodontic research findings. *Seminars in Orthodontics* **2**, 4–12.

Zachrisson, B.U. (2000a). Bonding in Orthodontics. In: Graber, T.M. & Vanarsdall, R.L., eds. *Orthodontics. Current Principles and Techniques*, 3rd edn. St. Louis: Mosby, Inc., pp. 557–645.

Zachrisson, B.U. (2000b). Orthodontic bonding to artificial tooth surfaces: clinical versus laboratory findings. *American Journal of Orthodontics and Dentofacial Orthopedics* **117**, 592–594.

Zachrisson, B.U. & Mjör, I.A. (1975). Remodelling of teeth by grinding. *American Journal of Orthodontics* **68**, 545–553.

Zachrisson, B.U., Nyøygaard, L. & Mobarak, K. (2007). Dental health assessed more than 10 years after interproximal enamel reduction of mandibular anterior teeth. *American Journal of Orthodontics and Dentofacial Orthopedics* **131**, 162–169.

Zachrisson, B.U., Stenvik, A. & Haanæs, H.R. (2004). Management of missing maxillary anterior teeth with emphasis on autotransplantation. *American Journal of Orthodontics and Dentofacial Orthopedics* **126**, 284–288.

Zuccati, G. & Bocchieri, A. (2003). Implant site development by orthodontic extrusion of teeth with poor prognosis. *Journal of Clinical Orthodontics* **37**, 307–311.

Chapter 58

Implants Used for Orthodontic Anchorage

Marc A. Schätzle and Niklaus P. Lang

Introduction, 1280
Evolution of implants for orthodontic anchorage, 1281
Prosthetic implants for orthodontic anchorage, 1282
    Bone reaction to orthodontic implant loading, 1282
    Indications of prosthetic oral implants for orthodontic
        anchorage, 1283
    Prosthetic oral implant anchorage in growing orthodontic
        patients, 1283
Orthodontic implants as temporary anchorage devices, 1284
    Implant designs and dimensions, 1284

Insertion sites of palatal implants, 1286
Palatal implants and their possible effect in growing
    patients, 1286
Clinical procedures and loading time schedule for palatal
    implant installation, 1288
Direct or indirect orthodontic implant
    anchorage, 1288
Stability and success rates, 1290
Implant removal, 1290
Advantages and disadvantages, 1290

Introduction

Anchorage is one of the limiting factors in orthodontics and its control is essential for successful orthodontic treatment. The term orthodontic anchorage was first introduced by Angle (1907) and later defined by Ottofy (1923). Orthodontic anchorage denoted the nature and degree of resistance to displacement of teeth offered by an anatomic unit when used for the purpose of tooth movement. The principle of orthodontic anchorage was implicitly explained in Newton's third law (1687) according to which an applied force can be divided into an *action* component and an equal and opposite *reaction* moment. In orthodontic treatment, reciprocal effects must be evaluated and controlled. The goal is to maximize desired tooth movement and minimize undesirable effects.

Basically, each tooth has its own anchorage potential as well as a tendency to move when force is applied towards the tooth. When teeth are used as anchorage, inappropriate movements of the anchoring units may result in a prolonged treatment time, and unpredictable or less-than-ideal outcomes.

Orthodontic anchorage is oriented to the quality of the biologic anchorage of the teeth. This is influenced by a number of factors such as the size of the root surfaces available for periodontal attachment, the height of the periodontal attachment, the density and structure of the alveolar bone, the turnover rate of the periodontal tissues, the muscular activity, the occlusal forces, the craniofacial morphology, and

the nature of the tooth movement planned for the intended correction (Diedrich 1993). To maximize tooth-related anchorage, techniques such as differential torque (Burstone 1982), placing roots into the cortex of the bone (Ricketts 1976), and distal inclination of the molars (Tweed 1941; Begg & Kesling 1977) may be used. If the periodontal anchorage is inadequate with respect to the intended treatment goal, additional intraoral and/or extraoral anchorage may be needed to avoid negative effects. While the teeth are the most frequent anatomic units used for anchorage in orthodontic therapy, other structures, such as the palate, the lingual mandibular alveolar bone, the occipital bone, and the neck, are also alternatives.

Additional anchorage such as extraoral and intraoral forces are visible and hence, compliance-dependent, and are associated with the risk of undesirable effects such as tipping of the occlusal plane, protrusion of mandibular incisors, and extrusion of teeth.

Implants, miniscrews and ankylosed teeth, as they are in direct contact with bone, do not possess a normal periodontal ligament. As a consequence, they do not move when orthodontic forces are applied (Melsen & Lang 2001) and hence, can be used for "absolute anchorage" that is independent of the patient's compliance.

The aim of this chapter is to present implants to be integrated into orthodontic treatment as "absolute anchorage", thereby avoiding the disadvantages listed above.

Evolution of implants for orthodontic anchorage

The first attempt to achieve skeletal anchorage was made in 1945. Gainsforth and Higley (1945) placed vitallium screws and stainless steel wires into the ramus of dog mandibles and applied elastics that extended from the screw to the hook of a maxillary arch wire to distally tip/retract the canine by immediate orthodontic loading (Fig. 58-1). Even though the authors did not describe the development of infection, failures encountered may be attributed to infection and the lack of antibiotics at that time, as well as the early dynamic loading of the screws. Although minor tooth movement was accomplished using basal bone anchorage in two animals, an effective orthodontic force could not be maintained for more than 31 days.

A generation later, skeletal anchorage systems have evolved from two directions. One such development originated from orthognatic fixation techniques used in maxillofacial surgery. As pioneers, Creekmore and Eklund (1983) used a vitallium bone screw to treat one patient with a deep impinging overbite. The screw was inserted in the anterior nasal spine to intrude and correct the upper incisors using an elastic thread from the screw to the incisors 10 days after the screw had been placed. Subsequently, Kanomi (1997) described a miniscrew specially designed for orthodontic use.

The second development originated from applications in implant dentistry. Linkow (1969) used blade implants for rubber band anchorage to retract teeth, but never presented long-term outcomes. Later, endosseous implants for orthodontic anchorage were suggested (Ödman *et al.* 1988; Saphiro & Kokich 1988). As indicated in various animal studies, osseointegrated titanium implants remained positionally stable under orthodontic loading and thus could be used for orthodontic anchorage (Sherman 1978; Turley *et al.* 1980, 1988; Roberts *et al.* 1984, 1989; Wehrbein & Dietrich 1993; Wehrbein 1994; Wehrbein *et al.* 1998; De Pauw *et al.* 1999; Majzoub *et al.* 1999) (Figs. 58-2, 58-3). This resulted in the development of specially designed implants in the retromolar area (Roberts *et al.* 1990) and the palatal site of the maxilla

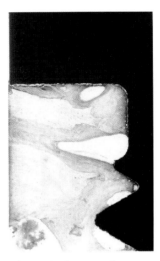

Fig 58-2 Detail of an orthodontic implant 11 months *in situ* in the mandibular retromolar area. Tight contact between the implant shoulder and crestal bone. Signs of remodeling are visible in the peri-implant bone (zones of darker and lighter staining). Toluidine/McNeal stain. Original magnification 20×. From Wehrbein *et al.* (1998) *Clinical Oral Implants Research*.

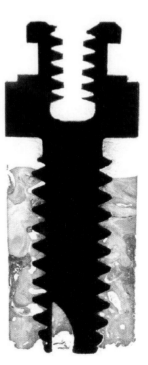

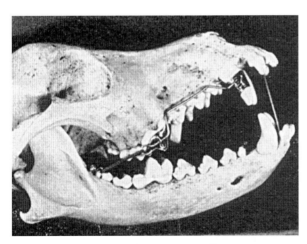

Fig. 58-1 Orthodontic appliance using vitallium screw anchorage. (Courtesy of Gainsforth, B.L. & Higley, L.B. (1945). A study of orthodontic anchorage possibilities in basal bone, *American Journal of Orthodontics and Oral Surgery* **31**, 406–417. Reproduced with permission, copyright © Elsevier.)

Fig. 58-3 Longitudinal section of an orthodontic implant after 2 years *in situ*. The implant is well osseointegrated. The shoulder, however, is not in direct contact with the bone surface. Toluidine/McNeal stain. Original magnification 6.6×. From Wehrbein *et al.* (1998) *Clinical Oral Implants Research*.

(Triaca *et al.* 1992). Both applications are used for direct or indirect anchorage (see below).

From a clinical point of view, it is of relevance whether implants are to be used only as temporary anchorage devices (TAD) (Daskalogiannakis 2000) or subsequently to be used as abutment for supporting prosthetic appliances. These aspects determine insertion sites, implant types and dimensions, as well as type of orthodontic anchorage. Moreover, the fact that these devices may have to be placed in a growing patient is of particular importance. Only TADs are suitable for such a purpose.

Prosthetic implants for orthodontic anchorage

The insertion site of prosthetic implants for orthodontic anchorage is determined by the subsequent use of the implant as a prosthetic abutment. The dimensions in length and diameter are dependent on the later prosthetic use. The positions within the alveolar process and the number of implants, however, have to be selected with reference to prospective final tooth position and space after orthodontic treatment.

To determine the location of the prosthetic implants before orthodontic therapy may often be confusing. This is especially true if the teeth are moving towards or away from the implant during orthodontic treatment. In these situations, the presumptive outcomes must be predetermined to achieve the proper implant location and the correct size of the crowns and pontics on the implant-supported prosthesis. In order to use oral implants both for both orthodontic anchorage as well as the subsequent restorative therapy, protocols have been developed for determining the accurate placement of dental implants for prosthetic reconstruction before orthodontic therapy (Smalley 1995; Smalley & Blanco 1995). A plastic placement guide is constructed and used by the clinician to determine proper implant location. The placement guide is based on information derived from a diagnostic wax-up. Therefore, it is necessary to construct the set-up casts from an exact duplicate of the tooth and base portions of the original dental casts. The bases are used as a reference for the proposed position of the implant.

An orthodontic attachment is then either fixed to the provisional crown or to a prefabricated bonding base (Figs. 58-4, 58-5). The orthodontic force acts at the implant suprastructure. The reactive moments and forces are then directly transmitted to the implant and its adjacent bone (direct implant anchorage).

Bone reaction to orthodontic implant loading

Dental implants should not only fulfill prosthetic stability but also withstand the stress and strain applied during orthodontic treatment. There are substantial

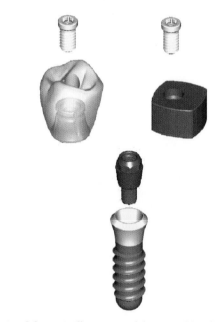

Fig. 58-4 Schematic illustration of the assembly of an orthodontic base on a oral implant designated for prosthetic use after the orthodontic treatment.

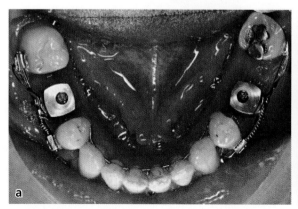
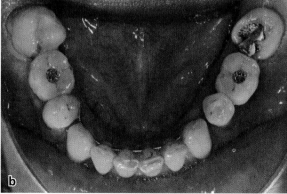

Fig. 58-5 Use of oral implants designated for prosthetic reconstruction as anchorage for orthodontic treatment. (a) Prefabricated orthodontic base as anchorage element. (b) Reconstruction of teeth 35 and 45 on oral implants following orthodontic treatment. (Courtesy of P. Göllner and T. Liechti, Berne, Switzerland.)

Table 58-1 Turnover characteristics of alveolar bone in relation to the magnitude of strain applied (from Melsen & Lang 2001)

Strain values	Bone appositional surface (%)	Resting bone (homeostatic) surface (%)	Bone resorptive surface (%)
>6700 µ strain			
Mean	16.4	21.2	51.5
95% confidence interval	11–22	16–26	42–62
3400–6600 µ strain			
Mean	62.7	16.9	5.0
95% confidence interval	56–70	12–22	1–9
<3300 µ strain			
Mean	20.9	61.9	43.5
95% confidence interval	15–27	56–68	34–53

differences between orthodontic forces and occlusal loading. Orthodontic forces are continuous and horizontal, occlusal loads, in contrast, are discontinuous and mainly in the vertical direction of the implants/teeth.

The effect of orthodontic loading to the adjacent bone of the oral implant is of great interest, because the applied forces should not have a negative impact on the peri-implant bone and therefore, should not impair the long-term prognosis as a prosthetic abutment.

Specially designed oral implants were inserted in monkeys and subjected to well defined continuous loading (Melsen & Lang 2001) (Table 58-1). None of the implants had lost osseointegration after 11 weeks of loading, but loading significantly influenced the turnover of the alveolar bone in the vicinity of the implants. Bone apposition was most frequently found when the calculated strain varied between 3400 and 6600 microstrain. On the other hand, when the strain exceeded 6700 microstrain, the remodeling of the bone resulted in a net loss of bone.

These studies support the theory that apposition of bone around an oral implant is the biologic response to a mechanical stress below a certain threshold, whereas loss of marginal bone or complete loss of osseointegration may be the result of mechanical stress beyond this threshold.

Several other studies where orthodontic forces have been applied confirmed the apposition or increase in bone density rather than loss of bone surrounding an oral implant (Roberts *et al.* 1984; Wehrbein & Diedrich 1993; Asikainen *et al.* 1997; Akin-Nergiz *et al.* 1998).

Indications of prosthetic oral implants for orthodontic anchorage

Orthodontic anchorage provided by prosthetic oral implants may be indicated in partially edentulous adult patients with intra-arch malposition of teeth to correct over-eruption, infra-eruption or tipping of teeth, to retract anteriorly displaced frontal teeth, and intra-arch protraction of teeth that are positioned dis-

tally to reduce a multi-tooth gap or improve tooth position in edentulous spaces (Fig. 58-6). Prosthetic oral implants might also be used for the correction of inter-arch malocclusion of single teeth or the whole dentition.

The most important factor of the entire process is interdisciplinary communication and planning. It is critically important for the orthodontist, periodontist, and restorative dentist to work closely as a team during the planning and treatment to achieve the best possible final result (Kokich 1996).

Prosthetic oral implant anchorage in growing orthodontic patients

The use of prosthetic oral implants in growing individuals has been studied in both clinical (Ödman *et al.* 1988; Thilander *et al.* 1994, 1999) and animal studies (Ödman *et al.* 1991; Thilander *et al.* 1992; Sennerby *et al.* 1993). Like ankylosed teeth (Fig. 58-7), oral implants do not follow the developmental changes of the alveolar processes encountered in combination with continuous eruption of adjacent teeth (Fig. 58-8). Moreover, the osseointegrated implants will not be able to be displaced in all dimensions during growth of the jaws (Thilander *et al.* 1994; Iseri & Solow 1996) and hence, would impair the development of the surrounding bony structures and even that of adjacent teeth.

Implant therapy in young individuals with residuous growth potential has been addressed in several studies and yielded major impairment in esthetic outcomes, especially in anterior implant-borne restorations. To assess remaining facial growth potential, hand–wrist radiographs have been proposed for evaluation, but appear not to be specific enough. The best method of evaluating the completion of facial growth is based on the superimposition of sequential cephalometric radiographs. It is, therefore, advisable to await the completion of adolescent body growth in height. At that point, a cephalometric radiograph should be taken. Another radiograph should be taken at least 6 months to a year later. If these radiographs are superimposed with no changes revealed in

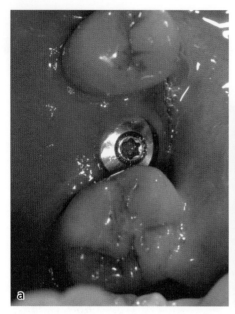
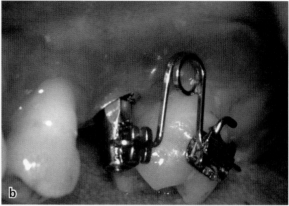

Fig. 58-6 (a) Occlusal view of an oral implant replacing tooth 26, 3 months after installation. Tooth 27 has tipped mesially rendering prosthetic reconstruction of tooth 26 impossible. (b) Following prosthetic abutment connection, the implant is used as anchorage for uprighting tooth 27, hereby providing adequate space for the installation of a single crown.

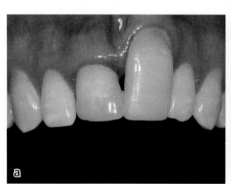
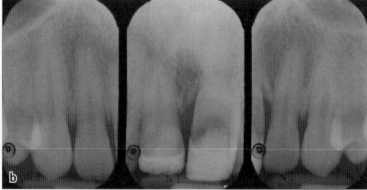

Fig. 58-7 (a) Ankylosed tooth 21 after trauma and on-going composite adaptation over several years. Tooth 21 has not followed the changes associated with alveolar process growth. (b) Radiographic documentation 6 years following trauma of tooth 21 yielding the development of the alveolar process with concomitant ankylosis of tooth 21.

vertical facial height (nasion to menton), the completion of the facial growth may be assumed. The installation of an oral implant at that time may no longer be associated with significant eruption of adjacent teeth (Kokich 2004).

In most adult patients, completion of facial growth is assumed but residual growth and ageing changes affecting the alveolar process may be encountered. This was documented in a retrospective study (Bernard *et al*. 2004) supporting the assumption that mature adults may also exhibit major vertical steps after anterior restorations were inserted on osseointegrated implants.

Orthodontic implants as temporary anchorage devices

Fundamental differences exist with respect to implant dimensions, insertion sites, type of implant anchor-

age, and intended duration of implant use. The most important difference is that a temporary anchorage device is to be removed after completion of intended orthodontic tooth movement (Daskalogiannakis 2000).

Implant designs and dimensions

As regular orthodontic patients do not display edentulous alveolar bony ridges for the insertion of an implant, implants for orthodontic anchorage must be placed in areas other than the usual topographical locations foreseen for the replacement of missing teeth. Besides the installation of orthodontic anchorage implants into the retromolar area of the mandible (Roberts *et al*. 1990; Higuchi & Slack 1991), the midsagittal palatal region (Triaca *et al*. 1992; Block & Hoffmann 1995; Wehrbein *et al*. 1996a) was initially proposed.

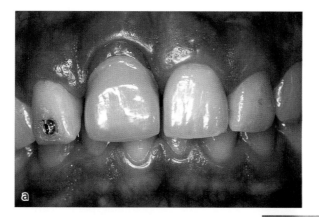

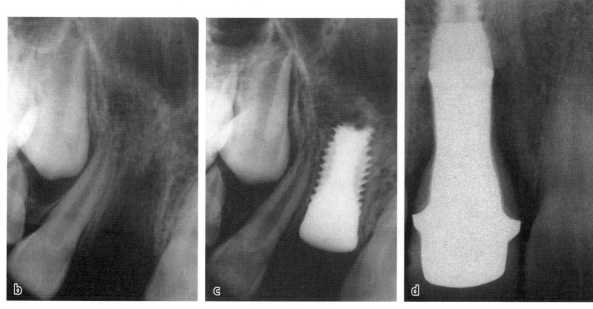

Fig. 58-8 (a) Oral implant placed prematurely (at age 9 years) in a growing patient. The implant did not follow the growth development of the alveolar process resulting in the need for multiple (three times) replacement of the prosthetic reconstruction until adolescence. Unsatisfactory esthetic outcomes persist. Radiographic documentation: (b) Following traumatic loss of tooth 11 at age 9 years. (c) Implant placement in the growing maxilla. (d) Oral implant 9 years after placement and third single tooth crown reconstruction (Courtesy of G.E. Salvi, Berne, Switzerland.)

The introduction of diameter-reduced temporary orthodontic anchorage devices such as miniscrews (<2 mm) in various lengths (Kanomi 1997; Costa *et al.* 1998) and titanium pins (Bousquet *et al.* 1996), as well as L-shaped miniplates with the long arm exposed into the oral cavity (Umemori *et al.* 1999) and the zygomatic anchors (De Clerck *et al.* 2002) both fixed by bone screws, offered new additional insertion sites: (1) the inter-radicular septum (Bousquet *et al.* 1996; Kanomi 1997); (2) the supra-apical and infra-zygomatic area (Kanomi 1997; Costa *et al.* 1998; Umemori *et al.* 1999; De Clerck *et al.* 2002); and (3) the mandibular symphysis (Costa *et al.* 1998). It must be pointed out, however, that the retention of miniscrews and titanium pins constitutes only a mechanical fixation of the devices and, hence, is not based on the principle of osseointegration.

Length-reduced orthodontic anchorage devices, such as titanium flat screws (Triaca *et al.* 1992), resorbable orthodontic implant anchors (Glatzmaier *et al.* 1995), T-shaped orthodontic implants (Wehrbein *et al.* 1996) (Orthosystem®, Institut Straumann, Waldenburg, Switzerland) and the Graz implant-supported pendulum (Byloff *et al.* 2000), were subsequently introduced.

Another device, the Onplant® (Block & Hofmann 1995), placed subperiostally, is a smooth titanium disc with a hydroxyapatite-coated surface that is supposed to connect to the bone. Owing to the submerged installation, monitoring of the healing process of these Onplants® may be troublesome, and their osseointegration may be questioned (Celenza & Hochman 2000).

The most widely used orthodontic anchorage system is the Orthosytem® (Institut Straumann, Basel, Switzerland). This titanium implant consists of three distinct features (Fig. 58-9): (1) the self-tapping endosseous body, 4.2 mm long and either 4.1 mm or 4.8 mm in diameter, designed to be inserted into bone; (2) a smooth neck portion (4.8 mm in diameter and 1.8 mm long) as the transmucosal part; and (3) the trigonal head to serve as the orthodontic appliance fixation.

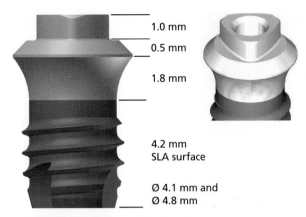

1.0 mm
0.5 mm
1.8 mm

4.2 mm
SLA surface

Ø 4.1 mm and
Ø 4.8 mm

Fig. 58-9 The Orthosystem® (Institut Straumann, Waldenburg, Switzerland) designed for orthodontic anchorage with an intraosseous SLA rough surface, a smooth transmucosal portion, and a trigonal orthodontic fixation base.

Insertion sites of palatal implants

The incomplete closure of the median palatal suture during childhood and early adolescence is a limiting factor for the installation of orthodontic implants in the midsagittal region for fully grown juveniles and adults. Therefore, the paramedian regions of the hard palate (Bernhart et al. 2000, 2001) represent a feasible alternative. With respect to the anatomic limitations, sites chosen for palatal orthodontic anchorage device insertion should be carefully evaluated to avoid perforations into the inferior nasal turbinate (Wehrbein et al. 1996b). Pre-implantation examinations of the anterior palate have shown that the vertical bone volume decreases from the anterior to the posterior region.

The presence of the palatal suture and the limited bone thickness of the hard palate available may be causes of concern for the achievement of stability of palatal implants. It may be useful to perform imaging diagnosis before palatal implant insertion. Dental computed tomography and/or lateral cephalograms have been recommended for evaluating the vertical bone volume of the hard palate presurgically.

Dental computed tomography of the alveolar process is well established for the evaluation of the alveolar bone volume before implant placement (Lindh et al. 1995). It may also be used to assess the vertical bone volume of the hard palate and is currently the most accurate method. The greatest mean thickness was identified to be about 6–9 mm posterior to the incisal foramen in the mid-sagittal plane (Bernhart et al. 2000). Avoiding the midpalatal suture, the area suitable for implant placement is, therefore, located 6–9 mm posterior to the incisal foramen and 3–6 mm lateral to the mid-sagittal plane. If the necessary bone volume for an orthodontic implant installation is defined as 4 mm or more (Bernhart et al. 2000). In a study, 95% of the patients investigated had adequate vertical bone volume for accommodating

palatal implants, 4 mm in length; this is in agreement with other clinical reports (Schiel et al. 1996). It must be considered, however, that the patients examined showed a great range of variation of vertical bone volume so a detailed pre-operative diagnostic process is necessary in order to avoid perforation of the lower nasal duct.

Insisting on obtaining precise information for the intended implant sites before placing palatal implants on lateral cephalograms rather than CT examination was proposed (Wehrbein et al. 1999). Since the former are used for orthodontic diagnosis and treatment planning, patients are spared from additional radiation exposure. Furthermore, superimposition of structures in CT scans renders this methodology complicated, imprecise, and hazardous for the presurgical assessment of bone volumes for orthodontic anchorage implants.

On wire-marked skulls, the highest bony demarcation of the palatal complex seen radiographically largely coincided with the nasal floor rather than with the mid-sagittal nasal septum, which has additional vertical bone height (Wehrbein et al. 1999). Hence, it was suggested that the vertical bone heights in the anterior and middle thirds of the hard palate were at least 2 mm higher vertically than identified on lateral cephalograms. A safety level of at least 2 mm is, therefore, recommended when planning treatment on the basis of lateral cephalograms (Wehrbein et al. 1999). It must be realized that even though some implants may project beyond the nasal floor in lateral cephalograms, they may represent false-positive results and may not be related to actual penetrations into the nasal cavity (Crismani et al. 2005c). If the palatal complex is perforated, intra-operative probing with a periodontal probe or a sinus probe must be performed for verification.

In addition to the palatal bony morphology, the implant's antero-posterior location and its inclination must also take into account both the pre-treatment and planned final position of the maxillary central incisor, when the implant is placed mid-sagittally (Fig. 58-10).

A distinction has to be made between the vertical bone volume in the mid-sagittal and the paramedian regions, as the indication for implant treatment in the mid-sagittal plane should be limited to adults and fully grown juveniles due to possible developmental disturbances of the palatal suture (Glatzmaier et al. 1995; Wehrbein et al. 1996b).

Palatal implants and their possible effects in growing patients

During growth, maxillary expansion in a transverse direction is the result of two processes: appositional remodeling of the alveolar process and growth of the palatal suture (Björk & Skieller 1974). While the remodeling process leads to the expansion of the dental arches, the growth in the median suture leads

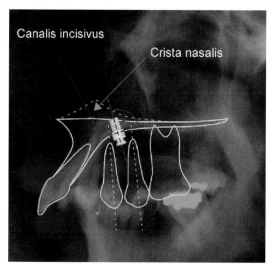

Fig. 58-10 Most palatal implants are installed satisfactorily when the location of entry into the cortical bone is at the antero-posterior level of the maxillary first and second premolars – perpendicular to the palatal surface. From Männchen & Schätzle (2008).

(a)

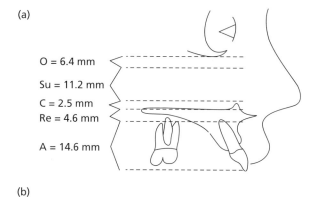

O = 6.4 mm
Su = 11.2 mm
C = 2.5 mm
Re = 4.6 mm
A = 14.6 mm

(b)

VERTICAL GROWTH 4 YEARS – ADULT

O   Apposition, floor of orbit
Su   Sutural lowering of maxilla
C   Apposition at the infrazygomatic crest
Re   Amount of resorptive lowering of the nasal floor
A   Apposition, increasing height of the alveolar process

Fig. 58-11 Vertical growth related changes encountered from age 4 years to adulthood. From Björk & Skieller (1977), with permission from the British Orthodontic Society.

to the expansion of the palate that represents the most important factor in the development of the maxillary width. An average growth in maxillary width of 3 mm was demonstrated between the ages of 10 and 18 years (Björk & Skieller 1977). Since the median or paramedian anterior palate may be chosen as insertion sites for palatal implants, the question arises whether or not the implantation of an orthodontic anchorage device may affect normal transverse palatal growth. Palatal implants affected normal transverse growth in an animal study (Asscherickx *et al*. 2005). It could be shown that implant placement resulted in less transverse sutural growth.

Deficient transverse maxillary width may also cause maxillary arch length discrepancies, as demonstrated for canine impaction (McConnell *et al*. 1996). Therefore, all interventions that might cause a restriction in normal transverse maxillary growth should be avoided. Because it has been shown that the insertion of implants in the median palatal suture in adolescent beagle dogs could cause restriction in normal transverse development of the palate (McConnell *et al*. 1996), the installation of the orthodontic palatal implants is better performed in paramedian areas in growing individuals. Moreover, studies have suggested that the installation of orthodontic implants in the midpalatal suture of growing patients is contraindicated because of the questionable quality of bone to provide adequate primary stability (Bernhart *et al*. 2001; Lioubavina-Hack *et al*. 2006). The paramedian region of the anterior palate is largely stable from a growth point of view (Thilander 1995).

The most important vertical growth changes are the result of the displacement of the maxillary complex and surface remodeling processes. The

sutural lowering of the maxillary complex as well as the apposition at the orbital floor and at the infrazygomatic crest will not be affected by implant installation in the palate. The resorptive lowering of the nasal floor, however, and the increase of the maxillary alveolar bone height might be influenced. The mean degree of growth from the age of 4 years to adulthood has been identified (Björk & Skieller 1977). The nasal floor appears to drift 4.6 mm caudally, and the height of the maxillary alveolar bone appears to increase 14.6 mm. Assuming that about one third of these growth changes take place from the age of 12 years to adulthood implies a residual vertical growth of about 1.5 mm in the palate and of about 5 mm in maxillary alveolar bone height (Fig. 58-11).

Osseointegrated implants are in direct contact with bone, do not possess a periodontal ligament and hence, behave like ankylosed teeth. Therefore, an osseointegrated palatal implant would remain 1.5 mm behind its surrounding bone, whereas an implant placed in the alveolar bone would produce an infra-occlusion of 5 mm during the same period. Consequently, palatal implants directly or indirectly attached to teeth would lead to an infra-eruption of a single tooth, several teeth or the whole upper dentition, respectively. By influencing the maxillary vertical growth dimension the horizontal displacement of the mandible will also be affected and would, therefore, cause a closing effect on the mandibular plane angle (anterior mandible rotation). It must be considered, however, that palatal implants as temporary orthodontic anchorage devices usually remain 1–2 years *in situ*. Thus, potential vertical and transversal growth impairment are likely to be limited to values of less than 1 mm.

Clinical procedures and loading time schedule for palatal implant installation

Patient stress during implantation and/or explantation and subsequent wound healing may be minimized by applying a minimally traumatic surgical technique. Under palatal local anesthesia, the palatal mucosa is perforated to the cortical bone using a mucosal punch or a system-compatible trephine during explantation and removed with an elevator or a curette (Fig. 58-12a). After smoothing the exposed bone surface to prevent the profile drill from slipping, the centre of the implant site is marked with a round bur (Fig. 58-12b). The implant bed is then prepared to the required depth using a series of pilot and twist drills (Fig. 58-12c). The drilling axis perpendicular to the bone surface is defined based on the pre-surgical cephalometric analysis. While preparing the insertion site intermediate drilling and cooling of the drilling channel continuously with pre-cooled physiologic saline or Ringer's solution should be performed. The implant is then hand-installed as far as possible, and a ratchet is used to tighten the implant to its final position (Fig. 58-12d). The implant is covered with the healing cap to prevent the inner screw well of the implant from clogging up and from being covered by hyperplastic mucosal tissue (Fig. 58-12e). After insertion, the palatal Orthosystem® implant is allowed to heal *in situ* for 12 weeks during which it should not be loaded.

In some cases, there may be a premature loss of the implant prior to orthodontic load. This loss may be caused by the lack of adequate primary stability. Such insufficient primary stability, causes inappropriate healing and the possible premature loss of the implant (Friberg *et al.* 1991; Lioubavina-Hack *et al.* 2006). Therefore, it is generally recommended to use the 4.1 mm diameter palatal Orthosystem® implant. The 4.8 mm diameter device should only be used if the prerequisite of primary stability cannot be achieved with the smaller (regular 4.1 mm) diameter implant.

Following the placement of an endosseous implant, primary mechanical stability is gradually replaced by biologic bonding. The transition from primary mechanical stability, provided by the implant design, to biologic stability, provided by the osseointegration process, occurs during the first month of wound healing (Berglundh *et al.* 2003). During this critical time, the orthodontic implant should not be used as anchorage.

The installation of implants as absolute anchorage devices facilitates and accelerates orthodontic therapy (Trisi & Rebaudi 2002), even though an inactive waiting time of at least 3 months after insertion (12 week healing time) remains (Wehrbein *et al.* 1996a, 1998; Keles *et al.* 2003; Crismani *et al.* 2005a,b). Especially in adult patients, there is a growing need to reduce this inactive waiting time and to reduce the risk for implant failure during early loading.

There are several studies that have reported a successful outcome of early/immediate loaded conventional dental implants placed in the alveolar ridge (Calandriello *et al.* 2003; Rocci *et al.* 2003; Bischof *et al.* 2004; Gallucci *et al.* 2004; Glauser *et al.* 2004; Jaffin *et al.* 2004). However, as of today there is only one study evaluating early loaded palatal orthodontic implants in humans by means of resonance frequency analysis (RFA). On this basis, the possibility of loading palatal orthodontic implants earlier than recommended in the aforementioned literature was suggested with caution (Crismani *et al.* 2006).

There is still a lack of histologic documentation about adequately termed healing periods before loading orthodontic implants in the palatal region and no attempts have been made to document sequential histologic changes of the transition from primary stability to the process of osseointegration. Further studies are needed to define shorter appropriate healing periods.

After the recommended inactive healing period, an impression is taken for the construction of the transpalatal arch (TPA) connection (Fig. 58-12f,g). After integration of the TPA, the implant-related orthodontic treatment is begun. Depending on the treatment goal, schedule, and TPA design, different palatal arches may be necessary during the course of treatment in the same patient.

Direct or indirect orthodontic implant anchorage

Reliable three-dimensional attachment of orthodontic wires to the orthodontic implant is of crucial importance. There are two principles in using implants for orthodontic anchorage:

- Orthodontic forces are applied at anchorage teeth that are not to be moved and are kept in position through a rigid connection (e.g. transpalatal arch, lingual arch) with the implant (*indirect anchorage*) (Wehrbein *et al.* 1996b). The element connected directly to teeth may limit tooth movements and need adaptation or refabrication of the TPA by a dental technician (Fig. 58-12f).
- If force systems act directly between the teeth to be moved and the implant (*direct anchorage*), then the TPA may be adapted more easily by adjusting the active sectional wires (Männchen 1999). It must be considered, however, that the implant should be placed paramedian on the same side in order to keep the torque moments as low as possible, if a direct unilateral sagittal force is applied to the implant (Fig. 58-12g).

The three-dimensional attachment of the orthodontic wire to the implant may be guaranteed by using a clamping cap, a welding or soldering cap or a post cap with a pre-lased wire.

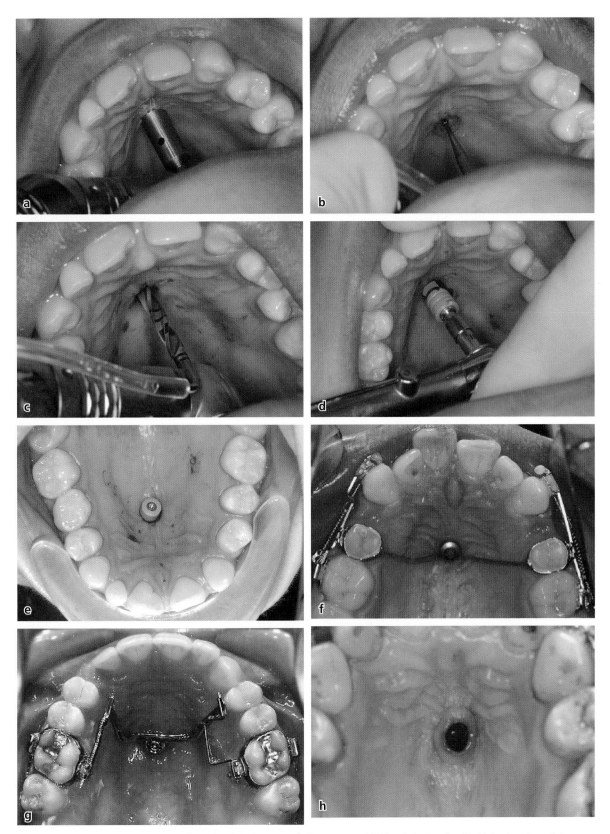

Fig. 58-12 Clinical procedures to install a palatal Orthosystem® (Straumann AG, Basel, Switzerland). (a) Perforation of the palatal mucosa using a system compatible punch or trephine. (b) Marking the center of the intended implant site with a round bur. (c) Preparation of the implant bed at the location determined presurgically and perpendicular to the bone surface. (d) Tightening of the orthodontic implant using a ratchet. (e) Covering the device with a healing cap. (f) Affixation of the transpalatal arch (TPA) for indirect loading (from Wehrbein *et al*. 1998) and (g) for direct loading (according to Männchen 1999). (h) Palatal orthodontic anchorage site after explantation.

Besides offering reliable fixation of the connecting element to the implant abutment, the connecting element must be sufficiently rigid to prevent deflection. A mean loss of anchorage of approximately 1 mm by retracting or torquing of incisors to the buccal segment has been reported (Wehrbein *et al.* 1999a). This contradiction was probably due to deformation of the TPA and/or a slight rotational play of the supraconstruction. Although this anchorage loss might be clinically irrelevant, the pre-activation of the connecting element in the opposite direction may help to avoid this side effect.

It is clear that implant-supported teeth receive continuous loading stimulation. Unfavorable jiggling forces on anchor teeth, as found in compliance-dependent anchorage aids, might be reduced or avoided. This may play a more decisive role in cases with reduced periodontal anchorage.

Stability and success rates

Despite the small dimensions, orthodontic implant anchoring devices must maintain positional stability under orthodontic loading in order to serve as absolute anchorage. As connective tissue encapsulation would initiate implant dislocation, osseointegration is a prerequisite. Histologic examination of explanted human orthodontic implant bone specimens inserted palatally revealed that osseointegration is maintained during long-term orthodontic loading under clinical conditions (Figs. 58-2, 58-3). The percentage of implant-to-bone contact in patients varied between 34% and 93% with an average of 75% (Wehrbein *et al.* 1998), obviously an adequate anchorage to withstand orthodontic loading.

There is only one retrospective cohort study reporting the success rate of a large number of inserted palatal Orthosystem® implants (Männchen & Schätzle 2008). Only three out of 70 inserted palatal implants (4.3%) did not successfully osseointegrate. Of these, two implants were lost due to inadequate primary stability. These were replaced after a short healing period with implants of a greater dimension and osseointegrated successfully thereafter. One implant was placed penetrating the incisal canal and was lost spontaneously. Of the 67 successfully osseointegrated implants loaded actively and/or passively for approximately 19 months, only one implant (1.5%) was lost after 5 months of unilateral heavy active loading (Männchen & Schätzle 2008). This report documented success rates for palatal implants after orthodontic loading comparable to those reported for conventional oral implants (Berglundh *et al.* 2002; Pjetursson *et al.* 2007).

Implant removal

No reports exist on "sleeping orthodontic palatal implants". As a consequence, they have to be removed after completion of the orthodontic treatment. By means of a system-compatible trephine, the peri-implant bone is separated from the device. Then, the implant may be explanted together with the surrounding bone by slow rotations with a extraction forceps. As a variation, the implant–bone contact may be broken by turning the ratchet used for seating the implant counter-clockwise, applying a torque of up to 40 N/cm, and a mechanical torque wrench The implant is then retrieved (Fig. 58-12h). After explantation, possible oro-antral communication must be verified and treated if necessary.

Full recovery at the original anchorage site may be observed 3–4 weeks after implant removal.

Advantages and disadvantages

Even though the orthodontic treatment may be completed faster and with more predictability, patients have to undergo two minor surgical procedures. Additionally, an inactive waiting time after implant installation remains. The extra cost for placing a palatal orthodontic implant must be balanced against other treatment options. Besides cooperation and esthetic aspects to be considered, the costs of orthognathic surgery and/or prosthetic reconstruction may be avoided or reduced by installation of an implant for orthodontic anchorage. In cases in which the palatal implant is directly loaded, bonding of the whole jaw or the entire dentition may not be necessary (Fig. 58-13). The main risks encountered with the use of orthodontic implant anchorage are the development of peri-implant infection, oro-antral connection, and/or implant loss prior to completion of orthodontic treatment.

Conclusions

Osseointegrated implants are providing absolute orthodontic anchorage and hence, are considered to be superior to any orthodontic tooth-borne anchorage device. Indications for orthodontic implant anchorage include: inadequate periodontal anchorage; non-compliant patients for extra- and/or intraoral anchorage aids; prevention of potential side effects of conventional anchorage devices; esthetic aspects; or avoidance of orthognathic surgery after growth completion. Moreover, prosthetic reconstruction may be avoided. The simplicity in use, minimal stress during surgical implant installation and removal, as well as the reliable success rates are prerequisites for the high acceptance of this treatment by orthodontic patients. It must be kept in mind, however, that treatment objectives may be achieved by several treatment plans. Proper orthodontic anchorage should be chosen according to the preceeding diagnosis and to fit the appropriate treatment plan.

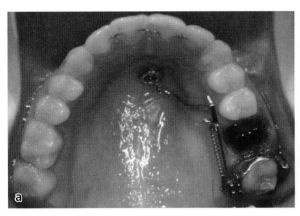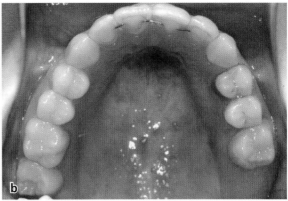

Fig. 58-13 Absolute anchorage by means of a palatal orthodontic implant avoiding the need for bonding the entire maxillary dentition with fixed orthodontic appliances. (a) After the extraction of tooth 26, protraction of tooth 27 was initiated by direct implant loading. (b) At implant and orthodontic appliance removal, the gap between teeth 25 and 27 has been completely closed, thereby avoiding the placement of a fixed partial denture. (Courtesy of R. Männchen, Winterthur, Switzerland.)

References

Akin-Nergiz, N., Nergiz, I., Schulz, A., Arpak, N. & Niedermeier, W. (1998). Reactions of peri-implant tissues to continuous loading of osseointegrated implants. *American Journal of Orthodontics and Dentofacial Orthopedics* **114**, 292–298.

Angle, E.H. (1907). *Treatment of Malocclusion of Teeth*, 7th edn. S. S. White Dental Manufacturing Comp., Philadelphia.

Asikainen, P., Klemetti, E., Vuillemin, T., Sutter, F., Rainio, V. & Kotilainen, R. (1997). Titanium implants and lateral forces. An experimental study with sheep. *Clinical Oral Implants Research* **8**, 465–468.

Asscherickx, K., Hanssens, J. L., Wehrbein, H. & Sabzevar, M.M. (2005). Orthodontic anchorage implants inserted in the median palatal suture and normal transverse maxillary growth in growing dogs: a biometric and radiographic study. *The Angle Orthodontist* **75**, 826–831.

Bantleon, H.P., Bernhart, T., Crismani, A.G. & Zachrisson, B.J. (2002). Stable orthodontic anchorage with palatal osseointegrated implants. *World Journal of Orthodontics* **3**, 109–116.

Begg, P.R. & Kesling, P.C. (1977). The differential force method of orthodontic treatment. *American Journal of Orthodontics* **71**, 1–39.

Berglundh, T., Abrahamsson, I., Lang, N.P. & Lindhe, J. (2003). De novo alveolar bone formation adjacent to endosseous implants. *Clinical Oral Implants Research* **14**, 251–262.

Berglundh, T., Persson, L. & Klinge, B. (2002). A systematic review of the incidence of biological and technical complications in implant dentistry reported in prospective longitudinal studies of at least 5 years. *Journal of Clinical Periodontology* **29**, 197–202.

Bernard, J.P., Schatz, J.P., Christou, P., Belser, U. & Kiliaridis, S. (2004). Long-term vertical changes of the anterior maxillary teeth adjacent to single implants in young and mature adults. A retrospective study. *Journal of Clinical Periodontology* **31**, 1024–1028.

Bernhart, T., Freudenthaler, J., Dortbudak, O., Bantleon, H.-P. & Watzek, G. (2001). Short epithetic implants for orthodontic anchorage in the paramedian region of the palate – a clinical study. *Clinical Oral Implants Research* **12**, 624–631.

Bernhart, T., Vollgruber, A., Gahleitner, A., Dortbudak, O. & Haas, R. (2000). Alternative to the median region of the palate for placement of an orthodontic implant. *Clinical Oral Implants Research* **11**, 595–601.

Bischof, M., Nedir, R., Szmukler-Moncler, S., Bernard, J.P. & Samson, J. (2004). Implant stability measurement of delayed and immediately loaded implants during healing. *Clinical Oral Implants Research* **15**, 529–539.

Björk, A. & Skieller, V. (1974). Growth in width of the maxilla studied by the implant method. *Scandinavian Journal of Plastic and Reconstruction Surgery* **8**, 26–33.

Björk, A. & Skieller, V. (1977). Growth of the maxilla in three dimensions as revealed radiographically by the implant method. *British Journal of Orthodontics* **4**, 53–64.

Block, M.S. & Hoffman, D.R. (1995). A new device for absolute anchorage for orthodontics. *American Journal of Orthodontics and Dentofacial Orthopedics* **3**, 251–258.

Bousquet, F., Bousquet, P., Mauran, G. & Parguel, P. (1996). Use of an impacted post for anchorage. *Journal of Clinical Orthodontics* **30**, 261–265.

Burstone, C.J. (1982). The segmented arch approach to space closure. *American Journal of Orthodontics* **82**, 361–378.

Byloff, F.K., Karcher, H., Clar, E. & Stoff, F. (2000). An implant to eliminate anchorage loss during molar distalization: a case report involving the Graz implant-supported pendulum. *International Journal of Adult Orthodontics and Orthognathic Surgery* **15**, 129–137.

Calandriello, R., Tomatis, M. & Rangert, B. (2003). Immediate functional loading of Brånemark Systems implants with enhanced initial stability: a prospective 1 to 2 year clinical & radiographic study. *Clinical Implant Dentistry and Related Research* **5** (Suppl 1), 10–20.

Celenza, F. & Hochman, M.N. (2000). Absolute anchorage in orthodontics: direct and indirect implant-assisted modalities. *Journal of Clinical Orthodontics* **34**, 397–402.

Costa, A., Raffaini, M. & Melsen, B. (1998). Miniscrews as orthodontic anchorage: a preliminary report. *International Journal of Adult Orthodontics and Orthognathic Surgery* **13**, 201–209.

Creekmore, T.D. & Eklund, M.K. (1983). The possibility of skeletal anchorage. *Journal of Clinical Orthodontics* **17**, 266–269.

Crismani, A.G., Bernhart, T., Bantleon, H.-P. & Cope, J.B. (2005a). Palatal implants: the straumann orthosystem. *Seminars in Orthodontics* **11**, 16–23.

Crismani, A.G., Bernhart, T., Bantleon, H.-P. & Kucher, G. (2005b). An innovative adhesive procedure for connecting transpalatal arches with palatal implants. *European Journal of Orthodontics* **27**, 226–230.

Crismani, A.G., Bernhart, T., Schwarz, K., Čelar, A.G., Bantleon, H.-P. & Watzek, G. (2006). Ninety percent success in palatal implants loaded 1 week after placement: a clinical evaluation by resonance frequency analysis. *Clinical Oral Implants Research* **17**, 445–450.

Crismani, A.G., Bernhart, T., Tangl, S., Bantleon, H.P. & Watzek, G. (2005c). Nasal cavity perforation by palatal implants:

false-positive records on the lateral cephalogram. *International Journal of Oral and Maxillofacial Implants* **20**, 267–273.

Daskalogiannakis, J. (2000). *Glossary of Orthodontic Terms.* Quintessence Publishing Co., Leipzig.

De Clerck, H., Geerinckx, V. & Siciliano, S. (2002). The Zygoma Anchorage System. *Journal of Clinical Orthodontics* **36**, 455–459.

De Pauw, G.A., Dermaut, L., De Bruyn, H. & Johansson, C. (1999). Stability of implants as anchorage for orthopedic traction. *The Angle Orthodontist* **69**, 401–407.

Diedrich, P. (1993). Different orthodontic anchorage systems. A critical examination. *Fortschritte der Kieferorthopädie* **54**, 156–171.

Friberg, B., Jemt, T. & Lekholm, U. (1991). Early failures in 4,641 consecutively placed Brånemark dental implants: a study from stage 1 surgery to the connection of completed prostheses. *International Journal of Oral and Maxillofacial Implants* **6**, 142–146.

Gainsforth, B.L. & Higley, L.B. (1945). A study of orthodontic anchorage possibilities in basal bone, *American Journal of Orthodontics and Oral Surgery* 31, 406–417.

Gallucci, G.O., Bernard, J.P., Bertosa, M. & Belser, U.C. (2004). Immediate loading with fixed screwretained provisional restorations in edentulous jaws: the pickup technique. *International Journal of Oral and Maxillofacial Implants* **19**, 524–533.

Glatzmaier, J., Wehrbein, H. & Diedrich, P. (1995). Die Entwicklung eines resorbierbaren Implantatsystems zur orthodontischen Verankerung. *Fortschritte der Kieferorthopädie* **56**, 175–181.

Gedrange, T., Bourauel, C., Köbel, C. & Harzer, W. (2003). Three-dimensional analysis of endosseous palatal implants and bones after vertical, horizontal, and diagonal force application. *European Journal of Orthodontics* **25**, 109–115.

Glauser, R., Sennerby, L., Meredith, N., Ree, A., Lundgren, A., Gottlow, J. & Hämmerle, C.H. (2004). Resonance frequency analysis of implants subjected to immediate or early functional occlusal loading. Successful vs. failing implants. *Clinical Oral Implants Research* **15**, 428–434.

Higuchi, K.W. & Slack, J.M. (1991). The use of titanium fixtures for intraoral anchorage to facilitate orthodontic tooth movement. *International Journal of Oral and Maxillofacial Implants* **6**, 338–344.

Iseri, H. & Solow, B. (1996). Continued eruption of maxillary incisors and first molars in girls from 9 to 25 years, studied by the implant method. *European Journal of Orthodontics* **18**, 245–256.

Jaffin, R.A., Kumar, A. & Berman, C.L. (2004). Immediate loading of dental implants in the completely edentulous maxilla: a clinical report. *International Journal of Oral and Maxillofacial Implants* **19**, 721–730.

Kanomi, R. (1997). Mini-implant for orthodontic anchorage. *Journal of Clinical Orthodontics* **31**, 763–767.

Keles, A., Erverdi, N. & Sezen, S. (2003). Bodily distalization of molars with absolute anchorage. *The Angle Orthodontist* **73**, 471–482.

Kokich, V.G. (2004). Maxillary lateral incisor implants planning with the aid of orthodontics. *Journal of Oral and Maxillofacial Surgery* 62 (Suppl 2), 48–56.

Kokich, V.G. (1996). Managing complex orthodontic problems: the use of implants for anchorage. *Seminars in Orthodontics* **2**, 153–160.

Linkow, L.I. (1969), The endosseous blade implant and its use in orthodontics. *International Journal of Orthodontics* 7 149–154.

Lindh, C., Petersson, A. & Klinge, B. (1995). Measurements of distances related to the mandibular canal in radiographs. *Clinical Oral Implants Research* 6, 96–103.

Lioubavina-Hack, N., Lang, N.P. & Karring, T. (2006). Significance of primary stability for osseointegration of dental implants. *Clinical Oral Implants Research* **17**, 244–250.

Majzoub, Z., Finotti, M., Miotti, F., Giardino, R., Aldini, N.N. & Cordioli, G. (1999). Bone response to orthodontic loading of endosseous implants in the rabbit calvaria: early continuous distalizing forces. *European Journal of Orthodontics* **21**, 223–230.

Männchen, R. (1999). A new supraconstruction for palatal orthodontic implants. *Journal of Clinical Orthodontics* **33**, 373–382.

Männchen, R. & Schätzle, M. (2008). Success rates of palatal orthodontic implants. A prospective longitudinal study. *Clinical Oral Implants Research* (accepted).

McConnell, T.L., Hoffman, D.L., Forbes, D.P., Janzen, E.K. & Weintraub, N.H. (1996). Maxillary canine impaction in patients with transverse maxillary deficiency. *ASDC Journal of Dentistry for Children* **63**, 190–195.

Melsen, B. & Lang, N.P. (2001). Biological reactions of alveolar bone to orthodontic loading of oral implants. *Clinical Oral Implants Research* **12**, 144–152.

Ödman, J., Grondahl, K., Lekholm, U. & Thilander, B. (1991). The effect of osseointegrated implants on the dento-alveolar development. A clinical and radiographic study in growing pigs. *European Journal of Orthodontics* **13**, 279–286.

Ödman, J., Lekholm, U., Jemt, T., Brånemark, P.I. & Thilander, B. (1988). Osseointegrated titanium implants – a new approach in orthodontic treatment. *European Journal of Orthodontics* **10**, 98–105.

Ödman, J., Lekholm, U., Jemt, T. & Thilander, B. (1994). Osseointegrated implants as orthodontic anchorage in the treatment of partially edentulous adult patients. *European Journal of Orthodontics* **16**, 187–201.

Ottofy, L. (1923). *Standard Dental Dictionary.* Laird and Lee, Inc, Chicago, IL.

Pjetursson, B.E., Brägger, U., Lang, N.P. & Zwahlen, M. (2007). Comparison of survival and complication rates of tooth-supported fixed dental prostheses (FDPs) and implant-supported fixed dental prostheses and single crowns (SCs). *Clinical Oral Implants Research* **18** (Suppl 3), 97–113.

Ricketts, R.M. (1976). Bioprogressive therapy as an answer to orthodontic needs. Part II. *American Journal of Orthodontics* **70**, 359–397.

Roberts, W.E., Helm, F.R., Marshall, K.J. & Gongloff, R.K. (1989). Rigid endosseous implants for orthodontic and orthopedic anchorage. *The Angle Orthodontist* **59**, 247–256.

Roberts, W.E., Marshall, K.J. & Mozsary, P.G. (1990). Rigid endosseous implant utilized as anchorage to protract molars and close an atrophic extraction site. *The Angle Orthodontist* **60**, 135–152.

Roberts, W.E., Smith, R.K., Zilberman, Y., Mozsary, P.G. & Smith, R.S. (1984). Osseous adaptation to continuous loading of rigid endosseous implants. *American Journal of Orthodontics* 86, 95–111.

Rocci, A., Martignoni, M., Burgos, P.M., Gottlow, J. & Sennerby, L. (2003). Histology of retrieved immediately and early loaded oxidized implants: light microscopic observations after 5 to 9 months of loading in the posterior mandible. *Clinical Implant Dentistry and Related Research* **5** (Suppl 1), 88–98.

Schiel, H.J., Klein, J. & Widmer, B. (1996). Das enosssle Implantat als kieferorthopädisches Verankerungselement. *Zeitschrift für Zahnärztliche Implantologie* **12**, 183–188.

Sennerby, L., Ödman, J., Lekholm, U. & Thilander, B. (1993). Tissue reactions towards titanium implants inserted in growing jaws. A histological study in the pig. *Clinical Oral Implants Research* **4**, 65–75.

Shapiro, P.A. & Kokich, V.G. (1988). Uses of implants in orthodontics. *Dental Clinics of North America* 32, 539–550.

Sherman, A.J. (1978). Bone reaction to orthodontic forces on vitreous carbon dental implants. *American Journal of Orthodontics* **74**, 79–87.

Smalley, W. (1995). Implants for orthodontic tooth movement. Determining implant location and orientation. *Journal of Esthetic Dentistry* **7**, 62–72.

Smalley, W. & Blanco, A. (1995). Implants for tooth movement: A fabrication and placement technique for provisional restorations. *Journal of Esthetic Dentistry* **7**, 150–154.

Stöckli, P.W. (1994). Postnataler Wachstumsverlauf, Gesichts-Kieferwachstum und Entwicklung der Dentition. In: Stöckli, P.W. & Ben-Zur, E.D., eds. *Zahnmedizin bei Kindern und Jugendlichen*. 3. Aufl., Georg Thieme Verlag, Stuttgart, pp. 5–67.

Thilander, B. (1995). Basic mechanisms in craniofacial growth. *Acta Orthopaedica Scandinavica* **53**, 144–151.

Thilander, B., Ödman, J., Grondahl, K. & Friberg, B. (1994). Osseointegrated implants in adolescents. An alternative in replacing missing teeth? *European Journal of Orthodontics* **16**, 84–95.

Thilander, B., Ödman, J., Grondahl, K. & Lekholm, U. (1992). Aspects on osseointegrated implants inserted in growing jaws. A biometric and radiographic study in the young pig. *European Journal of Orthodontics* **14**, 99–109.

Thilander, B., Ödman, J. & Jemt, T. (1999). Single implants in the upper incisor region and their relationship to the adjacent teeth. An 8-year follow-up study. *Clinical Oral Implants Research* **10**, 346–355.

Triaca, A., Antonini, M. & Wintermantel, E. (1992). Ein neues Titan-Flachschrauben-Implantat zur orthodontischen Verankerung am anterioren Gaumen. *Informationen aus Orthodontie und Kieferorthopädie* **24**, 251–257.

Trisi, P. & Rebaudi, A. (2002). Progressive bone adaptation of titanium implants during and after orthodontic load in humans. *International Journal of Periodontics and Restorative Dentistry* **22**, 31–43.

Turley, P.K., Kean, C., Schur, J., Stefanac, J., Gray, J., Hennes, J. & Poon, L.C. (1988). Orthodontic force application to titanium endosseous implants. *The Angle Orthodontist* **58**, 151–162.

Turley, P.K., Shapiro, P.A. & Moffett, B.C. (1980). The loading of bioglass-coated aluminium oxide implants to produce sutural expansion of the maxillary complex in the pigtail monkey (*Macaca nemestrina*). *Archives of Oral Biology* **25**, 459–469.

Tweed, C.H. (1941). The applications of the principles of the edgewise arch in the treatment of malocclusions. *The Angle Orthodontist* **11**, 12–67

Umemori, M., Sugawara, J., Mitani, H., Nagasaka, H. & Kawamura, H. (1999). Skeletal anchorage system for open-bite correction. *American Journal of Orthodontics and Dentofacial Orthopedics* **115**, 166–174.

Wehrbein, H. (1994). Endosseous titanium implants as orthodontic anchoring elements. Experimental studies and clinical application. *Fortschritte der Kieferorthopädie* **55**, 236–250.

Wehrbein, H. & Diedrich, P. (1993). Endosseous titanium implants during and after orthodontic load – an experimental study in the dog. *Clinical Oral Implants Research* **4**, 76–82.

Wehrbein, H., Feifel, H. & Diedrich, P. (1999a). Palatal implant anchorage reinforcement of posterior teeth a prospective study. *American Journal of Orthodontics and Dentofacial Orthopedics* **116**, 678–686.

Wehrbein, H., Glatzmaier, J., Mundwiller, U. & Diedrich, P. (1996a). The Orthosystem – a new implant system for orthodontic anchorage in the palate. *Journal of Orofacial Orthopedics* **57**, 142–153.

Wehrbein, H., Merz, B.R. & Diedrich, P. (1999b). Palatal bone support for orthodontic implant anchorage – a clinical and radiological study. *European Journal of Orthodontics* **21**, 65–70.

Wehrbein, H., Merz, B.R., Diedrich, P. & Glatzmaier, J. (1996b). The use of palatal implants for orthodontic anchorage. Design and clinical application of the orthosystem. *Clinical Oral Implants Research* **7**, 410–416.

Wehrbein, H., Merz, B.R., Hämmerle, C.H. & Lang, N.P. (1998). Bone-to-implant contact of orthodontic implants in humans subjected to horizontal loading. *Clinical Oral Implants Research* **9**, 348–353.

Part 18: Supportive Care

59   Supportive Periodontal Therapy (SPT), 1297
     Niklaus P. Lang, Urs Brägger, Giovanni E. Salvi, and Maurizio S. Tonetti

See also:

41   Treatment of Peri-implant Lesions, 875
     Tord Berglundh, Niklaus P. Lang, and Jan Lindhe

Chapter 59

Supportive Periodontal Therapy (SPT)

Niklaus P. Lang, Urs Brägger, Giovanni E. Salvi, and Maurizio S. Tonetti

Definitions, 1297
Basic paradigms for the prevention of periodontal disease, 1297
Patients at risk for periodontitis without SPT, 1300
SPT for patients with gingivitis, 1302
SPT for patients with periodontitis, 1302
Continuous multi-level risk assessment, 1303
  Subject risk assessment, 1303
  Tooth risk assessment, 1309
  Site risk assessment, 1310

Radiographic evaluation of periodontal disease
  progression, 1312
Clinical implementation, 1312
Objectives for SPT, 1313
SPT in daily practice, 1314
  Examination, re-evaluation, and diagnosis (ERD), 1314
  Motivation, reinstruction, and instrumentation (MRI), 1315
  Treatment of reinfected sites (TRS), 1315
  Polishing, fluorides, determination of recall interval (PFD), 1317

Clinical trials on the long-term effects of treatment of periodontitis have clearly demonstrated that post-therapeutic professional maintenance care is an integral part of the treatment. This also constitutes the only means of assuring the maintenance of long-term beneficial therapeutic effects. Reinfection could be prevented or kept to a minimum in most patients, mainly through rigid surveillance involving professional visits at regular intervals. However, the maintenance systems presented in various studies do not allow the presentation of a clear concept with general validity for the frequency of professional maintenance visits and the mode of maintenance therapy. A danger for supervised neglect of reinfection and recurrent disease in some patients coexists with a tendency for overtreatment in others.

Objective criteria for assessing the patient's individual risk for recurrent disease have been the focus of attention of recent years. However, the evaluation of the patient's individual risk still has to be based on a probability estimation based on the analysis of patient, tooth or tooth site risk assessments.

The purpose of this chapter is to discuss the basics of continuous patient monitoring following active periodontal therapy in order to prevent reinfection and the continued progression of periodontal disease following therapy. The mode and extent of interceptive therapeutic measures needed to achieve this goal will also be evaluated.

Definitions

Periodontal treatment includes:
1. Systemic evaluation of the patient's health
2. A cause-related therapeutic phase with, in some cases
3. A corrective phase involving periodontal surgical procedures
4. Maintenance phase.

The 3rd World Workshop of the American Academy of Periodontology (1989) renamed this treatment phase "supportive periodontal therapy" (SPT). This term expresses the essential need for therapeutic measures to support the patient's own efforts to control periodontal infections and to avoid reinfection. Regular visits to the therapist should serve as a positive feedback mechanism between the patient and the therapist with the purpose of ensuring that patients have the opportunity to maintain their dentitions in a healthy status for the longest possible time. An integral part of SPT is the continuous diagnostic monitoring of the patient in order to intercept with adequate therapy and to optimize the therapeutic interventions tailored to the patient's needs.

Basic paradigms for the prevention of periodontal disease

Periodontal maintenance care, or SPT, follows the paradigms of the etiology and pathogenesis of periodontal disease and – at present – must consider the fact that these diseases are coping with the result of the host defense on an opportunistic infection.

Almost 40 years ago, a cause–effect relationship between the accumulation of bacterial plaque on teeth and the development of gingivitis was proven (Löe *et al.* 1965). This relationship was also documented by the restoration of gingival health following plaque removal. Ten years later, a corresponding relationship between plaque accumulation and the development of periodontal disease, characterized by loss of connective tissue attachment and resorption of alveolar bone, was shown in laboratory animals (Lindhe *et al.* 1975). Since some of these animals did not develop periodontal disease despite a persistent plaque accumulation for 48 months, it must be considered that the composition of the microbiota or the host's defense mechanisms or susceptibility for disease may vary from individual to individual. Nevertheless, in the study mentioned, the initiation of periodontal disease was always preceded by obvious signs of gingivitis. Hence, it seems reasonable to predict that the elimination of gingival inflammation and the maintenance of healthy gingival tissues will result in the prevention of both the initiation and the recurrence of periodontal disease. In fact, as early as 1746, Fauchard stated that "little or no care as to the cleaning of teeth is ordinarily the cause of all diseases that destroy them" (Fauchard 1746).

From the clinical point of view, the above-mentioned results must be translated into the necessity for proper and regular personal plaque elimination, at least in patients treated for or susceptible to periodontal disease. This simple principle may be difficult to implement in all patients; however, interceptive professional supportive therapy at regular intervals may, to a certain extent, compensate for the lack of personal compliance with regard to oral hygiene standards.

These aspects have been imitated in a beagle dog model with naturally occurring periodontal disease (Morrison *et al.* 1979). Two groups of animals were used. The test group was subjected to initial scaling and root planing and, subsequently, plaque was eliminated by daily toothbrushing and biweekly polishing with rubber cups for a period of 3 years. In the control group, no initial scaling and no oral hygiene practices were performed during the same period of time. Every 6 months, however, the teeth in two diagonally opposed jaw quadrants in both test and control animals were scaled and root planed. The results showed that the reduction of probing depth and the gain of probing attachment, obtained after the initial scaling and root planing in the test animals, were maintained throughout the entire course of the study irrespective of whether or not repeated scaling and root planing had been performed. The control animals, on the other hand, continued to show increasing probing depths and loss of attachment in

all quadrants irrespective of whether or not repeated scaling and root planing had been performed. However, in the jaw quadrants where the teeth were repeatedly instrumented every 6 months, the progression of periodontal destruction was significantly less pronounced (Fig. 59-1). These results indicate that professional supportive therapy, performed at regular intervals, may, at least to a certain extent, compensate for a "suboptimal" personal oral hygiene standard. In this respect, it has been demonstrated that following root instrumentation, the subgingival microbiota is significantly altered in quantity and quality (Listgarten *et al.* 1978), and that the re-establishment of a disease-associated, subgingival microbiota may take several months (Listgarten *et al.* 1978; Slots *et al.* 1979; Mousquès *et al.* 1980; Caton *et al.* 1982; Magnusson *et al.* 1984).

In a number of longitudinal, clinical studies on the outcome of periodontal therapy, the crucial role of SPT in maintaining successful results has been documented (Ramfjord *et al.* 1968, 1975; Lindhe & Nyman 1975, 1984; Rosling *et al.* 1976; Nyman *et al.* 1977; Knowles *et al.* 1979, 1980; Badersten *et al.* 1981, 1987; Hill *et al.* 1981; Lindhe *et al.* 1982a,b; Pihlström *et al.* 1983; Westfelt *et al.* 1983a, 1985; Isidor & Karring 1986; Kaldahl *et al.* 1988). In all these studies, probing depths and clinical attachment levels were maintained as a result of a well organized professional maintenance care program (recall intervals varying between 3 and 6 months) irrespective of the initial treatment modality performed. In one of the studies (Nyman *et al.* 1977) an alarming result was that patients treated for advanced periodontal disease involving surgical techniques, but not incorporated in a supervised maintenance care program, exhibited recurrent periodontitis including loss of attachment at a rate three to five times higher than documented for natural progression of periodontal disease in population groups with high disease susceptibility (Löe *et al.* 1978, 1986). Within this area, the effect of negligence in providing adequate supportive maintenance care following periodontal treatment has been studied over a 6-year period by Axelsson and Lindhe (1981a). Following presurgical root instrumentation and instruction in oral hygiene practices, all study patients were subjected to modified Widman flap procedures. During a 2-month healing period, professional toothcleaning was performed every 2 weeks. Following this time period, baseline clinical data were obtained and one out of every three patients was dismissed from the clinic, while the other two were incorporated in a professionally conducted maintenance program with a recall once every 3 months. These patients maintained excellent oral hygiene and consequently yielded a very low frequency of bleeding sites. In addition, probing depths and probing attachment levels were maintained unchanged over the 6-year period. In contrast, the non-recalled patients demonstrated obvious signs of recurrent periodontitis at the 3-year and 6-year

(a) Reduction (+) or Increase (-) in Pocket Depth

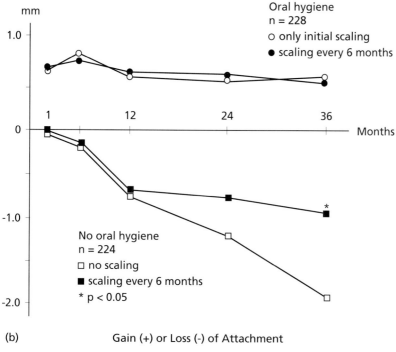

(b) Gain (+) or Loss (-) of Attachment

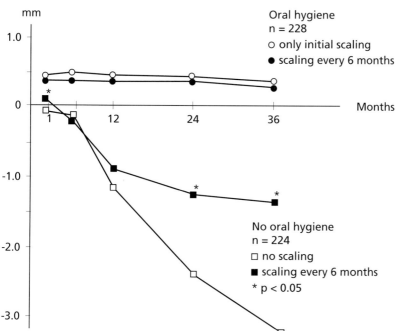

Fig. 59-1 (a) Mean probing depth reduction (+) or increase in probing depth (−) in millimeters with or without repeated scaling and root planing in experimental (oral hygiene) and control (no oral hygiene) animals relative to baseline means. (b) Mean gain (+) or loss (−) of probing attachment with or without repeated scaling and root planing in experimental (oral hygiene) and control (no oral hygiene) animals relative to baseline means. (Data from Morrison *et al.* 1979.)

re-examinations. Further evidence for the likelihood of recurrent disease in patients not subjected to professional maintenance care was presented by Kerr (1981). Five years after successful treatment, 45% of the patients presented with periodontal conditions similar to their status before treatment. Supportive therapy had only been provided at intervals varying between 9 and 18 months.

Similar results have been described for private practice patients who decided not to participate in an organized maintenance care program following active periodontal therapy (Becker *et al.* 1984). Subse-

quent examinations revealed clear signs of recurrent periodontal disease including increased probing depths and involvements of furcations of multi-rooted teeth concomitant with tooth loss. Also, loss of alveolar bone observed in radiographs and tooth loss have been reported for a group of patients in whom post-therapeutic supportive maintenance care was provided less frequently than once every 12 months (De Vore *et al.* 1986). From all these studies it is evident that periodontal treatment is ineffective in maintaining periodontal health if supportive maintenance care is neglected, denied or omitted.

Even though the number of well controlled longitudinal clinical trials is rather limited for patients who, in addition to periodontal treatment, have undergone extensive reconstructive therapy, it should be realized that the concept of professional maintenance care has unrestricted validity. In a longitudinal study of combined periodontal and prosthetic treatment of patients with advanced periodontal disease, periodontal health could be maintained over a study period of 5–8 years with regular recall appointments scheduled every 3–6 months (Nyman & Lindhe 1979). Similar results have been presented by Valderhaug and Birkeland (1976) and by Valderhaug (1980) for periods of up to 15 years. Another study of 36 patients who received extensive poly-unit cantilevered bridgework following periodontal therapy, confirmed the maintenance of periodontal health over 5–12 years (Laurell et al. 1991). More recent studies on the long-term maintenance over 10 and 11 years of periodontal patients who, following successful treatment of chronic periodontitis, were reconstructed with extensive fixed reconstructions revealed that regularly performed SPT resulted in periodontal stability. Only 1.3% (Hämmerle et al. 2000) and 2.0% (Moser et al. 2002) of the abutments showed some minor attachment loss during these long periods of observation. In contrast, a report of insurance cases who were not regularly maintained by SPT yielded a recurrence rate for periodontitis of almost 10% after an observation of 6.5 years (Randow et al. 1986).

Summary: The etiology of gingivitis and periodontitis is fairly well understood. However, the causative factors, i.e. the microbial challenge which induces and maintains the inflammatory response, may not be completely eliminated from the dentogingival environment for any length of time. This requires the professional removal of all microbial deposits in the supragingival and subgingival areas at regular intervals, since recolonization will occur following the debridement procedures, leading to a reinfection of the ecologic niche and, hence, giving rise to further progression of the disease process. Numerous well controlled clinical trials, however, have documented that such a development can be prevented over very long periods of time only by regular interference with the subgingival environment which aims at removal of the subgingival bacteria.

Patients at risk for periodontitis without SPT

The effect of an omission of SPT in patients with periodontitis may best be studied either in untreated populations or patient groups with poor compliance.

One of the few studies documenting untreated periodontitis-susceptible patients reported on the continuous loss of periodontal attachment as well as teeth in Sri Lankan tea plantation workers receiving no dental therapy (Löe et al. 1986). In this – for the western world – rather unique model situation, an average loss of 0.3 mm per tooth surface and year was encountered. Also, the laborers lost between 0.1 and 0.3 teeth per year as a result of periodontitis. In another untreated group in the United States, 0.61 teeth had been lost per year during an observation period of 4 years (Becker et al. 1979). This is in dramatic contrast to reports on tooth loss in well maintained patients treated for periodontitis (e.g. Hirschfeld & Wasserman 1978; McFall 1982; Becker et al. 1984; Wilson et al. 1987). Such patients were either completely stable and lost no teeth during maintenance periods ranging up to 22 years or lost only very little periodontal attachment and only 0.03 teeth (Hirschfeld & Wasserman 1978) or 0.06 teeth (Wilson et al. 1987), respectively.

Non-complying, but periodontitis-susceptible patients receiving no SPT following periodontal surgical interventions continued to lose periodontal attachment at a rate of approximately 1 mm per year regardless of the type of surgery chosen (Nyman et al. 1977). This is almost three times more than would have to be expected as a result of the "natural" course of periodontal disease progression (Löe et al. 1978, 1986).

In a British study of a private practice situation (Kerr 1981) where the patients were referred back to the general dentist after periodontal therapy, 45% of the patients showed complete reinfection after 5 years.

Probably the most impressive documentation of the lack of SPT in disease-susceptible individuals arises from a clinical trial in which one third of the patients had been sent back to the referring general practitioner for maintenance, while two thirds of the patients received SPT in a well organized maintenance system (Axelsson & Lindhe 1981a). The 77 patients were examined before treatment, 2 months after the last surgical procedure and 3 and 6 years later. The 52 patients on the carefully designed SPT system visited the program every 2 months for the first 2 years and every 3 months for the remaining 4 years of the observation period. The results obtained from the second examination (2 months after the last surgery) showed that the effect of the initial treatment was good in both groups. Subsequently, the recall patients were able to maintain proper oral hygiene and unaltered attachment levels. In the non-recall group, plaque scores increased markedly from the baseline values, as did the number of inflamed gingival units (Fig. 59-2a). Concomitantly, there were obvious signs of recurrent periodontitis. The mean values for pocket depth and attachment levels at the 3-year and 6-year examinations were higher than at baseline (Fig. 59-2b). In the recall group, approximately 99% of the tooth surfaces showed either improvement, no change or less than 1 mm loss of attachment, compared to 45% in the non-recall group

(Table 59-1). In the latter patients, 55% of the sites showed a further loss of attachment of 2–5 mm at the 6-year examination, and 20% of the pockets were 4 mm deep or more (Tables 59-1, 59-2).

Summary: Patients susceptible to periodontal disease are at high risk for reinfection and progression of periodontal lesions without meticulously organized and performed SPT. Since all patients who were treated for periodontal diseases belong to this risk category by virtue of their past history, an adequate maintenance care program is of utmost importance for a beneficial long-term treatment outcome. SPT has to be aimed at the regular removal of the subgingival microbiota and must be supplemented by the patient's efforts for optimal supragingival plaque control.

Table 59-1 Percentage of sites showing various changes in probing attachment level between baseline examination, 2 months after completion of active periodontal therapy, and at follow-up examination 6 years later (adapted from Axelsson & Lindhe 1981b)

Change in attachment level	Percentage of surfaces showing change	
	Recall	Non-recall
Attachment level improved	17	1
No change	72	10
Attachment level worse by:		
≥1 mm	10	34
2–5 mm	1	55

Table 59-2 Percentage of various probing depths in recall and non-recall patients at the initial examination, 2 months after active periodontal treatment, and at 3- and 6-year follow-up visits (adapted from Axelsson & Lindhe 1981b)

Examinations	Percentage of pockets of various depths					
	≤3 mm		4–6 mm		≥7 mm	
	Recall	Non-recall	Recall	Non-recall	Recall	Non-recall
Initial	35	50	58	38	8	12
Baseline	99	99	1	1	0	0
3 years	99	91	1	9	0	0
6 years	99	80	1	19	0	1

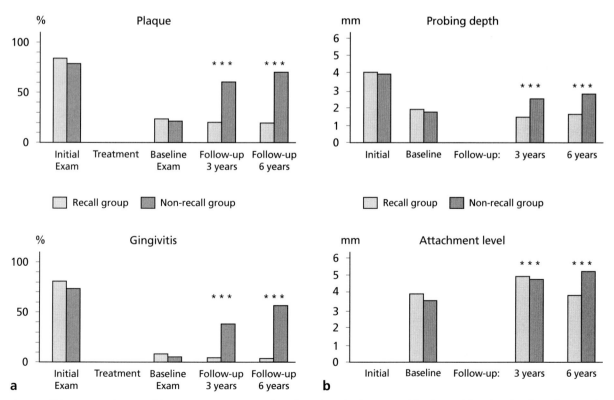

Fig. 59-2 Histograms showing (a) average percentages of tooth surfaces harboring visible plaque (above) and inflamed gingival units (bleeding on probing) (below), and (b) average probing depth (above) and probing attachment levels (below), at initial, baseline and follow-up examinations. (Data from Axelsson & Lindhe 1981b.)

SPT for patients with gingivitis

Several studies, predominantly in children, have documented that periodic professional prophylactic visits in conjunction with reinforcement of personal oral hygiene are effective in controlling gingivitis (Badersten *et al.* 1975; Poulsen *et al.* 1976; Axelsson & Lindhe 1981a,b; Bellini *et al.* 1981). This, however, does not imply that maintenance visits in childhood preclude the development of more severe disease later in life. It is obvious that SPT, therefore, must be a lifelong commitment of both the patient and the profession.

Adults whose effective oral hygiene was combined with periodic professional prophylaxis were clearly healthier periodontally than patients who did not participate in such programs (Lövdal *et al.* 1961; Suomi *et al.* 1971). One particular study of historic significance was performed on 1428 adults from an industrial company in Oslo, Norway (Lövdal *et al.* 1961). Over a 5-year observation period, the subjects were recalled two to four times per year for instruction in oral hygiene and supragingival and subgingival scaling. Gingival conditions improved by approximately 60% and tooth loss was reduced by about 50% of what would be expected without these efforts.

In another study (Suomi *et al.* 1971) loss of periodontal tissue support in young individuals with gingivitis or only loss of small amounts of attachment was followed over 3 years. An experimental group receiving scaling and instruction in oral hygiene every 3 months yielded significantly less plaque and gingival inflammation than the control group in which no special efforts had been made. The mean loss of probing attachment was only 0.08 mm per surface in the experimental as opposed to 0.3 mm in the control group.

When adult patients with gingivitis were treated with scaling and root planing, but did not improve their oral hygiene procedures, the gingival condition did not improve compared with individuals receiving prophylaxes at 6-month intervals (Listgarten & Schifter 1982).

Summary: The available information indicates that the prevention of gingival inflammation and early loss of attachment in patients with gingivitis depends primarily on the level of personal plaque control, but also on further measures to reduce the accumulation of supragingival and subgingival plaque.

SPT for patients with periodontitis

As mentioned previously, a series of longitudinal studies on periodontal therapeutic modalities was performed over the past 25 years, first at the University of Michigan, later at the University of Gothenburg, Sweden, and also at the Universities of Minnesota, Nebraska, and Loma Linda. These studies always incorporated the patients into a well orga-

nized maintenance care system with recall visits at regular intervals (generally 3–4 months). Although the patients performed plaque control with various degrees of efficacy, the SPT resulted in excellent maintenance of post-operative attachment levels in most patients (Knowles 1973; Ramfjord *et al.* 1982).

On average, excellent treatment results with maintained reduced probing depths and maintained gains of probing attachment were documented for most of the patients in the longitudinal studies irrespective of the treatment modality chosen (Ramfjord *et al.* 1975; Lindhe & Nyman 1975; Rosling *et al.* 1976; Nyman *et al.* 1977; Knowles *et al.* 1979, 1980; Badersten *et al.* 1981, 1987; Hill *et al.* 1981; Lindhe *et al.* 1982a; Pihlström *et al.* 1983; Westfelt *et al.* 1983a,b, 1985; Isidor & Karring 1986).

In a study on 75 patients with extremely advanced periodontitis, who had been successfully treated for the disease with cause-related therapy and modified Widman flap procedures (Lindhe & Nyman 1984), recurrent infection occurred in only very few sites during a 14-year period of effective SPT. However, it has to be realized that recurrent periodontitis was noticed at completely unpredictable time intervals, but was concentrated in about 25% of the patient population (15 out of 61). This suggests that, in a periodontitis-susceptible risk population, the majority of patients can be "cured" provided an optimally organized SPT is performed, while a relatively small proportion of patients (20–25%) will suffer from occasional episodes of recurrent periodontal reinfection. It is obviously a challenge for the diagnostician to identify such patients with very high disease susceptibility and to monitor the dentitions for recurrent periodontitis on a long-term basis.

As opposed to the study by Lindhe and Nyman (1984) which exclusively involved patients with advanced periodontitis, another study on 52 patients with generalized mild to moderate adult periodontitis addressed the efficacy of SPT 8 years following completion of cause-related periodontal therapy (Brägger *et al.* 1992). Full-mouth intraoral radiographs were used to assess changes in the radiographic alveolar bone height as a percentage of the total tooth length. As a result of cause-related therapy, a gain in probing attachment followed by a loss of 0.5–0.8 mm over the following 8 years was observed. The radiographic loss of alveolar bone height in the same time period was less than 2% and thus clinically insignificant. In this patient group initially presenting with mild to moderate periodontitis, the frequency of SPT rendered per year did not affect the rate of progression of periodontal desease. However, patients seeking SPT less than once per year over 8 years lost further periodontal attachment during the period of observation. From these studies it is evident that patients having experienced periodontitis need some kind of SPT. Obviously, the frequency of SPT visits has to be adapted to the risk of susceptibility for the disease. Patients with advanced periodontitis may need SPT at a regular and rather short time interval (3–4 months), while for mild to moderate forms of periodontitis, one annual visit may be enough to prevent further loss of attachment.

More recently, the effect of a plaque-control-based maintenance program on tooth mortality, caries, and periodontal disease progression was presented after 30 years of SPT in a private dental office (Axelsson *et al.* 2004). This prospective controlled cohort study initially included 375 test and 180 control patients that received traditional maintenance care (by the referring dentist once to twice a year). After 6 years, the control group was discontinued. The test group was subjected to prophylactic visits every second month for the first 2 years and every 3–12 months (according to their individual needs) during years 3–30. The prophylactic visits to the dental hygienist included plaque disclosure and professional mechanical tooth cleaning, including the use of a fluoride-containing dentifrice. During the 30 years of maintenance, very few teeth were lost (0.4–1.8%), and these were predominately lost because of root fractures. Within 30 years of maintenance, 1.2–2.1 new carious lesions (>80% secondary caries) were found. With the exception of buccal sites, no sites demonstrated any loss of periodontal attachment during this period. On approximal sites, there was even some gain of attachment. This unique study clearly demonstrated that SPT based on plaque control tailored to the individual needs of the patient will result in very low tooth mortality, minimal recurrent caries, and almost complete periodontal stability.

Summary: SPT is an absolute prerequisite to guarantee beneficial treatment outcomes with maintained levels of clinical attachment over long periods of time. The maintenance of treatment results for the majority of patients has been documented up to 14 years, and in a private practice situation even up to 30 years, but it has to be realized that a small proportion of patients will experience recurrent infections with progression of periodontal lesions in a few sites in a completely unpredictable mode. The continuous risk assessment at subject, tooth and tooth site levels, therefore, represents a challenge for the SPT concept.

Continuous multi-level risk assessment

As opposed to an initial periodontal diagnosis which considers the sequelae of the disease process, i.e. documents the net loss of periodontal attachment and the concomitant formation of periodontal pockets and the existence of inflammation, clinical diagnosis during SPT has to be based on the variations of the health status obtained following successful active periodontal treatment. This, in turn, means that a new baseline will have to be established once the treatment goals of active periodontal therapy (i.e.

phases 1–3) are reached and periodontal health is restored (Claffey 1991). This baseline includes the level of clinical attachment achieved while the inflammatory parameters are supposed to be under control. Under optimal circumstances, supportive periodontal care would maintain clinical attachment levels obtained after active therapy for the years to come. The relevant question would, therefore, be which clinical parameters may serve as early indicators for a new onset or recurrence of the periodontal disease process, i.e. reinfection and progression of periodontal breakdown of a previously treated periodontal site.

From a clinical point of view the stability of periodontal conditions reflects a dynamic equilibrium between bacterial aggression and effective host response. As such, this homeostasis is prone to sudden changes whenever one of the two factors prevails. Hence, it is evident that the diagnostic process must be based on continuous monitoring of the multi-level risk profile. The intervals between diagnostic assessments must also be chosen based on the overall risk profile and the expected benefit. To schedule patients for supportive periodontal therapy on the basis of an individual risk evaluation for recurrence of disease has been demonstrated to be cost effective (Axelsson & Lindhe 1981a,b; Axelsson *et al.* 1991).

By virtue of their previous disease predisposition, all patients under a periodontal maintenance program represent a population with a moderate to high risk for recurrent periodontal infection. As opposed to the general population without such a history, periodontal patients need to participate in a well organized recall system which should provide both continuous risk assessment and adequate supportive care. Without this, the patients are likely to experience progressive loss of periodontal attachment (Axelsson & Lindhe 1981a; Kerr 1981; Becker *et al.* 1984; Cortellini *et al.* 1994, 1996). On the other hand, it is important to determine the level of risk for progression in each individual patient in order to be able to determine the frequency and extent of professional support necessary to maintain the attachment levels obtained following active therapy. The determination of such risk level would thus prevent undertreatment, and also excessive overtreatment, during SPT (Brägger *et al.* 1992).

Subject risk assessment

The patient's risk assessment for recurrence of periodontitis may be evaluated on the basis of a number of clinical conditions whereby no single parameter displays a more paramount role. The entire spectrum of risk factors and risk indicators ought to be evaluated simultaneously. For this purpose, a functional diagram has been constructed (Fig. 59-3) (Lang & Tonetti 2003) including the following aspects:

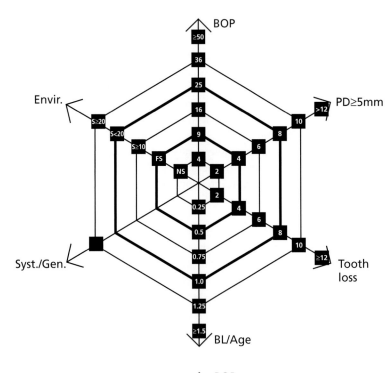

Fig. 59-3a Functional diagram to evaluate the patient's risk for recurrence of periodontitis. Each vector represents one risk factor or indicator with an area of relatively low risk, an area of moderate risk, and an area of high risk for disease progression. All factors have to be evaluated together and hence the area of relatively low risk is found within the center circle of the polygon, while the area of high risk is found outside the periphery of the second polygon in bold. Between the two rings in bold, there is the area of moderate risk.

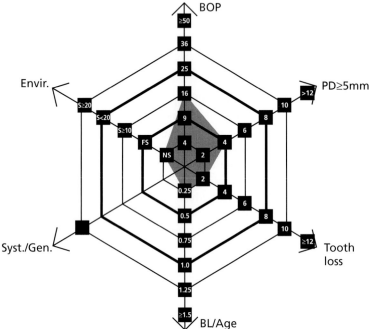

Fig. 59-3b Functional diagram of a low-risk maintenance patient. BOP is 15%, four residual pockets ≥5 mm are diagnosed, two teeth have been lost, the bone factor in relation to the age is 0.25, no systemic factor is known and the patient is a non-smoker.

1. Percentage of bleeding on probing
2. Prevalence of residual pockets greater than 4 mm
3. Loss of teeth from a total of 28 teeth
4. Loss of periodontal support in relation to the patient's age
5. Systemic and genetic conditions
6. Environmental factors such as cigarette smoking.

Each parameter has its own scale for minor, moderate, and high-risk profiles. A comprehensive evaluation, the functional diagram will provide an individualized total risk profile and determine the frequency and complexity of SPT visits. Modifications may be made to the functional diagram if additional factors become important from future evidence.

Compliance with recall system

Several investigations have indicated that only a minority of periodontal patients comply with the prescribed supportive periodontal care (Wilson *et al.* 1984; Mendoza *et al.* 1991; Checchi *et al.* 1994; Demetriou *et al.* 1995). Since it has been clearly established that treated periodontal patients who comply with regular periodontal maintenance appointments have a better prognosis than patients who do not comply (Axelsson & Lindhe 1981a; Becker *et al.* 1984; Cortellini *et al.* 1994, 1996), non-compliant or poorly compliant patients should be considered at higher risk for periodontal disease progression. A report that investigated the personality differences of patients

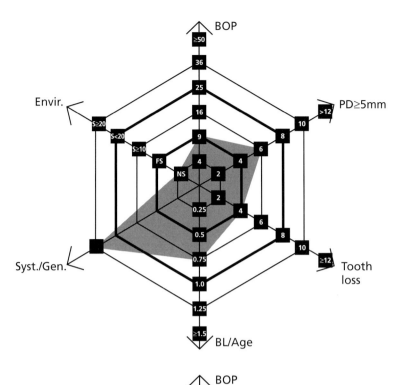

Fig. 59-3c Functional diagram of a medium-risk maintenance patient. BOP is 9%, six residual pockets ≥5 mm are diagnosed, four teeth have been lost, the bone factor in relation to the age is 0.75, the patient is a type I diabetic, but a non-smoker.

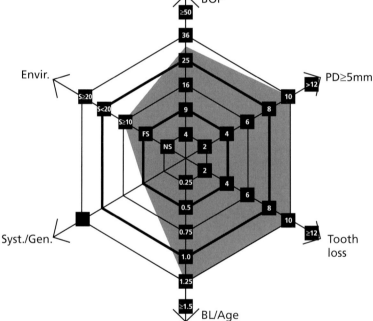

Fig. 59-3d Functional diagram of a high-risk maintenance patient. BOP is 32%, ten residual pockets ≥5 mm are diagnosed, ten teeth have been lost, the bone factor in relation to the age is 1.25, no systemic factor is known, and the patient is an occasional smoker.

participating in a regular recall program as compared to patients who did not, revealed that patients who did not take part in a maintenance program following periodontal therapy had higher incidences of stressful life events and less stable personal relationships in their lives (Becker *et al.* 1988).

Oral hygiene

Since bacterial plaque is by far the most important etiologic agent for the occurrence of periodontal diseases (for review see Kornman and Löe 1993), it is evident that the full-mouth assessment of the bacterial load must have a pivotal impact in the determination of the risk for disease recurrence. It has to be

realized, however, that regular interference with the microbial ecosystem during periodontal maintenance will eventually obscure such obvious associations. In patients treated with various surgical and non-surgical modalities, it has been clearly established that plaque-infected dentitions will yield recurrence of periodontal disease in multiple locations, while dentitions under plaque control and regular supportive care maintain periodontal stability for many years (Rosling *et al.* 1976; Axelsson & Lindhe 1981a,b). Studies have thus far not identified a level of plaque infection compatible with maintenance of periodontal health. However, in a clinical set-up, a plaque control record of 20–40% might be tolerable by most patients. It is important to realize that the full-mouth plaque score has to be related to the host response of the patient, i.e. compared to inflammatory parameters.

Percentage of sites with bleeding on probing

Bleeding on gentle probing represents an objective inflammatory parameter which has been incorporated into index systems for the evaluation of periodontal conditions (Löe & Silness 1963; Mühlemann & Son 1971) and is also used as a parameter by itself. In a patient's risk assessment for recurrence of periodontitis, bleeding on probing (BOP) reflects, at least in part, the patient's compliance and standards of oral hygiene performance. Although there is no established acceptable level of prevalence of BOP in the dentition above which a higher risk for disease recurrence has been established, a BOP prevalence of 25% has been the cut-off point between patients with maintained periodontal stability for 4 years and patients with recurrent disease in the same timeframe in a prospective study in a private practice (Joss et al. 1994) (Fig. 59-4). Further evidence of BOP percentages between 20% and 30% determining a higher risk for disease progression originates from studies of Claffey et al. (1990) and Badersten et al. (1990).

In assessing the patient's risk for disease progression, BOP percentages reflect a summary of the patient's ability to perform proper plaque control, the patient's host response to the bacterial challenge, and the patient's compliance. The percentage of BOP, therefore, is used as the first risk factor in the functional diagram of risk assessment (Fig. 59-3). The scale runs in a quadratic mode with 4, 9, 16, 25, 36, and >49% being the divisions on the vector.

Individuals with low mean BOP percentages (<10% of the surfaces) may be regarded as patients with a low risk for recurrent disease (Lang et al. 1990), while patients with mean BOP percentages >25% should be considered to be at high risk for reinfection.

Prevalence of residual pockets greater than 4 mm

The enumeration of the residual pockets with probing depths greater than 4 mm represents, to a certain extent, the degree of success of periodontal treatment rendered. Although this figure per se does not make much sense when considered as a sole parameter, the evaluation in conjunction with other parameters, such as BOP and/or suppuration, will reflect existing ecologic niches from and in which reinfection might occur. It is, therefore, conceivable that periodontal stability in a dentition would be reflected in a minimal number of residual pockets. Presence of high fre-

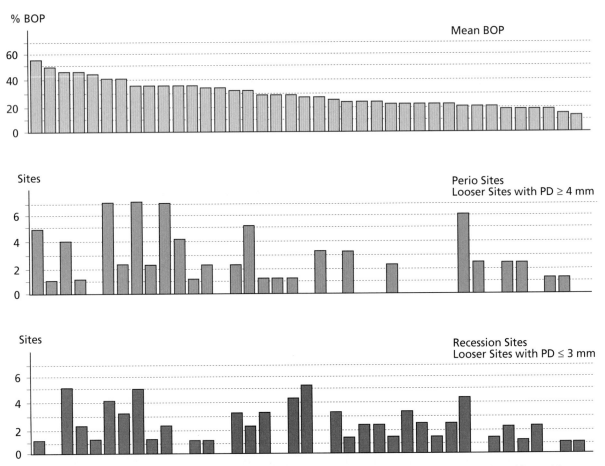

Fig. 59-4 Distribution of "looser" sites (probing depth (PD) ≥4 mm) due to periodontal disease progression with or without concomitant recession, dependent on the mean bleeding on probing (BOP) percentage during an observation period of 4 years. Patients are sorted by decreasing mean BOP percentages. Patients with <20% BOP have a significantly lower risk for disease recurrence. (Data from Joss et al. 1994.)

quencies of deep residual pockets and deepening of pockets during supportive periodontal care has, in fact, been associated with high risk for disease progression (Badersten *et al.* 1990; Claffey *et al.* 1990). On the other hand, it has to be realized that an increased number of residual pockets does not necessarily imply an increased risk for reinfection or disease progression, since a number of longitudinal studies have established the fact that, depending on the individual supportive therapy provided, even deeper pockets may be stable without further disease progression for years (e.g. Knowles *et al.* 1979; Lindhe & Nyman 1984).

Nevertheless, in assessing the patient's risk for disease progression, the number of residual pockets with a probing depth of ≥5 mm is assessed as the second risk indicator for recurrent disease in the functional diagram of risk assessment (Fig. 59-3). The scale runs in a linear mode with 2, 4, 6, 8, 10, and ≥12% being the divisions on the vector.

Individuals with up to four residual pockets may be regarded as patients with a relatively low risk, while patients with more than eight residual pockets may be regarded as individuals with high risk for recurrent disease.

Loss of teeth from a total of 28 teeth

Although the reason for tooth loss may not be known, the number of remaining teeth in a dentition reflects the functionality of the dentition. Mandibular stability and individual optimal function may be assured even with a shortened dental arch of premolar to premolar occlusion, i.e. 20 teeth. The shortened dental arch does not seem to predispose the individual to mandibular dysfunction (Witter *et al.* 1990, 1994). However, if more than eight teeth from a total of 28 teeth are lost, oral function is usually impaired (Käyser 1981, 1994, 1996). Since tooth loss also represents a true end-point outcome variable reflecting the patient's history of oral diseases and trauma, it is logical to incorporate this risk indicator as the third parameter in the functional diagram of risk assessment (Fig. 59-3). The number of teeth lost from the dentition without the third molars (28 teeth) is counted, irrespective of their replacement. The scale runs also in a linear mode with 2, 4, 6, 8, 10, and ≥12% being the divisions on the vector.

Individuals with up to four teeth lost may be regarded as patients in low risk, while patients with more than eight teeth lost may be considered as being in high risk.

Loss of periodontal support in relation to the patient's age

The extent and prevalence of periodontal attachment loss (i.e. previous disease experience and susceptibility), as evaluated by the height of the alveolar bone on radiographs, may represent the most obvious indicator of subject risk when related to the patient's age. In light of the present understanding of periodontal disease progression, and the evidence that both onset and rate of progression of periodontitis might vary among individuals and during different timeframes (van der Velden 1991), it has to be realized that previous attachment loss in relation to the patient's age does not rule out the possibility of rapidly progressing lesions. Therefore, the actual risk for further disease progression in a given individual may occasionally be underestimated. Hopefully, the rate of progression of disease has been positively affected by the treatment rendered and, hence, previous attachment loss in relation to patient's age may be a more accurate indicator during SPT than before active periodontal treatment. Given the hypothesis that a dentition may be functional for the most likely life expectancy of the subject in the presence of a reduced height of periodontal support (i.e. 25–50% of the root length), the risk assessment in treated periodontal patients may represent a reliable prognostic indicator for the stability of the overall treatment goal of keeping a functional dentition for a lifetime (Papapanou *et al.* 1988).

The estimation of the loss of alveolar bone is performed in the posterior region on either periapical radiographs, in which the worst site affected is estimated gross as a percentage of the root length, or on bite-wing radiographs in which the worst site affected is estimated in millimeters. One millimeter is equated with 10% bone loss. The percentage is then divided by the patient's age. This results in a factor. As an example, a 40-year-old patient with 20% of bone loss at the worst posterior site affected would be scored BL/Age = 0.5. Another 40-year-old patient with 50% bone loss at the worst posterior site scores BL/Age = 1.25.

In assessing the patient's risk for disease progression, the extent of alveolar bone loss in relation to the patient's age is estimated as the fourth risk indicator for recurrent disease in the functional diagram of risk assessment (Fig. 59-3). The scale runs in increments of 0.25 of the factor BL/Age, with 0.5 being the division between low and moderate risk and 1.0 being the division between moderate and high risk for disease progression. This, in turn, means that a patient who has lost a higher percentage of posterior alveolar bone than his/her own age is at high risk regarding this vector in a multi-factorial assessment of risk.

Systemic conditions

The most substantiated evidence for modification of disease susceptibility and/or progression of periodontal disease arises from studies on type I and type II (insulin-dependent and non-insulin-dependent) diabetes mellitus populations (Gusberti *et al.* 1983; Emrich *et al.* 1991; Genco & Löe 1993).

It has to be realized that the impact of diabetes on periodontal diseases has been documented in patients with untreated periodontal disease, while, as of today, no clear evidence is available for treated patients. It is reasonable, however, to assume that the influence of systemic conditions may also affect recurrence of disease.

In recent years, genetic markers have become available to determine various genotypes of patients regarding their susceptibility for periodontal diseases. Research on the interleukin-1 (IL-1) polymorphisms has indicated that IL-1 genotype-positive patients show more advanced periodontitis lesions than IL-1 genotype-negative patients of the same age group (Kornman et al. 1997). Also, there is a trend to higher tooth loss in the IL-1 genotype-positive subjects (McGuire & Nunn 1999). In a retrospective analysis of over 300 well maintained periodontal patients, the IL-1 genotype-positive patients showed significantly higher BOP percentages and a higher proportion of patients which yielded higher BOP percentages during a 1-year recall period than the IL-1 genotype-negative control patients (Lang et al. 2000). Also, the latter group had twice as many patients with improved BOP percentages during the same maintenance period, indicating that IL-1 genotype-positive subjects do indeed represent a group of hyper-reactive subjects even if they are regularly maintained by effective SPT (Lang et al. 2000). In a prospective study over 5 years on Australian white collar and blue collar workers on a University campus, the IL-1 genotype-positive age group above 50 years showed significantly deeper probing depth than their IL-1 genotype-negative counterparts, especially when they were non-smokers.

In assessing the patient's risk for disease progression, systemic factors are only considered, if known, as the fifth risk indicator for recurrent disease in the functional diagram of risk assessment (Fig. 59-3). In this case, the area of high risk is marked for this vector. If not known or absent, systemic factors are not taken into account for the overall evaluation of risk.

Research on the association and/or modifying influence in susceptibility and progression of periodontitis of physical or psychologic stress is sparse (Cohen-Cole et al. 1981; Green et al. 1986; Freeman & Goss 1993). The hormonal changes associated with this condition, however, are well documented (Selye 1950).

Cigarette smoking

Consumption of tobacco, predominantly in the form of smoking or chewing, affects the susceptibility and the treatment outcome of patients with adult periodontitis. Classical explanations for these observations have included the association between smoking habits and poor oral hygiene as well as lack of awareness of general health issues (Pindborg 1949; Rivera-Hidalgo 1986). More recent evidence, however, has established that smoking per se represents not only a risk marker, but probably a true risk factor for peri-

odontitis (Ismail et al. 1983; Bergström 1989; Bergström et al. 1991; Haber et al. 1993). In a young population (19–30 years of age), 51–56% of periodontitis was associated with cigarette smoking (Haber et al. 1993). The association of smoking and periodontitis has been shown to be dose-dependent (Haber et al. 1993). It has also been shown that smoking will affect the treatment outcome after scaling and root planing (Preber & Bergström 1985), modified Widman flap surgery (Preber & Bergström 1990), and regenerative periodontal therapy (Tonetti et al. 1995). Furthermore, a high proportion of so-called refractory patients has been identified as consisting of smokers (Bergström & Blomlöf 1992). The impact of cigarette smoking on the long-term effects of periodontal therapy in a population undergoing supportive periodontal care has been reported. Smokers displayed less favorable healing responses both at re-evaluation and during a 6-year period of supportive periodontal care (Baumert-Ah et al. 1994). In spite of the paucity of evidence relating cigarette smoking to impaired outcomes during supportive periodontal care, it seems reasonable to incorporate heavy smokers (>20 cigarettes/day) in a higher risk group during maintenance.

In assessing the patient's risk for disease progression, environmental factors such as smoking must be considered as the sixth risk factor for recurrent disease in the functional diagram of risk assessment (Fig. 59-3). While non-smokers (NS) and former smokers (FS) (more than 5 years since cessation) have a relatively low risk for recurrence of periodontitis, the heavy smokers (HS), as defined by smoking more than one pack per day, are definitely at high risk. Occasional (OS; <10 cigarettes a day) and moderate smokers (MS) may be considered at moderate risk for disease progression.

Calculating the patient's individual periodontal risk assessment (PRA)

Based on the six parameters specified above, a multifunctional diagram is constructed for the PRA. In this diagram, the vectors have been constructed on the basis of the scientific evidence available. It is obvious that ongoing validation may result in slight modifications.

- A low periodontal risk (PR) patient has all parameters within the low-risk categories or at the most one parameter in the moderate-risk category (Fig. 59-3b).
- A moderate PR patient has at least two parameters in the moderate category, but at most one parameter in the high-risk category (Fig. 59-3c).
- A high PR patient has at least two parameters in the high-risk category (Fig. 59-3d).

Based on a 4-year prospective cohort study, the application of the multi-functional diagram for the subject-based PRA was validated (Persson *et al.* 2003) and, indeed, yielded complete periodontal stability after individually tailored recall intervals for all patients with a negative IL-1 gene polymorphism. For the IL-1 genotype-positive patients, however, the PRA resulted only in periodontal stability for 90% of the patients.

Summary: The subject risk assessment may estimate the risk for susceptibility for progression of periodontal disease. It consists of an assessment of the level of infection (full-mouth bleeding scores), the prevalence of residual periodontal pockets, tooth loss, an estimation of the loss of periodontal support in relation to the patient's age, an evaluation of the systemic conditions of the patient, and finally, an evaluation of environmental and behavioral factors such as smoking and stress. All these factors should be contemplated and evaluated together. A functional diagram (Fig. 59-3) may help the clinician in determining the risk for disease progression on the subject level. This may be useful in customizing the frequency and content of SPT visits.

Tooth risk assessment

Tooth position within the dental arch

Early clinical surveys have associated the prevalence and severity of periodontal diseases with malocclusion and irregularities of tooth position (Ditto & Hall 1954; Bilimoria 1963). However, many subsequent studies using clinical evaluation methods could not confirm these conclusions (Beagrie & James 1962; Geiger 1962; Gould & Picton 1966). Although a relationship between crowding and increased plaque retention and gingival inflammation has been established (Ingervall *et al.* 1977; Buckley 1980; Griffith & Addy 1981; Hörup *et al.* 1987), no significant correlation between anterior overjet and overbite (Geiger *et al.* 1973), crowding and spacing (Geiger *et al.* 1974) or axial inclinations and tooth drifts (Geiger & Wasserman 1980) and periodontal destruction, i.e. attachment loss subsequent to gingival inflammation, could be established. It is evident from the literature mentioned that crowding of teeth might eventually affect the amount of plaque mass formed in dentitions with irregular oral hygiene practices, thus contributing to the development of chronic gingivitis, but, as of today, it remains to be demonstrated whether tooth malposition within the dental arch will lead to an increased risk for periodontal attachment loss.

Furcation involvement

It is evident that multi-rooted teeth with periodontal lesions extending into the furcation area have been the subject of intensive therapeutic studies for many years (Kalkwarf & Reinhardt 1988). Retrospective analyses of large patient populations in private periodontal practices of periodontal specialists (Hirschfeld

& Wasserman 1978; McFall 1982) have clearly established that multi-rooted teeth appear to be at high risk for tooth loss during the maintenance phase. The most impressive long-term documentation maintained 600 patients for an average duration of 22 years, and 10% of these patients were even maintained for more than 30 years (Hirschfeld & Wasserman 1978). While 83% of the patients could be considered "well maintained" and had lost only 0–3 teeth during the observation period, a patient group of 4% (25) was identified with an extreme risk for disease progression and had lost between 10 and 23 teeth during a regularly scheduled maintenance program. Irrespective of the patient group of low, moderate, and high risk for disease progression during maintenance, the majority of the teeth lost were furcation-involved molars (Hirschfeld & Wasserman 1978). Similar results were obtained in a study on 100 treated periodontal patients maintained for 15 years or longer (McFall 1982).

Prospective studies on periodontal therapy in multi-rooted teeth have also revealed significant differences between non-molar sites and molar flat surfaces on the one hand and molar furcation sites on the other, when looking at the treatment outcomes evaluated as bleeding frequency, probing depth reductions, and levels of attachment (Nordland *et al.* 1987). Again, teeth with furcation involvement and original probing depths >6 mm had reduced treatment outcomes.

The assumption that the prognosis for single-rooted teeth and non-furcation-involved multi-rooted teeth is better than the prognosis for furcation-involved multi-rooted teeth was also confirmed by Ramfjord *et al.* (1987) in a prospective study over 5 years. It has to be realized, however, that these results are not intended to imply that furcation-involved teeth should be extracted, since all the prospective studies have documented a rather good overall prognosis for such teeth if regular supportive care is provided by a well organized maintenance program.

Iatrogenic factors

Overhanging restorations and ill fitting crown margins certainly represent an area for plaque retention, and there is an abundance of association studies documenting increased prevalence of periodontal lesions in the presence of iatrogenic factors (for review see Leon 1977). Depending on the supragingival or subgingival location of such factors, their influence on the risk for disease progression has to be considered. It has been established that slightly subgingivally located overhanging restorations will, indeed, change the ecologic niche, providing more favorable conditions for the establishment of a Gram-negative anaerobic microbiota (Lang *et al.* 1983). There is no doubt that shifts in the subgingival microflora towards a more periodontopathic microbiota, if unaffected by treatment, represent an increased risk for periodontal breakdown.

Residual periodontal support

Although many clinicians believe that teeth with reduced periodontal support are unable to function alone and should be extracted or splinted, there is clear evidence from longitudinal studies that teeth with severely reduced, but healthy, periodontal support can function either individually or as abutments for many years without any further loss of attachment (Nyman & Lindhe 1979; Nyman & Ericsson 1982; Brägger *et al.* 1990). Hence, successfully periodontally treated teeth can be maintained over decades and function as abutments in fixed bridgework or as individual chewing units irrespective of the amount of residual periodontal support, provided that physiologic masticatory forces do not subject such teeth to a progressive trauma which may lead to spontaneous extraction. Obviously, by virtue of the already reduced support, should disease progression occur in severely compromised teeth, this may lead to spontaneous tooth exfoliation.

Mobility

In light of the discussion of abutment teeth with severely reduced but healthy periodontal support, tooth mobility may be an indicator for progressive traumatic lesions, provided that the mobility is increasing continuously (Nyman & Lang 1994). When assessing tooth mobility, it has to be realized that two factors may contribute to hypermobility: (1) a widening of the periodontal ligament as a result of unidirectional or multidirectional forces to the crown, high and frequent enough to induce resorption of the alveolar bone walls; and (2) the height of the periodontal supporting tissues. If this is reduced due to prior periodontal disease, but the width of the periodontal ligament is unchanged, the amplitude of root mobility within the remaining periodontium is the same as in a tooth with normal height, but the leverage on the tooth following application of forces to the crown is changed. Therefore, it has to be realized that all teeth that have lost periodontal support have increased tooth mobility as defined by crown displacement upon application of a given force. Nevertheless, this hypermobility should be regarded as physiologic (Nyman & Lindhe 1976).

Since tooth mobility is probably more frequently affected by reduced periodontal height rather than unidirectional or multidirectional application of forces on the tooth, its significance for the evaluation of the periodontal conditions has to be questioned. Several studies have indicated that tooth mobility varies greatly before, during, and after periodontal therapy (Persson 1980, 1981a,b). From these studies it can be concluded that periodontally involved teeth show a decrease in mobility following non-surgical

and/or surgical periodontal procedures. However, following surgical procedures, tooth mobility may temporarily increase during the healing phase and may resume decreased values later on. Provisional splinting as an adjunct to non-surgical or surgical therapy does not seem to affect the final result of tooth mobility.

Summary: The tooth risk assessment encompasses an estimation of the residual periodontal support, an evaluation of tooth positioning, furcation involvements, presence of iatrogenic factors, and a determination of tooth mobility to evaluate functional stability. A risk assessment at tooth level may be useful in evaluating the prognosis and function of an individual tooth and may indicate the need for specific therapeutic measures during SPT visits.

Site risk assessment

Bleeding on probing

Absence of bleeding on probing (BOP) is a reliable parameter to indicate periodontal stability if the test procedure for assessing BOP has been standardized (Lang *et al.* 1990). Presence of bleeding upon standardized probing will indicate presence of gingival inflammation. Whether or not repeated BOP over time will predict the progression of a lesion is, however, questionable (Lang *et al.* 1986, 1990; Vanooteghem *et al.* 1987). Nevertheless, a 30% probability for attachment loss to occur in the future may be predicted for sites repeatedly positive for BOP (Fig. 59-5) (Badersten *et al.* 1985, 1990; Lang *et al.* 1986; Vanooteghem *et al.* 1987, 1990; Claffey *et al.* 1990).

Obviously, BOP is rather sensitive to different forces applied to the tissues. An almost linear relationship (R = 0.87) existed between the probing force

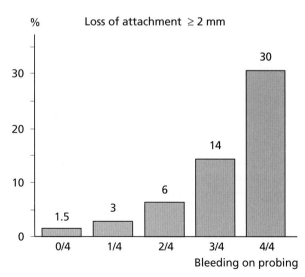

Fig. 59-5 Positive predictive values for loss of probing attachment of ≥2 mm in 2 years in sites which bled on probing 0, 1, 2, 3 or 4 times out of four SPT visits in a total of 48 patients following active periodontal therapy. (Data from Lang *et al.* 1986.)

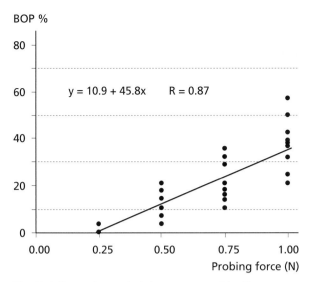

Fig. 59-6 Regression analysis between mean bleeding on probing (BOP) percentage and probing forces applied in young dental hygiene students with a healthy gingiva and normal anatomy. A very high correlation coefficient (R = 0.87) and an almost linear correlation between probing force and BOP percentage was found. (Data from Lang *et al.* 1991.)

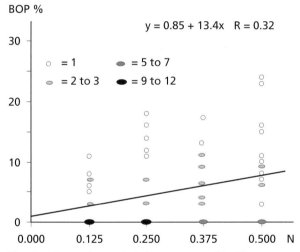

Fig. 59-7 Regression analysis between mean bleeding on probing (BOP) percentage and probing forces applied in subjects with successfully treated periodontitis: a reduced, but healthy, periodontium. (Data from Karayiannis *et al.* 1991.)

applied and the percentage of bleeding sites in a study on healthy young adults (Fig. 59-6) (Lang *et al.* 1991). If the probing force exceeded 0.25 N (25 g), the tissues were traumatized and bleeding was provoked as a result of trauma, rather than as a result of tissue alterations due to inflammation. To assess the "true" percentage of bleeding sites due to inflammation, a probing force of 0.25 N or less should be applied, which clinically means a light probing force. This has also been confirmed for patients who have experienced loss of attachment, i.e. with successfully treated advanced periodontitis (Fig. 59-7) (Karayiannis *et al.* 1991; Lang *et al.* 1991).

Since absence of BOP at 0.25 N indicated periodontal stability with a negative predictive value of 98–99% (Lang *et al.* 1990), this clinical parameter is the most reliable for monitoring patients over time in daily practice. Non-bleeding sites may be considered periodontally stable. On the other hand, bleeding sites seem to have an increased risk for progression of periodontitis, especially when the same site is bleeding at repeated evaluations over time (Lang *et al.* 1986; Claffey *et al.* 1990).

It is, therefore, advisable to register the sites with BOP in a dichotomous way using a constant force of 0.25 N. This allows the calculation of the mean BOP for the patient, and also yields the topographic location of the bleeding site. Repeated scores during maintenance will reveal the surfaces at higher risk for loss of attachment.

Probing depth and loss of attachment

Clinical probing is the most commonly used parameter both to document loss of attachment and to establish a diagnosis of periodontitis. There are, however, some sources of error inherent in this method which contribute to the variability in the measurements. Among these are (1) the dimension of the periodontal probe; (2) the placement of the probe and obtaining a reference point; (3) the crudeness of the measurement scale; (4) the probing force; and (5) the gingival tissue conditions.

In spite of the recognized method errors inherent in clinical probing, this diagnostic procedure has not only been the most commonly used but is also the most reliable parameter for the evaluation of the periodontal tissues. It has to be realized that increased probing depth and loss of probing attachment are parameters which reflect the history of periodontitis rather than its current state of activity. In order to obtain a more realistic assessment of the disease progression or, more commonly, the healing following therapy, multiple evaluations should be performed. Obviously, the first evaluation prior to therapy will yield results confounded by greater measurement error than evaluations following therapy. The reference point (cemento-enamel junction) may be obstructed by calculus or by dental restorations, and the condition of the gingival tissues may allow an easy penetration of the periodontal probe into the tissues, even though the probe position and force applied are standardized. These biologic variables (tissue conditions and calculus) may be minimized following initial periodontal therapy, and hence, repeated periodontal evaluations using probing will improve the metric assessment. The first periodontal evaluation after healing following initial periodontal therapy should, therefore, be taken as the baseline for long-term clinical monitoring (Claffey 1994).

Suppuration

In a proportion of periodontal lesions, pus will develop and may drain through the orifice of a pocket. This criterion of suppuration may be recognized while clinically probing the lesion, or preferably, by using a ball burnisher (Singh *et al.* 1977). Several longitudinal studies on the results of periodontal therapy have evaluated clinical parameters, including suppuration, for the prediction of future loss of attachment (Badersten *et al.* 1985, 1990; Claffey *et al.* 1990). In all these studies, the presence of suppuration increased the positive predictive value for disease progression in combination with other clinical parameters, such as BOP and increased probing depth. Hence, following therapy a suppurating lesion may provide evidence that the periodontitis site is undergoing a period of exacerbation (Kaldahl *et al.* 1990).

Summary: The tooth site risk assessment includes the registration of BOP, probing depth, loss of attachment, and suppuration. A risk assessment on the site level may be useful in evaluating periodontal disease activity and determining periodontal stability or ongoing inflammation. The site risk assessment is essential for the identification of the sites to be instrumented during SPT.

Radiographic evaluation of periodontal disease progression

As a consequence of the clinical risk assessments the decision may be made to gather radiographic information on the periodontal conditions as well (Hirschmann *et al.* 1994). The task may be related to a generalized pattern of disease progression or a localized monitoring. Not only periodontal aspects, but a comprehensive approach, should influence the choice of the radiographic technique (Rohlin & Akerblom 1992). Periodic radiographic surveys not based on clinical signs and symptoms should not be scheduled simply to confirm health.

Radiographic perception of periodontal changes is characterized by a high specificity, but a low sensitivity, with underestimation of the severity of a periodontal defect (Hämmerle *et al.* 1990; Åkesson *et al.* 1992). Undetectability of minute changes at the alveolar crest is related to overprojections and variations in projection geometry when taking repeated radiographs (Lang & Hill 1977; Goodson *et al.* 1984; Jenkins *et al.* 1992). This may result in mimicked variations in the alveolar bone height, obscured furcation status, etc. In addition, film processing variations may result in unreliable assessments of alveolar bone density changes (Rams *et al.* 1994).

The standard procedure for periodontal evaluations is based on a filmholder system with an alignment for long-cone paralleling technique (Rushton & Horner 1994). With the addition of simple pins to the filmholders as a repositioning reference, the methodologic error was impressively reduced (Carpio *et al.* 1994).

It is a fact that, in general, the standards in oral radiology related to agreement in the choice of a technique, the quality of film processing and the agreement in the diagnosis need to be improved (Brägger 1996).

Clinical implementation

The *three levels* of risk assessment presented represent a logic sequence of clinical evaluation to be performed prior to rendering treatment during maintenance. The information gathered from a stepwise evaluation should not impinge on, but should rather improve, the efficacy of secondary prophylactic periodontal care and treatment. A logical sequence of checks and examinations may be easily obtained in a short period of time and at no extra cost for laboratory tests. The information obtained from clinical monitoring and multi-level risk assessment facilitates an immediate appreciation of the periodontal health status of an individual and the possible risk for further infection and/or disease progression.

Most longitudinal studies published to date have been based on single-level, i.e. site or tooth, risk assessment, rather than accounting for the most evident factor in risk assessment: the patient. Ample evidence indicates that a minority of patients will continue to present problems and hence, differ completely from the maintenance pattern visualized in the majority of the patients. Even in the studies where this fact has been explicitly addressed (Hirschfeld & Wasserman 1978), the factors which determined whether or not a patient belonged to a well maintained group or to a group with continuous loss of periodontal attachment have not been identified.

Summary: It is suggested that patients be evaluated on the *three different levels* mentioned. At the patient level, loss of support in relation to patient age, full mouth plaque and/or bleeding scores, and prevalence of residual pockets are evaluated, together with the presence of systemic conditions or environmental factors, such as smoking, which can influence the prognosis. The clinical utility of this first level of risk assessment influences primarily the determination of the recall frequency and time requirements. It should also provide a perspective for the evaluation of risk assessment conducted at the tooth and site levels.

At the tooth and tooth site levels, residual periodontal support, inflammatory parameters and their persistence, presence of ecologic niches with difficult access such as furcations, and presence of iatrogenic factors have to be put into perspective with the patient overall risk profile (Fig. 59-8). The clinical utility of tooth and site risk assessment relates to rational allocation of the recall time available for therapeutic intervention to the sites with higher risk, and possibly to the selection of different forms of therapeutic intervention.

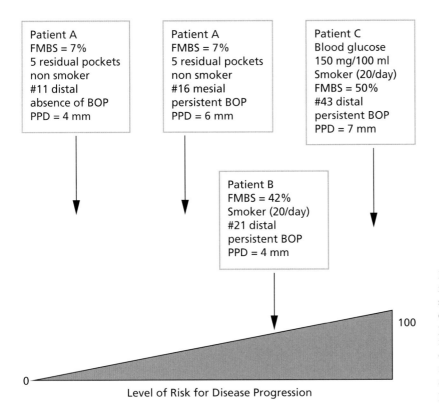

Patient A
FMBS = 7%
5 residual pockets
non smoker
#11 distal
absence of BOP
PPD = 4 mm

Patient A
FMBS = 7%
5 residual pockets
non smoker
#16 mesial
persistent BOP
PPD = 6 mm

Patient C
Blood glucose
150 mg/100 ml
Smoker (20/day)
FMBS = 50%
#43 distal
persistent BOP
PPD = 7 mm

Patient B
FMBS = 42%
Smoker (20/day)
#21 distal
persistent BOP
PPD = 4 mm

100

0

Level of Risk for Disease Progression

Fig. 59-8 Continuous multiple level risk assessment. Subject, tooth, and site parameters are combined to establish the clinical risk for disease progression. Note that different sites in the same patient may have a different level of risk. Subject-based risk factors are used to put the tooth and/or site risk assessment in perspective.

Objectives for SPT

The objective of maintenance care must be the continued preservation of gingival and periodontal health, obtained as a result of the active periodontal treatment. Irrespective of whether or not additional treatment such as prosthetic reconstructions or placement of implants has been rendered, the regular and adequate removal of supragingival plaque by the patient is, therefore, a prerequisite for a good long-term prognosis. In order to reach these goals, regular clinical re-evaluations with appropriate interceptive treatment, continued psychologic support and encouragement of the patient, and a lifelong commitment by the therapists are required.

General rules regarding frequency of maintenance care visits are difficult to define. However, there are a few aspects to consider in this respect: the patient's individual oral hygiene standard, the prevalence of sites exhibiting bleeding on probing, and the pre-therapeutic attachment level and alveolar bone height. This in turn means that patients with suboptimal plaque control and/or concomitant high prevalence of bleeding sites should be recalled more frequently than patients exhibiting excellent plaque control and healthy gingival tissues. Nevertheless, patients with healthy gingival conditions, but with a severely reduced height of periodontal support, should also be recalled with short time intervals (not exceeding 3–4 months) in order to exclude or at least reduce the risk of additional tooth loss. In most of the longitudinal studies referred to above, positive treatment results were maintained with regular maintenance care provided at 3–6-month intervals. It seems

reasonable to commence post-therapeutic maintenance with recall visits once every 3–4 months and then shorten or prolong these intervals in accordance with the aspects discussed above.

Since clinical attachment levels are usually stable 6 months following active periodontal therapy, it has been suggested that the first 6 months after completion of therapy be considered a healing phase (Westfelt *et al.* 1983b) during which frequent professional tooth-cleaning has been recommended. Following this healing phase, it is generally agreed to recall patients treated for periodontal disease at intervals of 3–4 months in a well organized system of SPT. It has to be realized that tissue contours may be subjected to remodeling processes despite stable clinical attachment levels and, hence, morphologic changes may still improve the accessibility of all tooth surfaces to oral hygiene practices for months and years. Proper oral hygiene practices appear to be the most important patient factor to guarantee long-term stability of treatment results (Knowles *et al.* 1979; Ramfjord *et al.* 1982, 1987; Lindhe & Nyman 1984). This, in turn, necessitates optimization of the patient's skills and continuous motivation and reinforcement to perform adequate mechanical oral hygiene practices, although chemical agents, such as the potent antiseptic chlorhexidine, may substitute and later complement the patient's efforts during the healing phase, when mechanical practices are difficult (Westfelt *et al.* 1983a). It is obvious that regular recall visits for SPT should be scheduled soon after completion of cause-related therapy, even if periodontal surgical procedures are still to be performed following a careful re-evaluation of the tissue response. To postpone the organization of a maintenance care program until corrective procedures such as surgery, endodontic, implant, operative or reconstructive therapy have been performed may reinforce a possible misconception of the patient that the professional visits to a therapist or hygienist guarantee positive treatment outcomes and optimal long-term prognosis rather than the patient's own regular performance of individually optimal and adequate oral hygiene practices.

SPT in daily practice

The recall hour should be planned to meet the patient's individual needs. It basically consists of four different sections which may require various amounts of time during a regularly scheduled visit:

1. Examination, re-evaluation, and diagnosis (ERD)
2. Motivation, reinstruction, and instrumentation (MRI)
3. Treatment of reinfected sites (TRS)
4. Polishing of the entire dentition, application of fluorides, and determination of future SPT (PFD).

The SPT recall hour (Fig. 59-9) is generally composed of 10–15 minutes of diagnostic procedures (ERD) followed by 30–40 minutes of motivation, reinstruction, and instrumentation (MRI) during which time the instrumentation is concentrated on the sites diagnosed with persistent inflammation. Treatment of reinfected sites (TRS) may include small surgical corrections, applications of local drug delivery devices or just intensive instrumentation under local anesthesia. Such procedures, if judged necessary, may require an additional appointment. The recall hour is normally concluded with polishing of the entire dentition, application of fluorides and another assessment of the situation, including the determination of future SPT visits (PFD). Approximately 5–10 minutes have to be reserved for this section.

Examination, re-evaluation, and diagnosis (ERD)

Since patients on SPT may experience significant changes in their health status and the use of medications, an update of the information on general health issues is appropriate. Changes in health status and medications should be noted. In middle-aged to elderly patients, especially, these aspects might influence the future management of the patient. An extra-oral and intraoral soft tissue examination should be performed at any SPT visit to detect any abnormalities and to act as a screening for oral cancer. The lateral borders of the tongue and the floor of the mouth should be inspected in particular. An evaluation of the patient's risk factors will also influence the choice of future SPT and the determination of the recall interval at the end of the maintenance visit. Following the assessment of the subject's risk factors,

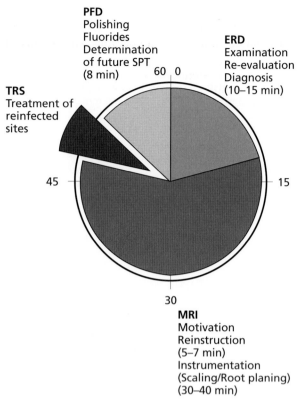

Fig. 59-9 The SPT recall hour is divided into four sections. (1) Examination, re-evaluation and diagnosis (ERD) providing information on stable and inflamed sites. This segment uses 10–15 minutes. (2) Motivation, reinstruction of oral hygiene where indicated, and instrumentation (MRI) will use the bulk of the recall hour (30–40 minutes). Sites which were diagnosed as not stable are instrumented. (3) Treatment of reinfected sites (TRS) may require a second appointment. (4) Polishing all tooth surfaces, application of fluorides and determination of the future recall interval (PFD) conclude the recall hour (5–10 minutes).

the tooth site-related risk factors are evaluated. As indicated above, the diagnostic procedure usually includes an assessment of the following:

1. The oral hygiene and plaque situation
2. The determination of sites with bleeding on probing, indicating persistent inflammation
3. The scoring of clinical probing depths and clinical attachment levels. The latter is quite time-consuming and requires the assessment of the location of the cemento-enamel junction as a reference mark on all (six) sites of each root. Therefore, an SPT evaluation usually only includes scoring of clinical probing depths
4. The inspection of reinfected sites with pus formation
5. The evaluation of existing reconstructions, including vitality checks for abutment teeth
6. The exploration for carious lesions.

All these evaluations are performed for both teeth and oral implants. Occasionally, conventional dental radiographs should be obtained at SPT visits. Especially for devitalized teeth, abutment teeth and oral implants, single periapical films exposed with a parallel and preferably standardized technique are of great value. Bite-wing radiographs are of special interest for caries diagnostic purposes. They also reveal plaque-retentive areas such as overhanging fillings and ill fitting crown margins. Since only approximately 10–15 minutes are available for this section, these assessments have to be performed in a well organized fashion. It is preferable to have a dental assistant available to note all the results of the diagnostic tests unless a voice-activated computer-assisted recording system is used.

Motivation, reinstruction, and instrumentation (MRI)

This aspect uses most of the available time of the SPT visit. When informed about the results of the diagnostic procedures, e.g. the total percentage of the BOP score or the number of pockets exceeding 4 mm, the patient may be motivated either in a confirmatory way in the case of low scores or in a challenging fashion in the case of high scores. Since encouragement usually has a greater impact on future positive developments than negative criticism, every effort should be made to acknowledge the patient's performance.

Patients who have experienced a relapse in their adequate oral hygiene practices need to be further motivated. Especially if the personal life situation has influenced the performance, positive encouragement is appropriate. Standard "lecturing" should be replaced by an individual approach.

Occasionally, patients present with hard tissue lesions (wedge-shaped dental defects) which suggest overzealous and/or faulty mechanical tooth cleaning (Fig. 59-10). Such habits should be broken and the patient reinstructed in toothbrushing techniques which emphasize vibratory rather than scrubbing movements.

Since it appears impossible to instrument 168 tooth sites in a complete dentition in the time allocated, only those sites which exhibit signs of inflammation and/or active disease progression will be re-instrumented during SPT visits. Hence, all the BOP-positive sites and all pockets with a probing depth exceeding 5 mm are carefully rescaled and root planed. Repeated instrumentation of healthy sites will inevitably result in mechanically caused continued loss of attachment (Lindhe *et al.* 1982a).

Similar observations were made in clinical studies by Claffey *et al.* (1988) where loss of clinical attachment levels immediately following instrumentation was observed in 24% of the sites. It is also known from regression analyses of several longitudinal studies (e.g. Lindhe *et al.* 1982b) that probing attachment may be lost following instrumentation of pockets below a "critical probing depth" of approximately 2.9 mm. Instrumentation of shallow sulci is, therefore, not recommended. As it has been shown

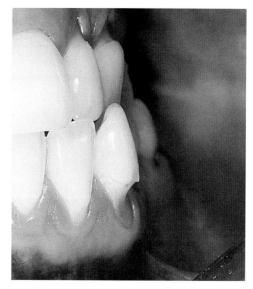

Fig. 59-10 Wedge-shaped defects apical to the cemento-enamel junction following recession of the gingival tissues resulting from overzealous or faulty toothbrushing.

in several studies that non-bleeding on probing sites represent stable sites (Lang *et al.* 1986, 1990; Joss *et al.* 1994), it appears reasonable to leave non-bleeding sites for polishing only and concentrate on periodontal sites with a positive BOP test or probing depths exceeding 5 mm. To protect the hard tissues, root planing should be performed with great caution. The deliberate removal of "contaminated" cementum during SPT is no longer justified (Nyman *et al.* 1986, 1988; Mombelli *et al.* 1995). During SPT visits, root surface instrumentation should be aimed especially at the removal of subgingival plaque rather than "diseased" cementum. This may require a more differentiated approach than hitherto recommended. In this respect, the use of ultrasonics may have to be re-evaluated.

Treatment of reinfected sites (TRS)

Single sites, especially furcation sites or sites with difficult access, may occasionally be reinfected and demonstrate suppuration. Such sites require a thorough instrumentation under anesthesia, the local application of antibiotics in controlled-release devices or even open debridement with surgical access. It is evident that such therapeutic procedures may be too time-consuming to be performed during the routine recall hour, and hence, it may be necessary to reschedule the patient for another appointment. Omission of thorough retreatment of such sites or only performing incomplete root instrumentation during SPT may result in continued loss of probing attachment (Kaldahl *et al.* 1988; Kalkwarf *et al.* 1989).

Treatment choices for reinfected sites should be based on an analysis of the causes most likely responsible for the reinfection.

Generalized reinfections are usually the result of inadequate SPT. Although not all sites positive for

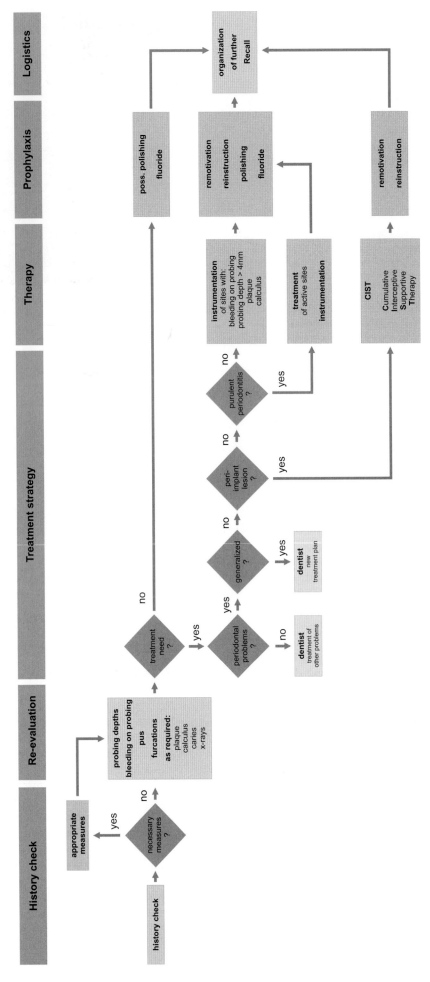

Fig. 59-11 Flow sheet of supportive periodontal therapy (SPT) with strategic decision tree for the recall visit.

BOP may further progress and lose attachment, high BOP percentages call for more intensive care and more frequent SPT visits. Sometimes, a second visit 2–3 weeks after the recall may be indicated to check the patient's performance in oral home care. It is particularly important to supervise patients closely for advanced periodontitis if they have a high subject risk assessment (Westfelt *et al.* 1983b; Ramfjord 1987).

Local reinfections may either be the result of inadequate plaque control in a local area or the formation of ecologic niches conducive to periodontal pathogens. The risk assessment on the tooth level may identify such niches which are inaccessible for regular oral hygiene practices. Furcation involvements often represent special periodontal risk factors which may require additional therapy to be performed following diagnosis in the regular SPT visit.

Polishing, fluorides, determination of recall interval (PFD)

The recall hour is concluded with polishing the entire dentition to remove all remaining soft deposits and stains. This may provide freshness to the patient and facilitates the diagnosis of early carious lesions. Following polishing, fluorides should be applied in high concentration in order to replace the fluorides which might have been removed by instrumentation from the superficial layers of the teeth. Fluoride or chlorhexidine varnishes may also be applied to prevent root surface caries, especially in areas with gingival recession. The determination of future SPT visits must be based on the patient's risk assessment.

Summary: Figure 59-11 provides a flowchart for SPT. The SPT recall hour is divided into four sections. While the first 10–15 minutes are reserved for examination, re-evaluation and diagnosis, the second and most time-consuming section of 30–40 minutes is devoted to reinstruction and instrumentation of sites at risk identified in the diagnostic process. Some reinfected sites may require further treatment, and hence, the patient may have to be rescheduled for an additional appointment. The recall hour is concluded by polishing the dentition, applying fluorides and determining the frequency of future SPT visits.

References

Åkesson, L., Håkonsson, J. & Rohlin, M. (1992). Comparison of panoramic and intraoral radiography and pocket probing for the measurement of alveolar bone. *Journal of Clinical Periodontology* **19**, 326–332.

Axelsson, P. & Lindhe, J. (1981a). Effect of controlled oral hygiene procedures on caries and periodontal disease in adults. Results after 6 years. *Journal of Clinical Periodontology* **8**, 239–248.

Axelsson, P. & Lindhe, J. (1981b). The significance of maintenance care in the treatment of periodontal disease. *Journal of Clinical Periodontology* **8**, 281–294.

Axelsson, P., Lindhe, J. & Nyström, B. (1991). On the prevention of caries and periodontal disease. Results of a 15-year longitudinal study in adults. *Journal of Clinical Periodontology* **18**, 182–189.

Axelsson, P., Nyström, B. & Lindhe, J. (2004). The long-term effect of a plaque control program on tooth mortality, caries and periodontal disease in adults. Results after 30 years of maintenance. *Journal of Clinical Periodontology* **31**, 749–757.

Badersten, A., Egelberg, J. & Koch, G. (1975). Effects of monthly prophylaxis on caries and gingivitis in school children. *Community Dentistry and Oral Epidemiology* **3**, 1–4.

Badersten, A., Nilvéus, R. & Egelberg, J. (1981). Effect of non-surgical periodontal therapy. I. Moderately advanced periodontitis. *Journal of Clinical Periodontology* **8**, 57–72.

Badersten, A., Nilvéus, R. & Egelberg, J. (1985). Effect of non-surgical periodontal therapy. (VII) Bleeding, suppuration and probing depths in sites with probing attachment loss. *Journal of Clinical Periodontology* **12**, 432–440.

Badersten, A., Nilvéus, R. & Egelberg, J. (1987). Effect of non-surgical periodontal therapy. (VIII) Probing attachment changes related to clinical characteristics. *Journal of Clinical Periodontology* **14**, 425–437.

Badersten, A., Nilvéus, R. & Egelberg, J. (1990). Scores of plaque, bleeding, suppuration and probing depth to predict probing attachment loss. *Journal of Clinical Periodontology* **17**, 102–107.

Baumert-Ah, M., Johnson, G., Kaldahl, W., Patil, K. & Kalkwarf, K. (1994). The effect of smoking on the response to periodontal therapy. *Journal of Clinical Periodontology* **21**, 91–97.

Beagrie, G. & James, G. (1962). The association of posterior tooth irregularities and periodontal disease. *British Dental Journal* **113**, 239–243.

Becker, B., Karp, C., Becker, W. & Berg, L. (1988). Personality differences and stressful life events. Differences between treated periodontal patients with and without maintenance. *Journal of Clinical Periodontology* **15**, 49–52.

Becker, W., Becker, B.E. & Berg, L.E. (1984). Periodontal treatment without maintenance. A retrospective study in 44 patients. *Journal of Periodontology* **55**, 505–509.

Becker, W., Berg, L.E. & Becker, B.E. (1979). Untreated periodontal disease: A longitudinal study. *Journal of Periodontology* **50**, 234–244.

Bellini, H., Campi, R. & Denardi, J. (1981). Four years of monthly professional tooth cleaning and topical fluoride application in Brazilian school children. *Journal of Clinical Periodontology* **8**, 231–238.

Bergström, J. (1989). Cigarette smoking as a risk factor in chronic periodontal disease. *Journal of Clinical Periodontology* **17**, 245–247.

Bergström, J. & Blomlöf, L. (1992). Tobacco smoking a major risk factor associated with refractory periodontal disease. *Journal of Dental Research* **71** (spec issue), 297 #1530 (IADR Abstr).

Bergström, J., Eliasson, S. & Preber, H. (1991). Cigarette smoking and periodontal bone loss. *Journal of Periodontology* **62**, 242–246.

Bilimoria, K. (1963). Malocclusion – Its role in the causation of periodontal disease. *Journal of the All-India Dental Association* **35**, 293–300.

Brägger, U. (1996). Radiographic diagnosis of periodontal disease progression. *Current Opinions in Dentistry* 3, 59–67.

Brägger, U., Håkanson, D. & Lang, N.P. (1992). Progression of periodontal disease in patients with mild to moderate adult periodontitis. *Journal of Clinical Periodontology* 19, 659–666.

Brägger, U., Nyman, S., Lang, N.P., von Wyttenbach, T., Salvi, G. & Schürch, Jr. E. (1990). The significance of alveolar bone in periodontal disease. A long-term observation in patients with cleft lip, alveolus and palate. *Journal of Clinical Periodontology* 17, 379–384.

Buckley, L. (1980). The relationship between irregular teeth, plaque, calculus and gingival disease. A study of 300 subjects. *British Dental Journal* 148, 67–69.

Carpio, L.C., Hausmann, E., Dunford, R.G., Allen, R.M. & Christensson, L.A. (1994). Evaluation of a simple modified radiographic alignment system for routine use. *Journal of Periodontology* 65, 62–67.

Caton, J.G., Proye, M. & Polson, A.M. (1982). Maintenance of healed periodontal pockets after a single episode of root planing. *Journal of Periodontology* 53, 420–424.

Checchi, L., Pellicioni, G., Gatto, M. & Kelescian, L. (1994). Patient compliance with maintenance therapy in an Italian periodontal practice. *Journal of Clinical Periodontology* 21, 309–312.

Claffey, N. (1991). Decision making in periodontal therapy. The re-evaluation. *Journal of Clinical Periodontology* 18, 384–389.

Claffey, N. (1994). Gold Standard clinical and radiographical assessment of disease activity. In: Lang, N. & Karring, T., eds. *Proceedings of the 1st European Workshop on Periodontology*. London: Quintessence, pp. 42–53.

Claffey, N., Loos, B., Gantes, B., Martin, M., Heins, P. & Egelberg, J. (1988). The relative effects of therapy and periodontal disease on loss of probing attachment after root debridement. *Journal of Clinical Periodontology* 15, 163–169.

Claffey, N., Nylund, K., Kiger, R., Garrett, S. & Egelberg, J. (1990). Diagnostic predictability of scores of plaque, bleeding, suppuration, and probing pocket depths for probing attachment loss. 3½ years of observation following initial therapy. *Journal of Clinical Periodontology* 17, 108–114.

Cohen-Cole, S., Cogen, R., Stevens, A., Kirk, K., Gaitan, E., Hain, J. & Freeman, A. (1981). Psychosocial, endocrine and immune factors in acute necrotizing ulcerative gingivitis. *Psychosomatic Medicine* 43, 91.

Cortellini, P., Pini Prato, G. & Tonetti, M. (1994). Periodontal regeneration of human infrabony defects. V. Effect of oral hygiene on long term stability. *Journal of Clinical Periodontology* 21, 606–610.

Cortellini, P., Pini Prato, G. & Tonetti, M. (1996). Long term stability of clinical attachment following guided tissue regeneration and conventional therapy. *Journal of Clinical Periodontology* 23, 106–111.

Cullinan, M.P., Westermann, B., Hamlet, S.P., Palmer J.E., Faddy, M.J., Lang, N.P. & Seymour, G.J. (2001). A longitudinal study of interleukin-1 gene polymorphisms and periodontal disease in a general adult population. *Journal of Clinical Periodontology* 28, 1137–1144.

Demetriou, N., Tsami-Pandi, A. & Parashis, A. (1995). Compliance with supportive periodontal treatment in private periodontal practice. A 14-year retrospective study. *Journal of Periodontology* 66, 145–149.

De Vore, C.H., Duckworth, J.E., Beck, F.M., Hicks, M.J., Brumfield, F.W. & Horton, J.E. (1986). Bone loss following periodontal therapy in subjects without frequent periodontal maintenance. *Journal of Periodontology* 57, 354–359.

Ditto, W. & Hall, D. (1954). A survey of 143 periodontal cases in terms of age and malocclusion. *American Journal of Orthodontics* 40, 234–243.

Emrich, L., Schlossman, M. & Genco, R. (1991). Periodontal disease in non-insulin dependent diabetes mellitus. *Journal of Periodontology* 62, 123–130.

Fauchard, P. (1746). *Le Chirurgien Dentiste, au Traité des Dents*. Chap. XI. Paris: P-J Mariette, pp. 177–182.

Freeman, R. & Goss, S. (1993). Stress measures as predictors of periodontal disease – a preliminary communication. *Community Dentistry and Oral Epidemiology* 21, 176–177.

Geiger, A. (1962). Occlusal studies in 188 consecutive cases of periodontal disease. *American Journal of Orthodontics* 48, 330–360.

Geiger, A. & Wassermann, B. (1980). Relationship of occlusion and periodontal disease. Part XI. Relation of axial inclination (mesial-distal) and tooth drift to periodontal status. *Journal of Periodontology* 51, 283–290.

Geiger, A., Wasserman, B. & Turgeon, L. (1973). Relationship of occlusion and periodontal disease. Part VI. Relation of anterior overjet and overbite to periodontal destruction and gingival inflammation. *Journal of Periodontology* 44, 150–157.

Geiger, A., Wassermann, B. & Turgeon, L. (1974). Relationship of occlusion and gingival inflammation. *Journal of Periodontology* 45, 43–49.

Genco, R. & Löe, H. (1993). The role of systemic conditions and disorders in periodontal disease. *Periodontology 2000* 2, 98–116.

Goodson, J.M., Haffajee, A.D. & Socransky, S.S. (1984). The relationship between attachment level loss and alveolar bone loss. *Journal of Clinical Periodontology* 11, 348–359.

Gould, M. & Picton, D. (1966). The relation between irregularities of teeth and periodontal disease. *British Dental Journal* 121, 20–23.

Green, L., Tryon, W., Marks, B. & Huryn, J. (1986). Periodontal disease as a function of life events stress. *Journal of Human Stress* 12, 32–36.

Griffith, G. & Addy, M. (1981). Effects of malalignment of teeth in the anterior segments on plaque accumulation. *Journal of Clinical Periodontology* 8, 481–490.

Gusberti, F.A., Syed, S.A., Bacon, G., Grossman, N. & Loesche, W.J. (1983). Puberty gingivitis in insulin-dependent diabetic children. I. Cross-sectional observations. *Journal of Periodontology* 54, 714–720.

Haber, J., Wattles, J., Crowley, M., Mandell, R., Joshipura, K. & Kent, R. (1993). Evidence for cigarette smoking as a major risk factor for periodontitis. *Journal of Periodontology* 64, 16–23.

Hämmerle, C.H.F., Ingold, H-P. & Lang, N.P. (1990). Evaluation of clinical and radiographic scoring methods before and after initial periodontal therapy. *Journal of Clinical Periodontology* 17, 255–263.

Hämmerle, C.H.F., Ungerer, M.C., Fantoni, P.C., Brägger, U., Bürgin, W. & Lang, N.P. (2000). Long-term analysis of biological and technical aspects of fixed partial dentures with cantilevers. *International Journal of Prosthodontics* 13, 409–415.

Hill, R.W., Ramfjord, S.P., Morrison, E.C., Appleberry, E.A., Caffesse, R.G., Kerry, G.J. & Nissle, R.R. (1981). Four types of periodontal treatment compared over two years. *Journal of Periodontology* 52, 655–677.

Hirschfeld, L. & Wasserman, B. (1978). A long-term survey of tooth loss in 600 treated periodontal patients. *Journal of Periodontology* 49, 225–237.

Hirschmann, P.N., Horner, K. & Rushton, V.E. (1994). Selection criteria for periodontal radiography. *Journal of Clinical Periodontology* 176, 324–325.

Hörup, N., Melsen, B. & Terp, S. (1987). Relationship between malocclusion and maintenance of teeth. *Community Dentistry and Oral Epidemiology* 15, 74–78.

Ingervall, B., Jacobsson, U. & Nyman, S. (1977). A clinical study of the relationship between crowding of teeth, plaque and gingival conditions. *Journal of Clinical Periodontology* 4, 214–222.

Isidor, F. & Karring, T. (1986). Long-term effect of surgical and non-surgical periodontal treatment. A 5-year clinical study. *Journal of Periodontal Research* 21, 462–472.

Ismail, A.L., Burt, B.A. & Eklund, S.A. (1983). Epidemiologic patterns of smoking and periodontal disease in the United

States. *Journal of the Alabama Dental Association* **106**, 617–621.

Jenkins, S.M., Dammer, P.M. & Addy, M. (1992). Radiographic evaluation of early periodontal bone loss in adolescents. An overview. *Journal of Clinical Periodontology* **19**, 363–366.

Joss, A., Adler, R. & Lang, N.P. (1994). Bleeding on probing. A parameter for monitoring periodontal conditions in clinical practice. *Journal of Clinical Periodontology* **21**, 402–408.

Kaldahl, W.B., Kalkwarf, K.L., Patil, K.D., Dyer, J.K. & Bates, R.E. (1988). Evaluation of four modalities of periodontal therapy. Mean probing depth, probing attachment level and recession changes. *Journal of Periodontology* **59**, 783–793.

Kaldahl, W., Kalkwarf, K., Patil, K.D. & Molvar, M. (1990). Evaluation of gingival suppuration and supragingival plaque following 4 modalities of periodontal therapy. *Journal of Clinical Periodontology* **17**, 642–649.

Kalkwarf, K.L., Kaldahl, W.B., Patil, K.D. & Molvar, M.P. (1989). Evaluation of gingival bleeding following 4 types of periodontal therapy. *Journal of Clinical Periodontology* **16**, 601–608.

Kalkwarf, K. & Reinhardt, R. (1988). The furcation problem: current controversies and future directions. *Dental Clinics of North America* **22**, 243–266.

Karayiannis, A., Lang, N.P., Joss, A. & Nyman, S. (1991). Bleeding on probing as it relates to probing pressures and gingival health in patients with a reduced but healthy periodontium. A clinical study. *Journal of Clinical Periodontology* **19**, 471–475.

Käyser, A.F. (1981). Shortened dental arches and oral function. *Journal of Oral Rehabilitation* **8**, 457–462.

Käyser, A.F. (1994). Limited treatment goals – shortened dental arches. *Periodontology 2000* **4**, 7–14.

Käyser, A.F. (1996). Teeth, tooth loss and prosthetic appliances. In: Øwall, B., Käyser, A.F. & Carlsson, G.E., eds. *Prosthodontics: Principles and Management Strategies*. London: Mosby-Wolfe, pp. 35–48.

Kerr, N.W. (1981). Treatment of chronic periodontitis. 45% failure rate. *British Dental Journal* **150**, 222–224.

Knowles, J.W. (1973). Oral hygiene related to long-term effects of periodontal therapy. *Journal of the Michigan State Dental Association* **55**, 147–150.

Knowles, J.W., Burgett, F.G., Morrison, E.C., Nissle, R.R. & Ramfjord, S.P. (1980). Comparison of results following three modalities of periodontal therapy related to tooth type and initial pocket depth. *Journal of Clinical Periodontology* **7**, 32–47.

Knowles, J.W., Burgett, F.G., Nissle, R.R., Shick, R.A., Morrison, E.C. & Ramfjord, S.P. (1979). Results of periodontal treatment related to pocket depth and attachment level. Eight years. *Journal of Periodontology* **50**, 225–233.

Kornman, K. & Löe, H. (1993). The role of local factors in the etiology of periodontal dieases. *Periodontology 2000* **2**, 83–97.

Kornman, K.S., Crane, A., Wang, H.Y., di Giovine, F.S., Newman, M.G., Pirk, F.W., Wilson, T.G. Jr., Higginbottom, F.L. & Duff, G.W. (1997). The interleukin-1 genotype as a severity factor in adult periodontal disease. *Journal of Clinical Periodontology* **24**, 72–77.

Lang, N.P., Adler, R., Joss, A. & Nyman, S. (1990). Absence of bleeding on probing. An indicator of periodontal stability. *Journal of Clinical Periodontology* **17**, 714–721.

Lang, N.P. & Hill, R.W. (1977). Radiographs in periodontics. *Journal of Clinical Periodontology* **4**, 16–28.

Lang, N.P., Joss, A., Orsanic, T., Gusberti, F.A. & Siegrist, B.E. (1986). Bleeding on probing. A predictor for the progression of periodontal disease? *Journal of Clinical Periodontology* **13**, 590–596.

Lang, N.P., Kiel, R. & Anderhalden, K. (1983). Clinical and microbiological effects of subgingival restorations with overhanging or clinically perfect margins. *Journal of Clinical Periodontology* **10**, 563–578.

Lang, N.P., Nyman, S., Senn, C. & Joss, A. (1991). Bleeding on probing as it relates to probing pressure and gingival health. *Journal of Clinical Periodontology* **18**, 257–261.

Lang, N.P. & Tonetti, M.S. (2003). Periodontal risk assessment for patients in supportive periodontal therapy (SPT). *Oral Health and Preventive Dentistry* **1**, 7–16.

Lang, N.P., Tonetti, M.S., Suter, J., Duff, G.W. & Kornmann, K.S. (2000). Effect of interleukin-1 gene polymorphisms on gingival inflammation assessed by bleeding on probing in a periodontal maintenance population. *Journal for Periodontal Research* **35**, 102–107.

Langer, B., Stein, S.D. & Wagenberg, B. (1981). An evaluation of root resections: A ten-year study. *Journal of Periodontology* **52**, 719–722.

Laurell, K., Lundgren, D., Falk, H. & Hugoson, A. (1991). Long-term prognosis of extensive poly-unit cantilevered fixed partial dentures. *Journal of Prosthetic Dentistry* **66**, 545–552.

Leon, A. (1977). The periodontium and restorative procedures. A critical review. *Journal of Oral Rehabilitation* **21**, 105–117.

Lindhe, J., Hamp, S-E. & Löe, H. (1975). Plaque induced periodontal disease in beagle dogs. A 4-year clinical, roentgenographical and histometric study. *Journal of Periodontal Research* **10**, 243–253.

Lindhe, J. & Nyman, S. (1975). The effect of plaque control and surgical pocket elimination on the establishment and maintenance of periodontal health. A longitudinal study of periodontal therapy in cases of advanced disease. *Journal of Clinical Periodontology* **2**, 67–79.

Lindhe, J. & Nyman, S. (1984). Long-term maintenance of patients treated for advanced periodontal disease. *Journal of Clinical Periodontology* **11**, 504–514.

Lindhe, J., Nyman, S. & Karring, T. (1982a). Scaling and root planing in shallow pockets. *Journal of Clinical Periodontology* **9**, 415–418.

Lindhe, J., Socransky, S.S., Nyman, S., Haffajee, A. & Westfelt, E. (1982b). "Critical probing depths" in periodontal therapy. *Journal of Clinical Periodontology* **9**, 323–336.

Lindhe, J., Westfelt, E., Nyman, S., Socransky, S.S., Heijl, L. & Bratthall, G. (1982c). Healing following surgical/non-surgical treatment of periodontol disease. A clinical study. *Journal of Clinical Periodontology* **9**, 115–128.

Listgarten, M.A. & Helldén, L. (1978). Relative distribution of bacteria at clinically healthy and periodontally diseased sites in humans. *Journal of Clinical Periodontology* **5**, 115–132.

Listgarten, M.A. & Levin, S. (1981). Positive correlation between the proportions of subgingival spirochetes and motile bacteria and susceptibility of human subjects to periodontal deterioration. *Journal of Clinical Periodontology* **8**, 122–138.

Listgarten, M.A., Lindhe, J. & Helldén, L. (1978). Effect of tetracycline and/or scaling on human periodontal disease. Clinical, microbiological and histological observations. *Journal of Clinical Periodontology* **5**, 246–271.

Listgarten, M.A. & Schifter, C. (1982). Differential darkfield microscopy of subgingival bacteria as an aid in selecting recall intervals: Results after 18 months. *Journal of Clinical Periodontology* **9**, 305–316.

Löe, H., Ånerud, Å., Boysen, H. & Smith, M. (1978). The natural history of periodontal disease in man. The role of periodontal destruction before 40 years. *Journal of Periodontal Research* **49**, 607–620.

Löe, H., Ånerud, Å., Boysen, H. & Morrison, E.C. (1986). Natural history of periodontal disease in man. Rapid, moderate and no loss of attachment in Sri Lankan laborers 14–46 years of age. *Journal of Clinical Periodontology* **13**, 431–440.

Löe, H. & Silness, J. (1963). Periodontal disease in pregnancy. I. Prevalence and severity. *Acta Odontologica Scandinavia* **21**, 533–551.

Löe, H., Theilade, E. & Jensen, S.B. (1965). Experimental gingivitis in man. *Journal of Periodontology* **36**, 177–187.

Lövdal, A., Arnö, A., Schei, O. & Waerhaug, J. (1961). Combined effect of subgingival scaling and controlled oral hygiene on the incidence of gingivitis. *Acta Odontologica Scandinavia* **19**, 537–553.

Magnusson, I., Lindhe, J., Yoneyama, T. & Liljenberg, B. (1984). Recolonization of a subgingival microbiota following scaling in deep pockets. *Journal of Clinical Periodontology* **11**, 193–207.

McFall, W.T. (1982). Tooth loss in 100 treated patients with periodontal disease in a long-term study. *Journal of Periodontology* **53**, 539–549.

McGuire, M.K. & Nunn, M.E. (1999). Prognosis versus actual outcome. IV. The effectiveness of clinical parameters and IL-1 genotype in accurately predicting prognoses and tooth survival. *Journal of Periodontology* **70**, 49–56.

Mendoza, A., Newcomb, G. & Nixon, K. (1991). Compliance with supportive periodontal therapy. *Journal of Periodontology* **62**, 731–736.

Mombelli, A., Nyman, S., Brägger, U., Wennström, J. & Lang, N.P. (1995). Clinical and microbiological changes associated with an altered subgingival environment induced by periodontal pocket reduction. *Journal of Clinical Periodontology* **22**, 780–787.

Morrison, E.C., Lang, N.P., Löe, H. & Ramfjord, S.P. (1979). Effects of repeated scaling and root planing and/or controlled oral hygiene on the periodontal attachment level and pocket depth in beagle dogs. I. Clinical findings. *Journal of Periodontal Research* **14**, 428–437.

Moser, P., Hämmerle, C.H.F., Lang, N.P., Schlegel-Bregenzer, B. & Persson, R.G. (2002). Maintenance of periodontal attachment levels in prosthetically treated patients with gingivitis or moderate chronic periodontitis 5–17 years post therapy. *Journal of Clinical Periodontology* **29**, 531–539.

Mousquès, T., Listgarten, M.A. & Phillips, R.W. (1980). Effect of scaling and root planing on the composition of the human subgingival microbial flora. *Journal of Periodontal Research* **15**, 144–151.

Mühlemann, H.R. & Son, S. (1971). Gingival sulcus bleeding – a leading symptom in initial gingivitis. *Helvetica Odontologica Acta* **15**, 107–113.

Nordland, P., Garret, S., Kiger, R., Vanooteghem, R., Hutchens, L.H. & Egelberg, J. (1987). The effect of plaque control and root debridement in molar teeth. *Journal of Clinical Periodontology* **14**, 231–236.

Nyman, S. & Ericsson, I. (1982). The capacity of reduced periodontal tissues to support fixed bridgework. *Journal of Clinical Periodontology* **9**, 409–414.

Nyman, S. & Lang, N.P. (1994). Tooth mobility and biological rationale for splinting teeth. *Periodontology 2000* **4**, 15–22.

Nyman, S. & Lindhe, J. (1976). Persistent tooth hypermobility following completion of periodontal treatment. *Journal of Clinical Periodontology* **3**, 81–93.

Nyman, S. & Lindhe, J. (1979). A longitudinal study of combined periodontal and prosthetic treatment of patients with advanced periodontal disease. *Journal of Periodontology* **50**, 163–169.

Nyman, S., Lindhe, J. & Rosling, B. (1977). Periodontal surgery in plaque-infected dentitions. *Journal of Clinical Periodontology* **4**, 240–249.

Nyman, S., Rosling, B. & Lindhe, J. (1975). Effect of professional tooth cleaning on healing after periodontal surgery. *Journal of Clinical Periodontology* **2**, 80–86.

Nyman, S., Sarhed, G., Ericsson, I., Gottlow, J. & Karring, T. (1986). The role of "diseased" root cementum for healing following treatment of periodontal disease. *Journal of Periodontal Research* **21**, 496–503.

Nyman, S., Westfelt, E., Sarhed, G. & Karring, T. (1988). Role of "diseased" root cementum in healing following treatment of periodontal disease. A clinical study. *Journal of Clinical Periodontology* **15**, 464–468.

Papapanou, P., Wennström, J. & Gröndahl, K. (1988). Periodontal status in relation to age and tooth type. A cross-sectional radiographic study. *Journal of Clinical Periodontology* **15**, 469–478.

Persson, G.R., Matulienė, G., Ramseier, C.A., Persson, R.E., Tonetti, M.S. & Lang, N.P. (2003). Influence of interleukin-1 gene polymorphism on the outcome of supportive periodontal therapy explored by a multi-factorial periodontal risk assessment model (PRA). *Oral Health and Preventive Dentistry* **1**, 17–27.

Persson, R. (1980). Assessment of tooth mobility using small loads. II. Effect of oral hygiene procedures. *Journal of Clinical Periodontology* **7**, 506–515.

Persson, R. (1981a). Assessment of tooth mobility using small loads. III. Effect of periodontal treatment including a gingivectomy procedure. *Journal of Clinical Periodontology* **8**, 4–11.

Persson, R. (1981b). Assessment of tooth mobility using small loads. IV. The effect of periodontal treatment including gingivectomy and flap procedures. *Journal of Clinical Periodontology* **8**, 88–97.

Pihlström, B.L., McHugh, R.B., Oliphant, T.H. & Ortiz-Campos, C. (1983). Comparison of surgical and non-surgical treatment of periodontal disease. A review of current studies and additional results after 6½ years. *Journal of Clinical Periodontology* **10**, 524–541.

Pindborg, J. (1949). Correlation between consumption of tobacco, ulcero-membraneous gingivitis and calculus. *Journal of Dental Research* **28**, 461–463.

Poulsen, S., Agerbaek, N., Melsen, B., Korts, D., Glavind, L. & Rölla, G. (1976). The effect of professional tooth cleaning on gingivitis and dental caries in children after 1 year. *Community Dentistry and Oral Epidemiology* **4**, 195–199.

Preber, H. & Bergström, J. (1985). The effect of non-surgical treatment on periodontal pockets in smokers and nonsmokers. *Journal of Clinical Periodontology* **13**, 319–323.

Preber, H. & Bergström, J. (1990). Effect of cigarette smoking on periodontal healing following surgical therapy. *Journal of Clinical Periodontology* **17**, 324–328.

Ramfjord, S.P. (1987). Maintenance care for treated periodontitis patients. *Journal of Clinical Periodontology* **14**, 433–437.

Ramfjord, S.P., Caffesse, R.G., Morrison, E.C., Hill, R., Kerry, G.J., Appleberry, E., Nissle, R.R. & Stults, J. (1987). Four modalities of periodontal treatment compared over 5 years. *Journal of Clinical Periodontology* **14**, 445–452.

Ramfjord, S.P., Knowles, J.W., Nissle, R.R., Shick, R.A. & Burgett, F.G. (1975). Results following three modalities of periodontal therapy. *Journal of Periodontology* **46**, 522–526.

Ramfjord, S.P., Morrison, E.C., Burgett, F.G., Nissle, R.R., Shick, R.A., Zann, G.J. & Knowles, J.W. (1982). Oral hygiene and maintenance of periodontal support. *Journal of Periodontology* **53**, 26–30.

Ramfjord, S.P., Nissle, R.R., Shick, R.A. & Cooper, H. (1968). Subgingival curettage versus surgical elimination of periodontal pockets. *Journal of Periodontology* **39**, 167–175.

Rams, T.E., Listgarten, M.A. & Slots, J. (1994). Utility of radiographic crestal lamina dura for predicting periodontal disease activity. *Journal of Clinical Periodontology* **21**, 571–576.

Randow, K., Glantz, P-O. & Zöger, B. (1986). Technical failures and some related clinical complications in extensive fixed prosthodontics. *Acta Odontologica Scandinavia* **44**, 241–255.

Rivera-Hidalgo, F. (1986). Smoking and periodontal disease. *Journal of Periodontology* **57**, 617–624.

Rohlin, M. & Akerblom, A. (1992). Individualized periapical radiography determined by clinical and panoramic examination. *Dental and Maxillofacial Radiology* **21**, 135–141.

Rosling, B., Nyman, S., Lindhe, J. & Jern, B. (1976). The healing potential of the periodontal tissues following different techniques of periodontal surgery in plaque-free dentitions. *Journal of Clinical Periodontology* **3**, 233–250.

Rushton, V.E. & Horner, K. (1994). A comparative study of radiographic quality with five periapical techniques in general dental practice. *Dental and Maxillofacial Radiology* **23**, 37–45.

Selye, H. (1950). *The Physiology and Pathology of Stress: a treatise based on the concepts of the general-adaptation-syndrome and the diseases of adaptation.* Montreal: Acta Medical Publishers, pp. 203.

Singh, S., Cianciola, L. & Genco, R. (1977). The suppurative index: an indicator of active periodontal disease. *Journal of Dental Research* **56**, 200, #593.

Slots, J., Mashimo, P., Levine, M.J. & Genco, R.J. (1979). Periodontal therapy in humans. I. Microbiological and clinical effects of a single course of periodontal scaling and root planing, and of adjunctive tetracycline therapy. *Journal of Periodontology* **50**, 495–509.

Suomi, J.D., Greene, J.C., Vermillion, J.R., Doyle Chang, J.J. & Leatherwood, E.C. (1971). The effect of controlled oral hygiene procedures on the progression of periodontal disease in adults: Results after third and final year. *Journal of Periodontology* **42**, 152–160.

Tonetti, M., Pini Prato, G. & Cortellini, P. (1995). Effect of cigarette smoking on periodontal healing following GTR in infrabony defects. A preliminary retrospective study. *Journal of Clinical Periodontology* **22**, 229–234.

Valderhaug, J. (1980). Periodontal conditions and carious lesions following the insertion of fixed prostheses: a 10-year follow-up study. *International Dental Journal* **30**, 296–304.

Valderhaug, J. & Birkeland, J.M. (1976). Periodontal conditions in patients 5 years following insertion of fixed prostheses. *Journal of Oral Rehabilitation* **3**, 237–243.

Vanooteghem, R., Hutchens, L.H., Bowers, G., Kramer, G., Schallhorn, R., Kiger, R., Crigger, M. & Egelberg, J. (1990). Subjective criteria and probing attachment loss to evaluate the effects of plaque control and root debridement. *Journal of Clinical Periodontology* **17**, 580–587.

Vanooteghem, R., Hutchens, L.H., Garrett, S., Kiger, R. & Egelberg, J. (1987). Bleeding on probing and probing depth as indicators of the response to plaque control and root debridement. *Journal of Clinical Periodontology* **14**, 226–230.

van der Velden, U. (1991). The onset age of periodontal destruction. *Journal of Clinical Periodontology* **18**, 380–383.

Westfelt, E., Bragd, L., Socransky, S.S., Haffajee, A.D., Nyman, S. & Lindhe, J. (1985). Improved periodontal conditions following therapy. *Journal of Clinical Periodontology* **12**, 283–293.

Westfelt, E., Nyman, S., Lindhe, J. & Socransky, S.S. (1983a). Use of chlorhexidine as a plaque control measure following surgical treatment of periodontal disease. *Journal of Clinical Periodontology* **10**, 22–36.

Westfelt, E., Nyman, S., Socransky, S.S. & Lindhe, J. (1983b). Significance of frequency of professional tooth cleaning for healing following periodontal surgery. *Journal of Clinical Periodontology* **10**, 148–156.

Wilson, T.G., Glover, M.E., Malik, A.K., Schoen, J.A. & Dorsett, D. (1987). Tooth loss in maintenance patients in a private periodontal practice. *Journal of Periodontology* **58**, 231–235.

Wilson, T., Glover, M., Schoen, J., Baus, C. & Jacobs, T. (1984). Compliance with maintenance therapy in a private periodontal practice. *Journal of Periodontology* **55**, 468–473.

Witter, D.J., Cramwinckel, A.B., van Rossum, G.M. & Käyser, A.F. (1990). Shortened dental arches and masticatory ability. *Journal of Dentistry* **18**, 185–189.

Witter, D.J., De Haan, A.F.J., Käyser, A.F. & van Rossum, G.M. (1994). A 6-year follow-up study of oral function in shortened dental arches. *Journal of Oral Rehabilitation* **21**, 113–125.

Part 19: Halitosis

60 Halitosis Control, 1325
Edwin G. Winkel

Chapter 60

Halitosis Control

Edwin G. Winkel

Introduction, 1325
  Epidemiology, 1325
  Odor characteristics, 1326
  Pathogenesis of intraoral halitosis, 1326
  Pathogenesis of extraoral halitosis, 1327
Diagnosis, 1328
  Flowchart in a halitosis practice, 1328
  Before first consultation, 1328
  At the first examination, 1328
  Classification of halitosis, 1333

Therapy, 1333
  Pseudo-halitosis and halitophobia, 1333
  Temporary halitosis, 1334
  Extraoral halitosis, 1334
  Intraoral halitosis, 1334
  Physiologic halitosis, 1335
  Treatment planning, 1335
  Adjustment of therapy, 1337
  Future perspectives, 1337

Introduction

Offensive body odor is one of the greatest taboos in our society. Conditions that are associated with body odors are bromidrosis, the secretion of foul-smelling sweat, body odor also known as osmidrosis or kakidrosis (Leyden 1981; Lukacs 1991; Guillet *et al.* 2000), flatulence, excessive production of bowel gases (Suarez *et al.* 1999; Bell 2000), and bad breath (Attia & Marshall 1982; Delanghe *et al.* 1997; van Steenberghe 1997). One factor these conditions have in common is that bacteria play an essential role in the etiology.

This chapter will focus on bad breath. Several terms like breath malodor, oral malodor, *fetor ex ore*, *fetor oris*, bad or foul breath, and halitosis are used to prescribe noticeably unpleasant odors exhaled in breathing. Halitosis is a technical term for bad breath and originates from the Latin "halitus" meaning "breath" and the Greek "osis" meaning "abnormal" or "diseased". Knowledge of this condition dates back to ancient cultures. The Talmud, a collection of ancient rabbinical writings dating back more than 2 millennia, states that bad breath is a major disability. The marriage license (the Ketuba) may be legally broken in the case of halitosis of one of the partners (Shifman *et al.* 2002). The theme is also discussed in ancient writings from China, Greek, Roman, early Christian, and Islamic cultures. For example, Islamic theology stresses the importance of the Siwak or Miswak, a stick obtained from a plant called Salvadore Persica, to clean the teeth and the tongue. Prior to the late 1930s, most references pertaining to halitosis consisted mainly of anecdotal statements that have been perpetuated in the literature. In 1934, Fair and Wells developed the osmoscope, an instrument for measuring the intensity of odors. Later, this apparatus was used for breath analysis (Brening *et al.* 1938). During the last 40 years, our scientific knowledge about the source and causes of halitosis has become much greater.

Several non-oral pathologic conditions have been related to oral malodor, including infection of the upper and lower respiratory tracts, the gastrointestinal tract, and some metabolic diseases involving the kidneys and the liver (Manolis 1983). However, clinical surveys have shown that over 90% of all bad breath odors originate in the mouth (Delanghe *et al.* 1997; van Steenberghe 1997).

Epidemiology

Information regarding the prevalence of oral halitosis is scarce due to the lack of epidemiologic studies. An early study from The Netherlands among 11 625 individuals revealed a prevalence of approximately 25% in subjects older than 60 years (de Wit 1966). In subjects under 20 years, the prevalence of oral halitosis was 10%, indicating that the prevalence of this condition increases with age. In Japan the prevalence of individuals with complaints of halitosis is approximately 14% (National Survey 1999). In the USA, it is estimated that 10–30% of the adult population have an appreciable problem with bad breath (Meskin 1996). Recently, in China the incidence of oral halitosis was surveyed in a sample of 2000 individuals aged 15–64 years. Oral halitosis was measured in 27.5% of the subjects with organoleptic measurements

Table 60-1 Breath volatile sulphur compounds and some amines, together with some of their known odor characteristics

Formula	Name	Odor qualification	100% odor recognition concentration (ppb)
H_2S	Hydrogen sulfide	Rotten eggs	1000
CH_3SH	Methyl mercaptan	Pungent, rotten cabbage	35
CH_3SCH_3	Dimethyl sulfide	Unpleasantly sweet	100
CH_3SSCH_3	Dimethyl disulfide	Pungent	7
$CH_2{=}CHCH_2SH$	Allyl mercaptan	Garlic-like	0.05
$CH_2{=}CHCH_2SCH_3$	Allyl methyl sulfide	Garlic-like	Unknown
$CH_3CH_2CH_2SH$	Propyl mercaptan	Unpleasant, pungent	0.7
$CH_3CH_2CH_2SCH_3$	Methyl propyl sulfide		Unknown
CS_2	Carbon disulfide	Slightly pungent	900
NH_3	Ammonia	Pleasantly sweet	55 000
$(CH_3)_2NH$	Dimethylamine	Fishy, ammoniacal	6000
$(CH_3)_3N$	Trimethylamine	Fishy, ammoniacal	4000

24 ppb = 1 nmol/l (at room temperature).
Adapted from Tangerman (2002).

(Liu *et al.* 2006). However, only a few patients visit dental clinics to seek help for this condition.

Odor characteristics

Together with some of their known odor characteristics, the most common odorous volatile sulfur compounds and some amines found in the breath of patients with halitosis of different origin are shown in Table 60-1 (Verschueren 1983; Tangerman 2002). The 100% odor recognition threshold is the concentration at which 100% of the odor panel defined the odor as being representative of the odorant being studied. The unsaturated mercaptans (allyl mercaptan in garlic) and the unsaturated sulfides (allyl methyl sulfide in garlic) are the most odorous, followed by saturated mercaptans (propyl mercaptan in onion, methyl mercaptan in bad breath), disulfides (dimethyl disulfide), and sulfides (methyl propyl sulfide in onion and dimethyl sulfide and hydrogen sulfide in bad breath).

For a proper diagnosis and therapy and/or referral to a physician or specialist, it is important for the general practitioner to clearly differentiate between halitosis from oral and non-oral origin. Therefore, in this chapter the term *intraoral halitosis* (oral malodor) will be used to define halitosis with a cause within the oral cavity, whereas *extraoral halitosis* is used for halitosis of non-oral cause.

Pathogenesis of intraoral halitosis

Intraoral halitosis may be indicative of either oral diseases, such as periodontal diseases, or the presence of excessive bacterial reservoirs on the tongue. The pathogenesis of intraoral halitosis is associated with the bacterial degradation of sulfur-containing amino acids (methionine, cystine, and cysteine) into volatile sulfur compounds (VSCs) of which methyl mercaptan (CH_3SH) and hydrogen sulfide (H_2S) are

the major compounds. It appears that methyl mercaptan is the predominant causative factor of malodor (Tangerman 2002; Awano *et al.* 2004; Tangerman & Winkel 2007). Despite the strong evidence that VSCs are the major causative factors in intraoral halitosis, several research groups still suggest that other volatile compounds such as cadaverine, indole, skatole, and butyric acid may influence oral halitosis (Rosenberg & McCulloch 1992; Goldberg *et al.* 1994; Rosenberg 1996; Greenman *et al.* 2004). No data of the presence of smellable concentrations of such volatiles in mouth air have ever been shown. Therefore, no evidence exists of such a relationship. On the contrary, Tonzetich (1977) clearly showed that diamines, such as cadaverine, inhibited odor formation. It was also stated that indole and skatole, although emanating an objectionable odor in pure state, did not impart an odor to saliva under conditions approximating those of the oral cavity. He ascribed this to their extremely low volatility. The same holds for butyric acid. Due to their low volatilities these compounds have a low odor potential. This is in strong contrast with the VSCs which have a very high odor potential (Verschueren *et al.* 1983).

Formation of volatile sulfur compounds

Gram-negative, proteolytic bacteria are believed to play an essential role in the formation of VSCs, although Gram-positive bacteria such as *Peptostreptococcus* species have also shown ability to produce VSCs *in vitro* (McNamara *et al.* 1972; Persson 1989; Claesson 1990; Persson *et al.* 1990). The most active producers of VSCs *in vitro* are shown in Table 60-2. In our clinic we selected over 100 patients with halitosis but without a history of periodontitis. By culturing periodontal pathogens we found meanly *Fusobacterium* species and low levels of *Prevotella intermedia* (unpublished data), which was in accordance with findings of Loesche and Kazor (2002). This

Table 60-2 Microorganisms with a high capability of generating volatile sulfur compounds *in vitro*

H₂S from serum	CH₃SH from serum	H₂S from cysteine	CH₃SH from methionine
Porphyromonas gingivalis	*Porphyromonas gingivalis*	*Bacteroides* spp.	*Bacteroides* spp.
Porphyromonas endodontalis	*Porphyromonas endodontalis*	*Selenomonas* spp.	*Porphyromonas endodontalis*
Prevotella loescheii		*Fusobacterium* spp.	*Fusobacterium* spp.
Treponema denticula		*Peptostreptococcus* spp.	*Eubacterium* spp.
Prevotella intermedia		*Prevotella intermedia*	
		Tannerella forsythensis	
		Eubacterium spp.	
		Centipedia periodontii	

Adapted from Persson *et al.* (1990).

suggested that the indigenous tongue flora is distinct from the periodontal flora. Therefore, microbiologic information about patients with halitosis should clearly differentiate between patients with or without (a history of) periodontitis.

Periodontium

In patients with periodontal disease, methyl mercaptan was found to be the most abundant VSC (Yaegaki & Sanada 1992c). The role of hydrogen sulfide (H_2S) and methyl mercaptan (MM) in the etiology of periodontitis is unclear. VSCs are potentially capable of altering the permeability of the gingival tissues, including inflammatory responses. By modulating the functions of gingival fibroblasts, VSCs may play a role in the pathogenesis of gingivitis and periodontitis (Ratkay *et al.* 1995; Ratcliff & Johnson 1999; Torresyap *et al.* 2003). In an *in vitro* study, it was shown that MM had a more pronounced effect on the permeability of mucosa than a similar concentration of H_2S (Johnson 1992; Ng 1984). MM has also been shown to act synergistically with both lipopolysaccharide (LPS) and interleukin 1-beta (IL-1β) to increase secretion of prostaglandin E_2 and collagenase, important mediators of inflammation and tissue destruction (Ratkay *et al.* 1995). In fact, increased VSCs in mouth air are related to deep periodontal pockets (Coil & Tonzetich 1992; Yaegaki & Sanada 1992a,c). However, it has also become clear that intraoral halitosis may also occur in individuals with a healthy periodontium (Kaizu *et al.* 1978; Bosy *et al.* 1994; Winkel *et al.* 2003). In patients with periodontitis, Yeagaki and Sanada (1992c) found six times more tongue coating than in those who were periodontally healthy.

Tongue

The tongue has the largest bacterial load of any oral tissue and makes the greatest contribution to bacteria found in the saliva. It is believed that the bacterial mass located at the posterior dorsum of the tongue is the principal site where malodorous compounds are produced (Bosy *et al.* 1994; De Boever *et al.* 1994). Individuals that suffer from intraoral halitosis have a significantly higher bacterial load on the dorsum of the tongue in comparison to individuals without intraoral halitosis (De Boever & Loesche 1995; Yaegaki & Sanada 1992a). In addition, the rough surface of the tongue provides an ideal habitat for anaerobic bacteria, which flourish under a continually forming tongue coating of food debris, dead cells, and hundreds of thousands of bacteria, both living and dead.

Pathogenesis of extraoral halitosis

Approximately 10% of cases of halitosis are caused by extraoral halitosis (Delanghe *et al.* 1998; Tangerman & Winkel 2007).

Examples of extraoral halitosis of the upper respiratory tract are chronic sinusitis, nasal obstruction, nasopharyngeal abscess, and carcinoma of the larynx. Examples of the lower respiratory tract are bronchitis, bronchiectasis, pneumonia, pulmonary abscess, and carcinoma of the lungs (Attia & Marshall 1982; Lu 1982; Durham *et al.* 1993; McDowell & Kassebaum 1993).

Extraoral halitosis might also be a manifestation of a serious systemic disease, such as hiatus hernia, hepatic cirrhosis, or diabetes mellitus. These diseases may produce specific smells (Tangerman 2002) (Table 60-3). For example, *fetor hepaticus* in liver cirrhosis is a type of severe bad breath caused by dimethyl sulfide (Tangerman *et al.* 1994). While intraoral halitosis is largely caused by MM and to a lesser extent by H_2S (Tangerman 2002; Awano *et al.* 2004; Tangerman & Winkel 2007), these components cannot be found in blood-borne halitosis (Tangerman 2002). A new finding is outlined in a study by Tangerman and Winkel (2007) where they found that the majority of extraoral blood-borne halitosis was caused by a hitherto unknown metabolic disorder resulting in elevated odorous levels of dimethyl sulfide in blood and breath. Unpleasant odor from the lower gastrointestinal tract is only detectable during belching or vomiting, because the oesophagus is normally collapsed (Attia & Marshall 1982). The stomach is therefore not considered to contribute to halitosis, except in rare circumstances (Rosenberg 1996).

Table 60-3 Odorous volatiles in the breath of patients with extraoral blood-borne halitosis

Causes of blood-borne halitosis	Odorant
Systemic diseases	
Hepatic failure/liver cirrhosis	Dimethyl sulfide
Uremia/kidney failure	Dimethylamine, trimethylamine
Diabetic ketoacidosis, diabetes mellitus	Acetone
Metabolic disorders	
Isolated persistent hypermethioninemia	Dimethyl sulfide
Fish odor syndrome, trimethylaminuria	Trimethylamine
Medication	
Disulfiram	Carbon disulfide
Dimethylsulfoxide	Dimethyl sulfide
Cysteamine	Dimethyl sulfide
Food	
Garlic	Allyl methyl sulfide
Onion	Methyl propyl sulfide

Adapted from Tangerman (2002).

Table 60-4 Organoleptic scoring scale

Score	Category	Description
0	Absence of halitosis	Odor cannot be detected
1	Questionable halitosis	Odor is detectable, although the examiner could not recognize it as halitosis
2	Slight halitosis	Odor is deemed to exceed the threshold of halitosis recognition
3	Moderate halitosis	Halitosis is definitely detected
4	Strong halitosis	Strong halitosis is detected, but can be tolerated by examiner
5	Severe halitosis	Overwhelming halitosis is detected and cannot be tolerated by examiner (examiner instinctively averts the nose)

Adapted from Yaegaki & Coil (2000).

Diagnosis

Flowchart in a halitosis practice

There are no accepted clinical protocols for the diagnosis of patients with halitosis.

In practice, the flowchart in Fig. 60-1 is suggested for patients with complaints of halitosis. The techniques and strategies for diagnosis and treatment that are described below have been drawn from the research methods and results of important workers in the field of halitosis (Tonzetich 1977; Preti *et al.* 1992; Rosenberg 1995; Richter 1996; van Steenberghe & Rosenberg 1996; Yaegaki & Coil 1999; Sanz *et al.* 2001; Coil *et al.* 2002; Quirynen *et al.* 2002b) and from the experience of the author in treating patients with chief complaints of halitosis for more than 10 years.

Before first consultation

Before the first appointment all patients receive detailed medical and halitosis questionnaires as well as written instructions (Fig. 60-2). The general medical questionnaire, which includes questions about e.g. systemic diseases, allergy, asthma, rhinitis, sinusitis, and medication, has to be filled in before the appointment and can be discussed beforehand with the physician if needed. Additionally a specific halitosis questionnaire is given to the patient (Fig. 60-3).

At the first examination

The questionnaires form the basis for the consultation. The various points and their implications are discussed with the patient. These points include the

unreliability of the patient's self assessment. One's own breath odor is often undetectable due to habituation. Many patients link bad breath with bad taste (metallic, sour, fecal, etc.). From the start of the consultation it must be made clear to the patient that you are treating *bad breath* and not *bad taste* and that the presence of a bad taste does not mean that the patient also has bad breath. Nor does a fresh taste imply fresh breath. The opinion of the patient about the level of halitosis is thus unreliable.

It is important to start the examination by firstly carrying out both subjective and objective assessment of the degree of halitosis and then start the intraoral examination. In this way, the severity of the halitosis is assessed before any changes in the degree of halitosis can occur.

Organoleptic measurements

Sniffing of expelled air of the patient by using the nose of the examiner, organoleptic scoring, is the usual technique for halitosis examination in daily practice (Schmidt *et al.* 1978; Rosenberg & McCulloch 1992; van Steenberghe 1997). Differentiation between intraoral and extraoral halitosis can easily be done by comparing mouth breath with nose breath (Durham *et al.* 1993; Richter 1996; Rosenberg 1996).

Examination: For the organoleptic evaluation, participants are instructed to close their mouth for 1 minute, then to slowly exhale air out of the mouth at a distance of approximately 10 cm from the nose of the examiner (Fig. 60-4). For evaluation of extraoral halitosis, patients are also asked to slowly exhale air out of the nose, also at a distance of approximately 10 cm from the nose of the examiner. Full mouth and nose organoleptic odor assessments are used, on a scale of 0 to 5 (Table 60-4) (Rosenberg *et al.* 1991b; Yaegaki & Coil 2000).

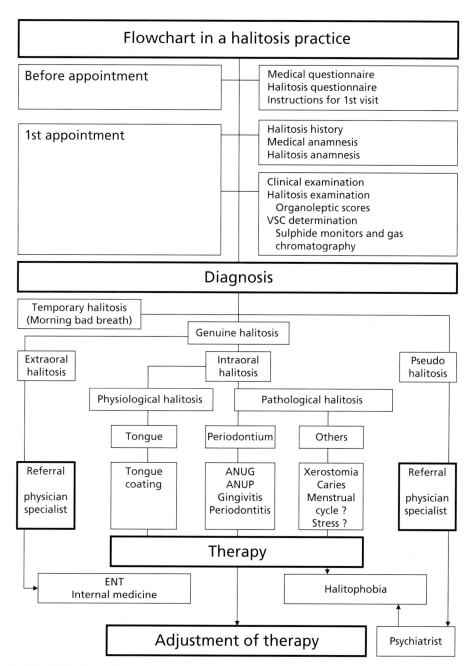

Fig. 60-1 Flowchart in a halitosis practice.

Sulfide monitor

Dental practices and breath clinics now use portable sulfide monitors. For example the Breathtron™ (Sopapornamorn 2006) and the Halimeter™ (Rosenberg et al. 1991a) can test the breath air for levels of sulphur emissions. The Halimeter (Fig. 60-5) has a high sensitivity for hydrogen sulfide but a lower sensitivity for methyl mercaptan, which is a significant contributor to halitosis. Certain foods such as garlic and onions produce sulfur in the breath for as long as 48 hours and may result in false readings. The Halimeter is also very sensitive to alcohol, so one should avoid drinking alcohol or using alcohol-containing mouthwashes for at least 12 hours prior to being tested.

The Halimeter is unsuitable for measuring patients with extraoral halitosis from dimethyl sulfide (Tangerman & Winkel 2007).

Examination: The Halimeter needs to be calibrated to zero on ambient air prior to each measurement. First, the disposable straw, connected to the Halimeter, is placed in the opening of the nose of the patient. Then the patient is asked to blow slowly through to the nose. The maximum peak value of VSCs is recorded. Second, the patient is asked to close the mouth for 1 minute. Then the patient is asked to open the mouth and protrude the tongue. The straw is placed at the dorsal posterior mid part of the tongue and fixed until again the maximum peak value of VSCs is recorded. Peak VSC levels are registered in parts per billion (ppb) (Fig. 60-6a). According to

Instructions for 1st visit

In these instructions, subjects are asked **not** to:

1) take antibiotics for <u>8 weeks</u> before assessment;

2) consume food containing onions, garlic or hot spices for <u>48 hours</u> before the baseline measurements;

3) drink alcohol or smoke in the previous <u>12 hours</u>;

4) eat and drink in the previous <u>8 hours</u> (drinking water up to <u>3 hours</u> before examinations is allowed);

5) perform oral hygiene, including tooth brushing, interdental and tongue cleaning, and not to use mouthrinses <u>the morning of the examination</u>;

6) use scented cosmetics or after-shave lotions <u>on the morning of the examination</u>.

If the patient has any condition like diabetes, which will be aggravated by fasting for the period of time indicated, please contact the dentist about alternative methods of preparation.

Fig. 60-2 Instructions for first visit.

the manufacturer, human standard ("normal") Halimeter readings range between 80 and 110 ppb (http://www.halimeter.com/halcal.htm). Values over 160 ppb are considered to identify a patient with true halitosis (Fig. 60-6b).

Gas chromatography

Gas chromatography is by far the most appropriate method to detect halitosis of different origins and should be considered as the gold standard. It is an objective means of obtaining exact values for the various odorous volatiles (Tonzetich 1967; Furne et al. 2002; Tangerman 2002). New technology is now appearing in the form of portable gas chromatography machines such as the OralChroma™ (Fig. 60-7), which is specifically designed to digitally measure molecular levels of the three major VSCs (hydrogen sulfide, methyl mercaptan, and dimethyl sulfide) in a sample of breath air. It is extremely sensitive and produces visual results in graph form via computer interface (Fig. 60-8a).

Examination: Insert the 1-ml plastic syringe half-way into the oral cavity and ask the patient to hold the syringe between the lips (Fig. 60-8b). Ask the patient not to touch the syringe with the tongue nor the palate. Wait 1 minute, then slowly pull the plunger, push it in again, and pull it for a second time before removing the syringe out of the oral cavity. Avoid saliva in the syringe. If the top of the syringe is wet, wipe it dry with a tissue, attach the needle and eject the air to 0.5 ml and then insert the needle in the injection port of the gas chromatograph (Fig. 60-8c). The apparatus will process the sample in 8 minutes.

Oral inspection

During the first visit, extensive soft tissue, hard tissue, and periodontal examinations are performed in order to determine whether the patient has other oral health problems. Specific attention is paid to the tongue and the presence of tongue debris is noted using a tongue-coating index.

Index systems for tongue coating

A variety of index systems has been developed over the years (Miyazaki et al. 1995; Gomez et al. 2001; Winkel et al. 2003; Lundgren et al. 2007). Miyazaki et al. (1995) divides the tongue into three sections and the presence or absence of tongue coating is registered as follows: score 0 = none visible; 1 = less than one third of tongue dorsum is covered; 2 = between one and two thirds; 3 = more than two thirds. Gomez et al. (2001) divides the tongue into nine different sections, whilst Winkel et al. (2003) divides the tongue into six sections, three in the posterior and three in the anterior part of the tongue. Each sextant is categorized as: score 0 = no coating present; 1 = presence of a light coating; 2 = presence of a distinct coating. The resulting Winkel tongue coating index (WTCI) is obtained by adding all six scores (Winkel et al. 2003) (Fig. 60-9).

The tongue is normally pink (Fig. 60-10) but a very thin whitish coating can also be considered normal. Having a coating on your tongue does not necessarily mean that you have bad breath (Fig. 60-11), although heavy tongue coatings are usually positively related to halitosis (Fig. 60-12).

Halitosis questionnaire

Do you suffer from a dry mouth?

Do you breathe through your mouth?

How many drinks do you have per day (include **all** beverages)?

How many cups of coffee do you drink per day?

How many units of alcohol do you drink per day?

Do you often have a bad taste in your mouth?

Is this related to your bad breath?

What time of day do you have problems with bad breath?

From who have you heard that you have bad breath?

Over how many years have you had a problem with bad breath?

How would you assess the severity of your bad breath?

How do others assess the severity of your bad breath?

How have you consulted a doctor over this problem?

Do you have problems with phlegm in the back of your throat (post nasal drip)?

Do you think that there is a relationship between your bad breath and stomach troubles?

Do you smoke? If so, how many per day and over how long a period? (pack/years)

Do you ever brush your tongue?

Do you use a tongue scraper?

Do you use a mouthwash? If so, what sort of mouthwash do you use?

Do you move away from other people because of your bad breath? If so what is the minimal distance that you are comfortable with?

Do you use sweets (e.g. mints or chewing gum) to disguise your bad breath?

Fig. 60-3 Halitosis questionnaire.

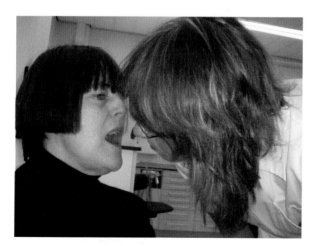

Fig. 60-4 Organoleptic scores. Examiner at 10 cm distance from patient.

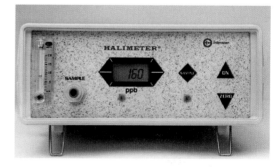

Fig. 60-5 Halimeter™.

(a)

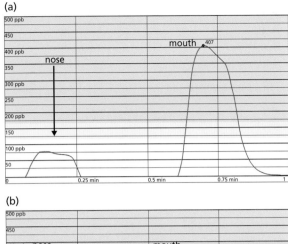

(b)

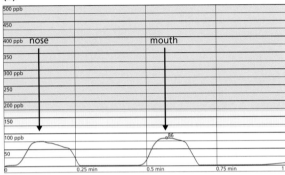

Fig. 60-6 (a) Halimeter computer readout from nose and mouth from patient with intraoral halitosis. (b) Halimeter computer readout from nose and mouth from patient with no halitosis, extraoral halitosis, or after successful therapy or with possible pseudo-halitosis or halitophobia.

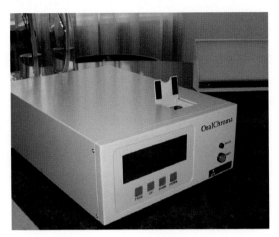

Fig. 60-7 OralChroma™ apparatus.

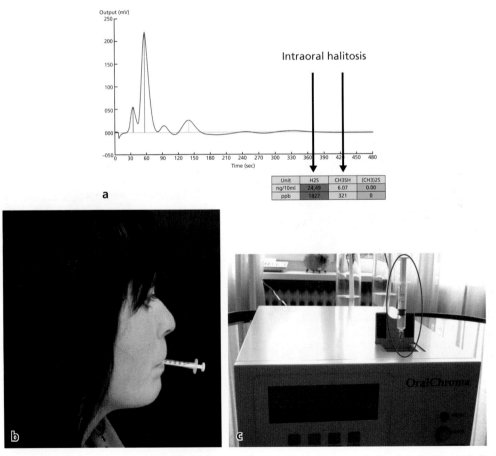

Intraoral halitosis

Unit	H2S	CH3SH	(CH3)2S
ng/10ml	24,49	6.07	0.00
ppb	1827	321	0

a

b

c

Fig. 60-8 (a) OralChroma graphic from patient with intraoral halitosis. (b) Syringe in mouth for air collection with OralChroma. (c) Syringe in OralChroma.

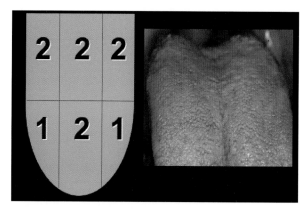

Fig. 60-9 Winkel Tongue Coating Index (WTCI).

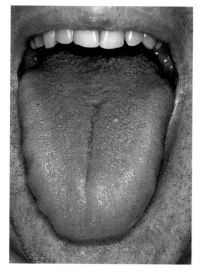

Fig. 60-11 Tongue with light tongue coating.

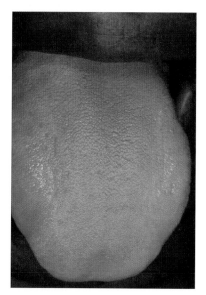

Fig. 60-10 Normal tongue (without coating).

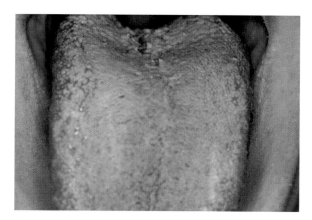

Fig. 60-12 Tongue with heavy tongue coating.

Classification of halitosis

In 1999, Miyazaki and co-workers classified halitosis as *"genuine" halitosis, pseudo-halitosis*, and *halitophobia* (see Fig. 60-1). One year later genuine halitosis was subclassified as *physiologic halitosis* or *pathologic halitosis*. In physiologic halitosis there is no apparent disease or pathologic condition, whereas pathologic halitosis occurs as a consequence of an infection of the oral tissues. *Pseudo-halitosis* is a condition in which halitosis is non-existent but the patients are convinced that they have halitosis. *Halitophobia* can occur when there is no physical or social confirmation to suggest that halitosis is present, which can persist after therapy for either genuine halitosis or pseudo-halitosis (Yaegaki & Coil 2000).

Temporary or transient halitosis is a term for a very common temporary condition caused by such things as oral dryness, hunger (ketosis), stress, eating certain foods such as garlic (Suarez *et al.* 1999) and onions, smoking, or poor oral hygiene. *"Morning bad breath"* is a common example of temporary halitosis and is attributed to physiologic causes, such as reduced salivary flow during sleep.

Therapy

Pseudo-halitosis and halitophobia

Pseudo-halitosis must be considered if halitosis cannot be detected organoleptically from the patient complaining of bad breath, if higher than normal VSCs cannot be demonstrated instrumentally and if the patient cannot provide reliable third-party verification (confidant) of an odor problem. If after treatment for genuine halitosis or pseudo-halitosis the patient still believes that he or she has halitosis, the diagnosis should be halitophobia (Yaegaki & Coil 2000) and the patient might be referred to a psychiatrist. The therapeutic recommendation is never to advise the patient to use certain products against halitosis, because the patient will think that this therapist has finally found something and the patient may be a constant problem in your practice. Patients with the experience of tonsilloliths also can develop a halitophobia. A tonsillolith, also called *tonsil stone* or *calculus of the tonsil*, is a calcified structure that develops in the tonsillar crypts (Fletcher & Blair 1988;

Tsuneishi *et al.* 2006). These deposits break away from the tonsils and are coughed up as small stones that have an unpleasant smell. Patients often wrongly assume that they have halitosis based on this experience.

Patients with pseudo-halitosis and halitophobia might be advised to visit a clinical psychologist. However, few of these patients are willing to follow this advice. Again, it is very important that such patients are not treated for halitosis because there are no benefits in this course of action.

Temporary halitosis

Temporary halitosis gradually disappears on its own by eating, by not smoking, and not using garlic, onions or spicy food.

Morning bad breath

Morning bad breath in healthy subjects is a cosmetic problem analogous to body malodor. Morning bad breath develops during sleep when the saliva flow rate and the oxygen availability are at their lowest, promoting anaerobic formation of VSCs. This would explain why halitosis is generally most severe upon arising in the morning.

To reduce morning bad breath one could advise the patient to use a tongue scraper in the evening before sleeping (Tonzetich & Ng 1976; Faveri *et al.* 2006). Mouth rinses (Roldan *et al.* 2003a) are also advocated to reduce morning bad breath (see below). After drinking and eating in the morning the halitosis will most likely disappear.

Extraoral halitosis

Nose and throat

Extraoral halitosis associated with respiratory problems, e.g. rhinitis, sinusitis, tonsillitis, pharyngitis or foreign bodies (unilateral), is characterized by bad breath arising from the nose and not or limited from the mouth, i.e. the organoleptic score for nose breath is higher than that for mouth breath. Halimeter and gas chromatographic scores are usually low. Chronic infection of the nasal cavity and paranasal sinuses leads to changes in the cleansing action of the respiratory epithelium, allowing bacterial overgrowth and stasis of the secretions to occur.

These patients should be sent to an ENT specialist. Post-nasal drip may also give rise to unpleasant odors but seems to be difficult to treat. Dental treatment such as root canal therapy and dental extractions may violate the maxillary sinus and cause infections necessitating further dental intervention.

Systemic conditions

Extraoral halitosis associated with pulmonary problems (blood-borne halitosis) is characterized by bad

Table 60-5 Some drugs associated with halitosis

Tobacco
Alcohol
Chloral hydrate
Nitrites and nitrates
Dimethyl sulfoxide
Disulfiram
Cytotoxic agents
Phenothiazines
Amphetamines

Adapted from Porter & Scully (2006).

breath arising from both nose and the mouth, i.e. the organoleptic score for nose breath and mouth breath are about the same. The Halimeter readings are low in both cases because H_2S and MM are not present. Gas chromatography may show high dimethyl sulfide (DMS) values and low or zero H_2S and MM levels (Tangerman & Winkel 2007).

Medication
It is important to note that some medications for allergy and high blood pressure, antidepressants, and sinus medication can give rise to blood-borne halitosis (Table 60-5) (Porter & Scully 2006). Metabolites of many drugs have been found to be excreted via the lungs. A good example is disulfiram (Antabuse), a drug used in treating alcoholism, which is metabolized to carbon disulfide (Manolis 1983). Antineoplastic medications may indirectly contribute to halitosis due to mucosites, ulceration, and increased gingival inflammation. Some drugs may induce xerostomia (see below).

Trimethylaminuria: the fish malodor syndrome
The fish malodor syndrome, also known as the fish odor syndrome and trimethylaminuria, is a metabolic disorder characterized by the presence of abnormal amounts of dietary-derived trimethylamine, in the urine, sweat, expired air, and other bodily secretions. Trimethylamine itself has the powerful aroma of rotten fish, resulting in a highly objectionable body odor, which can be destructive to the personal, social, and work life of the affected individual. Therapy for this syndrome is limited. It appears that dietary management might be most effective in mild to moderate forms of fish odor syndrome but not in all cases (Mitchell 2005). Fortunately, cases of trimethylaminuria are very rare.

Treatment planning

Patients with these forms of extra-oral halitosis are referred to the appropriate specialist. Halitosis associated with medication need to be discussed with the patient's physician.

Intraoral halitosis

In a halitosis practice most patients (±90%) have intraoral halitosis (Delanghe *et al.* 1998; Seemann *et al.* 2006). Intraoral halitosis is characterized by a low or non-existant score for nose breath combined with a high organoleptic score for mouth breath. The Halimeter gives similar results. The gas chromatograph shows high levels of H_2S and MM and low levels of DMS. Occasionally, the levels of VSCs registered by the Halimeter are unusually low due to low levels of H_2S whilst the organoleptic scores are high. This is usually associated with halitosis with high levels of MM.

Pathologic halitosis

Periodontium

According to a majority of authors, halitosis is more closely associated with tongue coating than with the severity of periodontal disease (Tonzetich & Ng 1976; Bosy *et al.* 1994). Causes of halitosis such as periodontitis (Sulsur *et al.* 1939; Sato *et al.* 1980; Delanghe *et al.* 1998), pericoronitis, dry socket, necrotizing periodontitis, necrotizing ulcerative gingivitis (NUG), oral infection, and dental caries (Sulsur *et al.* 1939) should be treated accordingly by the dentist and/or periodontist.

Xerostomia

Xerostomia is defined as a subjective complaint of dry mouth that may result from a decrease in the production of saliva (Guggenheimer 2003). Studies have found this condition in approximately 20% of sampled populations (Nederfors 1997). There seems to be a strong correlation between medication (Table 60-6) and dry mouth (Guggenheimer 2003; Nederfors 1997). Dental caries is a major complication of xerostomia. Patients with symptoms associated with a dry mouth and/or medication require further investigation by the appropriate practitioner/specialist.

Menstrual cycles
Elevated VSCs were found in mouth air during mid-cycle and around menstruation (Tonzetich *et al.* 1978; Queiroz 2002).

Stress
Stressful situations can be a predisposing factor for the increase of VSCs in mouth air, but the mechanism cannot be simply explained by the reduction of the salivary flow (Queiroz 2002).

Physiologic halitosis

Tongue coating

It has been shown that mechanical tongue cleaning has a significant reducing effect on the VSC levels in mouth air (Yaegaki & Sanada 1992a; Danser *et al.* 2003). Tongue scraping seems to be the most effective hygienic procedure to reduce morning bad breath in periodontally healthy subjects (Faveri *et al.* 2006), even more than interdental flossing. Tongue scrapers seem to be a little bit more effective than toothbrushes (Seemann *et al.* 2001; Outhouse *et al.* 2006). Cleaning the surface of the tongue with a hard toothbrush wetted with chlorhexidine also seems to be effective in reducing halitosis (Bosy *et al.* 1994; De Boever & Loesche 1995; Cicek *et al.* 2003).

Treatment planning

Tongue scraper

Mechanical cleansing is recommended in patients with tongue coating. Both tongue brushing (Gross *et al.* 1975) and tongue scraping (Fig. 60-13) have been advocated as a means of removing the tongue coating (Quirynen 2004). It is important to clean the back of the tongue as far as possible, because the posterior portion of the tongue is loaded with most coating. A recommended regime for patients with severe halito-

Table 60-6 Some drugs associated with xerostomia

Anticholinergic agents
Antidepressant agents
Antipsychotic agents
Diuretic agents
Antihypertensive agents
Sedative agents
Muscle relaxant agents
Analgesic agents
Antihistamines
Anticonvulsants
Anorexiants
Anti-incontinence agents
Antiparkinsonian agents
Smoking cessation

Adapted from Guggenheimer (2003).

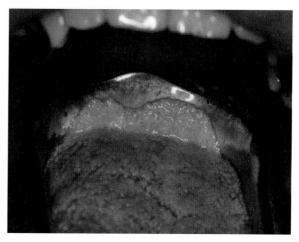

Fig. 60-13 Tongue scraping.

sis is to use five strokes of the tongue scraper twice a day. Care must be taken not to irreversibly damage the tongue. Tongue cleaning reduces the substrate for putrefaction (Gross *et al.* 1975; Quirynen 2004), rather than the bacterial load (Menon & Coykendall 1994; Quirynen 2004). Moreover, tongue scraping improved the taste sensation more than tongue brushing (Quirynen 2004).

Dentifrice

It was shown that brushing the dorso-posterior surface of the tongue with a dentifrice was more effective than brushing the teeth in reducing VSCs (Tonzetich & Ng 1976). In volunteers, dentifrices with triclosan have been shown to reduce organoleptic scores significantly (Gerlach *et al.* 1998; Niles *et al.* 1999; Sharma *et al.* 1999; Nogueira-Filho *et al.* 2002; Hu *et al.* 2003; Vazquez *et al.* 2003; Farrell *et al.* 2006). Also dentifrices with baking soda (Brunette *et al.* 1998), essential oils (Olshan *et al.* 2000), and stannous fluoride (Gerlach *et al.* 1998) seem to be effective. The delivery of an antimicrobial agent via a dentifrice may not be as efficient in reducing intraoral halitosis as the same agent delivered in a mouth rinse (Loesche & Kazor 2002).

Mouth rinses

In addition to tongue scraping, the use of mouth rinses has been advocated (Nachnani 1997; Roldan *et al.* 2003a). Active components in these rinses include antibacterial compounds such as: cetylpyridinium chloride (Yaegaki & Sanada 1992b; Rosenberg *et al.* 1992; Kozlovsky *et al.* 1996; Silwood *et al.* 2001; van Steenberghe *et al.* 2001; Borden *et al.* 2002; Quirynen *et al.* 2002a, 2005; Winkel *et al.* 2003; Carvalho *et al.* 2004; Roldan *et al.* 2004, 2005); chlorhexidine (Rosenberg *et al.* 1992; Bosy *et al.* 1994; De Boever & Loesche 1995; Quirynen *et al.* 1998, 2002a, 2005; van Steenberghe *et al.* 2001; Winkel *et al.* 2003; Roldan *et al.* 2003b, 2004, 2005; Carvalho *et al.* 2004); essential oils (Pitts *et al.* 1981, 1983; Rosenberg *et al.* 1992; Yaegaki & Sanada 1992b; Kozlovsky *et al.* 1996; Silwood *et al.* 2001; Borden *et al.* 2002; Carvalho *et al.* 2004); chlorine dioxide (Frascella *et al.* 1998, 2000; Silwood *et al.* 2001; Borden *et al.* 2002); metal ions, such as zinc lactate and zinc chloride (Schmidt & Tarbet 1978; van Steenberghe *et al.* 2001; Young *et al.* 2001; Borden *et al.* 2002; Quirynen *et al.* 2002a; Winkel *et al.* 2003; Codipilly *et al.* 2004; Roldan *et al.* 2004, 2005); triclosan (Carvalho *et al.* 2004); and hydrogen peroxide (Suarez *et al.* 2000). Most of these studies demonstrated that these products are effective in reducing oral malodor.

Despite the recommendations of the various manufacturers of these oral rinses, the efficacy of these products on intraoral halitosis is not clear. The main reason for this is that the duration and the number of controlled clinical trials is limited. The other problem with the studies which are available is that the patient groups in the studies are rarely patients with a definite diagnosis of intraoral halitosis. The mouth rinses are tested in students (Rosenberg *et al.* 1992; van Steenberghe *et al.* 2001; Quirynen *et al.* 2002a; Carvalho *et al.* 2004) and volunteers (Pitts *et al.* 1981, 1983; Yaegaki & Sanada 1992b; Kozlovsky *et al.* 1996; Suarez *et al.* 2000; Silwood *et al.* 2001; Borden *et al.* 2002; Codipilly *et al.* 2004; Roldan *et al.* 2004; Quirynen *et al.* 2005) without any complaints of halitosis. It is questionable if the results of these studies in "normal" patients and/or patients with Halimeter values within the normal range (80–110 ppb) are applicable for the treatment of patients with real halitosis. Only a limited amount of studies were performed in subjects with a complaint of "bad breath" or with high objectionable levels of VSCs. These are case report studies with 0.2% chlorhexidine (Bosy *et al.* 1994), 0.12% chlorhexidine (De Boever & Loesche 1995), and 0.05% chlorhexidine, 0.05% cetylpyridinium chloride and 0.14% zinc lactate (Roldan *et al.* 2005) with a 3-month follow-up. A dual centre, placebo-controlled, double-blind, randomized controlled clinical trial with 0.05% chlorhexidine, 0.05% cetylpyridinium chloride, and 0.14% zinc lactate was performed by Winkel *et al.* (2003) and Roldan *et al.* (2003). The mouth rinse used in this study (Halita) was specifically formulated to treat halitosis. This mouth rinse contains ingredients with low concentrations of the active components without alcohol and has therefore limited side effects for long-term use. The results indicated significant improvements in organoleptic and VSC scores in the test group.

Quirynen *et al.* (1998) found a reduction in organoleptic scores in periodontitis patients with and without complaints of oral halitosis, after scaling and root planing of all pockets within 24 hours together with the application of chlorhexidine. Despite the demonstrated efficacy of 0.2% and 0.12% chlorhexidine, long-term use of these solutions cannot be recommended because of the side effects (Gagari & Kabani 1995). Some of these adverse effects are lost taste and discoloration of the teeth and the tongue. More suitable agents are mouth rinses with low concentrations of active ingredients. Based on the double-blind placebo-controlled study (Winkel *et al.* 2003) a recommended regime for severe halitosis patients is gargling twice a day for 1 minute with 15 ml of Halita with the tongue out. By gargling, instead of rinsing, the cleansing agents can reach the dorsal surface of the back of the tongue.

Antibiotics

Currently, no research data are available about the use of antibiotics in patients with halitosis. In our clinic some patients with halitosis had used systemic antibiotics for other medical reasons. For a limited

---

Instructions for recall visit

In these instructions, subjects are asked **not** to:

1)   consume food containing onions, garlic or hot spices for 48 hours
     before recall visit;

2)   drink alcohol or smoke in the previous 12 hours;

3)   use scented cosmetics or after-shave lotions on the morning of the
     recall visit.

Patient should perform oral hygiene, including tooth brushing, interdental and
tongue cleaning, and use mouthrinses according to the treatment protocol.

Fig. 60-14 Instructions for recall visit.

time there was a reduction of intraoral halitosis but after a few weeks, halitosis recurred. A possible explanation is that patients with intraoral halitosis based on tongue coating have commensal bacteria (Van Winkelhoff & Winkel 1997), e.g. *Fusobacterium nucleatum*. These commensal bacteria are suppressed by the antibiotics for a short period of time but re-colonize up to a normal level after some weeks.

Use of a confidant

Previous research has demonstrated that patients with halitosis are generally unable to rate the intensity of their own halitosis (Rosenberg *et al.* 1995). Therefore, patients cannot reliably assess the effectiveness of the prescribed therapy. The recommended course of action is to ask them to use another person as a confidant. A confidant could be a spouse, a family member or close friend, who is willing to smell the patient's breath and provide straightforward feedback.

Adjustment of therapy

All patients with the diagnosis of intraoral halitosis should come back for a recall visit and adjustment of therapy (Fig. 60-14). At the first visit, patients are seen in the "worst" condition to make a proper diagnosis. At the re-examination patients are asked to present themselves in the "best" condition, meaning proper oral hygiene and correctly following the advised treatment protocol for patients with halitosis. The purpose of the recall visit is to adjust the therapy based on the results of this re-examination. Organoleptic scores, measurement with the sulphide monitor and gas chromatography are performed. The first question to the patient is: "Did the therapy work?" Although, most of the time the therapy for intraoral halitosis is very successful, some patients will answer "No". The reason is that most of these patients still have a bad taste and think that the pres-

ence of a bad taste means that they have a bad breath, which is not necessarily the case. A confidant is of paramount importance for this group of patients. Another important question is about the "comfort range". The result is compared with the comfort range from the first examination. If the comfort range is the same and the halitosis is well treated, the patient could develop halitophobia and needs to seek professional help.

Future perspectives

In a preliminary study, Burton *et al.* (2005) showed that replacement of bacteria implicated in halitosis by colonization with competitive bacteria (probiotica) such as *S. salivarius* may provide an effective strategy to reduce the severity of halitosis.

Conclusions

Social relationships are one of the pillars of the quality of life (Elias & Ferriani 2006). In that respect, halitosis can be a crippling social problem and therefore needs to be considered a serious problem. Extraoral halitosis might be a manifestation of a serious disease. It is of paramount importance to differentiate between extra- and intraoral halitosis.

Although there is an effective treatment of intraoral halitosis, many physicians, dentists, and dental hygienists do not recognize intraoral halitosis as a manageable condition. Since in most of the cases of halitosis the oral cavity is *the place of origin*, health professionals in medicine and dentistry should be knowledgeable about diagnosis and therapy of this disorder. In most cases intraoral halitosis can be treated by tongue scraping and the use of chemical solutions with low concentrations of zinc ions, chlorhexidine, and cetylpyridinium chloride. The dental hygienist, dentist, and periodontist are the most appropriate professionals to diagnose and to treat this condition.

References

Attia, E.L. & Marshall, K.G. (1982). Halitosis. *Canadian Medical Association Journal* **126**, 1281–1285.

Awano, S., Koshimune, S., Kurihara, E., Gohara, K., Sakai, A., Soh, I., Hamasaki, T., Ansai, T. & Takehara, T. (2004). The assessment of methyl mercaptan, an important clinical marker for the diagnosis of oral malodor. *Journal of Dentistry* **32**, 555–559.

Bell, A. (2000). Managing bloating, flatus and flatulence. *The Practitioner* **244**, 301–311.

Borden, L.C., Chaves, E.S., Bowman, J.P., Fath, B.M. & Hollar, G.L. (2002). The effect of four mouthrinses on oral malodor. *Compendium of Continuing Education in Dentistry* **23**, 531–536, 538, 540.

Bosy, A., Kulkarni, G.V., Rosenberg, M. & McCulloch, C.A. (1994) Relationship of oral malodor to periodontitis: evidence of independence in discrete subpopulations. *Journal of Periodontology* **65**, 37–46.

Brening, R.H., Sulser, G.F. & Fosdick, L.S. (1938) The determination of halitosis by use of the osmoscope and cryoscopic method. Meeting of the International Association for Dental Research, Minneapolis, Minnesota, pp. 127–132.

Brunette, D.M., Proskin, H.M. & Nelson, B.J. (1998) The effects of dentifrice systems on oral malodor. *Journal of Clinical Dentistry* **9**, 76–82.

Burton, J., Chilcott, C. & Tagg, J. (2005). The rationale and potential for the reduction of oral malodour using *Streptococcus salivarius* probiotics. *Oral Diseases* **11**, 29–31.

Carvalho, M.D., Tabchoury, C.M., Cury, J.A., Toledo, S. & Nogueira-Filho, G.R. (2004). Impact of mouthrinses on morning bad breath in healthy subjects. *Journal of Clinical Periodontology* **31**, 85–90.

Cicek, Y., Orbak, R., Tezel, A., Orbak, Z. & Erciyas, K. (2003). Effect of tongue brushing on oral malodor in adolescents. *Pediatrics International* **45**, 719–723.

Claesson, R. (1990). Production of volatile sulfur compounds by various *Fusobacterium* species. *Oral Microbiology and Immunology* **5**, 137–142.

Codipilly, D.P., Kaufman, H.W. & Kleinberg, I. (2004). Use of a novel group of oral malodor measurements to evaluate an anti-oral malodor mouthrinse (TriOral™) in humans. *Journal of Clinical Dentistry* **15**, 98–104.

Coil, J.M. & Tonzetich, J. (1992). Characterization of volatile sulphur compounds production at individual gingival crevicular sites in humans. *Journal of Clinical Dentistry* **3**, 97–103.

Coil, J.M., Yaegaki, K., Matsuo, T. & Miyazaki, H. (2002). Treatment needs (TN) and practical remedies for halitosis. *International Dental Journal* **52** (Suppl 3), 187–191.

Danser, M.M., Gomez, S.M. & Van der Weijden, G.A. (2003). Tongue coating and tongue brushing: a literature review. *International Journal of Dental Hygiene* **1**, 151–158.

De Boever, E.H., De, U.M. & Loesche, W.J. (1994). Relationship between volatile sulfur compounds, BANA-hydrolyzing bacteria and gingival health in patients with and without complaints of oral malodor. *Journal of Clinical Dentistry* **4**, 114–119.

De Boever, E.H. & Loesche, W.J. (1995). Assessing the contribution of anaerobic microflora of the tongue to oral malodor. *Journal of the American Dental Association* **126**, 1384–1393.

de Wit, G. (1966). Foetor ex ore. *Nederlands Tijdschrift voor Tandheelkunde* **110**, 1689–1692.

Delanghe, G., Bollen, C., van Steenberghe, D. & Feenstra, L. (1998). Halitosis, foetor ex ore. *Nederlands Tijdschrift voor Tandheelkunde* **105**, 314–317.

Delanghe, G., Ghyselen, J., van Steenberghe, D. & Feenstra, L. (1997). Multidisciplinary breath-odour clinic. *The Lancet* **350**, 187.

Durham, T.M., Malloy, T. & Hodges, E.D. (1993). Halitosis: knowing when 'bad breath' signals systemic disease. *Geriatrics* **48**, 55–59.

Elias, M.S. & Ferriani, M.D. (2006). Historical and social aspects of halitosis. *Revista Latino-Americana de Enfermagem* **14**, 821–823.

Farrell, S., Baker, R.A., Somogyi-Mann, M., Witt, J.J. & Gerlach, R.W. (2006). Oral malodor reduction by a combination of chemotherapeutical and mechanical treatments. *Clinical Oral Investigations* **10**, 157–163.

Faveri, M., Hayacibara, M.F., Pupio, G.C., Cury, J.A., Tsuzuki, C.O. & Hayacibara, R.M. (2006). A cross-over study on the effect of various therapeutic approaches to morning breath odour. *Journal of Clinical Periodontology* **33**, 555–560.

Fletcher, S.M. & Blair, P.A. (1988). Chronic halitosis from tonsilloliths: a common etiology. *The Journal of the Louisiana State Medical Society* **140**, 7–9.

Frascella, J., Gilbert, R. & Fernandez, P. (1998). Odor reduction potential of a chlorine dioxide mouthrinse. *Journal of Clinical Dentistry* **9**, 39–42.

Frascella, J., Gilbert, R.D., Fernandez, P. & Hendler, J. (2000). Efficacy of a chlorine dioxide-containing mouthrinse in oral malodor. *Compendium of Continuing Education in Dentistry* **21**, 241–244, 246, 248.

Furne, J., Majerus, G., Lenton, P., Springfield, J., Levitt, D.G. & Levitt, M.D. (2002). Comparison of volatile sulfur compound concentrations measured with a sulfide detector vs. gas chromatography. *Journal of Dental Research* **81**, 140–143.

Gagari, E. & Kabani, S. (1995). Adverse effects of mouthwash use. A review. *Oral Surgery, Oral Medicine, Oral Pathology, Oral Radiology and Endodontics* **80**, 432–439.

Gerlach, R.W., Hyde, J.D., Poore, C.L., Stevens, D.P. & Witt, J.J. (1998). Breath effects of three marketed dentifrices: a comparative study evaluating single and cumulative use. *Journal of Clinical Dentistry* **9**, 83–88.

Goldberg, S., Kozlovsky, A., Gordon, D., Gelernter, I., Sintov, A. & Rosenberg, M. (1994). Cadaverine as a putative component of oral malodor. *Journal of Dental Research* **73**, 1168–1172.

Gomez, S.M., Danser, M.M., Sipos, P.M., Rowshani, B., van der Velden, U. & van der Weijden, G.A. (2001). Tongue coating and salivary bacterial counts in healthy/gingivitis subjects and periodontal patients. *Journal of Clinical Periodontology* **28**, 970–978.

Greenman, J., Duffield, J., Spencer, P., Rosenberg, M., Corry, D., Saad, S., Lenton, P., Majerus, G., Nachnani, S. & El-Maaytah, M. (2004). Study on the organoleptic intensity scale for measuring oral malodor. *Journal of Dental Research* **83**, 81–85.

Gross, A., Barnes, G.P. & Lyon, T.C. (1975). Effects of tongue brushing on tongue coating and dental plaque scores. *Journal of Dental Research* **54**, 1236.

Guggenheimer, J. (2003). Xerostomia: etiology, recognition and treatment. *Journal of the American Dental Association* **134**, 61–69.

Guillet, G., Zampetti, A. & Ballain-Colloc, M.L. (2000). Correlation between bacterial population and axillary and plantar bromidrosis: study of 30 patients. *European Journal of Dermatology* **10**, 41–42.

Hu, D., Zhang, Y.P., Petrone, M., Volpe, A.R., DeVizio, W. & Proskin, H.M. (2003). Clinical effectiveness of a triclosan/copolymer/sodium-fluoride dentifrice in controlling oral malodor: a three-week clinical trial. *Compendium of Continuing Education in Dentistry* **24**, 34–41.

Johnson, P. (1992). Effect of volatile thiol compounds on protein metabolism by human gingival fibroblasts. *Journal of Periodontal Research* **27**, 553–561.

Kaizu, T., Sato, H., Shiozaki, A., Tsunoda, M. & Aoki, H. (1978). Reduction of bad breath from the periodontal patients by dilute hydrogen peroxide solution (author's transl). *Nippon Shishubyo Gakkai Kaishi* **20**, 260–266.

Kozlovsky, A., Goldberg, S., Natour, I., Rogatky-Gat, A., Gelernter, I. & Rosenberg, M. (1996). Efficacy of a 2-phase oil: water mouthrinse in controlling oral malodor, gingivitis, and plaque. *Journal of Periodontology* **67**, 577–582.

Leyden, J. (1981). The microbiology of the human axilla and its relationship to axillary odor. *Journal of Investigative Dermatology* **77**, 413–416.

Liu, X.N., Shinada, K., Chen, X.C., Zhang, B.X., Yaegaki, K. & Kawaguchi, Y. (2006). Oral malodor-related parameters in the Chinese general population. *Journal of Clinical Periodontology* **33**, 31–36.

Loesche, W.J. & Kazor, C. (2002). Microbiology and treatment of halitosis. *Periodontology 2000* **28**, 256–279.

Lu, D.P. (1982). Halitosis: an etiologic classification, a treatment approach, and prevention. *Oral Surgery, Oral Medicine and Oral Pathology* **54**, 521–526.

Lukacs, A. (1991). Do cutaneous coryneform bacteria produce short-chain fatty acids in vitro? *Dermatologica* **182**, 32–34.

Lundgren, T., Mobilia, A., Hallström, H. & Egelberg, J. (2007). Evaluation of tongue coating indices. *Oral Diseases* **13**(2), 177–180.

Manolis, A. (1983). The diagnostic potential of breath analysis. *Clinical Chemistry* **29**, 5–15.

McDowell, J.D. & Kassebaum, D.K. (1993). Diagnosing and treating halitosis. *Journal of the American Dental Association* **124**, 55–64.

McNamara, T.F., Alexander, J.F. & Lee, M. (1972). The role of microorganisms in the production of oral malodor. *Oral Surgery, Oral Medicine and Oral Pathology* **34**, 41–48.

Menon, M.V. & Coykendall, A. (1994). Effect of tongue scraping. *Journal of Dental Research* **73**, 1492.

Meskin, L.H. (1996). A breath of fresh air. *Journal of the American Dental Association* **127**, 1282, 1284, 1286.

Mitchell, S. (2005). Trimethylaminuria (fish-odour syndrome) and oral malodour. *Oral Diseases* **11** (Suppl 1), 10–13.

Miyazaki, H., Arao, M., Okamura, K., Kawaguchi, Y., Tyofuku, A. & Hoshi, K. (1999). Tentative classification of halitosis and its treatment needs. *Niigata Dental Journal* **32**, 7–11.

Miyazaki, H., Sakao, S., Katoh, Y. & Takehara, T. (1995). Correlation between volatile sulphur compounds and certain oral health measurements in the general population. *Journal of Periodontology* **66**, 679–684.

Nachnani, S. (1997). The effects of oral rinses on halitosis. *Journal of the California Dental Association* **25**, 145–150.

National Survey (1999). Ministry of Health and Welfare, Japan.

Nederfors, T. (1997). Prevalence of perceived symptoms of dry mouth in an adult Swedish population – relation to age, sex and pharmacotherapy. *Community Dentistry and Oral Epidemiology* **25**, 211–216.

Ng, W. (1984). Effect of hydrogen sulfide and methyl mercaptan on the permeability of oral mucosa. *Journal of Dental Research* **63**, 994–997.

Niles, H.P., Vazquez, J., Rustogi, K.N., Williams, M., Gaffar, A. & Proskin, H.M. (1999) The clinical effectiveness of a dentifrice containing triclosan and a copolymer for providing long-term control of breath odor measured chromatographically. *Journal of Clinical Dentistry* **10**, 135–138.

Nogueira-Filho, G.R., Duarte, P.M., Toledo, S., Tabchoury, C.P. & Cury, J.A. (2002). Effect of triclosan dentifrices on mouth volatile sulphur compounds and dental plaque trypsin-like activity during experimental gingivitis development. *Journal of Clinical Periodontology* **29**, 1059–1064.

Olshan, A.M., Kohut, B.E., Vincent, J.W., Borden, L.C., Delgado, N., Qaqish, J., Sharma, N.C. & McGuire, J.A. (2000). Clinical effectiveness of essential oil-containing dentifrices in controlling oral malodor. *American Journal of Dentistry* **13**, 18C–22C.

Outhouse, T.L., Al-Alawi, R., Fedorowicz, Z. & Keenan, J.V. (2006). Tongue scraping for treating halitosis. *Cochrane Database of Systematic Reviews* CD005519.

Persson, S. (1989). The capacity of subgingival microbiotas to produce volatile sulfur compounds in human serum. *Oral Microbiology and Immunology* **4**, 169–172.

Persson, S., Edlund, M-B., Claesson, R. & Carlsson, J. (1990). The formation of hydrogen sulfide and methyl mercaptan by oral bacteria. *Oral Microbiology and Immunology* **5**, 195–201.

Pitts, G., Brogdon, C., Hu, L., Masurat, T., Pianotti, R. & Schumann, P. (1983). Mechanism of action of an antiseptic, anti-odor mouthwash. *Journal of Dental Research* **62**, 738–742.

Pitts, G., Pianotti, R., Feary, T.W., McGuiness, J. & Masurat, T. (1981). The in vivo effects of an antiseptic mouthwash on odor-producing microorganisms. *Journal of Dental Research* **60**, 1891–1896.

Porter, S.R. & Scully, C. (2006). Oral malodour (halitosis). *British Medical Journal* **333**, 632–635.

Preti, G., Clark, L., Cowart, B.J., Feldman, R.S., Lowry, L.D., Weber, E. & Young, I.M. (1992). Non-oral etiologies of oral malodor and altered chemosensation. *Journal of Periodontology* **63**, 790–796.

Queiroz, C. (2002). Relationship between stressful situations, salivary flow rate and oral volatile sulfur-containing compounds. *European Journal of Oral Sciences* **110**, 337–340.

Quirynen, M. (2004). Impact of tongue cleansers on microbial load and taste. *Journal of Clinical Periodontology* **31**, 506–510.

Quirynen, M., Avontroodt, P., Soers, C., Zhao, H., Pauwels, M., Coucke, W. & van Steenberghe, D. (2002a) The efficacy of amine fluoride/stannous fluoride in the suppression of morning breath odour. *Journal of Clinical Periodontology* **29**, 944–954.

Quirynen, M., Mongardini, C. & van Steenberghe, D. (1998). The effect of a 1-stage full-mouth disinfection on oral malodor and microbial colonization of the tongue in periodontitis. A pilot study. *Journal of Periodontology* **69**, 374–382.

Quirynen, M., Zhao, H., Soers, C., Dekeyser, C., Pauwels, M., Coucke, W. & van Steenberghe, D. (2005). The impact of periodontal therapy and the adjunctive effect of antiseptics on breath odor-related outcome variables: a double-blind randomized study. *Journal of Periodontology* **76**, 705–712.

Quirynen, M., Zhao, H. & van Steenberghe, D. (2002b). Review of the treatment strategies for oral malodour. *Clinical Oral Investigations* **6**, 1–10.

Ratcliff, P.A. & Johnson, P.W. (1999). The relationship between oral malodor, gingivitis, and periodontitis. A review. *Journal of Periodontology* **70**, 485–489.

Ratkay, J.G., Waterfield, J.D. & Tonzetich, J. (1995). Stimulation of enzyme and cytokine production by methyl mercaptan in human gingival fibroblast and monocyte cell cultures. *Archives of Oral Biology* **40**, 337–344.

Richter, J.L. (1996). Diagnosis and treatment of halitosis. *Compendium of Continuing Education in Dentistry* **17**, 370–376.

Roldan, S., Herrera, D., O'Connor, A., Gonzalez, I. & Sanz, M. (2005). A combined therapeutic approach to manage oral halitosis: a 3-month prospective case series. *Journal of Periodontology* **76**, 1025–1033.

Roldan, S., Herrera, D., Santa-Cruz, I., O'Connor, A., Gonzalez, I. & Sanz, M. (2004). Comparative effects of different chlorhexidine mouth-rinse formulations on volatile sulphur compounds and salivary bacterial counts. *Journal of Clinical Periodontology* **31**, 1128–1134.

Roldan, S., Herrera, D. & Sanz, M. (2003a). Biofilms and the tongue: therapeutical approaches for the control of halitosis. *Clinical Oral Investigations* **7**, 189–197.

Roldan, S., Winkel, E.G., Herrera, D., Sanz, M. & Van Winkelhoff, A.J. (2003b). The effects of a new mouthrinse containing chlorhexidine, cetylpyridinium chloride and zinc lactate on the microflora of oral halitosis patients: a dual-centre, double-blind placebo-controlled study. *Journal of Clinical Periodontology* **30**, 427–434.

Rosenberg, M. (1995). *Bad Breath*. Tel Aviv: Ramot Publishing.

Rosenberg, M. (1996). Clinical assessment of bad breath: current concepts. *Journal of the American Dental Association* **127**, 475–482.

Rosenberg, M., Gelernter, I., Barki, M. & Bar-Ness, R. (1992). Day-long reduction of oral malodor by a two-phase oil: water mouthrinse as compared to chlorhexidine and placebo rinses. *Journal of Periodontology* **63**, 39–43.

Rosenberg, M., Kozlovsky, A., Gelernter, I., Cherniak, O., Gabbay, J., Baht, R. & Eli, I. (1995). Self-estimation of oral malodor. *Journal of Dental Research* **74**, 1577–1582.

Rosenberg, M., Kulkarni, G.V., Bosy, A. & McCulloch, C.A. (1991a). Reproducibility and sensitivity of oral malodor measurements with a portable sulphide monitor. *Journal of Dental Research* **70**, 1436–1440.

Rosenberg, M. & McCulloch, C.A. (1992). Measurement of oral malodor: current methods and future prospects. *Journal of Periodontology* **63**, 776–782.

Rosenberg, M., Septon, I., Eli, I., Bar-Ness, R., Gelernter, I., Brenner, S. & Gabbay, J. (1991b). Halitosis measurement by an industrial sulphide monitor. *Journal of Periodontology* **62**, 487–489.

Sanz, M., Roldan, S. & Herrera, D. (2001). Fundamentals of breath malodour. *Journal of Contemporary Dental Practice* **2**, 1–17.

Sato, H., Ohkushi, T., Kaizu, T., Tsunoda, M. & Sato, T. (1980). A study of the mechanism of halitosis occurrence in periodontal patients. *Bulletin of Tokyo Dental College* **21**, 271–278.

Schmidt, N.F., Missan, S.R., Tarbet, W.J., Cooper, A.D. & Vernon, M. (1978). The correlation between organoleptic mouth-odor ratings and levels of volatile sulfur compounds. *Oral Surgery, Oral Medicine and Oral Pathology* **45**, 560–567.

Schmidt, N.F. & Tarbet, W.J. (1978). The effect of oral rinses on organoleptic mouth odor ratings and levels of volatile sulfur compounds. *Oral Surgery, Oral Medicine and Oral Pathology* **45**, 876–883.

Seemann, R., Bizhang, M., Djamchidi, C., Kage, A. & Nachnani, S. (2006). The proportion of pseudo-halitosis patients in a multidisciplinary breath malodour consultation. *International Dental Journal* **56**, 77–81.

Seemann, R., Kison, A., Bizhang, M. & Zimmer, S. (2001). Effectiveness of mechanical tongue cleaning on oral levels of volatile sulfur compounds. *Journal of the American Dental Association* **132**, 1263–1267.

Sharma, N., Galustians, H.J., Qaquish, J., Galustions, A., Rustogi, K.N., Petrone, M.E., Chaknis, P., Garcia, L., Volpe, A.R. & Proskin, H.M. (1999). The clinical effectiveness of a dentifrice containing triclosan and a copolymer for controlling breath odor measured organoleptically twelve hours after toothbrushing. *Journal of Clinical Dentistry* **10**, 131–134.

Shifman, A., Orenbuch, S. & Rosenberg, M. (2002). Bad breath – a major disability according to the Talmud. *The Israel Medical Association Journal* **4**, 843–845.

Silwood, C.J., Grootveld, M.C. & Lynch, E. (2001). A multifactorial investigation of the ability of oral health care products (OHCPs) to alleviate oral malodour. *Journal of Clinical Periodontology* **28**, 634–641.

Sopapornamorn, P. (2006). Association between oral malodor and measurements obtained using a new sulfide monitor. *Journal of Dentistry* **34**, 770–774.

Suarez, F., Springfield, J., Furne, J. & Levitt, M. (1999). Differentiation of mouth versus gut as site of origin of odoriferous breath gases after garlic ingestion. *American Journal of Physiology* **276**, G425–G430.

Suarez, F.L., Furne, J.K., Springfield, J. & Levitt, M.D. (2000). Morning breath odor: influence of treatments on sulfur gases. *Journal of Dental Research* **79**, 1773–1777.

Sulsur, G.F., Brening, R.H. & Fosdick, L.S. (1939). Some conditions that effect the odor concentration of breath. *Journal of Dental Research* **18**, 355–359.

Tangerman, A. (2002). Halitosis in medicine: a review. *International Dental Journal* **52** (Suppl 3), 201–206.

Tangerman, A., Meuwese-Arends, M.T. & Jansen, J.B. (1994). Cause and composition of foetor hepaticus. *The Lancet* **343**, 483.

Tangerman, A. & Winkel, E.G. (2007). Intra- and extra-oral halitosis: finding of a new metabolic disorder in extra-oral halitosis. *Journal of Clinical Periodontology* **34**, 748–755.

Tonzetich, J. (1977). Production and origin of oral malodor: a review of mechanisms and methods of analysis. *Journal of Periodontology* **48**, 13–20.

Tonzetich, J. (1967). Volatility as a factor in the inability of certain amines and indole to increase the odour of saliva. *Archives of Oral Biology* **12**, 1167–1175.

Tonzetich, J. & Ng, S.K. (1976). Reduction of malodor by oral cleansing procedures. *Oral Surgery, Oral Medicine and Oral Pathology* **42**, 172–181.

Tonzetich, J., Preti, G. & Huggins, G.R. (1978). Changes in concentration of volatile sulphur compounds of mouth air during the menstrual cycle. *The Journal of International Medical Research* **6**, 245–254.

Torresyap, G., Haffajee, A.D., Uzel, N.G. & Socransky, S.S. (2003). Relationship between periodontal pocket sulfide levels and subgingival species. *Journal of Clinical Periodontology* **30**, 1003–1010.

Tsuneishi, M., Yamamoto, T., Kokeguchi, S., Tamaki, N., Fukui, K. & Watanabe, T. (2006). Composition of the bacterial flora in tonsilloliths. *Microbes and Infection* **8**, 2384.

van Steenberghe, D. (1997). Breath malodor. *Current Opinion in Periodontology* **4**, 137–143.

van Steenberghe, D. & Rosenberg, M. (1996). *Bad Breath. A Multidisciplinary Approach*. Leuven: Leuven University Press.

van Steenberghe, D., Avontroodt, P., Peeters, W., Pauwels, M., Coucke, W., Lijnen, A. & Quirynen, M. (2001). Effect of different mouthrinses on morning breath. *Journal of Periodontology* **72**, 1183–1191.

Van Winkelhoff, A.J. & Winkel, E.G. (1997). Systemic antibiotic therapy in severe periodontitis. *Current Opinion in Periodontology* **4**, 35–40.

Vazquez, J., Pilch, S., Williams, M.I. & Cummins, D. (2003). Clinical efficacy of Colgate Total Advanced Fresh and a commercially available breath-freshening dentifrice in reducing mouth-odor-causing bacteria. *Compendium of Continuing Education in Dentistry* **24**, 20–24.

Verschueren, K. (1983). *Handbook of Environmental Data on Organic Chemicals*. 2nd edn, pp. 52–59. New York, Cincinnati, Toronto, London, Melbourne: Van Nostrand Reinhold Company.

Winkel, E.G., Roldan, S., Van Winkelhoff, A.J., Herrera, D. & Sanz, M. (2003). Clinical effects of a new mouthrinse containing chlorhexidine, cetylpyridinium chloride and zinc-lactate on oral halitosis. A dual-center, double-blind placebo-controlled study. *Journal of Clinical Periodontology* **30**, 300–306.

Yaegaki, K. & Coil, J.M. (1999). Clinical application of a questionnaire for diagnosis and treatment of halitosis. *Quintessence International* **30**, 302–306.

Yaegaki, K. & Coil, J.M. (2000). Examination, classification, and treatment of halitosis; clinical perspectives. *Journal of the Canadian Dental Association* **66**, 257–261.

Yaegaki, K. & Sanada, K. (1992a). Biochemical and clinical factors influencing oral malodor in periodontal patients. *Journal of Periodontology* **63**, 783–789.

Yaegaki, K. & Sanada, K. (1992b). Effects of a two-phase oil-water mouthwash on halitosis. *Clinical Preventive Dentistry* **14**, 5–9.

Yaegaki, K. & Sanada, K. (1992c). Volatile sulfur compounds in mouth air from clinically healthy subjects and patients with periodontal disease. *Journal of Periodontal Research* **27**, 233–238.

Young, A., Jonski, G., Rolla, G. & Waler, S.M. (2001). Effects of metal salts on the oral production of volatile sulfur-containing compounds (VSC). *Journal of Clinical Periodontology* **28**, 776–781.

Index

Note: page numbers in *italics* refer to
figures and boxes, those in **bold** refer to
tables.

Aae protein adhesin 217, 237
abortion, spontaneous 161–2, 480
abrasive agents 740–1
abscess
    periapical
        diabetes mellitus 309
        drainage 851, *852*
    see also periodontal abscess
absorbable collagen sponge (ACS) 1093
abutments
    angulated 1198–9
    ceramic 1233
    implant-supported restorations 1225–
        6, *1227*, 1231
    Zirconia 1233
access therapy 783–820
    distal wedge procedures 794–7
    periodontal pocket surgery
        techniques 783–94
    periodontal surgery
        guidelines 797–812
        outcome 812–20
accessory canals 507–8, 510, *511*
acellular freeze-dried dermal matrix
        (ADM) allografts 966–7
acetylsalicylic acid burn 396
aciclovir 379
Actinobacillus actinomycetemcomitans see
        Aggregatibacter
        actinomycetemcomitans
Actinomyces
    biofilm composition 238, 239
    colonization 246
    peri-implant infections 273
    plaque formation 185, *186*, 212
Actinomyces naeslundii
    biofilm on implant surfaces 268–71
    coaggregation 246
Actinomyces viscosus 212
active threshold determination 115,
        117
acute necrotizing ulcerative gingivitis
        (ANUG) 210, 211
    etiology 212
    microbial invasion 294
    smokers 317
    spirochetes 221

adhesins 231, 245–6
adhesion molecules 289
adolescents
    palatal implants 1286–7
    periodontal tissue breakdown 1243
    plaque removal 1243
    prosthetic oral implant anchorage for
        orthodontics 1283–4
    see also puberty
adrenal function disorders, surgery
        contraindication 800
advanced flap procedure, root
        coverage 972, 975–80
advanced glycation end-products
        (AGEs) 310, 311, 487
afferent nerve fibers 109
age
    aggressive periodontitis 447–8
    attachment loss 144
    chronic periodontitis risk 424
    implant patient 639–40
    necrotizing periodontal disease 470
    periodontal disease 143–4
    periodontal support loss 1307
    see also adolescents; children
Aggregatibacter actinomycetemcomitans
        145–6, *148*, *149*
    aggressive periodontitis 438–40, 441,
        448, 449
        elimination 449–51
    antibiotics 450–1
        local delivery 893
        microbiologic tests 890
        susceptibility 886–7
        synergism 887
        systemic 889
    antibodies in aggressive
        periodontitis 445
    antibody response 217
    antibody titers 303–4
    association studies 438
    bacteriocin production 244, 247
    cardiovascular disease 157, 158
    carotid endarterectomy 157
    clonal subset 216
    connective tissue invasion 440
    diabetes mellitus 245
    elimination by extraction of all
        teeth 274
    growth inhibition factors 243, 247
    HIV infection 244

    immune response 438–9
    interbacterial antagonism 243–4
    invasion 248
    leukotoxins **214**, 216, 248, 294, 438,
        440
    linear gingival erythema 382
    metronidazole with amoxicillin
        combination 889
    oral cavity colonization 217
    peri-implant infection 272–3, 274
        periodontal disease history 276–7
    periodontal infection 213, **214**, 215–
        17, 243
    periodontal lesions in diabetes 310
    polymicrobial microbiota 226
    prevalence in periodontal disease
        331
    serotypes 216–17
    smoking association 319
    subgingival peri-implant
        infections 639
    suppression 883
    transmission 236, 237
    virulence 243
aggressive periodontitis 331–2, 428–52
    age at onset 447–8
    A. actinomycetemcomitans 438–40, 441,
        448, 449–51
    alveolar bone loss *450–1*
    antibodies 441, 445, 449
    associated medical conditions 446
    attachment loss 429, 433, 446, 448,
        450–1
    bacterial etiology 437–41
    candidate genes 444–5
    classification 429–31
    clinical diagnosis 445–8
    clinical syndromes 429–31
    crevicular fluid prostaglandin E_2
        levels 449
    dentition
        permanent 432–3
        primary 432
    diabetes mellitus 446
    diagnosis 445–9
    differential diagnosis 447
    drug-induced granulocytopenia 446
    environmental factors 445, *446*
    epidemiology 431–3
    etiology 437–41
    familial aggregation 447

aggressive periodontitis (*continued*)
 forms 428
 furcation involvement 657–67
 generalized 428, 429, 430, 431, 440,
  441, 447
 genetic diagnosis 449
 genetic factors 441–5
 heritability 331–2
 HIV infection 446
 host defense evaluation 448–9
 host response to bacterial
  pathogens 440–1
 host susceptibility 441–5
 hypophosphatasia 446
 implants 661
  planning 680–2
 inheritance 442–5
 leukemia 446
 leukocyte adhesion deficiency 446
 local inflammatory responses 441
 localized 140–1, 213, 215–17, 428, 429,
  430–1, 437–41, 447
 microbiologic diagnosis 445–8
 microbiologic testing 451–2
 orthodontic therapy 662, *665*
 palmo-plantar keratitis 446
 pathogenesis 441–5
 pathogenic flora elimination/
  suppression 449–52
 periodontal probing 437
 periodontium rate of destruction
  447
 permanent dentition 432–3
 polymorphonuclear leukocytes 441
 P. gingivalis 440, 441, 448
 primary dentition 432
 prosthetic treatment 661
 restorative therapy 662, *665*
 restorative treatment 661
 screening 433–7
 sibling monitoring 448
 smoking *432–3*, 445, *446*
 surgery 661, *663*
 therapeutic intervention 449–52
 treatment 657–67
agranulocytosis, surgery
  contraindication 800
AIDS *see* HIV infection
alcohol abuse, implant patient 645
alcohol consumption, necrotizing
  periodontal disease 470
alexidine, plaque control 744
allele frequencies *330*
allergic reactions 393, 690
 oral mucosa 392–4
 periodontium 849
alloplastic grafts 552–3
alveolar bone 3, 27–8, 34–42, 86–95
 blood vessels 45, 46
 dehiscence 36
  gingival recession 961, 1267, 1269
 deposition 42
 destruction *510*
 fenestration 36
 formation 39, 86
 healing 88–9
 height 657
 loss 86, 92–3
  aggressive periodontitis *450–1*
  children 140–1
  diabetes mellitus 488
  osseous surgery 795
  P. gingivalis 219
  radiographic assessment 131
  risk assessment 1307
  smokers 318
  trauma from occlusion 360
 membrane barriers 94, 95
 necrosis 462
 neurovascularization 109–10

orthodontic loading 363–5
osteoclast activity 41
osteoporosis 89–91
patient examination 583
radiographic analysis *576*, 583
regrowth 542
remodeling 42
renewal *40*, 41
repair 94–5
resorption 41, 42, 66, 67
 periodontitis 440
 pulpal inflammatory response 506,
  508
 turnover with orthodontic
  loading 364
alveolar bone proper 3, 4, 5, 36, 38, 42
 lamellar bone 37
 periodontal ligament 28
  fibers 30, *32*, 33, 42
 resorption 63
 Sharpey's fibers 38, 42
 tooth attachment 37
 tooth extraction *55*
 tooth socket healing 63, 64, 65
alveolar crest 28
 distance to cemento-enamel
  junction 434–7
 fibers 28
 outline 657
 preparation for implant
  placement 1072
 recontouring 832
 width determination 1068–9
alveolar crestal height (ACH) 90
alveolar mucosa 5, 7–8, 15
 necrotizing periodontal disease 462,
  463, *464*
 transplanted *24*, *25–7*
alveolar nerve, inferior 48
 tooth extraction 120
alveolar plexus, superior 48
alveolar process 3, 27, *28*, 34–5
 adaptation after tooth extraction
  1059
 bone 86–95
  cancellous 1063
  lamellar 37, 54
  loss 86
  spongy 54
 cortical plates 53, 54
 CT 1286
 edentulous alveolar ridge 50, *51*, 52–3
 formation 37
 mineralization 37
 resorption rate 1089
 tooth extraction 54–5, *56*, 57, *58–9*, 60,
  61, 62–6
 topography 53–4, *55*
alveolar pyorrhea, trauma from
  occlusion association 349–50
alveolar ridge
 augmentation 1011–17, *1018–19*, 1020,
  1021–3
  clinical concepts 1088–92
  dehiscence defects 1090–1
  differentiation factors 1093
  extraction sockets 1089–90
  growth factors 1093
  horizontal defects 1091–2
  horizontal tooth movement 1264–5,
   1267, *1268*
  long-term results 1087–8
  materials 1085–7
  procedures 1083–94
  vertical defects 1092
  vertical tooth movement 1263–4,
   1265, *1266*
 defects
  correction 1010–11
  dehiscence 1090–1

 horizontal 1091–2
 regeneration 1084
 soft tissue grafts 1089
 vertical 1092
 extraction sockets 1089–90
 healed following tooth loss 1063
 preservation 1088–9
alveolar ridge, edentulous 50–67
 atrophy following tooth loss 1060–1
 augmentation 1011–17, *1018–19*, 1020,
  1021–3
 bone gain 53
 bone loss 53
 bone marrow 67
 bundle bone 63, *64*
 classification of remaining bone 53
 defect correction 1010–11
 deformed 1008–17, *1018–19*, 1020,
  1021–3
 extra-alveolar processes 62–6
 free graft procedures 1013–17, *1018–
  19*, 1020, *1021–3*
 gingivoplasty soft tissue
  sculpting 1020, *1021–3*
 implant placement 1055–6, *1057*,
  1058–61, *1062*
 interpositional graft procedures 1014,
  1015, *1016*
  combined with onlay grafts 1020
 intra-alveolar processes 54–5, *56*, 57,
  58–9, 60, *61*, 62
 lamellar bone 67
 onlay graft procedures 1015–17,
  1018–19, 1020, *1021–3*
  combined with interpositional
   grafts 1020
 osseointegration 99
 pedicle grafts 1011–13
 pontic contours 1020, *1021–3*
 pouch graft procedures 1013–14
 remaining bone 52–3
 soft tissue collapse
  prevention 1009–10
 soft tissue grafts 1010–11
 surgical procedures for
  augmentation 1011–17, *1018–19*,
  1020, *1021–3*
 topography 66–7
amalgam tattoo 398
ameloblasts 16
amine alcohols, plaque control 746–7
amine fluoride 746
amino acids, sulfur-containing 1326
amoeba 209
amoxicillin 450, 451, 886
 metronidazole combination 889
 peri-implant lesions 878
amphotericin B 752
amyloglucosidase, plaque control 744
analgesia 691
anchorage
 orthodontic
  absolute 1280–90, *1291*
  implants as temporary
   devices 1284–8, *1289*, 1290,
   1291
  indications for implants 1283,
   1284
  length-reduced devices 1285
  skeletal systems 1281
  temporary devices 1282
anchoring fibers 12, *13*
androgens 408
anemia, surgery contraindication 800
angina pectoris, surgery
  contraindication 799
angiogenesis 60
angular bone
 defects 351, 360
 destruction 358, 359

ankylosis 547
external inflammatory root
resorption 871
functional 99
implants 1228
maxillary anterior single-tooth
replacement 1159, *1160*, 1161
replacement root resorption 868
antiadhesive agents, chemical plaque
control 739
antibiotics 882–94
adjunctive systemic 251, 252
adverse reactions 887–8
aggressive periodontitis 450–1
biofilm protection of bacteria 884
carriers 885–6
controlled delivery 886
controlled release 879–80
cumulative interceptive supportive
therapy 879–80
delivery routes 884–6
evaluation 886–94
halitosis treatment 1336–7
local delivery/application 885–6, 886
clinical practice 893–4
clinical trials 890–2
microbiologic tests 889–90
minimal inhibitory concentration
885
necrotizing periodontal disease 471
peri-implant lesions 878, 879–80
periodontal abscesses 497, 500–1,
502
periodontal dressings 811
periodontal therapy 251
plaque control 743–4
pre-operative prophylaxis 799
principles of therapy 882–6
prophylactic
bacterial endocarditis 688–9
patients on
immunosuppressants 800
reconstructive therapy 914
reconstructive therapy 914
resistance 248, 744, 883, 890
biofilms 228–9
systemic 884–5
clinical practice 889–90
clinical trials 888–90
antibodies
aggressive periodontitis 441, 445,
449
avidity 301
evasion by pathogens 247–8
innate defense systems 440
production 301
response 303–4
anticalculus agents 741
anticaries agents 736
anticoagulants
implants 641–2
surgery contraindication 799
treatment planning 689, 690
anticonvulsants, gingival
overgrowth 410
antigen presentation 299–300
antigen presenting cells 299–300
humoral immune response 304
antigingivitis agents 734, 754
antimicrobial agents
plaque control 734, 743–4, 754
chemical 739–40
systemic 743–4
uptake measurements 755
see also antibiotics
antimicrobial tests 755, 756
antineoplastic drugs 392
antioxidants 311
antipathogenic agents, plaque
control 740

antiplaque agents 734, 740, 742–60
evaluation 754–60
antiseptics
cumulative interceptive supportive
therapy 878
peri-implant lesions 878
plaque control 742–3, 744, 747
resistance 248
see also chlorhexidine
alpha-1 antitrypsin 295
antiviral drugs, herpetic
gingivostomatitis 379
anxiety
control 690–1
non-surgical therapy 774
apically repositioned flap 788–9
Arg1-protease 294
ARG-gingipain 249
arterial hypertension, surgery
contraindication 799
articulation
implants 628
problems and oral stereognostic
ability 118–19
aspirators 805
atheromatous plaque 157
atherosclerosis 156–9
risk with periodontitis 477, 478, 479
attachment
bony defect diagnosis 902–3
creeping 995
gingival augmentation 957
guided tissue regeneration 1260
level changes 816–17
orthodontic intrusion 1259–60
see also clinical attachment level
(CAL); probing attachment level
(PAL)
attachment apparatus 4
loss 857
see also alveolar bone proper;
cementum; connective tissue,
attachment re-establishment;
periodontal ligament
attachment loss 134
age 144
aggressive periodontitis 429, 433, 446,
448, *450–1*
chronic periodontitis 423
diabetes mellitus 308–9, 488
endodontic lesions 858
gingival inflammation 422
incidental 433, 448
intrusion of plaque-infected
teeth 1259
percentile plots 133
periodontitis 440, 1300
probing pocket depth *579*
pulp infection 517
risk assessment 1311
autoimmune disorders, implant
patient 643–4
autoinducer-2 228
azathioprine 392, *393*

B cells
adaptive defense system 299
regulation process 301–2
smoking effects 321
bacteria/bacterial infections 184
adhesion 185
to calculus 199
antagonism 243
antibiotic resistance 228–9, 248, 774,
883, 890
attachment 228, 271
bacterial endocarditis 688–9
bacterial vaginosis 481
beneficial species 243
bridging species 222, 232, 246

cardiovascular disease 157, 158
cell-to-cell recognition 231, *233*
challenge to host 156–7
coaggregation 222, 231–2, *233*, 246
colonizing species 232, *233*
host defense mechanisms 247–8
commensal 1337
in maxillary sinus 1101
complex formation in biofilm 231–2
deposits on implants 629
endodontic origin lesions 511–12
fibrils 228
fimbriae 228
gingival disease 377
gingivitis 145–6, *147–8*, 148
necrotizing 466
plaque-induced 408
halitosis 1325, 1326
insulin resistance 309
interbacterial relationships 246–7
antagonism 243
intraoral transmission 275
invasion of periodontal tissue
210–11
linear gingival erythema 382
metabolic products 189–90
migration along stitch canal 1037–8
mixed anaerobic 211–12
nutritional conditions 185
periodontitis 145–6, *147–8*, 148, 208,
209
plaque 203
formation 188–90, 241
rapid/slow formers 241
subgingival 192, *193*, 194, *195*,
198
pneumonia 488, 491
primary colonization 185–6
root canal infection 512–14
smoking effects 319
tissue reactions around
sutures 1037–8
tongue 1327
transmission 236–8
transport in dentinal tubules 520
volatile sulfur compound
formation 1326–7
see also biofilms
bacteriocin 244, 247
Bacteroides
black-pigmented group 217–18
fusiform 219
Bacteroides forsythus see Tannerella
forsythia
Bacteroides melaninogenicus see Prevotella
intermedia
barrier epithelium 73, 74
barrier membranes 905–7, 945
bioabsorbable materials 930, 937, 948,
1084
pedicle soft tissue graft for root
coverage 981–2
ridge augmentation 1084, 1086
combined procedures 940, *941*, 942–3
furcation involvement 906, *908*, 932–7
gingival dehiscence 915
intrabony defects 906, *908*, 930–2, **933**
lateral bone augmentation for
posterior implants 1184, *1185*
materials 1093–4
regenerative surgery 928, 930–8
maxillary anterior single-tooth
replacement 1157
modified papilla preservation
technique 917–18, *919*, *920*, *921*
non-absorbable materials 928, 930–2,
933, 937, 945, 948, 1084
pedicle soft tissue graft for root
coverage 980–1, *983*
ridge augmentation 1084, 1085–6

barrier membranes (*continued*)
  oral hygiene 937
  pedicle graft procedure for root
      coverage 980–1, *983*
  removal 937–8
  ridge augmentation 1084, 1085–6
basal cells 12, *13*
basal lamina 16
basement membrane 12
basic periodontal examination
      (BPE) 656
  system code 656–7
Bass technique of toothbrushing 708
behavior, discrepancy development 698
behavioral change
  counseling 695–6
  oral hygiene 700–2, 707
benign mucous membrane pemphigoid
      (BMMP) 387, 388–9
benzalconium chloride 744
beta-lactamase 227, 229, 886
beveled flap 789, *790*
bioabsorbable materials 928
biofilms 183–4, 208
  antibiotic resistance 228–9
  antimicrobial agents 187
  bacteria
    attachment 228, 271
    coaggregation 231–2, *233*
    detection/enumeration 229
    enzymes 294
    growth rate 228, 229
    transmission 236–8
  climax community 226, 271–3
  communication 226
  complexity 230, 271–3
  composition
    subgingival 232, 234–9
    supragingival 238–9, *240*
  dental plaque 226–32, *233*, 234–9, *240*,
      241–2
  epithelial cell-associated 231
  exopolymer matrix 228–9
  exopolysaccharides 227
  extracellular enzymes 229
  formation 185, 187
  genetic information exchange 227–8
  glycocalyx 229
  health sites 234
  host factors 234, 235–6
  implant surfaces 268–71
  local environment 234, 235–6
  major perturbations 226
  microbial complexes 231–2
  microcolonies 227, 228, 230
  nutrients 227, 230
  oral hygiene 242
  orange complex species
    adjunctive systemic antibiotics 252
    peri-implant infections 273
    periodontal infections 234, 239,
      252
  peri-implant infections 273, 277–9
  periodontal disease 229–31
    status 232, 234
  pH 227
  physiological heterogeneity 227
  pioneer species 241
  properties 227–9
  protection against antibiotics 884
  quorum sensing 227–8
  red complex species
    adjunctive systemic antibiotics 252
    peri-implant infections 273
    periodontal infections 234, 235,
      239, 252
  shear force 227
  structure 226–7
  subgingival 232, 234–8
    composition *234*, 238–9

development 239, 241–2
  therapy effects 249–52, *253*
supragingival
  composition 238–9, *240*
  development 239, 241–2
  tooth cleaning 242
  water channels 227, 230
  yellow complex species 273
bio-glass grafts 557
biologic width establishment 1162
biologically active regenerative
      materials 905, 908–9, 938–40
  modified papilla preservation
      technique 918, *922*
  see also enamel matrix derivatives
      (EMD)
Bio-Oss® grafts 942
bisbiguanide antiseptics 744
bisphosphonates 90, *91*
  implant patient 640–1
  osteonecrosis 591
bite force, implant-supported
      restorations 1228
black triangle, interdental 996, 1155,
      1156, 1162
bleaching agents 741, 746, 870, 871
bleeding on probing (BoP)
  basic periodontal examination 656,
      657
  gingival 574–7
  patient examination 585
  peri-implant 630, 876
  risk assessment *1304*, *1305*, 1306,
      1310–11
BMP4 gene 341
body mass index (BMI),
      periodontitis 153–4
body odor 1325
bonding of artificial tooth surfaces
      1248
bone 86–95
  anti-resorptive agents 90, *91*
  augmentation for implants 608, *609*,
      610, 1083–94
  available for implants 610, *611*
  biology 86–9
  bundle 63, 64, 65
  contouring 903
  cortical and orthodontic tooth
      movement 1253, *1256*
  cyclic load reaction 368
  dehiscence 1253, *1256*, 1267
    gingival recession 1269
  destruction in periodontitis 296–7
  diabetes mellitus 91–3
  emergency type 1264
  endochondral formation 86
  functional loading 365, *366*
  healing 89–95
  height for implants 601–2, 607, 608,
      609, *610*, 636
    residual 1100
  induction with autotransplantation of
      teeth 1267
  intramembranous formation 86
  lamellar 62
    edentulous alveolar ridge 67
    osseointegration 107
  loss
    cyclic loading 368
    endodontic lesions 854–5
    horizontal 1256
    peri-implant 1058–9
    peri-implantitis 533, 534, 535
  metabolic disorders 89–93, 643
  modeling 87
    implant placement 1056, *1057*,
      1058
    osseointegration 104–5
  parallel-fibered 62

preparation for implant
      placement 1071–2
  quality 1068, *1069*
  reaction to orthodontic implant
      loading 1282–3
  recontouring for crown-
      lengthening 1000, 1002, *1003*
  regeneration 93–5, 542, *543*
    autogenous grafts 553
    peri-implant 1046–7
    trauma from occlusion 1128–9
  remodeling 87–8
    adaptive 368
    implant placement 1056, *1057*, 1058
    osseointegration 107
  repair inhibition 92–3
  resorption 41, 42, 866
    active 357, 358
    direct 354
    endodontic lesions 514
    indirect 354
    therapeutic strategies *91*
    woven bone 62
  smoking effects 322
  static load reaction 368
  surgical site 1068–70
  systemic loss 90
  volume 89–93, 1068, *1069*
  width for implants 607, 608, *609*, *610*,
      636
  wound healing *87*
  woven
    osseointegration 104–5, *106*, 107
    peri-implant loss 1058–9
    resorption 62
    tooth socket healing *56*, 57, *58*, 60,
      61, 62, 63, 64, *65*
  see also alveolar bone; guided bone
      regeneration (GBR)
bone cells 86–7
  regenerative capacity 547
bone chips 1156
  lateral bone augmentation for
      posterior implants 1184, *1185*
bone chisels 805
bone defects
  angular 351, 818–20, 854, 855
    deep pocket probing depths 858
    forced tooth eruption 1004, *1005*
    iatrogenic root perforation 858, *859*
    intrusion of plaque-infected
      teeth 1259
    trauma from occlusion 1125
  classification 901–3
  diagnosis 901–3
  horizontal 1084
  implant placement planning 1070
  morphology 911–12
  periodontal attachment
      restoration 903
  regenerative periodontal
      therapy 911–12
  vertical 1084–5
  see also intrabony defects
bone fill, angular bone defects 818–20
bone grafts 93–4
  allogeneic 552, 554–5, 938
  autogenous 552, 553–4
    cortico-cancellous 1087
    horizontal ridge defects 1091–2
    maxillary anterior single-tooth
      replacement 1157
    maxillary sinus floor elevation
      1107
  materials 94
  maxillary sinus floor elevation 1107,
      1115–16
  osteoconductive 544, 546
  osteoinductive 546
  osteoproliferative 544

regenerative therapy 544–5, 546–7,
    907–8, *909*
ridge augmentation 1086–7
simplified papilla preservation
    flap 922, *925*
tissue regeneration 551–7
types 552
vertical bone defects 1084–5
vertical ridge defects 1092
xenogeneic 552, 555–6
bone lining cells 86
bone marrow
    edentulous alveolar ridge 67
    osseointegration 107
    tooth socket healing 62, 64
bone mineral density 89, 90
bone morphogenetic proteins
    (BMPs) 87, 93, 341, 559
    alveolar bone healing 89
    collagen carrier 1093
    expandable polytetrafluoroethylene
        membrane effect 1093–4
    ridge augmentation 1093
bone multicellular unit (BMU) 41, 88
bone removal instruments 805
bone replacement grafts, regenerative
    therapy 905, 907–8, *909*, 938
bone substitute materials
    horizontal ridge defects 1092
    maxillary anterior single tooth
        replacement 1156
    maxillary sinus floor
        elevation 1107–8
    ridge augmentation 1086–7
    vertical bone defects 1084–5
    xenogenic 1087
bone-added osteotome sinus floor
    elevation (BAOSFE) 1111
bovine bone-derived biomaterials 555
Braun Oral-B Plaque Remover 713
Breathtron™ 1329
bridges, tooth mobility 1134–6
bridging, healing phenomenon 995
bruxism 829
    implant failure 591
buccal artery 43
buccal bone plate, height reduction after
    extraction 52
buccal nerve 48
bucco-lingual thickness, gingival
    recession 1269, 1271
Buerger disease, *Campylobacter rectus*
    association 223
bundle bone *see* alveolar bone proper
bupropion 322
burns, thermal 397–8
burs 804, 805
burst hypothesis of disease
    progression 424
butyric acid 1326

cadaverine 1326
calcitonin 88
calcium 314–15
calcium channel blockers, gingival
    hyperplasia/overgrowth 410–11,
    641, 800
calculus, dental 183–4, 197, 199–203
    attachment to tooth surfaces/
        implants 200–1
    carbon fiber curettes 876
    clinical appearance 197, 199–200
    clinical implications 202–3
    composition 201–2
    detection 766–8
    diagnosis 197, 199–200
    distribution 197, 199–200
    formation rate 199
    lipopolysaccharide 766
    mineralization 201–2

periodontitis in adults 133, 134, 202–3
removal 766–72
    complete 767
    non-surgical root
        debridement 767–72
    structure 201–2
    subgingival 585
    supragingival 585
Caldwell–Luc technique 1102
    modified 1109
Campylobacter rectus 160
    aggressive periodontitis 438
    atherosclerosis association 223
    cardiovascular disease 158
    diabetes mellitus 310
    fetal effects 223
        growth restriction 482
    leukotoxin 223
    linear gingival erythema 382
    periodontal infection 222–3
    pregnancy adverse outcomes 223, 482
    smoking association 319
cancer chemotherapy 392
    implants 641
cancrum oris 459
Candida albicans (candidiasis)
    chlorhexidine use 752–3
    diabetes mellitus 308
    gingival disease 380–1
    linear gingival erythema 382
    pseudomembranous 381
    smoking association 319
canines, periodontal abscesses *500*
cantilever units
    extensions 1213
    fixed partial dentures 588, *590*, 1182–
        3, *1184*, 1213–15
    implant restorations 1182–3, *1184*
Capnocytophaga
    aggressive periodontitis 438
    periodontal lesions in diabetes 310
CARD15(NOD2) gene
    polymorphisms 338, *339*
cardiovascular disease 156–9
    patient health protection 688
    periodontitis
        risk with 476–80
        treatment 489
    Porphyromonas gingivalis 157, 158,
        479–80
    surgery contraindication 799
    treatment complications 690
caries, dental 208
    high-risk patients 753
carotid artery, intima media thickness
    (IMT) 157, 158
carotid endarterectomy 157
cathepsin C 332, 333
    gene mutations 645
CD4 lymphocyte count 154, 155
    HIV infection 412
    necrotizing periodontitis 469
CD4-positive cells 301
CD8 marker 300, 301
CD14–260 gene polymorphism 338,
    339
cellulase 227
cemented multiple-unit posterior
    implant prostheses 1197–8
cementoblasts 4, 5, 21, 32
    cementum intrinsic fiber system 33
cementocytes 32–3
cemento-enamel junction 6, 17, 28, *29*
    clinical attachment level 130
    distance to alveolar crest 434–7
    implant planning 1225
    implant shoulder sink depth 1150
    leveling *1005*
    tissue regeneration 544, *545*
cementoid 4–5

cementum 4, 31–4
    acellular, extrinsic fiber 31–2, *32*, 33,
        34
    bone grafting *546*, 547
    cellular
        intrinsic fiber 32–3, 34
        mixed stratified 31, *32*, 34
    components 31
    damage 516, *517*
    dental pulp
        infection 516, *517*
        protection 516
    deposition 32, 33–4
    extrinsic fiber system 33
    formation of new 542
        autogenous grafts 553
        enamel matrix derivative use 558,
            559
    incremental lines 34
    intrinsic fiber system 33
    lipopolysaccharide 766
    mineralization 34
    peri-implant mucosa 76–7
    tooth attachment 37
    types 31, *32*
    see also root cementum
central nervous system (CNS),
    sensitization 521
cephalosporins 886
cerebrovascular disease 156–9
cervical lymph nodes, deep 47
cetylpyridinium chloride 741
    antimicrobial activity 742–3
    halitosis treatment 1336
    plaque control 744–5
Charters technique of
    toothbrushing 709
checkerboard DNA–DNA
    hybridization 213, *214*
    Eubacterium 224
    peri-implant infection 274–5, 277, 278
    Tannerella forsythia 220
Chediak–Steinbrinck–Higashi
    syndrome 446
chemical injury 396
chewing comfort *1140*, 1141, 1143
chewing gum 742
    allergic reactions 393
chewing sticks 736
chickenpox 379–80
children
    aggressive periodontitis 432, 433, *434*,
        435
    cemento-enamel junction distance to
        alveolar crest 434–7
    gingival recession defects 971, *972*
    necrotizing periodontal disease 460
    palatal implants 1286–7
    prosthetic oral implant anchorage for
        orthodontics 1283–4
chlorhexidine 414, 734, 748–54
    anti-discoloration system 750
    antimicrobial activity 742–3, *756*
    chewing gum 742
    clinical uses 751–4
    full-mouth disinfection 776
    gels 751
    halitosis treatment 1335, 1336
    irrigation 717
    irrigators 742
    local application 886
    mechanism of action 750
    mouth rinses 741, 751
        side effects 748–50
    mucosal desquamation induction 396
    necrotizing periodontal disease
        treatment 471–2
    oral hygiene 752
    oral ulceration 753
    plaque control 744

chlorhexidine (*continued*)
post-regenerative surgery 925, 926
products 750–1
professional prophylaxis 752
professional tooth cleaning 925
regenerative surgery 947
safety 748–9
side effects 748–50
slow-release vehicles 751
sodium fluoride synergism 753
sprays 741–2, 751
staining 749
structure *748*
subgingival irrigation 753
toothpaste content 741, 751
toxicology 748–9
use 752
chlorhexidine gluconate in gelatin
chip 892
chorioamnionitis 481
chromosomes *329, 330*
chronic obstructive pulmonary
disease 488–9
cigarette smoking *see* smoking
ciprofloxacin 886
circular fibers 22, *23*
circumferential supracrestal fiberotomy
(CSF) technique 1274
citric acid demineralization 557–8, 973
guided tissue regeneration
combination 942–3
clavulanic acid 886
clear cells 11–12, 13
clenching 829
implant failure 591
clindamycin 889
clinical attachment level (CAL) 130
regenerative therapy 944, 948
supportive periodontal
therapy 1313–14
clinical trials
antibiotics
local 890–2
systemic 888–90
blindness 758
controls 758–9
plaque control 757–60
randomization 758
study groups 759–60
clonal expansion 299
Clostridium difficile 888
clotting mechanisms 689
cocaine burn 396
col region 7
collagen
bioabsorbable barrier membrane
1086
formation after orthodontic
extrusion 1264
growth factor carriers 1093
loss in gingivitis 290, 292
collagen fibers 21, 28, *29*
dento-alveolar 73, 76–7
dento-gingival 73, 76–7
lamina propria 19
orientation 22, *23*, 28–9
periosteum 40
production 32
see also periodontal ligament,
principal fibers
collagen fibrils 29
collagenase 249
collagen-like platelet aggregation
associated proteins (PAAP) 479
communication skills
Community Periodontal Index for
Treatment Needs (CPITN) 131,
132–3, 135, 140, 437
complement 298, 301
innate defense systems 440

computed tomography (CT) 605, 606,
609, 610
alveolar process 1286
confounding 143
congenital heart lesions, surgery
contraindication 799
connective tissue 5, *9*, 10
attachment re-establishment 544, *545,*
546, 547
periodontal ligament cells 548–9
dental pulp infection 515
diabetes mellitus 310–11
disorders in implant patients 643–4
fibers 21–2
gingiva 19–24
regenerative capacity 547–8
transplant 25
inflammatory cell infiltrate *580*
invasion by *A.*
actinomycetemcomitans 440
jiggling trauma 357
loss with orthodontic forces 354
matrix 23–4
osseointegration 104, *105*
papillae 9–10
peri-implant 73
smoking effects 321
supracrestal fiber severing 1005, *1006*
tooth socket healing 55, *56,* 57, *58,* 60,
61
transmucosal attachment 75
connective tissue grafts 985–7, *988–9,*
990
combined with coronally advanced
flap *985,* 986, *988,* 989
envelope technique 987, *989*
papilla reconstruction 997, *998*
trap door approach 986, 987, *988*
tunnel technique 987, 990
connectors for implants 1184
contraceptives, periodontal effects 312,
316
copper salts 746
coral skeleton 555–6
coronally advanced flaps *985,* 986, *989,*
990, 991–2
healing 994–5
coronary heart disease (CHD)
acute coronary syndrome with milleri
streptococci 225
periodontal infection 158
Prevotella intermedia 222
cortisone 690
craters, interproximal 902
C-reactive protein (CRP) 157, 159, 479
creeping attachment 995
critical probing depth 816–17
Crohn's disease 394
crown(s)
dental pulp diseases 505
displacement (*see* tooth mobility)
length-to-width ratio 595–6
crown length
increase
with gingivectomy 1275, *1276*
with orthodontic intrusion 1256
orthodontic intrusion 1256, 1260
crown-lengthening procedures 997,
999–1000, *1001,* 1002–6, *1007,*
1008
ectopic tooth eruption 1005–6, *1007,*
1008
excessive gingival display 997, 999–
1000, *1001,* 1002
exposure of sound tooth
structure 1002–5, *1006*
sutures *1040*
crown–root ratio 587
crown–root–alveolar bone relationships,
crown-lengthening 999

CTSC gene mutation 332–3
cumulative implant survival rate
(CISR) 1213
cumulative interceptive supportive
therapy (CIST) 878–80
curettes 804–5
carbon fiber 876
root debridement 768–70, *771*
cuticle 191–2
cyanoacrylates, periodontal
dressings 811
cyclosporin, gingival hyperplasia/
overgrowth 392, 410, 411, 641,
800
cytokines 296
alveolar bone healing 88–9
diabetes mellitus 310
systemic bone loss 90
cytomegalovirus (CMV)
necrotizing periodontal disease 466
periodontal infection 225

debridement
peri-implant lesions
mechanical 877, 878
non-surgical 876
see also root debridement
decalcified freeze-dried bone allogeneic
grafts 554–5
delmopinol 739, 746–7
demineralization, root surface 557–8,
559, 973
demineralized bone matrix (DBM) 93
demineralized freeze-dried bone
allografts 904, 938, 940, **941,** 942
dental arch, shortened (SDA) 1139
dental artery 43
dental follicle 4, 5
dental lamina 3
dental nerve 48
dental organ 3, 4
dental papilla 4
dental restorative materials
allergic reactions 393
foreign body reactions 398
see also restorative dentistry
dental status
stereognostic ability 118
tactile function 116–17
dental tape 714–15
dental team, infection protection 687–8
dental water jet 717
dentifrices 396, 414, 718
halitosis treatment 1336
soft tissue abrasion 719
see also toothpaste
dentilisin 221
dentin
abrasion 741
bone formation at surface 868
dehydration in root-filled teeth 861
etching by dietary components 521
formation 4, 5
hypersensitivity 518, 520–2, 741
nerve fiber response to exposure 520
permeability to
microorganisms 505–6
removal in periodontal treatment 518
reparative 506, *507*
dentinal tubules
bacteria transport 520
infection in root-filled teeth 858
invasion by subgingival bacteria 193
natural occlusion 521
open 520
pulp infection 516, *517*
dentin–pulp complex 4
dento-gingival epithelium 16–19
gingivitis 290, *291*
invasion by pathogens 294

proliferation in trauma from
    occlusion 359
dento-gingival fibers 22, *23*
dento-gingival interface probing 79
dento-gingival plexus *44*, 45
dento-gingival plexus, protein
    exudate 286, 287
dento-gingival region 17
dento-periosteal fibers 22, *23*
denture stomatitis *630*
    chlorhexidine use 753
dentures
    removable 50
        partial 1177
    see also fixed partial dentures (FPD);
        overdentures
denudation procedure 965–6, 968–9
deproteinized bovine bone mineral
    (DBBM) 1087, 1092
desensitizing agents 741
desmosomes 13–14
    epithelial cell rests 30, *31*
detergents
    plaque control 746
    toothpaste 396, 741
developing countries, necrotizing
    periodontal disease 460
dextranase 740, 744
diabetes mellitus 307–12
    aggressive periodontitis 446
    alveolar bone loss 488
    attachment loss 308–9, 488
    bone effects 91–3
    chronic periodontitis 425
    clinical symptoms 308
    control 309–10, 690
    gingival disease 411
    glycemic control 308
    halitosis 1327
    host response effects 310–11
    host susceptibility to disease 245
    host–bacteria relationship
        modification 310–11
    implant patient 642–3
    metabolic control 151, 153, 162
    oral effects 308–9
    periodontal effects 308–9
    periodontal treatment 311–12
    periodontitis 92, 151, *152–3*, 153, 162,
        486–8
        treatment effects 490–1
    risk assessment 1307–8
    surgery contraindication 800
    treatment considerations 690
    type 1 91–2, 307–8
    type 2 92, 307–8
diamines 1326
diet, dentin etching 521
dietary habits, motivational
    interviewing 698
dietary proteins, allergic reactions 394
differentiation factors, ridge
    augmentation 1093
digital volume tomography 605, 606–7,
    610
dimethylsulfoxide 1327
disclosing agents 720–1, *722*
discoid lupus erythematosus 391
disease predictors 142
disease-modifying genes 328
    implant failures 340–2
    peri-implant infections 340–2
    periodontitis 333–40
disinfection, full-mouth 717–18, 776
distal wedge procedures 794–5
distance between implant shoulder and
    mucosal margin (DIM
    measurements) 1150
DNA *329*
DNA hybridization 229

Down syndrome, implant patients 645
doxycycline 886
    controlled delivery *886*
    regenerative surgery 947
doxycycline hyclate in biodegradable
    polymer 891
dressings
    light-cured 811, 812
    periodontal 811–12
drug-induced disorders
    chronic periodontitis 425
    gingival 410–11
    granulocytopenia 446
    halitosis 1334
    mucocutaneous 392
    see also medications
dual energy X-ray absorptiometry
    (DXA) 89

ectomesenchyme 3, 4, 5
    differentiation 32
Eikenella corrodens 223
    aggressive periodontitis 438
elastase 227, 296
elastic fibers 21, 22, *23*, 30
electric pulp testing 854
electric stimulation 854
empathy 697, 698
enamel 4, 16, 17, 18, 19
    matrix proteins 558, *559*
    mesio-distal reduction 1271–2, *1273*,
        1274
enamel matrix derivatives (EMD) 558,
    559
    Bio-Oss® graft comparison 942
    free soft tissue graft healing 995–6
    furcation defects 843
    intrabony defects 908–9, 939–40
    modified papilla preservation
        technique 918, *922*
    outcomes 945
    pedicle graft procedure for root
        coverage 981–2
    regenerative therapy 908–9, 938, 939–
        40, 942, 948
    simplified papilla preservation
        flap 922, *925*
endodontic lesions 504–22, 849–51, *852*,
    853–9
    bacteria 511–12
    drainage 851, *852*
    periodontitis differential
        diagnosis 851, 853–6
    pulp vitality testing 851, 853–6, *857*
    vertical root fractures 859–63, *864*,
        865
endodontic treatment 858
    iatrogenic root perforation 858–9, *860*
    inflammatory exudate access to root
        canal 514
    root separation and resection 837
endonucleases 236
endopeptidases 295
endo–perio lesions 848
    diagnosis/treatment 856–8
endothelial dysfunction, periodontal
    therapy 159
endothelial leukocyte adhesion
    molecule 1 (ELAM-1) 289, 302–3
endotoxins 294
    necrotizing periodontal disease 467
Enterobacter agglomerans 225
Enterobacter cloacae 225
enzyme-linked immunosorbent assay
    (ELISA) 229
enzymes, plaque control 740, 744
epidemiology of periodontal
    disease 129–63
    age 143–4
    atherosclerosis 156–9

causal relationship 141–2
cigarette smoking 148, *149–50*, 151
confounding 143
diabetes mellitus 151, *152–3*, 153
exposure 142–3
frequency distribution 133
health survivor effect 141
HIV infection 154–5
index systems 129–31
initiation factors 156
methodology 129–33
microbiology 145–6, *147–8*, 148
necessity of condition 141
non-modifiable background
    factors 143–5
obesity 153–4
osteopenia/osteoporosis 154
pregnancy complications 159–62
prevalence 133–5, *136–7*, 138, *139–40*,
    140–1
progression factors 156
psychosocial factors 155
risk factors 141–6, *147–8*, 148, *149–50*,
    151, *152–3*, 153–6
selection bias 141
sufficiency of condition 141
systemic disease risk 156–62
epilepsy, surgery contraindication 800
epithelial cell rests of Mallassez 30, 31,
    516
epithelial cells
    gingivitis 289–90, *291*, 292, *293*
    pathogen invasion 247
    see also oral epithelium
epithelial rete pegs 290
    gingivitis 289
epithelial ridges *9*, 10, 11
epithelial root sheath 4
epithelial sheath of Hertwig 31–2
epithelial strands 516
epithelialized soft tissue graft, root
    coverage 982, *984*, 985, **990**
Epstein–Barr virus (EBV) 225
epulis 314
erythema multiforme 390–1
erythrocytes, implant wound
    chamber 104
erythrosine 720–1
Escherichia coli, smoking association 319
essential oils
    halitosis treatment 1336
    plaque control 745
esthetics
    anterior single-tooth
        replacement 1149–57, *1158*, 1159,
        1160, 1161
    cantilever pontics for fixed partial
        dentures 1213
    checklist 1147
    implant 1146–70
        direction 1075
        maxillary anterior
            restorations 1148–9
        multiple-unit anterior fixed
            restorations 1161–5
        patient 594–7, 597, **598**
        placement 1064, *1065*
        scalloped design 1165–6
        segmented fixed restorations 1166,
            1167–70, 1170
        tooth movement 1263–5, *1266*, 1267
    implant-supported restorations 630–
        2, 1233–4
    missing tooth replacement *1142*, 1144
    objective criteria 1147
    orthodontic treatment *1244*, *1246–7*,
        1248
        tooth movement 1263–5, *1266*,
            1267
    principles 1147–8

esthetics (*continued*)
  single-tooth problem 683, *684–5*
  treatment goal 655
  treatment modality review 1148
estradiol 312
estriol 312
estrogen 312
  bone resorption treatment *91*
  chronic periodontitis 425
  gingival disease 408
  hormonal contraceptives 316
  pregnancy 313–14
  smokers 315
  tissue response 316
ethnicity *see* race/ethnicity
Eubacterium 224
exopeptidases 295
exopolysaccharides 227
Extent and Severity Index (ESI) 130–1,
    135
extraction of teeth
  cortical plasticity 121
  neuroplasticity 121
  periodontal ligament receptors 108–9,
    113, 116, *117*
  phantom tooth phenomenon 121
  sensory amputation 119–20
  sensory nerve damage 120
extravascular circulation 46, *47*

facial artery 43, 44
factor VIIc 316
factor XIIc 316
famciclovir 379
familial aggregation, aggressive
    periodontitis 447, 449
Fc gamma receptors (FcγR) gene
    polymorphisms 336, *337*, 338
FcγRIIa polymorphisms 336, *337*, 338
fetal growth restriction, *Campylobacter
    rectus* 482
fetal–placental unit 481
fetor hepaticus 1327
fever, necrotizing periodontal
    disease 463
fiberotomy
  forced tooth eruption 1005, *1006*
  with orthodontic treatment 1274
fibrin 104
fibrinogen 479
fibroblast growth factor (FGF) 87
  alveolar bone healing 89
  ridge augmentation 1093
fibroblasts 19, 33
  dental pulp infection 515
  smoking effects 321
fibroplasia 60
  osseointegration 104, *105*
fish malodor syndrome 1334
fixed partial dentures (FPD) 676–7, 679–
    80, 683, 1208–18
  abutments 1223–4
    fractures 1224
  avoidance with implants 1177
  cantilever pontics 1213–15
  cantilever units 588, *590*, 1182–3, *1184*
  cantilevered 588, *590*
  cast post 1223
  cement-retained 1233
  complete-arch fixed complete
    denture *1210*, 1211
  complications 1211, 1222–4, 1235
  diagnostic waxing 1212
  dowels 1223
  forces during function 1211–12
  full-arch tooth replacement 1210–11
  high risk 1177, **1178**
  implant-supported 676–7, 679–80,
    683, 1181, 1182
    biomechanical risk reduction 1212

clinical success assessment 1215–16
  immediate provisionalization 1215
  success/survival rate 1234–5
implant-to-implant supported 1208,
    1211–16
long-term success 1223–4
partially edentulous tooth
    replacement therapy 1211–16
patient assessment 1208–9
prosthesis design 1210–16
retention loss 1224
screw-retained 1213, 1233
splinted metal–ceramic 1186
straight 683
success/survival rate 1234–5
support with implant and natural
    teeth combination 1183–4
survival rate 1223–4
tooth-implant supported 1208,
    1216–18
  complications 1217, 1218
  implant loss risk 1217
  maintenance 1218
  natural tooth intrusion 1217–18
tooth-supported 1125–36, 1175–6,
    1179
treatment planning 1209–11
flap handling instruments 805
flap margin recession *842*
flap procedures 786–93
  apically positioned 1000, *1001*, 1002,
    1003
  ectopic tooth eruption 1006, 1008
  apically repositioned 788–9, 813–14
  beveled 789, *790*
  clinical outcomes 931–2, **933**
  coronally advanced flaps *985*, 986,
    988, **990**
  envelope flap 987, *989*, 1014, *1015*
  hard tissue pockets 807–8
  healing 813–14
  implants 1054–5
  modified operation 787–8
  mucoperiosteal flaps 786, 787, 788,
    1073
    maxillary anterior single-tooth
      replacement 1157
    maxillary sinus floor elevation
      1102
  operation with/without osseous
    surgery 806
  rotational **990**
  soft tissue lesion excision 817
  soft tissue pockets 806, *807*
  suturing 808–11
  tension elimination 992
flexible spiral wire (FSW) retainer *1245*,
    1246, 1248–9, *1250–1*
floss holders 715
flossing 714–15
  instruction 725
  traumatic lesions 396, *397*
fluoride
  anticaries action 736
  chlorhexidine synergism 753
  crystals in woodsticks 715
  halitosis treatment 1336
  plaque control 746
  toothpaste 741
foam brushes 718
foods, allergic reactions 394
forced tooth eruption 1002, 1003–5,
    1006
  with fiberotomy 1005, *1006*
  procedure 596
foreign body
  impaction 497
  reactions 398
formaldehyde dehydrogenase 229
formaldehyde lyase 229

free graft procedures, edentulous
    ridge 1013–17, *1018–19*, 1020,
    1021–3
free soft tissue graft procedures
  epithelialized **990**
  gingival augmentation 966, *967*
  healing 995–6
  interpositional grafts 1014, *1015*, *1016*
  pouch graft procedures 1013–14
  ridge augmentation 1013–17, *1018–
    19*, 1020, *1021–3*
  root coverage 972, 982, *984*, 985–7,
    988–9, 990, **990**, 991–2
    thickness 992
freeze-dried bone allogeneic grafts
    (FDBA) 554–5
frenectomy 1274–5
frenotomy with orthodontic
    treatment 1274–5
fungal infection
  chlorhexidine activity 748
  gingival disease 380–3
  linear gingival erythema 382
  see also Candida albicans (candidiasis)
furcated region 823
furcation
  definition 823
  incisors 826
  mandibular molars 825–6
  mandibular premolars 826, *827*
  maxillary molars 824, *825*
  maxillary premolars 825
  probing 828
furcation defects
  degree III 936–7
  guided tissue regeneration 904
  mandibular degree II 933–6, 942
  maxillary degree II 936
  regenerative therapy 840–3, *844*, 904,
    932–7
  techniques 942
furcation entrance 823, *824*
  exposure *842*
  molars 828
furcation fornix 823, *824*
furcation involvement
  aggressive periodontitis 657–67
  anatomy 824–6
  assessment 580–3
  automated probing systems 580
  barrier membranes 906, *908*, 932–7
  basic periodontal examination 657
  chronic periodontitis 575, 667, *668*,
    669–73
  classification 827
  degree 582
  diagnosis 826–8, *829*
  differential diagnosis 829–30
  extraction of tooth 843
  guided tissue regeneration 840–3, 913
  implant planning 682–3
  molar uprighting 1262–3
  occlusal interference 353, 829–30
  orthodontic treatment 1262–3
  papilla preservation flaps 916, *917*
  prognosis 843, 845–6
  radiography 828, *829*, *830*
  regeneration of defects 840–3, 903
  regenerative procedures 541–2
    barrier membranes 932–7
  risk assessment 1309
  root debridement 773
  root separation and resection 832–5,
    836, 837–8, *839*, 840, **845**
  root surface biomodification 557
  terminology 823–4
  trauma from occlusion 353
  treatment 823–46
    goal 655
  tunnel preparation 832

furcation plasty 830–1
fusiforms 209–10, 211
Fusobacterium
 necrotizing gingivitis 466
 necrotizing periodontal disease 466
 plaque formation 185
 root canal infection 512–13
Fusobacterium nucleatum 222
 adherence 248
 biofilm
  content 242
  implant surfaces 268–71
 bridging species function 222, 232,
  246
 diabetes mellitus 245
 HIV infection 244
 linear gingival erythema 382
 peri-implant infection 272, 277
 periodontal abscesses 498
 plaque formation *186*
 smoking association 319
 suppression by antibiotics 1337
fusospirochetal infections 211

gas chromatography 1330, *1332*
gastrointestinal disease 394
gender in periodontal disease 144
gene(s) *329–30*
 disease-modifying 328, 333–42
 horizontal transfer 237–8
gene polymorphisms *329–30*
 aggressive periodontitis 445
 chronic periodontitis 426
 miscellaneous 340, *341*
 periodontitis 144–5, 333–40
genetic markers, risk assessment 1308
genetic risk factors
 aggressive periodontitis 441–5
 chronic periodontitis 425
 periodontal disease 331
genetic traits/disorders, implant
  patient 644–5
genotype frequencies *330*
gingiva 3, 5–27, 69–71
 abrasion by toothbrushes 711, 719,
  720, 958
 adequate zone 956
 after implants 73
 attached 6
 biologic width 69
 biotypes 70, 71
 bleeding
  damage from interdental
   cleaning 714
  on probing 574–7
 blood supply 43, 44–5, 77–8
 buccal tissue dimensions 69–70, 80–1
 cleft removal 1275
 clinically healthy 286–7
 connective tissue 19–24, 25
  inflammatory cell infiltrate *580*
  regenerative capacity 547–8
 contour 795
 dento-gingival epithelium 16–19
 dimensions 956–8, 962
  biologic width 69
  restorative therapy 964–5
  width *7, 8*, 69
 enlargement 800
  drug-induced 392, 410–11, 641,
   800
  hereditary 413
  leukemia-associated 412
 epithelial mesenchymal
   interaction 24–7
 excessive display 997, 999–1000, *1001*,
  1002
 flat 70, 71
 free 6
 health 956–8

height 959–60
 increase 1269
 recession defects 959, 960–1
 root coverage 992
inadequate zone 956
innervation 48, 49
interdental, cleaning 714
invagination removal 1275
keratinization reduction in
  pregnancy 313–14
laceration 396
lamina propria 19–24
linear erythema 381–2, 412
macroscopic anatomy 5–8
microbial challenge response 286–7
microscopic anatomy 8–27
 oral epithelium 8–15
overgrowth 410–11
patient examination 574–7
periodontal mechanoreceptor
  activation 117
periodontal protection 956–7
pigmentation 1000
pink tissue 1000
probing 78–9, 81
pronounced scallop 70, 71
prosthesis 1271
smokers 318
stippling *7, 10, 11*
stretching in orthodontic
  treatment 963
transplanted *24*, 25–7
traumatic lesions 396–8
width *7, 8*
 biologic 69
see also gingival margin; gingival
  pocket/crevice
gingival augmentation 955–70
 denudation procedure 965–6, 968–9
 grafting procedures 966–7
  healing after 969–70
 healing 968–70
 indications 965
 periosteal retention procedure 965–6
 procedures 965–70
 root coverage 970–82, *983–4, 985–7,
  988–9, 990–6*
 split flap procedure 965–6, 968–9
 vestibular/gingival extension 965–6
  healing after 968–9
gingival crevice fluid (GCF) 246, 286
 flow rate 319
 gingivitis 287, 289, 290
 immunoglobulins 301
 innate mechanisms 298
 prostaglandin E$_2$ levels in aggressive
  periodontitis 449
 smoking 319, 320–1
 see also gingival pocket/crevice
gingival disease
 allergic reactions 392–4
 bacterial origin 377
 candidosis 380–1
 classification criteria 405–6, *407*
 clinical signs 405–6, *407*
 drug-induced 392, 410–11, 641, 800
 endogenous hormones 408
 exudate alterations in gingivitis *290*
 fungal origin 380–3
 genetic origin 383–4, 413
  pemphigus 389
 hereditary fibromatosis 383–4, 413
 herpes virus infections 378–80
 histoplasmosis 382–3
 inflammation/inflammatory
  lesions 287, *288*, 289, 406, *407*,
   408, 415
  attachment loss 422
  leukemia associated 412
  non-plaque induced 377–98

 plaque induced 405–15
 prevalence 738
 tooth loss 422
linear gingival erythema 381–2
malnutrition 412–13
mucocutaneous disorders 384, *385–6,*
  387–92
non-plaque-induced 377–98
plaque-induced 405–15
 treatment 414
pregnancy-associated 313, 409–10
scurvy 412–13
sex steroid hormones 408, *409*
spectrum 405
systemic diseases 384, *385–6*, 387–96
 association 411–12
 manifestations 394–6
ulcerative lesions 413–14
viral origin 378–80
see also gingivitis
gingival graft, regenerated interdental
  tissue 915
gingival groove, free *6, 7*
gingival hyperplasia *see* gingiva,
  enlargement
Gingival Index (GI) 130, *290*
gingival margin
 apical displacement 963
 endodontic lesion drainage 851
 forced tooth eruption 1003, *1004*
 free 5, 6, 7
 maxillary anterior teeth 1248, *1259*
 orthodontic intrusion 1260
 orthodontic treatment 1248, *1259*
 plaque-induced gingivitis 408
 position alteration 960
 recession
  limitation 905
  orthodontic treatment 961–4
  thickness 964
 root coverage 992
 sinus tracts 861, *863*
 supra-erupted teeth 1260
gingival pocket/crevice 6
 biofilms 231
 depth 234
 incidence 133, 134
 innate mechanisms 298
 leukocytes 286, *288*
 microbial growth environment 246
 neutrophils 286, *288, 291*
 probing 78–80
 smokers 318
 systemic humoral immune
   response *303*
gingival recession 541
 alveolar bone dehiscence 961, 1267
 bucco-lingual thickness 1269, 1271
 children 971, *972*
 defects 959–60
  classification 971
  orthodontic therapy 971, *973*
 inflammation control 960
 interdental 1271–2, *1273,* 1274
  treatment options 1271
 labial 1267, 1269, *1270*
 marginal tissue 958–61
  limitation 905
  orthodontic treatment 961–4
  thickness 964
 orthodontic forces 354
 predictors 963–4
 soft tissue thickness 963
 tooth abrasion 719, *720*
 tooth movement 1267, 1269, *1270,*
  1271–2, *1273, 1274*
  direction 962–3
  favorable 1269
  unfavorable 1269, 1271
toothbrush trauma 958

gingival recession (*continued*)
  treatment comparison 817–18
  see also root coverage
gingival sulcus 17
  subgingival plaque 194
Gingival Sulcus Bleeding Index 130
gingivectomy
  beveled 1000, *1001*
    internal 805, *806*
  healing 812–13
  with orthodontic treatment 1275,
    1276
  procedures 784–6
  surgical technique 805, *806*
gingivitis
  artefacta 397
  bacterial flora 408
  chronic 735
  chronic periodontitis risk 422
  clinical signs/symptoms 408
  collagen loss 290, 292
  control agents **743**
  dento-gingival epithelium 290, *291*
  diabetes mellitus-associated 411
  diagnosis 583–4
  epithelial cells 289–90, *291*, 292, *293*
  experimental studies 756–7
  foreign body 398
  histopathological features 287, *288*,
    289
  hormonal contraceptive use 316
  immune reactions 286–7
  index systems 574–5
  inflammation 289
  inflammatory reaction 286–7
  lesions 289–90, *291*, 292, *293*–4
  leukemia-associated 411–12
  lymphocytes 289
  menstrual cycle-associated 409
  microbiology 145–6, *147–8*, 148
  necrotizing 459
    acute form 463–4
    chronic form 463–4
    diagnosis 464–5
    histopathology 465–6
    host response 468
    interproximal craters 461–2
    lesion development 460–1
    recurrent 464
    traumatic ulcerative gingival lesion
      differential diagnosis 396–7
    treatment 472
    ulcerative 413–14, 426
  neutrophils 286, *288*, *293*
  oral contraceptive-associated 411
  periodontitis in adults 133, 134
  plaque removal 710
  plaque-induced 406, **407**, 407–8, 422,
    1298
  plasma cells 292, *293*
  polymorphonuclear leukocytes 289
  pregnancy 313, 314, 409–10
  prevalence 738, 739
  prevention in periodontitis
    prevention 426
  progression to periodontal
    disease 414–15
  puberty-associated 312, 408–9
  smoking 319
  spectrum of disease 405
  spirochetes 221
  supportive periodontal therapy 1302
  supragingival plaque
    accumulation 735, 736
  susceptibility 423
  treatment goal 655
  see also acute necrotizing ulcerative
    gingivitis (ANUG)
gingivoplasty 805
  soft tissue sculpting 1020, *1021–3*

gingivostomatitis, herpetic
  necrotizing periodontal disease
    differential diagnosis 463, 464–5
  primary 378–9, 464–5
glucose intolerance 153
  see also diabetes mellitus
glucose oxidase, plaque control 744
glutathione 311
glycoprotein pellicle 188
glycoproteins 23
glycosaminoglycans 23
glycosyl-phosphatidyl-inositol
    (GPI) *337*
Good Clinical Practice Guidelines 757–8
Gore Tex Periodontal Material® 928
grafting procedures
  free gingival 1008
  gingival augmentation 966–7
  interpositional 1014, *1015*, *1016*
    combined with onlay grafts 1020
  maxillary sinus floor
    elevation 1107–8
  onlay grafts 1015–17, *1018–19*, 1020,
    1021–3
    combined with interpositional
      grafts 1020
  roll flap procedure 1011–13
  soft tissue for ridge defects 1010–11,
    1089
  see also free soft tissue graft
    procedures; pedicle graft
    procedures
granulation tissue
  interpositional grafts 1014
  peripheral inflammatory root
    resorption 869, 870
  tooth socket healing 55, *56*, 57, *58*, 60
growth factors 559
  alveolar bone healing 88–9
  delivery systems 1093
  osteoinductive/osteopromotive 87
  ridge augmentation 1093
  tooth socket healing 57, 60
growth hormone (GH) 88
guided bone regeneration (GBR) 1083–5
  augmentation materials 1085–7
  bone grafts 1084–5, 1086–7
  bone morphology 1084–5
  bone substitute materials 1084–5,
    1086–7
  clinical concepts 1088–92
  long-term results 1087–8
  patient selection 1084
  soft tissue morphology 1085
guided tissue regeneration (GTR) 555,
    559–61, 793
  aggressive periodontitis 661, *663*
  attachment 1260
  barrier membranes 905–7
  bioabsorbable materials 930
  citric acid demineralization
    combination 942–3
  clinical outcomes 931–2, **933**
  combined procedures 940, *941*, 942–3
  with demineralized freeze-dried bone
    allograft 940, **941**, 942
  enamel matrix derivative
    comparison 558
  evaluation 562
  furcation
    defect regeneration 840–3, *844*, 904,
      932–7
    involvement 913
  healing 914
  intrabony defects 903, 905, *906*, *907*,
    910
    membranes 930–2
  oral hygiene 1261
  orthodontic tooth movement 1261–2
  pedicle soft tissue graft with barrier

membrane for root
  coverage 980–1, *983*
peripheral inflammatory root
  resorption 871
post-operative morbidity 926–8
root coverage **990**, 992
  healing 995
gum-wing profile 997

Halimeter™ 1329, *1331*, *1332*
halitophobia 1332, 1333
  therapy 1333–4
halitosis
  blood-borne 1327, 1334
  chlorhexidine use for oral
    malodor 753
  classification 1333
  confidant use 1337
  control 1325–37
  diagnosis 1328–30, *1331–2*, 1333
  drug-induced 1334
  epidemiology 1325–6
  extraoral 1327, **1328**, 1334–5, 1337
  instructions for patient 1328, *1330*
  intraoral 1326–7, 1335–7
  morning 1334
  odor characteristics 1326
  oral inspection 1330, *1332*, *1333*
  organoleptic evaluation *1331*
  organoleptic measurements 1328
  pathogenesis 1326–7, **1328**
  pathologic 1335
  practice flowchart 1328, *1329*
  prevalence 1325–6
  questionnaire 1328, *1331*
  sulfide monitor 1329–30, *1331*, *1332*
  temporary 1333, 1334
  treatment 1333–7
    adjustment 1337
    planning 1334–5, 1335–7
hand instruments, root
  debridement 768–70, *771*
hard tissue
  replacement 556
  resorption mechanisms 865–6
  see also alveolar bone; bone
Haversian canals 38, 39, *40*, 41
health education 695–6
health survivor effect 141
heart disease, postmenopausal
  women 315
heat necrosis, implants 614–15
hematologic disorders
  chronic periodontitis 425
  gingival manifestations 395–6
  implant patient 644
  surgery contraindication 800
hemidesmosomes 12–13, 14, 16, 18
  epithelial cell rests 30, *31*
  junctional epithelium attachment 19
hemiseptal defects 901–2
hemoglobin, glycated (HbA1c) 162
hemostasis, local 801
hepatitis, dental team protection 687
hepatitis B infection, chlorhexidine
  activity 748
herb extracts, plaque control 745–6
hereditary gingival fibromatosis 383–4,
    413
herpes simplex virus (HSV)
  dental team protection 687
  erythema multiforme 390
  gingival disease 378–9
  periodontal infection 225
herpes virus infections 378–80
  primary gingivostomatitis 463, 464–5
herpes zoster 379–80
Hertwig's epithelial root sheath 4
  fragmentation 32
  remnants 30

hexetidine 747
high-strength all-ceramic implant
    restorations 1199–200
histiocytosis X
    aggressive periodontitis 446
    chronic periodontitis 425
histoplasmosis, gingival disease 382–3
HIV infection
    aggressive periodontitis 446
    chlorhexidine activity 748
    chronic periodontitis 425, 426
    herpetic gingivostomatitis 379
    host susceptibility to disease 244
    implant patient 642
    linear gingival erythema 382, 412
    necrotizing periodontal disease 460,
        462, 463, 464, 468–9, 471–2
    necrotizing stomatitis 462, 464
    periodontitis 154–5
    plaque accumulation 412
homing 304
hormonal contraceptives
    gingivitis 411
    periodontal effects 312, 316
hormone replacement therapy 315
    periodontal effects 312
hormones
    endogenous in gingival disease 408
    sex steroid 408, 409, 425
    see also estrogen; progesterone
host defense mechanisms 208, 209
    adaptive defense system 299–304
    enhancement for plaque control 744
    humoral immune response 301
    immune defense system 299–304
    innate 297–9
    pathogens overcoming 247–8
    periodontal infections 295–304
host response
    evaluation in aggressive
        periodontitis 448–9
    necrotizing periodontal disease 468–9
    pathogens 440–1
    smoking 319–22
host susceptibility to disease 244–5
    aggressive periodontitis 441–5
    environmental factors 445
    plaque formation 738, 739
host-compatibility 243
Howship's lacunae 41
humoral immune response 301
    antigen presenting cells 304
hyaline layer 32
hydrogen peroxide 247
    bleaching 746, 870
    halitosis treatment 1336
    necrotizing periodontal disease
        treatment 472
    plaque control 746
    production by bacterial beneficial
        species 243
    tooth whitening 746, 870
hydrogen sulfide 249, 1326, 1327
hydroxyapatite 39, 556
    crystals 34, 37
    porous 556
hyperglycemia 310
hyperinsulinemia 92
hypoglycemia 690
hypophosphatasia 446
hypothiocyanite 744

I-Brush® 718
IL1 gene 334–6, 341
IL1 gene polymorphisms 145, 336
    composite genotype 335–6
    genetic marker 1308
    implant failures 341, 342
    implant patient 644
    peri-implant bone loss 589

peri-implantitis 590
    severe periodontal disease
        susceptibility 589–90
    smoking 589, 591
IL1A gene 334, 335
    implant failures 341, 342
IL1B gene 334–5
    implant failures 341, 342
IL1RN gene 334, 335
    implant failures 341, 342
IL10 gene polymorphisms 339–40
iliac crest marrow grafts 553–4
illumination
    loupes 1032
    microscope 1034
    microsurgery 1030, 1034–5
image plate systems 618, 620
image-guided surgery 620, 621
immune memory 299
immune pathology 248
immune reactions
    gingivitis 286–7
    periodontal infections 285
    protective role 302–3
immune receptors, innate 338, 339
immune system
    innate 297–9
        gingival crevicular fluid
            antibodies/complement 440
        microbial modulation 299
    necrotizing periodontal disease 468
    periodontal infections 299–304
    smoking 320
    suppression by pathogens 248
immunodeficient patients
    herpetic gingivostomatitis 379
    see also HIV infection;
        immunosuppression
immunofluorescence techniques, biofilm
        bacterial
        detection/enumeration 229
immunoglobulin(s) 301
    maxillary sinus 1101
    pemphigoid 389
immunoglobulin A (IgA) 301
immunoglobulin G (IgG) 301–2
    Fc receptors 337
    necrotizing periodontal disease 468
    smoking effects 321
immunoglobulin M (IgM) 468
immunosuppressants
    chronic periodontitis 425
    gingival overgrowth 410, 411
    implants 642
    prophylactic antibiotics 800
immunosuppression
    chlorhexidine use 753
    chronic periodontitis 425, 426
    implant patients 642
    see also HIV infection
implant(s)
    abutment
        material 75
        for prosthetic appliances 1282
    abutment-level impression 1196–7
    adjacent teeth condition 631
    aggressive periodontitis 661, 680–2
    alveolar bone loss in diabetes 92–3
    anatomic landmarks with potential
        risk 1072–3
    anatomic structure avoidance 637
    angle 1225–6
    angulation 1231–2
    ankylosis 1228
    anterior single-tooth
        replacement 1149–57, 1158, 1159,
        1160, 1161
    articulation 628
    bacterial deposits 629
    biological differences from teeth 637

bone
    apposition 364, 365
    augmentation 608, 609, 610
    available 610, 611
    height/width 601–2, 603, 607, 608,
        609, 610, 636
    loss 533, 534
    modeling/remodeling 1056, 1057,
        1058
    preparation 1071–2
    reaction to orthodontic
        loading 1282–3
bony borders 602, 603
buccal–lingual dimensions 1074–5
calculus attachment 201, 202
chewing comfort 1140, 1141, 1143
classification 1054
clinical inspection/
    examination 625–6
clinical test of mobility 629
color shades 632
completed soft tissue coverage of
    tooth socket 1061–2
complications 626–8
connectors 1184
crater-formed defects 532, 533
cumulative implant survival
    rate 1213
cutting 101–2, 103
cyclic loads 366, 368
dehiscence defects 1090–1
direction 1074–6
distally shortened arch 1180–7
early stability 637
endosseous receptors 119–20
esthetic zone 1146–70
extraction sockets 1089–90
failures and disease-modifying
    genes 340–2
fixed prostheses 587
flap
    closure 1054–5
    elevation 1071
flapless insertion 1071
function analysis 628
functional differences from teeth 637
furcation involvement 682–3
healing time 1076–7
heat necrosis 614–15
horizontal defects 1091–2
identification of presence 623, 624,
    625
image-guided surgery 620, 621
inclination 1074–6
incorrectly placed 615, 616
indications 1139, 1140, 1141, 1142,
    1143–5
infection 199
insertion torque 1077
installation 99–100
interarch distance 1194
interdental contact line 1155
interdental space assessment 630, 631
length 607
loading 363, 1076–7
    excessive 363, 365–6, 367
    functional 365, 366
    loss of osseointegration 368–9
    maxillary anterior single tooth
        replacement 1156
    overloading 363
    static 366, 368
long axis 1154
long-term performance 588–9
loss 533–4
malpositioned 1225–6, 1234
marginal hard tissue defect 1045–6,
    1064
masticatory occlusal forces 369–70
materials 1199–200

implant(s) (*continued*)
  maxillary anterior
      restorations 1148–9
    multiple-unit fixed 1161–5
  mechanical stimuli perception 119
  mechanical stress 364
  mesio-distal orientation 1075, *1076*
  model-based guided surgery 1071
  molars *1140*, 1141, 1143
  multiple adjacent restorations 596
  natural tooth substance
      preservation *1142*, 1143–4
  neuropathies 1072
  non-cutting 100–1
  number 1074
  oral mucosa 71–8
  oro-facial position 1154
  orthodontic anchorage 1203, 1280–90,
      1291
    advantages 1290, *1291*
    direct 1288, *1289*, 1290
    disadvantages 1290
    forces 1288, *1289*, 1290
    growing patients 1283–4
    indications 1283, *1284*
    indirect 1288, *1289*, 1290
    length-reduced devices 1285
    loading 1288, *1289*
    removal *1289*, 1290
    stability 1290
    success rate 1290
    temporary devices 1284–8, *1289*,
      1290, *1291*
  osteoporosis 90–1
  outcomes 1065
  overloading 363
  palatal 1290, *1291*
    clinical procedures 1288, *1289*
    growing patient effects 1286–7
    insertion sites 1286
    loading time schedule 1288, *1289*
  palpation 629
  papilla
    assessment 630
    dimensions 81–3, *84*
    tissue loss 594–5
  patient satisfaction 1147
  periodontally compromised
      patients 587–90
  periosteal receptors 120
  phonetics 628
    disturbances 595–6
  placement 593, 602, 637
    alveolar ridge healing 1063
    clinical concepts 1063–5
    completed soft tissue coverage of
      tooth socket 1061–2
    fresh extraction sockets 1064
    guiding concept 1071
    planning 1069–70
    ridge corrections 1055–6, *1057*,
      1058–61
    substantial bone fill in extraction
      socket 1062–3
    therapy aims 1063–5
    timing 1053–65
  plaque formation 196–7
  position 1073–4
    sites with limited vertical
      bone 1192, *1193*
  posterior dentition 1175–204
    abutment-level impression 1196–7
    angulated abutments 1198–9
    cemented multiple-unit posterior
      implant prostheses 1197–8
    clinical applications 1193–201,
      1202, 1203
    combination with natural tooth
      support 1183–4
    concepts 1175–7

    controversial issues 1179
    distally shortened arch 1180–7
    distribution 1180–2
    early fixed restorations 1203–4
    fixed implant-supported
      prostheses 1180–7
    high-strength all-ceramic implant
      restorations 1199–200
    immediate fixed
      restorations 1203–4
    indications 1176, 1177–80
    lateral bone augmentation 1184–6
    multiple-unit tooth-bound
      restorations 1187–90, *1191*
    number 1180–2
    occlusal considerations 1200–1,
      1202, 1203
    orthodontic considerations 1200–1,
      1202, 1203
    restoration with cantilever
      units 1182–3, *1184*
    screw-retained restorations 1193–6
    shoulder-level impression 1196–7
    single-tooth replacement 1191–2,
      1193
    sites with anterior sinus floor
      proximity 1184–7
    sites with extended horizontal bone
      volume deficiencies 1184–7
    size 1180–2
    splinted *versus* single-unit
      restorations 1189–90, *1191*
    technique 1176–7
    treatment planning 1175–6
  posterior segment 676–7, *678*
  premolars *1140*, 1141, 1143
  psychophysical testing 114–15, 121,
      122
  recipient site 1074
  re-innervation 120
  rejuvenation at contaminated
      surface 1047
  removable prostheses 587
  replacement of teeth
    diseased 587
    strategically important
      missing 1144–5
  resonance frequency analysis 629
  restoration-driven 1156
  restorative dentistry 1138–45
  ridge augmentation
      procedures 1083–94
  risk indicators 635–6
  risk predictors 636
  rotation–symmetrical 1165
  safety zone 611–12, *613*
  scalloped design 1165–6
  screw-retained suprastructure 1154–5
  screws 627
    component complications 1230–1
    diameter 594
    solid 103
  segmented fixed restorations 1166,
      1167–70, 1170
  self-tapping 101–2, *103*
  sensory motor interactions 121–2
  short 1117–18
  shoulder
    depth in relation to labial mucosal
      margin 1154
    distance to plane of occlusion
      1194
    microgap 1162
    sink depth 1150
    submucosal 1165
  shoulder-level impression 1196–7
  single-tooth 596
  smoking risk 589, 591
  soft tissue 629–30, 636
    grafts 1089

    loss 1214–15
    stability 1147
  splinting 1189–90, *1191*
  stability 1077
    placement immediately after
      extraction 1061
  static loads 366, 368
  submucosal shoulder position 1165
  success criteria 635
  supportive care 676
  surface quality 1048, *1049*, 1050
  surgical site 1068–77
  survival rate 639
    maxillary sinus floor
      elevation 1110, 1116–17
  system components 626, 627–8
  tactile capacity 121–2
  technical failures 626–8
  tilted *1100*
  tissue biotype 1064–5
  tissue injury 99–100
  titanium 600
  tooth lengthening 590
  trap door procedure *1185*
  treatment spectrum 604–5
  treatment success 1065
  vertical distance requirement 594
  vertical ridge defects 1092
  vibrotactile capacity 121, 122
  wide-diameter/wide-platform 1182
  wound chamber 103–4, *105*
  wound healing 100
  see also maxillary sinus floor
      elevation; osseointegration;
      peri-implantitis
implant pass 623, *624*
implant patient
  age 639–40
  alcohol abuse 645
  anamnestic information 625
  autoimmune disorders 643–4
  clinical conditions 596
  clinical inspection 625–6
  communication problems 645–6
  connective tissue disorders 643–4
  diabetes mellitus 642–3
  endodontic infection 639
  esthetic implication sites 594–7, **598**
  esthetics and tooth movement 1263–
      5, *1266*, 1267
  examination 587–97, **598**
    clinical 596–7, 601, 625–6
    components 636
    extraoral 591–2
    implant-supported
      restorations 623–32
    intraoral 592–7
    local 591–7
    radiographic 592, *593*, 596–7,
      600–21
  expectations 646
  failure-associated complications 635
  history 590–1
  immunosuppression 642
  implant placement 593
  lack of understanding 645–6
  local conditions 637–9
  medications 640–2
  oral hygiene 645, 646
  oral infections 637–9
  orthodontic pretreatment 593, *594*
  osteoporosis 643
  pass 623, *624*
  periodontitis 638–9
  post-surgical infection
      minimizing 636–7
  post-treatment care/maintenance
      program 646
  prognosis 675–6
  psychiatric/psychological issues 645

questionnaire 625
radiography
    examination 592, *593*, 596–7,
        600–21
    treatment monitoring 614–16, *617*,
        618, *619*–20
risk assessment 597, **598**, 634–46
    behavioral considerations 645–6
    clinical information 636
    principles 634–7
risk factors
    local 637–9
    systemic 639–45
satisfaction 1147
smoking 640, 645
substance use/abuse 645
technical procedures to minimize
    risk 636–7
tissue damage minimization 637
treatment
    planning 601–7, 675–84, *685*
        radiographic monitoring 614–16,
        617, 618, *619*–20
implant recognition software 625
implant stability quotient (ISQ) 629,
    1077
implant-supported restorations
    abutments 1225–6, *1227*, 1231
        materials 1233
    bite force 1228
    butt-joint interface 1230
    cement-retained 1233
    clinical
        inspection/examination 625–6
    complications 626–8, 1222–35
        abutment-related 1231
        biologic 1224–6
        clinical 1224–31
        implant screw-related 1230–1
        mechanical 1226–31
        overdenture 1226–8
        peri-implant 1224–5
        prosthetic 1231–5
        surgical 1224
    diagnostic waxing 1225
    esthetics 630–2, 1233–4
    external hex 1230–1, 1232
    implants 628–9
        angulation 1231–2
        loss 1224
        malpositioned 1225–6, 1234
    internal hex 1232
    load resistance 1232
    marginal defects 1225
    material failures 1228–9
    midline fracture 1229
    occlusal wear 1229
    one-piece implant designs 1232
    overdentures 1226–8, 1232
    patient examination 623–32
    restorative veneer fracture 1228
    screw-retained 1233
    soft tissues 629–30
        responses 1234
    success/survival rate 1234–5
    surgical guide 1225, *1226*
    technical failures 626–8
    treatment planning 1225
    see also fixed partial dentures (FPD)
impressions, master model 1154
incisive foramen width 607
incisors
    crowded 1274
    furcations 826
    overlapping 1274
    papillae 1248
indole 1326
infection 184
    control
        for implant placement 676

self-performed 798–9
    in surgery 815
dental pulp 504–8, *509*, 510–16, *517*
dental team protection 687–8
dissemination 502
endodontic 639
focal 476
maxillary sinus 1106
medical conditions
        predisposing 752–3
opportunistic 184
oral in implant patients 637–9
periodontium of endodontic
        origin 849–51, *852*, 853–8
post-surgical 636–7
preterm birth 481
root-filled teeth 858
soft tissues around implants 629,
    630
systemic diseases 476
treatment complication 688–9
see also bacteria/bacterial infections;
        fungal infection; gingivitis;
        pathogens; peri-implantitis;
        periodontal abscess;
        periodontitis; root canal infection;
        stomatitis; viral infections
infection plaque 856
inflammation
    gingival 287, *288*, 289, 406, *407*, 408,
        415
        attachment loss/tooth loss 422
    gingivitis lesion 289
    innate immune process 298–9
    orthodontic therapy 963
    periodontal tissue assessment 130
inflammatory cells 20, 21
    infiltrate *580*
inflammatory mediators, preterm
    birth 481
inflammatory processes
    dental pulp 506, *507*, *508*, *509*
    periodontal infections 295
inflammatory response
    aggressive periodontitis 441
    clinically healthy gingiva 286–7
    dental pulp 505–6, *507*, *508*, *509*
    gingivitis 286–7
    innate immune mechanism 297
    leukocyte migration 302
    peri-implant mucosa 531
    peri-implantitis 534, *535*
    periodontal infections 285
    periodontium 850–1
    smoking 320
    sutures 1037–8
infrabony defects 901, *902*
    orthodontic tooth movement 1252–3
infrabony pockets 351
    orthodontic intrusion 1256
    trauma from occlusion 352
infraorbital artery 43
infraorbital nerve 48
initial tooth mobility (ITM) 1125–7
innate defense systems 297–9
    gingival crevicular fluid antibodies/
        complement 440
    microbial modulation 299
innate immunity receptors, gene
    polymorphisms 338, *339*
insertion/deletion polymorphisms *329*
instrument tray 803
instrumentation, hard tissue
        trauma 882
instruments
    maxillary sinus floor elevation 1099
    microsurgery 1030, 1035
    root debridement 768–70, *771*
    surgery 802–5
insulin 92

insulin resistance 91, 92, 308
    bacterial infection 309
insulin-like growth factor (IGF) 87,
    559
    alveolar bone healing 89
    ridge augmentation 1093
insulin-like growth factor 1 (IGF-1)
    311
intercellular adhesion molecule 1
        (ICAM-1) 302–3
    leukocyte adhesion deficiency 320
intercellular adhesion molecule, soluble
        (sICAM) 320
interdental brushes 714, 716–17, 727
    efficacy 736
    hard tissue damage *720*
interdental cleaning 714–17, 735, 736
    efficacy 736
    mechanical for plaque build-up
        prevention 414
interdental papilla *see* papilla
interdental recession 1271–2, *1273*,
    1274
    prevention 1272
interdental septum 53, *54*, *55*
interdental space, assessment 630, *631*
interdental support, root coverage 991
interferon γ (IFN-γ) 300
interleukin(s) 296
interleukin 1 (IL-1)
    bone loss
        peri-implant 341
        systemic 90
    late implant failures 342
    see also IL1 gene
interleukin 1α (IL-1α) 296
interleukin 1β (IL-1β) 249, 296, 310
interleukin 2 (IL-2) 300
interleukin 6 (IL-6) 90
interleukin 10 (IL-10) gene
        polymorphisms 339–40
intermicrobial matrix 189–91
international normalized ratio
        (INR) 642
interpositional graft procedure 1014,
    1015, *1016*
    combined with onlay grafts 1020
interproximal brushes 714, 716–17, 727
intrabony defects 551, *552*
    barrier membranes 906, *908*
    enamel matrix derivatives 908–9,
        939–40
    guided tissue regeneration 903, 905,
        906, *907*, **910**
    membranes 930–2, **933**
    papilla preservation flaps 916–17,
        918
    regenerative therapy strategy 948
    surgical access 945
intracellular adhesion molecule 1
        (ICAM-1) 289, *291*
intracoronal bleeding, peripheral
        inflammatory root resorption 870
intradental A-delta fibers 520
intradental nerve 48
intraseptal artery 43, 46
iodine tincture, vertical root fracture
        diagnosis 863
irradiation geometry 618, *620*
irrigation
    full-mouth disinfection 776
    subgingival 753
irrigators 742
    pulsating 717

jaw
    bone defects 36
        implant placement planning 1070
    fixation and chlorhexidine use 752
    shape variation 1073
    see also mandible; maxilla

jiggling-type trauma 354–7, 358, 360, *361*
  anchor teeth 1290
  orthodontic treatment *1246, 1250–1,* 1262
  zones of co-destruction 359
jugulodigastric lymph nodes 47
junctional epithelium 8, *9*, 16, 17, 18, 19

Kaposi's sarcoma *464*
keratin synthesis 15
keratinization 11, 15
keratinocytes 12, 14–15
  cytotoxic immune reaction 390
  differentiation 14, 15
keratin-producing cells 11
keratohyalin bodies 14–15
Klebsiella oxytoca 225
Klebsiella pneumoniae 225
knives 803–4
Koch's postulates 213

lactoferrin 296, 298
lamellar bone 62
  edentulous alveolar ridge 67
  osseointegration 107
lamina dura 27, *28*, 36
lamina propria 5, 19–24
Langerhans cells 11, 12
laser therapy, ablative 771, 772
leptin 88
leukemia
  aggressive periodontitis 446
  chronic periodontitis 425
  gingival manifestations 395–6
  gingivitis 411–12
  necrotizing periodontal disease 465, 468
  necrotizing ulcers 465
  surgery contraindication 800
leukocyte(s)
  gingival crevice 286, *288*
  implant wound chamber 104
  migration 302
  necrotizing periodontal disease 468
  peri-implant mucosa 531
  periodontal abscesses 499
  pocket epithelium 292
  recruitment 304
  subgingival plaque 192, *193*, 194, *198*
leukocyte adhesion deficiency (LAD) 320
  aggressive periodontitis 446
leukoplakia, oral 393
leukotoxins **214**, 216, 223, 248, 294
  A. actinomycetemcomitans **214**, 216, 294, 438, 440
  aggressive periodontitis bacteria 438, 440
lichen planus 384, *385–6*, 387
lichenoid lesions, oral 387
lighting 1030
linear gingival erythema 381–2, 412
lingual artery 1072, *1073*
lingual nerve 48
  block 802
linkage analysis, aggressive periodontitis inheritance 442–3
lipopolysaccharide 156, 249, 294
  A. actinomycetemcomitans 439–40
  in calculus 766
  on cementum 766
  host receptor recognition 298
  preterm birth 481–2
lipopolysaccharide-binding protein 298
lipoteichoic acids 294
liver disease 689
  fetor hepaticus 1327
local anesthesia
  individual variability 801–2

  mechanism of action 800
  surgery 800–2
  techniques 802
  types 801
localized aggressive periodontitis (LAP) 140–1, 213
  A. actinomycetemcomitans 215–17, 243
  Eikenella corrodens 223
  lesion long-term stability 243–4
long tooth syndrome 595–6
loupes 1030–2
  advantages 1034–5
  convergence angle *1031*, 1032
  disadvantages 1034–5
  field of view *1031*, 1032
  illumination 1032
  interpupillary distance 1032
  selection 1032, **1033**
  viewing angle *1031*, 1032
  working distance/range 1031
low birthweight 480
  periodontal disease 482, **483**, 484, **485**, 486
lupus erythematosus 391–2
lymph nodes 47
  swelling 463
lymphatics, periodontium 47
lymphocytes *20*, 21
  adaptive defense system 299
  gingivitis 289
  host defense 248
  smoking effects 321
lymphogranulomatosis, surgery contraindication 800
lymphoreticular disorders, implant patient 644
LYS-gingipain 249
lysozymes 1101

alpha-2 macroglobulin 295
macrophages 19, 20
  diabetes mellitus 310
  host defense 248
  implant wound chamber 104
  migration 301
  tooth socket healing *59*, 60
MadCAM-1 homing receptor 304
magnetic resonance imaging, functional (fMRI) 114
Maillard reactions 749
maintenance care visits 1313
major histocompatibility complex (MHC) 300
malnutrition
  gingival disease 412–13
  necrotizing periodontal disease 469
malocclusion, incisor crown shape 1274
mandible
  incisive canal bundle 110
  local anesthesia 802
  neuroanatomy 110–11, *112*
  opening amplitude 592
  premolars 826, *827*
  see also molars, mandibular
mandibular canal
  identification 1069
  implant planning 611–12, *613*, 614
mandibular overdentures 370
marginal tissue 629–30
  recession 632, 958–61
mast cells 19–20
master model, impressions 1154
matrix metalloproteinases (MMPs) 295–6
  polymorphisms 644–5
maxilla
  alveolar process 6
  anterior teeth gingival margins 1248, *1259*

edentulous 1166, *1167–70*, 1170
local anesthesia 802
neuroanatomy 110, *112, 113*
segmented fixed implant restorations 1166, *1167–70*, 1170
width growth 1287
see also molars, maxillary; premolars, maxillary
maxillary anterior single-tooth replacement 1149–57, *1158*, 1159, *1160*, 1161
  sites with extended horizontal deficiencies 1156–7, *1158*
  sites with localized horizontal deficiencies 1156
  sites with major vertical tissue loss 1157, 1159, *1160*, 1161, *1162*
  sites without significant tissue deficiencies 1152–5, *1156*
maxillary arch, length discrepancies 1287
maxillary complex displacement 1287
maxillary multiple-unit anterior fixed implant restorations 1161–5
  sites with extended horizontal deficiencies 1164–5
  sites with major vertical tissue loss 1165
  sites without significant tissue deficiencies 1163–4
maxillary sinus
  anatomy 1100–1
  blood supply 1101
  drainage 1101
  infection 1106
  membrane perforation 1106
  respiratory epithelium 1101
  septa 1101
maxillary sinus floor
  elevation 1099–119
  augmentation 1100
  clinical decisions 1118, *1119*
  crestal approach 1099, 1110–17
    implant placement 1111–14, *1115*
    implant survival 1116–17
    indications 1111
    outcome 1116–17
    post-surgical care 1115
    success 1116–17
    surgical technique 1111–14
  delayed (two-stage) 1104, 1109, *1110*
  grafting materials 1107–8, 1115–16
  lateral approach 1099, 1100–10
    complications 1106
    contraindications 1102
    implant survival 1108–10
    indications 1102
    outcome 1108–10
    post-surgical care 1105–6
    pre-surgical examination 1101–2
    success 1108–10
    techniques 1102–5
  one-stage with implant installation 1104, *1105*, 1109
  osteotome technique 1110–17
    with grafting material 1114, *1115*
  short implants 1117–18
  sinus membrane perforation 1106
  sinusitis 1106
  treatment options 1099–100
  two-stage 1104, 1109, *1110*
mechanical stimulation 854
mechanoreceptors 109
mechano-transduction mediators 1264
medications
  chronic periodontitis 425
  drug interactions 690
  gingival disease 410–11
  gingival enlargement 392, 410–11, 641, 800

implant patients 591, 640–2
mucocutaneous disorders 392
patient examination 574
melanocytes 11–12, 14
Melkersson–Rosenthal syndrome 394
membrane-associated CD14 298
menopause
chronic periodontitis 425
periodontal effects 314–15
menstruation
gingivitis 409
halitosis 1335
periodontal effects 312
mental artery 43
Merkel's cells 11, 12
mesio-distal enamel reduction 1271–2, *1273*, 1274
mesio-distal gap
implant placement 1213
optimization of dimensions 1201
metal salts, plaque control 746
methicillin-resistant *Staphylococcus aureus* (MRSA) 744
methotrexate 392
methyl mercaptan 1326, 1327
methylene blue, root fracture diagnosis 863
metronidazole 450, 451, 471, 886
activity 889
amoxicillin combination 889
controlled delivery *886*
gel 891–2
healing after guided tissue regeneration 914
peri-implant lesions 878
microarrays 249
microbe-associated molecular patterns (MAMPs) 299
microbiota, healthy sites 234
Micromonas micros
cardiovascular disease 158
peri-implant infections 639
microorganisms
changing concepts 212–13
complex formation in biofilm 231–2
control 210
dentin permeability 505–6
endodontic 512–14
host-compatible 243
interactions 243
periodontal infections 208, 209–13
persistence 882–3
regrowth 882–3
screw-retained implant restoration colonization 1193
subgingival 883
subgingival plaque 192–3, 194, *195*, *198*
see also bacteria/bacterial infections;
fungal infection; *named organisms*;
viral infections
micro-satellites *329–30*
microscope, surgical 1030, 1032–4
advantages 1034–5
binocular tubes 1033, *1034*
disadvantages 1034–5
eyepieces 1033–4
lighting unit 1034
magnification changer 1033
objective lenses 1033
microsurgery 1029–42
clinical indications 1039–40
comparison to conventional interventions 1040, *1041*, 1042
concepts 1030–9
illumination 1030, 1034–5
instruments 1030, 1035
limitations 1039–40
magnification 1030–5, 1038, 1039
needle for suturing 1036, **1037**

practice requirements 1039
root coverage *1041*, 1042
suture materials 1035–8
sutures 1035–8, *1040*
teamwork 1038–9
techniques 1029–30
training 1038–9
microsurgical triad 1030
Miller class I–II defects **990**, **991**
mineral trioxide aggregate (MTA) 859
minimal inhibitory concentration (MIC) 885
minimally invasive surgical technique (MIST) 1039–40
miniplates, L-shaped 1285
miniscrews 1285
minocycline 886
microspheres 880, 891
ointment 891
miscarriage 161–2, 480
MMP gene polymorphisms 644–5
modified flap operation 787–8
molars
accessory canals 508
banding 1248
bonding 1248
implants *1140*, 1141, *1143*
mandibular 825–6
furcation defect regeneration *844*
furcation entrance 828
furcation plasty *831*
root separation and resection 835, 837, *837*, *839*, *842*
vertical fractures 861
maxillary 824, *825*
furcation entrance 828
root separation and resection 834–5, *836*, 837–8, *839*, *842*
periodontal abscesses 497, *499*
single-tooth restoration 1191–2, *1193*
uprighting and furcation involvement 1262–3
vertical root fracture diagnosis 863
monocytes
diabetes mellitus 310
implant wound chamber 104
necrotizing gingivitis 466
periodontal abscesses 499
motivational interviewing 695–702
advice giving 700
communication 698–700
definition 697
development 696–7
evidence for 697–8
implementation 698–700
oral hygiene 700–2
smoking cessation 702–3
mouth, hematoma of floor 1072–3
mouth rinses 737
alcoholic 741
allergic reactions 393
halitosis treatment 1336
home use studies 757
morning bad breath 1334
plaque control 741
standards 738
triclosan 745
see also chlorhexidine
mucocutaneous disorders
drug-induced 392
gingival disease 384, *385–6*, 387–92
mucogingival junction 6, 7, 8
ectopic tooth eruption 1006, *1007*, 1008
mucogingival margin/line 5, 6
mucogingival therapy 955–1023
crown-lengthening procedures 997, 999–1000, *1001*, 1002–6, *1007*, 1008

deformed edentulous ridge 1008–17, *1018–19*, 1020, *1021–3*
gingival augmentation 955–70
interdental papilla reconstruction 996–7
root coverage 970–82, *983–4*, *985–7*, *988–9*, 990–6
mucoperiosteal flaps 786, 787, *788*
deep dissection 1073
maxillary anterior single-tooth replacement 1157
maxillary sinus floor elevation 1102
mucosa *see* oral mucosa
mucositis
probing 80
see also peri-implant mucositis
multiple sclerosis, surgery contraindication 800
mutanase 740, 744
mutilated dentition treatment 1138–45
Mycobacterium chelonae 377
Mycoplasma pneumoniae 390
myocardial infarction (MI)
Peptostreptococcus micros association 224
risk with periodontitis 158, 476–7
surgery contraindication 799

nasal–maxillary complex alteration 1102
nasopalatine canals 111, *113*
bone augmentation *609*
width 607
nasopalatine foramen 111, *113*
necrotizing periodontal disease 459–72
acute phase treatment 470–2
age 470
alcohol consumption 470
alveolar mucosa 462, *463*, *464*
clinical characteristics 460–4
communicability 467–8
diagnosis 464–5
endotoxins 467
fever 463
gingival defect elimination 472
gingivitis pre-existence 469
histopathology 465–6
HIV infection 460, 462, *463*, *464*, 471–2
host response 468–9
inadequate sleep 469–70
interproximal craters 461–2
lesion development 460–1
leukemia 465, 468
lymph node swelling 463
maintenance phase treatment 472
malnutrition 469
microbiology 466–8
oral hygiene 463, *464*, 469, 471–2
pathogenesis 466–8
plaque control 472
predisposing factors 468–9
prevalence 460
previous history 469
racial factors 470
sequestrum formation 462
smoking 470
stress 469
systemic disease 468–9
treatment 470–2
necrotizing stomatitis 459, 462, *463*, *464*
diagnosis 464–5
necrotizing ulcerative gingivitis (NUG) 209–10, 413–14, 459
chronic periodontitis 426
needle, microsurgical suturing 1036, **1037**
Neisseria gonorrhoeae, gingival disease 377
nerve fibers, dentin exposure response 520

Neumann flap 787
neural crest 3
neurologic disorders, surgery
  contraindication 800
neutrophils 20, 21
  gingival crevice 286, *288, 291*
  gingivitis 286, *288, 293*
    necrotizing 466, *467*
  implant wound chamber 104
  peri-implant mucosa healing 76
  periodontal abscesses 499
  tooth socket healing *59, 60*
new attachment procedures 542, 551
NF-kappa B pathway *339*
nicotine 320
  absorption 317
nicotine replacement therapy 322
nifedipine, gingival overgrowth 392,
  410–11
nitro-imidazoles 886
nociceptors 109
non-specific plaque hypothesis 211
nutritional deficiencies
  chronic periodontitis 425
  malnutrition 412–13, 469
nystatin 752

obesity
  biofilm composition 235
  periodontitis 153–4
occlusal concept, implant-specific 1203
occlusal interference 829–30
occlusal relationships, crown-
  lengthening 1000, 1002
occlusion
  assessment 592
  masticatory forces 369–70
  trauma 353, 1125
    bone regeneration 1128–9
    orthodontic treatment *1246, 1250–1,*
    1262
    tooth mobility 1128
octenidine, plaque control 744
octopinol 746
odds ratio 143
odontoblasts 4
odontoplasty 831, *833*
onlay graft procedures 1015–17, *1018–*
  19, 1020, *1021–3*
  combined with interpositional
    grafts 1020
  donor site/tissue 1015, 1016–17
Onplant® 1285
open flap curettage technique 789–92
opsonization 301
oral contraceptives
  gingivitis 411
  periodontal effects 312, 316
oral epithelium 8–15
  barrier function 297
  basal layer 12
  cell layers 11
  clear cells 11–12, 13, 14
  dento-gingival region 17
  glycogen content in pregnancy 314
  junctional 8, *9,* 16, 17, 18, 19
  keratinized 73
  keratin-producing cells 11
  migration 16
  progenitor cell compartment 12
  reduced 16
  stratum spinosum 13
  subsurface *9, 10,* 11
  wound healing role 549–50
  see also dento-gingival epithelium
oral health
  motivational interviewing 698
  patient responsibility 720
oral hygiene
  access for devices 834

adherence 695–6
adjunctive aids 717–18
barrier membranes 937
behavior change 700–2, 707
biofilms 242
guided tissue regeneration 1261
implant patient 645, 646
instruction 720–2
interdental cleaning 714–17
motivation 706–7
motivational interviewing 700–2
necrotizing periodontal disease 463,
  464, 469, 471–2, *472*
orthodontic treatment of adults 1243–
  4, 1248
patient examination 573, 584–5
plaque build-up prevention 414
post-regenerative therapy 925–6
programs 721
psychosocial factors 738
public awareness 707
regenerative surgery 947
risk assessment 1305–6
root coverage 991
self-performed plaque control 706–19
side effects 718–19
tongue cleaning 717–18
see also chlorhexidine; toothbrushes;
  toothbrushing
oral hygiene products 737–8
  allergic reactions 393
  chemical injury 396
  see also dentifrices; mouth rinses;
    toothpaste
oral leukoplakia 393
oral lichenoid lesions 387
  allergic reactions 393
oral malodor, chlorhexidine use 753
oral mucosa 5
  allergic reactions 392–4
  buccal soft tissue dimensions 80–1
  keratinized 630, 631
  lining 5
  margin 629–30
    receding 632, 958–61
  masticatory 5–6
  peri-implant 71–8, 629, *630*
    receding margins 632
  periodontal mechanoreceptor
    activation 117
  ridge 530
  specialized 5
  tissue-matched shades 1214
  see also peri-implant mucosa
oral sepsis 476
oral sulcular epithelium 8, *9,* 10, 17, 18
oral tumors
  maxillary sinus 1102
  periodontal abscess differential
    diagnosis 500
Oral-B Sonic Complete® toothbrush
  713
OralChroma™ 1330, *1332*
organ transplantation, surgery
  contraindication 799–800
organic acids 247
organoleptic evaluation 1328, *1331*
oro-antral fissure, necrotizing
  stomatitis 462
orofacial granulomatosis 394
orofacial region neuroplasticity 121
orthodontic appliances
  bonding 1248
  chlorhexidine use 753
  implants for abutment 1282
  periodontally compromised
    patients 1244–5, *1246–7,* 1248
  retention *1242, 1244, 1245, 1246–7,*
    1248–9, *1250–1*
  steel ligatures *1245, 1246–7,* 1248

orthodontic forces, root surface
  resorption 867–8
orthodontic loading, alveolar
  bone 363–5
orthodontic tilting movements 354
orthodontic trauma 353–4
orthodontic treatment
  aggressive periodontitis 662, *665*
  anchorage 1280–90, *1291*
  bodily tooth movement 354
  esthetics *1244, 1246–7,* 1248
  extrusion of single teeth 1255–6,
    1257–8, 1259, 1263, *1265–6, 1266*
    collagen formation 1264
  furcation involvement 1262–3
  gingival margins 1248, *1259*
  gingival recession 961–4
  hopeless teeth as anchorage *1251,*
    1252
  implant anchorage 1203, 1280–90,
    1291
  intrusion 1256, 1259–60
  jiggling *1246, 1250–1,* 1262
  legal aspects 1249, 1252
  minor surgery 1274–5, *1276*
  oral hygiene 1243–4, 1248
  periodontal disease 1243–5, 1248
  peripheral inflammatory root
    resorption 870
  recession defects 971, *973*
  retention *1242, 1244, 1245, 1246–7,*
    1248–9, *1250–1*
  risk management 1249, 1252
  splinting 1249
  tooth inflammation 963
  tooth movement in adults 1252–3,
    1254, 1255–6, 1257–8, 1259–65,
    1266, 1267
  traumatic occlusion *1246, 1250–1,*
    1262
  see also tooth movement, orthodontic
orthokeratinization 11
Orthosystem® 1285, *1286, 1289,* 1290
osseointegration 99–107, 363
  bone remodeling 107
  definition 99
  excessive occlusal load 366, **367**
  failure 618, *619*
  functional loading 365
  loss 364
    excessive loading 368–9
    peri-implant 1058–9
  osteoporosis 90–1
  process 103–5, *106,* 107
  quality assessment 629
  wide marginal defects 1045–6
  wound chamber 103–4, *106,* 107
  wound cleansing 104
  see also implant(s); re-osseointegration
osseoperception
  neurophysiology 109–11, *112, 113*
  peri-implant 108–11, *112,* 119–22
osseous defects *see* bone defects
ostectomy 796–7
osteitis, necrotizing stomatitis 462
osteoblasts 5, 21, 39, 40, 86
  bone deposition 42
  bone multicellular unit 41, 88
  bone resorption 866
  communication with osteocytes 39
  differentiation 92
  proliferation 92
osteocalcin, diabetes mellitus 91
osteoclasts 41, 42, 87
  activation 296
  bone multicellular unit 88
  bone resorption 359
    indirect 354
    treatment *91*
  jiggling forces 358

osteoconduction 93, 94
osteocytes 38–9, 86
  communication with osteoblasts 39
  cytoplasmic processes 40–1
osteogenesis 93
  malpositioned tooth movement 1253, *1256*
osteoid 39
  formation 60
osteoinduction 93, 94
osteoinductive factors 559
osteomyelitis
  bisphosphonate-associated 591
  periodontal abscess differential diagnosis 500
osteonecrosis
  bisphosphonate-associated 591, 640–1
  implant failure 640–1
  of the jaw 90
osteons 37–9
  primary 62, *106*, 107
  secondary 62, 107
  tooth socket healing 62
osteopenia 89–91
  periodontitis 154
osteoplasty 796
osteoporosis 89–91
  chronic periodontitis 425
  fractures 315
  implant patient 643
  periodontal effects 314–15
  periodontitis 154
  smoking 315, 322
  treatment 315
osteoprogenitor cells 86–7
osteoprotegrin 91, 296, 297
osteoradionecrosis, implant patient 642
osteotome, tapered 1099, *1100*
osteotome technique of maxillary sinus floor elevation 1110–17
overdentures 1075
  implant angulation 1232
  implant-supported restoration complications 1226–8
  mandibular and occlusal force distribution patterns 370
oxidation–reduction potential (Eh)
  pathogen growth conditions 247
  periodontal infections 209
oxygen
  bacterial growth 185
  pathogen requirements 247
oxygenating agents 746
oxytalan fibers 21, 22, 30

pain
  control during treatment 690–1
  non-surgical treatment 773–4
  post-operative control 812
  scaling and root planing 773
  vertical root fracture 861, *862*, *864*
pain syndromes
  root dentin hypersensitivity 518, 520
  treatment goal 655
palatal nerve
  block 802
  greater 48
palate, hard 5, 6
palatine artery, greater 43
palatine canal, greater 43
palmo-plantar keratitis, aggressive periodontitis 446
papilla 6, 7
  classification system 996
  defects 1271
  dimensions 71
    between adjacent implants 82–3, *84*
    between teeth and implants 81–2
  height
    classification 996

  loss 996, 997
  inter-implant 82–3, *84*, 594–5
  maxillary incisors 1248
  reconstruction 996–7, *998*
  surgical techniques 997, *998*
  tissue loss 594–5, 1274
papilla preservation flap 792–3, 916–17
  e-PTFE combination 945
  intrabony defects 916–17, *918*
  modified 916
  outcomes 945
  simplified 920–2, *923*, *924*, *925*, 945, 948
    minimally invasive surgery 922–3
papilla preservation technique, modified 917–18, *919*, *920*, *921*, *922*, 945
  barrier membranes 917–18, *919*, *920*, *921*
  biologically active regenerative materials 918, *922*
  enamel matrix derivative 918, *922*
  minimally invasive surgery 922–3
papillomavirus, periodontal infection 225
Papillon–Lefèvre syndrome (PLS) 332–3
  aggressive periodontitis 446
  implant patients 645
paraformaldehyde 396
parakeratinization 11
parathyroid hormone (PTH) 88
  ridge augmentation 1093
Parkinson's disease, surgery contraindication 800
parodontitis interradicularis 584
parodontitis profunda 584
parodontitis superficialis 583–4
passive threshold determination 115, *116*, *117*
pathogen-associated molecular patterns (PAMPs) *339*
pathogenicity mechanisms 245–9
pathogen-related oral spirochetes 221
pathogens 208
  adherence 248
  antibiotic susceptibility 886–7
  antibody evasion 247–8
  bridging species 222, 232, 246
  climax community complexity 271–3
  coaggregation 222, 231–2, *233*, 246
  colonization 245–9, *246*
    antagonistic substances 247
    host defense mechanisms 247–8
  criteria for defining 213
  elimination in aggressive periodontitis 449–52
  genome sequences 249
  host response 440–1
  host-compatible 243
  immune pathology 248–9
  immune suppression 248
  interbacterial relationships 246–7
  interfamily transmission 237
  intraoral transmission 275
  invasion 248–9
  mixed infections 225–6
  multiplication 246
  necrotizing periodontal disease 466–8
  new putative 225
  nutrient requirements 246
  oxygen requirements 247
  peri-implant infections 268–79
    climax community complexity 271–3
    edentulous subjects 273–5
    implant exposure timing 271–3
  periodontal 145–6, *147–8*, 148, 184
  polymicrobial microbiota 226
  prevalence in periodontitis patients 331

  regulons 244
  resistance
    to antiseptics/antibiotics 248
  source 208
  specific suppression 883
  tissue damage 248, 249
  transmission 236–8
    intraoral 275
  types 213, *214*, 215–26
  virulence mechanisms 249
  virulent 243
  see also bacteria/bacterial infections; fungal infection; viral infections
patient(s)
  affirming 699
  giving advice 700
  health protection 688
  history for implant therapy 590–1
  reflection of communication 699
  responsibility for oral health 720
  see also implant patient
patient examination
  alveolar bone 583
  chief complaint 573, 590
  compliance 591
  dental history 573, 590–1
  expectations 573, 590
    implant success 646
  family history 573, 590
  functional disturbance screening 585
  furcation involvement assessment 580–3
  gingiva 574–7
  habits 591
  hard tissue assessment 592
  implant therapy 590–1
    candidate 587–97, **598**
  implant-supported restorations 623–32
  medical history/medications 574, 591
  motivation 591
  occlusion assessment 592
  oral hygiene 573, 584–5
  periodontal disease 573–85
    signs/symptoms 574–83
  periodontal lesion diagnosis 583–4
  periodontal ligament 577–83
  radiographic 592
  root cementum 577–83
  smoking history 574
  social history 573, 590
  tooth mobility assessment 580, 582
pattern recognition receptors (PRRs) 299
pedicle graft procedures
  double 1005–6, *1007*
  gingival augmentation 966
  healing 993–5
  roll flap procedure 1011–13
  root coverage 972, 974–82, *983*
    combined with barrier membrane 980–1, *983*
    enamel matrix derivatives 981–2
peer-abutment 1179
pemphigoid 387–9
pemphigus vulgaris 389–90
penicillins 886
  adverse reactions 887
Peptostreptococcus, root canal infection 512–13
Peptostreptococcus micros 223–4
  peri-implant infection 275, 277
  smoking association 319
perception, periodontal tactile 108–11, *112*
  neurophysiology 109–11, *112*, *113*
  peri-implant osseoperception 108–11, *112*
  psychophysical assessment 114–15
  testing 113–15

periapical abscess
  diabetes mellitus 309
  drainage 851, *852*
pericytes 87
  bone multicellular unit 88
peri-implant crevicular fluid (PICF)
      analysis 1150
peri-implant lesions 875–80
  bone defects 877
  cumulative interceptive supportive
      therapy 878–80
  diagnosis 875
  mechanical debridement 877
  non-surgical debridement 876
  regenerative therapy 880
  resective therapy 880
  resolution 877–8
  surgical therapy 876–7
  treatment strategies 875–8
peri-implant mucosa 71–8, 529
  barrier epithelium 73, 74
  biologic width 72–6
  buccal soft tissue dimensions 80–1
  collagen fibres 76
  connective tissue quality 76–7
  dimensions 82
  healing 76
  inflammatory response 531
  morphogenesis of attachment 76
  probing 79–80, 81
  thin/thick periodontal biotypes 81,
      82
  vascular system 78
peri-implant mucositis 530, 531–2, 876,
      877
  plaque formation 530–2
peri-implant tissues 363–72
  load/loading
    bone reactions to functional 365
    cyclic 366, 368
    excessive occlusal 365–6, *367*
    orthodontic 363–5
    osseointegration loss 368–9
    static 366, 368
  masticatory occlusal forces 369–70
  osseoperception 108–11, *112*
  tooth–implant supported
      reconstructions 370–2
peri-implantitis 199, 268–79, 529–37
  bone loss 533, 534, 535
  climax community complexity 271–3
  clinical features 532, *533*
  disease-modifying genes 340–2
  edentulous subjects 273–5
  granulation tissue pathogens 277–8
  histopathology 534–7
  IL1 gene polymorphisms 590
  implant exposure timing 271–3
  implant-supported restorations 1225
  inflammatory response 534, *535*
  management 878
  microbiota of infection sites 277–9
  P. gingivalis 218
  partially edentulous subjects 275–6
  periodontal disease history 276–7
  pocket formation 535–6
  prevalence 532–4
  probing 80
  progression 536–7
  re-osseointegration 1046–8, *1049*,
      1050
  risk 589
  risk factors **635**
  soft tissues around implants 629, *630*
  treatment 877
periodontal abscess 496–502
  classification 496–7
  complications 501–2
  diabetes mellitus 309
  diagnosis 498–500

differential diagnosis 499–500
histopathology 497–8
infection dissemination 502
microbiology 498
non-periodontitis-related 496, 497
pathogenesis 497–8
periodontitis-related 496
peripheral inflammatory root
    resorption 869
post-therapy 496–7
prevalence 497
signs/symptoms 499, 500
sites 497, *499, 500*
tooth loss 501
treatment 500–1, **502**
vertical root fracture 861, *862*
periodontal disease
  age 143–4
  animal experiments *356, 357*
  assessment 135
  biofilms 229–31
  characteristics *576*
  definition 738
  destructive 218
    agents **215**
    gingival recession 959
  examination methods 129–31
  gender 144
  genetic component 328, 331
  genetic risk factors 331, 332–4
  index systems 129–31
  initiation 242–5
  lesion diagnosis 583–4
  low birthweight 482, *483*, 484, **485**,
      486
  maintenance care 1300
  orthodontic treatment 1243–5,
      1248
  patient examination 573–85
  peri-implant microbiota 276–7
  plaque-associated 358–60, *361*
  pre-eclampsia 486
  preterm birth 482, **483**, 484
  prevalence 133–5, *136–7*, 138, *139–40*,
      140–1
  prevention 1297–300
  probing assessments 132
  progression 134–5, 242–5, 331
    radiographic evaluation 1312
  pulp influence 516–18, *519*
  race/ethnicity 144, 471
  recurrent 1299–300
  screening 656–7
  sibling relationship 332
  signs/symptoms 574–83
  smokers 317–19
  susceptibility 735
  systemic disease risk 475–91
  tooth mobility 1127
  vaccines 210
  volatile sulfur compounds 1327
Periodontal Disease Index 130
periodontal dressings 811–12
Periodontal Index 130
periodontal innervation 112–13
  neural feedback 119
periodontal ligament 3, 4, 27–31
  blood supply 43, 46
  blood vessels 45
  collagen fiber bundles 31–2
  epithelial cells 30
  fibroblasts 33
  formation 5
  innervation 48, 49
  mechanoreceptors 108–9, 112–13, 116,
      117, 119
    activation 117
  patient examination 577–83
  principal fibers 28, 29, 30, *32*, 33, 36,
      42

re-establishment in re-implanted
    roots 547
tooth attachment 37
trauma from occlusion 357, 359
vascular plexus 77–8
widening 357, 359
  increased tooth mobility 1128–9
periodontal ligament cells 30
  periodontal regeneration 547
  regenerative capacity 548–9
periodontal pockets
  antibiotic actions 884
  antibiotic delivery 890
  bacterial infection 185, 884
  deep with peri-implant lesions 876
  depth
    reduction with forced tooth
        eruption 1004
    residual and regenerative
        surgery 931
  distal wedge procedures 794–5
  elimination 797
  endodontic lesion 855–6
  epithelium 292
  flap procedures 786–93
  gingivectomy procedures 784–6
  hard tissue 807–8
  iatrogenic root perforation 858,
      859
  microbial growth environment
      246
  periodontal abscesses 499
  probeable depth 797
  regenerative procedures 793–4
  residual 1306–7
  root debridement 770
  soft tissue 806, *807*
  spirochetes 220
  subgingival bacterial deposit 192–3,
      195, 197, 234, *238*
  subgingival calculus 197
  surgery
    healing 812–14
    techniques 783–94
  volatile sulfur compounds 1327
periodontal probes *578, 582*
periodontal probing
  aggressive periodontitis
      screening 437
  automated systems 580, *581*
  dento-gingival interface 79
  depth
    critical 816–17
    non-surgical treatment 774–5
    periodontal disease after scaling
        and root planing 1298, *1299*
    smoking 318, 321
  furcation involvement
      assessment 582
  peri-implant mucosa 79–80, 81
  peri-implantitis 80
  periodontal tissue assessment 130,
      132
    patient assessment 577–83
    regeneration 561–2
periodontal receptors 108–9, 112–13
  activations 117
  oral stereognosis 119
  reduction 116, *117*
periodontal risk assessment (PRA)
      calculation 1308–9
periodontal support
  interdental 991
  loss in relation to age 1307
  residual 1310
periodontal tactile function 115–17
  active threshold determination 115,
      117
  passive threshold determination 115,
      116, 117

periodontal tissues 349–60, *361*
  breakdown and orthodontic tooth
      movement 1241, *1242*, 1243–5,
      1246–7, 1248–9, *1250–1*, 1252
  fibrous reunion 544, *545*
  regeneration 541–62
    assessment 542, 561–2
    concepts 550–61
    grafting procedures 551–7
    growth regulatory factors 559
    histologic studies 562
    root surface biomodification 557–8,
        559
    wound healing 542–4, *545*, 546–50
periodontitis 90, 207–52, *253*
  adaptive defense system 299–304
  adult 133–5, *136–7*, 138, *139–40*, 140–
      1, 332
    assessment for implants *588*
  advanced 584
  age 143–4
  alveolar bone resorption 440
  alveolar process change 52
  apical 511
  attachment loss 440, 1300
  biofilms 208
  BMI 153–4
  bone destruction 296–7
  buccal migration of tooth *576*
  calculus association 133, 134, 202–3
  cardiovascular disease 476–80
    risk 476–80
    treatment effects 489
  characteristics 883–4
  chronic 332, 420–6
    attachment loss 423
    characteristics 420, *421*, 422
    clinical features 420
    etiology 669
    furcation involvement *575*, 667,
        668, 669–73
    gingivitis as risk 422
    heritability 332
    prevalence 423
    progression 423–4
    risk factors 424–6
    single implant 683, *684–5*
    stress 425–6
    susceptibility 422–3
    treatment 426, 667, *668*, 669–73
  chronic obstructive pulmonary
      disease 488–9
  classification 428
  colonization 208
  complexity 328
  course 208
  dental plaque association 212–13
  diabetes mellitus 151, *152–3*, 153, 162,
      245, 308
    association 92, 486–8
    control 309–10
    treatment effects 490–1
  diagnosis 583–4
  disease-modifying genes 333–40
  early onset 331–2, 428, 431–2
  endodontic lesion differential
      diagnosis 851, 853–6
  etiologic agents 208, 209, 212
  etiology 212
  FcγRIIa polymorphisms 338
  fixed partial denture loss 1224
  frequency distribution 133
  furcation area 584
  gender 144
  gene mutation 332–3
  gene polymorphisms 144–5, 333–40
  genetic component 328–9, 426
  genetic risk factors 331, 332–4
  genetics role 331–2
  glucose intolerance 153

heritability
  aggressive disease 331–2
  chronic disease 332
historical aspects 209–13
HIV infection 154–5, 244
host defense processes 295–304
host factors 234, 235–6
  susceptibility 244–5
host–parasite relationship 208–9, 294
  modification in diabetes
      mellitus 310
immune defense system 299–304
immune reactions 285
implant patients 638–9
inflammatory processes 295
inflammatory reactions 285
initiation 242–5
  factors 156
innate immune processes 298–9
invasion by pathogens 248–9
juvenile 193, *196*, *197*, 331–2
lesions 289–90, *291*, 292, *293–4*
ligature-induced 218
local environment 243–4
microbial invasion 294
microbiology 145–6, *147–8*, 148, 183–4
mixed infections 225–6
necrotizing 459
  acute form 463–4
  chronic form 463–4
  diagnosis 464–5
  interproximal craters 461–2
  Kaposi's sarcoma *464*
  recurrent 464
obesity 153–4
osteopenia 154
osteoporosis 154
pathogenesis 285–304
pathogenicity mechanisms 245–9
pathogens 208
  virulent 243
patients at risk 1300–2
periodontic/orthodontic
    treatment 1241, *1242*, 1243, *1244*,
    1245, *1246–7*, *1250–1*
phenotype 144–5
population at risk 331
pregnancy adverse outcomes 480–2,
    483, 484, **485**, 486
prepubertal 140–1, 333
prevalence 738
progression 134, 153, 242–5
  factors 156
proteases 295
psychosocial factors 155
race/ethnicity 144, 470
recurrent 1302–3
regenerative periodontal therapy 911
respiratory infection risk 488–9
risk assessment *1304*
risk factors 141–6, *147–8*, 148, *149–50*,
    151, *152–3*, 153–6, 655
severity 135, 153
  variability 286
sibling relationship 332
similarities to other infections 207–8
smoking 148, *149–50*, 151, 224, 235,
    245
spirochetes 221
stress 155
supportive periodontal
    therapy 1302–3
susceptibility 328–43
systemic disease
  risk 156–62
  treatment impact 489–91
tooth loss 141
trauma from occlusion 352–3
triclosan-containing toothpaste 745
unique features 208–9

virulence factors 243, 294
viruses 225
volatile sulfur compounds 1327
see also aggressive periodontitis
periodontium/periodontal tissue 3
  allergic reactions 849
  alveolar bone anatomy 34–42
  anatomy 3–49
  bacterial damage 440
  bacterial invasion 210–11
  blood supply 43–6, *47*
  development 3–5
  endodontic origin and infectious
      processes 849–51, *852*, 853–8
  endodontic treatment of lesions 858
  extravascular circulation 46, *47*
  function 3
  gingiva anatomy 5–27
  halitosis 1327, 1335
  healthy
    jiggling-type trauma 354–7
    reduced height 355–7
  inflammation assessment 130
  inflammatory lesions 850–1
  lymphatic system 47
  nerves 48–9
  neural feedback 119
  orthodontic single-tooth
      extrusion 1256, *1259*
  overt lesions 849
  periodontal ligament anatomy 27–31
  potential infection 208
  preservation 797
  rate of destruction 447
  regeneration 793–4
  root cementum anatomy 31–4
  smoking cessation 151
  support loss assessment 130–1
  toxic reactions 849
Periodontometer 1126
periosteal retention procedure 965–6
periosteum 40
  mechanoreceptors 121
    activation 117
Periotest® 1126–7
  implants 629
peroxyborate/peroxycarbonate 746
pH
  biofilms 227
  pathogen growth conditions 247
  periodontal infections 209
phagocytes
  defects in aggressive
      periodontitis 449
  endodontic lesions 514
phagocytosis *198*, 301
  pulp inflammatory response 507, *509*
  subgingival plaque 194
phantom tooth phenomenon 121
phenols, plaque control 745
phenytoin
  gingival enlargement 392, 410, 641,
      800
  surgery contraindication 800
phonetics with implants 628
  disturbances 595–6
physically handicapped people,
    chlorhexidine use 752
plant extracts, plaque control 745–6
plaque, atheromatous 157
  bacterial 192, *193*
plaque, dental 183–4
  accumulation with orthodontic
      appliances 1245, 1248
  Actinomyces-induced 185, *186*, 212
  bacteria 194, *195*, *198*, 199, 203
    rapid/slow former 241
    smoking effects 319
  biofilms 226–31, 238–9, *240*, 241–2
    mechanical debridement 772–3

plaque, dental (*continued*)
  carbohydrate content 191
  chemical control agents 742–60
    evaluation 754–60
  chronic periodontitis
    risk 424
    role 422
  conditioning film 185
  control 203
    bacterial tests 755
    clinical trials 757–60
    instruction 719–29
    motivation 719–29
    self-performed 522, 798–9
    study methods 755–7
    uptake measurements 755
  etiology 212
  experimental studies 756
  fibrillar component 190, *191*
  formation 185–7
  gingival disease 405–15
    treatment 414
  gingival margin accumulation 186–7
  gingival recession 958–9
  gingivitis 406, **407**, 407–8, 422, 1298
  glycoprotein pellicle 188
  HIV infection 412
  host susceptibility 738, 739
  immune response suppression 314
  infection 856
    association 212–13
    non-specific plaque hypothesis 211
  inflammatory response 415
  inhibitory agents 734, 754
  intermicrobial matrix 189–91
  lipids 191
  mechanical debridement 772–3
  microbial complexes 231–2, *233*, 234–8
  mineralization 199–200
  non-specific plaque hypothesis of infection 211
  oxygen levels 247
  patient examination 584–5
  peri-implant 196–7
  peri-implant mucosa response 530–2
  periodontitis in adults 133, 134
  reducing agents 734, 754
  removal
    adolescents 1243
    agents 740
    brushing force 718–19
    gingivitis control 710
    insufficient 735
    peri-implant 876
    self-performed 705, 706–19
  retentive factors 585
  smoking effects on bacteria 319
  structure 187–94, *195*, 196–7
  subgingival 191–4, *195*, 196, *198*, 199
    biofilm 231
    debridement 772–3
    Eubacterium 224
    pathogens 225
  supragingival 187–91, 199
    biofilm 230
    chemical agents 742–60
    chemical control 734–5, 737–60
    control 736–7
    debridement 772–3
    mechanical control 705–29, 735, 736–7
    removal 705–6
    vehicles for delivery of chemical agents 740–3
  treatment comparisons 815, *816*
Plaque Index (PLI) 130, *290*
plaque-inhibitory agents 742–60
  evaluation 754–60

plasma cells *20*, 21
  adaptive defense system 299
  aggressive periodontitis 441
  antibody production 301, *302*
  gingival *302*
  gingivitis 292, *293*
    necrotizing 466
plasma immunoglobulins 301
plasmatic circulation 969, 970
plastic surgery *see* microsurgery; mucogingival therapy
platelet-derived growth factor (PDGF) 87, 559, 938–9
  alveolar bone healing 89
  ridge augmentation 1093
platelets
  aggregation 479
  tooth socket healing 57, *59*
pneumonia, bacterial 488, 491
pocket probing depth (PPD) 575–6
  endodontic lesions 856, *857*
    angular bone defects 858
  peri-implant lesions 877
  regenerative therapy 948
  risk assessment 1311
  single-tooth replacement 1150
  soft tissue around implants 630
polyethylene glycol (PEG)
  hydrogel membranes 1094
  PTH carrier 1093
polyglycolic acid 930, 1084
  bioabsorbable barrier membrane 1086
polylactic acid 930, 1084
  bioabsorbable barrier membrane 1086
polymer grafts 556
polymerase chain reaction (PCR) 213
  biofilm bacterial detection/ enumeration 229
polymorphonuclear leukocytes (PMNs) *20*, 21
  aggressive periodontitis 441, 443–4
  chronic periodontitis risk 425
  dental pulp infection 514–15
  diabetes mellitus 310
  gingival crevice 286
  gingivitis 289
  host defense 248
    processes 296, *297*
  migration 301, 311
  peri-implantitis 534
  pocket epithelium 292
  pulp inflammatory response 506, 507, *509*
  smoking 320
polyphosphates 741
polytetrafluoroethylene, expanded (e-PTFE) 928, 945, 948, 1084
  BMP effects 1093–4
  lateral bone augmentation for posterior implants 1184
  maxillary anterior single-tooth replacement 1157
  papilla preservation flap combination 945
  pedicle soft tissue graft for root coverage 980
  ridge augmentation 1084, 1085–6
pontic
  central 1181, 1182
  contour refinement 1020, *1021–3*
porcelain-fused-to-metal alloys 1199
Porphyromonas, root canal infection 512–13
Porphyromonas gingivalis 145–6, *147–8*, *150*, 184
  adherence 248
  aggressive periodontitis 440, 441, 448
  alveolar bone loss 219
  antibiotics

local delivery 893
  microbiologic tests 890
  susceptibility 886–7
  systemic 889
antibody titers 303–4
Arg1-protease production 294
biofilm 231, 232
  composition 235–6, *237*, 239
  content 242
  implant surfaces 268–71
cardiovascular disease 157, 158, 479–80
carotid endarterectomy 157
destructive periodontal disease **215**, 218
diabetes mellitus 245
elimination by extraction of all teeth 274
endothelial cell invasion 479
HIV infection 244
immune response 218
immunization studies 218–19
infection 217–19
  mixed with *T. forsythia* 226
invasion 248
iron levels in environment 244
linear gingival erythema 382
pathogenic potential 243
peri-implant infection 271–3, 274, 275–6, 279
  periodontal disease history 276–7
  subgingival 639
periodontal abscesses 498
periodontal lesions in diabetes 310
polymicrobial microbiota 226
pregnancy exposure 482
prevalence in periodontal disease 331
protease production 249
smoking association 319
suppression 883
transmission 236
virulence factors 479
posterior dentition implants 1175–204
  clinical applications 1193–201, *1202*, 1203
  distally shortened arch 1180–7
  fixed implant-supported prostheses 1180–7
  multiple-unit tooth-bound restorations 1187–90, *1191*
  screw-retained restorations 1193–6
  single-tooth replacement 1191–2, *1193*
potassium salts
  desensitizing 741
  root dentin hypersensitivity 522
pouch graft procedures 1013–14
povidone iodine, plaque control 747
predentin 34
pre-eclampsia 480
  periodontal disease 486
pregnancy
  adverse outcomes with periodontitis 480–2, **483**, 484, **485**, 486
  complications 159–62
  gingival disease 409–10
  gingival keratinization reduction 313–14
  gingivitis 313, 409–10
  loss 161–2, 480
  medications 314
  periodontal effects 312–14
  periodontal treatment 314, 489–90
  periodontitis 480–2, **483**, 484, **485**, 486
    treatment effects 489–90
  plaque immune response suppression 314
pregnancy granuloma 314
pregnancy tumor 409–10

pre-medication 690–1
premolars
    implants *1140*, 1141, 1143
    mandibular 826, *827*
    maxillary 825
        root anatomy variation 828
        root separation and resection 835, *836*
        single-tooth restoration 1191, 1192, *1192, 1193*
        vertical root fracture diagnosis 863
presbyopia 1030
pressure zones 353, 354, 357, 358
preterm birth 159–60, 480–1
    infection 481
    periodontal disease 482, **483**, 484
Prevotella
    aggressive periodontitis 438
    root canal infection 512–13
Prevotella intermedia 211–12, 221–2
    biofilm
        content 242
        implant surfaces 268–71
    coronary heart disease 222
    diabetes mellitus 245, 310
    HIV infection 244
    linear gingival erythema 382
    necrotizing periodontal disease 466, 467, 468
    peri-implant infection 272–3, 274, 275–6, 279
        periodontal disease history 276–7
        subgingival 639
    periodontal abscesses 498
    plaque formation *186*
    pregnancy gingivitis 313
    prevalence in periodontal disease 331
    pubertal gingivitis 312
    smoking association 319
    virulence 222
Prevotella melaninogenica 498
Prevotella nigrescens 221–2
    peri-implant infection 277–8, 279
prism loupes 1031
probing *see* periodontal probing
probing attachment level (PAL) 130
    assessment 577
    basic periodontal examination 657
    inherent errors 577–80
    measurement errors 580
    peri-implant soft tissue 630
    periodontal disease after scaling and root planing 1298, *1299*
    periodontal tissue regeneration assessment 562
    supportive periodontal therapy *1301*
probing pocket depth (PPD) 130
    assessment 577, *578, 579*
    attachment loss *579*
    basic periodontal examination 656, 657
    inherent errors 577–80
    measurement errors 579–80
    reduction 655
        treatment comparisons 816
    trauma from occlusion 353
progesterone 312
    hormonal contraceptives 316
    pregnancy 312, 313–14
    tissue response 316
progestins, gingival disease 408
prognostic factors 142
pro-inflammatory mediators 479
prostaglandin E₂ 310
    crevicular fluid levels in aggressive periodontitis 449
    pregnancy 482
    preterm birth 481
prostaglandins 296
prosthetic components of implants 626

protease inhibitors 295
proteases 249, 294
    periodontal infections 295
    plaque control 744
proteoglycans 23, 24
proteolytic enzymes 209
pseudo-halitosis 1333
    therapy 1333–4
pseudomembrane 460
Pseudomonas aeruginosa 225
    antibiotic resistance 229
    biofilm 229
pseudopockets 583
psychiatric/psychological issues, implant patient 645
psychosocial factors, periodontitis 155
puberty
    gingivitis 312, 408–9
    periodontal effects 312
    see also adolescents
pulp, dental
    accessory canal communication 508, *510, 511*
    defense potential 505
    disease
        causes 504–5
        processes 504–8, *509*, 510–16, 849
        progression 505–7
    dynamic events 505–7
    exposure to oral environment 506
    fibrosis 518
    infection 504–8, *509*, 510–16, *517*
    inflammatory processes 506, *507, 508, 509*
        root canal system infection 510–16
    inflammatory responses 505–6
    intra-pulpal mineralizations 518
    necrosis 506–7, *509*
    periodontal disease influence 516–18, *519*
    periodontal treatment effects 518, *520*
    sensibility 854
    tissue necrosis 505
    vitality 505
        lost 849, 850
        testing 851, 853–6
pulpal axons, terminal branch sprouting 520
pulpal pathosis 829
pyogenic granuloma, pregnancy-associated 409–10
pyrophosphates 741

quaternary ammonium compounds 744–5
questions, open-ended 699
quorum sensing, biofilms 227–8

race/ethnicity
    factors in necrotizing periodontal disease 470
    periodontal disease 144
radiation detectors 618, *620*
radiation therapy, implant patient 642
radiographic analysis
    alveolar bone *576*, 583
    periodontal regeneration assessment 561, 562
radiography
    abutment placement 615–16
    aggressive periodontitis 659, 666, *667*
    ALARA principle *601*, 606
    alveolar crest for implant placement 1072
    bone loss 616, *618*
    chronic periodontitis 668, *673*
    condition of remaining teeth 602–3
    dosage *601*
    furcation involvement 828, *829, 830*

    implant patient 592, *593*, 596–7, 600–21
        treatment monitoring 614–16, *617*, 618, *619*–20
    implant planning 603–7
        lower jaw imaging 610–12, *613*, 614
        placement 1069–70
        upper jaw imaging 607–8, *609*, 610
    intraoral 604, 616, *617*
        radiation detectors 618, *620*
    necessary information 601–3
    osseointegration failure 618, *619*
    osseous lesions 902
    palatal implant insertion sites 1286
    panoramic 604, 615
    periodontal disease progression 1312
    reference 616
    root resorption 866, *867*
    surgical site 1068–9
    threaded implants 616, *617*
RANKL *91*, 296–7
reactive oxygen species 311, 321
reattachment procedures 542
receptor activator of nuclear factor-kappa beta (RANK) 296–7
receptors for advanced glycation endproducts (RAGEs) 487
reduced dental epithelium 16
re-entry operations, periodontal regeneration assessment 561, 562
reflection 699
regenerative periodontal surgery 541, 542, 903, 913–48
    bacterial contamination control 947
    barrier materials 928, 930–8
        furcation involvement 932–7
    barrier membranes 937–8
    biologically active materials 938–40
    bone replacement grafts 905, 907–8, *909*, 938
    complications 928
    coverage of regenerated tissue 915
    crestal incision 945
    furcation defects 840–3, *844*
        barrier membranes 904, 932–7
    infection control regime 926
    minimally invasive technique 922–5, *926, 927, 928, 929*
    modified papilla preservation technique 945
    oral hygiene 925–6, 947
    orthodontic tooth movement 1261–2
    outcomes 945
    papilla preservation flap 792–3, 916–17
        intrabony defects 916–17, *918*
        modified 916
        simplified 920–2, *923, 924, 925*, 945, 948
    papilla preservation modified technique 917–18, *919, 920, 921, 922*, 945
    post-operative morbidity 926–8
    post-operative regime 925–6
    suturing approach 945, 947
regenerative periodontal therapy 793–4, 901–48
    barrier membranes 905–7
    benefits 903–5
    biologically active regenerative materials 905, 908–9
    bone grafts 544–5, 546–7
        replacement 905, 907–8, *909*
    clinical efficacy 905–9
    clinical strategies 944–5, *946*, 947–8
    defect factors 911–12
    effectiveness 905–9
    enamel matrix derivatives 908–9
    evidence-based strategy 945
    indications 903

regenerative periodontal therapy
        (continued)
    long-term effects 903–5
    material selection 945
    patient factors 911
    PDGF 938–9
    periodontal infection 911
    prognostic factors 909, **910**, 911–13
    smoking 911
    surgical approach 913–48
    tooth factors 912–13
    tooth survival 904–5
    see also root surface, biomodification
regulons 244
relative risk 143
removable partial dentures (RPD) 1177
re-osseointegration 1046–8, *1049*, 1050
    definition 1046
    implant surface quality 1048, *1049*,
        1050
resonance frequency analysis,
        implants 629
respiratory burst 321
respiratory tract
    infections and periodontitis 488–9
    upper and extraoral halitosis 1327,
        1334
restorative dentistry
    defective margins 585
    dental pulp diseases 505
    gingival dimensions 964–5
    implants 1138–45
    shortened dental arch complex 1139
    treatment
        concepts 1138–9
        goals 1139
retainers 1248–9
rete pegs 10
retention assessment 755–6
reticulin fibers 21, 22
rheumatic endocarditis, surgery
        contraindication 799
ridge mucosa 530
risk assessment
    alveolar bone loss 1307
    attachment loss 1311
    bleeding on probing 1306, 1310–11
    calculation 1308–9
    continuous multi-level 1303–12, *1313*
    furcation involvement 1309
    iatrogenic factors 1309–10
    oral hygiene 1305–6
    periodontitis *1304*, *1305*
    pocket probing depth 1311
    process 142
        clinical implementation 1312
    recall system compliance 1304–5
    relative risk 143
    site 1310–12
    smoking 1308
    subject 1303–4
    systemic disease 1307–8
    tooth 1309–10
        loss 1307
        mobility 1310
risk factors for periodontal disease 141–
        6, *147–8*, 148, *149–50*, 151, *152–3*,
        153–6
    potential/putative 142, 143
    true 142
roll flap procedure 1011–13
roll with resistance 698
rongeurs 805
root
    coefficient of separation 823, *824*
    degree of separation 823, *824*
    development 4
    divergence 823, *824*
    iatrogenic perforation 858–9
        sealing 859, *860*

intra-alveolar displacement 1126
mechanical cleaning of surfaces 882
morphology alterations 497
resorption 547, 548, 550
    clinical presentation 866, *867*
    external 865–72
    external inflammatory 869, 871–2
    forms 866–72
    identification 866, *867*
    peripheral inflammatory 869–71
    replacement 868–9
    surface 866–8
    trigger mechanism 866
sensitivity with non-surgical
        treatment 773–4
stability 834
support remaining 834
trunk 823
    length 832
vertical fractures 859–63, *864*, *865*
    clinical expressions 861–2
    diagnosis 862–3
    incidence 861
    mechanisms 860–1
    treatment 863
see also furcated region; furcation
root canal infection 510–16, 850–1
    bacteria 512–14
    endodontic lesions 856, *857*
    periodontal tissue response 512
    treatment 856
root canal system, accessory
        canals 507–8, 510
root cementum 3, *29*
    patient examination 577–83
    periodontal ligament 28
root complex 823
root cones
    divergence 832, *833*
    fusion between 823–4, 833–4
    length 832–3
    shape 832–3
root coverage 970–82, *983–4*, *985–7*,
        988–9, *990*–6
    advanced flap procedure 972, 975–80
    clinical outcome 990–2
    connective tissue graft 985–7, *988–9*,
        990
    conventional surgery *1041*, 1042
    coronally advanced flaps 975–80, *981*,
        982, 985, 986, *989*, **990**, 991–2
        healing 994–5
        for multiple recessions 978–9,
            981
    double papilla flap 974
    epithelialized soft tissue graft *982*,
        984, 985, **990**
    exposed root surface treatment 973
    extent 990–2
    flap tension elimination 992
    free soft tissue graft procedure 972,
        982, *984*, 985–7, *988–9*, 990, 991–2
        epithelialized **990**
        healing 995–6
        thickness 992
    gingival margin position 992
    guided tissue regeneration **990**, 992
        healing 995
    interdental support 991
    microsurgery *1041*, 1042
    pedicle graft procedures 972, 974–82,
        983
        combined with barrier
            membrane 980–1, *983*
        with enamel matrix
            derivatives 981–2
        healing 993–5
    procedures 971–82, *983–4*, *985–7*,
        988–9, 990
    rotational flap procedure 972, 974–5

semilunar coronally repositioned flap
        procedure 976, 979–80, *982*
    soft tissue healing 992–6
root debridement
    ablative laser therapy 771, 772
    calculus removal 767–8
    full-mouth disinfection 776
    furcation involvement 773
    hand instrumentation 768–70, *771*
    method selection 771–2
    non-surgical methods 768–72
    reciprocating instruments 770–1
    sonic scalers 770, 771
    subgingival biofilm influence 772–3
    ultrasonic scalers 770, 771
root dentin hypersensitivity 518, 520–2
root planing
    chlorhexidine use 752
    see also scaling and root planing
root separation and resection 832–5,
        836, 837–8, *839*, 840, **845**
    mandibular molars 837, *839*, *842*
    maxillary molars 834–5, *836*, 837–8,
        839, *842*
    maxillary premolars 835, *836*
    periodontal surgery 838, 840
    prosthetic restoration 840, *841*
    treatment sequence 837–8, *839*, 840
root surface
    biomodification 557–8, *559*, 808, 943
    conditioning 808
    demineralization 557–8, *559*, 973
    exposed 973
    instrumentation 808
    tetracycline biomodification 943
root-filled teeth
    dentin dehydration 861
    fracture propensity 860
    infection 858
    moisture content 860–1
rotational flap procedure, root
        coverage 972, 974–5

salifluor 747
saline
    antimicrobial activity *756*
    sterile physiologic 805
saliva, innate mechanisms 298
sanguinarine 745
sarcoidosis 394
saucerization 1162
scalers 804–5
    sonic/ultrasonic 770, 771
scaling
    necrotizing periodontal disease 472
    periodontal abscesses 496–7
    periodontal therapy 251, *253*
    Tannerella forsythia control 219–20
scaling and root planing *253*
    attachment gain 817
    chronic periodontitis 671
    full-mouth disinfection 776
    furcation involvement 830
    impaired access 797–8
    local antibiotic delivery
        comparison 891
    new attachment 550–1
    pain 773
    periodontal disease prevention 1298,
        1299
    periodontal therapy 251
    systemic antibiotics 889
    Tannerella forsythia control 219–20
scanograms 615
scars, dental pulp diseases 505
Schwartzman reaction 467
scleroderma, implant patient 643
screw-retained restorations 1193–6
    transocclusal 1193–5
    transverse 1195–6

scurvy 412–13
    chronic periodontitis 425
selection bias 141
selective estrogen receptor modulators
    (SERMs) 91
Selenomonas 224
    necrotizing periodontal disease 466
self-efficacy, support 698
self-inflicted injuries 397, *398*
semilunar ganglion 48
sensibility tests 854, 855
sex steroid hormones
    chronic periodontitis 425
    gingival disease 408, *409*
    see also estrogen; progesterone
Sharpey's fibers 30, *32*, 33, 36
    alveolar bone proper 38, 42
    mineralization 34
shear force, biofilms 227
shortened dental arch (SDA) 1139
simple tandem repeats (STRs) *330*
single nucleotide polymorphisms
    (SNPs) *329*
sinusitis 1102
    maxillary sinus floor elevation
        1106
size discrimination 117, 118
Sjögren's syndrome
    biofilm composition 235
    implant patient 644
skatole 1326
skeletal anchorage systems 1281
sleep, inadequate 469–70
small-for-gestational-age births 484
smile line assessment 592
smoking 316–22
    alveolar bone loss 318
    antibiotic therapy regimens 890
    biofilm composition 235
    bone effects 322
    cessation 151, 322, 691, 696
        motivational interviewing 697–8,
            702–3
    counseling 691
    estrogen levels 315
    Eubacterium infection 224
    gingiva 318
    gingival crevice fluid effects 320–1
    gingivitis 319
    healing effects 321–2
    host response 319–22
    host susceptibility to disease 245
    IL1 gene polymorphisms 589, 591
    immune system effects 320
    implant patient 640, 645
    implant risks 589, 591
    inflammatory system effects 320
    inhalation 317
    maxillary sinus floor elevation 1102
    osteoporosis effects 315, 322
    patient examination 574
    periodontal disease 317–19
        necrotizing 470
    periodontitis 148, *149–50*, 151, 224,
        235, 245
        aggressive *432–3*, 445, *446*
        chronic 424, 669
    probing depth 318, 321
    regenerative periodontal therapy
        911
    risk assessment 1308
    smoke composition/exposure 317
    surgery contraindication 800
    vascular effects 321
socioeconomic status in
    periodontitis 144
socket former 1099
sodium chlorite, acidified 747
sodium fluoride, chlorhexidine
    synergism 753

sodium lauryl sulfate 741
    antimicrobial activity *756*
    plaque control 746
sodium valproate, gingival
    overgrowth 410
soft tissue
    damage from interdental
        cleaning 714
    morphology for bone
        regeneration 1085
    recession 683
    see also gingiva
soft tissue curettage 550–1
soft tissues, peri-implant 629–30
    evaluation 636
somatosensory system, oral 108, 109
    functional testing 117–19
specific plaque hypothesis 184
sphenopalatine nerve, long 48
spirochetes 209, 211, 220–1
    biofilm 231
    decrease with periodontal infection
        treatment 221
    invasion 249
    necrotizing gingivitis 466, *467*
    peri-implant infection 272
    periodontal abscesses 498
splinting
    implants 1189–90, *1191*
    orthodontic treatment 1249
    tooth mobility 1130, 1133, 1135–6,
        1249
split flap procedure 965–6, 968–9
spongy bone 27, *28*
sprays 741–2
    chlorhexidine 741–2, 751
stannous fluoride 746
    halitosis treatment 1336
Staphylococcus, peri-implant
    infections 639
Staphylococcus epidermidis 184
stereognosis, oral 118
    compromising factors 118–19
    receptor activation 119
stillbirth, periodontal treatment 161–2
stomatitis
    denture *630*
        chlorhexidine use 753
    necrotizing 459, 462, *463*, *464*
        diagnosis 464–5
stratum corneum 15
stratum germinativum 12
stratum granulosum 14, 15
streptococci 210
    bacterial coaggregation 232
    biofilm formation 241
    colonization 246
    dental plaque development 237
    "milleri" 224–5
Streptococcus anginosus 224, 225
Streptococcus constellatus 224
Streptococcus intermedius 224, 225
    peri-implant microbiota 275
Streptococcus mitis 237
    biofilm formation 241
Streptococcus mutans 753
Streptococcus oralis 241
Streptococcus sanguinis **241**
    coaggregation 246
    growth inhibition 247
    hydrogen peroxide production 247
    plaque formation 185, *186*
    virulence factors 479
stress
    chronic periodontitis 425–6
    dental procedures 690
    halitosis 1335
    hypoglycemia 690
    necrotizing periodontal disease 469
    periodontitis 155

stripping, mesio-distal enamel
    reduction 1271–2, *1273*, 1274
stroke, periodontal infection 158
strontium salts 741
subepithelial plexus *44*, 45
subgingival irrigation 753
sublingual artery 43, 1072, *1073*
sublingual nerve 48
sublingual region 1072, *1073*
submandibular lymph nodes 47
submandibular region 1072, *1073*
submental artery 1072, *1073*
submental lymph nodes 47
substance use/abuse, implant
    patient 645
sulfide monitor 1329–30, *1331*, *1332*
Summers technique 1111
supportive periodontal therapy 501,
    663, 1297–317
    clinical attachment level 1313–14
    clinical implementation 1312
    continuous multi-level risk
        assessment 1303–12, *1313*
    in daily practice 1314–15, *1316*,
        1317
    examination, re-evaluation and
        diagnosis (ERD) 1314–15, *1316*
    gingivitis 1302
    lack in disease-susceptible
        individuals 1300–1
    maintenance care visits 1313
    motivation, reinstruction and
        instrumentation (MRI) 1314,
        1315, *1316*
    objectives 1313–14
    periodontitis 1302–3
    polishing, fluorides, determination of
        recall interval (PFD) 1314, *1316*,
        1317
    treatment of reinfected sites
        (TRS) 1314, 1315, *1316*, 1317
suppuration, risk assessment 1311–12
suprabony defects 901
supraperiosteal blood vessels
    gingiva 44–5, 77
    peri-implant mucosa 78
surgery
    access therapy 783–820
    aggressive periodontitis 661, *663*
    attachment gain 817
    bone fill in angular bone
        defects 818–20
    chlorhexidine use 752
    chronic periodontitis 671–2
    comparison with non-surgical
        treatment 814–20
    contraindications 799–800
    distal wedge procedures 794–5
    edentulous ridge augmentation 1011–
        17, *1018–19*, *1020*, *1021–3*
    guidelines 797–812
    healing 812–14
    image-guided *620*, 621
    indications 797–9
        techniques 805–6
    infection control 815
    instrumentation 802–5
    local anesthesia 800–2
    minor with orthodontic
        treatment 1274–5, *1276*
    objectives 797
    osseous 795–7
    outcomes 812–20
    patient cooperation 799
    periodontal abscesses 497
    periodontal dressings 811–12
    post-operative care 812
    post-operative pain control 812
    pre-operative chlorhexidine rinsing/
        irrigation 753

surgery (*continued*)
root separation and resection 838, 840
root surface conditioning/
biomodification 808
suturing 808–11
technique selection 805–8
visibility in field of operation 805
wound stability 812
see also flap procedures;
gingivectomy; grafting
procedures; microsurgery;
mucogingival therapy;
regenerative periodontal surgery;
sutures/suturing
surgical guide 1225, *1226*
surgical site for implants 1068–77
anatomic landmarks with potential
risk 1072–3
clinical examination 1068
healing time 1076–7
implant placement 1071–2
direction/inclination 1074–6
position of implant 1073–4
radiographic examination 1068–9
sutures/suturing 808–11
bacteriostat-coated 1038
continuous 810–11
interrupted dental 809
intraoral tissue reactions 1037–8
microsurgery 1035–8, *1040*
modified mattress 809–10
needle 1036, **1037**
non-resorbable 1037, 1038
removal 812
resorbable 1036–7
suspensory 810
technique 809–11
swabs 718
systemic disease
aggressive periodontitis
association 446
chronic periodontitis risk 424–5
extraoral halitosis 1334
gingival disease association 411–12
halitosis 1327
historical concepts 475–6
oral infections 476
periodontal disease 475–91
manifestation 446
necrotizing 468–9
risk 156–62, 475–91
periodontitis 156–62
aggressive 446
chronic 424–5
treatment effects 489–91
risk assessment 1307–8
treatment considerations 690
see also diabetes mellitus; leukemia
systemic lupus erythematosus
(SLE) 391
implant patient 643–4

T cell receptors (TCRs) 300
T cells
adaptive defense system 299
aggressive periodontitis 441
migration 302
smoking effects 321
T helper (Th) cells 300, 301
tactile function 115–17
dental status 116–17, 118
oral stereognosis 118
testing 113–15
Tannerella forsythia 145–6, *147–8*, 148,
150, 219–20
aggressive periodontitis 440
biofilm 231, 232
composition 239
cardiovascular disease 157, 158
carotid endarterectomy 157

destructive periodontal disease **215**
invasion 248
mixed infection with *P. gingivalis*
226
peri-implant infection 271, 272, 278
periodontal disease history 276–7
periodontal abscesses 498
polymicrobial microbiota 226
prevalence 219
serum antibodies 220
S-layer 219
smoking association 319
tea tree oil 745–6
temporary anchorage devices
(TAD) 1282
temporomandibular joint (TMJ)
receptors 119
tension zones 353, 354, 357, 358
tetracycline 886
activity 889
adverse reactions 887–8
controlled-release 880, *886*
non-resorbable plastic
co-polymer 892
root surface biomodification 943
therapeutic alliance 697
thermal stimulation 854
thermoreceptors 109
thiocyanate 744
tin salts 746
titanium pins 1285
TNFA gene 336
TNFA R-alleles 336
toll-like receptors (TLRs) 298, 299
gene polymorphisms 338, *339*
tomography 604
conventional 605
incorrectly placed implants 615, *616*
lower jaw 611, *613*
vertical root fractures 861–2
see also computed tomography (CT);
digital volume tomography (CT)
tongue
bacterial load 1327
cleaning 1335
tongue cleaners 717–18, 729
tongue coating 1327, 1335
index systems 1330, *1333*
tongue scraper 1334, 1335–6
tonofilaments 13, 14
tonsilloliths (tonsil stone) 1333–4
tooth
abrasion 719
autotransplantation 1267
bodily movement 353–4
cleaning
biofilms 242
professional 925
eruption 8, 16–17, 29
ectopic 1005–6, *1007*, 1008
forced 596, 1002, 1003–5, *1006*
hopeless 1249, *1251*, *1252*
extrusion 1256, *1266*
orthodontic extraction 1263, *1265*,
1266
innervation 48
lengthening 590
periodontal infections 208, 209
position within dental arch 1309
pre-therapeutic single tooth
prognosis *659*, 660, 669
risk assessment 1309–10
single and implant decisions 679–80
esthetic zone 683, *684–5*
strategically important
missing 1144–5
survival with regenerative
periodontal therapy 904–5
total clearance 141
tooth bud 28, *29*

tooth extraction
alveolar process adaptation 1059
alveolar ridge healing 1063
bone resorption 52
implant placement immediately
following 1055–6, *1057*, 1058–61,
1062, 1064
intra-alveolar processes 54–5, *56*, 57,
58–9, 60, *61*, 62
multiple 50, *51*
socket
bone fill 1062–3
changes 55
completed soft tissue
coverage 1061–2
healing 55, *56*, 57, *58–9*, 60, *61*, 62
soft tissue collapse
prevention 1009–10
tooth germ 3, 4
tooth loss
alveolar ridge atrophy 1060–1
gingival inflammation 422
periodontal abscesses 501
periodontal disease 331
prevalence 135
periodontitis 141
risk assessment 1307
tooth mobility 28
automated probing systems 580
basic periodontal examination 657
bridges 1132
mobility increase 1134–6
clinical assessment 1127–8
horizontal forces 1128
increased
increased periodontal ligament
width 1128–9
normal periodontal ligament
width 1129–30
initial 1125–7
mechanisms 1125–6
pathologic 1127
patient examination 580, 582
periodontal disease 1127
physiologic 1127, 1132
progressive 353, 355, 357, 1125, 1128
reduced periodontal ligament 1132
regenerative periodontal therapy 913
risk assessment 1310
secondary 1125–7
splinting 1130, 1133, 1135–6, 1249
trauma from occlusion 352, 353, 1125,
1128
treatment 667, 668, 669–73, 1128–30,
1131, 1132–6
tooth movement
direction 962
gingival recession 962–3, 1267, 1269,
1270, 1271–2, *1273*, *1274*
implant esthetics 1263–5, *1266*, 1267
orthodontic
adults 1252–3, *1254*, 1255–6, *1257–*
8, 1259–65, *1266*, 1267
adults with periodontal tissue
breakdown 1241, *1242*, 1243–5,
1246–7, 1248–9, *1250–1*, 1252
compromised bone areas 1253,
1254–5
forced tooth eruption 1003–5, *1006*
infrabony pockets 1252–3
regenerative procedures 1261–2
single teeth extrusion/
intrusion 1255–6, *1257–8*,
1259–60
through cortical bone 1253, *1256*
pathologic 1243, *1244*, *1245*, 1246–7
periodontally compromised
patient 1241–76
root surface resorption 868
tooth powders 737

tooth size discrepancies (TSD)
    correction 1272
tooth socket
    bone fill 1062–3
    changes 55
    completed soft tissue
        coverage 1061–2
tooth socket healing 55, *56, 57, 58–9*, 60,
        61, 62
    blood clot formation 55, *56, 57, 58–9*
    bone marrow 62, 64
    bundle bone 63, 64, 65
    connective tissue 55, *56, 57, 58*, 60, *61*
    edentulous alveolar ridge
        topography 66–7
    fibrinolysis of blood clot 57
    granulation tissue 55, *56, 57, 58*, 60
    hard tissue cap 62, *63*
    lamellar bone 62
    osteoid formation 60
    osteons 62
    tissue formation *56*, 60, *61*, 62
    wound cleansing *59*, 60
    woven bone *56, 57, 58*, 60, *61*, 62, *63*,
        64, *65*
tooth towelettes 718
toothbrush trauma 711, 719, *720*
    gingival recession 958
toothbrushes 706, *707–12*
    abrasion 719, *720*
    chemical 740
    electric 712–13, 718, 724
        efficacy 736–7
    electrically active 713–14
    end-tufted 717, 728
    filaments 711
        end-rounding 711
        tapering 712
        wear 712
    foam 718
    instruction 723
    ionic 713–14
    manual 723
    replacement 711–12
    single-tufted 717, 728
    sonic 713
    wear 711–12
toothbrushing 706, 735, 736
    Bass technique 708
    circular 708
    duration 710–11, 736
    efficacy 708, 736
    force 718–19
    frequency 710, 736
    gingival lesions 396, *397*
    horizontal 708
    ineffective 720
    instruction 720
    methods 708–10
    modified Bass/Stillman
        technique 709
    plaque build-up prevention 414
    roll technique 709
    scrubbing 708
    sulcular 708
    vertical 708
    vibratory technique 709
tooth–implant supported
        reconstructions 370–2
toothpaste 414, 718, 737–8
    abrasives 740–1
    abrasivity 737, 738, 741
    active ingredients 741
    allergic reactions 393
    chemical agent delivery 740–1
    chlorhexidine 741, 751
    detergents 396, 741
    flavors 741
    fluoride 741
    home use studies 757

humectants 741
    potassium-containing 522
    standards 737–8, 741
    sweeteners 741
    thickeners 741
    triclosan-containing 745
    see also dentifrices
toothpicks 715
total tooth clearance 141
toxic reactions in periodontium 849
transeptal fibers 22–3
transforming growth factor β (TGF-β)
    alveolar bone healing 89
    hereditary gingival fibromatosis 384
    ridge augmentation 1093
transmucosal attachment 72, 75
transpalatal arch (TPA) 1288, *1289*,
        1290
transposon transfer 228
trauma
    dental pulp diseases 505
    foreign body reactions 398, 497
    gingival lesions 396–8
    gingival recession 958
    hard tissue 719, *720*
    instrumentation 882
    mechanical cleaning 882
    non-surgical therapy 773
    orthodontic 353–4
    physical injury 396–7, *398*
    root resorption
        peripheral inflammatory 870
        surface 867
    self-inflicted injuries 397, *398*
    thermal injury 397–8
    toothbrush 711, 719, *720*, 958
    ulcerative gingival lesion 396, *397*
    see also jiggling-type trauma
trauma from occlusion 349–60, 353, *361*,
        1125
    alveolar bone loss 360
    alveolar pyorrhea association 349–50
    angular bony defects 351
    animal experiments 353–60, *361*
    bone regeneration 1128–9
    clinical trials 352–3
    Glickman's concept 350–1
    human autopsy material 350–2
    infrabony pockets 351, 352
    jiggling-type 354–7
    orthodontic treatment *1246, 1250–1,*
        1262
    orthodontic-type 353–4
    peri-implant tissues 363–72
    periodontal ligament 357, 359
    periodontitis 352–3
    plaque-associated periodontal
        disease 358–60, *361*
    primary 349
    secondary 349
    tooth mobility 352, 353, 1125, 1128
    Waerhaug's concept 351–2
    zone of co-destruction 350, 351, 359
    zone of irritation 350, 351, 359
treatment *253*
    aggressive periodontitis 657–67
    allergic reactions 690
    anxiety control 690–1
    bleeding risk 689, 690
    cardiovascular disease effects 489
    cardiovascular incidents 690
    case presentation 659–64, *665–6, 667,*
        670
    cause-related 670–1
    complications prevention 688–90
    corrective phase 656, 661–2
    definitions 1297
    dentin removal 518
    diabetes mellitus 311–12
    drug interactions 690

effectiveness 251
    evaluation of non-surgical
        therapy 775–6
    furcation-involved teeth 823–46
    gingival recession 817–18
    goals 655
    infectious complications 688–9
    initial phase 656, 660–1
    maintenance phase 656, 662–3
    needs assessment 131
    non-surgical 765–76
        discomfort 773–4
        outcome prediction 775–6
        pain 773–4
        probing measurements 774–5
        re-evaluation 774–5
        root debridement 767–74
        root sensitivity 773–4
        surgery comparison 814–20
        tissue trauma 773
        treatment evaluation 775–6
    outcome parameters 655
    pain control 690–1
    planning 655, 658–91
        chronic periodontitis 669–73
        implants in periodontally
            compromised patient 676–84, *685*
        initial 658–60
    pregnancy 314
        outcomes 489–90
    pre-medication 690–1
    pre-therapeutic single tooth
        prognosis *659*, 660, 669
    prognosis *659*, 660
    pulp effects 518, *520*
    re-evaluation
        after corrective phase 662
        non-surgical therapy 774–5
    spontaneous abortion 161–2
    stillbirth 161–2
    supportive 656, 663, 673
    systemic disease 690
    systemic phase 655–6, 660, 687–91
    Tannerella forsythia control 219–20
    see also supportive periodontal
        therapy; surgery
tremor, microsurgeons 1039
Treponema, necrotizing periodontal
        disease 466
Treponema denticola 146, *147–8*, 148
    biofilm 231, 232
        composition 235–6, *237*, 239
        implant surfaces 268–71
    cardiovascular disease 157, 158
    peri-implant infection 278
        periodontal disease history 276–7
    peri-implant microbiota 275
    periodontal disease 221
Treponema pallidum 377
Treponema socranskii 268–71
beta-tricalcium phosphate (β-TCP) 556
triclosan
    antimicrobial activity *756*
    halitosis treatment 1336
    plaque control 745
    suture coating 1038
trigeminal nerve 48
    neurophysiology 109–11, *112, 113*
    neurosensory pathway 109
trigeminal somatosensory evoked
        potentials (RSEP) 113–14
trimethylaminuria 1334
tropocollagen 21
tuberculosis, dental team protection 687
tumor necrosis factor α (TNF-α) 296,
        300
    diabetes mellitus 309, 310
    genes *335, 336*
    pregnancy 482
    preterm birth 481

tunnel preparation 832
two-point discrimination 117–18

ulcerative lesions
  gingival disease 413–14
  recurrent 753
  traumatic gingival 396, *397*

vaccines, periodontal disease 210
vaginosis, bacterial 481
valaciclovir 379
variable number of tandem repeats
      (VNTR) *329*
varicella-zoster 379–80
varnishes 742
  chlorhexidine 751
vasoconstrictors 801
VDR gene polymorphisms 338–9,
      340
Veillonella, plaque formation 185
verapamil, gingival overgrowth 410–11
vibrio corroders 223
Vincent's angina 209–10, 459
  see also necrotizing ulcerative
      gingivitis (NUG)
viral infections 225
  chlorhexidine activity 748
  gingival disease 378–80
  necrotizing periodontal disease 466
  see also HIV infection
virulence factors 208

aggressive periodontitis bacteria 438
  environmental effects on
      expression 244
  expression 244
  immune pathology 248
  killing other pathogens 247
  periodontal infections 243, 294
  tissue damage 249
visual acuity 1030
vitamin C deficiency 412–13
  chronic periodontitis 425
vitamin D receptor gene
      polymorphisms 338–9, *340*
vitamin K 312
volatile sulfur compounds 1326, 1335
  formation 1326–7
  measurement 1329–30, *1331, 1332*
Volkmann's canals 36, 38, 46, 49, *55*

water jet, dental 717
whitening agents 741, 870, 871
  hydrogen peroxide 746
Widman flap 786–7
  healing 814
  modified 789–92, 814, 819
Winkel Tongue Coating Index
      (WTCI) 1330, *1333*
woodsticks 714, 715–16
  use 726
World Health Organization (WHO),
      periodontal treatment needs 131

wound cleansing
  osseointegration 104
  tooth socket healing *59*, 60
wound healing
  bone cell regenerative capacity 547
  enamel matrix derivatives 940
  epithelium role 549–50
  gingival connective tissue cells
      547–8
  impairment 311
  implants 100
  onlay graft procedures 1020
  PDGF 938–9
  periodontal 542–4, *545*, 546–50
  periodontal ligament cells 548–50
  root resorption 550
woven bone
  osseointegration 104–5, *106*, 107
  peri-implant loss 1058–9
  resorption 62
  tooth socket healing *56, 57, 58*, 60, *61,
      62, 63, 64, 65*

xenografts 552, 555–6
xerostomia 308
  halitosis 1335
  implant patient 644

zinc salts 745, 746
Zirconia 1233
zygomatic anchors 1285